SONOGRAPHY IN OBSTETRICS AND GYNECOLOGY

Principles & Practice

Sixth Edition

SONOGRAPHY IN OBSTETRICS AND GYNECOLOGY

Principles & Practice

Sixth Edition

Edited by

Arthur C. Fleischer, MD
Professor of Radiology and Radiologic Sciences
Professor of Obstetrics and Gynecology
Chief, Diagnostic Sonography
Vanderbilt University Medical Center
Nashville, Tennessee

Frank A. Manning, MD
Professor
Department of Obstetrics and Gynecology
Montefiore Medical Center
Bronx, New York

Philippe Jeanty, MD, PhD
Director, Diagnostic Sonography
Chief Fetustician
Women's Health Alliance
Nashville, Tennessee

Roberto Romero, MD
Chief, Perinatology Research Branch, NICHD/NIH
Professor, Obstetrics and Gynecology
Department of Obstetrics and Gynecology
Wayne State University/Hutzel Hospital
Detroit, Michigan

McGraw-Hill
Medical Publishing Division

New York   St. Louis   San Francisco   Auckland   Bogotá   Caracas   Lisbon   London
Madrid   Mexico City   Milan   Montreal   New Delhi   San Juan   Singapore   Sydney   Tokyo   Toronto

McGraw-Hill

A Division of The McGraw·Hill Companies

SONOGRAPHY IN OBSTETRICS AND GYNECOLOGY
Principles & Practice, Sixth edition

Copyright © 2001 by **The McGraw-Hill Companies, Inc.** Fetal Biometry, Neck and Chest Fetal Anomalies, Fetal Syndromes, Ultrasound Detection of Chromosomal Anomalies, and Sonography of Multiple Gestations © 2001 by Philippe Jeanty. Copyright © 1996, 1991 by Appleton & Lange. Copyright © 1985, 1980, 1977 by Appleton-Century-Crofts. All rights reserved. Except as permitted under the United States Copyright Act of 1976, no part of this publication may be reproduced or distributed in any form or by any means, or stored in a data base or retrieval system, without the prior written permission of the publisher.

1234567890 IMP/IMP 09876543210

ISBN 0-8385-8614-7

This book was set in Times Roman by York Graphic Services, Inc.
The editors were Andrea Seils, Nicky Panton, and Kitty McCullough.
The production supervisor was Phil Galea.
The cover designer was Aimeé Nordin.
The index was prepared by Jerry Ralya.

Printed and bound through Imago (U.S.A.), Inc., in China.

This book is printed on acid-free paper.

Library of Congress Cataloging-in-Publication Data
Sonography in obstetrics and gynecology: principles & practice / edited by Arthur C. Fleischer ... [et al.].— 6th ed.
    p.; cm.
  Includes bibliographical references and index. [ADJUST 008?]
  ISBN 0-8385-8614-7
    1. Ultrasonics in obstetrics. 2. Generative organs, Female—Ultrasonic imaging.
  I. Fleischer, Arthur C.
    [DNLM: 1. Pregnancy Complications—ultrasonography. 2. Genital Diseases, Female—ultrasonography. WQ 240 S699 2001]
  RG527.5.U48 S66 2001
  618′.047543—dc21   00-051532

Dedication

To our families who provide constant support
for major undertakings such as the completion of this tome.

Contents

Contributors

Alfred Z. Abuhamad, MD
Professor of Obstetrics and Gynecology
Director, Maternal Fetal Medical Division
East Virginia Medical Center
Department of Obstetrics & Gynecology
Norfolk, Virginia
[*Chapter 1*]

Carol B. Benson, MD
Associate Professor of Radiology
Harvard Medical School
Director of Ultrasound and Co-Director of
High Risk Obstetrical Ultrasound
Brigham and Women's Hospital
Boston, Massachusetts
[*Chapter 19*]

Stanley M. Berry, MD
Associate Professor of Obstetrics & Gynecology
Vice Chair of Obstetrical Services
Director, Maternal-Fetal Medicine Fellowship
Maternal-Fetal Medicine Division
Department of OB/GYN
Hutzel Hospital/Wayne State University
Detroit, Michigan
[*Chapter 29*]

Katherine Bianco, MD
Visiting Fellow

Perinatology Research Branch, NICHD/NIH
Wayne State University/Hutzel Hospital
Department of Obstetrics & Gynecology
Division of Maternal-Fetal Medicine
Detroit, Michigan
[*Chapter 15*]

Sean Blackwell, MD
Fellow
Wayne State University/Hutzel Hospital
Department of Obstetrics & Gynecology
Division of Maternal-Fetal Medicine
Detroit, Michigan
[*Chapter 29*]

Luciano Bovicelli, MD
Director
Azienda Ospedaliera di Bologna
Policlinico S. Orsola-Malpighi
Bologna, Italy
[*Chapter 16*]

James D. Bowie, MD
Reed and Martha Rice Professor of Radiology
Assistant Professor of Obstetrics & Gynecology
Duke University Medical Center
Department of Radiology
Durham, North Carolina
[*Chapter 18*]

Albert L. Bundy, MD, JD
Partner, Boston Ultrasound Consultants, P.C.
Brookline, Massachusetts
[*Chapter 51*]

Alessandra Capponi, MD
Associate Professor
Department of Obstetrics & Gynecology
Ospedale GB Grassi
Rome, Italy
[*Chapter 9*]

Peter S. Cartwright, MD
Vice Chairman
Department of Obstetrics & Gynecology
Director of Gynecology
Meharry Medical Service Foundation
Nashville, Tennessee
[*Chapter 6*]

Werther Adrian Clavelli, MD
11 de Septiembre 1745
Piso 7
Department A
Codigo Postal 1426 Republica
Capital Federal
Buenos Aires, Argentina
[*Chapter 22*]

David Cosgrove, MBChB
Professor of Clinical Ultrasound
Imperial College of Medicine
Consultant Radiologist
Division of Radiology
Hammersmith Hospital
London, United Kingdom
[*Chapter 48*]

Jeanne A. Cullinan, MD
Associate Professor
University of Rochester
Department of Radiology
Rochester, New York
[*Chapter 36*]

Laura Detti, MD
Visitor Research Fellow
Department of Obstetrics & Gynecology
Yale University School of Medicine
New Haven, Connecticut
[*Chapter 12*]

Michael P. Diamond, MD
Director
Reproductive Endocrinology and Infertility

Wayne State University/Hutzel Hospital
Detroit, Michigan
[*Chapter 6*]

Edwin F. Donnelly, MD
Assistant Professor
Department of Radiology and Radiologic Sciences
Vanderbilt University Medical Center
Nashville, Tennessee
[*Chapter 50C*]

Peter M. Doubilet, MD, PhD
Associate Professor of Radiology
Harvard Medical School
Vice Chairman of Radiology
Brigham and Women's Hospital
Boston, Massachusetts
[*Chapter 19*]

Donald S. Emerson, MD
Professor of Radiology
Department of Radiology
University of Tennessee Sciences Center
Memphis, Tennessee
[*Chapter 14*]

Stephen S. Entman, MD
Professor and Chairman
Department of Obstetrics & Gynecology
Vanderbilt University Medical Center
Nashville, Tennessee
[*Chapters 35, 37*]

Arthur C. Fleischer, MD
Professor of Radiology and Radiologic Sciences
Professor of Obstetrics & Gynecology
Chief, Diagnostic Sonography
Vanderbilt University Medical Center
Nashville, Tennessee
[*Chapters 1, 3, 4, 6, 11, 32, 34, 35, 36, 37, 38, 39, 40, 41, 42, 44, 45, 50C*]

Sandro Gabrielli, MD
Consultant in Obstetrics & Gynecology
Azienda Ospedaliera di Bologna
Policlinico S. Orsola-Malpighi
Bologna, Italy
[*Chapter 16*]

Kathleen A. Gadwood, MD
Chief of Ultrasound
Bronson Medical Hospital
Michigan State University
Kalamazoo, Michigan
[*Chapter 33*]

Maria-Teresa Gervasi, MD
Fellow, Perinatology Research Branch
National Institute of Child Health and Human Development
National Institute of Health
Detroit, Michigan
[*Chapters 13, 28, 31*]

Fabio Ghezzi, MD
Assistant Professor
Department of Obstetrics & Gynecology
University of Insubria
Varese, Italy
[*Chapters 20, 28, 29*]

Luís F. Gonçalves, MD
Consultant in Fetal Medicine
Clinica de Medicina Materno-Fetal
Florianopolis, SC
Brazil
[*Chapters 13, 15, 24, 28*]

Lawrence P. Gordon, MD
Associate Pathologist
Crouse Hospital
Syracuse, New York
[*Chapter 10*]

Chris Harman, MD
Vice Chair
Department of Obstetrics & Gynecology
Director of Maternal & Fetal Medicine
Obstetrics, Gynecology, and Reproductive Sciences
University of Maryland School of Medicine
Baltimore, Maryland
[*Chapter 25*]

Barbara S. Hertzberg, MD
Professor of Radiology
Associate Professor of Obstetrics & Gynecology
Co-Director, Fetal Diagnostic Center
Duke University Medical Center
Department of Radiology
Durham, North Carolina
[*Chapter 18*]

Andrew D. Hull, MD
Assistant Professor
Department of Reproductive Medicine
Division of Perinatal Medicine
University of California San Diego
La Jolla, California
[*Chapter 49*]

Nadin Ochsenbein-Imhof, MD
Research Fellow
Department of Obstetrics & Gynecology
University of Zurich
Zurich, Switzerland
[*Chapter 47*]

Marcia C. Javitt, MD
Professor, Diagnostic Radiology
University of Maryland Medical System
Director of Women's Imaging
Mercy Medical Center
Baltimore, Maryland
[*Chapter 40*]

Philippe Jeanty, MD, PhD
Director, Diagnostic Sonography
Chief Fetustician
Women's Health Alliance
Nashville, Tennessee
[*Chapters 7, 8, 15, 17, 20, 21, 22, 24, 31*]

Howard W. Jones, III, MD
Professor of Obstetrics & Gynecology
Director
Division of Gynecologic Oncology
Department of Obstetrics & Gynecology
Vanderbilt University Medical Center
Nashville, Tennessee
[*Chapters 32, 39*]

Donna M. Kepple, RDMS
Chief Sonographer/Senior Technical Manager
Department of Radiology and Radiologic Sciences
Section of Ultrasound
Vanderbilt University Medical Center
Nashville, Tennessee
[*Chapters 3, 4, 36*]

Mark A. Kliewer, MD
Associate Professor of Radiology
Duke University Medical Center
Department of Radiology
Durham, North Carolina
[*Chapter 18*]

S. Kupesic, MD, PhD
Professor of Obstetrics & Gynecology
Department of Obstetrics & Gynecology
Medical School University of Zagreb
Sveti Duh Hospital
Zagreb, Croatia
[*Chapters 43, 50A*]

A. Kurjak, MD, PhD
Professor and Chair
Department of Obstetrics & Gynecology
Medical School University of Zagreb
Sveti Duh Hospital
Zagreb, Croatia
[*Chapters 43, 50A*]

J. Patrick Lavery, MD
Chief, Obstetrics and Gynecology Section
Bronson Methodist Hospital
Kalamazoo, Michigan
[*Chapter 33*]

Jodi P. Lerner, MD
Associate Clinical Professor of Obstetrics & Gynecology
Department of Obstetrics & Gynecology
Columbia University College of Physicians and Surgeons
New York, New York
[*Chapter 45*]

Jorge L. Londano, MD
Research Assistant
University of South Florida
Tampa, Florida
[*Chapter 44*]

Frank A. Manning, MD
Professor
Department of Obstetrics & Gynecology
Montefiore Medical Center
Bronx, New York
[*Chapters 5, 23, 26, 30*]

Giancarlo Mari, MD, FACOG
Director of Prenatal Diagnosis and Fetal Treatment
Department of Obstetrics & Gynecology
UVA Health System
Charlottesville, Virginia
[*Chapter 12*]

Eli Maymon, MD
Visiting Scientist
Perinatology Research Branch, NICHD/NIH
Wayne State University/Hutzel Hospital
Department of Obstetrics & Gynecology
Division of Maternal-Fetal Medicine
Detroit, Michigan
[*Chapters 13, 15, 20, 28, 29, 31*]

Ana Monteagudo, MD
Associate Professor
Department of Obstetrics & Gynecology
New York University Medical Center
New York, New York
[*Chapter 45*]

Thomas R. Nelson, Ph.D.
Professor
Department of Radiology
University of California San Diego
La Jolla, California
[*Chapter 49*]

William D. O'Brien, Jr., PhD
Director, Bioacustics Research Laboratory
Department of Electrical and Computer Engineering
University of Illinois Urbana-Champaign
Urbana, Illinois
[*Chapter 2*]

Percy Pacora, MD
Visiting Fellow
Perinatology Research Branch, NICHD/NIH
Wayne State University/Hutzel Hospital
Department of Obstetrics & Gynecology
Division of Maternal-Fetal Medicine
Detroit, Michigan
[*Chapters 13, 15, 20, 31*]

Helmut Pairleitner, MD
Krankenanstalt Rudolfsstiftung
Juchgasse 25, 1030
Vienna, Austria
[*Chapter 50B*]

Anna K. Parsons, MD
Associate Professor of Obstetrics & Gynecology
Director of Reproductive Ultrasound
University of South Florida College of Medicine
Department of Obstetrics & Gynecology
Tampa, Florida
[*Chapters 42, 44*]

Antonella Perolo, MD
Consultant in Obstetrics & Gynecology
Policlinico S. Orsola-Malpighi
Bologna, Italy
[*Chapters 8, 16*]

Gianluigi Pilu, MD
Consultant in Obstetrics & Gynecology
Azienda Ospedaliera di Bologna
Policlinico S. Orsola-Malpighi
Bologna, Italy
[*Chapters 8, 13, 16, 20*]

Daniela Prandstraller, MD
Consultant, Pediatric Cardiology
Cardiology Institute
Bologna, Italy
[*Chapter 8*]

Dolores H. Pretorius, MD
Professor
Department of Radiology
University of California San Diego
La Jolla, California
[*Chapter 49*]

Ronald R. Price, PhD
Professor of Radiology and Radiologic Sciences
Director, Radiologic Sciences Division
Vanderbilt University Medical Center
Nashville, Tennessee
[*Chapter 1*]

Martin Quinn, MD, MBChB
Senior Registrar in Obstetrics & Gynecology
Department of Obstetrics & Gynecology
University of Wales College of Medicine
Health Park
Cardiff, Wales
United Kingdom
[*Chapter 46*]

Mark Redman, MD
Fellow
Wayne State University/Hutzel Hospital
Department of Obstetrics & Gynecology
Division of Maternal Fetal Medicine
Detroit, Michigan
[*Chapters 28, 29*]

Jacqueline Reyes, MD
Sonologist
Department of Radiology
Instituto de Oncologia Dr. Heriberto Pieter
Santo Domingo, Dominican Republic
[*Chapter 24*]

Giuseppe Rizzo, MD
Associate Professor
University of Rome "Tor Vergata"
Division of Obstetrics & Gynecology
Ospedale Fatebenefratelli
Rome, Italy
[*Chapter 9*]

Carlo Romanini, MD
Professor
University of Rome "Tor Vergata"
Department of Obstetrics & Gynecology

Rome, Italy
[*Chapter 9*]

Silvia Susana Romaris, MD
11 de Septiembre 1745
Piso 7
Department A
Codigo Postal 1426 Republica
Capital Federal
Buenos Aires, Argentina
[*Chapter 22*]

Roberto Romero, MD
Chief, Perinatology Research Branch, NICHD/NIH
Professor, Obstetrics & Gynecology
Department of Obstetrics & Gynecology
Wayne State University/Hutzel Hospital
Detroit, Michigan
[*Chapters 13, 15, 16, 20, 28, 29, 31*]

David M. Sherer, MD
Professor of Obstetrics and Gynecology
Department of Obstetrics & Gynecology and
Women's Health
Albert Einstein College of Medicine
Bronx, New York
[*Chapter 5*]

Tariq A. Siddiqi, MD
Professor
Director of Maternal Fetal Medicine
Department of Obstetrics & Gynecology
University of Cincinnati Medical Center
Cincinnati, Ohio
[*Chapter 2*]

Sandra Rejane Silva, MD
Assistant Doctor
Maternal Fetal Medicine
Fetus—Centro de Diagnóstico Pré-natal e Medicina Fetal
São Paulo, Brazil
[*Chapters 21, 24*]

Beverly A. Spirt, MD
Professor of Radiology
State University of New York Upstate Medical University
Syracuse, New York
[*Chapter 10*]

Ilan E. Timor-Tritsch, MD
Professor of Obstetrics & Gynecology
Director, OB/GYN Ultrasound Unit
New York University Medical Center
New York, New York
[*Chapter 45*]

Jaime M. Vasquez, MD
Director
Center for Reproductive Health
Nashville, Tennessee
[*Chapter 42*]

Ronald J. Wapner, MD
Director
Division of Maternal & Fetal Medicine
Department of Obstetrics & Gynecology
Thomas Jefferson University
Philadelphia, Pennsylvania
[*Chapter 27*]

Thomas C. Wheeler, MD
Assistant Professor
Department of Obstetrics & Gynecology
Maternal Fetal Medicine Division
Vanderbilt University Medical Center
Nashville, Tennessee
[*Chapter 34*]

Josef Wisser, MD, PhD
Associate Professor
Department of Obstetrics
University of Zurich
Zurich, Switzerland
[*Chapter 47*]

Preface

As the new millennium begins, it is apparent that diagnostic sonography has become an integral part of the management of women and their obstetric and gynecologic disorders. Diagnostic sonography units have become "the stethoscope of the future," as Dr. Roy Filly said in an editorial 12 years ago. To paraphrase him, "they are used by many and understood by few." With the continued expanded utilization of diagnostic sonography, the future seems to be now. To obtain the most clinically pertinent information from sonography, sonographers and sonologists must be committed to provide the best service, combined with experience and practical "know-how."

One of the new developments since the last edition of this book involves the accredition of obstetric/gynecologic ultrasound practices by nationally and internationally recognized organizations (AIUM, ACOG, ACR). This is advocated by the editors as a means to ensure that the quality and interpretation of an obstetric/gynecologic sonogram meets certain minimal standards.

Another new development is the more extensive use of the Doppler technique in obstetrics to assess fetal–placental, utero-placental blood flow, and fetal blood flow, and fetal blood flow redistribution and in gynecology for assessment of malignancy and the vascularity of the endometrium, myometrium, and ovaries. Further investigation is needed before a more complete understanding of the correlation of blood flow to organ function is better known. Newer techniques such as three-dimensional reconstruction and use of contrast and harmonic imaging will enlighten us about this correlation.

Although the use of diagnostic sonography for endometrial assessment has become routine, the efficacy of screening for ovarian cancer remains a controversial issue. The use of contrast affords sonographic assessment of tubal patency. Sonography is also providing a means for more extensive use of guided procedures.

In obstetrics, sonography continues to play a pivotal role in both high and low risk pregnancies. Improved depiction of flow disturbances allows early detection of the fetus at risk for hypoxia. Although the initial enthusiasm for ultrasonographically guided fetal interventional procedures has waned somewhat, diagnostic sonography continues to be a means for facilitating new approaches to new and old fetal maladies.

Well, what's in store for this edition and ones to come? Probably more three-dimensional and specialized image processing and probably more on the use of contrast and blood flow. The only thing one can be certain of is that new applications will be added to those already tested and proven.

It is my sincere hope that we, as ultrasound enthusiasts and professionals, will continue the quest to improve the quality of life by the thoughtful applications of new technology. Personally, I find this both challenging and rewarding. I hope you do, too.

Arthur C. Fleischer, MD
Nashville, Tennessee

REFERENCE

1. Filly R. Ultrasound: The stethoscope of the future, alas. *Radiology.* 1988;167:400.

Acknowledgments

The authors would like to express their gratitude to Jane Licht, former Executive Editor at Appleton & Lange, whose professionalism and tenacity enabled the initiation of work on this revised edition. We are also grateful to Andrea Seils, Sponsoring Editor, Nicky Panton, Editing Supervisor, and Kitty McCullough, Developmental Editor at McGraw-Hill Companies, Inc., and others who contributed to the completion and distribution of this book. Sarah Campbell-Mackie, Theresa Thompson, and John Bobbit of Vanderbilt University Medical Center, are thanked for all of their efforts, on behalf of completing this book, too.

Sonographic Instrumentation and Operational Concerns

Ronald R. Price • Arthur C. Fleischer • Alfred Z. Abuhamad

Improvements in sonographic (ultrasound) instrumentation have primarily been the result of more complete integration of high-speed digital electronics. Special-purpose microcomputers are being used to steer and dynamically focus array transducers, allowing greater flexibility and control over image formation and producing images with both higher spatial and higher intensity resolution. Developments in real-time color Doppler systems have also been the product of high-speed, special-purpose microprocessors. Selection of a satisfactory scanner from the wide variety of equipment available can often be puzzling and time-consuming. It is difficult to obtain an unbiased opinion. Although there are no definite guidelines, some general considerations are presented here. Discussion will be restricted to those aspects of ultrasound imaging technology applicable to general abdominal and obstetric and gynecologic imaging.

In general, it is important to understand the principles of ultrasound and to have a fundamental knowledge of how the image is formed. In addition, the patient population to be scanned must be analyzed because this will determine the variety of examinations to be performed and the type of equipment needed.

The focus of this chapter will be to review each of the various categories of real-time scanners, to describe the relative advantages and disadvantages of each, and to discuss advances in each design. In addition, the features of the various types of transducer/probes relative to their clinical use will be emphasized.

SCANNER COMPONENTS

Real-time instruments rapidly sweep the ultrasound beam through a sector or rectangular area by either mechanical or electronic means. Frame rates greater than 15 frames per second are required to produce flicker-free images and to observe moving structures. Because real-time probes are usually not attached to a scanning arm, the sonographer has great flexibility in selecting the image plane orientation.

Ultrasound scanning systems typically consist of the following:

1. A mechanical or electronic means of moving the ultrasound beam through an image plane.
2. An electronic signal processing unit with controls for changing the transducer power output, overall receiver gain, and other operational parameters, such as time-gain compensation (TGC).

3. A gray-scale display unit equipped with controls for changing the image brightness and contrast.
4. A device for permanently recording the images, such as a Polaroid, multi-image format camera, video disc, or videotape.

Modern instruments should also have a keyboard for superimposing on the recorded image the patient identification, exam date, and study information.

TRANSDUCER DESIGNS

Transducers are characterized by their frequency, size (effective aperture in the case of arrays), and degree of focusing. Typically, the range of frequency for diagnostic ultrasound imaging is 3.5 to 10.0 MHz. The degree of focusing is either short (1 to 4 cm), medium (4 to 8 cm), or long (6 to 12 cm). Focusing is achieved internally by the crystal shape, externally by an acoustic lens, electronically by selective pulsing of individual elements of an array, or by a combination of these three methods. The length of the zone available for focusing (Fresnel zone) is governed by the effective transducer aperture and its operating frequency. In selecting a transducer that has the optimum combination of frequency, aperture size, and focal zone for a particular type of examination, the following general points should be considered:

1. Increasing transducer frequency generally results in enhanced axial resolution but at the expense of reduced tissue penetration. The highest frequency consistent with adequate tissue penetration should be used.
2. For a selected transducer frequency, decreasing the transducer aperture improves lateral resolution in the near field. The length of the Fresnel zone (useful working range of the transducer), however, is reduced; lateral resolution beyond this zone (the Fraunhofer zone) is degraded because of beam divergence. Decreasing the transducer aperture also decreases its sensitivity. It is important to note that many new array systems provide the capability of "dynamic aperture," which means that the effective aperture size can be changed by using smaller or larger subunit transducers depending on the depth of focus chosen.
3. Larger aperture transducers are more suited to lower frequencies so that good lateral resolution is preserved at depth; smaller apertures are better suited to higher frequency transducers to provide improved lateral resolution over the shorter range.
4. Focused transducers provide improved lateral resolution and sensitivity at the depth of the fo-

cal zone, which is limited by the length of the Fresnel zone. The choice of focal zone, therefore, depends on the depth of structures to be resolved.

ALTERNATIVES IN SCANNER DESIGN

The evolution of the real-time scanners has led to a development of a variety of types of real-time scanner designs and configurations. It is generally true that no single design provides maximum performance in all image parameters, but rather some image parameters are optimized at the expense of others. Examples of these are the trade-off of axial resolution obtained from higher frequencies with depth of penetration, good lateral resolution at a specific depth resulting from a large aperture transducer with decreased lateral resolution at other depths, the convenience of fully electronic scanners against less expensive mechanical scanners, and the large echo dynamic range of mechanically driven, single-element transducers against the more rapid multielement arrays that may have a more limited echo dynamic range. Real-time scanners can be grouped according to how they form the beam (focusing) and how the beam is steered (scanned) to form the image. In each case (focusing and steering), the task may be accomplished either mechanically or electronically. *Mechanical focusing* is the name frequently given to the use of acoustic lenses. Single-element transducers use mechanical means exclusively for beam focusing, whereas multielement arrays use pulse timing to bring about a convergent beam in the plane of the array and mechanical means to converge the beam in the "slice-thickness" direction (perpendicular to the array axis). Beam steering can be accomplished either by mechanically moving the transducer (or alternatively an acoustic mirror) or by electronic steering by means of pulse-timing sequences in multielement systems. Hybrid systems are also available that use a combination of array focusing and mechanical steering.

As noted earlier, new advances in real-time ultrasonic imaging are largely the result of the more complete integration of high-speed dedicated digital electronics (computers) into imaging systems. The term *computed sonography* is now being used to emphasize this increased dependence of the ultrasound image formation on the digital computer.

Single-Element Mechanically Steered Scanners

Most single-element mechanically steered scanners produce a sector (pie-shaped) format image. The sector's opening angles may range from 30 to 120 degrees (most are approximately 90 degrees). The ultrasonic beam may be steered by moving the transducer itself or by reflecting the beam from an oscillating "acoustic mirror." Because of the difficulty of maintaining adequate skin contact with either the moving transducer or moving mirror, most mechanically steered scanners use a fluid-filled case with an acoustically transparent window to contain the moving parts. In this manner, skin contact is made with the acoustic window case rather than directly with the moving components. This configuration ensures adequate acoustic coupling even at relatively large steering angles.

Mechanically steered scanners have two main advantages relative to electronically steered scanners:

1. The use of a single-element transducer requires less sophisticated electronics and generally allows for a more simple transducer head design.
2. There are fewer image artifacts due to side lobes and grating lobes (unique to electronically steered beams).

The disadvantages of mechanically steered arrays are:

1. The beam focus and beam pattern are fixed for a given transducer. To change the focus, one must change the entire transducer head.
2. The image framing rate depends on how rapidly the transducer is oscillated. The framing rate is governed by the line density needed to produce an image of diagnostic quality and by the depth of the field of view. The velocity of ultrasound in tissue is the ultimate factor governing the oscillation rate of the transducer. Thus, the framing rate may become quite low when large fields of view are chosen that require large excursions of the transducer element.
3. Field of view and image frame rates are in competition in sector format images when the total number of scan lines per image is kept constant. Thus, large opening angles are needed for large field sizes, and small opening angles are required for high resolution. In other words, the sector angle must decrease if higher line density is desired. This problem is not unique to mechanical scanners, however, and will be discussed again in regard to electronically steered scanners.

Although many variations on the mechanical oscillating transducer design have been designed and built, the most common design is a transducer that oscillates about a single fixed point and yields a sector-shaped image format (Fig. 1–1).

When a single-element "wobbler" transducer is placed in contact with the skin surface, it is rocked from side to side in a small arc by means of an electric motor. Each individual line of the B-mode image is produced and displayed as a radius of a circle, with the transducer at the center.

Beam formation in mechanical scanners is achieved through mechanical focusing by using either a shaped transducer (internal focus) or an acoustic lens that is attached to the transducer surface (external focus) (Fig. 1–2). One of the disadvantages of this design is that, to change to focal zone, one must physically replace the transducer and, consequently, the

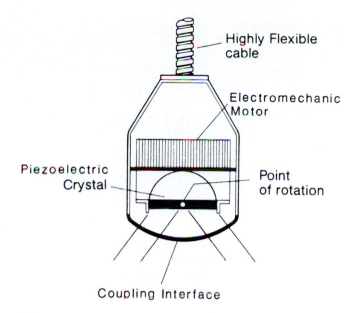

Figure 1–1. Mechanical sector real-time scanner of the oscillating single-element fixed-focus design.

focal zone cannot be conveniently changed during scanning. Electronically focused scanners achieve focusing by delayed pulse sequences, allowing the focal zone to be changed without physically altering the scanner.

An alternative approach to beam steering in a mechanical scanner is to keep the transducer stationary and to use an oscillating acoustic mirror to move the beam in a sector

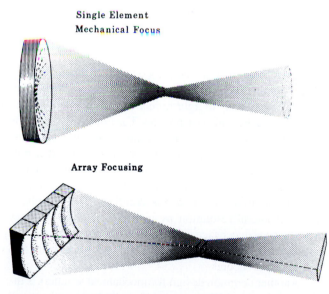

Figure 1–2. Single-element scanners require curved transducer crystals or an attached acoustic lens to achieve focusing *(top)*. Single-element transducers are thus focused to a specific depth (fixed focus). Array focusing is achieved by altering the times at which each subelement is pulsed, thus allowing multiple focal depths *(bottom)*.

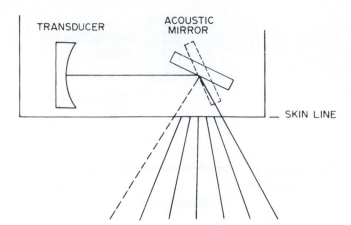

Figure 1–3. A mechanical sector scanner using an oscillating acoustic mirror for beam steering. Focal depth is determined by the mechanical focus of the transducer and is not affected by the presence of the mirror. Oscillating mirrors are also used to steer annular arrays in some systems.

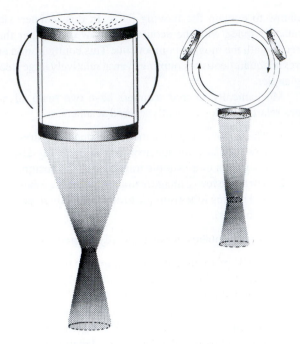

Figure 1–4. Rotating wheel mechanical scanners with multiple elements provide more rapid frame rates than single-element scanners and may also produce wider fields of view.

format (Fig. 1–3). This design requires that the mirror and transducer also be contained within a fluid-filled housing so that the moving mirror does not make direct contact with the patient.

The oscillating mirror design offer an advantage over the oscillating transducer design by eliminating the need to move an electrically active component (the transducer). In addition, the mirror is usually lighter and can be moved more easily and rapidly. The lighter mirror results in the need for a smaller motor, which results in a more compact and lighter transducer probe.

A plane mirror only changes the direction of the beam and does not affect the beam focus. Thus, the focal characteristics are entirely determined by the transducer and its mechanical construction. The angle at which the beam is reflected from the mirror surface is equal to the angle of beam incidence analogous to light reflection—with essentially no energy loss in the reflection process. The fluid-path length, by necessity, will be slightly longer (approximately 1 cm) than scanners that use an oscillating transducer without a mirror, thus making the image field of view more trapezoidal in format. This is not necessarily a disadvantage, however, because the additional offset of the skin line usually results in the better lateral resolution by moving the skin line away from the transducer face and closer to the focal zone of the transducer. Scanners of this design operate typically at 15 to 30 frames per second.

Another common design for mechanical scanners is the rotating wheel, which consists of multiple (usually three) transducers mounted on a wheel that is rotated by an external motor (Fig. 1–4). The wheel is rotated in the same direction, making the mechanical assembly much simpler. The wheel and transducer are housed in a fluid-filled case with an acoustic window at the lower surface, which makes contact with the

patient. As the transducers rotate, the output is switched from one transducer to the next in sequence, depending on which transducer has rotated in front of the acoustic window. This design allows for rapid framing without flicker—typically 30 frames per second. The design produces a sector-shaped field of view and allows a wide opening angle of 90 degrees or more.

Electronically Steered Scanners

Included in this category are linear phased arrays, multielement linear sequenced arrays, and multielement annular arrays. Through the proper phasing of the transmit-receive timing of the transducer elements that are used to fabricate the arrays, a composite ultrasonic beam can be created. In this manner, the beam can be focused and steered electronically. Fundamental to electronic focusing is the fact that each element of the array generates an ultrasonic wave, which has a definite phase relationship with the waves from the other elements. The ultrasonic waves generated by each element can be superimposed in a precise manner to create the effect of a single wave front.

Multielement linear sequenced arrays sequentially pulse subunits of transducers so as to produce a wave front that moves normally to the transducer face, thus yielding a rectangular field. In contrast, linear phased arrays pulse all of the available transducers for each line and thus must steer as well as focus (Fig. 1–5A). An interesting and valuable variation on this general field geometry is the field shape produced by "radial" or "convex" linear array transducers

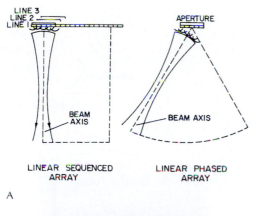

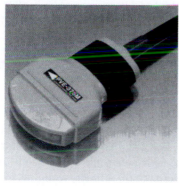

Figure 1–5. **(A)** Traditional linear sequenced arrays *(left)* produce rectangular fields of view and use both transmit and receive array focusing. Phased linear arrays *(right)* are steered to produce a sector-shaped field of view and also to use both transmit and receive focusing. **(B)** Radial or convex linear arrays provide increased field of view with depth without electronic scanning, thus reducing grating-lobe artifacts that accompany traditional phased arrays when large steering angles are used.

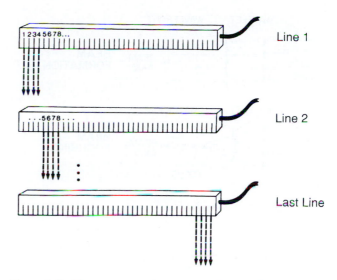

Figure 1–6. Linear sequenced arrays scan the beam by sequentially pulsing transducer subgroups along the length of the array; thus, only a small portion of the crystals is used to form any one line.

(Fig. 1–5B). Radial arrays operate in much the same way that conventional linear sequenced arrays operate, but rather than being aligned in a straight line, the transducer subelements are aligned along an arc. The advantages of this design are several: (1) by launching the ultrasound wave perpendicular to the transducer face and to the skin, better transmission is achieved; (2) beam steering is achieved geometrically rather than by pulse timing, thereby eliminating increased grating-lobe artifacts seen in phased arrays at large steering angles; and (3) there is increased field of view depth, unlike with conventional sequenced arrays that produce rectangular fields of view.

The transducer array is usually composed of many (typically 128 to 256) small piezoelectric crystals (**M**) arranged in a row (Fig. 1–6). Because the field from a single small crystal element diverges very rapidly, several elements (**N**) are driven simultaneously, and electronic focusing is used. In the subgroup of **N** crystals, the outer crystals may be pulsed first with the inner crystals delayed. In this circumstance, the

field from the **N** elements will be focused at a depth that depends on the magnitude (time interval) of the delays. By changing the magnitudes of the delays, the focal zone can be chosen for a specific depth. The elements may also be designed to be sensitive to the returning waves in a manner determined by the same delay factors used in transmission, thus constituting a focusing effect on the returning signals. A signal scan line in the real-time images is formed in this manner. The next adjacent scan line is generated by using another group of **N** crystals formed by shifting from the previous **N** crystals, one crystal position along the transducer array. The same transmit-receive pattern is then repeated for this set of **N** crystals and, subsequently, for all other sets of **N** crystals along the array in a cyclic manner. Focusing in the plane of the transducer elements improves lateral resolution sensitivity by increasing the amount of energy in the focal zone (constructive interference). Focusing in the plane perpendicular to the scan lines determines the slice thickness and is accomplished by the use of mechanically focused elements (double focusing, see Fig. 1–2).

The linear phased array is frequently termed an *electronic sector scanner* because the resulting field is pieshaped, with the field diverging as the distance from the transducers is increased. How this field shape is created is illustrated in Figure 1–7. The outside transducers are activated first, and the inner transducers are delayed in time, with the central transducer having the greater delay to yield a wave axis perpendicular to the plane of the transducer. By changing the order of the delay, the wave can be focused at a specified depth, and the wave axis can be scanned through a sector of 60 to 90 degrees. Properly selected delays can produce steering and focusing simultaneously. One distinction between linear sequenced arrays and linear phased arrays is that, in

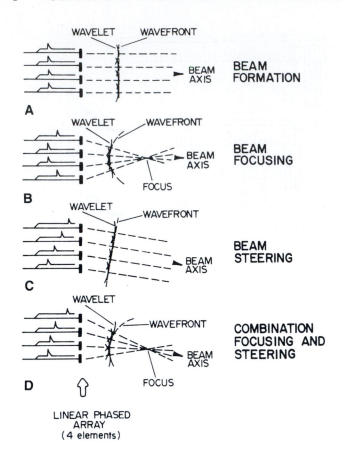

Figure 1–7. Phased arrays are capable of electronic beam formation **(A)**, beam focusing **(B)**, beam steering **(C)**, or any combination of focusing and steering **(D)**, allowing dynamic focusing and steering.

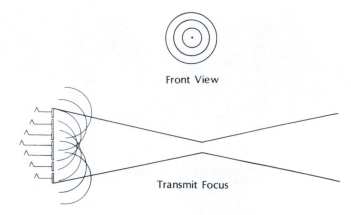

Figure 1–8. Phased annular arrays are also capable of dynamic focusing and offer the added advantage that the beam is focused in two dimensions, unlike linear arrays that are only capable of electronic focusing in the plane of the array. For linear arrays, focusing in the slice-thickness direction must be accomplished mechanically. Annular arrays, however, must be steered mechanically.

the phased array, every element is used to form the beam for each line. In the linear sequenced array, only a small subset of the transducers is used to create a given line.

The phased annular array scanner represents a hybrid system and possesses characteristics of both mechanical and electronic designs. The transducer is composed of a series of independent transducers. Each element has the shape of an annular ring, and multiple elements are arranged in concentric rings around central transducer element (Fig. 1–8).

Beam formation and focusing are achieved electronically by proper phasing of the transducer elements. An advantage of this design is readily recognized in that focusing is achieved in two dimensions as with a single focused element, but, unlike mechanical focusing, the focal zone can be changed without physically changing the transducer. Beam steering must be achieved mechanically. The beam is swept through a trapezoidal field of view with an oscillating mirror, or the transducer itself may be oscillated. As with other mechanically steered scanners, the transducers, the mirrors, or both are contained within a fluid-filled housing.

In the oscillating mirror design, the transducer may be quite large, typically 10 cm or more. A large transducer aperture can be used to achieve a long focal zone, which may be

appropriately positioned in the area of interest by choosing the fluid-path length properly. Because the fluid-path length is usually longer than the maximum depth of view in the patient, no reverberation artifacts resulting from echoes reflected back and forth between the patient's skin and the transducer face will be seen in the images. Because of the exceedingly long path length, however, the pulse repetition rate must be reduced relative to hand-held scanners. Typical frame rates are at 12 frames per second (128-line resolution) and high-resolution images at 1 frame per second.

Commercially available annular array scanners offer a variable focal zone option that allows the user to specify one of several focal zones. The systems also operate in a survey scan mode in which the transducers are cyclically scanned through the available focal zones while the operator observes the images. Once a particular depth of interest is specified, the operator terminates the survey scan and selects the appropriate focal zone for optimum visualization.

DISPLAY AND STORAGE OF REAL-TIME IMAGES

The number of gray shades displayed in the ultrasound image depends on the characteristics of the *scan converter* that translates the pressure change received by the transducer to electric impulses.

Most instruments for B-mode imaging use *digital* scan converters (Fig. 1–9). In these systems, the analog voltage levels, which correspond to the returning echo amplitudes for each line of the image, are digitized by an analog-to-digital converter. The generated array of numbers is then stored in a digital memory. The digital memory is divided into a number of picture elements or *pixels*. Typically, each pixel element depicts 1×1 mm of the image. The size of the memory

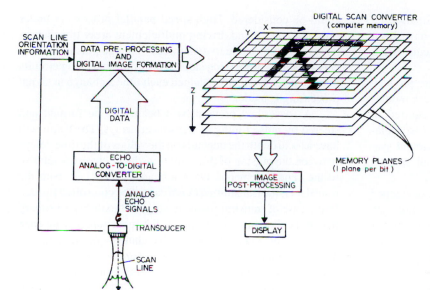

Figure 1–9. Block diagram of a digital ultrasound system. Echo signals detected by the transducer are digitized and then stored in a computer memory (digital scan converter), which is then read out to a video monitor.

can be described by the number of pixel elements, such as 512 × 512. Each pixel represents a region in the body whose size is equal to the image field of view divided by the number of pixels. For example, a 25-cm field of view imaged with a 512 × 512 pixel matrix would yield pixel sizes of approximately 0.5 × 0.5 mm. The memory can then be interrogated, and the image displayed on a video monitor. The brightness of the video signal representing each picture element is controlled by the value stored in the corresponding digital word. The number of shades of gray available is determined by the size of the digital word used to store the information for each picture element. The size of the word is measured in terms of the number of bits and is frequently referred to as the *depth* of the memory. Three bit words provide the capacity for displaying eight shades of gray, four bits provide 16 shades of gray, and five bits provide 32 shades of gray. Most digital memories used for real-time scanners are at least 512 × 512 by 8 bits deep (256 shades of gray).

The discreteness of both the spatial domain and the gray scale shades provides an image that is not as "smooth" as the analog image. The appearance of the image will be different, and the margin between picture elements (pixels) will be more definite than with analog displays. As the number of pixels increases and these become smaller, however, it becomes difficult to distinguish between the two types of images. Images are frequently processed by linear interpolation to produce more aesthetically pleasing images. Interpolation "fills in" between picture elements without altering the original image data; however, the digital system is more stable, does not drift, and is less sensitive to heat. This eliminates long start-up time and allows one to institute predigital and postdigital image processing.

Common methods for permanent archiving of ultrasound images are multi-image format film, video tape and a variety of digital storage systems usually including optical disks. Multiformat film imagers have become the recording device of choice not only for ultrasound but also for computed tomography, nuclear medicine, and magnetic resonance imaging (MRI). Due to the transportability of most ultrasound systems, multiformat cameras are usually chosen in the "compact" design. In most applications, the 9-on-1 format on 8 × 10 inch film is an adequate size for viewing and measuring. If larger recorded images are desired, the 6-on-1 format is also readily available.

Videotape recorders have also become very popular storage devices because of their ability to allow a real-time study to be recorded just as it was performed—often with superimposed audio from the operator for further study and clarification on orientation and other descriptive findings.

Video recorders using one-half inch VHS standard or super VHS videotape are relatively inexpensive and store several hours of video on a single tape with acceptable resolution. These units generally include slow/fast motion playback modes, still-frame replay mode, and automatic search capabilities. Care should be taken to recognize that in most units when still-frame imaging is used the number of displayed lines will be reduced to approximately one half of the real-time display resolution. One method to optimize the quality of the frozen taped image is to record the still-frame. When it is played back, double the number of lines are read compared with stopping a taped image.

PICTURE ARCHIVING AND COMMUNICATIONS SYSTEM

The Picture Archiving and Communications System (PACS), introduced in the early to mid-1980s, promises completely filmless operation through the use of digital image acquisition and display. At the present time there are relatively small numbers of large-scale institutions with PACSs. Small-scale systems, often called "mini-PCASs," however, have been successfully applied in ultrasound, nuclear medicine, MRI, neuroradiology, and intensive care units.

The fact that essentially all ultrasound units produce analog video has made ultrasound a particularly easy modality for connection to a mini-PACS. The interface required, in most cases, for connecting an image to the PACS is a relatively inexpensive video digitizer. In newer ultrasound systems, vendors are providing access to direct digital imagers by way of the ACR-NEMA DICOM format.

The ACR-NEMA digital data standard was developed to enable different system manufacturers to communicate with one another. The standard defines the specifications for the data format by which images and associated information are stored and by a set of protocols for transferring the data through an electronic interface.

Versions 1 and 2 of the ACR-NEMA standard were released in 1985 and 1988, respectively, and were designed primarily for point-to-point connections. Version 3, referred to as the digital interfacing and communications in medicine (DICOM) standard, is a much more flexible and complete standard. The DICOM standard is fully compatible with the earlier versions of the ACR-NEMA standard.

The most common use of PACS in ultrasound is providing centralized hard copies. Either the ultrasound machines are interfaced to a local area network (LAN) print manager that receives, stores, and organizes images by patient and prints the images, or each machine can be outfitted with an on-board removable digital storage medium (magnetic or optical disk) that is manually removed and loaded onto the print manager. Because ultrasound systems are often moved for portable studies, the latter option is often the most popular.

With a centralized imager, most usually a laser camera, the fact that each machine no longer has its own imager, the lack of a back-up system, and the possibility of a single-point failure should be considered. In addition, the rate at which films will be needed must be considered so that a single hardcopy printer does not result in a system bottleneck. In most cases, the most obvious advantage with a centralized printer is the reduction of the sonographer's workload by not having to handle and develop multiple small format film cassettes.

COMPUTED ULTRASOUND

In addition to the use of digital scan converters, which have become commonplace in real-time systems, several manufacturers have extended the use of digital technology by replacing many of the traditional analog portions of the system's pulsing and receiving hardware. In the past, it has been appreciated that digital components provide flexibility through software programmability that analog systems cannot; however, the price and speed of digital systems have only recently been such that the replacement of analog circuits

could be considered. High-speed parallel processors under program control and driving multielement array transducers have made it possible to dynamically change pulsing and receiving signal processing steps. This is unlike analog circuits that must be physically changed each time a change in signal processing is made.

As described previously, a beam can be formed and steered by pulse timing of transducer arrays. The beam will have a focal depth the depends on the values of the time delays between the pulsing of the outer transducer elements relative to the center elements. Once a beam is launched from the transducer, the transmitted beam cannot be controlled further. In the case of transmit focus, the digital flexibility's primary benefit is allowing one to choose the focal zone before each scan without having to physically change the transducers. This is an important practical benefit but does not change the resultant image quality relative to that of analog systems.

The most significant improvement in image quality that has resulted directly from the use of the digital system has been benefits derived from the dynamic signal processing on the returning echoes. This is often referred to as *receive focusing* or *dynamic focusing*. Even though the transmitted beam can have only a single focal zone, it is possible to selectively "listen" to the returning echoes. Because returning echoes from different depths arrive at different times, reflections from deeper sites. Accepting only those echoes that have the proper pattern of arrival times assures that the returning signals are in focus for each depth (Fig. 1–10). This

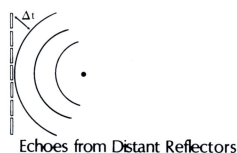

Echoes from Distant Reflectors

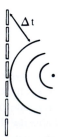

Echoes from Near Reflectors

Figure 1–10. Receive focus is carried out in real time by means of high-speed digital processors capable of monitoring the response received by each individual transducer element. By using predetermined time-delay patterns, the system can distinguish echoes that come from different depths by the relative time delays (Δt) observed by the array elements.

is the essence of dynamic focusing. To accomplish dynamic focusing, it is essential that the system have almost complete control over the pulsing and receiving of each individual transducer element. It is this fact that requires the power of high-speed parallel processing. Conventional multielement scanners sum the received signal with equal weights from the various elements to produce the echo signal. In the parallel processed systems, the gain of each element is controlled separately. This dynamically variable gain capability is referred to as *dynamic apodization*. Dynamic variations in the individual gains can be used to discard echoes from off-axis sites to minimize side-lobe and grating-lobe artifacts. The same technique can also be used to effectively change the size of the aperture during the scan, depending on whether or not one is scanning in the near or far field.

Another improvement in transducer technology is the use of broad band transducers. This method optimizes the frequencies used to image based on the depth within the body where the region of interest lies.

INTRALUMINAL TRANSDUCER PROBES

Advances in transducer designs have afforded development of transducers that can be mounted on probes to be placed in various lumina within the body. Specifically, the two major types of intraluminal probes that have gained clinical application include transvaginal transducer/probes (for imaging of the uterus, early pregnancy, and the adnexa) and transrectal transducer/probes (for imaging of the cervix and parametrium).

Because of the proximity of the organ of interest to the transducer, both transvaginal and transrectal probes can use high-frequency transducers, usually 5 or 7.5 MHz. In general, the use of these probes can contribute to increased diagnostic specificity through the improved resolution afforded by proximity of the transducer to the area of interest and by the higher transducer frequencies that can be used.

As illustrated in the chapters on early obstetric sonography and gynecologic infertility sonography, transvaginal transducer/probes significantly enhance the sonographic evaluation of the uterus and adnexa. At present, there are between 10 and 15 different types of commercially available probes (Table 1–1). The major types of transvaginal probes include those that use a single-element mechanical oscillating transducer, those with a curved linear array, those that use an electronically phased steering of multiple transducer elements, and those that are a single-element transducer that rotates (Fig. 1–11A and B).

In general, the field of view of most transvaginal probes is approximately 10 cm, with the focal ranging from 2 to 7 cm, depending on the type and design of the transducers. The sector of the field of view is typically 90 to 100 degrees, with some rotating wheel designs going as high as 240 degrees. The design of the actual probe housing ranges from a straight shaft, with a transducer mounted on the end, to some in which the transducer's face is inclined relative to the handle. Needle guides are available on several transvaginal transducer/probes and attach onto the shaft.

When selecting the type of transvaginal transducer/probe to be used, one should keep in mind that they differ according to the size of the actual imaging surface or "footprint," the size of the shaft, and the angle of the handle. Handles that assist the operator in determining probe orientation are preferred. Probes with the smallest shaft size may be preferred in virgins or young girls and in older women with atrophic vaginas.

Transrectal probes are used extensively for evaluation of the prostate in men (Fig. 1–12A and B). These probes usually contain one, or more than one, array of transducers. For imaging in the sagittal plane, a series of linear array elements with electronic or phased array focusing in usually used. For those probes that have two elements, the axial view is usually obtained by a single-element mechanically oscillated transducer, curved linear array, or phased array transducer array.

Static scanner biopsy probes have been largely replaced by real-time transducers with biopsy guide attachments. A unique advantage is the ability to select the needle path on a real-time, two-dimensional image and then to directly observe the needle penetrating the organ, tumor, or fluid collection.

DOPPLER SCANNERS

Doppler scanners have evolved from relatively simple continuous wave (CW) units, which yielded an audible frequency to the users' earphones, to pulsed Doppler systems that are capable of yielding color-coded flow images in real time. This evolution has been made possible in large part by the advent of relatively inexpensive high-speed parallel processing computers. The basic interaction of the Doppler effect has not changed over the years, but the ability to rapidly process and analyze the returning echo data has.

The general effect of sound that passes through the body is to be absorbed (a decrease in beam intensity of about 1 dB/cm/MHz) or reflected. Sound is reflected at each point along the beam where the relative acoustical impedance changes. If this reflecting interface is stationary, the frequency of the reflected wave will be identical to the incident beam. If the interface is moving, the reflected echo frequency will be shifted up or down (relative to the incident wave) by an amount proportional to the velocity along the beam direction. This shift Δf is the Doppler shift and is given by the following equation:

$$\Delta f = \pm \frac{2Vf}{c} \cos\theta \qquad [1]$$

where Δf the Doppler shift frequency (Hz), V is the velocity of the moving interface (cm/s), f_0 is the frequency of the incident sound (Hz), c is the velocity of sound in tissue (cm/s),

TABLE 1–1. TRANSVAGINAL TRANSDUCER/PROBE CHARACTERISTICS

Manufacturer	Frequency (MHz)	Focal Range (mm)	Sector Size (degree)	Type	Insertion Length (cm)	"Footprint" Diameter (cm)	Needle Guide	Color Doppler
Acuson	5.0	15–40	90	Phased array sector	16.0	0.8	Flush	+
ATL	5.0, 6.0, 7.5	40–50	90	Mechanical sector	16.0	1.9–2.5	Flush	++
	3.0	12–60	150	Curvilinear	13.0	1.9	Flush	++
	5–9	30–60	90		18.0	1.9		
Ausonics/Universal	5.0	20–40	90	Mechanical sector	17.0	1.2–2.5		
Bruel & Kjaer	7.5	10–60	115	Mechanical sector	7.2	2.1–3.8	Flush	
Cone Instruments/ Kretz	7.5	30–70	112	Mechanical sector	15.0	1.2–2.6	Outrigged	
	5.0	20–50	240					
Corometrics Medical Systems (Aloka)	5.0	15–45	60	Curvilinear (convex)	14.0	1.6–2.0		+
	5.0	15–50	88		17.9	1.9–2.7		
Diasonics	7.5	20–40	100	Mechanical sector	20.2	1.5–1.7	Outrigged	
Elscint	6.5	20–60	30–105	Mechanical sector	16.1	2.6	Outrigged	
GE Medical Systems	5.0	25–80	90	Phased array sector	19.2	1.0–2.5	Flush	
Hewlett-Packard	5.0	20–80	110	Mechanical sector	16.0	1.4–2.6	Outrigged	
International/ ESAOTE Biomedica	6.5	15–45	80	Curvilinear convex	14.0	1.6–2.0	Flush	
	5.0, 7.5	15–70	90	Annular array	14.0	1.8–2.2	Flush	
Philips Ultrasound International	5.0 / 7.5	30–70 / 20–65	90	Mechanical sector	15.0	2.3–3.3		
Picker International	3.5, 5, 7.5	20–40 (approx)	100 (approx)	Mechanical sector	23 (approx)	2.0		
Pie Medical USA	5.0	Sector: 40–120 / Linear: 40–80	Sector: 110 / Linear: 5 (cm)	Mechanical sector or linear	Sector: 15 / Linear: 19	Sector: 3.5 / Linear: 1.2–2.2		
	5.0	10–50	150	Annular array sector	20.0	2.0–2.3		
Siemens Medical Systems	5, 6, 7.5 Selectable	20–70	220	Mechanical sector	14.0	1.8	Flush	
Shimadzu	5.0	20–120 (autofocus)	115 / 90	Curvilinear convex or phased array sector	15.0	0.7		
Toshiba Medical Systems	5.0	50 (autofocus)	86	Curvilinear convex	20.0	2.2–2.7	Flush	+
	6.0	50 (autofocus)	120	Curvilinear	20	2.2	Flush	+

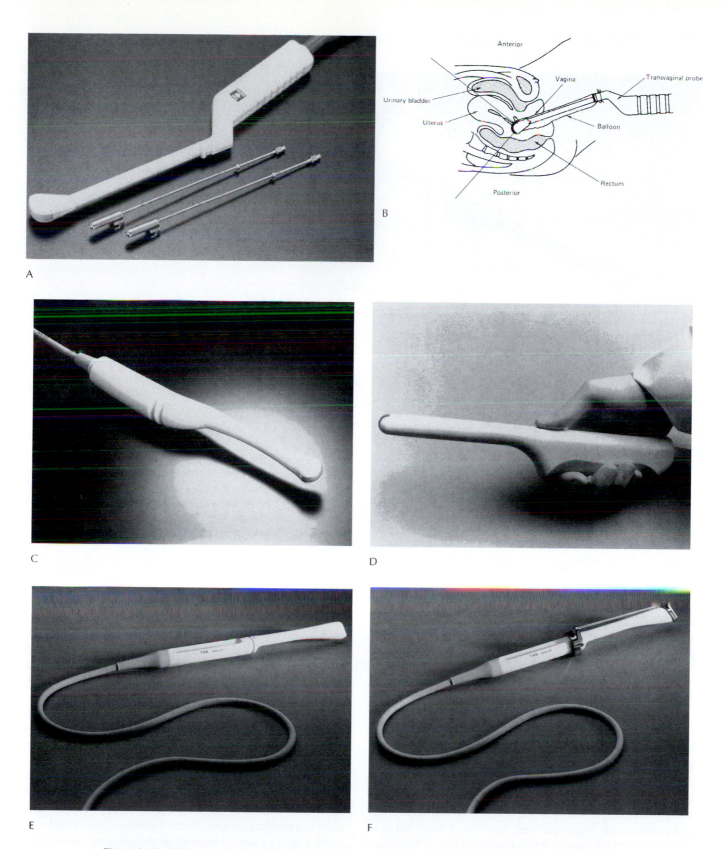

Figure 1-11. **(A)** Transvaginal proble of the curved linear array design shown with needle guide attachments. **(B)** Diagram of curved linear array transvaginal probe, illustrating approximate field of view. *(Courtesy of Toshiba, Inc.)* **(C)** "Tightly" curved transvaginal probe that uses 200 subelements with a central frequency of 6 MHz. *(Courtesy of Toshiba America US Inc.)* **(D)** ATL convex transvaginal probe which operates at 5–9 MHz. *(Courtesy of ATL, Inc.)* **(E)** Phased array transvaginal probe with a tilted "footprint." This probe allows imaging with selectable frequencies of 5.0, 6.5, or 7.5 MHz. *(Courtesy of Acuson, Inc.)* **(F)** Same probe as in **E** with needle guide attached. *(Courtesy of Acuson, Inc.)*

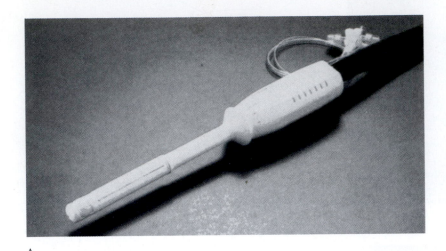

A

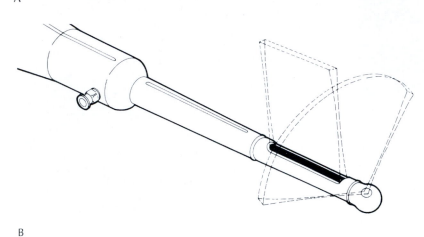

B

Figure 1–12. (A) Transrectal probe with biplanar capability (both linear and sector scanners incorporated into a single probe). **(B)** Diagram of field of view and scan plane orientations for the biplane dual-transducer transrectal probe. *(Courtesy of Toshiba and ATL, Inc.)*

and θ is the angle in degrees between the sound beam direction and the direction of the moving interface. The frequency shift may be either positive or negative relative to the incident frequency.

Thus, their actual received frequency (fr) from the moving interface would be

$$fr = f_0 \pm \Delta f \qquad [2]$$

When the impinging ultrasound beam passes through a blood vessel, scattering of the sound wave occurs. In this process, small amounts of sound energy are absorbed by each red cell and reradiated in all directions. If the red blood cell is moving with respect to the source, the backscattered energy returning to the receiving transducer will be shifted in frequency; the magnitude and direction of this shift are proportional to the velocity of the respective cell. If the ultrasound beam is considered to fill the entire lumen of a blood vessel, then the backscattered signal will consist of all the Doppler shifts produced by the red cells moving through the ultrasonic beam. Because there will always be a range of velocities present, from zero at the vessel wall to a peak value near the center of the vessel lumen, a spectrum of Doppler shift frequencies will always be present. The frequency spectrum is derived from the application of a mathematical operation called a Fourier transformation to the returning echo wave train. This spectrum can become quite complex, with pulsating blood flow and vessel wall motion, especially when blood flow disturbances due to anatomic defects are present. Vessel wall irregularity, ulcerated plaques, narrowed or partly occluded vessels, or such other abnormalities as stenotic heart valves cause velocity variation readily detected by differences in the frequency spectrum of the Doppler signal.

A number of imaging schemes have been devised to give the user information on vessel anatomy in addition to blood flow. The simplest of these uses a CW Doppler transducer fixed to a mechanical arm. As the transducer moves back and forth over a vessel of interest, an image is produced on a storage oscilloscope corresponding to each site of inquiry. A serious deficiency of this simple CW Doppler instrument is depth resolution.

The most practical way to add depth resolution to a Doppler instrument is to pulse the source and add a range gate to the receiver. Such pulsed Doppler devices are similar to a pulse echo instrument in that bursts of ultrasound are emitted at a regular repetition rate into the body tissue. A new pulse will not be transmitted until echoes from the previous pulse have ceased or significantly diminished. The depth of a pulse can be determined by noting the time of its flight to an interface and return. Relatively short bursts of approximately 0.5- to 1.0-second duration can be used to give high axial resolution for detection of the location and separation of interfaces within 1 mm or less.

The principle for the pulsed Doppler is actually quite different from that employed with a pulse echo instrument. To simultaneously determine the Doppler spectrum of a reflected wave from many depths in real-time requires extremely fast parallel processes to carry out the many Fourier transformations. To display these multidimensional data (flow magnitude, direction, and location), color-coded images are often used. In the image, color is used to encode direction and hue is used to encode relative magnitude.

A disadvantage of pulsed Doppler scanners is their inability to accurately determine rapid flow; this may present aliased results in which a high-flow location is actually presented as a low-flow location. The maximum flow that can be measured by a pulsed Doppler system is determined by the pulse repetition frequency (PRF) of the system. Specifically, the detected Doppler shift frequency (f) cannot be greater than PRF/2. To increase PRF to allow estimates of rapid flow unfortunately limits the field of view to very superficial structures and also adds the potential for range ambiguity errors. (Range ambiguity errors occur when echoes from previous lines are received as echoes from the current line.) Fortunately, flow aliasing can often be recognized and will not generally lead to mistaken diagnoses.

COLOR DOPPLER SONOGRAPHY

Color Doppler sonography (CDS) has many applications in obstetrics and gynecology. CDS allows assessment of blood flow to vital organs, such as the uterus, placenta, and ovary. It involves depiction of system shifts in a region of interest. The gray-scale depiction of interfaces is superimposed over areas of flow depicted in a variety of colors depending on the direction and velocity of flow. A variant of this technique, color velocity imaging (CVI), involves recognition of the speed of a particular "packet" of echoes and affords quantification of flow volume.

Color Doppler sonography involves intensities less than the suggested limit for FDA (94 mW/cm^2). It may actually decrease the intensities needed for Doppler interrogation by quicker identification of the vessel of interest rather than by the interrogation of relatively large fields of view required by pulsed Doppler techniques.

QUALITY CONTROL

The purpose of a quality assurance program is to ensure that the diagnostic quality of all ultrasonic images is maintained at the maximum attainable level. Part of this program must include monitoring procedures that will ensure the proper and consistent operation of all equipment. Equipment acceptance tests must be performed on delivery of new equipment and repeated whenever major equipment repairs are made. Quality assurance tests should be performed on a routine basis to detect deviations from the baseline acceptance tests. Quality assurance is the joint responsibility of physician, technician, and the service support personnel.

There are numerous test objects and instruments that are available for assessing the performance of ultrasonic equipment. A number of documents are also available that contain detailed protocols for establishing a quality assurance program. Probably the single most versatile and complete test object that can be used in these studies is the American Institute of Ultrasound in Medicine (AIUM) Standard 100-mm Test Object (Fig. 1–13A). (The standard AIUM test object is filled with a relatively nonattenuating medium. Phantoms with a similar configuration, but filled with an attenuating "tissue-equivalent" material, are also commercially available. These tissue-equivalent phantoms provide system beam-parameter measurements in a more patientlike environment.

A minimal quality assurance program should include routine monitoring of the performance of the gray-scale photography, image system sensitivity, axial resolution, and the accuracy and linearity of distance markers. In addition to evaluation of the gray-scale system, the AIUM Test Object may be used to assess each of the other system parameters. The minimal quality assurance program provides relative parameter values. Relative values are useful for detecting early changes in image system characteristics. Absolute measurements of system parameters are more difficult and may require additional test objects and equipment.

Of equal importance to the actual performance testing is the documentation of the test results. These recorded data are essential for accurate monitoring of equipment performance and are useful to both the equipment service personnel and the equipment manufacturer. It is also an incumbent possibility that this will be required by government regulatory and certifying agencies in the near future.

The initial camera settings and scan converter output controls depend largely on individual points of reference. Once a baseline has been established, a daily evaluation should be made to ensure that the same range of echo amplitudes can be seen as was present on previous test exposures.

Most systems now generate gray-scale bars displayed to one side or at the bottom of the image. This bar should be examined daily for consistency of step distribution and display. The comparison can be made either by visual inspection or with the aid of a densitometer, which is more quantitative.

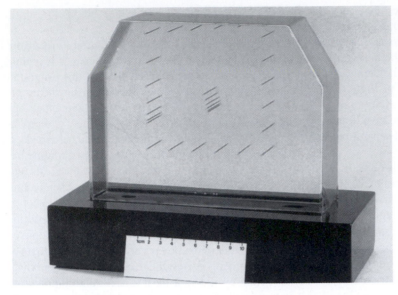

A

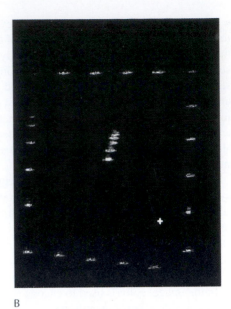

B

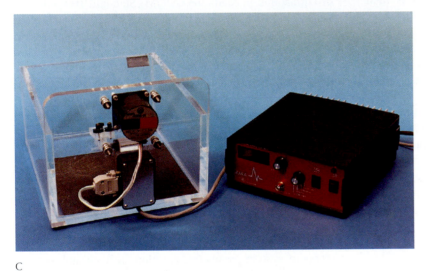

C

Figure 1–13. (A) Photograph of the AIUM Standard 100-mm Test Object. **(B)** Scan image of the AIUM phantom illustrates axial-resolution wire-set *(center)*, dead-zone wire-set *(top)*, and distance markers *(vertical and horizontal)*. **(C)** Photograph of a moving string phantom and a programmable control module. The control module can be programmed to provide a variety of velocity profiles (e.g., constant velocity and simulated arterial pulsatile flow). *(Figure continued.)*

A simple test for system sensitivity stability can be performed with the aid of the AIUM phantom. After carefully positioning the transducer directly above the reference wires, which are spaced 2 cm apart (making sure the transducer face is flat against the phantom surface), the system gain (attenuation or output) settings should be adjusted to display a one-division echo from the most distant wire. These gain settings should not change on subsequent recordings. Similarly, the minimum gain settings required to yield a discernible echo in the B-mode image should not change with time. By this method the stability of the instrumentation over time can be determined.

A single image of the AIUM phantom will provide data on axial resolution and on the accuracy and linearity of the distance markers. Axial resolution is assessed from the minimum resolvable spacing in the set of diagonal wires at the center of the phantom (Fig. 1–13B). Within this set, wire spac-

ings range from 5 to 1 mm. Most imaging systems should exhibit the ability to resolve 2-mm wire spacings, and this value should remain constant over time.

The accuracy and linearity of the system-generated distance markers can be evaluated by direct measurement of the distances of the vertical and horizontal wires from a B-mode image. The distance between the uppermost and bottom wires in the 2-cm spaced group is actually 10 cm, and this distance—as estimated by the markers—should not differ by more than 2 mm.

The increased use of Doppler and especially two-dimensional color Doppler imaging for diagnostic procedures makes it essential to extend ultrasound quality assurance programs to include Doppler instrumentation. Commercial Doppler flow phantoms of different designs have become available. Included in these are phantoms that provide true fluid flow through simulated vessels of different sizes and

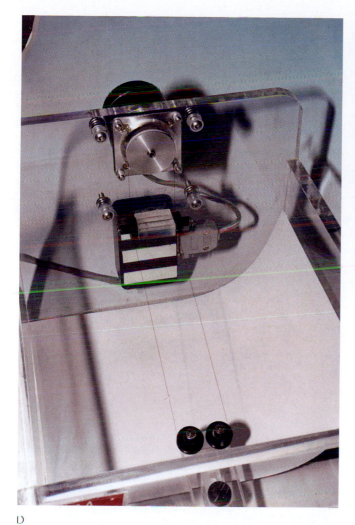

D

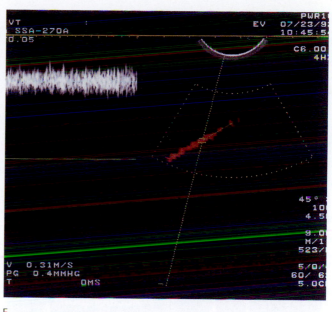

E

Figure 1–13. *(continued)* **(D)** Photograph of string and water bath. Chamber is filled with water for coupling purposes, and string is angulated with respect to horizontal to provide Doppler angle other than 90 degrees. **(E)** Photograph of a typical color Doppler image of the string phantom. Phantom image acquired with string running at a constant velocity of 30 cm/s. Doppler window over center of string image provides conventional Doppler velocity display.

orientations and phantoms that are based on a moving string (Figs. 1–13C, D). In each of these, known velocities corresponding to known Doppler shift frequencies can be used to evaluate instrument performance and stability. Phantoms can be used to provide a variety of flow profiles, from constant flow to highly pulsatile arterial flow. Figure 1–13E illustrates a typical color Doppler scan and conventional Doppler velocity time plot of a string phantom operating at a constant velocity of 30 cm/s.

Color Doppler Sonography

There are several ways to quantitate the Doppler waveform (Figs. 1–14A, B). The simplest is comparing systolic with diastolic velocities (S/D). However, calculation of true velocities requires factoring in the angle of incidence (Fig. 1–14C). Both the resistive (RI) and pulsatility (PI) indices are angle independent and unitless. They reflect the relative resistence to downstream flow. Other Doppler parameters, such as acceleration time and index reflect the time from the beginning of systole to systolic maximum velocities and deceleration time and time from maximum systolic velocity to end of diastolic

velocity, have clinical implications in conditions outside of obstetrics and gynecology such as in the evaluation for renal artery stenosis.

Color Doppler sonography combines gray-scale imaging with flow depiction (Figs. 1–14D, E). However, the same principles that are involved in CW or nongated Doppler affect color Doppler sonography. For example, if the area of interest is not sampled between 30 and 60 degrees of the transducer, significant error and dropout of signal occurs. No signal will be obtained if the incident beam is perpendicular to the flow. Aliasing may occur if the PRF is not sufficiently high. The PRF must be twice the frequency of the frequency shift to be detected.

Frequency-based (CDS) reflects velocity differences in the flowing blood (Fig. 1–14A). Differences in incident and received frequencies (Doppler shift) are proportional to the velocity of flow and the angle of flow relative to the incident beam. Typically, the color scale runs from red to blue depending on the direction of flow (red = toward transducer, blue = from transducer). Lighter shades of each color indicate higher velocities. Turbulence maps can be shown in shades of green.

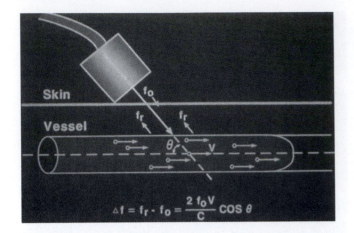

A

Figure 1–14. Principles of color Doppler sonography. **(A)** Diagram showing Doppler equation to calculate flow velocity. The change in emitted *(f_o)* and returned *(f_r)* frequency (Δf) is related to the angle of insonation (cos θ). *(Courtesy of W. Charboneau, MD.)* **(B)** Methods to quantitate flow from Doppler waveform. **(C)** Graph depicting percentage of error relative to the angle of insonation. There is minimal error in calculated velocity up to 60 degrees. **(D)** Diagram of the components of the color Doppler sonogram showing flow information obtained from moving targets recorded over a gray-scale depiction of interfaces. *(Figure continued.)*

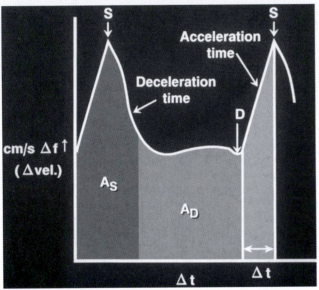

(B) left

Systolic/Diastolic	=	S/D
Resistive Index (R.I.)	=	$\frac{S-D}{S}$
Pulsatility Index (P.I.)	=	$\frac{S-D}{mean}$
Acceleration to peak (Acc)		$\frac{\text{vel. (max) - vel (min)}}{\text{t (beginning of systolic to max) - t (time to peak systole)}}$
Perfusion Index (Per I)	=	$\frac{\int \text{Area under curve during systole}}{\int \text{Area under curve during diastole}}$
Deceleration time (Dec)	=	$\frac{\Delta v}{\Delta t \text{ (First derivative decrease in diastole/time)}}$
Impedance Index (IMI)		$\frac{\text{S mean}}{D^2}$

(B) right

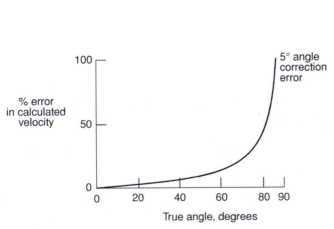

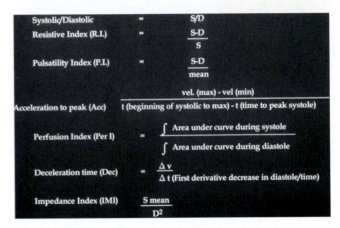

COLOR DOPPLER PRINCIPLES

C

D

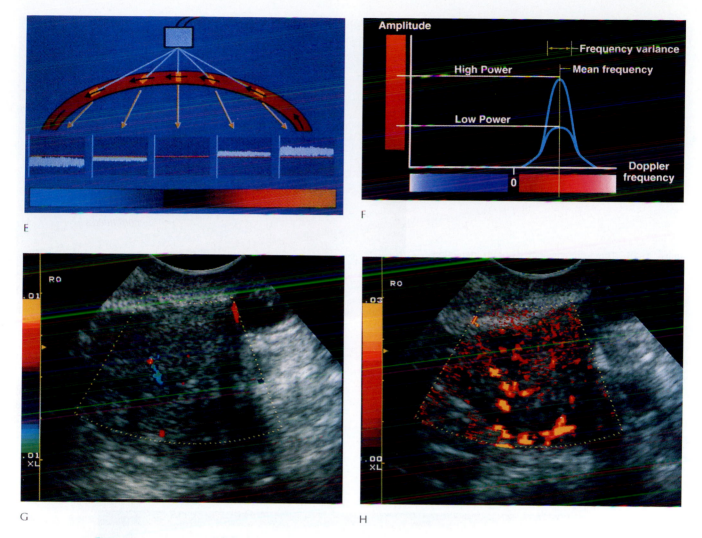

Figure 1–14. *(continued)* **(E)** Diagram showing color assignment of flow and waveform display. The waveform is depicted above the baseline if it is going toward the transducer, below if away. It is depicted in red if moving toward the transducer or blue if it is moving away. Doppler signals are not readily obtained perpendicular to the transducer and are shown as black. **(F)** Relation between frequency and amplitude or power CDS. Frequency-based CDS is based on differences in transmitted and received frequencies. The flow is coded with red if the flow is toward the transducer, with blue if it is away. Frequency CDS reflects changes in velocity as they relate to flow. Amplitude CDS reflects the number of blood elements or power flowing within a field of view. The Doppler shifts are coded in shades of orange. **(G)** Directional amplitude color Doppler sonography displays directional information (red = toward, blue = away) superimposed on flow. **(H)** Amplitude CDS of right ovary shown in **G** shows flow around a corpus luteum and is more sensitive to flow but does not discriminate its directional flow.

Amplitude CDS (a-CDS) reflects the number of blood elements flowing past the transducer. The color scale is usually in shades of orange (Figs. 1–14B, F). Directional a-CDS includes the directional information superimposed on the color scale.

Amplitude CDS is more sensitive to flow than frequency-based CDS, but it is degraded by motion. However, a-CDS is less angle dependent than frequency CDS.

The sensitivity of CDS to flow has recently improved with the clinical use of power or a-CDS. Whereas conventional CDS depends on changes in frequency as related to velocity of moving blood, a-CDS reflects the absolute number of blood elements flowing (Fig. 1–14F). Amplitude CDS is relatively angle independent but is degraded by motion. It also probably reflects venous flow due to an increased persistence. Amplitude CDS images are usually displayed in shades of

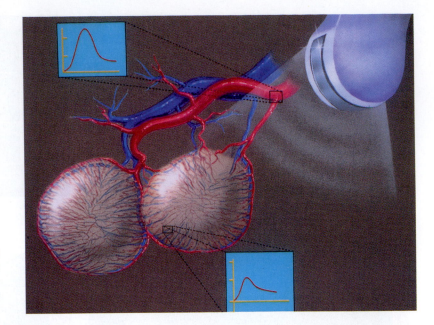

Figure 1–15. Three-dimensional diagram depicting different waveforms arising from a peripheral versus central vessels. The resistence in central vessels is typically less than in larger peripheral vessels. *(Drawing by Paul Gross, MS.)*

orange, whereas frequency-band CDS shows red as flow toward the transducer and blue as flow from the transducer (Figs. 1–14G, H).

Contrast media have been developed for CDS including ones consisting of microbubbles suspended in albumin (Albunex® Mallincrodkt, Inc., St. Louis, MO) and microbubbles suspended in sugar (Levovist®, Schering Inc., Berlin, Germany). These agents enhance the detection of blood flow and may allow time–activity calculations. Contrast is also used for the assessment of tubal patency.

Harmonic imaging improves the signal-to-noise ratio especially for CDS (Burns, 1995). It uses a multiple of the transmitter frequency to listen for returning signals. The combination of harmonic imaging, three-dimensional (3D) Ultrasonography, and contrast promises enhanced delineation of vascularity (Figs. 1–15 and 1–16).

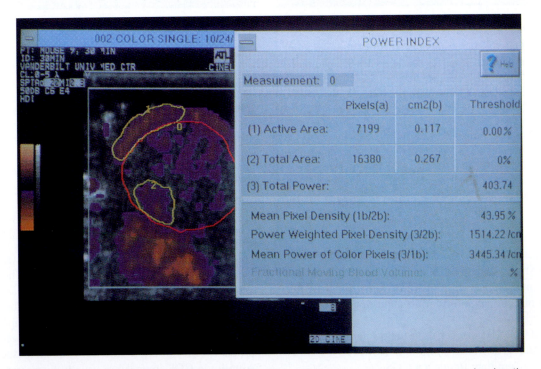

Figure 1–16. Two-dimensional CPA of a color Doppler angiogram implanted mouse tumor showing the power-weighted pixel density within the inner tumor to be 1514.22/cm².

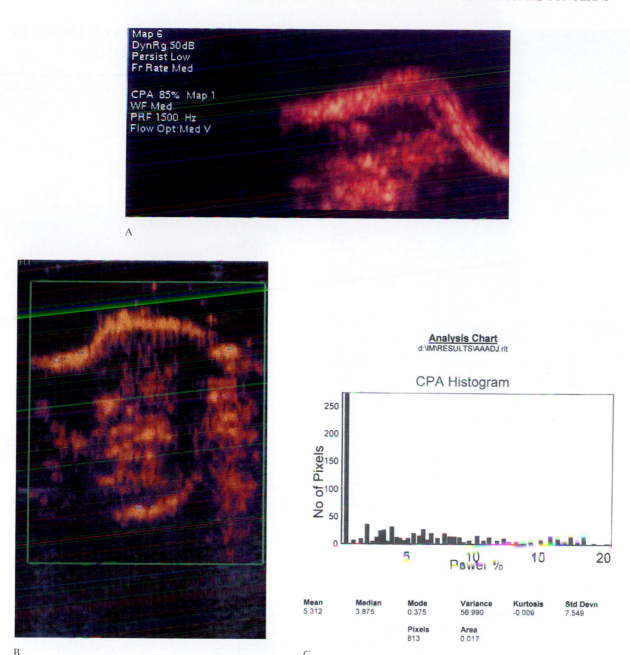

Figure 1–17. CDS quantification of flow. **(A)** A 3D CDS of an implanted mouse lung tumor. **(B)** One frame from a 3D CDS of a tumor in an axial plane. **(C)** Histogram of pixel densities from the image shown in **A**. Most were of low (<10%) power. *(Figure continued.)*

Blood Flow Quantification

Quantification of CDS has been studied as a means to objectively estimate vascularity (Figs. 1–16 and 1–17). One technique uses a software program to quantify a weighted pixel density, and researchers have reported a technique of determining "fractional blood flow" (Meyerowitz, 1996; Rubin, 1997). Determination of fractional blood volume depends on comparison with a known vessel with significant blood flow and allows for serial assessment. Flow determination by quantification of pixel density becomes more problematic as deeper structures are studied. Either method may allow calculation of time–activity curves, differ in benign and malignant lesions. Malignant lesions tend to peak faster and have longer dwell times than benign ones (Cosgrove, 1993).

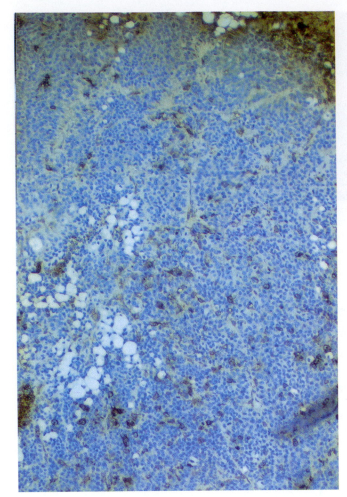

D

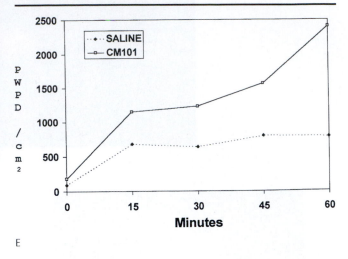

E

Figure 1–17. *(continued)* **(D)** Vessel stained specimen (200×) of tumor imaged in **A–C** shows peripheral arrangement of vessels, with several intratumor branches shown in brown. **(E)** Time–activity curve of saline versus extoxin (CM-101) over 60 minutes (CM-101), probably secondary to vasodilation caused by exotoxin injection.

Contrast Agents

Contrast agents have been used clinically in a variety of applications such as cardiac and renal sonography. There are a variety of contrast agents, from microbubbles suspended in human albumin (Albunex®) to those changing into gas when introduced into the body (Echogen) to galactose-coated microbubbles (Echovist®). All of these are either injected intravenously or instilled and provide enhanced delineation of tubal anatomy [Albunex®, Optison® Mallincrodkt, Inc., and Echovist®, cardiac function (Echovist®)], and improved visualization of hepatic masses. Injection of a contrast agent also affords determination of "enhancement kinetics" by generation of a time–activity curve. There will be many more new applications of ultrasonographic contrast in the near future for differentiation of normal from abnormal tissues.

Harmonic Imaging

One of the newest developments in sonographic instrumentation is the clinical use of harmonic imaging. This technique uses the harmonic principle to improve the signal-to-noise ratio, thereby improving image quality. Harmonic imaging is based on the principle that returned frequency at one or two multiples of the transmitter frequency has an improved signal-to-noise ratio and is more distinct over background noise. For example, when imaging a large patient with a 3.5 MHz transducer, harmonic imaging at 6 to 7 MHz could improve the image clarity.

Tissue harmonics are best perceived in the deeper tissue, which allows sufficient time for them to be generated. The signals are 1/100th of the incident beam. Thus, visualization of deeper structures such as in the abdomen seem to benefit most from the use of tissue harmonics.

This improvement is seen most frequently in the detection of subtle gallstones or common duct stones and of subtle masses in the kidney or liver. Harmonic imaging can also improve delineation of fetal and pelvic structures (Fig. 1–18).

Harmonic imaging can also improve the resolution when a contrast agent is used. This is particularly true when assessing arterial flow with a large organ such as the kidney. For gas-filled microsphere contrast, the energy from the incident

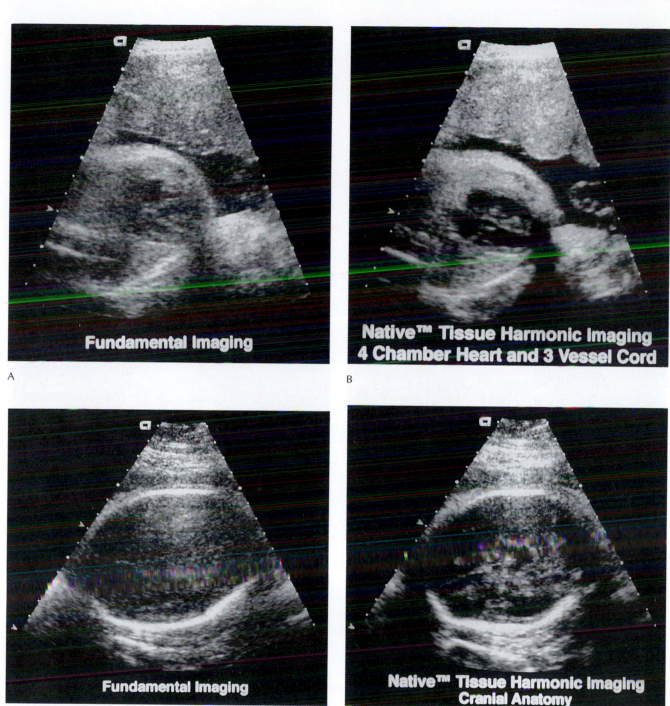

Figure 1–18. Harmonic imaging applications in obstetrics and gynecology. **(A)** Fundamental transverse sonogram of the fetal chest at 29 weeks of gestation in a difficult-to-image patient secondary to multiple abdominal scarring from prior surgeries. The presence of an anterior placenta and decreased amniotic fluid volume adds to the difficulty of this exam. In **A,** we are attempting to obtain a four-chamber view of the fetal heart. As seen, imaging is suboptimal and a four-chamber view of the fetal heart could not be obtained. **(B)** Images of the same patient shown in **A** in the same plane with Native Tissue Harmonic Imaging® *(Acuson, Inc.).* Now the four-chamber view is clearly imaged. A three-vessel transverse segment of the umbilical cord is also imaged within the amniotic fluid. **(C)** Fundamental transverse sonogram of the fetal head at 34 weeks of gestation in a difficult-to-image patient with severe oligohydramnios. In this case, we are attempting to image fetal intracranial anatomy, but imaging of the intracranial anatomy is suboptimal. **(D)** Images of the same patient in the same plane as in **C** with Native Tissue Harmonic Imaging®. The interhemispheric fissure, thalamus, and insula are now clearly seen. *(Figure continued.)*

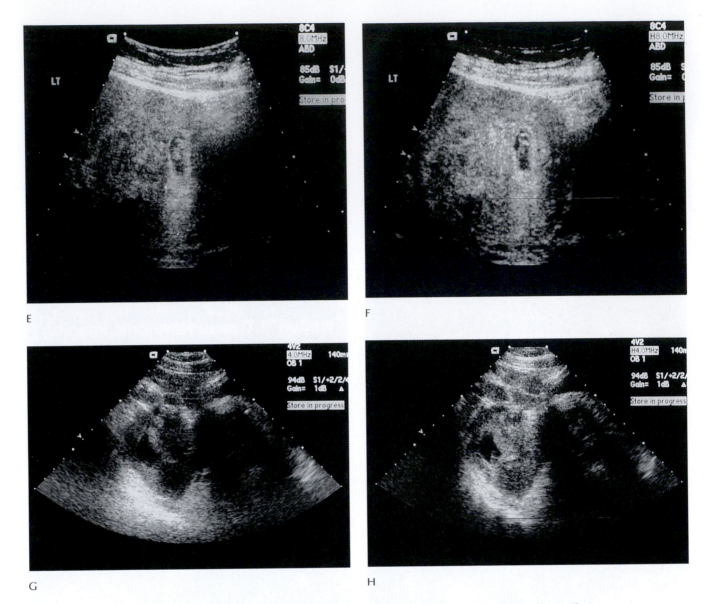

Figure 1–18. *(continued)* **(E)** Transabdominal fundamental sonogram of an elarged uterus in a patient presenting to the emergency room with abdominal pain and positive pregnancy test. Endovaginal sonography showed an enlarged uterus with a large fibroid. Due to the size of the uterus, the endometrial cavity could not be assessed, thus, an intrauterine pregnancy could not be confirmed by endovaginal scanning. On fundamental transabdominal sonography, a suspicion of an intrauterine gestation is present; however, a fetal pole and a yolk sac could not be confirmed. **(F)** Same as in **E** but with Native Tissue Harmonic Imaging®. Note the clear delineation of a yolk sac within the gestation, thus confirming an intrauterine pregnancy. **(G)** Transabdominal fundamental sonogram of a difficult-to-image patient referred with a positive pregnancy test. A fetal pole could not be documented by fundamental imaging. **(H)** Same as in **G** but with Native Tissue Harmonic Imaging®. A fetal pole is clearly seen within a gestation sac, and the patient was thus reassured.

ultrasonic waves deforms the shell of the microbubble, which then absorbs and releases vibrations at a multiple of the incident frequency. Harmonic imaging combined with contrast has the potential to obtain time–activity curves, thereby enabling assessment of overall flow.

Three-Dimensional Sonography

Several scanners have 3D capabilities. Some use reconstruction of a summated image as obtained by a sweep of the transducer (Fig. 1–17A). Other use a transducer holder that allows incremental movement in two orthogonal planes.

Thus far, the most common clinical application of 3D sonography in obstetrics is for the evaluation of fetal facial extremity and cardiac deformities.

The reader is referred to Chap. 49 for further details and examples of clinical applications.

PACS and Telesonography

The PACSs provide a means to display the sonographic images on a monitor and store the exam electronically (Fig. 1–19). These systems improve efficiency of the sonographer because films do not need to be developed and stored. Electronic display also affords manipulation of the image while on the screen for optimizing contrast and brightness.

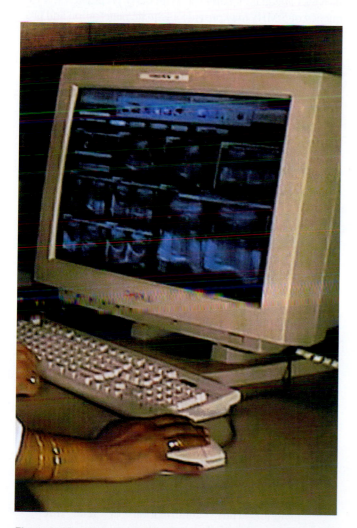

Figure 1–19. Ultrasound PACS. Several sonographic images are displayed on the monitor and stored electronically. The digital storage process allows manipulation and optimization of the images. Several scanners can be hooked up to this display module. The systems greatly enhance sonographer productivity and throughput because there is no need to take, process, or store films. *(Courtesy of ALI, Inc.)*

Films can be printed as needed for conference. Several manufacturers offer PACS as part of their systems.

Several institutions provide coverage remote from the central office by telesonography. The images are digitized and sent over telephone lines to a central facility. Sonographers can have real-time feedback while performing the sonogram at a remote site.

Facility Accreditation

The standards for operation of ultrasound facilities have been established by the (AIUM) and the American College of Radiology (ACR). Each of these societies has a specific process for accreditation, but the processes are very similar. The applicant facility undergoes a self-study that analyzes equipment, personnel, and qualification and experience of its personnel. Adequate handling of reports, documentation, and continuing medical education of the personnel are parameters that are assessed during the accreditation process.

Once a facility is accredited, the patient can be assured that the study performed is of sufficient quality for diagnosis, and the skill and experience of the personnel are at or above standard.

The AIUM has specific examination guidelines for standard sonographic procedures, specifically those in obstetrics and gynecology (Appendices A and B). In each of these guidelines, the parameters that should be assessed and documented are stated. This material is available to patients and their lawyers so that a standard examination is now well defined and universally applicable.

The specifics of the accreditation process and the various standards are available through the AIUM and ACR offices.

SUMMARY

This chapter has discussed and illustrated the pivotal and clinically pertinent principles involved in sonographic imaging.

REFERENCES

Physics

Christensen EE, Curry T, Dowdey J. *Introduction to the Physics of Diagnostic Radiology*, 3rd ed. Philadelphia: Lea & Febiger; 1984.

Kremkau FW. *Diagnostic Ultrasound Principles, Instrumentation and Exercises*, 2nd ed. New York: Grune & Stratton; 1984.

Powis R, Powis W. *A Thinker's Guide to Ultrasonic Imaging*. Baltimore: Urban & Schwarzenberg; 1984.

Price RR, Jones T, Fleischer AC, et al. Ultrasound basic principles. In: Coulam CM, Erickson JJ, Rollo FD, et al. *The Physical Basis of Medical Imaging*. New York: Appleton-Century-Crofts; 1981;155.

Doppler

Burns P. Harmonic imaging adds to ultrasound capabilities. *Diagn Imaging.* May 1995;AU7.

Cosgrove DO, Kedar R, Bamber J, et al. Breast diseases: Color Doppler US in differential diagnosis. *Radiology.* 1993;189:99.

Harmonic ultrasound. *Diagn Imaging.* June 1998; Supplement.

Merritt CRB. Imaging blood flow with Doppler. *Diagn Imaging.* November 1986;146.

Meyerowitz CB, Fleischer AC, Pickens DR, et al. Quantification of tumor vascularity and flow with amplitude color Doppler sonography in an experimental model: Preliminary results. *J Ultrasound Med.* 1996;15:827.

Phillips DJ, Hossack J, Beach KW, et al. Testing ultrasonic pulsed Doppler instruments with a physiologic string phantom. *J Ultrasound Med.* 1990;9:429–436.

Rubin JM, Adler RS, Fowlkes JB, et al. Fractional moving blood volume estimation using power Doppler imaging. *Radiology.* 1995;197:183.

Taylor KWJ. Going to the depths with duplex Doppler. *Diagn Imaging.* October 1987;106.

Taylor KJW, Morse SS, Rigsby CM, et al. Vascular complications in renal allografts. Detection with duplex Doppler ultrasound. *Radiology.* 1987;62:31–38.

Zagzebski JA. Physics and instrumentation of Doppler ultrasonography. *Semin Ultrasound.* 1981;11:246.

Intraluminal Probes

Berneschek G, Tatru G, Janisch H. Rectal sonography—A major advance in the diagnosis of recurrence of cervical malignancies. *Radiology.* 1985;155:557.

Platt LD. New look in ultrasound: The vaginal probe. *Contemp Obstet Gynecol.* October 1987;99–105.

Quality Assurance

Goldstein A. *Quality Assurance in Diagnostic Ultrasound: A Manual for the Clinical User.* Washington, DC: US Government Printing Office; 1980. HHS Publication FDA 81–8139.

Goldstein A, Madrazo BL. Slice-thickness artifacts in gray-scale ultrasound. *J Clin Ultrasound.* 1981;9:365–375.

Wolfman NT, Boehme JM, Choplin RH, et al. Evaluation of PACS in ultrasonography. *J Ultrasound Med.* 1992;11:217.

APPENDIX A
AIUM POLICY STATEMENT: ANTEPARTUM OBSTETRIC ULTRASOUND EXAMINATION GUIDELINES

These guidelines have been developed for use by practitioners of ultrasonography in the performance of obstetric ultrasound studies. It should be noted that these are guidelines for the examination, and in some cases additional or specialized examination will be necessary. Although it is not possible to detect all structural congenital anomalies with diagnostic ultrasound, adherence to the following guidelines will maximize chances of detecting conditions currently thought diagnosable.

Equipment

These studies should be conducted with real-time or a combination of real-time and static scanners, but never solely with a static scanner. A transducer of appropriate frequency (from 3 to 5 MHz) should be used.

Comment. Real time is necessary to confidently confirm the presence of fetal life through observation of cardiac activity, respiration, and active movement. Real-time studies simplify evaluation of the entire fetus and the task of obtaining the numerous measurements that must be made.

The choice of frequency is a trade-off between beam penetration and resolution. With modern equipment, 3 to 5 MHz allows beam penetration in nearly all patients and provides adequate resolution. With early pregnancies, a frequency of 5 MHz may provide adequate penetration and produce superior resolution.

Documentation

Adequate documentation of the study is essential for high-quality patient care and should include a permanent record of the ultrasound images with appropriate labeling. Whenever possible, an attempt should be made to demonstrate the measurement parameters and anatomic findings proposed below. A written report of the ultrasound findings should be included in the patient's medical record. The images should be labeled with the examination date, patient identification, and image orientation.

Guidelines for First Trimester

1. The location of the gestational sac should be documented. The embryo should be identified and the crown–rump length recorded.
   Comment. The crown–rump length is one of the most accurate indicators of fetal age. Comparison should be made with standard tables. Late in the first trimester, biparietal diameter and other fetal measurements may be used.

2. Presence or absence of fetal life should be reported.
   Comment. Real-time observation is critical in this diagnosis. Cardiac activity may be visible prior to 7 weeks as determined by crown–rump length. Thus, confirmation of fetal life may require follow-up evaluation.

3. Fetal number should be documented.
   Comment. Multiple embryos should be reported only in those instances in which the embryos themselves are demonstrated. Due to variability in fusion between the amnion and

chorion, the appearance of more than one sac-like structure in early pregnancy is often noted, but does not necessarily represent multiple gestations.

4. Evaluation of the uterus (including cervix) and adnexal structures should be performed.
   Comment. This will allow recognition of associated findings that may have clinical implications. The presence, location, and size of myomas and adnexal masses should be recorded.

Guidelines for Second and Third Trimesters

1. Fetal life, number, and presentation should be documented.
   Comment. Abnormal heart rate or rhythm should be reported. Multiple pregnancies require the reporting of additional information: placental number, sac number, and comparison of fetal size.

2. An estimate of the amount of amniotic fluid (increased, decreased, normal) should be reported.
   Comment. Although this evaluation is subjective, there is little difficulty in recognizing the extremes of amniotic fluid volume. Physiologic variation with stage of pregnancy must be taken into account.

3. The placental location should be recorded and its relation to the internal cervical os determined.

4. Assessment of gestation age in the second and third trimesters should be accomplished using at least two of the following parameters: biparietal diameter, head circumference, femur length, and abdominal circumference. If previous studies have been done, an estimate of the appropriateness of interval growth should be given.
   Comment. Third-trimester measurements may not accurately reflect gestational age. Determination of gestational age should be performed prior to 26 weeks whenever possible.

   A. Biparietal diameter at a standard reference level should be measured and recorded and should include the cavum septi pellucidi, the thalamus, or the cerebral peduncles to confirm that the appropriate level was selected.
   Comment. If the fetal head is dolichocephalic or brachycephalic, the biparietal diameter itself may be misleading. In such situations, the head circumference is required.

   B. Head circumference is measured at the same level as the biparietal diameter.

   C. Femur length should be measured routinely and recorded after the 12th week of gestation.
   Comment. As with biparietal diameter, considerable variation is present late in pregnancy.

   D. Abdominal circumference should be determined at the level of the junction of the umbilical vein and portal sinus.
   Comment. Abdominal circumference measurement may allow detection of asymmetrical growth retardation, a condition of the late second and third trimesters. Comparison of the abdominal circumference with the head circumference should be made. If the abdominal measurement is below that expected for the stated gestation, it is recommended that circumferences of head and body be performed, and head circumference and abdominal circumference ratio be reported. The use of circumferences is also suggested in those instances in which the shape of either the head or body is different from that normally encountered.

5. Evaluation of the uterus (including cervix) and adnexal structures should be performed.
   Comment. This will allow recognition of associated findings that may have clinical implications. The presence, location, and size of myomas and adnexal should be recorded

6. The study should include an attempt to demonstrate but not necessarily be limited to the following fetal anatomy: cerebral ventricles, spine, stomach, urinary bladder, umbilical cord insertion site, and renal regions.

Suspected abnormalities may require a specialized evaluation.

APPENDIX B
ACR STANDARD FOR PERFORMANCE OF THE ULTRASOUND EXAMINATION OF THE FEMALE PELVIS

Introduction
This standard has been developed to provide assistance to physicians performing ultrasound studies of the female pelvis. Ultrasound of the female pelvis should be performed only when there is a valid medical reason, and the lowest possible ultrasonic exposure settings should be used to gain the necessary diagnostic information. In some cases, additional or specialized examinations may be necessary. Although it

is not possible to detect every abnormality, adherence to the following standard will maximize the probability of detecting most of the abnormalities that occur.

Qualifications of Personnel

See the ACR Standard for Performing and Interpreting Diagnostic Ultrasound Examinations.

Equipment

Ultrasound examination of the female pelvis should be conducted with a real-time scanner, preferably using sector, curved linear, or endovaginal transducers. The transducer or scanner should be adjusted to operate at the highest clinically appropriate frequency, realizing that there is a trade-off between resolution and beam penetration. With modern equipment, studies performed from the anterior abdominal wall can usually use frequencies of 3.5 MHz or higher, and scans performed from the vagina should use frequencies of 5 MHz or higher.

All probes should be cleaned after use. Vaginal probes should be covered by a protective sheath before insertion. After the examination, the sheath should be disposed of and the probe cleaned in an antimicrobial solution. The type of solution and cleaning time depend on the manufacturer's and infectious disease recommendations.

Quality Control

Each facility should have documented policies and procedures for monitoring and evaluating the effective management, safety, and proper performance of imaging equipment. The quality control program should be designed to maximize the quality of the diagnostic information. Equipment performance should be monitored. This may be accomplished as part of routine preventative maintenance.

Quality Improvement

Procedures should be systematically monitored and evaluated as part of the overall quality improvement program of the facility. Monitoring should include the evaluation of the accuracy of interpretations and the appropriateness of the examination. Complications and adverse events should be recorded and periodically reviewed to identify opportunities to improve patient care. The data should be collected in a manner that complies with statutory and regulatory peer-review procedures to protect the confidentiality of the peer-review data.

Documentation

Adequate documentation is essential for high-quality patient care. There should be a permanent record of the ultrasound examination and its interpretation included in the medical record. Images of all appropriate areas, both normal and abnormal, should be recorded in an imaging or storage format. Variations from normal size should be accompanied by measurements. Images are to be appropriately labeled with the examination date, facility name, patient identification, date of last menstrual period, image orientation, and, whenever possible, the organ or area imaged. Retention of the permanent record of the ultrasound examination should be consistent with both clinical need and the relevant legal and local health care facility requirements. Reporting should be in accordance with the ACR Standard for Communication.

Ultrasound Examination of the Female Pelvis

The following standard describes the examination to be performed for each organ and anatomic region in the female pelvis. All relevant structures should be identified by the transabdominal or transvaginal approach. In many cases, both will be needed.

General Pelvic Preparation. For a pelvic sonogram performed transabdominally, the patient's urinary bladder should be adequately distended. For a transvaginal sonogram, the urinary bladder is usually empty. The vaginal transducer may be introduced by the patient, the sonographer, or the sonologist. It is recommended that a woman be present in the examining room during a transvaginal sonogram, as either an examiner or a chaperone.

Uterus. The vagina and uterus provide an anatomic landmark that can be used as a reference point for the remaining normal and abnormal pelvic structures. In evaluating the uterus, the following should be documented: (a) the uterine size, shape, and orientation; (b) the endometrium; (c) the myometrium; and (d) the cervix. The vagina should be imaged as a landmark for the cervix and lower uterine segment.

Uterine size can be obtained. Uterine length is evaluated in the long axis from the fundus to the cervix (the external os, if it can be identified). The depth of the uterus (anteroposterior dimension) is measured in the same long-axis view from its anterior to posterior walls, perpendicular to the length. The width is measured from the transaxial or coronal view. Cervical diameters can be similarly obtained.

Abnormalities of the uterus should be documented. The endometrium should be analyzed for thickness, echogenicity, and its position within the uterus. The myometrium and cervix should be evaluated for contour changes, echogenicity, and masses.

Adnexa (Ovaries and Fallopian Tubes). When evaluating the adnexa, an attempt should be made to identify the ovaries first because they can serve as the major point of reference for adnexal structures. Frequently the ovaries are situated anterior to the internal iliac (hypogastric) vessels, which serve as a landmark for their identification. The following ovarian findings should be documented: (a) size, shape, contour, and echogenicity; and (b) position relative to the uterus. The ovarian size can be determined by measuring the length in the long axis with the anteroposterior dimension measured perpendicular to the length. The ovarian width is measured in the transaxial or coronal view. A volume can be calculated.

The normal fallopian tubes are not commonly identified. This region should be surveyed for abnormalities, in particular dilated tubular structures.

If an adnexal mass is noted, its relation to the ovaries and uterus should be documented. Its size and echopattern (cystic, solid, or mixed) should be determined. A search for embryonic cardiac activity should be conducted when appropriate. Doppler or color Doppler ultrasound may be useful in select cases and can identify the vascular nature of tubular pelvic structures.

Cul-de-Sac. The cul-de-sac and bowel posterior to the uterus may not be clearly defined. This area should be evaluated for the presence of free fluid or a mass. If a mass is detected, its size, position, shape, echopattern (cystic, solid, or complex), and relation to the ovaries and uterus should be documented. Differentiation of normal loops of bowel from a mass may be difficult if only an abdominal examination is performed. A transvaginal examination may be helpful to distinguish a suspected mass from fluid and feces within the normal rec-

tosigmoid. An ultrasound water enema study or a repeat examination after a cleansing enema may also help distinguish a suspected mass from bowel.

REFERENCES

Laing FC. US analysis of adnexal masses: The art of making the correct diagnosis. *Radiology.* 1994;191:21.

Lin MC, Gosink BB, Wolf SI, et al. Endometrial thickness after menopause: Effect of hormone replacement. *Radiology.* 1991;180:427.

Mendelson EB, Bohm-Velez M, Joseph N, Neiman HL. Gynecologic imaging: Comparison of transabdominal and transvaginal sonography. *Radiology.* 1988;166:321.

Sheth S, Hamper UM, Kurman RJ. Thickened endometrium in the postmenopausal woman: Sonographic-pathologic correlation. *Radiology.* 1993;187:135.

Taylor KJW, Schwartz PE. Screening for early ovarian cancer. *Radiology.* 1994;192:1.

Tessler FN, Schiller VL, Perrella RR, et al. Transabdominal versus endovaginal pelvic sonography: Prospective study. *Radiology.* 1989;170:553.

Wolf SI, Gosink BB, Feldesman MR, et al. Prevalence of simple adnexal cysts in postmenopausal women. *Radiology.* 1991;180:65.

2

Obstetric Sonography: The Output Display Standard and Ultrasound Bioeffects

William D. O'Brien, Jr. • *Tariq A. Siddiqi*

The first ultrasonic devices for imaging the fetus *in utero* were developed almost a half-century ago.[1] These early instruments demonstrated the potential to provide high-resolution fetal images, information previously not available without hazard. Since then, diagnostic ultrasound not only has gained wide clinical acceptance because of its ease of use and patient comfort but has also profoundly influenced the general practice of medicine and especially obstetrics. It has been almost three decades since the first major efforts were made to assess the risk of ultrasonic energy.[2,3] Since then, there have been numerous safety-related reviews published.[1,4–37] Meanwhile, the use of diagnostic ultrasound in obstetrics continues to increase worldwide despite efforts by several national[11,14,16,25,28,31,34,37] and international[12,26,29,36] organizations and the RADIUS Study[38] to restrict its use to clinically indicated examinations. These recommended restrictions have occurred despite the fact that the studies necessary to support a reliable assessment of the risks associated with human exposure to ultrasound have not been undertaken. Nevertheless, this has not adversely impacted diagnostic ultrasound's necessary and valuable applications in clinical medicine.

There is a general belief in the medical community that diagnostic ultrasound does not pose any risk to mother or fetus, but academic and government research scientists continue to investigate and evaluate potential risks. Many of these investigators have argued that the appropriate research has not been performed to support a reliable assessment of risks associated with human exposure to ultrasound. By the same token, it has also been properly argued that there is always an insufficient database to "prove" a modality totally safe. The fact that there continues to be concern for the safety of ultrasound demonstrates a continued interest by the clinical and basic science community in ensuring that the use of this imaging modality remains safe. Continued research will also improve our database and increase our confidence. And, if a serious biological effect is identified (which has not yet been the case), such information will then be disseminated to the clinical community so that appropriate risk–benefit decisions can be made. Diagnostic ultrasound has an outstanding safety record to date, and the reason for such a remarkable safety record is the rigid non–safety-based regulatory control the US Food and Drug Administration (FDA) has exercised over this diagnostic modality, a level of control unmatched by any other radiologic imaging modality.[1]

This chapter reviews our understanding of ultrasound-induced biological effects relative to diagnostic ultrasound applications in fetal medicine and further examines issues of the *Standard for Real-Time Display of Thermal and Mechanical Acoustic Output Indices on Diagnostic Ultrasound Equipment* (commonly referred to as the Output Display Standard, or ODS)[39] in terms of fetal exposure.

ULTRASONIC BIOPHYSICS

Ultrasonic biophysics[40] is the study of mechanisms responsible for the interaction of ultrasound and biological materials. As shown in Figure 2–1, bioeffects studies investigate how ultrasound affects biological materials, whereas the study of how tissues affect the ultrasound waveform provides the basis for ultrasound imaging. Thus, an understanding of the interaction of ultrasound with tissue provides the scientific basis for understanding image production and risk assessment.

The emphasis of ultrasonic biophysics studies in this contribution is on mechanisms responsible for how ultrasound and biological materials interact, and research in this area has shown that ultrasound can produce changes in living systems. Such knowledge comes from fundamental laboratory studies that form the basis for an understanding of the known mechanisms by which ultrasound can affect living systems.[18,21,27,32,33,40,41] These mechanisms can be classified in terms of whether a temperature increase (thermal) or a mechanical effect (usually bubblelike or cavitationlike activity) is believed to be the principal cause for the given biologic effect.

When discussing bioeffects studies and biophysical mechanisms, whether thermal or mechanical, there are selected exposure quantities that need to be completely characterized.[42] The source of ultrasonic power can be completely characterized *in vitro* in a lossless medium, i.e., water, as is required of equipment manufacturers by the FDA.[43–46] In fact, depending on the intended clinical use, ultrasound equipment can be designed to specific acoustic output characteristics and tested to ensure performance within defined output limits. The relevance of this process and *in vitro* acoustic pressure data, obtained in a lossless medium, to *in situ* exposure levels remains uncertain. For regulatory purposes, the FDA uses a homogeneous tissue model (called a *derating factor*) where it is assumed that the ultrasonic attenuation coefficient of tissue between the ultrasound transducer and, for example, the conceptus, is 0.3 dB/(cm/MHz).[43–47] Although 0.3-dB/(cm/MHz) derating factor is believed to be conservative, thereby modeling the "maximum exposure" or "worst-case" risk, *in vivo* studies have shown that the *in vivo* minimum insertion loss value for human pregnancy at 20 weeks or less of gestation is 0.14 dB/(cm/MHz).[48] Thus, in certain cases, the FDA's derating factor could significantly underestimate acoustic exposures to sensitive embryonic or fetal tissues. This risk is further compounded by the recent FDA change in the maximum allowable derated spatial peak, temporal average intensity ($I_{SPTA.3}$) from 94 to 720 mW/cm^2 for obstetric ultrasound equipment.[45] The ".3" in the subscript denotes the specific derating factor of 0.3 dB/(cm/MHz).

When the FDA initiated the regulation of diagnostic ultrasound equipment in 1985,[43] application-specific intensity limits were set which manufacturers could not exceed (Table 2–1). For fetal imaging and other applications, the derated $I_{SPTA.3}$ could not exceed 46 mW/cm^2. Likewise, the derated spatial peak, pulse average intensity ($I_{SPPA.3}$), and derated maximum intensity ($I_{m.3}$) could not exceed 65 and 160 W/cm^2, respectively. These limits were (and are) *not* based on safety considerations but rather on the known maximum output limits of diagnostic ultrasound equipment at the time when the Medical Devices Amendments were enacted (May 28, 1976), hence the term *preamendments levels*. To emphasize FDA's date-based regulatory approach as opposed to a safety- and efficacy-based regulatory approach, the American Institute of Ultrasound in Medicine notified[49] the

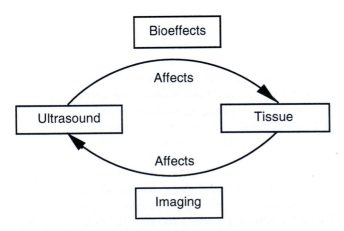

Figure 2–1. View of ultrasonic biophysics that includes ultrasonic bioeffects studies.

TABLE 2–1. FDA'S PREAMENDMENTS LEVELS OF DIAGNOSTIC ULTRASOUND DEVICES[43]

	Derated Intensity Values		
	$I_{SPTA.3}$ (mW/cm^2)	$I_{SPPA.3}$ (W/cm^2)	$I_{m.3}$ (W/cm^2)
Cardiac	430	65	160
Peripheral vessel	720	65	160
Ophthalmic	17	28	50
Fetal imaging and other[a]	46	65	160

[a]Abdominal, intraoperative, small organ (breast, thyroid, testes), neonatal cephalic, and adult cephalic.

TABLE 2–2. FDA'S PREAMENDMENTS LEVELS OF DIAGNOSTIC ULTRASOUND DEVICES[44]

	Derated Intensity Values		
	$I_{SPTA.3}$ (mW/cm^2)	$I_{SPPA.3}$ (W/cm^2)	$I_{m.3}$ (W/cm^2)
Cardiac	430	190	310
Peripheral vessel	720	190	310
Ophthalmic	17	28	50
Fetal imaging and other[a]	94	190	310

[a]Abdominal, intraoperative, small organ (breast, thyroid, testes), neonatal cephalic, and adult cephalic.

FDA in mid-1986 that there existed before May 28, 1976 at least two diagnostic preenactment ultrasound devices that had output intensity levels greater than those listed in Table 2–1. In early 1987, the FDA updated their diagnostic ultrasound guidance to the higher intensity levels[44] listed in Table 2–2. The date-based regulatory approach has been criticized by technical, scientific, and medical professionals and by the diagnostic ultrasound industry.[50] The implication is that these arbitrary limits are safety based and could limit future clinical benefits by preventing the development of more advanced diagnostic ultrasound systems and, hence, greater clinical benefit, that may require higher output levels. Further, it was observed[50] that limited diagnostic ultrasound capabilities may, in fact, be responsible for greater risk to the patient due to an inadequate diagnosis or to the need to use another diagnostic procedure with a defined risk.

All of these exposimetry quantities are defined in selected references.[13,22,51] When considering exposimetry quantities related to the interaction of ultrasound with tissues the intensity of the ultrasound beam is important because it has been the most commonly reported quantity in the bioeffects literature and because the FDA (see Tables 2–1 and 2–2 for examples) regulates diagnostic ultrasound equipment based on intensity. However, intensity is not a dosimetric quantity and is thus flawed as a predictor of heating and cavitation in tissue. Nontheless most of the contemporary and previous bioeffect literature has reported results in terms of intensity quantities, as will be seen in this chapter.

Diagnostic ultrasound manufacturers can still have their equipment approved through the application-specific limits listed in Table 2–2. Alternately, manufacturers can have their equipment approved under the provisions of the ODS.[39,45–47] Although the ODS does not specify upper limits, when FDA implemented the ODS into its regulatory process, it stipulated a regulatory upper limit of 720 mW/cm^2 for the derated $I_{SPTA.3}$.[45] Subsequently, the FDA replaced both the $I_{SPPA.3}$ and $I_{m.3}$ as regulated quantities with the mechanical index (MI; from the ODS[39]) and stipulated a regulatory upper limit of 1.9 for the MI. These FDA limits of 720 mW/cm^2 ($I_{SPTA.3}$) and 1.9 (MI) were for all clinical applications of ultrasound equipment. Then, in 1997, the FDA lowered the

regulated upper limits for ophthalmologic applications.[46] All of these FDA ultrasound exposure limits are date based, not safety based.

OUTPUT DISPLAY STANDARD

The purpose of the ODS[34,39] is to provide users of diagnostic ultrasound equipment the capability to operate their systems at intensities significantly higher than previously possible to improve their diagnostic capabilities. As a result, there is an increased potential of harm to patients, which requires that a quantitative method be devised for the user to specifically assess the possible biological consequences of the increased power output. The ODS[39] does this in part by providing calculated quantities that are based on biophysical indicators, namely indices that relate to the maximum tissue temperature increase in the beam (thermal indices, or TI) and an index that relates to the potential for producing cavitation (MI). Therefore, when any of these two biophysical indices are provided, the equipment operator has a real-time display of information to make appropriate clinical decisions, namely benefit versus risk, and to implement the ALARA (as low as reasonably achievable) principle.[34,52]

Thermal Index

Figure 2–2 shows the three thermal indices for three tissue models and two scan mode conditions. The three TIs are the soft-tissue thermal index (TIS), the bone thermal index (TIB), and the cranial bone thermal index (TIC). The unscanned mode is typically used clinically for spectral Doppler and M-mode, where the ultrasound beam remains stationary for a period of time. Also, the unscanned-mode TIS and the TIB are the only TI quantities that attempt to estimate temperature increase at locations other than at or near the source surface.

	Scanned Mode	Unscanned Mode
Soft Tissue	TIS at Surface	TIS Small Aperture Large Aperture
Bone at Focus	TIS at Surface	TIB
Bone at Surface	TIC	TIC

Figure 2–2. Thermal indices used for the three tissue models and two scanning conditions.

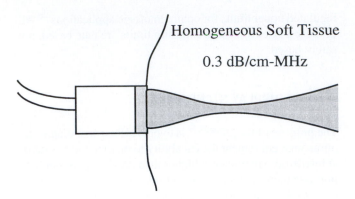

Figure 2–3. Homogeneous soft-tissue model.

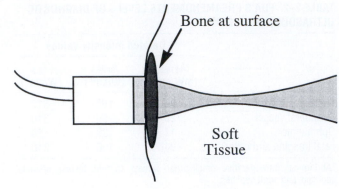

Figure 2–5. Bone-at-surface tissue model.

The others estimate temperature increase at or near the source surface.

The basic definition of all *TI*s is

$$TI = \frac{W_o}{W_{DEG}} \qquad [1]$$

where W_o is the source power of the diagnostic ultrasound system and W_{DEG} is the source power required to increase the tissue temperature 1°C under very specific and conservative conditions. Tissue perfusion is included in the W_{DEG} expressions.

Three tissue models were considered for implementing the ODS (Figs. 2–3, 2–4, and 2–5). The *homogeneous soft-tissue* model (Fig. 2–3) is typical of a scanning condition for which there is only soft tissue in the sound beam path. The assumption is that the soft tissue is homogeneous (in terms of both acoustic and thermal properties), with an attenuation coefficient (derating factor) of 0.3 dB/(cm/MHz). Figures 2–4 and 2–5 show the two cases in which bone is within the sound beam path. The *bone-at-focus* tissue model (Fig. 2–4) is typical of second- and third-trimester fetal imaging for which fetal bone is intercepted by the sound beam. In this case, the interposed tissue is assumed to have the same homogeneous properties as the soft-tissue model. The

bone-at-surface tissue model (Fig. 2–5) is typical of adult cephalic imaging.

Both scanned and unscanned modes (Fig. 2–6) are considered in the development of the W_{DEG} expressions for the estimate of the appropriate *TI*s. For the scanned mode, the *TI*s are based on calculations at or near the transducer surface. For the unscanned mode, the *TI*s are based on calculations at locations other than at or near the source surface, with the unscanned mode for *TIC* being the exception.

TIS at Surface (Scanned Mode)

Figure 2–7 shows a typical axial temperature increase profile for the homogeneous soft-tissue model under scanned-mode conditions. The maximum temperature increase occurs near the surface, usually within the first couple of centimeters of the skin surface.

Figure 2–8 shows a typical axial temperature increase profile for the bone-at-focus tissue model under scanned-mode conditions. The maximum temperature increase also occurs near the surface, usually within the first couple of centimeters of the skin surface. The same *TIS* calculation was made for both cases shown in Figures 2–7 and 2–8. The *TIS* calculation estimates the *TI* at the location where the temperature increase is a maximum value, namely at the surface.

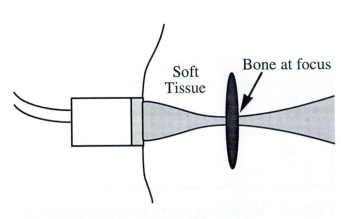

Figure 2–4. Bone-at-focus tissue model.

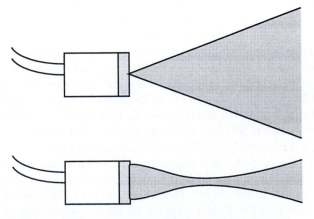

Figure 2–6. Scanned *(top)* and unscanned *(bottom)* modes.

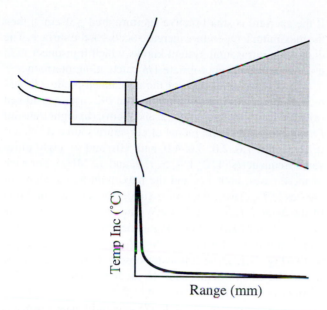

Figure 2–7. Axial temperature increase profile for the homogeneous soft-tissue model and scanned mode.

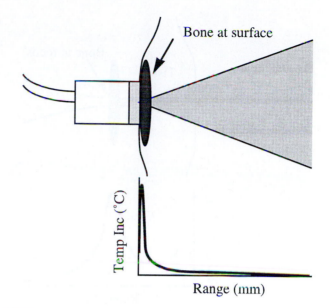

Figure 2–9. Axial temperature increase profile for the bone-at-surface tissue model and scanned mode.

TIC (Scanned and Unscanned Modes)

Figure 2–9 shows a typical axial temperature increase profile for the bone-at-surface tissue model under scanned-mode conditions. The maximum temperature increase occurs at the bone surface. Figure 2–10 shows a typical axial temperature increase profile for the bone-at-surface tissue model under unscanned-mode conditions. The maximum temperature increase also occurs at the bone surface. The same *TIC* calculation was made for both conditions shown in Figures 2–9 and 2–10. The *TIC* calculation estimates the *TI* at the location where the temperature increase is a maximum value, namely at the adult cranial bone surface.

TIB (Unscanned Mode)

Figure 2–11 shows a typical axial temperature increase profile for the bone-at-focus tissue model under unscanned-mode conditions. The maximum temperature increase occurs at the bone, not at the skin surface, although there might be a slight increase in temperature at the skin surface also. The *TIB* calculation estimates the *TI* at the location where the temperature increase is a maximum value, namely at the second or third trimester fetal bone.

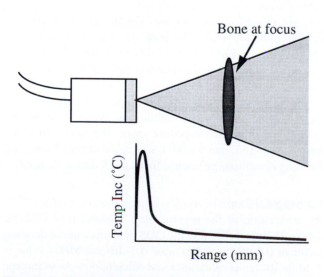

Figure 2–8. Axial temperature increase profile for the bone-at-focus tissue model and scanned mode.

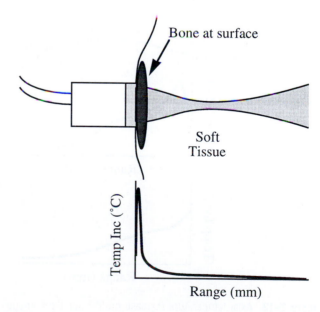

Figure 2–10. Axial temperature increase profile for the bone-at-surface tissue model and unscanned mode.

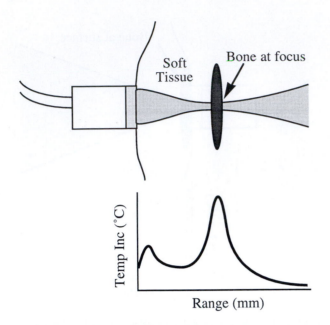

Figure 2–11. Axial temperature increase profile for the bone-at-focus tissue model and unscanned mode.

TIS: Small and Large Apertures (Unscanned Mode)

Figure 2–12 shows typical axial temperature increase profiles for the homogeneous soft-tissue model under unscanned-mode conditions. The axial temperature increase profile is slightly different depending on the size of the transducer aperture. If the aperture is large (active aperture area > 1 cm^2), then the maximum temperature increase occurs near, but not at, the surface, usually within the first couple of centimeters.

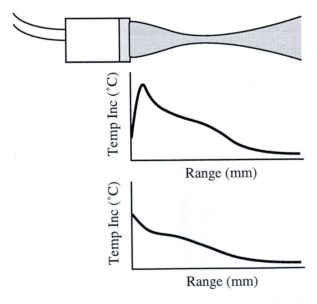

Figure 2–12. Axial temperature increase profiles for the homogeneous soft-tissue model and unscanned mode (*top:* large aperture; *bottom:* small aperture).

If the aperture is small (active aperture area ≤ 1 cm^2), then the maximum temperature increase occurs at the surface. The diagnostic ultrasound system knows which transducer is in use and makes the appropriate *TIS* calculation internally.

A detailed evaluation of the unscanned-mode *TIS* was recently completed for 192 cases.[53] The 192 cases considered (a) three source diameters (1, 2, and 4 cm), (b) eight transmit *f numbers* (ratio of the radius of curvature/source diameter: 0.7, 1.0, 1.3, 1.6, 2.0, 3.0, 4.0, and 5.0), and (c) eight ultrasonic frequencies (1, 2, 3, 4, 5, 7, 9, and 12 MHz). For each of these cases, both *TIS* and the maximum temperature increases ($\Delta T_{\max}$) were determined under the specific condition of the derated $I_{\text{SPTA.3}}$ at 720 mW/cm^2, the maximum value allowed by the FDA 510(k) diagnostic ultrasound equipment approval process. From the TIS–$\Delta T_{\max}$ pairs shown graphically (Fig. 2–13), the following observations can be made that are based on whether short-to-medium focusing (f/0.7 to f/2.0) or medium-to-long focusing (f/3.0 to f/5.0) conditions are used. The unscanned-mode *TIS* generally underestimates (is less than) $\Delta T_{\max}$ for *f numbers* ≤ 2, conditions for which $\Delta T_{\max} \leq 0.30°$C and $TIS \leq 0.40$. This suggests that for transmit *f numbers* ≤ 2, the unscanned-mode *TIS* would not need to be displayed according to the ODS display requirements (see display requirements below). Also, for *f numbers* ≥ 3, the unscanned-mode *TIS* generally tracks $\Delta T_{\max}$. This suggests that the unscanned-mode *TIS* is a reasonable indicator for estimating $\Delta T_{\max}$.

Specific ODS Obstetric Cases

A significant increase in intrauterine temperature has not been considered possible in a human clinical setting because the output levels of commercial systems and the methods of exposure have been considered to be significantly different than those employed in experimental studies. However, with the FDA's implementation of the regulatory $I_{\text{SPTA.3}}$ limit of 720 mW/cm^2, *in utero* temperature increases greater than 1°C are possible. Consider two cases, one for transvaginal exposure for which the homogeneous tissue model is applied (Fig. 2–14A) and the other for transabdominal exposure for which a layered model is applied (Fig. 2–14B). A well-described computational model[54] was used to calculate the tissue temperature increase for both exposure cases using $I_{\text{SPTA.3}} = 720$ mW/cm^2 conditions. As an example and to compare these two exposure cases, the same ultrasonic frequencies (1, 5, and 9 MHz), source diameter (2 cm), and focusing condition (geometric focus at 10 cm) were used.

Transvaginal Case. For typical human subjects *in situ*,[48,55–57] the attenuation of the myometrium is about 0.14 dB/(cm/MHz). Therefore, because the ODS procedure uses a derating factor of 0.3 dB/(cm/MHz), the 0.3-dB/(cm/MHz) value is used for the temperature increase calculations. As ultrasonic frequency increases, the temperature increase ΔT increases (Fig. 2–15A) and the maximum ΔT values ($\Delta T_{\max}$) for the

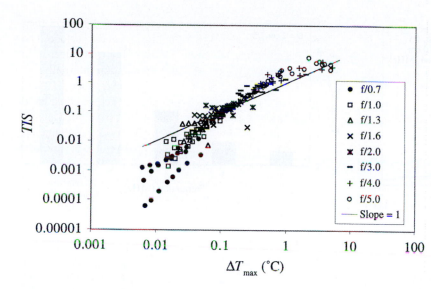

Figure 2–13. Unscanned soft-tissue thermal index (*TIS*) as a function of maximum steady-state temperature increase (ΔT_{max}) under the condition that the derated spatial peak, temporal average intensity ($I_{SPTA.3}$) is 720 mW/cm². The straight line denotes $TIS = \Delta T_{max}$.

higher frequencies exceed 1°C (Fig. 2–16A). The location of ΔT_{max} is close to the source and not near the geometric focus (at 10 cm).

Transabdominal Case. For typical human subjects *in situ*,[48,55–58] the thickness of the abdominal wall (d_{aw}) is about 2.5 cm and attenuation (A_{aw}) is about 1.4 dB/(cm/MHz), the thickness of the bladder ($d_{bladder}$) is about 5 cm, and the thickness of the myometrium is about 4 cm and attenuation (A_c) is about 0.14 dB/(cm/MHz). The region posterior to the bladder–myometrium boundary is referred to as the *conceptus* (Fig. 2–14B). Therefore, the following values are used:

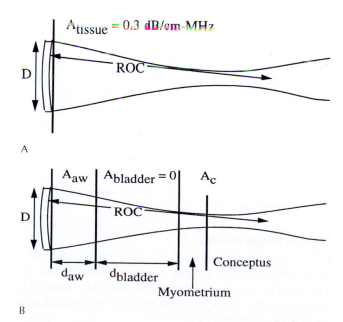

Figure 2–14. Two ultrasonic fetal exposure cases: **(A)** transvaginal exposure with the homogeneous tissue model and **(B)** transabdominal exposure with a layered model.

$d_{aw} = 0.5, 1.0,$ and 1.5 cm; $A_{aw} = 0.5$ and 1.0 dB/(cm/MHz); $d_{bladder} = 3.0$ and 7.0 cm; $A_{bladder} = 0$ dB/(cm/MHz); and $A_c = 0.3$ dB/(cm/MHz). As ultrasonic frequency increases, the temperature increase ΔT in the abdominal wall increases (Fig. 2–15B) and the maximum ΔT values (ΔT_{max}) for the higher frequencies exceed 1°C. In the conceptus (Fig. 2–17), the temperature increase in less than that in the abdominal wall but, for the higher frequencies, is also greater than 1°C.

These examples demonstrate that the temperature increase can exceed 1°C. However, the implementation of the ODS requires that the *TI* be displayed. Because the *TI* provides information about tissue temperature increase, the equipment operator has it available to provide an estimate of temperature increase. Thus, these examples are compared with the *TI* values.

The axial temperature increase profile for the large aperture (Fig. 2–12 *top*) resembles the calculated axial temperature increase profile shown in Fig. 2–15A. Also, the unscanned-mode *TIS* calculations can be related directly to the calculated temperature increases for both the transvaginal and transabdominal models shown in Fig. 2–15 through 2–17. The tissue temperature increases can exceed 1°C for these cases when the maximum permissible FDA intensity limit ($I_{SPTA.3} = 720$mW/cm²) is used. However, with the displayed *TI* value, the user has real-time feedback about the estimated output value (in terms of the unscanned-mode *TIS* for these cases).

For the transvaginal cases, the homogeneous tissue model was used. Figure 2–13 shows that the unscanned-mode *TIS* is a reasonable indicator for estimating ΔT_{max}.

For the transabdominal cases, the greatest abdominal wall thickness (d_{aw}) in these simulations was 1.5 cm, and the highest abdominal wall attenuation (A_{aw}) in these simulations was 1.0 dB/(cm/MHz). These maximum temperature increases (ΔT_{max}) are compared with what the *TIS* would be for these exposure conditions and are represented as the

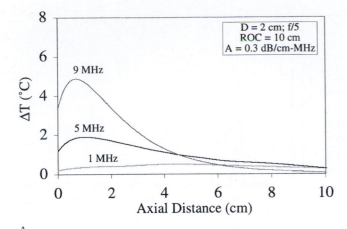

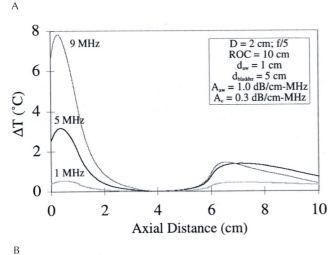

Figure 2–15. Temperature increase (ΔT) profiles along the beam axis for three ultrasonic frequencies (1, 5, and 9 MHz) for the two ultrasonic fetal exposure cases shown in Figure 2–14: **(A)** transvaginal exposure for the homogeneous tissue model and **(B)** transabdominal exposure for a layered model. The source diameter is 2 cm, for a long-focus condition (geometric focus at 10 cm).

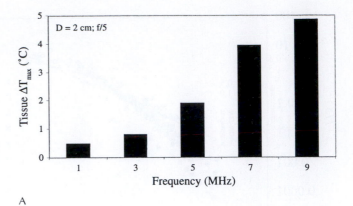

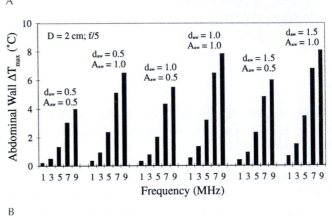

Figure 2–16. (A) Maximum tissue temperature increase (ΔT_{max}) as a function of frequency for the homogeneous tissue model that is used to model the transvaginal exposure case. **(B)** Maximum temperature increase (ΔT_{max}) in the abdominal wall as a function of frequency for the layered tissue model that is used to model the transabdominal exposure case. For all cases, the source diameter is 2 cm and the source is focused at 10 cm (*f number* is 5).

ratio $\Delta T_{max}/TIS$. The $\Delta T_{max}/TIS$ ratio remains less than 0.6 (Fig. 2–18), i.e., the TIS overestimates the ΔT_{max} of the conceptus. This suggests that the TIS is an adequate indicator for monitoring the maximum temperature increase in the myometrium and possibly the fetus under these simulated conditions and also demonstrates the clinical benefit of the TI values. It does not make any difference what the maximum output levels are, or even whether there are regulatory output limits. The TI provides the necessary information to the user as to what the system output is and provides this information as a valuable biophysical quantity.

Mechanical Index

The MI is defined as

$$MI = \frac{p_{r.3}}{\sqrt{f}} \qquad [2]$$

where $p_{r.3}$ is the derated peak rarefactional pressure (Fig. 2–19) in megapascals and f is the ultrasonic frequency in megaHertz. The derating factor (attenuation coefficient of the homogeneous soft-tissue model; see Fig. 2–3) is 0.3 dB/(cm/MHz). The MI represents the potential for cavitation in tissue, although there has never been a reported case in which cavitation has been known to occur from scanning a patient with diagnostic ultrasound equipment. The index is based on theoretical and *in vitro* laboratory experiments, not on tissue-based experiments.[37,59]

Display Requirements

If the diagnostic ultrasound equipment is capable of equaling or exceeding a TI of 1, then the appropriate TI (*TIS, TIC, TIB*) must be displayed in increments of no more than 0.2 for indices less than 1 and in increments of 1 or less for indices equal to or greater than 1.

If the diagnostic ultrasound equipment is capable of equaling or exceeding an MI of 1, then the appropriate MI must be displayed in increments of no more than 0.2 for

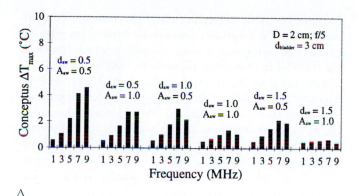

A

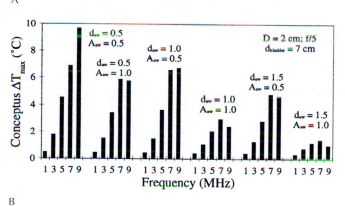

B

Figure 2–17. Maximum temperature increase ($\Delta T_{\max}$) in the conceptus as a function of frequency for the layered tissue model that is used to model the transabdominal exposure case. **(A)** Abdominal wall thickness is 3 cm. **(B)** Abdominal wall thickness is 7 cm. For all cases, the source diameter is 2 cm and the source is focused at 10 cm (*f number* is 5).

indices less than 1 and in increments of 1 or less for indices equal to or greater than 1.

In those cases where indices must be displayed, the index must be displayed from a value of 0.4. This allows the system operator to know when the appropriate index is approaching a critical value, say around 1, and then make the appropriate clinical decision.

All indices do not have to be displayed at the same time.

- The *MI* need only be displayed when the system is operating in B-mode imaging only.
- The *TIS* and *TIB* need not be displayed at the same time during an obstetric examination, but the system must have the capability for the operator to choose between the two indices to be displayed.
- The *TIC* must be provided when the system is intended solely for adult cephalic application.

The system must also have the capability to display the appropriate indices under combined modes of operation. This applies to the *TIs* where multiple modes of operation can produce a summation of heating from each mode.

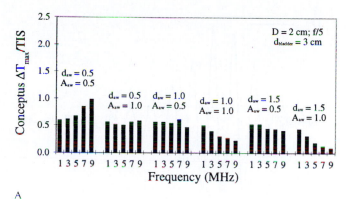

A

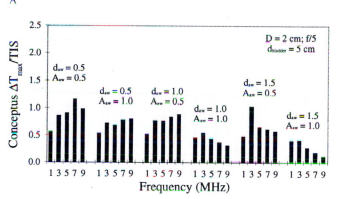

B

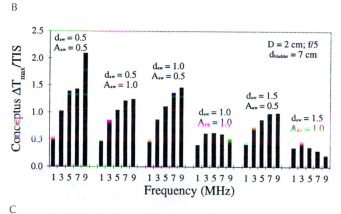

C

Figure 2–18. Ratio of the maximum temperature increase ($\Delta T_{\max}$) in the conceptus to the calculated *TIS* ($\Delta T_{\max}/TIS$) as a function of frequency for three different abdominal wall thicknesses (d_{aw}) and two different abdominal wall attenuation coefficients (A_{aw}). The three bladder thicknesses ($d_{bladder}$) are **(A)** 3 cm, **(B)** 5 cm, and **(C)** 7 cm. For all cases, the source diameter is 2 cm and the source is focused at 10 cm (*f number* is 5).

IN VIVO EXPOSIMETRY

The ODS[39] addresses one important aspect of ultrasound dosimetry. Diagnostic ultrasound equipment users are provided with quantitative indices that relate to temperature increase, the *TI*, and the potential for cavitation, the *MI*, from the diagnostic ultrasound field. In the development of the ODS, certain tissue characteristics were assumed to estimate

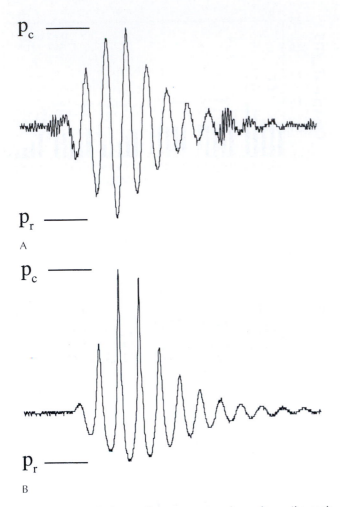

Figure 2–19. Typical acoustic pressure waveform shows the peak compressional pressure (p_c) and peak rarefactional pressure (p_r). **(A)** Is a lower pressure amplitude waveform than **(B)**.

in situ ultrasound exposure levels. Ultrasound exposimetry, a necessary component of ultrasound dosimetry, is thus concerned with the quantitative determination of ultrasonic exposure levels in biological materials because the development of quantitative tissue models is a necessary part of such studies.

Therefore, there is a need for realistic tissue models to predict *in situ* acoustic exposure levels from measurements of acoustic output made in water to have an improved basis for estimating risk. Both national[14,25,28,31,37,39] and international[26,29,36] organizations and research groups[48,55–57,60–65] have been evaluating and/or developing models and guidelines. For example, the FDA[43–47] uses a homogeneous tissue model, also referred to as a derating model, in their 510(k) process which is required by manufacturers and importers of diagnostic ultrasound devices in the United States to estimate *in situ* exposure levels.

In the past, reports by the FDA,[11] National Council on Radiation Protection (NCRP),[14,28] American Institute of Ultrasound in Medicine (AIUM),[25,31,37] World Federation for Ultrasound in Medicine and Biology (WFUMB),[26,29,36] and

National Institutes of Health (NIH)[16] have included recommendations for bioeffects research in those areas where a paucity of information was available, which included the study of fundamental mechanisms leading to bioeffects and postnatal studies in experimental animals after *in utero* exposure. Most animal studies have provided limited information that can be applied to the human based on the methods incorporated for the exposures (output parameters, length of exposures) and the substantial physiologic differences in scanning a small laboratory rodent versus a confined area of an adult human. Studies using nonhuman primates[32] can provide more relevant data because of anatomic and developmental similarities and the ability to control exposure conditions (i.e., number of examinations performed, time between each examination, stage of development, duration of exposure, length of time the beam is concentrated in a given area, output parameters of the ultrasound unit), thereby more accurately simulating the clinical setting.

One of the more central issues with regard to bioeffects has been quantitation of the "dose" the embryo or fetus receives during an ultrasound examination. This has become a monumental task based on the multitude of parameters that must be considered when attempting its assessment. Examples include factors related to attenuation (reported in decibels)[66] and the volume of tissue that must be traversed before the beam reaches the conceptus. The *in utero* ultrasonic intensities in both the gravid and nongravid human uterus have been estimated by mathematical techniques based on these variable tissue layers.[11,14,48,55–57] In these early studies, layers between the skin surface and gestational sac (i.e., muscle, fat, peritoneum, urinary bladder) yielded a total attenuation in the range of 2 to 20 dB at scanning frequencies between 2 and 5 MHz. The distances between the abdominal surface and the conceptus in early pregnancy were estimated to range between 2 and 11 cm. In more recent work, similar distances were estimated to be in the range of 2.6 cm,[62] whereas others have reported ranges between 4.4 and 12 cm.[48,57] Direct *in utero* intensity measurements have been obtained in the human adult female: the average attenuation was reported to be 6.2 ± 3.5 dB under full and 7.3 ± 4.9 dB under empty bladder conditions in the nongravid uterus[55–57] and 7.2 ± 3.7 dB under full and 9.3 ± 6.0 dB under empty bladder conditions in the gravid uterus.[48]

Further studies have applied the *fixed-path attenuation tissue model*[28,48,55,57,63] where attenuation is based on the assumptions that the ultrasonic attenuation between the skin surface and conceptus is linearly dependent on frequency and independent of distance. In this case, the *fixed-path* attenuation coefficient has been estimated experimentally to be 3.6 ± 2.2 dB/MHz and could be applied independent of bladder state (full versus empty), gestational age (between 7 and 20 weeks), and distance between skin surface and conceptus (between 4.4 and 12 cm).[48] The NRCP[28] has recommended the use of the *fixed-path* attenuation coefficient values of 1.0 and 0.75 dB/MHz for first- and second-trimester obstetric applications, respectively. These values are based on a worst-case ("maximum" exposure) approach but are not consistent with the experimental observations.[48,55,57]

The *overlying tissue model*[48,55–57,64] is based on the assumptions that the ultrasonic attenuation occurs uniformly within intact tissue *only* and that there is negligible attenuation from any intervening fluid path. The *overlying* attenuation coefficient has been experimentally estimated to be 0.82 ± 0.54 dB/(cm/MHz) and could be applied independent of gestational age (between 7 and 20 weeks); however, it is dependent on bladder state and distance between skin surface and conceptus (between 4.4 and 12 cm).[48,57]

The FDA's 510(k) equipment approval processes uses the *homogeneous tissue model*[17–43] where attenuation is based on the assumption that the ultrasonic attenuation occurs uniformly over the total distance between the skin surface and the conceptus. The *homogeneous* attenuation coefficient has been experimentally estimated to be 0.52 ± 0.33 dB/(cm/MHz) and could be applied independent of gestational age (between 7 and 20 weeks) and empty bladder state; however, it is dependent on distance between skin surface and conceptus for the full bladder state (between 4.4 and 12 cm).[48] The FDA[43–47] uses a value of 0.3 dB/(cm/MHz) as a factor for manufacturers in their 510(k) process (required for all ultrasound systems approved for marketing). Because the measured values for these tissue models are considerably greater than the values currently used by the FDA, it is apparent that the output requirements for ultrasound systems err on the side of safety. It is evident, however, that improved methods for estimating the attenuation that occurs *in vivo* will be required to more accurately assess the "dose" received by the second- and third-trimester fetus. This information will also help to confirm that the attenuation coefficient used by the FDA continues to remain relevant.

ULTRASONIC BIOEFFECTS: GENERAL OBSERVATIONS

Experimental studies of ultrasonic biologic effects can be classified into those that describe morphologic tissue alterations and those that describe functional tissue alterations.[40,67] Morphologic tissue damage is usually permanent, i.e., irreversible. Such studies have been essential to the understanding of the mechanisms responsible for ultrasonically induced alterations to biologic material. Ultrasound at high intensities can cause damage to tissue by heating or by a phenomenon called *cavitation,* a general term used to describe the growth and subsequent dynamic behavior of gaseous bubbles produced in tissue by ultrasound. The action by ultrasound on these bubbles causes them to respond by producing large shearing forces within the bubble vicinity. These forces in

turn can disrupt and destroy biologic tissues. Morphologic changes caused by both heating and cavitation have been identified and studied with very high ultrasonic intensities.

Biologic changes such as biochemical values, pH, function, activity, weight, and so forth, are termed *functional alterations.* These changes are not necessarily permanent. An example of a functional alteration is fetal weight change.[68–72] In general, much greater ultrasonic intensity levels are required to produce morphologic alterations than functional alterations. The I_{SPTA} and spatial average, temporal average (I_{SATA}) intensity levels used in the fetal weight studies were much less than those used for studying morphologic alterations. Had these higher intensity levels been used to expose the mouse fetuses *in utero,* irreversible damage to the fetuses, and perhaps death, would have been the result.

Scientists and clinicians tend to question research findings of others, whether they agree or disagree with them; *such questioning is essential in science.* However, it is interesting to observe that the content of scientific conflict changes as the intensity level of ultrasound diminishes, especially with respect to ultrasonic bioeffect studies. Morphologic alterations are produced by quite high levels of ultrasonic energy. There is no apparent conflict over whether or not the morphologic effect has occurred, but rather the scientific debate centers on what caused the alteration (i.e., heating, cavitation, or some other mechanism). These are the levels employed in the surgical application of ultrasound for which consistently well-defined, permanent biologic alterations can be produced. For example, three laboratories have independently confirmed that a highly focused ultrasonic beam can produce a lesion in mammalian (cat and rat) brain tissue.[73–76] Further, there is agreement that the effect has a threshold, and these investigators all agree as to the threshold. However, there is disagreement as to what degree the effect is caused by a thermal mechanism or by cavitation.

At lower ultrasonic levels, usually within the therapeutic range, there are conflicting viewpoints as to whether and to what degree morphologic alterations have occurred. Most of the mouse fetal weight studies have been conducted at intensities in the therapeutic range (I_{SATA}: 0.5–6 W/cm^2). There have been almost 3 dozen studies about the effect of *in utero* ultrasonic exposure on fetal weight in either rats or mice.[18,21,27] These studies have provided a number of perplexing and conflicting observations. For example, under identical exposure and experimental conditions, statistically significant fetal weight reduction was determined in one strain of mouse but not in another. Both of these observations have been further confirmed in independent laboratories. Thus, under biologic conditions that are not understood, consistent and confirmed observations have been obtained for both positive and negative effects.

For a third general category, at ultrasonic levels lower than those in the therapeutic range and sometimes into the diagnostic range (I_{SATA}: 0.1–100 mW/cm^2), there are conflicting data as to whether or not a functional alteration has occurred. This is aptly demonstrated in the numerous experimental studies that examined the effect of ultrasound on sister chromatid exchange (SCE) frequency (an indication of chromosome damage of which the biologic significance is unclear). Some of these studies have shown an effect when a diagnostic ultrasound device was used. However, others have reported no change in SCE frequency[15] at diagnostic levels and at levels much higher than those used in therapy. A study by Liebeskind and associates[77] appears to have received the greatest attention because it indicated an increase in human lymphocyte SCEs (a positive effect) from a diagnostic system. In another study by the same authors,[78] however, also with a diagnostic system, no change in SCEs was reported (a negative effect). In the latter study, two different types of cells were used. There have been two other positive observations[79,80] of increased SCEs, both with diagnostic levels of ultrasound. There have been at least 10 other studies, however, some at diagnostic levels (both pulsed and continuous wave exposure conditions) and some at levels within or higher than therapeutic levels, which have reported no increase in SCEs. These 14 studies have been carefully and thoroughly reviewed by the AIUM's Bioeffects Committee.[15] The committee's conclusion was that these studies do not suggest a hazard from exposure to diagnostic ultrasound.

One of the more controversial studies in the early 1970s of prenatal ultrasonic exposure of pregnant mice was conducted with a commercial fetal Doppler device.[81,82] Fetal abnormalities were observed in both the exposed and control groups, but the differences were not significant. However, the rate of fetal death was increased significantly in the exposed group. The same researchers[82–84] found a statistically significant increase in fetal abnormalities in a different mouse strain. In both of these studies, pregnant mice were given an initial dose of sodium nembutal that was effective for about 1 h, after which the animals awoke and struggled in their harness for 4 h; the ultrasound exposure duration was 5 h. Edmonds[85] drew attention to errors in the statistical analyses, the conclusions drawn, and the effective ultrasound power (about 280 mW). He concluded that the reported effects were related to a combination of prolonged binding of the mice and ultrasonic hyperthermia.

A significant reduction in the frequency of mitotic cells in surgically simulated rat liver from diagnostic-level, continuous-wave ultrasound (I_{SATA} of 60 mW/cm^2) has been reported.[86] However, this observation could not be confirmed under virtually the identical research protocol, even when I_{SATA} ranged from 60 mW/cm^2 up to 16 W/cm^2.[87]

These are a few of the many studies reporting ultrasonically induced biologic effects at I_{SATA} levels below 100 mW/cm^2 for which attempts at replication have failed. There are also many more studies for which no attempt has been made to replicate the original finding because, in general, research funding does not support this type of activity.

MECHANISMS RESPONSIBLE FOR ULTRASONIC BIOEFFECTS

Thermal Mechanism

When ultrasound is propagated into an attenuating material such as soft tissues, the amplitude of the ultrasonic wave decreases as it traverses deeper structures. This decrease in wave amplitude is due to either *absorption* or *scattering*. Absorption is a mechanism that represents that portion of the wave's energy that is lost by its conversion into heat; scattering can be thought of as that portion that changes direction, some of which is reflected as echoes that produce the images seen on the screen of the scanner.

Hyperthermia is a proven teratogen in experimental animals[88,89] and, although controversial,[90] is considered by some investigators to be a human teratogen under certain circumstances.[91] Because biologic tissues exposed to ultrasound are capable of absorbing energy, with the resultant production of heat, a temperature rise may occur when the rate at which heat is produced is greater than the rate at which heat is removed.[7,41] The increase in temperature produced by ultrasound can be calculated with mathematical modeling techniques[28,92–96] and has been estimated for a variety of exposure conditions *in vivo*.[14,24,28,54,58,98–104] It has been shown that temperature elevations between 2.5°C and 5.0°C or greater can occur with ultrasound after exposures of an hour or more.[25,31,105,106] Obstetric-based examples were described earlier in this chapter in the OUTPUT DISPLAY STANDARD section.

An evaluation of the world literature on the biological consequences of hyperthermia concluded that there is an absence of any thermally mediated effects on animals below 39°C.[106] However, the actual elevations that occur within embryonic or fetal tissues from diagnostic ultrasound equipment exposures have not been sufficiently evaluated *in utero*. The potential effects of any change in the basal temperature of specific areas of the conceptus (particularly if repetitive) are also not known.

Nonthermal (Mechanical) Mechanisms

In the past, this section would have discussed cavitation mechanisms.[35] However, because potentially significant biological effects have been identified that cannot be described by a thermal mechanism, the need to discuss the wider range of nonthermal mechanisms becomes more important. Any process that can produce a biological effect without a significant degree of heating, e.g., one producing a temperature increase of less than about 1°C above normal physiologic temperature, is a nonthermal mechanism.[37] Further, because any nonthermal mechanism is considered to produce an effect by mechanical actions or processes, a nonthermal mechanism is equivalent to a mechanical mechanism. There are two mechanical mechanism categories: cavitational and noncavitational. The former generally occurs in the presence of gas bodies and the latter does not, although the presence of gas bodies at the site of an observed bioeffect does not guarantee a cavitational mechanism. Gas bodies include naturally occuring microbubbles, e.g., gas in the lung, bowel, or other organ, and injected microbubbles, e.g., ultrasound contrast agents.[37]

The cavitation mechanism can be discussed under two general categories, namely *transient* and *stable* cavitation.[107] Transient cavitation (now termed *inertial cavitation*) refers to a relatively violent activity (i.e., bubble collapse) in which "hot spots" of high temperature and/or pressure occur in very short (microsecond) bursts. These bursts may be accompanied by localized shock waves or by the generation of highly reactive chemical species such as hydroxyl radicals. In contrast, a much less violent form is stable cavitation, which is associated with the vibration of these gas bodies. The nature of this form of cavitation consists of a micron-size gaseous body that, because of the presence of an ultrasound field, may oscillate or pulsate. The mechanisms by which a gas body (bubble) can affect nearby biological media are dependent on the amplitude of the acoustic field. Essentially all bubbles produce acoustic radiation forces[108] and microstreaming.[109] However, only the more strongly affected gas bodies from the higher-amplitude acoustic fields will exhibit the violent responses, e.g., shock wave generation or free radical production, characteristic of inertial cavitation.

The noncavitation mechanism can cause an ultrasound-induced biological effect under conditions when there is an absence of excess heating and an absence of gas bodies. The noncavitation mechanism is sometimes found to be in the form of radiation force or torque or of acoustic streaming.[110]

Although a known phenomenon with regard to ultrasound, the cavitation mechanism has been difficult to document in mammalian systems. Many studies have been performed with *Drosophila melanogaster* because of the natural presence of air in these organisms.[111] Although little work has been done regarding cavitation and the mammalian fetus, it has been shown that ultrasonically induced damage can occur *in vivo* in aerated lungs of adult mice.[112–116] These observations correlate with frequency-dependent *in vitro* cavitation experiments,[117] but the mechanism has not been directly linked to a bubble-related activity. In an effort to confirm whether the lung sensitivity observed in adult mice was related to the presence of air, *in utero* mouse fetuses were exposed to high peak ultrasonic pressures (20 MPa) on the 18th day of gestation.[113] Results indicated no significant effects on fetal tissues exposed *in situ* (including the lung); peak acoustic pressure levels were roughly 10 times the output required for damage in adults in previous studies.[112] As anticipated, marked intestinal and lung hemorrhages were noted in the dams of these fetuses at the higher exposures. These studies support the hypothesis that cavitation- or bubblelike activity may *not* be a significant concern in relation to the fetal lung, although the potential for cavitation nuclei in other regions of the fetus is unknown. However, if gas-containing ultrasound contrast agents are used, then a cavitation nuclei source has been introduced, and virtually no studies have been conducted to evaluate these implications on biological effect.

A major workshop sponsored by the AIUM dealt extensively with nonthermal mechanical bioeffects, and this document provides extensive discussion on all known bioeffects and mechanisms related to mechanical bioeffects.[37]

RESEARCH APPROACHES TO ULTRASONIC BIOEFFECTS

Dose–Effect Approach

Experimental studies consist of exposing the specimen to ultrasound and evaluating whether there have been any biologic changes that can be attributed directly to the exposure. The choice of exposure quantity and the type of biologic effect are critical elements of the experimental protocol. Exposure quantity variables include, but are not limited to, the following: pulsed or continuous wave conditions; frequency; power; I_{SATA}; I_{SPTA}; I_{SPPA}; p_r; unfocused or focused fields; and exposure duration. If a diagnostic system is the exposure source for the experiment, then its output quantities generally are not easy to control and quite challenging to measure. Only exposure duration can be easily changed with a diagnostic system because most of the other output quantities are fixed within the system. However, when specially designed exposure systems are used, virtually every exposure quantity is under the investigator's control. It is essential to have control over all exposure quantities because only then can dose–effect studies be properly planned and conducted.

What is meant by *dose?* It is quite difficult to determine the exposure time that the human fetal heart, for example, is undergoing during an examination, especially when the ultrasonic beam is rapidly scanning from the transducer assembly and the transducer assembly is also being moved. Under such conditions, the ultrasonic dose is quite difficult to quantify. Further, it is not known which of the various ultrasonic intensity quantities are relevant in terms of the dose determination. Consider the fact that the very high I_{SPPA} acts for only a millionth of a second and that this action repeats itself every thousandth of a second, whereas the very much lower I_{SATA} acts for quite a long period of time. Dose for the former is more than likely much lower than that for the latter, depending, of course, on how the dose quantity is defined.

Dose–effect studies are necessary for two important reasons: (a) they provide the capability to extrapolate the amount or kind of effect at the doses used experimentally to the dose generated by diagnostic systems (it is easier to determine what is generated than what a tissue receives), and

(b) they provide the fundamental basis from which the biophysic mechanisms causing the effect can be evaluated (i.e., was it due to heating, cavitation, or some other cause). To obtain measurable and highly repeatable biologic effects in experimental studies, the dose conditions are generally higher than those used diagnostically. The dose is changed over this higher range of values and the effect is evaluated. In this way, extrapolation to the lower diagnostic dose levels is placed on a scientific basis. Let us consider two examples. In one case, the effect might be proportional in such a way that, when extrapolated, it does not go to zero (or to a normal level) until the dose goes to zero. This would be considered a *no-threshold effect*. In another case, the experimental study could yield an effect that goes to zero (or a normal level) at some nonzero dose. This would be an example of a *threshold effect*. In the first case, the degree of the effect would have to be evaluated when extrapolated to diagnostic levels. In the latter, the evaluation would depend on where the threshold occurred.

Consider the mouse dose–effect fetal weight data shown in Figure 2–20. The laboratory observations that ultrasonic exposure *in utero* can cause weight reduction in mouse fetuses has been shown by three research groups using three different strains of mice.[68,70,71] Figure 2–20 graphically summarizes in a unified way the three published studies[68,70,71] that reported statistically significant effects of fetal weight reduction from *in utero* exposure to ultrasound wherein the results are represented by the percentage weight change (against sham) as a function of the calculated dose parameter I^2t. All three studies have graphically shown that as the value of I^2t increases, the fetal weight (against sham) generally decreases. These fetal weight studies have been summarized in greater detail.[27]

For example, if we were to apply dose–effect curve a[68] (Fig. 2–20) to a clinical exposure condition for purposes of assessing risk, then we would first examine the upper value of the dose parameter I^2t for pulse-echo scanners operating in B-mode only. For a single pulse, I_{SPPA} might be 500 W/cm^2 and the exposure time (in this case, pulse duration) about

1 microsecond, yielding an I^2t value of 0.25. For the time average case, I_{SPTA} could be 200 mW/cm^2 and the exposure time (in this case, length of the exam for maximum effect) would be about 30 mins, yielding an I^2t value of about 72. Of course, this latter case would require examining the same tissue volume for the entire length of time. This might not be the situation with pulse-echo scanner operating in B-mode only but is quite possible for spectral Doppler. The point made is that one is in a better position scientifically to examine what the effect might be under clinical conditions with a dose–effect model. The model would have to be validated for such applicability, of course.

Risk Assessment Approach

With our current understanding of ultrasonically induced biologic effects, it is difficult to argue against statements such as "diagnostic ultrasound is not harmful to the fetus." Experimental studies cannot be used to prove diagnostic ultrasound safe. Rather, what such studies will provide, if properly planned and executed, are data to aid in the overall assessment of risk associated with exposure to ultrasound. The term *safe* can imply the *complete* absence of an effect, i.e., the procedure involves no risk. It simply is not possible, however, to prove that ultrasound, or for that matter any agent, produces no effect whatsoever at the levels employed diagnostically. The actual use of the word *safe* in medicine is also vague because it almost never refers to the absence of an effect and the term can also imply the *apparent* absence of an effect. A more useful and workable approach, therefore, is to examine the *risk* associated with ultrasonic exposure.

Some 35 years after the Curies discovered piezoelectricity in 1880,[118] the first use of ultrasonic energy was developed: underwater acoustic echoes were bounced off submerged objects.[119,120] During the course of this work, the first reported observation was made that ultrasonic energy had a lethal effect on small aquatic animals.[1,121] The first extensive investigation of the phenomenon confirmed that ultrasonic energy could kill small fishes and frogs within a minute or

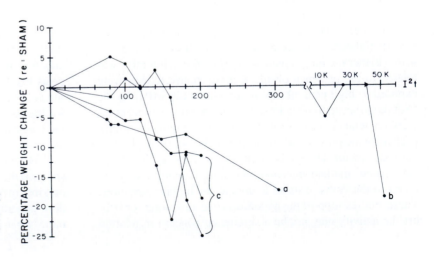

Figure 2–20. Summary of three mouse fetal weight studies in terms of the dose quantity I^2t. Curves a, b, and c represent data from references 68, 70, and 71, respectively.

two.[122] In perhaps the first review paper of ultrasonically induced biologic effects,[123] the physical, chemical, and biologic effects of ultrasound were evaluated. The effects on cells, isolated cells, bacteria, and tissues were summarized, with a view toward identifying the responsible mechanism. The ultrasonic exposure conditions in these early works were not well characterized, but the intensity levels were undoubtedly very much higher than what is currently in clinical usage.

In the early pioneering studies, where the ultrasonic exposure conditions were more carefully controlled and specified, sciatic nerve paralysis was easily produced in the frog[124,125] and lesions were produced in central nervous system tissue.[126] In addition, high-intensity ultrasound was employed to produce lesions in adult cat and rat brain,[73–76,126–128] adult rat and neonatal mouse spinal cord,[126,128,129] adult frog muscle,[130,131] rabbit blood vessel,[132] rabbit kidney and testicle,[133] and rabbit ocular tissue.[134–136] The ultrasonic intensities were very much higher than those used in diagnostic ultrasound, and for the most part these studies caused well-characterized and rather severe tissue damage. They have been extremely important in the elucidation of fundamental interaction processes. In terms of risk assessment, these studies have supported the view that diagnostic ultrasonic exposure conditions would more than likely not produce acute, gross irreversible damage.

These high-intensity studies also aided in recognizing the important fact that, at sufficient output levels, ultrasound is capable of destroying biologic material. An approach, therefore, to the question of assessing the risk from ultrasound is, (a) What biologic systems are most sensitive to ultrasound? and (b) What exposure levels impose a significant risk on these systems?

This approach unfortunately has its difficulties. How does one determine significant risk? *Significant risk* usually means risk that is greater than some upper limit of acceptability. A benefit-versus-risk analysis is simple in principle but is not so easily implemented in practice.

An important consideration with respect to the evaluation of risk is an estimate of the extent of ultrasonic exposure that the patient receives. However, this may not give a good indication as to the amount of ultrasonic energy that the patient population or a particular organ system receives because (a) the number of examinations a patient receives is generally unknown, (b) multiple examinations may be performed with different types of equipment, and (c) the amount of ultrasonic energy that a patient receives differs from exam type to exam type and from examiner to examiner. Whereas no recent statistically based survey is known to have documented the extent to which ultrasound is being used, a number of early indicators suggest that its use is increasing and that a large fraction of the human population will eventually be exposed, especially *in utero*. These earlier indicators were summarized in the previous edition of this chapter.[35] However, it is well recognized that the application of ultrasound in obstetrics and gynecology is essentially universal in modern

societies, and thus even the slightest risk could have a major impact.

EPIDEMIOLOGIC STUDIES

Human epidemiologic studies[137–145] and numerous *in vivo* studies in mammals have been performed to examine the many issues related to the use of diagnostic ultrasound with regard to safety. Overall, some conclusions can be drawn from these reports. For one, if ultrasound were a physical agent capable of inducing gross malformations, then a rise in the occurrence of birth defects would have been documented by now. This has not been the case, as epidemiologic studies have shown no correlations between a rise in its use and the incidence of congenital anomalies. However, based on the fact that results of experimental studies have proven inconsistent, it is clear that the interaction of ultrasound with biological systems, in particular those with rapidly dividing cells, is still not fully understood. What remains of concern are the subtle and long-term manifestations of frequent intrauterine exposure. These concerns remain pertinent due to a number of factors such as the continued rise in the percentage of the prenatal population that is exposed each year and advances in technology that can result in increased exposure (dose) to the fetus. The exposure time may also be increased as additional diagnostic information is sought. These points emphasize the need to pursue these questions in an effort to confirm that unwanted effects do not occur.

Although an increase in dyslexic children exposed to ultrasound *in utero* has been reported,[142] no differences between groups was observed in multiple neurologic and cognitive tests performed between 7 and 12 years of age. Other studies[138] have failed to confirm any significant effects related to exposure, no significant differences were found in head circumference at birth or in height and weight from birth to 6 years of age across 149 human sibling pairs, of which only one was exposed to ultrasound prenatally. Previous studies that have suggested the occurrence of growth retardation in the human population after exposure to ultrasound prenatally[139,142,144] may have been confounded by the population of infants incorporated in the analyses. It has also been suggested[139] that a relation may exist between the frequency of ultrasound exposure and reduced body weights; i.e., maternal and fetal risk factors rather than the ultrasound exposure may be the primary cause of the low body weights observed postnatally.

More recently reported[146] was an increased rate of intrauterine growth restriction in fetuses serially exposed to clinical ultrasound studies between 18 and 38 weeks of gestation (average of 5 examinations including placental arcuate and umbilical artery Doppler flow studies). Although these results are subject to significant criticism, fetal weight restriction as a result of ultrasound exposure has previously been reported in several animal models.[32] Thus, this is an area that requires continued attention given the conflicting epidemiologic data.

SPECIAL CONSIDERATIONS

First-Trimester Ultrasound Examinations

During human pregnancy, the period of greatest vulnerability is the first trimester, when embryonic cells are undergoing rapid mitotic division and differentiation. Organogenesis is more or less complete by the 12th week of gestation, and the potential for harm by teratogenic agents declines rapidly thereafter. Heat is a known teratogen, especially when the developing embryo is subjected to sustained temperature elevations at least 1.5°C (and probably higher) above the maternal core temperature for some finite period of time. Absorbed ultrasonic energy is converted to heat, and the resulting temperature increase has the potential to act as a human teratogen, especially during transvaginal scanning, when transducer heating may compound the effect. As shown in Figures 2–14A and 2–15A for transvaginal exposure conditions using a homogeneous tissue model and assuming an upper FDA $I_{SPTA.3}$ limit of 720 mW/cm^2, temperature elevations of approximately 2°C to 6°C are possible. However, as shown in Figures 2–11 and 2–12, the embryo may theoretically be exposed to these levels of temperature elevations only in the unscanned mode and only fleetingly because the examination in these situations is usually very brief. In the first trimester there is no ossification of any of the bones so that the example provided in Figure 2–11 would not apply at this stage, although it may be relevant to Doppler and pulsed Doppler studies performed later in gestation using the transvaginal approach. As a result, users are cautioned to not use color Doppler or pulsed Doppler modalities in the first trimester, especially during transvaginal examinations, unless the benefits clearly outweigh the risks. When use of these ultrasound modalities is necessary, the practitioner must remain cognizant of the importance of the ALARA principle.[34]

Gas-Carrier Ultrasound Contrast Agents in Obstetric Examinations

Gas-carrier contrast agents (GCAs) potentiate inertial cavitation and have been shown to increase tissue damage when mice were exposed to lithotripter fields.[37] There are no data available with regard to the safety of GCA use in pregnant women. Until such data are available, the use of GCAs is best avoided in the obstetric examination.

SUMMARY

The current scanning conditions and information available to date suggest that the perceived risk associated with the clinical use of ultrasound is low, provided that the length of the examination period and methods used for scanning pregnant patients are "prudent."[31,143] However, it must be emphasized that our knowledge regarding ultrasonic bioeffects and biophysical interactions with developing tissues is incomplete at this time. Several areas will require more rigorous investigations with appropriate animal models. Because of this apparent paradox, it is essential for clinicians and sonographers to be aware of the most up-to-date information on any perceived risks so that they can continue to render an informed benefit–risk judgment. The principal source of such data will be from relevant animal experimentation that can focus on defined effects and the respective mechanisms responsible for their occurrence.

ACKNOWLEDGMENTS

The author gratefully acknowledges the partial support by grants from the National Institutes of Health's National Cancer Institute (CA 09067), National Institute of Child Health and Health Development (HD21687, HD20748), and National Heart, Lung, and Blood Institute (HL 58218).

REFERENCES

1. O'Brien WD Jr. Assessing the risks for modern diagnostic ultrasound imaging (Invited). *Jpn J Appl Phys.* 1998;37: 2781.
2. Reid JM, Sikov MR, eds. *Interaction of Ultrasound and Biological Tissues Workshop Proceedings.* Washington, DC: US Government Printing Office; 1973. DHEW Publication FDA 73-8008 BRH-DBE.
3. O'Brien WD Jr, Shore ML, Fred RK, et al. On the assessment of risk of ultrasound. *IEEE Ultrasonics Symp Proc.* 1972;486.
4. Ulrick WD. Ultrasound dosage for nontherapeutic use on human beings-extrapolation from a literature survey. *IEEE Trans Biomed Eng.* 1974;BME-21:48.
5. Wells PNT. The possibility of harmful biological effects in ultrasonic diagnosis. In: Renemall RS, ed. *Cardiovascular Applications of Ultrasound.* New York: Elsevier; 1974:17.
6. Hazzard DG, Litz ML, eds. *Symposium on Biological Effects and Characterization of Ultrasound Sources Proceedings.* Washington, DC: US Government Printing Office; 1977. DHEW Publication FDA 78-8084.
7. O'Brien WD Jr. Safety of ultrasound. In: de Vlieger M, et al, eds. *Clinical Handbook of Ultrasound.* New York: Wiley; 1978:99.
8. Repacholi MH, Benwell DA, eds. *Ultrasound Short Course Transactions.* Canada: Radiation Protection Bureau, Health Protection Branch, National Health and Welfare; 1979.
9. Repacholi MH. *Ultrasound: Characteristics and Biological Action.* Ottawa, Canada: National Research Council of Canada; 1981 Publication NRCC 19244.
10. Dunn F, Frizzell LA. Bioeffects of ultrasound. In: Lehmann JF, ed. *Therapeutic Heat and Cold.* Baltimore, MD: Williams & Wilkins; 1982:386.

11. Stewart HF, Stratmeyer ME. *An Overview of Ultrasound: Theory, Measurement, Medical Applications, and Biological Effects*. Washington, DC: US Government Printing Office; 1982. HHS Publication FDA 82-8190.

12. *Environmental Health Criteria 22*. Geneva, Switzerland: World Health Organization; 1982.

13. *AIUM/NEMA Safety Standard for Diagnostic Ultrasound Equipment*. Laurel, MD: American Institute of Ultrasound in Medicine. *J Ultrasound Med*. 1983;(suppl):S1.

14. *Biological Effects of Ultrasound: Mechanisms and Clinical Implications*. Washington, DC: National Council on Radiation Protection and Measurement Document 74;1984.

15. Goss SA. Sister chromatid exchange and ultrasound. *J Ultrasound Med*. 1984;3:463.

16. *The Use of Diagnostic Ultrasound Imaging in Pregnancy*. National Institute of Child Health and Human Development. NIH Consensus Development Conference Process. Washington, DC: US Government Printing Office; 1984.

17. *Safety Considerations for Diagnostic Ultrasound*. Laurel, MD: American Institute of Ultrasound in Medicine Publication 316; 1984.

18. O'Brien WD Jr. Safety of ultrasound with selected emphasis for obstetrics. In: Raymond HW, Zwiebel WJ, eds. *Seminars in Ultrasound, 5*. Orlando, FL: Grune & Stratton; 1984: 105.

19. O'Brien WD Jr. Ultrasonic bioeffects: A view of experimental studies. *Birth*. 1984;11:143.

20. Nyborg WL. Optimization of exposure conditions for medical ultrasound. *Ultrasound Med Biol*. 1985;11:246.

21. O'Brien WD Jr, Withrow TJ. An approach to ultrasonic risk assessment and an analysis of selected experimental studies. In: Sanders RC, James AE Jr, eds. *Principles and Practices of Ultrasound in Obstetrics and Gynecology*. Norwalk, CT: Appleton-Century-Crofts, 1985:15.

22. O'Brien WD Jr. Biological effects of ultrasound: Rationale for the measurement of selected ultrasonic output quantities. *Echocardiogr Rev Cardiovasc Ultrasound*. 1986;3: 165.

23. Sikov MR. Effect of ultrasound on development: I: Introduction and studies in inframammalian species. *J Ultrasound Med*. 1986;5:577.

24. Sikov MR. Effect of ultrasound on development: II: Studies in mammalian species and overview. *J Ultrasound Med*. 1986;5:651.

25. *Bioeffects Consideration for the Safety of Diagnostic Ultrasound*. Laurel, MD: American Institute of Ultrasound in Medicine. *J Ultrasound Med*. 1988;7(suppl):S1.

26. *Second WFUMB Symposium on Safety and Standardization in Medical Ultrasound. Ultrasound Med Biol*. 1989;15(suppl 1):1.

27. O'Brien WD Jr. Ultrasound bioeffects related to obstetrical sonography. In: Fleischer AC, et al, eds. *The Principles and Practice of Ultrasonography in Obstetrics and Gynecology*, 4th ed. Norwalk, CT: Appleton and Lange; 1991;15.

28. *Exposure Criteria for Medical Diagnostic Ultrasound: I. Criteria Based on Thermal Mechanisms*. Bethesda, MD: National Council on Radiation Protection and Measurement Document 113; 1992.

29. *WFUMB Symposium on Safety and Standardization in Medical Ultrasound: Issues and Recommendations Regarding Thermal Mechanisms for Biological Effects of Ultrasound. Ultrasound Med Biol*. 1992;18;731.

30. Carstensen EL, Duck FA, Meltzer RS, et al. Bioeffects in echocardiography. *Echocardiography* 1992;6:605.

31. *Bioeffects and Safety of Diagnostic Ultrasound*. Laurel, MD: American Institute of Ultrasound in Medicine; 1993.

32. Tarantal AF, O'Brien WD Jr. Discussion of ultrasonic safety related to obstetrics. In: Sabbagha RE, ed. *Ultrasound Applied to Obstetrics and Gynecology*, 3rd ed. Philadelphia: JB Lippincott; 1994;45.

33. O'Brien WD Jr. A bioeffect produced at diagnostic levels. *Proc Soc Diagn Med Sonograph Conf*. 1994;305.

34. *Medical Ultrasound Safety*. Laurel, MD: American Institute of Ultrasound in Medicine; 1994.

35. O'Brien WD Jr. Ultrasound bioeffect issues related to obstetric sonography and related issues of the output display standard. In: Fleischer AC, et al, eds. *The Principles and Practice of Ultrasonography in Obstetrics and Gynecology*, 5th ed. Norwalk, CT: Appleton & Lange; 1995;17.

36. *WFUMB Symposium on Safety of Ultrasound in Medical. Ultrasound Med Biol*. 1998;24:S1.

37. *Nonthermal Mechanical Bioeffects*. Laurel, MD: American Institute of Ultrasound in Medicine; 1999.

38. Ewigman BG, Crane JP, Frigoletto FD, et al. Effect of prenatal ultrasound screening on prenatal outcome. RADIUS Study Group. *N Engl J Med*. 1993;329:821.

39. *Standard for Real-Time Display of Thermal and Mechanical Indices on Diagnostic Ultrasound Equipment*. Laurel, MD: American Institute of Ultrasound in Medicine; 1992, revised 1996.

40. Dunn F, O'Brien WD Jr, eds. *Ultrasonic Biophysics*. Stroudsburg, PA: Dowden, Hutchinson & Ross; 1976.

41. O'Brien WD Jr. Ultrasound dosimetry and interaction mechanisms. In Greene MW, ed. *Non-Ionizing Radiation: Proceedings of the Second International Non-Ionizing Radiation Workshop*. Vancouver, BC: Canadian Radiation Protection Association; 1992;151.

42. Raum K, O'Brien WD Jr. Pulse-echo field distribution measurement technique of high-frequency ultrasound sources. *IEEE Trans Ultrasonics Ferroelectr Freq Control*. 1997;44: 810.

43. *501(k) Guide for Measuring and Reporting Acoustic Output of Diagnostic Ultrasound Medical Devices*. Rockville, MD: Center for Devices and Radiological Health, US Food and Drug Administration; 1985.

44. *Diagnostic Ultrasound Guidance Update*. Rockville, MD: Center for Devices and Radiological Health, US Food and Drug Administration; 1987.

45. *Revised 510(k) Diagnostic Ultrasound Guidance for 1993*. Rockville, MD: Center for Devices and Radiological Health, US Food and Drug Administration; 1993.

46. *Information for Manufacturers Seeking Marketing Clearance of Diagnostic Ultrasound Systems and Transducers*. Rockville, MD: Center for Devices and Radiological Health, US Food and Drug Administration; 1997.

47. *Use of Mechanical Index in Place of Spatial Peak, Pulse Average Intensity in Determining Substantial Equivalence*. Rockville, MD: Center for Devices and Radiological Health, US Food and Drug Administration; 1994.

48. Siddiqi TA, O'Brien WD Jr., Meyer RA, et al. *In situ* human

obstetrical ultrasound exposimetry: Estimates of derating factors for each of three different tissue models. *Ultrasound Med Biol.* 1995;21:397.

49. Letter from AIUM President and AIUM Standards Committee Chair to Director, FDA's CDRH Office of Device Evaluation and Acting Director, FDA's CDRH Office of Science and Technology; June 23, 1986.

50. Merritt CRB. Ultrasound safety: What are the issues? *Radiology.* 1989;173:304.

51. *Acoustic Output Measurement and Labeling Standard for Diagnostic Ultrasound Equipment.* Laurel, MD: American Institute of Ultrasound in Medicine; 1992.

52. *Implementation of the Principle of as Low as Reasonably Achievable (ALARA) for Medical and Dental Personnel.* Bethesda, MD: National Council on Radiation Protection and Measurement Document 107;1990.

53. O'Brien WD Jr, Ellis DS. Evaluation of the soft-tissue thermal index. *IEEE Trans Ultrasonics Ferroelectr Freq Control.* 1999;46:1459.

54. Ellis DS, O'Brien WD Jr. The monopole-source solution for estimating tissue temperature increases for focused diagnostic ultrasound. *IEEE Trans Ultrasonics Ferroelectr Freq Control.* 1996;43:88.

55. Siddiqi TA, O'Brien WD Jr, Meyer RA, et al. *In situ* exposimetry: The ovarian ultrasound examination. *Ultrasound Med Biol.* 1991;17:257.

56. Siddiqi TA, O'Brien WD Jr, Meyer RA, et al. Human *in situ* dosimetry: Differential insertion loss during passage through abdominal wall and myometrium. *Ultrasound Med Biol.* 1992;18:681.

57. Siddiqi TA, Miodovnik M, Meyer RA, et al. I. *In vivo* ultrasound exposimetry: Human tissue-specific attenuation coefficients in the gynecologic examination. *Am J Obstet Gynecol.* 1999;180:866.

58. O'Brien WD Jr. Temperature increase estimates for transabdominal obstetrical exposures. *IEEE Ultrasonics Symp Proc.* 1998;1405.

59. Apfel RE, Holland CK. Gauging the likelihood of cavitation from short-pulse, low-duty cycle diagnostic ultrasound. *Ultrasound Med Biol.* 1991;17:179.

60. Smith SW, Stewart HF, Jenkins DP. A plane layered model to estimate *in situ* ultrasound exposures. *Ultrasonics.* 1985;23:31.

61. Akaiwa A. Ultrasonic attenuation character estimated from backscattered radio frequency signals in obstetrics and gynecology. *Yonago Acta Med.* 1989;32:1.

62. Carson PL, Rubin JM, Chiang EH. Fetal depth and ultrasound path lengths through overlying tissues. *Ultrasound Med Biol.* 1989;15:629.

63. Carson PL. Constant soft tissue distance model in pregnancy. *Ultrasound Med Biol.* 1989;15:27.

64. Daft CMW, Siddiqi TA, Fitting DW, et al. *In vivo* fetal ultrasound exposimetry. *IEEE Trans Ultrasonics Ferroelectr Freq Control.* 1990;37:501.

65. Ramnarine KV, Nassiri DK, Pearce JM, et al. Estimation of *in situ* ultrasound exposure during obstetric examinations. *Ultrasound Med Biol.* 1993;19:319.

66. Zagzebski JG. Physics and instrumentation. In: Sabbagha RE, ed. *Ultrasound Applied to Obstetrics and Gynecology,* 3rd ed. Philadelphia: JB Lippincott; 1994:3.

67. Sarvazyan AP. Some general problems of biological action of ultrasound. *IEEE Trans Sonics Ultrasonics.* 1983;SU-30:2.

68. O'Brien WD Jr. Dose-dependent effect of ultrasound on fetal weight in mice. *J Ultrasound Med.* 1983;2:1.

69. O'Brien WD Jr. Ultrasonically induced fetal weight reduction in mice. In: White D, Barnes R, eds. *Ultrasound in Medicine.* New York: Plenum; 1976:531.

70. Stolzenberg SC, Torbit CA, Edmonds PD, et al. Effects of ultrasound on the mouse exposed at different stages of gestation: Acute study. *Radiat Environment Biophys.* 1980;17:245.

71. Fry FJ, Erdmann WA, Johnson LK, et al. Ultrasonic toxicity study. *Ultrasound Med Biol.* 1978;3:351.

72. Kim HL, Picciano MF, O'Brien WD Jr. Influence on maternal dietary protein and fat levels on fetal growth in mice. *Growth.* 1981;45:8.

73. Fry FJ, Kossoff G, Eggleton RC, Dunn F. Threshold ultrasonic dosages for structural changes in the mammalian brain. *J Acoust Soc Am.* 1970;48:1413.

74. Pond JB. The role of heat in the production of ultrasonic focal lesions. *J Acoust Soc Am.* 1970;47:1607.

75. Dunn F, Fry FJ. Ultrasonic threshold dosages for the mammalian central nervous system. *IEEE Trans Biomed Eng.* 1971:BME-18:253.

76. Robinson TC, Lele PP. An analysis of lesion development in the brain and in plastics by high-intensity focused ultrasound at low-megahertz frequencies. *J Acoust Soc Am.* 1972;51:1333.

77. Liebeskind D, Bases R, Mendex F, et al. Sister chromatid exchanges in human lymphocytes after exposure to diagnostic ultrasound. *Science.* 1979;205:1273.

78. Liebeskind D, Bases R, Elequin F, et al. Diagnostic ultrasound: Effects on the DNA and growth patterns of animal cells. *Radiology.* 1979;131:177.

79. Haupt M, Martin AO, Simpson JL, et al. Ultrasonic induction of sister chromatid exchanges in human lymphocytes. *Hum Genet.* 1981;59:221.

80. Ehlinger CA, Katayama KP, Roesler MR, et al. Diagnostic ultrasound increases sister chromatid exchange. Preliminary report. *Wisconsin Med J.* 1981;80:21.

81. Shoji K, Momma E, Shimizu T, et al. An experimental study on the effect of low-intensity ultrasound on developing mouse embryos. *J Faculty Sci Ser VI.* 1971;18:51.

82. Shoji R, Momma T, Shimizu T, Matsuda S. Experimental studies on the effect of ultrasound on mouse embryos. *Teratology.* 1972;6:119.

83. Shoji R, Murakami U, Shimizu T. Influence of low-intensity ultrasonic irradiation on prenatal development of two inbred mouse strains. *Tetratology.* 1975;12:227.

84. Shimizu T, Shoji R. Experimental safety-study on mice exposed to low-intensity ultrasound. Presented at the Second Congress on Ultrasonics in Medicine; June 1973, Rotterdam, The Netherlands.

85. Edmonds PD. Further skeptical comment of reported adverse effects of alleged low-intensity ultrasound. *Proceedings of 1980 AIUM Conference.* New Orleans: 1980:50.

86. Kremkau FW, Witkofski RL. Mitotic reduction in rat liver exposed to ultrasound. *J Clin Ultrasound.* 1974;2:123.

87. Miller MW, Kaufman GE, Cataldo FL, Carstensen EL. Absence of mitotic reduction in regenerating rat livers exposed to ultrasound. *J Clin Ultrasound.* 1976;4:169.

88. Edwards MJ. Hyperthermia as a teratogen: A review of experimental studies and their clinical significance. *Teratogen Carcinogen Mutagen.* 1986;6:563.

89. Edwards MJ, Wanner RA. Extremes of temperature. In: Wilson JG, Fraser FC, eds. *Handbook of Teratology, Vol. 1. General Principles and Etiology.* New York: Plenum Press; 1977:421.

90. Warkany J. Teratogen update: Hyperthermia. *Teratology.* 1986;33:365.

91. Shepard TH. Human teratogenicity. *Adv Pediatr.* 1986;33:225.

92. Cavicchi TJ, O'Brien WD Jr. Heat generated by ultrasound in an absorbing medium. *J Acoust Soc Am.* 1984;70:1244.

93. Cavicchi TJ, O'Brien WD Jr. Heating distribution color graphics for homogeneous lossy spheres irradiated with plane wave ultrasound. *IEEE Trans Sonics Ultrasonics.* 1985;SU-32:17.

94. Lerner RM, Carstensen EL, Dunn F. Frequency dependence of thresholds for ultrasonic production of thermal lesions in tissue. *J Acoust Soc Am.* 1973;54:504.

95. Nyborg WL. Heat generation by ultrasound in a relaxing medium. *J Acoust Soc Am.* 1981;70:310.

96. Nyborg WL, Steele RB. Temperature elevation in a beam of ultrasound. *Ultrasound Med Biol.* 1983;9:611.

97. Herman BA, Harris GR. Theoretical study of steady-state temperature rise within the eye due to ultrasound insonation. *IEEE Trans Ultrasonics Ferroelectr Freq Control.* 1999;46:1566.

98. Nyborg WL, O'Brien WD Jr. An alternative simple formula for temperature estimate. *J Ultrasound Med.* 1989;8:653.

99. Ellis DS, O'Brien WD Jr. A computational comparison of ultrasonically induced tissue heating between circular and rectangular apertures. *IEEE Ultrasonics Symp Proc.* 1991;1133.

100. Ellis DS, O'Brien WD Jr. Evaluation of the soft tissue thermal index and the maximum temperature increase for homogeneous and layered tissues. *IEEE Ultrasonics Symp Proc.* 1992;1271.

101. Ellis DS, Siddiqi TA, O'Brien WD Jr. et al. In situ exposimetry, part II: Maximum in situ temperature at the location of specific fetal parts. Presented at the Thirty-Eighth Annual Meeting of the American Institute of Ultrasound in Medicine; March 20–23, 1994, Baltimore, MD.

102. Siddiqi TA, O'Brien WD Jr, Ellis DS, et al. Ultrasound dosimetry Part I: Maximum *in situ* dosage during routine obstetric sonography. Presented at the Seventh Congress of the World Federation for Ultrasound in Medicine and Biology; July 17–22, 1994, Sapporo, Hokkaido, Japan.

103. Smith NB, Webb AG, Ellis DS, et al. Experimental verification of theoretical *in vivo* ultrasound heating using cobalt detected magnetic resonance. *IEEE Trans Ultrasonics Ferroelectr Freq Control.* 1995;42:489.

104. O'Brien WD Jr, Ellis DS. Comparison of the output display standard's TIS estimates with independently determined maximum temperature increase calculations. *IEEE Ultrasonics Symp Proc.* 1996;1171.

105. Lele PP. Safety and potential hazards in the current applications of ultrasound in obstetrics and gynecology. *Ultrasound Med Biol.* 1979;5:307.

106. Miller MW, Ziskin MD. Biological consequences of hyperthermia. *Ultrasound Med Biol.* 1989;15:707.

107. Flynn HG. Physics of acoustic cavitation in liquids. In: Mason WP, ed. *Physical Acoustics, Vol. 1B.* New York: Academic Press; 1964;57.

108. Coakley WT, Nyborg WL. Cavitation: dynamics of gas bubbles; applications. In: Fry FJ, ed. *Ultrasound: Its Application in Medicine and Biology.* New York: Elsevier; 1978;77.

109. Nyborg WL. Acoustic streaming. In: Mason WP, ed. *Physical Acoustics, Vol. 1B.* New York: Academic Press; 1965;265.

110. Nyborg WL. Physical principles of ultrasound. In: Fry FJ, ed. *Ultrasound: Its Application in Medicine and Biology.* New York: Elsevier; 1978;1.

111. Carstensen EL, Campbell DS, Hoffman D, et al. Killing of *Drosophila* larvae by the fields of an electrohydroulic lithotripter. *Ultrasound Med Biol.* 1990;16:687.

112. Child SZ, Hartman CL, Schery LA, Carstensen EL. Lung damage from exposure to pulsed ultrasound. *Ultrasound Med Biol.* 1990;16:817.

113. Hartman, C, Child SZ, Mayer R, et al. Lung damage from exposure to the fields of an electrohydraulic lithotripter. *Ultrasound Med Biol.* 1990;16:675.

114. O'Brien WD Jr, Zachary JF. Mouse lung damage from exposure to 30 kHz ultrasound. *Ultrasound Med Biol.* 1994;20:287.

115. O'Brien WD Jr, Zachary JF. Comparison of mouse and rabbit lung damage exposure to 30 kHz ultrasound. *Ultrasound Med Biol.* 1994;20:299.

116. Zachary JF, O'Brien WD Jr. Lung hemorrhage induced by continuous and pulsed wave (diagnostic) ultrasound in mice, rabbits, and pigs. *Vet Pathol.* 1995;32:43.

117. Apfel RE, Holland CK. Gauging the likelihood of cavitation from short pulse, low duty cycle diagnostic ultrasound. *Ultrasound Med Biol.* 1991;17:179.

118. Cady WG. *Piezoelectricity, Vol 1.* New York: Dover; 1946.

119. Urick RJ. *Principles of Underwater Sound for Engineers.* New York: McGraw-Hill; 1967.

120. Van Went JM. *Ultrasonic and Ultrashort Waves in Medicine.* New York: Elsevier; 1954.

121. Graber P. Biological actions of ultrasonic waves. In: Lawrence JH, Tobias CA, eds. *Advances in Biological Physics, Vol 3.* New York: Academic; 1953:191.

122. Wood RW, Loomis AL. The physical and biological effects of high-frequency sound-waves of great intensity. *Phil Mag.* 1927;4:417.

123. Harvey EN. Biological aspects of ultrasonic waves: A general survey. *Biol Bull.* 1930;59:306.

124. Fry WJ, Wulff VJ, Tucker D, et al. Physical factors involved in ultrasonically induced changes in living systems: I: Identification of non-temperature effects. *J Acoust Soc Am.* 1950;22:867.

125. Fry WJ, Tucker D, Fry FJ, et al. Physical factors involved in ultrasonically induced changes in living systems. II. Amplitude duration relations and the effect of hydrostatic pressure for nerve tissue. *J Acoust Soc Am.* 1951;23:365.

126. Fry WJ. Intense ultrasound in investigation of the central nervous system. *Adv Biol Med Phys.* 1958;6:281.

127. Hueter TF, Ballantine HT Jr, Cotter WC. Production of lesions in the central nervous system with focused ultrasound. A study of dosage factors. *J Acoust Soc Am.* 1956;28:192.

128. Dunn F. Physical mechanisms of the action of intense ultrasound on tissue. *Am J Phys Med.* 1958;37:148.

129. Taylor KJW, Pond J. The effects of ultrasound on varying frequencies on rat liver. *J Pathol.* 1969;100:287.

130. Eggleton RC, Kelly E, Fry FJ, et al. Morphology of ultrasonically irradiated skeletal muscle. In: Kelly E, ed. *Ultrasonic Energy.* Urbana: University of Illinois Press; 1965;117.

131. Ravitz MJ, Schnitzler RM. Morphological changes induced in the frog semitendinosus muscle fiber by localized ultrasound. *Exp Cell Res.* 1970;60:78.

132. Fallon JT, Stephens WF. Effect of ultrasound on arteries. *Arch Pathol.* 1972;94:380.

133. Frizzell LA, Linke CA, Carstensen EL, et al. Thresholds for focal ultrasonic lesions in rabbit kidney, liver and testicle. *IEEE Trans Biomed Eng.* 1977;BME-24:393.

134. Coleman DJ, Lizzi F, Burt W, et al. Ultrasonically induced cataract. *Am J Ophthalmol.* 1971;71:1284.

135. Sokollu A. Destructive effect of ultrasound on ocular tissue. In: Reid JM, Sikov M, eds. *Interaction of Ultrasound and Biological Tissue.* Washington, DC: US Government Printing Office; 1972. DHEW Publication FDA 73-8008:129.

136. Lizzi FL, Parker AJ, Coleman DJ. Experimental cataract production by high frequency ultrasound. *Ann Ophthalmol.* 1978;10:934.

137. Hellman LM, Duffus GM, Ronald I, et al. Safety of diagnostic ultrasound in obstetrics. *Lancet.* 1970;1:1133.

138. Lyons EA, Dyke C, Toms M, et al. *In utero* exposure to diagnostic ultrasound: A 6-year follow-up. *Radiology.* 1988;166:687.

139. Moore RM, Diamond EL, Cavalieri RL. The relationship of birth weight and intrauterine diagnostic ultrasound exposure. *Obstet Gynecol.* 1988;71:513.

140. Mukubo M. Epidemiological study: Safety of diagnostic ultrasound during pregnancy on fetus and child development. *Ultrasound Med Biol.* 1986;12:691.

141. Scheidt PC, Stanley F, Bryla DA. One-year follow-up of infants exposed to ultrasound *in utero. Am J Obstet Gynecol.* 1978;131:743.

142. Stark CR, Orleans M, Haverkamp AD, et al. Short- and long-term risks after exposure to diagnostic ultrasound *in utero. Obstet Gynecol.* 1984;63:194.

143. Ziskin MC, Petitti DB. Epidemiology of human exposure to ultrasound: A critical review. *Ultrasound Med Biol.* 1988;14:91.

144. Moore RMJ, Barrick KM, Hamilton TM. Effect of sonic radiation on growth and development. *Proceedings of the Meeting of the Society of Epidemiologic Research.* Cincinnati, OH; 1982:571.

145. Salvesen KA, Vatten LV, Bakketeig LS, Eik-Nes SH. Routine ultrasonography *in utero* and speech development. *Ultrasound Obstet Gynecol.* 1994;4:101.

146. Newnham JP, Evans SF, Michael CA, et al. Effects of frequent ultrasound during pregnancy: A randomised controlled trial. *Lancet.* 1993;342:887.

3

Normal Pelvic Anatomy as Depicted with Transvaginal Sonography

Arthur C. Fleischer • Donna M. Kepple

Transvaginal sonography (TVS) affords improved resolution of the uterus and ovaries over that which can be obtained with the conventional transabdominal approach (TAS). Although the proximity of the transducer/probe to the pelvic organs allows their more detailed depiction, it may be more, rather than less, difficult for the sonographer to become oriented to the images obtained on a TVS when compared with conventional TAS because of the limited field of view and unusual scanning planes depicted with TVS. As one develops a systematic approach to the examination of the uterus and adnexal structures with TVS, however, the examination becomes much easier to perform. In this chapter, the sonographic appearances of the uterus, ovary, and other adnexal and pelvic structures will be described, with particular emphasis on how they are best depicted in a real-time TVS examination.

SCANNING TECHNIQUE AND INSTRUMENTATION

The three scanning maneuvers that are used in TVS include:

1. Vaginal insertion of the probe with side-to-side movement within the upper vagina for sagittal imaging.

2. Transverse orientation of the probe for imaging in various degrees of semiaxial to semicoronal planes.
3. Variation in depth of probe insertion for optimal imaging of the fundus to the cervix by gradual withdrawal of the probe into the lower vagina for imaging of the cervix.

In contrast to conventional TAS, bladder distention is not necessary for TVS. In fact, overdistention can hinder TVS by placing the desired field of view outside the optimal focal range of the transducer. Minimal distention is useful in a patient with a severely anteflexed uterus to straighten the uterus relative to the imaging plane.

As is true for conventional sonographic equipment, one should select the highest-frequency transducer possible that allows adequate penetration and depiction of a particular region of interest. Thus, 5.0- and 7.5-MHz transducers are preferred, but these higher-frequency transducers limit the field of view to within only 6 cm of the probe.

The major types of transducer/probes that are used for TVS include those that contain a single-element oscillating transducer, multiple small transducer elements that are arranged in a curved linear array, and those that consist of multiple small elements steered by an electronic phased array.

All of these depict the anatomy in a sector format that usually encompasses 100 to 120 degrees. In our experience, the greatest resolution is achieved with a curved linear array that contains multiple (up to 200) separate transmit–receive elements. Mechanical sector transducers may be subject to minor image distortions at the edges of the field due to the hysteresis (lag in effect when stopping and starting) that occurs with an oscillating transducer. Reverberation artifacts can be created by suboptimal coupling of the condom/probe/vagina surfaces. Although degradation of image quality by side-lobe artifacts can occur in the far field in a phased array transducer, they do not significantly degrade the image in the near field. Therefore, phased array transducers have similar resolution capabilities to sector as curved linear array transducers for use in transvaginal examinations.

After completely covering the transducer/probe with a condom and securing the condom to the shaft of the probe with a rubber band, the transducer is lubricated on its tip and periphery and then inserted into the vagina and manipulated around the cervical lips and into the fornix to depict the structures of interest in best detail. When the transducer is oriented in the longitudinal or sagittal plane, the long axis of the uterus can usually be depicted by slight angulation off midline. The uterus is used as a landmark for depiction of other adnexal structures. Once the uterus is identified, the transducer can be angled to the right or left of midline in the sagittal plane to depict the ovaries. The internal iliac artery and vein appear as tubular structures along the pelvic side wall. Low-level blood echoes can occasionally be seen streaming within these vessels. The ovaries typically lie medial to those vessels. After appropriate images are obtained in the sagittal plane, the transducer can be turned 90 degrees counterclockwise to depict these structures in their axial or semicoronal planes.

Particularly in larger patients, it is helpful for the sonographer to use one hand to scan while the other is used for gentle abdominal palpation to move structures, such as the ovaries, as close as possible to the transducer/probe.

UTERUS

Examination of the uterus (Fig. 3–1) begins with its depiction in long axis. The endometrial interface, which is typically echogenic, is a useful landmark to depict in long axis. Once the endometrium is identified in long axis, images of the uterus can be obtained in the sagittal and semiaxial/coronal planes.[1]

It may be difficult to determine the flexion of the uterus on the hard-copy images obtained solely from transvaginal scanning except in extreme cases of anteflexion or retroflexion; however, one can obtain an impression of uterine flexion during the examination by the relative orientation of the transducer/probe needed to obtain the most optimal images of the uterus. For example, retroflexed uteri are best depicted when the probe is in the anterior fornix and angulated in a

posterior direction. The fundus of the anteflexed uterus is directed to the upper left corner of the image. Conversely, the retroflexed uterus will demonstrate the fundus directed to the inferior right corner of the image.

The endometrium has a variety of appearances depending on its stage of development. In the proliferative phase, the endometrium measures 5 to 7 mm in anterior–posterior (AP) dimension. This measurement includes two layers of endometrium. A hypoechoic interface can be seen within the luminal aspects of echogenic layers of endometrium in the periovulatory phase and probably represents edema and increased glycogen and mucous in the inner layers of endometrium. In the few days after ovulation, a small amount of secretion into the endometrial lumen can be seen. During the secretory phase the endometrium typically measures between 6 and 12 mm in bilayer thickness, is homogenously echogenic, most likely as a result of multiple interfaces resulting from stromal edema, and is surrounded by a hypoechoic band, representing the inner layer of the myometrium. This inner layer of myometrium appears hypoechoic on TVS and corresponds roughly to the "junctional zone" seen on magnetic resonance imaging (MRI). The junctional zone, however, may be thicker than the hypoechoic band seen in TVS, perhaps because of different physical interaction with the myometrium in this area.[2] This layer is hypoechoic probably due to the longitudinal arrangement of the myometrial fibers.

Endometrial volume may be calculated by measuring its long axis and multiplying by the AP and transverse dimension.[3] One can use the axial plane landmark where the endometrium invaginates into the area of ostia in the region of the uterine cornu.

Because of the proximity of the transducer/probe to the cervix, the cervix is not as readily depicted as the remainder of the uterus. If one withdraws the probe into the vagina, however, images of the cervix can be obtained. The mucus within the endocervical canal usually appears as an echogenic interface. This interface may become hypoechoic during the periovulatory period because the cervical mucus has a higher fluid content.

OVARIES

Ovaries (Fig. 3–2) are typically depicted as oblong structures measuring approximately 3 cm in long axis and 2 cm in AP and transverse dimensions. On angled long-axis scans, they are immediately medial to the pelvic vessels. They are particularly well depicted when they contain a mature follicle that is typically in the 1.5- to 2.0-cm range. It is not unusual to depict multiple immature or atretic follicles in the 3- to 7-mm range.

The size of an ovary is related to the patient's age and phase of follicular development. When the ovary contains a mature follicle, it can become twice as large in volume as one that does not contain mature follicles. The greatest dimension

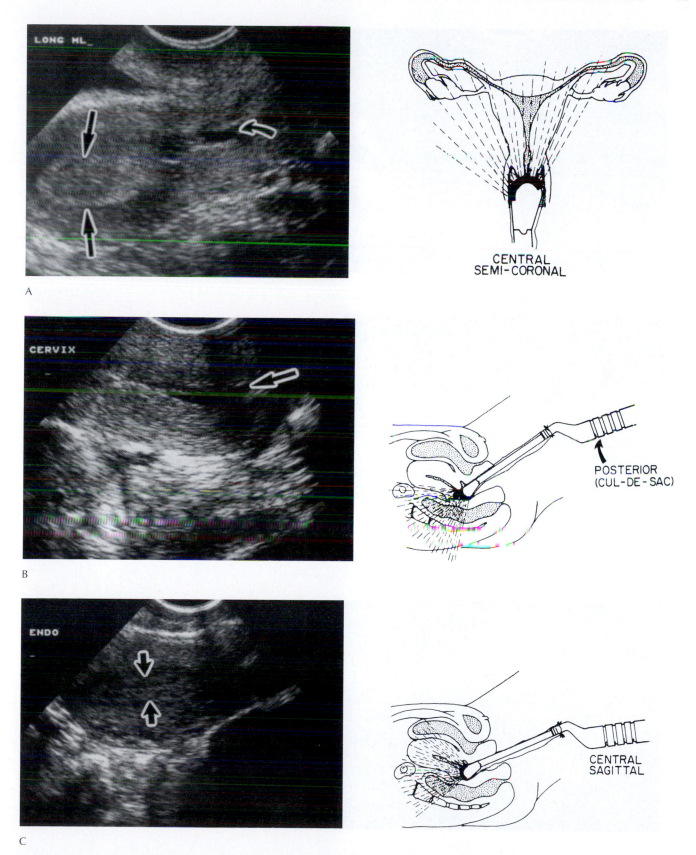

Figure 3–1. Uterus, endometrium, and cervix. Drawings depict plane of section. **(A)** Long axis of uterus in semicoronal plane showing the endometrium *(arrows)* and the cervix. There is a small amount of fluid *(curved arrow)* within the endocervical canal. **(B)** Same patient after withdrawing the probe into the midvagina. The endocervical canal with its fluid mucus *(arrow)* is clearly seen. **(C)** Long axis of endometrium *(arrowheads)* during the proliferative phase. It is relatively hypoechoic at this state. *(Figure continued.)*

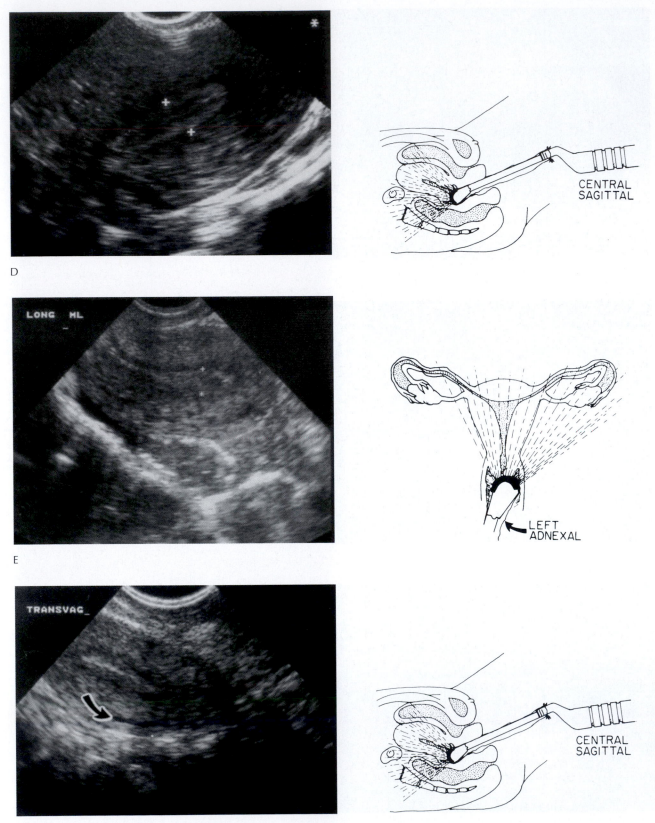

D

E

F

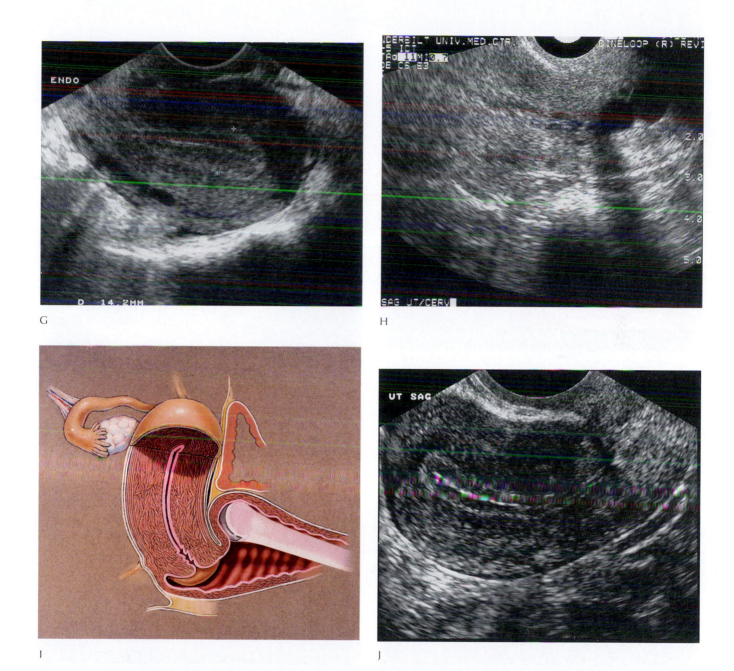

Figure 3–1. *(continued)* **(D–J)** Uterus, endometrium, and cervix. Drawings depict plane of section. **(D)** Long axis of the endometrium during the periovulatory phase showing hypoechoic inner layer. The multilayered endometrium is clearly seen between the +'s. **(E)** Long axis of endometrium (between +'s) in secretory phase, appearing as echogenic tissue (reversed orientation with uterine fundus to right of image). **(F)** Oblique image showing arcuate veins *(arrow)* within outer myometrium. **(G)** TVS of retroflexed uterus with distended arcuate veins. The endometrium (between *cursors*) shows a typical secretory phase pattern. **(H)** TVS showing two large cervical inclusion cysts. **(I)** Transducer/probe motion to enhance depiction of the uterus and endometrium in an anteflexed uterus. The probe is placed in the anterior vaginal fornix and directed anteriorly. **(J)** Complete delineation of the multilayered endometrium in long axis. *(Figure continued.)*

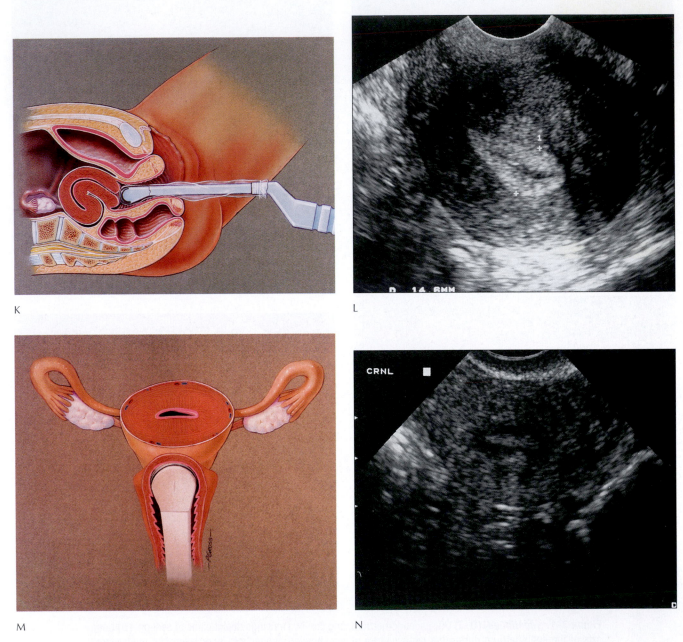

Figure 3–1. *(continued)* **(K)** Transducer probe showing direction of probe used to enhance depiction of a retroflexed uterus. **(L)** Corresponding TVS of drawing shown in **K** showing retroflexed uterus with secretory phase endometrium (between cursors). **(M)** Diagram showing "short-axis" image of endometrium. **(N)** Corresponding TVS of image plane in **M** showing short-axis view of the endometrium with surrounding hypoechoic inner myometrium.

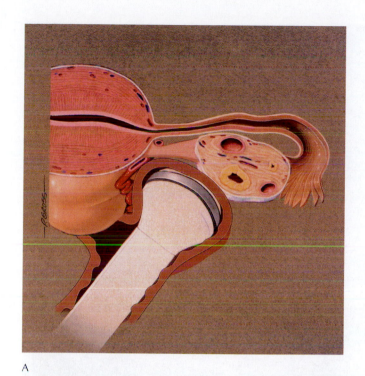

A

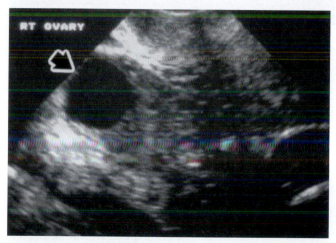

B

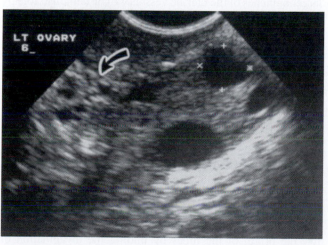

C

Figure 3–2. **(A)** Ovaries diagram showing transducer probe direction of depiction of the ovary and tube. **(B)** Right ovary containing a mature follicle *(arrow)* in a spontaneous cycle. **(C)** Left ovary containing a fresh corpus luteum (+'s). The wall is thick and irregular secondary to luteinization. Some pericervical vessels *(curved arrow)* are also seen. *(Figure continued.)*

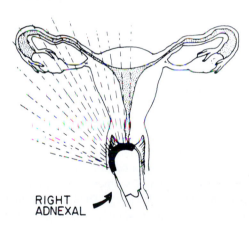

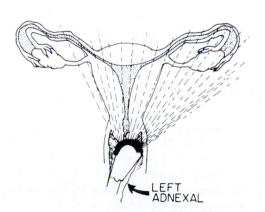

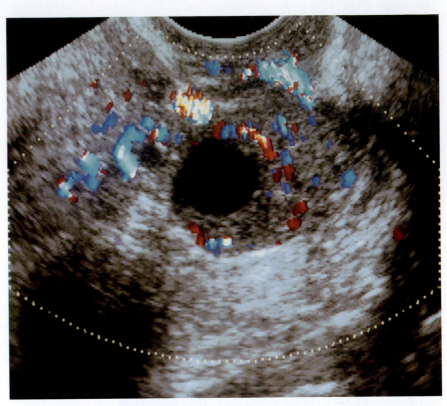

Figure 3–2. *(continued)* **(D)** TV–color Doppler sonogram of a mature follicle showing blood flow within the ovary.

D

of a normal ovary, however, is typically less than 3 cm.[4] The ovaries of postmenopausal women may be difficult to recognize because they are relatively small and usually do not contain follicles that enhance their sonographic recognition.

Ovarian volumes can be estimated by measurement of the greater transverse, longitudinal, and AP dimensions. The average ovarian volumes measured in menstruating women were 9.8 cm^3, postmenopausal women were 5.8 cm^3, and premenarchal females were 3.0 cm^3.[5] There is a gradual decrease in ovarian volume after menopause except in women receiving hormone replacement.[6] Echogenic foci can be seen on TVS within the center and/or periphery of the ovary. Most of the central foci are due to tiny cysts or calcifications within atretic follicles. Those that are peripherally located are of no clinical significance and represent calcified foci within superficial epithelial inclusion cysts.[9]

OTHER PELVIC STRUCTURES

Transvaginal sonography can depict several other pelvic structures (Fig. 3–3) besides the uterus and ovaries. These include bowel loops within the pelvis, iliac vessels, and occasionally distended fallopian tubes. Even small amounts (1 to 3 cc) of intraperitoneal fluid can be detected in the cul-de-sac or surrounding the uterus.

The pelvic vessels appear as straight tubular structures on either pelvic side wall. The internal iliac arteries have a typical width of between 5 and 7 mm and tend to pulsate with expansion of both walls. The iliac vein is larger (approximately 1 cm) but does not demonstrate this pulsation. Occasionally, low-level blood echoes will be seen streaming within the vein. The transducer can be manipulated or pivoted to demonstrate these vessels in their long axis. Occasionally, a distended distal ureter may have this appearance but does not demonstrate pulsations. The distal ureter and urethra course toward the base of the urinary bladder. In most patients, the larger branches of the uterine vessels will be demonstrable by TVS as tubular structures coursing in the paracervical area.

Distended uterine veins can be traced back into the myometrium, where the arcuate veins that course in the outer third of the myometrium lie. Ovarian veins tend to be located superior to the ovary. When normal, these vessels do not measure more than 5 mm. When there is valvular incompetency, however, the ovarian vein can be distended (over 5 mm) (Fig. 3–3E). Whether or not this finding is associated with a distinct clinical entity, such as "pelvic congestion syndrome," is controversial because many women with distended veins do not experience pain.

The nondistended fallopian tube is difficult to depict on TVS, which is probably related to its small intraluminal size and serpiginous course. Occasionally, one can identify the origin of the tubes by finding the invagination of

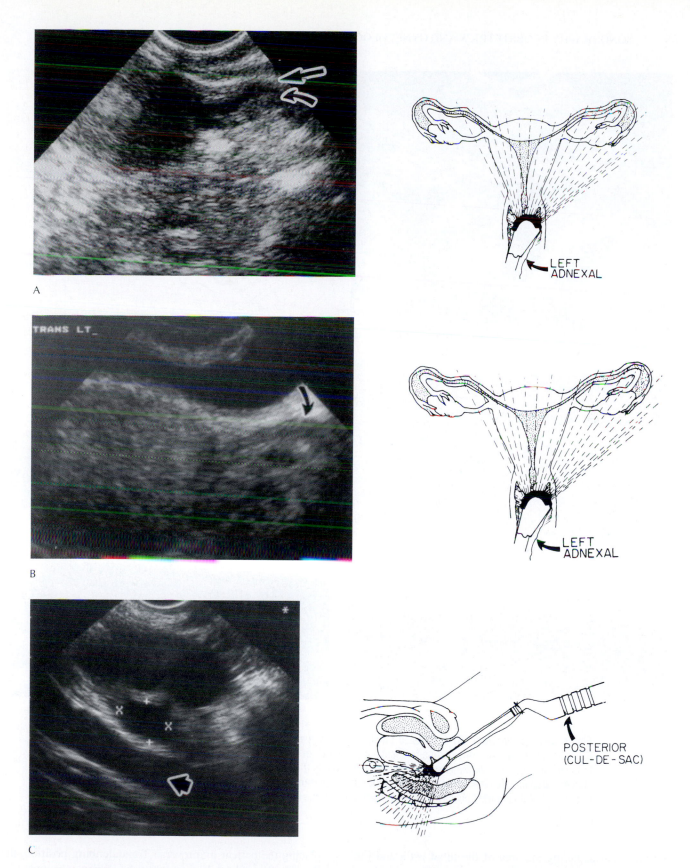

Figure 3–3. Other pelvic structures. Drawings depict plane of section. **(A)** Normal left tube *(curved arrow)* arising from cornual area adjacent to the uterine attachment of the round ligament *(straight arrow)*. **(B)** Normal left uterine tube *(curved arrow)* extending from left uterine corpus. **(C)** Internal iliac vein *(arrow)* and artery in long axis adjacent to a follicle-containing ovary. *(Figure continued.)*

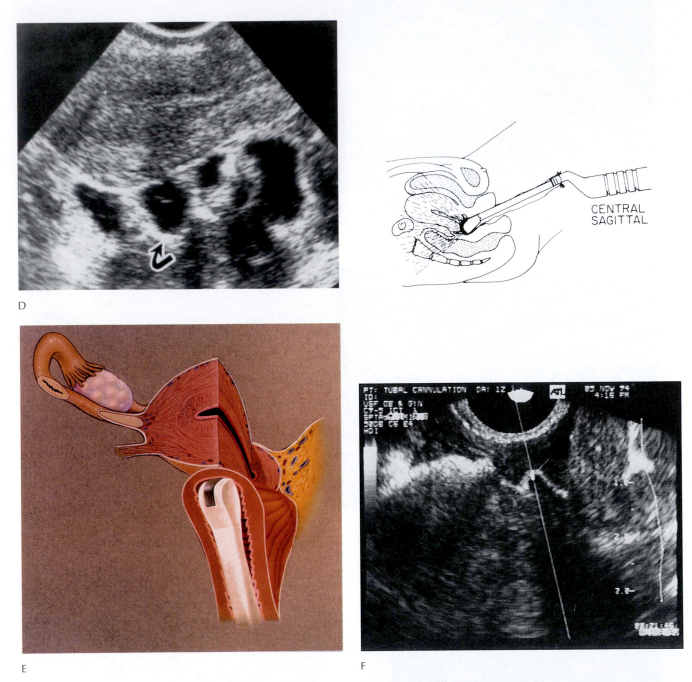

Figure 3–3. *(continued)* **(D)** Fluid-filled small bowel *(curved arrow)* surrounded by intraperitoneal fluid. **(E)** To evaluate the tube, one begins by identifying the area of the tubal ostia. The endometrium can be seen to invaginate into the uterine cornua, particularly when it is thick and echogenic in the luteal phase. **(F)** TVS showing area of tube. The actual lumen and tube cannot be routinely depicted on TVS without the use of saline or contrast. With contrast injection, the tortuous course of the tube is depicted. *(Courtesy of A. Parsons, MD.)*

endometrium depicting the area of the tubal ostia and following these structures laterally in the axial or coronal plane. The ovarian and infundibulopelvic ligaments usually cannot be depicted.

Sonographic delineation of the tubes is facilitated by intraperitoneal fluid that may be present in the cul-de-sac.[7] By placing the patient in a reverse Trendelenburg position, the fluid can be collected around the tube. When surrounded by fluid, the normal tube appears as a 0.5- to 1-cm wide tubular echogenic structure that usually comes from the lateral aspect of the uterine cornu posterolaterally into the adnexal regions and cul-de-sac. The flaring of the fimbriated end of the tube can be appreciated in some patients because it approximates its nearby ovary. Transvaginal sonographic depiction of the tubes is also facilitated when they contain intraluminal fluid. Rarely, small (smaller than 1 cm) rounded structures can be seen projecting from the fimbriated end of the tube representing cysts of Morgagni.[8]

The transvaginal sonographic appearances of the round ligaments are somewhat similar to that arising from a nondistended tube, except that its course is straighter and more parallel to the uterine cornu.

The bowel typically can be recognized as a fusiform structure that frequently contains intraluminal fluid and changes in configuration due to active peristalsis. If there is fluid within the lumen, periodic intraluminal projections—resulting from the valvulae conniventes—can be recognized from small bowel or the haustral indentations that are characteristic of large bowel. Nondistended bowel appears as a fusiform structure that consists of an echogenic center, representing mucus and enteric contents, surrounded by a hypoechoic rim, representing the muscularis of the bowel wall.

SUMMARY

Transvaginal sonography affords detailed depiction of the uterus and ovaries; however, it requires a systematic evaluation of these pelvic structures for their complete delineation because of the limited field of view of transvaginal transducer/probes. This can be achieved by understanding the anatomic relations of these structures from previous experience with TAS combined with anticipated findings from prior palpation of these structures during pelvic examination.

REFERENCES

1. Fleischer AC, Mendleson E, Bohm-Velez M. Sonographic depiction of the endometrium with transabdominal and transvaginal scanning. *Semin Ultrasound CT MRI.* 1988;9:81.
2. Mitchell DG, Schonholz L, Hilpert PL, et al. Zones of the uterus. Discrepancy between US and MR images. *Radiology.* 1990;174:827–831.
3. Fleischer AC, Herbert CM, Hill GA, et al. Transvaginal sonography of the endometrium during induced cycles. *J Ultrasound Med.* 1991;10:93–95.
4. Granberg S, Wikland M. Comparison between endovaginal and transabdominal transducers for measuring ovarian volume. *J Ultrasound Med.* 1987;16:649–654.
5. Cohen HS, Tice HM, Mandel FS. Ovarian volumes measured by US: Bigger than we think. *Radiology.* 1990;177:189–192.
6. Andolf E, Jorgensen C, Svalenius E, et al. Ultrasound measurement of the ovarian volume. *Acta Obstet Gynecol Scand.* 1987;66:387–389.
7. Timor-Tritsch IE, Rottem S. Transvaginal ultrasonographic study of the fallopian tube. *Obstet Gynecol.* 1987;70:424–428.
8. Schiebler ML, Dotters D, Baudoin L, et al. Sonographic diagnosis of hydatids of Morgagni of the fallopian tube. *J Ultrasound Med.* 1992;11:115–116.
9. Kupfer M, Ralls P, Fu Y. Transvaginal sonographic evaluation of multiple peripherally distributed echogenic foci of the ovary: Prevalence and histologic correlation. *AJR.* 1998;171:483–486.

4

Transvaginal Sonography of Early Intrauterine Pregnancy

Arthur C. Fleischer • *Donna M. Kepple*

Transvaginal sonography (TVS) has become the method of choice for the detection and evaluation of early pregnancy. It affords detailed delineation of the choriodecidua and embryo/fetus and separates living from nonliving embryos/fetuses by establishing the presence of heart motion. Most of the sonographic milestones used for assessment of early pregnancy can be established 1 week earlier with TVS than with conventional transabdominal sonography (TAS).[1]

This chapter discusses the role of TVS in the evaluation of a first-trimester pregnancy that is within the uterus. Chap. 6 is devoted to the sonographic evaluation of ectopic pregnancy.

CLINICAL INDICATIONS

Transvaginal sonography has several clinical indications in the first trimester of pregnancy. The majority of these involve the establishment of the location of the pregnancy and the detection of embryonic/fetal life. Other indications concern establishing the cause of bleeding and the prognostic effect on the pregnancy.

Approximately 20% to 50% of patients may experience bleeding in the first few weeks of pregnancy.[2] This bleeding has been attributed to the anchoring of the choriodecidua as it burrows into the decidualized endometrium. This bleed-

ing is usually limited and not associated with cramping. On the other hand, 20% to 30% of patients with bleeding will progress to a threatened abortion.[2] This condition is probably related to an extension of a retrochorionic hemorrhage to involve more of the implantation size. The size of the retrochorionic hemorrhage can be correlated to clinical outcome.[3]

Transvaginal sonography has a major role in evaluating patients with suspected ectopic pregnancy. Most importantly, TVS can accurately establish that the pregnancy is intrauterine, virtually excluding the possibility it is ectopic. This can be accomplished best by transvaginal scanning that can document an intrauterine pregnancy (IUP) as early as 4 to 5 postmenstrual weeks.[4,5]

Thus, the major indications for TVS in the first trimester include

1. Establishment of intrauterine pregnancy, particularly when ectopic pregnancy is suspected.
2. Evaluation of complicated early pregnancy, such as retrochorionic hemorrhage, incomplete abortion, early pregnancy failure with resorption, or completed abortion.
3. Detection of embryonic/fetal life.
4. Precise localization of intrauterine devices (IUDs) associated with early pregnancy.

5. Detection of multiple gestations when clinically suspected.

INSTRUMENTATION AND SCANNING TECHNIQUE

In most cases, TVS is the method of choice over TAS for evaluation of first-trimester pregnancies. This is primarily because of its improved resolution of the intrauterine contents and increased patient acceptance.[4] Because of the theoretic potential for ascending infection, TVS should not be used when there is active bleeding and a dilated external cervical os. Transabdominal sonography still is an accurate means for confirmation of location and confirmation of a live pregnancy greater than 8 to 10 weeks, and it can be used solely or in conjunction with TVS.

The technique for TVS begins with placing some ultrasonic coupling gel within a condom and covering the disinfected transducer with the condom. The transducer is lubricated and then inserted through the introitus and into the midvagina. When placed within the vagina, the transducer can be manipulated in the semicoronal and sagittal planes for delineation of the uterus and in the adnexa in long and short axes. A slightly distended bladder may assist in placing a very anteflexed uterus to a more neutral or horizontal position; however, greater degrees of bladder filling may displace the uterus away from the focal zone of the transducer, making detailed examination of the embryo and choriodecidua difficult.

On a routine first trimester TVS, certain structures should be clearly documented. These landmarks can be correlated to a specific range of β-human chorionic gonadotropin (β-hCG) values.[6–8] Included in the evaluation are the position and regularity of the choriodecidua of the gestational sac, the presence or absence of a yolk sac, embryo, or both, and the evaluation of the adnexa and cul-de-sac. When an embryo is identified, its crown–rump length (CRL) should be measured accurately. If an embryo cannot be delineated, gestational sac dimensions are useful alternative parameters for measurement to determine gestational duration.[9] For this measurement, the three inner-to-inner dimensions (long, short, and anterior–posterior) are obtained and then averaged. Prior to depicting an embryo, the sonographic documentation of a yolk sac within the gestational sac is a reliable means to confirm that the pregnancy is indeed intrauterine.[10]

Although TVS is usually sufficient in early pregnancy, occasionally structures that are superior to the uterus and outside the field of view of the transducer may be difficult to image. For these, a routine transabdominal scan with a fully distended bladder may be helpful.

Normal First-Trimester Pregnancy

This discussion of normal development is divided into discussions of 4 to 6 weeks, 7 to 8 weeks, and 9 to 11 weeks.

During the embryonic period, all of the main viscera are formed. In the fetal period, these formed structures grow and complete their functional development. This distinction is somewhat arbitrary and is based on terminology used in embryology. The terms used by embryologic texts, specifically *gestational age,* differ in meaning from those used clinically. Embryologic texts typically describe development in terms of the time from conception (gestational age), whereas menstrual age is used in a clinical setting because it dates from a recordable event. Although there is usually a 2-week interval between the time of fertilization and the last day of menses, this can vary by ±8 days. The events described in this chapter are classified by their menstrual dates.

Four to Six Weeks. The midembryonic period of development can generally be defined from the fourth to sixth menstrual weeks (Figs. 4–1 and 4–2). The embryonic anatomy present in early embryonic development is generally below the resolution of most currently available systems. Variations in the time of ovulation (up to 12 days) and implantation (up to 3 days) may influence what is depicted on a transvaginal scan in this early stage of pregnancy.

Using TVS, one of the first signs of an IUP is a hypoechoic complex within the thickened decidualized endometrium. This complex measures only a few millimeters. The gestational sac can be identified as early as 4 weeks and 3 days but should be routinely detected by TVS after 5 weeks.[11] Within the sac, a double sac structure measuring a few millimeters, which represents the developing primary yolk sac and extraembryonic coelom (double bleb), can be seen surrounded by the echogenic layer of choriodecidua at 5 weeks.[12] This configuration is only present for 2 to 3 days. The embryo, which is not visible at this stage, is termed a *trilaminar embryo* because, microscopically, three distinct layers (endoderm, mesoderm, and ectoderm) are present.

Because TVS is a relatively new clinical modality, additional experience with it is needed before absolute standards for sac size relative to yolk sac/embryo visualization are established. Using data collected from patients undergoing in vitro fertilization, one study has indicated that a gestational sac can be seen routinely between 4 and 5 weeks of menstrual age.[11] Our experience indicates that a gestational sac can be identified as early as 4 weeks and 2 days menstrual age. In general, a yolk sac can usually be demonstrated within the gestational sac by TVS when the sac is approximately 1 cm in size; an embryo/yolk sac is usually seen in sacs that average 1.5 cm.[13] Similarly, preliminary experience has suggested that the β-hCG level at which early gestational sacs are seen by TVS is in the range of 500 to 800 mIU (the second international standard). The most recent international standard is 1500 to 2400 mIU. This is significantly lower than the level reported with TAS (1800 to 3000 mIU).[8,13] The gestational sac itself grows approximately 1 to 2 mm in size each day at this time and can usually be delineated within the

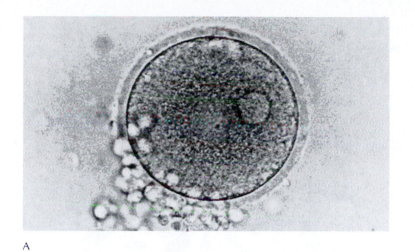

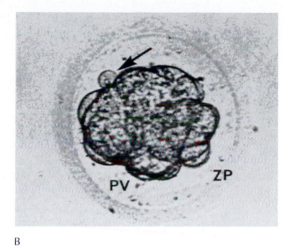

A

B

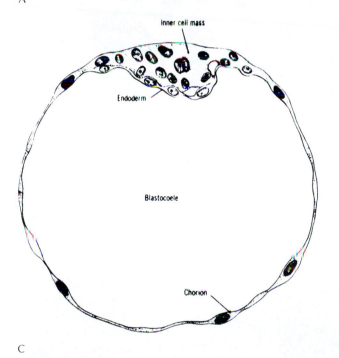

inner cell mass

Endoderm

Blastocoele

Chorion

C

Figure 4–1. Diagrammatic representation of embryonic/early fetal development. **(A)** Human oocyte in process of fertilization (×420). **(B)** A preimplantation baboon embryo (similar to the human) as the morula is transforming into a blastocyst. Arrow, column segmentation cavity; PV, perivitelline space; ZP, zona pellucida. **(C)** Line drawing of blastocyst showing early inner cell mass and trophoblast. *(Reprinted with permission from Davies J. Human Developmental Anatomy. New York: Ronald; 1963.)* **(D)** Section of 11-day human embryo showing cellular and syncytial trophoblast. *(Reprinted with permission from Arey B. Developmental Anatomy. Philadelphia: Saunders; 1962.) (Figure continued.)*

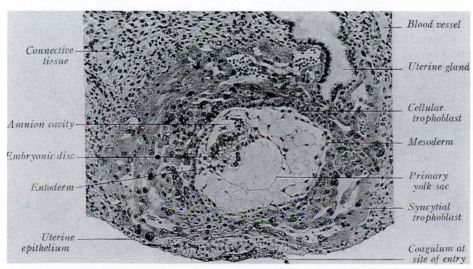

Connective tissue

Amnion cavity

Embryonic disc

Entoderm

Uterine epithelium

Blood vessel

Uterine gland

Cellular trophoblast

Mesoderm

Primary yolk sac

Syncytial trophoblast

Coagulum at site of entry

D

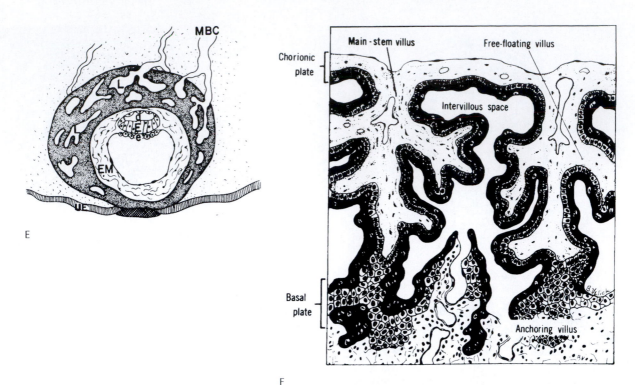

E

F

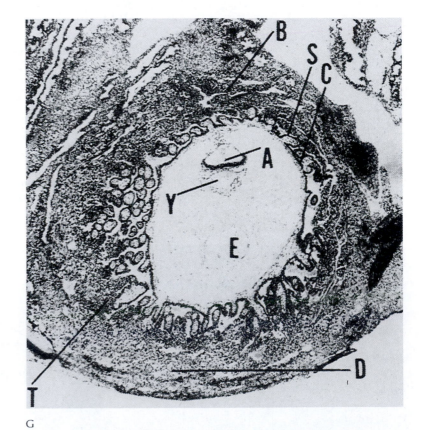

Figure 4–1. *(continued)* (E) 12-day implanted embryo. a, Amnion and amniotic cavity; E, embryonic ectoderm; e, embryonic entoderm; EM, extraembryonic mesenchyme; L, maternal blood lacuna in the trophoblast; Ue, uterine epithelium; MBC, maternal blood circulation. *(Redrawn by Panigel. In: Grasse, ed. Traité de Zoologie Masson; 1976. Reprinted with permission from Hertig and Rock and from Starck.)* **(F)** Cross section of early human placenta that demonstrates portions of the villous tree and stem villi anchored to the decidua basalis. *(Reprinted with permission from Davies J. Human Developmental Anatomy. New York: Ronald; 1963.)* **(G)** Cross section through an early (16-day) gestational sac. B, Decidual basalis; D, decidual capsularis; T, cytotrophoblast; C, chorion; S, secondary villus; A, amnion; Y, yolk sac; E, exocoelomic cavity. *(Reprinted with permission from Gruenwald P. The Placenta, 1st ed. Baltimore: University Park; 1975.)* *(Figure continued.)*

G

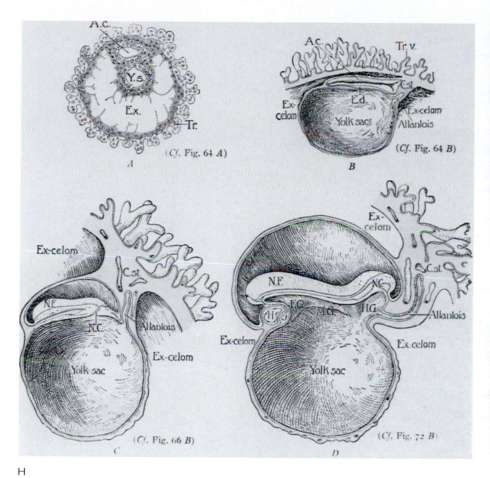

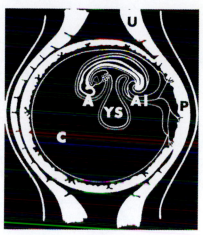

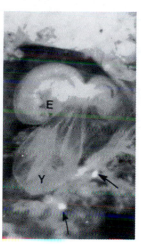

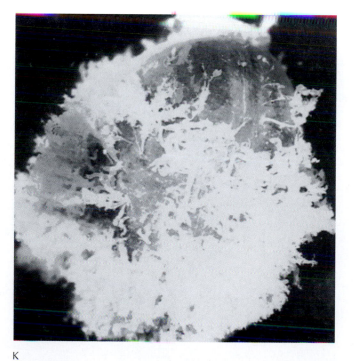

Figure 4–1. *(continued)* **(H)** Diagrams showing progressive growth (A through D) of the amniotic sac, yolk sac, and embryo. *(Reprinted with permission from Arey B.* Developmental Anatomy. *Philadelphia: Saunders; 1962:89.)* **(I)** Diagram of **J** showing 10-mm human embryo with its membranes and surrounding villous trophoblast. C, Amniotic cavity; P, placenta; U, uterus; YS, yolk sac. **(J)** E, 10-mm embryo; Y, yolk sac; and the chorionic villi *(arrows).* **(K)** The external surface of a human chorionic sac showing both the chorion frondosum and chorion laeve areas. *(Figure continued.)*

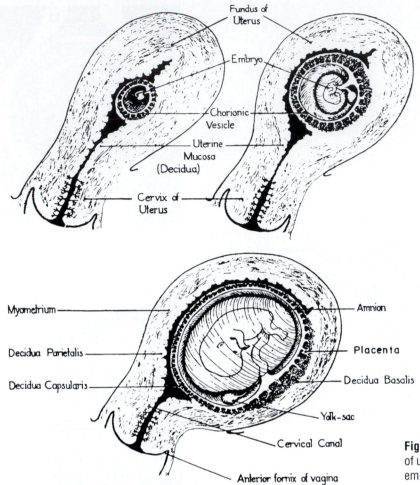

Figure 4–1. *(continued)* **(L)** Diagrams in cross section of uterus at 6, 8, and 10 weeks' menstrual age showing embryonic membranes and their development.

L

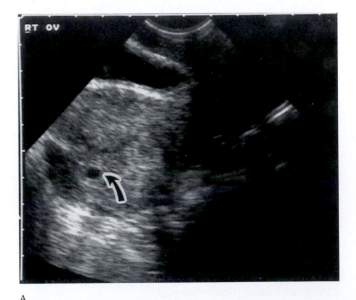

A

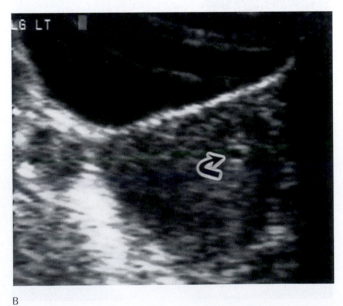

B

Figure 4–2. Normal 5-week intrauterine pregnancy (IUP). **(A)** Transvaginal (TV) sonogram of 4-week, 6-day pregnancy demonstrating 5-mm anechoic sac *(arrow)* within decidua. **(B)** Transabdominal (TA) sonogram of 5-week IUP *(arrow)* as depicted on magnified transverse scan. Normal 5-week IUP. *(Figure continued.)*

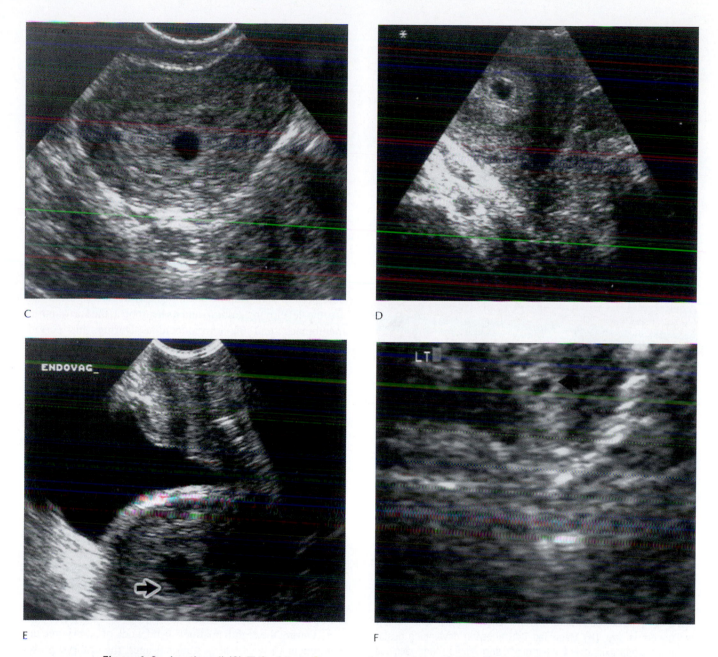

Figure 4–2. *(continued)* **(C)** TVS of 7- to 8-mm sac *(arrow)* of 5-week IUP. **(D)** TVS US of 5-week IUP appearing as anechoic area within the thickened decidualized endometrium. **(E)** TVS of 5-week, 6-day intrauterine pregnancy in a retroflexed uterus, demonstrating an embryo/yolk sac complex *(arrowhead)*. **(F)** Magnified transverse TAS of 5- to 6-week IUP showing concentric layers of decidua *(arrow)* and a "double bleb." *(Figure continued.)*

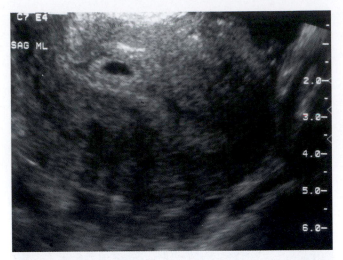

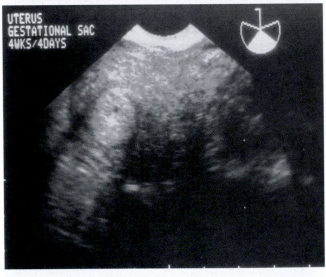

Figure 4–2. *(continued)* **(G)** TVS of 4-week IUP. The endometrium has undergone decidualization and the "chorionic sac" is just a few millimeters in size. **(H)** Magnified TVS showing developing gestational sac of approximately 4 × 6 mm and surrounding choriodecidua in this 5-week pregnancy.

thickened decidua vera. Changes in the gestational sac can be seen within 3 to 5 days of the initial screen.

During the middle of the fifth postmenstrual week (3 1/2 weeks of gestational age), the embryo measures between 2 and 5 mm and is located adjacent to the relatively prominent secondary yolk sac, which appears as a rounded hypoechoic structure between 3 and 4 mm in size. An enlarged yolk sac (over 6 mm) is associated with embryonic demise as well as those that are compromised and small.[14] The embryo/yolk sac complex lies adjacent to the edge of the gestational sac and has been described as forming a "double bleb," representing

the amniotic sac-embryo/yolk sac complex.[12] By the end of the first half of the embryonic period, the choriodecidua forms the boundaries of the gestational sac, which appears as an echogenic ring of tissue. At 4 weeks of menstrual age, the gestational sac measures only 3 to 5 mm in diameter and grows to approximately 1 cm at 5 weeks.

During the early embryonic period the embryo may be barely visible on TVS. Although many of the structures are present, they cannot be resolved sonographically. The neural tube is closed in its midportion but open at its rostral and caudal ends. Brachial arches form, and the somites develop as rounded surface elevations. Forty-two or forty-four somites form; these paired structures eventually give rise to the axial skeleton and associated musculature.

Seven to Eight Weeks. During the latter half of the embryonic period, sonographic scanning can depict a gestational sac, the developing embryo and its heart beat, the surrounding membranes, and the choriodecidua. During this period, organogenesis of the major body viscera occurs (Figs. 4–3 to 4–6).

On both TVS and TAS, heart pulsations can be depicted during this period of gestation. Transvaginal sonography is most precise in depicting early heart pulsation after 6 postmenstrual weeks, when the developing embryo forms from two enfolding fusiform tubes and begins contractile activity.

During the seventh postmenstrual week (fifth week of gestational age), the developing embryo grows from 6 to 11 mm in CRL. During this phase of development, the head growth is extensive and results primarily from rapid development of the brain. A cystic area can be identified in the brain, representing the rhombencephalon.[15] The yolk sac is relatively large, measuring less than 6 mm inner-to-inner dimensions, and floats within the gestational sac between the chorion and amnion, attached to the developing umbilical cord.

During the eighth postmenstrual week of embryonic development (6 weeks of gestational age), the embryo grows from 14 to 21 mm in length. The head remains a large and prominent structure and is bent over the heart prominence. The yolk sac becomes progressively smaller, and the intestines enter the base of the umbilical cord, beginning the normal process of umbilical herniation. By the end of the ninth postmenstrual week (seventh week of gestational age), the embryo has attained human features.[16] The head, body, and extremities can be identified sonographically. The intestine is still within the proximal portion of the umbilical cord. Occasionally, this physiologic umbilical herniation of bowel is particularly well depicted with TVS. Because this process of physiologic herniation of bowel into the umbilical cord is normal, abnormalities of the ventral wall should be suspected only if the bowel remains outside of the abdomen at 12 weeks or beyond.

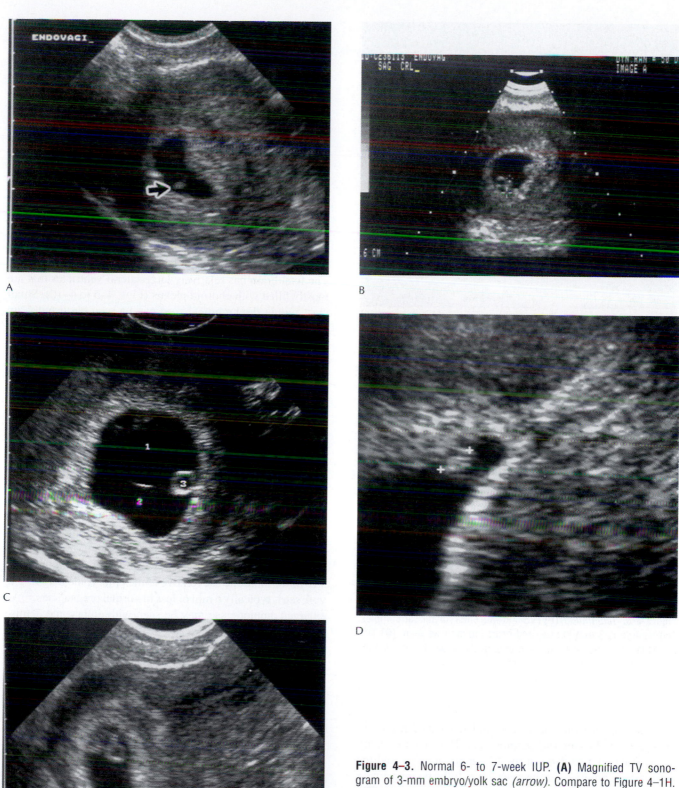

Figure 4–3. Normal 6- to 7-week IUP. **(A)** Magnified TV sonogram of 3-mm embryo/yolk sac *(arrow)*. Compare to Figure 4–1H. **(B)** TV sonogram of 6-week IUP with 6-mm embryo *(between x's)* adjacent to the yolk sac. **(C)** Magnified TV scan of 6-week IUP demonstrating embryo within embryonic cavity (1), extraembryonic coelom (2), and yolk sac (3). **(D)** Magnified TV sonogram of 6-week IUP demonstrating embryo/yolk sac complex and decidua capsularis and vera. Compare to Figure 4–1L. **(E)** Yolk sac/embryo surrounded by choriodecidual layers. *(Figure continued.)*

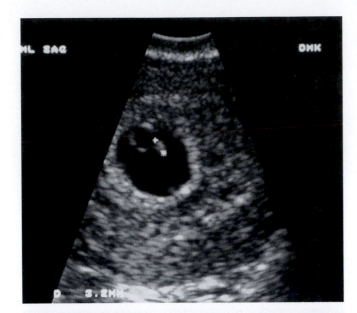

F

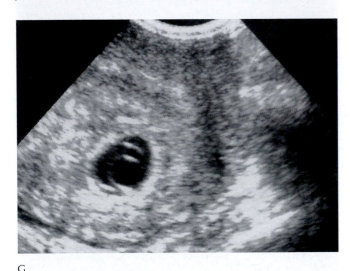

G

Figure 4–3. *(continued)* **(F)** TVS showing embryo/yolk sac complex. The embryo is 3 mm in size, and heart motion was seen. **(G)** TVS of "deflated" gestational sac with enlarged yolk sac but no definite embryo. This is consistent with embryonic demise.

Another structure that can be depicted in the late embryonic period is the amniotic membrane.[17] The amniotic cavity forms from an area deep in the trilaminar embryo, and the amniotic membrane can be seen on a fully floating linear interface in the outer portion of the amniotic cavity. The amnion approximates with the chorion only late in the first trimester of pregnancy (14 to 18 weeks).[18] At 6 to 8 weeks, the membrane can be seen as a thin rounded structure that encircles the embryo/fetus on TVS. Prior to this, the amniotic membrane may appear as a linear echogenic interface projected within the gestational sac in proximity to the embryo.

Besides depiction of the embryo/fetus, the choriodecidua is seen as it begins to thicken at the implantation site during the late embryonic and early fetal period. The anatomic and functional fusing of decidua basalis and chorion frondosum forms the future placenta.

Certain parameters provide useful prognostic signs, including the heart rate and the relative size of the embryo to the amniotic sac.

Nine to Eleven Weeks. After 9 weeks, the fetus is clearly depicted both with TAS and TVS. Nomograms for measurement of the embryo and fetus have been established.[19] The fetus begins to move its trunk and extremities, and it can be seen to do an occasional somersault within the uterus. Movement is rapid in nature and often appears convulsive. Upper extremity movement is followed by lower extremity. The fetal brain has relatively large lateral ventricles that are mostly filled with choroid plexus (Figs. 4–5 to 4–10). Small cysts within the umbilical cord can be seen but usually are resolved by 12 weeks.[20] Herniated bowel returns into the abdomen by 12 weeks also. Before 12 weeks, however, the physiologically herniated bowel can measure up to 1.5 times the umbilical cord at its abdominal insertion. Color Doppler sonography may be used to assess the size of the herniated bowel in relation to the cord.

Heart rate progressively increases to 120 to 160 beats per minute after 6 to 7 weeks.[21] Heart rates of less than 85 beats per minute have been associated with pregnancy failure and necessitate follow-up songrams.[21] In another study, heart rates of less than 90 beats per minute in the first trimester were associated with a dismal diagnosis.[22] Clearly, however, one could give the fetus the benefit of the doubt if slow heart rates are seen and confirm this finding on a follow-up study rather than terminate based on one abnormal examination.[32] Another parameter that seems to have prognostic value is the size of the amniotic sac relative to the embryonic length. The yolk sac is typically 6 mm or less in normal pregnancies.[23] An enlarged amniotic sac may be seen with embryonic demise as calculated by $CRL - D_a > 0.8$ cm (diameter of the amnionitic cavity).[24] In normal pregnancies, the amniotic sac minus embryonic length should be greater than 5 mm.[22] This measurement is less helpful because it may be difficult to completely visualize the amnion at this early stage of development.

Several studies have shown a gradual increase in velocity and diastolic flow in choriodecidual (spiral) arteries in early pregnancies.[28,29] However, the actual Doppler indices do not discriminate between viable and nonviable pregnancies. Increased venous flow within the choriodecidua can be seen in nonviable pregnancies associated with embryonic or early fetal demise.

Failed or failing early pregnancies seem to be more vascular than normal gestation.[30] Thus, color Doppler sonography (CDS) may help define the etiologic mechanism for early pregnancy failure. However, uncomplicated involution

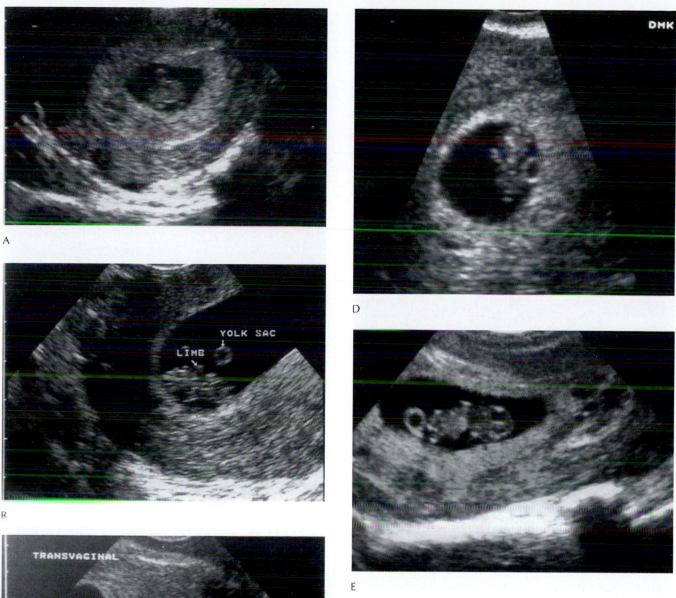

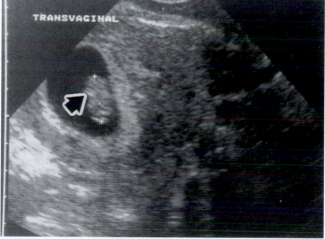

Figure 4–4. Normal embryo at 7 to 8 weeks. **(A)** TVS of 8-mm embryo with a yolk sac adjacent to embryo. **(B)** Ten-millimeter embryo demonstrating limb and yolk sac. **(C)** TV scan of 8-week embryo in coronal plane, demonstrating early ossification of clavicle *(arrow)*. **(D)** Seven-week embryo with adjacent yolk sac. The arm buds are seen. **(E)** Eight- to nine-week pregnancy showing the developing head (rhombencephalon). The choriodecidua now is intact.

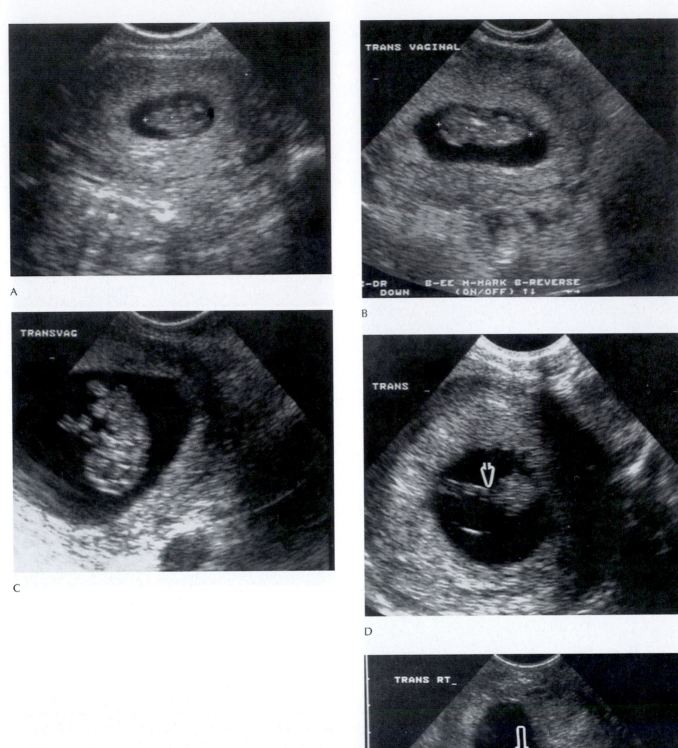

Figure 4–5. Normal fetal anatomy. **(A)** TVS of 17-mm embryo demonstrating prominent cystic area of brain corresponding to rhombencephalon. **(B)** TVS of 28-mm fetus. **(C)** TV scan of 10-week fetus demonstrating arms and legs. **(D)** Transverse of same fetus showing umbilical cord insertion within some physiologic herniation of bow into base of umbilical cord. **(E)** TVS showing hands on or near face of 11-week fetus. *(Figure continued.)*

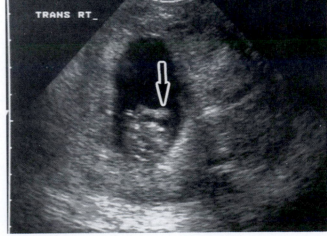

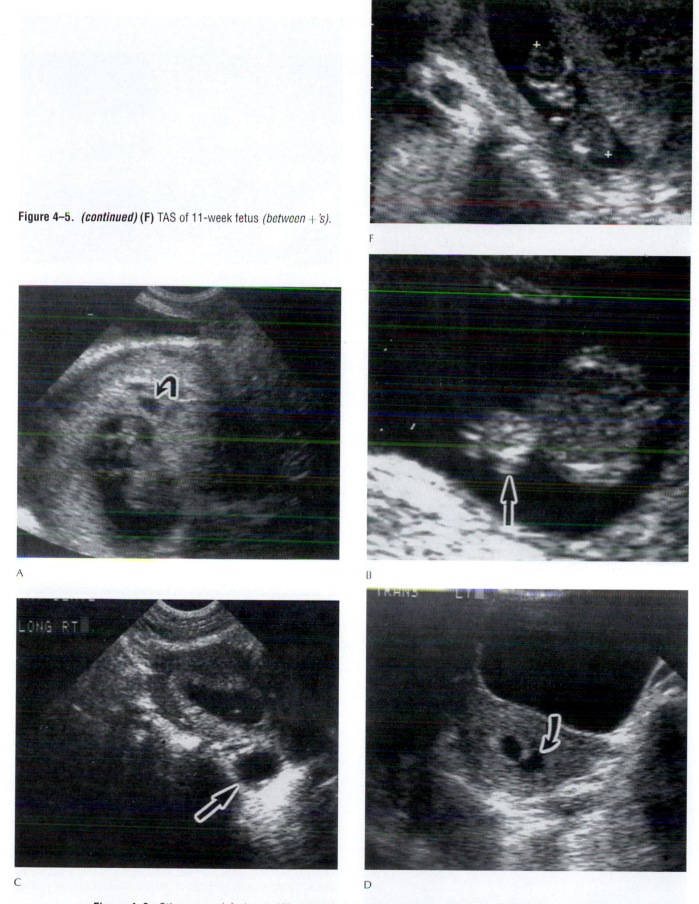

Figure 4–5. *(continued)* **(F)** TAS of 11-week fetus *(between + 's).*

F

A

B

C

D

Figure 4–6. Other normal features. **(A)** Hypoechoic lacunae *(curved arrow)* around decidual basalis of 10-week IUP. **(B)** Magnified TVS of 11-week fetus with bowel herniated into base of cord. **(C)** TAS of corpus luteum cyst of pregnancy. **(D)** TAS showing unoccupied lumen *(curved arrow)* at 6 weeks. *(Figure continued.)*

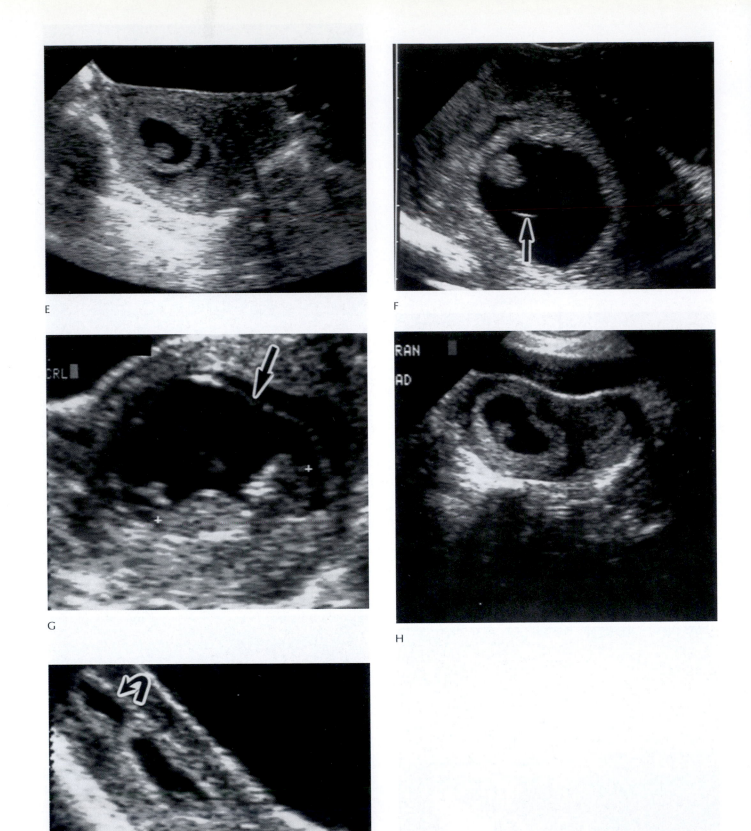

Figure 4–6. *(continued)* **(E)** Same patient as shown in **D**, 1 week later, showing embryo within sac and persistence of unobliterated lumen. **(F)** TVS showing amnion *(arrow)* surrounding 6-week embryo. **(G)** Unfused chorioamnion at 10 weeks shown on this magnified TAS. **(H)** TAS of 6-week IUP within the right cornu of a bicornuate uterus. **(I)** TAS showing prominent retrochorionic blood pool *(curved arrow)*.

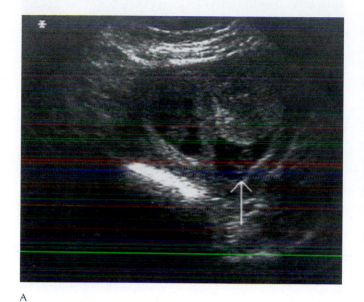

A

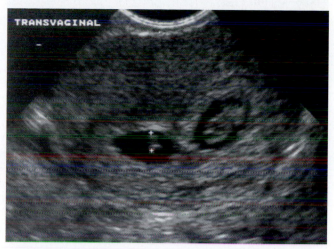

B

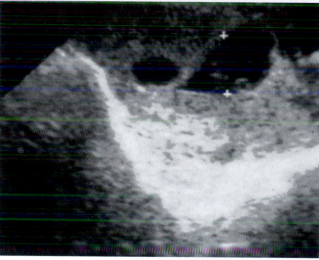

C

Figure 4–7. Multifetal pregnancy. **(A)** TAS of normal 7-week diamniotic, dichorionic twin IUP. **(B)** TVS of demised embryo *(+'s)* adjacent to living twin at 7 weeks. **(C)** TAS of "vanished" twin within an empty sac adjacent to a living embryo with an intact sac *(between +'s)*. **(D)** Diamniotic/dichorionic twin gestation showing thick interface between gestational sacs. **(E)** Triplet intrauterine pregnancy showing thick membrane between sacs most likely representing trichorionic. *(Figure continued.)*

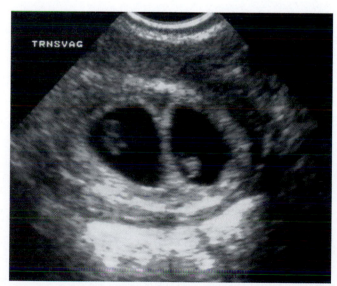

D

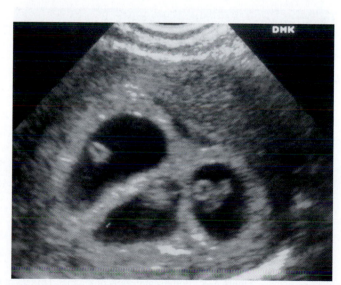

E

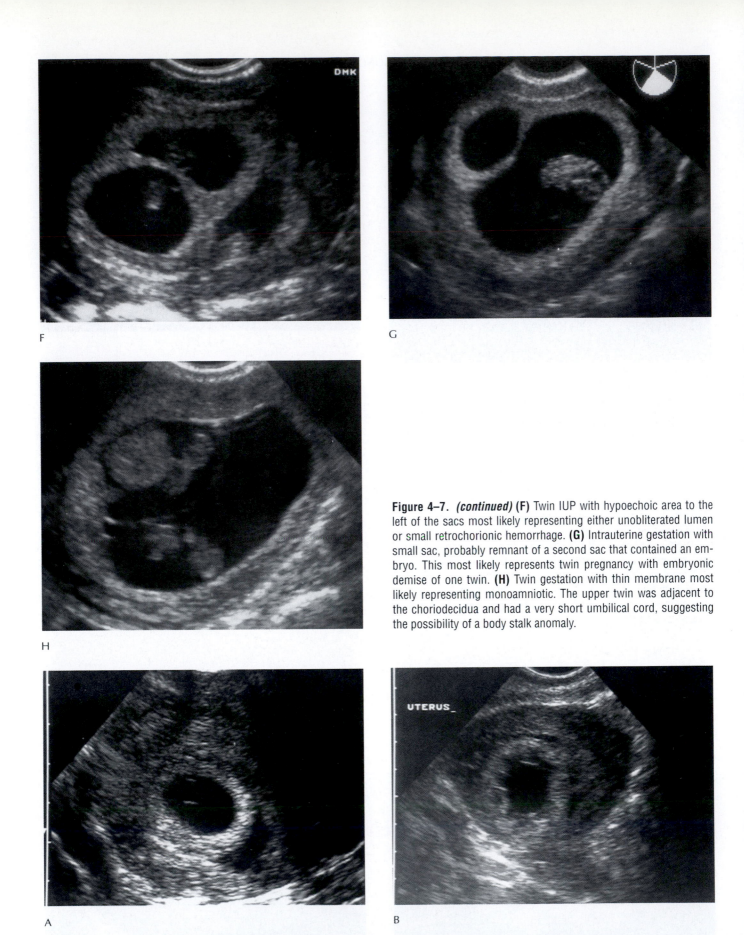

Figure 4–7. *(continued)* **(F)** Twin IUP with hypoechoic area to the left of the sacs most likely representing either unobliterated lumen or small retrochorionic hemorrhage. **(G)** Intrauterine gestation with small sac, probably remnant of a second sac that contained an embryo. This most likely represents twin pregnancy with embryonic demise of one twin. **(H)** Twin gestation with thin membrane most likely representing monoamniotic. The upper twin was adjacent to the choriodecidua and had a very short umbilical cord, suggesting the possibility of a body stalk anomaly.

Figure 4–8. Complicated early pregnancy. **(A)** TVS of an embryonic demise. **(B)** Semi-axial TVS of incomplete abortion with irregular choriodecidua and deflated sac. *(Figure continued.)*

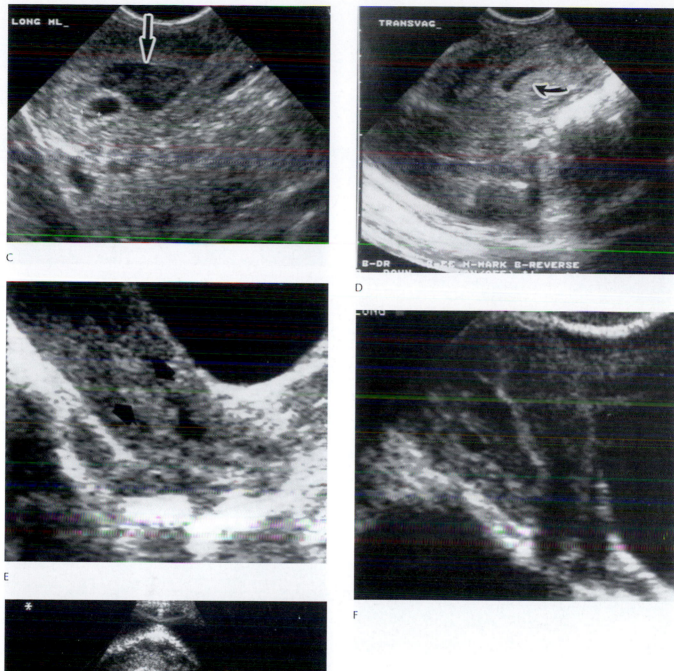

Figure 4–8. *(continued)* (C) TVS of retrochorionic hemorrhage *(arrow)* surrounding normal gestational sac with a living fetus. **(D)** TV sonogram of retained choriodecidua within lower uterine lumen *(curved arrow).* **(E)** TAS showing sloughed decidua *(between arrows)* in lower uterine lumen. **(F)** TAS of extremely irregular sac. On repeat scan 2 weeks later, a living fetus was found. **(G)** TVS of septated uterus with clot within right uterine lumen. The fetus *(between +'s)* within left side of uterus was living. *(Figure continued.)*

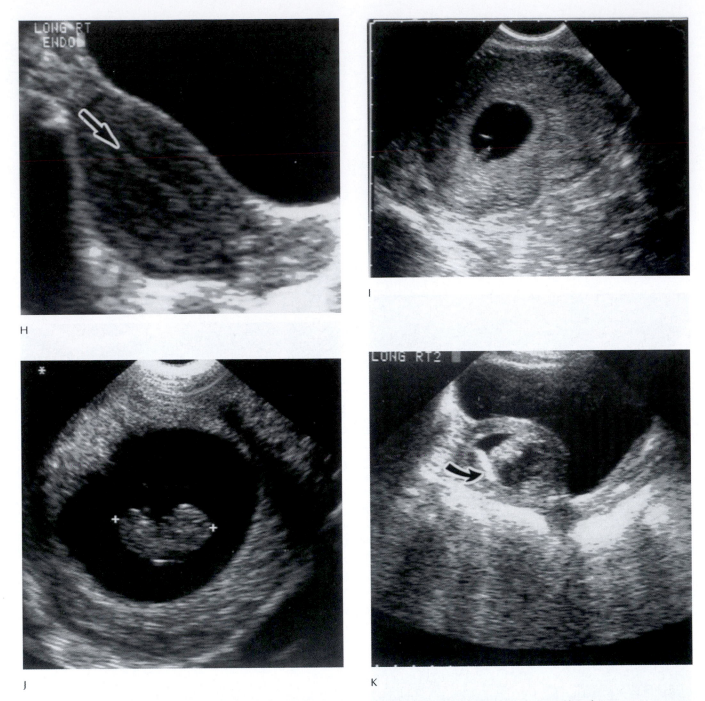

Figure 4–8. *(continued)* **(H)** TAS of completed abortion. Note thinness and regularity of endometrial interfaces *(arrow)*. **(I)** TVS of embryonic demise at 6 weeks. No heart activity was detected. **(J)** TV scan of fetal demise at 9 weeks. No heart motion was detected. **(K)** TAS showing retrochorionic hemorrhage surrounding an IUD *(curved arrow)*. The deflated sac is seen inferior to the IUD. *(Figure continued.)*

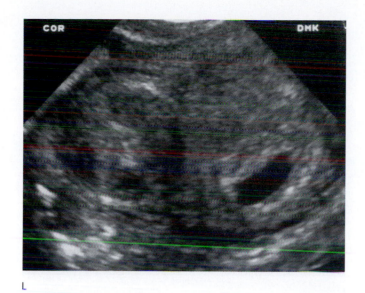

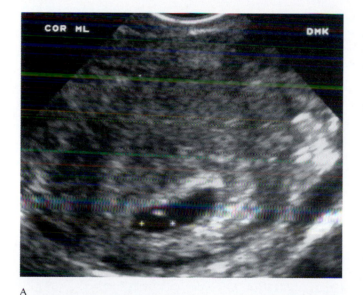

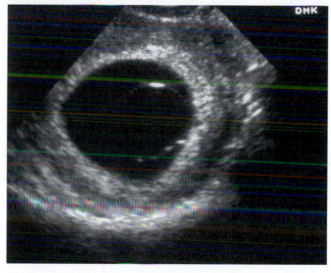

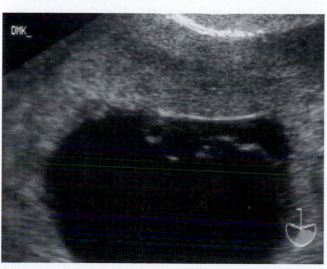

Figure 4–8. *(continued)* **(L)** TVS showing large fibroid on maternal right and normal gestational sac to the left of midline.

Figure 4–9. Gestational sac anomalies. **(A)** Yolk sac within an overall small gestation sac. **(B)** Large gestational sac. The amnion could be seen within the sac but no definite embryo. These are two ends of the spectrum seen in intrauterine fetal demise. **(C)** Vitelline duct leading to a deflated yolk sac. *(Figure continued.)*

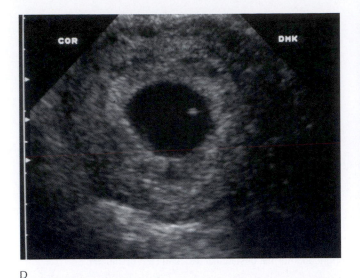

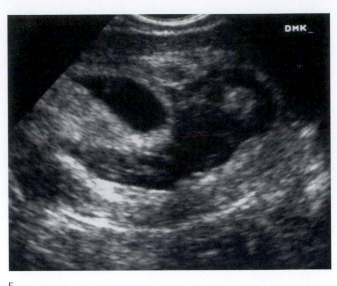

D

E

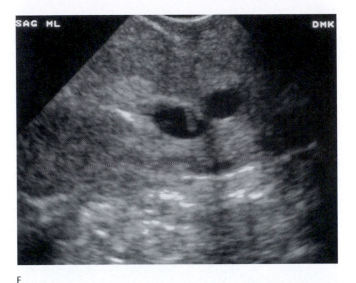

F

Figure 4–9. *(continued)* **(D)** Large sac size with deflated yolk sac indicating embryonic demise. **(E)** Large area of retrochorionic hemorrhage that extends behind the choriodecidua. **(F)** TVS of a cervical inclusion cyst adjacent to gestational sac and embryo in a spontaneous abortion.

of the uterus may contain echogenic material with low-impedance flow.[31] Thus, the role of CDS in evaluation of early pregnancy is yet to be determined.

Another study has reported that pregnancy failure is more common when the retrochorionic hemorrhagic is over two-thirds the size of the gestational sac, when the patient is over 35 years old, and when the pregnancy is less than 8 weeks.

COMPLICATED EARLY INTRAUTERINE PREGNANCY

As stated previously, it is not unusual for the pregnant patient to experience painless spotting in the first few weeks of pregnancy. This probably is related to trophoblastic implantation within the decidualized endometrium. As the gestational sac develops, small (2- to 5-mm) hypoechoic areas may be seen

immediately beneath the echogenic choriodecidua that probably represent areas of blood pools or lacunae (see Fig. 4–8).

On transvaginal color Doppler sonography (TV-CDS), arterial and venous flow can be seen within the choriodecidua prior to sonographic visualization of the embryo (Fig. 4–11). Arterial velocities within the choriodecidua gradually increase.

Failing or failed IUPs tend to demonstrate an increase in venous flow beneath the choriodecidua (see Fig. 4–11). There does not seem to be a statistically significant difference in their arterial velocities in normal versus abnormal early pregnancies, however.

Patients who present with extensive bleeding may have retrochorionic hemorrhage. In this disorder, there is more extensive bleeding behind the chorion, which appears as a hypoechoic area surrounding the gestational sac. Using the formula for a prolate ellipse volume (cc): length (cm) × width (cm) × height (cm) × 0.5, the relative size of the retrochorionic hemorrhage can be quantified in relation to the size of the gestational sac itself. It has been shown that the relative size of the retrochorionic hemorrhage has some implications as to whether or not the pregnancy will progress.[25] When the area of the retrochorionic hemorrhage is less than one-fourth of the gestational sac or less than 60 mL, it is likely that the pregnancy will progress.[3]

In spontaneous incomplete abortions, there is usually passage of the fetus or embryo with retained choriodecidua. This tissue typically appears as echogenic material within the uterine lumen. The choriodecidua is irregular, and the gestational sac itself appears "deflated" or irregular in shape.

In cases of failed embryonic development, there is a failed or abnormal development of the embryo and its associated umbilical cord and body stalk. Thus, even though a gestational sac may appear normally formed, no embryo or, on occasion, no yolk sac will be identified within the uterus. An early pregnancy failure is usually a reflection of a chromosomally aberrant conceptus.

Embryonic demise can be documented by TVS when there is lack of heart motion in an embryo that measures

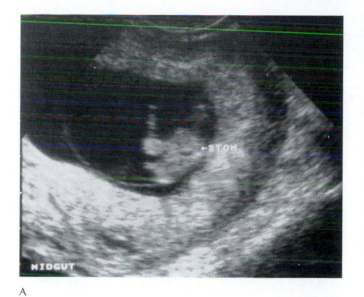

A

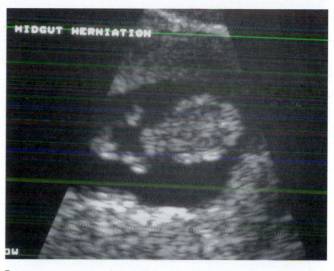

B

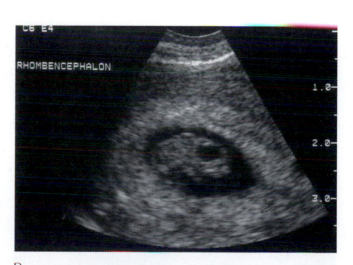

C

D

Figure 4–10. Normal anatomy of embryo/fetus in first trimester of pregnancy. **(A)** The stomach and umbilical cord seen in this 9-week pregnancy. There is herniation of some bowel into the cord. **(B)** Transverse TVS showing herniated bowel into the base of the cord, which is a physiologic process up to 12 weeks. **(C)** TVS showing normal configuration of the abdominal wall of this 10- to 12-week fetus after bowel has returned into the abdomen. **(D)** The rhombencephalon is seen in this 8-week fetus. *(Figure continued.)*

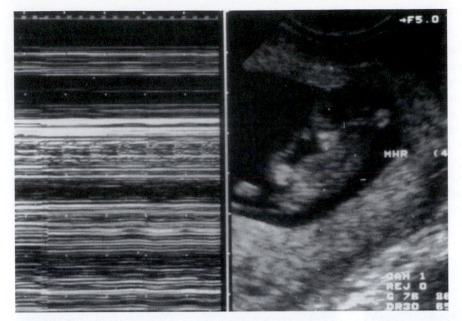

E

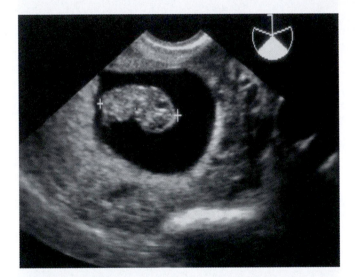

F

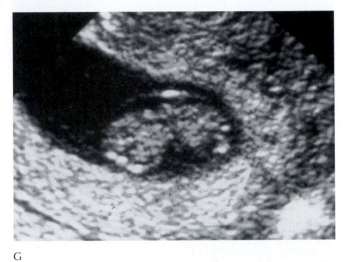

G

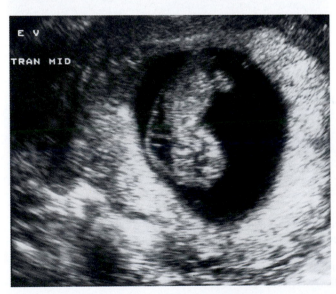

H

Figure 4–10. *(continued)* **(E)** Fetal heart motion detected in this normal fetus. **(F)** Rhombencephalon seen in this 9-week embryo showing measurement of crown-rump length. **(G)** Amnion surrounding embryo should not to be mistaken for nuchal thickening. **(H)** TVS of nuchal membrane. Although this multiloculated nuchal fluid collection looked like a cystic hystroma, it regressed and the karyotype was normal.

over 6 mm in length. In general, heart motion can usually be detected if an embryo can be delineated.[26] In some cases of failed embryonic development, amorphous internal debris can be present within the sac. They probably represent strands of blood or sloughed decidual tissues.

In completed miscarriages, there is close apposition of relatively thin and regular endometrial interfaces. Although one might argue that ectopic pregnancies may demonstrate this appearance, correlation with β-hCG values may be helpful in confirming a completed miscarriage. In completed miscarriage, serial β-hCG values will typically fall precipitously, whereas in ectopic pregnancy this value slowly decreases or reaches a plateau.[27] In induced abortions, β-hCG was detectable from 16 to 60 days with a mean of 30 days after

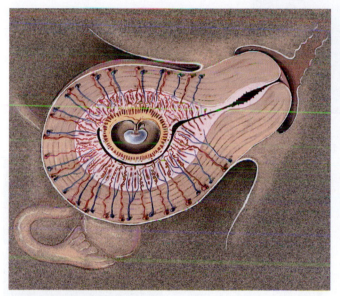

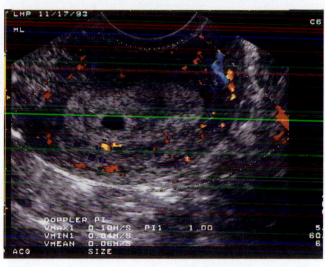

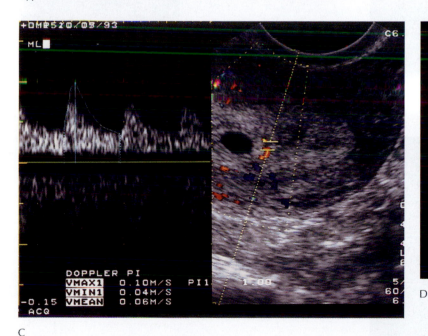

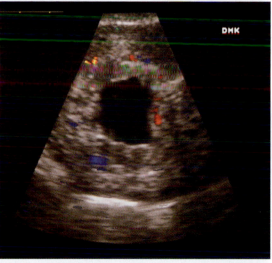

Figure 4–11. TV-CDS of early intrauterine pregnancy. **(A)** Diagram showing arterial and venous flow to the choriodecidua. The arcuate vessels branch into the radials, which traverse the myometrium ending in the spiral vessels within the choriodecidua. **(B)** TV-CDS of a normal 5-week IUP showing flow in the arcuate vessels and a form within the choriodecidua adjacent to the chorionic sac. **(C)** TV-CDS showing low impedance arterial flow within the choriodecidua in same patient as in **B**. **(D)** TV-CDS of abnormal or failed IUP. *(Figure continued.)*

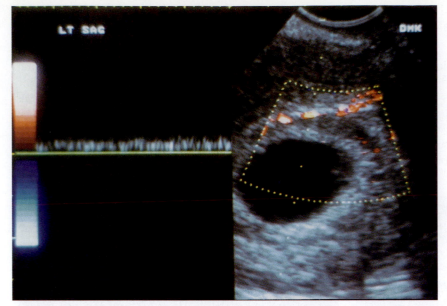

E

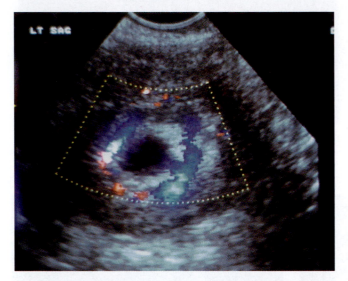

F

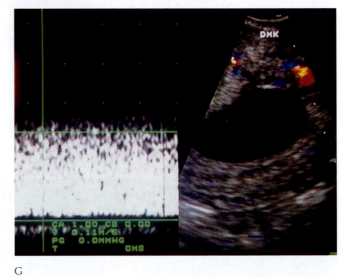

G

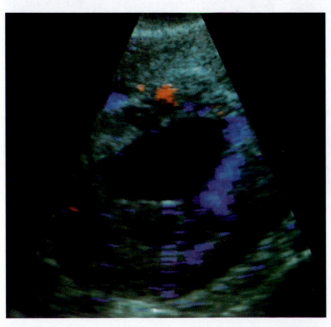

H

Figure 4–11. *(continued)* **(E)** TV-CDS showing increased venous flow between choriodecidua and myometrium. **(F)** TV-CDS of failed IUP with circumferential subchorionic hemorrhage. **(G)** TV-CDS of embryonic demise showing high-velocity venous flow. **(H)** TV-CDS of embryonic demise with increased subchorionic venous flow. *(Figure continued.)*

84

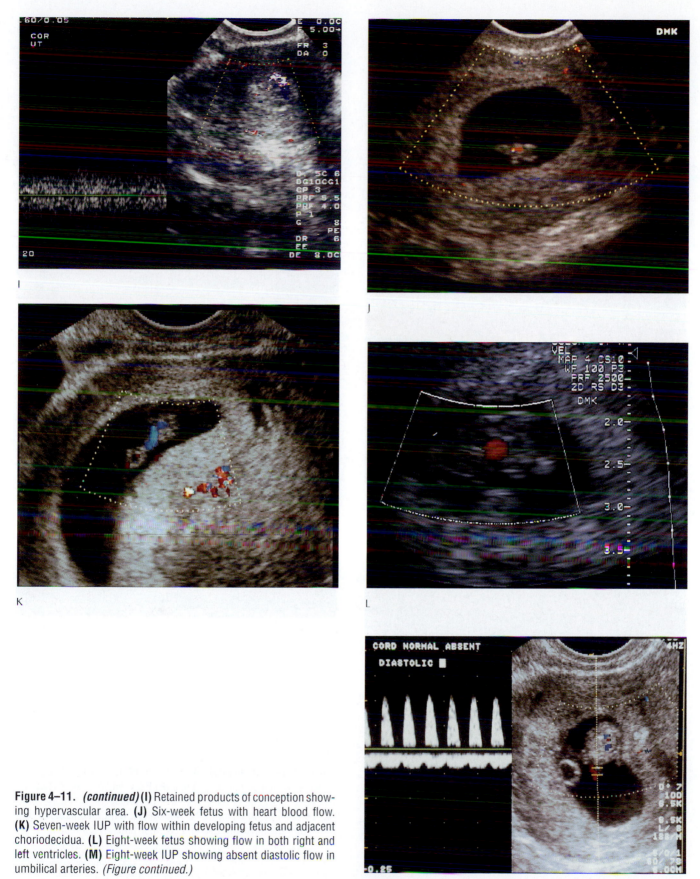

Figure 4–11. *(continued)* **(I)** Retained products of conception showing hypervascular area. **(J)** Six-week fetus with heart blood flow. **(K)** Seven-week IUP with flow within developing fetus and adjacent choriodecidua. **(L)** Eight-week fetus showing flow in both right and left ventricles. **(M)** Eight-week IUP showing absent diastolic flow in umbilical arteries. *(Figure continued.)*

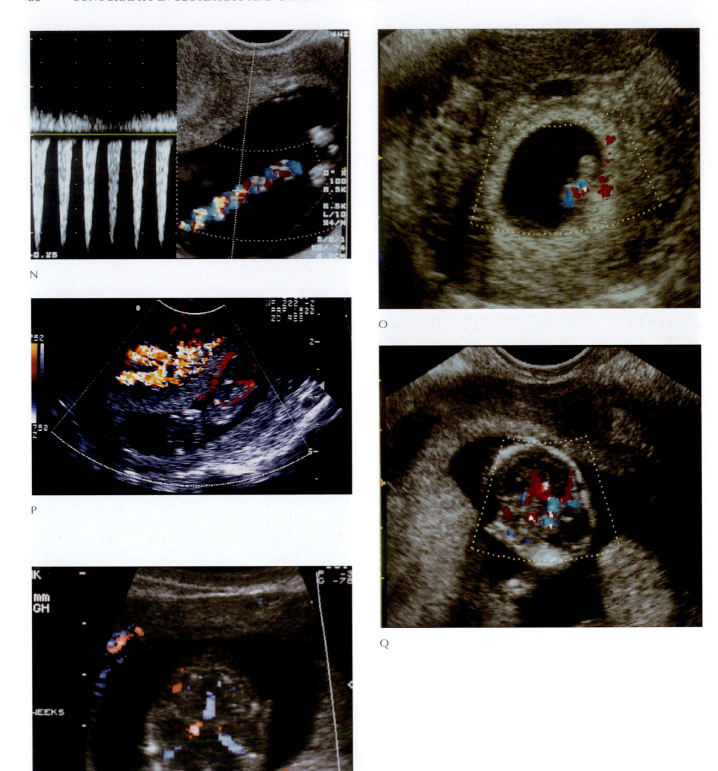

Figure 4–11. *(continued)* **(N)** Same as **M** at 10 weeks. **(O)** Flow within developing decidua basalis. **(P)** Flow within myometrium adjacent to placenta in 11-week IUP. *(Courtesy of C. Peery, MD.)* **(Q)** Cerebral blood flow in a 12-week fetus. **(R)** Cerebral blood flow in major intracranial arteries in a 13-week fetus. *(Figure continued.)*

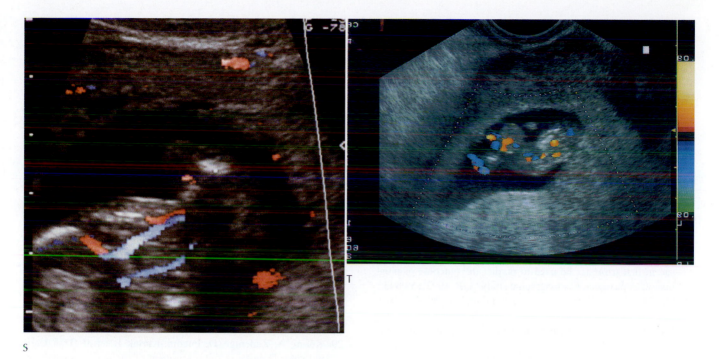

Figure 4–11. *(continued)* **(S)** Same as **R** showing internal carotid. **(T)** TV-CDS showing physiologic herniation of bowel adjacent to cord.

uterine evaluation, as opposed to spontaneous abortions where it was detectable from 9 to 35 days with a mean of 19 days, and in ectopic pregnancies, it was detectable for 1 to 31 days with a mean of 8 days, 5 days after laparoscopic tubal removal.[27]

OTHER APPLICATIONS

It is important in some patients with IUDs and complicated pregnancies to confirm the presence of an IUD and establish its location relative to the gestational sac in the developing choriodecidua. Clearly, IUDs that are implanted superior to the gestational sac are more difficult to extract than those that are inferior. The amount of retrochorionic hemorrhage associated with an IUD can also be quantified using TVS.

Transvaginal sonography may also be helpful in the evaluation of first trimester pregnancies complicated by trophoblastic disease. Although large hydropic villi may not be present in trophoblastic disease at this stage, the abnormal tissue can be diagnosed as well as its relative amount. Trophoblastic tissue, however, frequently has the sonographic appearance of retained choriodecidua. This disorder is discussed in detail in Chap. 32.

SUMMARY

The recent development of TVS as a has been discussed in this chapter. Transvaginal sonography primarily has a role

in the diagnosis of early intrauterine pregnancy in patients suspected of ectopic pregnancy and in detecting embryonic or fetal life in those patients with extensive bleeding, cramping, or both in the first trimester.

REFERENCES

1. Pennell RG, Needleman L, Pajak T, et al. Prospective comparison of vaginal and abdominal sonography in normal early pregnancy. *J Ultrasound Med.* 1991;10:63–67.
2. Pritchard L, MacDonald PC, Gant NF, eds. *Williams Obstetrics,* 16th ed. Norwalk, CT: Appleton-Century-Crofts; 1985.
3. Sauerbrei EE, Pham DH. Placental abruption and subchorionic hemorrhage in the first half of pregnancy: US appearance and clinical outcome. *Radiology.* 1986;160:109–112.
4. Pennell RG, Baltarowich OH, Kurtz AB, et al. Complicated first-trimester pregnancies: Evaluation with endovaginal US versus transabdominal technique. *Radiology.* 1987;165:79–83.
5. Timor-Tritsch IE, Rottem S, Thaler I. Review of transvaginal ultrasonography: A description with clinical application. *Ultrasound Q.* 1988;6(1):1–34.
6. Batzer FR, Weiner S, Corson SL. Landmarks during the first forty-two days of gestation demonstrated by the β subunit of human chorionic gonadotrophin and ultrasound. *Am J Obstet Gynecol.* 1983;146:973.
7. Nyberg DA, Filly RA, Mahony BS, et al. Early gestation: Correlation of hCG levels and sonographic identification. *AJR.* 1985;144:951.
8. Bree RL, Edwards M, Böhm-Vélez M, et al. Transvaginal

sonography in the evaluation of normal early pregnancy: Correlation with hCG level. *AJR.* 1989;153:75–79.

9. Daya S, Woods S, Ward S, et al. Early pregnancy assessment with transvaginal ultrasound scanning. *Can Med Assoc J.* 1991;144(4):441–446.

10. Nyberg DA, Mac LA, Harvey D, et al. Value of the yolk sac in evaluating early pregnancies. *J Ultrasound Med.* 1988; 7:129–135.

11. de Crespigny L, Cooper D, McKenna M. Early detection of intrauterine pregnancy with ultrasound. *J Ultrasound Med.* 1988; 7:7–10.

12. Yeh HC, Rabinowitz JG. Amniotic sac development: Ultrasound features of early pregnancy—The double bleb sign. *Radiology.* 1988;166:97–103.

13. Timor-Tritsch IE, Rottem S. *Transvaginal Sonography.* New York: Elsevier; 1988;98.

14. Kurtz A, Needleman L, Pennell P, et al. Can detection of yolk sac in first trimester be used to predict the outcome of pregnancy? A prospective sonographic study. *AJR.* 1992;158:843.

15. Cyr D, Mack L, Nyberg D, et al. Fetal rhombencephalon: Normal US findings. *Radiology.* 1988;166:691–692.

16. Moore K. *The Developing Human.* Philadelphia: Saunders; 1987.

17. Jeanty P. Sonographic appearance of normal amnion. *J Ultrasound Med.* 1982;1:243.

18. Torpin R. Fetal malformations caused by amnion rupture during gestation. In: Torpin R, ed. *The Human Placenta.* Springfield, IL: Thomas; 1968:1–76.

19. Lasser DM, Peisner DB, Vollebergh J, et al. First-trimester fetal biometry using transvaginal sonography. *Ultrasound Obstet Gynecol.* 1993;3:104–108.

20. Skibo LK, Lyons EA, Levi CS. First-trimester umbilical cord cysts. *Radiology.* 1992;182:719–722.

21. Laboda LA, Estroff JA, Benacerraf BR. First trimester bradycardia: A sign of impending fetal loss. *J Ultrasound Med.* 1989;8:561–563.

22. Bromley B, Harlow BL, Laboda LA, et al. Small sac size in the first trimester: A predictor of poor fetal outcome. *Radiology.* 1991;178:375–377.

23. Kurtz A, Needleman L, Pennell R, et al. Can detection of the yolk sac in the first trimester be used to predict the outcome of pregnancy? A prospective sonographic study. *AJR.* 1992;158:843.

24. Horrow MM. Enlarged amniotic cavity: A new sonographic sign of early embryonic death. *AJR.* 1992;158:359–362.

25. Pedersen JF, Mantoni M. Prevalence and significance of subchorionic hemorrhage in threatened abortion: A sonographic study. *AJR.* 1990;154:535–537.

26. Levi CS, Lyons EA, Zheng XH, et al. Endovaginal US: Demonstration of cardiac activity in embryos of less than 5.0 mm in crown-rump length. *Radiology.* 1990;176:71–74.

27. Steier JA, Bergsjo P, Myking OL. Human chorionic gonadotrophin in maternal plasma after induced abortion, spontaneous abortion, and removed ectopic pregnancy. *Obstet Gynecol.* 1984;64:391.

28. Arduini D, Rizzo G, Romanini C. Doppler ultrasonography in early pregnancy does not predict adverse pregnancy outcome. *Ultrasound Obstet Gynecol.* 1991;1:180–185.

29. Kurjak A, Zudenigo D, Funduk-Kurjak B, et al. Transvaginal color Doppler in the assessment of the uteroplacental circulation in normal early pregnancy. *J Perinat Med.* 1992;21: 25–34.

30. Jaffe R, Warsof SL. Color Doppler imaging in the assessment of uteroplacental blood flow in abnormal first trimester intrauterine pregnancies: An attempt to define etiologic mechanisms. *J Ultrasound Med.* 1992;11:41–44.

31. Dillon EH, Case CQ, Ramos IM, et al. Endovaginal US and Doppler findings after first-trimester abortion. *Radiology.* 1993;186:87–91.

32. Benson CB, Doubilet PM: Slow embryonic heart rate in early first trimester: Indicator of poor pregnancy outcome. *Radiology.* 1994;192:343–344.

First-Trimester Nuchal Translucency Screening for Fetal Aneuploidy

David M. Sherer • Frank A. Manning

Many structural anomalies strongly associated with specific fetal aneuploidies may be diagnosed during second- or third-trimester ultrasonographic assessment. Such structural anomalies include the double bubble, reflecting duodenal atresia or endocardial cushion defect, both seen in association with fetal trisomy 21, or holoprosencephaly, median facial cleft defects, and overriding digits seen with fetal trisomies 13 and 18.[1–5] Depiction of such structural anomalies has led to amniocentesis and thus precise confirmation of possible underlying fetal aneuploidy[1–5] in women otherwise not at increased risk for fetal aneuploidy. For example, Nyberg et al.[1] reported the presence of major structural defects in 33% of trisomy 21 fetuses. These defects included cardiac abnormalities, duodenal atresia, cystic hygroma, omphalocele, hydrops, and hydrothorax.[1]

Similarly, attention has been drawn to the midtrimester finding of cystic hygroma, septated cystic projections at the posterior lateral of the fetal neck (considered to result from nuchal lymphatic obstruction), and a high incidence of associated chromosomal abnormalities, often 45,X.[6,7] Moreover, this sign is considered a poor prognostic indicator of survival. In a large series of 153 cases, Abramowicz et al.[8] noted that there were no survivors among such fetuses with abnormal karyotypes and only an overall 2 to 3% survival rate of in-tact survivors when fetuses with cystic hygroma diagnosed *in utero*.

After the introduction of first-trimester transvaginal ultrasonography toward the late 1980s, certain fetal structural anomalies could be diagnosed at this early gestational age.[9] With increasing application of first-trimester and especially transvaginal ultrasound, attention was drawn to fetuses exhibiting a translucency projected from the posterior aspect of the fetal neck, which at times extended caudally toward the fetal lumbar sacral area (Fig. 5–1). With the previously established knowledge of the association between mid-trimester cystic hygroma and fetal aneuploidy, early amniocentesis was often performed. Initial reports suggested a higher incidence of fetal chromosomal abnormalities among septated versus nonseptated cystic hygromata.[10,11] At times, the nonseptated cystic lesion was noted to have resolved spontaneously.[11] Irrespective of the fetal karyotype, the early sonographic finding of an extensive translucency extending caudally toward the sacrum was recognized as an ominous sign because many of these fetuses succumbed, with fetal demise being confirmed at ultrasound follow-up, often within days.

Subsequently, over the recent decade a growing body of evidence has been accumulated regarding first-trimester fetal nuchal translucency and fetal aneuploidy (Figs. 5–2 and

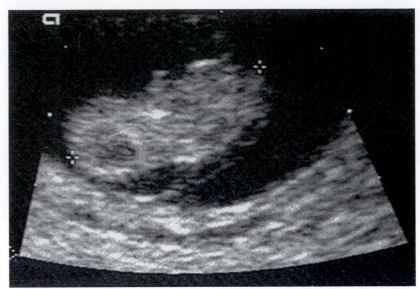

Figure 5–1. Marked nuchal and extended translucency extending caudally and involving the entire fetal back. *(Reproduced with permission from Sherer DM, Manning FA. Am J Perinatol. 1999;16:103.)*

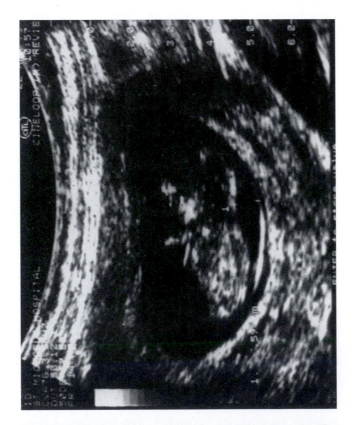

Figure 5–2. Ultrasound scan at 11 weeks of gestation demonstrating 6-mm nuchal translucency (scan has been rotated 90 degrees to the left to be comparable with Fig. 5–3). Chorionic villus sampling revealed trisomy 18. *(Reproduced with permission from Jackson S, Porter H, Vyas S. Ultrasound Obstet Gynecol. 1995;5:55.)*

5–3). As a result of this volume of data, first-trimester fetal nuchal translucency is currently being investigated (in conjuction with various first-trimester maternal serum analytes) as a possible early screening tool for populations at low risk for fetal aneuploidy.

This chapter will present current data pertaining to nuchal translucency, including definition of the finding, accuracy and effect of confounding factors on this ultrasonographic measurement, nomograms, effect of various ethnic origin, suggested possible pathophysiologic mechanisms, increased associated incidence of fetal cardiac anomalies, arrhythmias, and other structural anomalies, Doppler velocimetry (ductus venosus flow and umbilical artery velocimetry), lethality (or spontaneous subsequent miscarriage), implications of nuchal translucency in twin gestations, and potential effect of nuchal translucency screening on subsequent midtrimester maternal serum screening for fetal aneuploidy. All studies screening large populations (more than 500 participants) at either high or low risk for fetal chromosomal abnormalities with first-trimester nuchal translucency will be presented.

DEFINITION

Nuchal translucency pertains to the ultrasonographic depiction of a single nonseptated sonolucency projecting from the posterior aspect of the fetal neck (Figs. 5–2 and 5–4). This finding is not to be confused or interchanged with nuchal thickness or nuchal fold, which pertains to the mid-trimester

MEASUREMENT

First-trimester nuchal translucency may be obtained by either transabdominal or transvaginal ultrasonography. After precise calculation of gestational age by crown–rump length (CRL), the maximal nuchal translucency thickness is visualized in the mid-sagittal plane of the fetal neck. The width of the sonolucent area between the inner skin outline echo and the outer border of the soft tissues overlying the cervical spine is measured after placement of electronic calipers (see Figs. 5–2 and 5–4). In addition, care must be exercised to correctly identify septa within the translucency. To delineate ultrasonographic differences between nuchal translucency and cystic hygroma, Bonilla-Musoles et al.[17] rescanned 25 fetuses (13 with nuchal translucency and 12 with cystic hygroma) using transvaginal and three-dimensional ultrasonography. This retrospective analysis showed that the most striking difference was the presence of bullae in addition to greater irregularity and amplitude of the membrane in cases of cystic hygromas compared with cases of nuchal translucency. Fetuses with simple nuchal translucency had a more homogeneous linear membrane. Mahieu-Caputo et al.[18] demonstrated that the aneuploidy rate was significantly higher in cases in which the translucency involved the entire fetal trunk (65%) (see Fig. 5–1) than in cases in which translucency was confined to the nuchal area (16%).

Potential Pitfalls

Although measurement of first-trimester nuchal translucency is straightforward and usually uncomplicated, a number of potential pitfalls have been recognized, each that may, if undetected, contribute to incorrect measurement of this novel ultrasonographic parameter. Potential complicating factors that may be encountered include (a) approximation of the amnion, (b) fetal neck positioning, and (c) the presence of a nuchal cord.

When the fetus is located adjacent to the amnion, which in the late first trimester is not yet fused with the chorion, the fetus may be mistaken for the outer skin layer and may lead to an erroneous assessment of increased nuchal translucency. When this common occurrence is correctly identified, the operator may either wait for spontaneous fetal movement away from the amniotic membrane or actively assist in separating the two structures by tapping the maternal abdomen or asking the patient to cough slightly.

Variation Due to Fetal Head Positioning

Either fetal neck flexion or extension may result in poor measurement repeatability.[19,20] Whitlow et al.[20] determined the influence of the precise position of the fetal neck on nuchal translucency measurement. The mean extended nuchal translucency was 0.62 mm greater than the mean neutral nuchal translucency value, and the mean flexed nuchal translucency

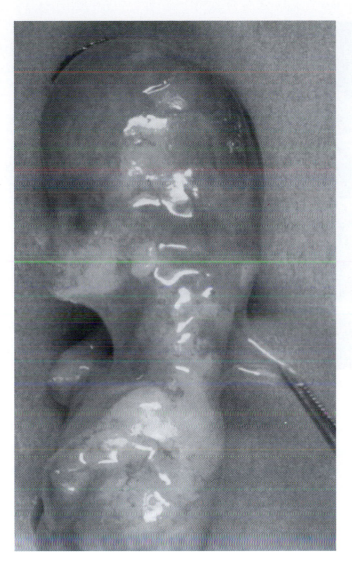

Figure 5–3. Same fetus as shown in Figure 5–2 after termination of pregnancy, demonstrating loose edematous skin over the neck, accounting for the nuchal translucency on ultrasound scanning. *(Reproduced with permission from Jackson S, Porter H, Vyas S. Ultrasound Obstet Gynecol. 1995;5:55.)*

ultrasonographic finding described by Benacerraf and others.[12–14] Whereas nuchal thickness is considered to represent the excessive nuchal skin that 80% of infants with trisomy 21 are known to exhibit,[15] a completely different spectrum of potential etiologies has been suggested for first-trimester nuchal translucency and will be discussed later in this chapter. In addition, first-trimester nuchal translucency should not be confused with cystic hygromas that, although usually noted as a mid-trimester finding, may be depicted earlier in the latter part of the first trimester (Fig. 5–5). In contrast to first-trimester nuchal translucency, cystic hygromas are considered to be the result of congenital lymphatic obstruction.[16]

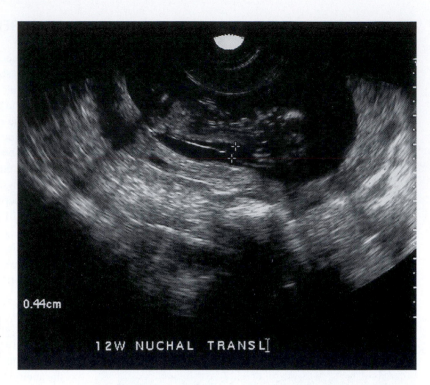

Figure 5–4. Transvaginal nuchal translucency at 12 weeks of gestation in a fetus with trisomy 21. *(Reproduced with permission from Sherer DM, Manning FA. Am J Perinatol. 1999;16:103.)*

was 0.40 mm less than the mean neutral nuchal translucency (both $P \leq 0.00001$). In addition, repeatability of measurements are more accurate with the fetal neck in the neutral position. These authors concluded that fetal neck position can make a significant difference to nuchal translucency measurements.[20]

The presence of a nuchal cord or a loop of umbilical cord within the vicinity of the posterior aspect of fetal neck may create an artifact. Schaefer et al.[21] determined the incidence of nuchal cord measurement and its possible effect on nuchal translucency between 10 and 14 weeks of gestation. Of 316 consecutive transabdominal nuchal translucency measurements, 26 (8.23%) fetuses were noted to have the umbilical cord around the neck. Inadvertent inclusion of the umbilical cord (which, other than the thin vessel wall, is sonolucent), measured with the nuchal translucency, adds a mean of 0.8 mm to the actual measurement. When the thickness of the umbilical cord was subtracted, the measurements of nuchal translucency did not differ from those of the overall population examined. These authors suggested that utilization of color Doppler imaging could decrease the false-positive rate in first-trimester screening for fetal aneuploidy (Figs. 5–6 and 5–7).[21]

Transabdominal versus Transvaginal Ultrasonography

Both transabdominal and transvaginal ultrasonographic modalities may be used to assess first-trimester nuchal translucency. Braithwaite et al.[19] prospectively assessed the abilities of transabdominal and transvaginal ultrasonography in measuring nuchal translucency. All 242 patients included

in the study underwent examinations with both ultrasonographic modalities. Nuchal translucency measurements were obtained in 92% and 90% of fetuses using abdominal and vaginal ultrasonography, respectively, and in 100% of patients combining the two methods. A significant overmeasuring of nuchal translucency was noted with transabdominal ultrasound (mean difference $\pm 0.10 \pm 0.29$ mm). Repeatability coefficients were 0.40 mm and 0.22 mm for transabdominal and transvaginal ultrasonography, respectively. These authors advocated that both ultrasonographic modalities should be available in laboratories performing such measurements.[19] Furthermore, cases in which nuchal translucency measurements obtained with transabdominal ultrasonography approach threshold values for screening positive should be followed with transvaginal ultrasonographic measurement because of the overmeasuring that has been documented with transabdominal ultrasound. In a larger study of 1,707 women, also by Braithwaite et al.,[22] similar repeatability coefficients for transabdominal and transvaginal ultrasonographic assessment of nuchal translucency were 0.44 mm and 0.23 mm, respectively.

Repeatability

Various studies have specifically addressed accuracy and repeatability of this ultrasonographic measurement. Pandya et al.[23] demonstrated that 95% of the time the intraobserver, interobserver, and caliper placement repeatability of measuring fetal nuchal translucency were less than 0.54 mm, 0.62 mm, and 0.58 mm, respectively. These authors also demonstrated that repeatability was unrelated to the size of

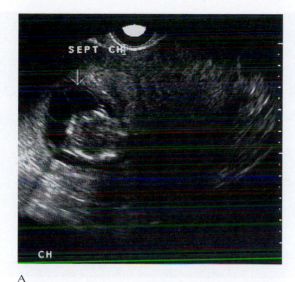

A

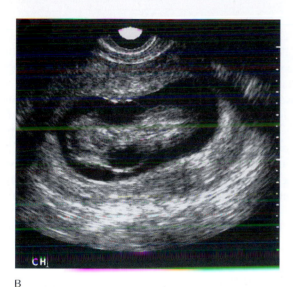

B

Figure 5–5. Transvaginal ultrasonographic depiction of a fetus with a septated first-trimester cystic hygroma. Subsequent genetic analysis demonstrated 45,X. **(A)** Transverse view of septated cystic hygroma. Note two fine, yet distinct, sepatations. **(B)** Coronal view of fetus. Note marked lateral projections of septated cystic hygroma. *(Reproduced with permission from Sherer DM, Manning FA. Am J Perinatol.* 1999;16:103.)

the nuchal translucency.[23] Herman et al.[24] demonstrated that nuchal translucency image magnification does not contribute to reproducibility of the measurement (Fig. 5–8). Despite significantly smaller mean values obtained from magnified images compared with regular-sized measurements, those differences do not justify modification of the criteria for caliper placement on magnified images. These authors recommended blind repeated measurements on either regular-sized or magnified images as a tool for self-assessment, quality control, and training.[24] Braithwaite et al.[25] proposed

training methods, standards, and criteria to serve as the basis for training sonographers in nuchal translucency measurements. Although trainees were quickly able to measure first-trimester nuchal translucency consistently with transabdominal ultrasonography (40 to 60 scans), more training was required for transvaginal assessment (more than 80 scans). Limited probe maneuverability was recognized as a reason for difficulty in obtaining correct transvaginal nuchal translucency measurements, especially if the fetus was in an unfavorable position. When difficulties were encountered with the transabdominal approach, these usually reflected patient habitus, poor resolution, and retroverted uterus. These authors suggested that measuring first-trimester nuchal translucency is not as easy as obtaining a CRL measurement. Herman et al.[26] evaluated the feasibility and reproducibility of a novel image-scoring method of first-trimester nuchal translucency measurement as an objective tool of ongoing audit and training. In this study, 105 consecutive singleton pregnancies undergoing first-trimester screening were scored according to the following criteria: section (oblique, 0; midsagittal, 2), caliper placing (misplaced, 0; proper, 2), skin line (nuchal only, 0; nuchal and back, 2), image size (unsatisfactory, 0; satisfactory, 1), amnion (not visualized, 0; visualized 1), and head position (flexion/hyperextension, 0; straight 1). The final score was then categorized into one of four quality groups: excellent (between 8 and 9), reasonable (between 4 and 7), intermediate (between 2 and 3), and unacceptable (between 0 and 1). Distributions of the four quality groups were similar across three reviewers: 11.4% were classified as excellent, 57.1% as reasonable, 25.7% as intermediate, and 5.7% as unacceptable. Interreviewer agreement showed identical classification by each pair of reviewers, from 65.7 to 74.3%, and partial agreement to neighboring quality groups, from 25.7 to 34.3% of cases. In none of the cases did the reviewers differ in categorizing cases to remarkably different quality groups. Application of the described audit method to the examiners demonstrated a similar distribution to the various quality groups and similar mean final scores. These authors suggested that this novel audit method may be employed by ultrasound centers in an independent fashion with minimal resources and regardless of the method of risk assessment.

Nuchal Translucency Nomograms

Pajkrt et al.[27] determined the normal range for the nuchal translucency measurement in chromosomally and phenotypically normal fetuses. These authors demonstrated a physiologic variation in the nuchal translucency measurement between 9 and 14 weeks of gestation. The nuchal translucency was measured in 771 women with singleton chromosomally normal fetuses and was found to increase from 0.7 mm at 10 weeks of gestation to 1.5 mm at 13 weeks of gestation (Fig. 5–9). Although a measurement greater than 2.5 mm was found in 4.6% of fetuses at 10 weeks, this

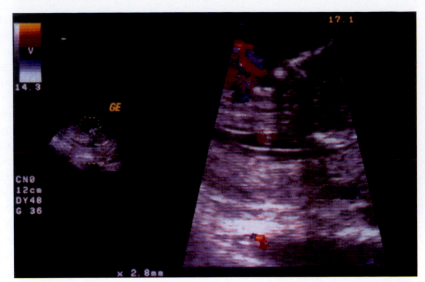

Figure 5–6. Sagittal plane of a 12-week fetus showing a nuchal cord visualized by color Doppler. Note the separate amnion. *(Reproduced with permission from Schaefer M, Laurichesse-Delmas H, Ville Y. Ultrasound Obstet Gynecol. 1998;11:271.)*

incidence increased to 8.7% at 14 weeks of gestation (Fig. 5–10). These authors suggested implementation of a gestational age-dependent cutoff point that may reduce the incidence of false-positive test results. Similarly, Braithwaite et al.[22] studied nuchal translucency in 1,707 women (1,685 singleton and 22 twin gestations) with chromosomally normal fetuses between 9 and 14⁶/₇ weeks of gestation. Of this general population, 4.2% had a nuchal translucency measurement larger than 2.5 mm, and this proportion differed significantly between gestational age groups. Cross-sectional data demonstrated an increase in nuchal translucency measurement between 9 and 12 weeks of gestation, followed by a decrease at 13 to 14 weeks. Longitudinal data available in 136 fetuses studied confirmed an incremental increase of nuchal translucency with increasing gestational age. These authors

negated using a single threshold nuchal translucency measurement value throughout the first-trimester and proposed gestational age-generated reference ranges. Pajkrt et al.[28] subsequently performed longitudinal assessment of the measurement in 64 normal fetuses, confirming that in 94% of cases an increase in nuchal translucency measurement (from 0.7 mm at 70 days of gestation to 1.7 mm at 91 days of gestation) was followed by a decline (to 1.0 mm at 105 days of gestation) (Fig. 5–11). The timing of peak thickening of the nuchal translucency appeared to be fetus specific. Yagel et al.[29] constructed appropriate gestational age-specific reference intervals for nuchal translucency with transvaginal ultrasound in 180 women at low risk for fetal aneuploidy (younger than 35 years) with normal fetuses between 9 and 14 weeks of gestation (between 60 and 105 days of gestation) (Figs. 5–12

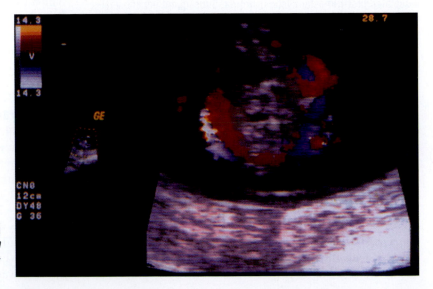

Figure 5–7. Cross-section of the fetal neck showing a complete nuchal cord. *(Reproduced with permission from Schaefer M, Laurichesse-Delmas H, Ville Y. Ultrasound Obstet Gynecol. 1998;11:271.)*

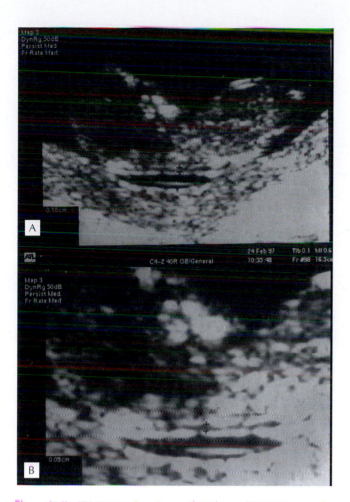

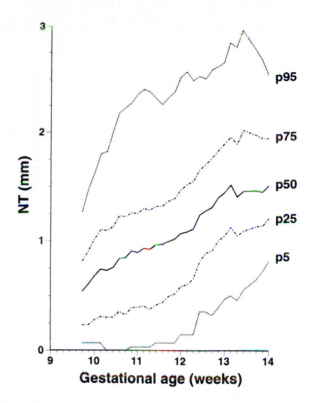

Figure 5–9. Smoothed curves of the 5th, 25th, 50th, 75th, and 90th percentiles (p) of the nuchal translucency (NT) measurements in normal (n) fetuses, measured in millimeters, as a function of gestational age. *(Reproduced with permission from Pajkrt E, Bilardo CM, van Lith JMM, et al. Obstet Gynecol. 1995;86:994.)*

Figure 5–8 **(A)** Electronic calipers placed over the nuchal translucency. Note the separate amnion adjacent to the nuchal translucency. **(B)** Magnified image of **(A)**. Note the similar measurement. *(Reproduced with permission from Herman A, Maymon R, Dreazen E, et al. Ultrasound Obstet Gynecol. 1998;11:266.)*

and 5–13; Table 5–1). In addition, these reference intervals were compared with the traditional threshold of 3 mm in 287 women scheduled for amniocentesis or chorionic villus sampling (CVS). Both methods had the same sensitivity of 85.7% and negative predictive value of 99.6% in predicting fetal chromosomal abnormalities. However, the specificity of gestational age-related reference intervals tended to be higher than that of the 3-mm threshold: 94.6% versus 87.9%. The positive predictive value of the gestational age-related reference values were higher than the 3-mm cutoff, 28.6% versus 15%, respectively. Application of gestational age reference intervals may save a significant number of unnecessary invasive diagnostic procedures.

Whitlow and Economides,[30] in a prospective cross-sectional study of 1288 women from an unselected population, determined the optimal gestational age for performing nuchal translucency assessment. The ability to measure nuchal translucency was similar from 10 to 13 weeks (100%,

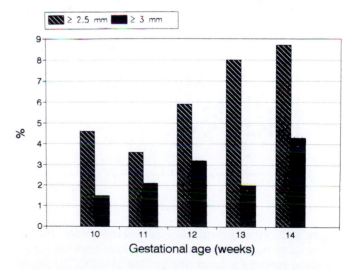

Figure 5–10. Incidence of nuchal translucency measurements greater than 2.5 mm and greater than 3 mm in normal fetuses in relation to gestational age. *(Reproduced with permission from Pajkrt E, Bilardo CM, van Lith JMM, et al. Obstet Gynecol. 1995;86:994.)*

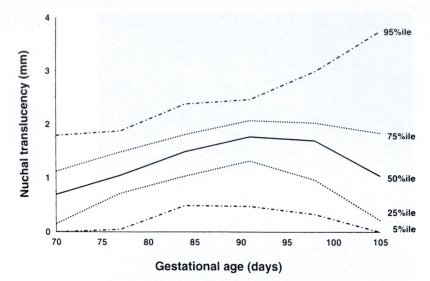

Figure 5–11. The 5th, 25th, 50th, 75th, and 95th percentiles (%ile) of nuchal translucency measurements in all fetuses, measured in millimeters, as a function of gestational age. *(Reproduced with permission from Pajkrt E, de Graaf IM, Mol BWJ, et al. Obstet Gynecol. 1998;91:208.)*

98%, 98% and 98% success rates, respectively) but fell to 90% at 14 weeks of gestation. Similarly, visualization of fetal anatomy improved with increasing gestational age (6%, 75%, 96%, and 98% of cases could be visualized at 10, 11, 12, and 13 weeks of gestation, respectively). Furthermore, the need for transvaginal ultrasonography steadily decreased with increasing gestational age (100%, 42%, 21%, 15%, and 11% at 10, 11, 12, 13, and 14 weeks of gestation, respectively). These authors concluded from these data that the optimal gestational age to measure nuchal translucency in the first trimester is at 13 weeks of gestation.

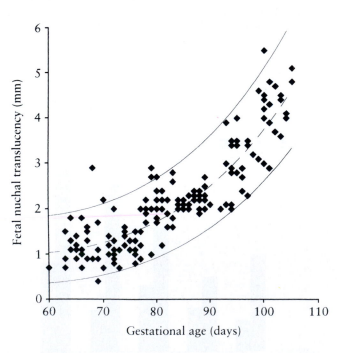

Figure 5–12. Fetal nuchal translucency by gestational age. The normal range for nuchal translucency was calculated from 180 women on whom the model is based (younger than 35 years). The dashed line represents the predicted value of nuchal translucency thickness, and solid lines represent 95% confidence intervals. *(Reproduced with permission from Yagel S, Anteby EY, Rosen L, et al. Ultrasound Obstet Gynecol. 1998;11:262.)*

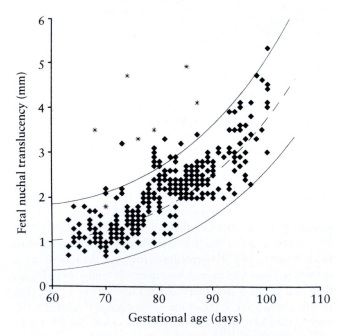

Figure 5–13. Fetal nuchal translucency by gestational age. Measurements were obtained from 280 women older than 35 years who gave birth to normal babies. Those seven women whose babies had chromosomal abnormalities are represented by stars. The dashed line represents the predicted value of the nuchal translucency thickness, and the solid lines represent 95% confidence intervals. *(Reproduced with permission from Yagel S, Anteby EY, Rosen L, et al. Ultrasound Obstet Gynecol. 1998;11:262.)*

TABLE 5–1. REFERENCE INTERVALS FOR NUCHAL TRANSLUCENCY (IN MILLIMETERS) BY DAYS

Days	Lower	Predicted	Upper
60	0.35650	1.03417	1.84865
61	0.36709	1.04690	1.86395
62	0.37940	1.06169	1.88174
63	0.39346	1.07858	1.90204
64	0.40927	1.09759	1.92488
65	0.42688	1.11875	1.95031
66	0.44629	1.14209	1.97836
67	0.46755	1.16764	2.00907
68	0.49069	1.19545	2.04249
69	0.51574	1.22555	2.07868
70	0.54274	1.25800	2.11768
71	0.57173	1.29285	2.15956
72	0.60276	1.33014	2.20438
73	0.63587	1.36994	2.25222
74	0.67113	1.41232	2.30315
75	0.70858	1.45733	2.35725
76	0.74829	1.50505	2.41461
77	0.79031	1.55557	2.47532
78	0.83473	1.60895	2.53948
79	0.88161	1.66529	2.60720
80	0.93102	1.72468	2.67858
81	0.98305	1.78722	2.75374
82	1.03780	1.85301	2.83282
83	1.09534	1.92217	2.91594
84	1.15578	1.99481	3.00325
85	1.21921	2.07106	3.09489
86	1.28577	2.15105	3.19103
87	1.35554	2.23491	3.29182
88	1.42867	2.32280	3.39746
89	1.50528	2.41486	3.50812
90	1.58550	2.51130	3.62401
91	1.66949	2.61224	3.74533
92	1.75739	2.71789	3.87231
93	1.84937	2.82844	4.00519
94	1.94560	2.94411	4.14420
95	2.04627	3.06509	4.28962
96	2.15156	3.19164	4.44171
97	2.26167	3.32399	4.60078
98	2.37683	3.46240	4.76713
99	2.49726	3.60713	4.94109
100	2.62319	3.75849	5.12301
101	2.75489	3.91678	5.31325
102	2.89261	4.08231	5.51220
103	3.03665	4.25543	5.72028
104	3.18730	4.43650	5.93790
105	3.34489	4.62590	6.16554

Reproduced with permission from Yagel S, Anteby EY, Rosen L, et al. Ultrasound Obstet Gynecol. *1998;11:26.*

Schuchter et al.[31] obtained nuchal translucency measurements in 561 women with singleton fetuses not affected by trisomy 21. Nuchal translucency measurements increased by approximately 17% for each additional gestational week. These authors expressed the results as a multiple of the median (MOM) nuchal translucency for a given CRL, allowing for this increase with gestational age, and yielded a distribution of values that was approximately Gaussian.[31] About 96% of values were between 0.5 and 2.0 MOM. The variance and therefore the false-positive rate of nuchal translucency were significantly reduced by recording several measurements and using the average. These authors suggested that estimating the distribution of nuchal translucency in MOM values would assist in specifying the statistical parameters to be applied in screening for trisomy 21 and that the use of averaged repeated nuchal translucency measurements may have a useful effect on reducing the false-positive rate at any given MOM cutoff level.

Ethnic Origin and Nuchal Translucency

The possibility of ethnic origin affecting nuchal translucency measurements has not been widely assessed. In the only study regarding this potential complicating issue, Thilaganathan et al.[32] determined the influence of ethnic origin on access to and equity of nuchal translucency measurements. In a multiple regression analysis of 1944 women attending a hospital antenatal clinic, these authors noted a small but significant difference in nuchal translucency measurement between fetuses of different ethnic origin. These differences were too small to require correction when nuchal translucency was applied as a screening tool for trisomy 21.

SUGGESTED PATHOPHYSIOLOGIC MECHANISMS OF FIRST-TRIMESTER NUCHAL TRANSLUCENCY

The precise underlying mechanism explaining the presence of nuchal translucency in both normal and abnormal fetuses is unclear. In cases of cystic hygroma, obstructed lymph is considered the underlying etiology; this appears not to be the case in association with increased nuchal translucency.[10,16] Jackson et al.,[33] for example, demonstrated the striking absence of endothelial lining (by immunohistochemical staining for both factor VIII–related antigen and CD34) in tissue from the back of the neck in a fetus with trisomy 18 diagnosed after increased first-trimester nuchal translucency. In addition to lack of precise knowledge as to the etiology of nuchal translucency, it is unclear why in most cases (with normal or at times abnormal chromosomes) spontaneous resolution of the nuchal translucency will occur, usually within 4 weeks of diagnosis.[10,16] Potential etiologies of increased nuchal translucency include:

1. fetal cardiac abnormalities
2. a possible protective decompression mechanism that guards the developing central nervous system
3. abnormal skin collagen

Each of these potential pathophysiologic mechanisms are presented separately.

Fetal Structural Cardiac Abnormalities

Hyett et al.[34] performed pathology examinations in 36 fetuses with trisomy 21 confirmed by CVS after first-trimester ultrasonographic depiction of nuchal translucency of 3 mm or greater at routine ultrasonography. Perimembranous ventricular and atrioventricular septal defects were common and were detected in 20 of 36 fetal hearts (55.5%). A septal defect was observed in 1 of the 11 fetuses with nuchal translucency of 3 mm and in 19 of 25 fetuses with nuchal translucency of 4 mm or greater. These findings confirm that the incidence of perimembranous ventricular and atrioventricular septal defects is much higher in fetuses with trisomy 21 and increased nuchal translucency than in liveborn infants with this chromosomal abnormality. Furthermore, the incidence of cardiac septal defects increases with increasing nuchal translucency thickness. Hyett et al.[35] similarly reported the association of fetal trisomy 18 and cardiac defects in 19 fetuses with trisomy 18 and increased nuchal translucency between 11 and 14 weeks of gestation. In all cases, trisomy 18 was confirmed by CVS after first-trimester ultrasonographic depiction of increased nuchal translucency. All 19 fetuses had cardiac abnormalities. Septal and valvular defects were the most common, with each of these abnormalities seen in 16 (84%) fetuses. In contrast, 50 control cases exhibited normal heart and great vessels. In 14 of the 16 cases with valvular abnormalities, more than one valve was affected. Great vessels were available for assessment in 18 of the 19 cases. In 10 cases, a hypoplastic aortic isthmus or pulmonary trunk was noted. In 6 cases, a persistent left superior vena cava was demonstrated. These authors postulated that hemodynamic changes due to the valvular abnormalities (imperforate valves and hypoplasia of the great vessels) may be the underlying mechanism for the increased nuchal translucency of trisomic fetuses.[35] Hyett et al.[36] assessed morphologic parameters of the great vessels in 30 of 34 fetuses with trisomy 21 confirmed by CVS after first-trimester detection of increased nuchal translucency. In 16 cases, a septal cardiac defect was documented. In 24 cases, all measurements of the great vessels were obtained. Morphometric analysis of the great vessels demonstrated that the diameter of the isthmus was narrower, whereas the aortic valve and ascending aorta were wider in fetuses with trisomy 21 and increased nuchal translucency than in normal fetuses. Furthermore, a significant increase in the ratio of the distal ductus arteriosus diameter to that of the aortic isthmus was detected (Figs. 5–14 and 5–15). The degree of narrowing of the aortic isthmus is greater in fetuses with high nuchal translucency. The fact that the narrowing of the aortic isthmus in

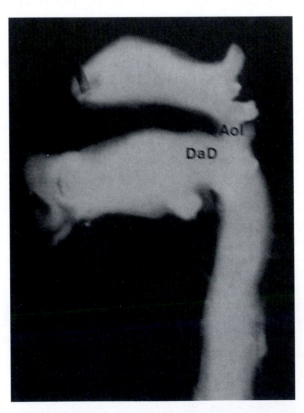

Figure 5–14. Photomicrograph of the great vessels in a 14-week fetus with trisomy 21 in which the diameter of the aortic isthmus (AoI) is narrow in comparison with that of the distal ductus arteriosus (DaD). Scale; 1 mm = 16 mm. *(Reproduced with permission from Hyett J, Moscoso G, Nicolaides KH. Hum Reprod. 1995;10:3049.)*

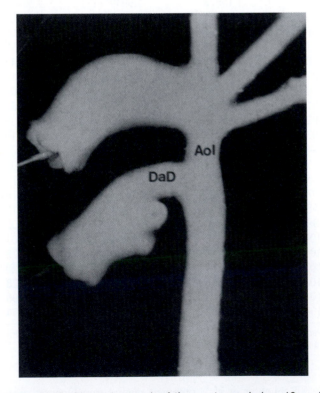

Figure 5–15. Photomicrograph of the great vessels in a 12-week fetus with normal karyotype. At this gestational age, the diameter of the aortic ishmus (AoI) is similar to that of the distal ductus arteriosus (DaD). Scale: 1 mm = 14 mm. *(Reproduced with permission from Hyett J, Moscoso G, Nicholaides KH. Hum Reprod. 1995;10:3045.)*

these fetuses is accompanied by widening of the aortic valve and ascending aorta is suggestive that narrowing of the isthmus is the primary event. Widening of the ascending aorta with narrowing of the aortic isthmus may be the etiology of increased nuchal translucency in these fetuses, manifesting as subcutaneous edema as a result of overperfusion of head and neck tissues. With advancing gestational age, the diameter of the aortic isthmus increases more rapidly than the aortic valve and distal ductus.[37] Therefore, hemodynamic effects of aortic isthmic narrowing may decrease. These authors suggested that this hypothesis may explain the gestational age-related spontaneous resolution observed in fetuses with trisomy 21, in which abnormal nuchal translucency decreases from 80 to 30% of such fetuses from 11 to 20 weeks of gestation. This phenomenon may also explain the transient finding of increased nuchal translucency in euploid fetuses. This same group of investigators in a subsequent study[38] assessed hearts and great vessels of fetuses exhibiting increased nuchal translucency in the presence of normal chromosomes. In 19 of 21 cases, abnormalities were documented. The most common finding was narrowing of the aorta at the isthmus and immediately above the aortic valve in contrast to fetuses with trisomy 21 in whom narrowing of the aortic isthmus was associated with an increased aortic valve diameter. Nevertheless, this study suggested that abnormalities of the heart and great vessels also may be implicated in the pathogenesis of increased nuchal translucency in chromosomally normal fetuses. If confirmed, increased nuchal translucency may be used as a potential first-trimester ultrasonographic marker for fetal cardiac abnormalities.[38]

In an "extended study," Hyett et al.[39] assessed the prevalence of cardiac and great vessel abnormalities among 112 fetuses with trisomies 21, 18, and 13 and monosomy 45,X diagnosed after first-trimester ultrasonographic depiction of increased nuchal translucency and confirmed by CVS. The most common lesions in trisomy 21 consisted of septal defects. Trisomy 18 was associated with ventricular defects and/or polyvalvular abnormalities, trisomy 13 with septal defects, valvular abnormalities, and either narrowing of the isthmus or truncus arteriosus, and 45,X was associated with severe narrowing of the whole aortic arch. Fetuses with these chromosomal abnormalities exhibited an aortic isthmus significantly narrower than that seen in normal fetuses with increased nuchal translucency. These results were thought to support the hypothesis that narrowing of the aortic isthmus may be the underlying mechanism causing nuchal translucency (Fig. 5–16).[39]

Matias et al.[40] described three cases of increased nuchal translucency between 12 and 13 weeks of gestation in three fetuses with trisomies 13, 18, and 21. All three fetuses exhibited anomalous venous return with Doppler ultrasonography. Severe hemodynamic compromise consisting of high retrograde flow in the inferior vena cava, a very low velocity or reversed flow during the atrial contraction phase, and a dicrotic pulsatile flow in the umbilical vein were depicted.

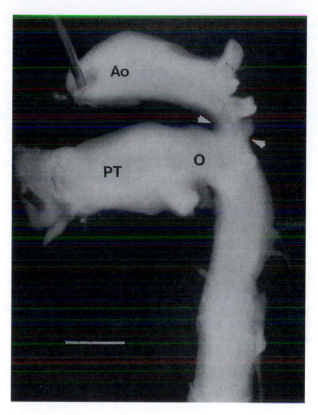

Figure 5–16. Photomicrograph of the great vessels in a 14 week trisomy 21 in which the diameter of the aortic isthmus (AoI) is normal compared with that of the distal ductus arteriosus (DaD) which is mildly dilated. Scale 1 mm = 1.6 cm. *(Reproduced with permission from Hyett J, Moscoso G, Nicolaides K. Hum Reprod. 1995;10:3049.)*

These results also support first-trimester nuchal translucency as an early marker for cardiac malformations.

Transient abnormal ductus venosus flow (as manifested by reversed flow during the atrial contraction phase) in a trisomy 18 fetus at 13 weeks with increased nuchal translucency that reverted to normal at 20 weeks of gestation, at which time normal ductus venosus flow was noted, was reported by Huisman and Bilardo.[41] This finding supports the concept of transient cardiac strain as an etiology of first-trimester nuchal translucency. On this basis, one could speculate that due to various reasons (probably anatomical) nuchal translucency is the way first-trimester fetuses express or manifest nonimmune hydrops. If the condition worsens, the degree of nuchal translucency increases, increasing the likelihood of immediate fetal demise. Similarly, if the condition is transient with pick-up of growth of the aortic isthmus, cardiac strain will resolve with concurrent resolution of the nuchal translucency.

Hyett et al.[42] assessed the prevalence of cardiac anomalies in 1427 chromosomally normal fetuses in whom first-trimester ultrasonography depicted increased nuchal translucency to establish the value of this sonographic finding as a marker in screening for major cardiac defects. The prevalence of major cardiac defects was 17 per 1000 (24 of 1427 fetuses) and increased to 5.5 per 1000 in the presence of nuchal translucency between 2.5 and 3.4 mm and to 233 per 1000 for nuchal translucency of 5.5 mm or greater. These findings strongly support that nuchal translucency between 10 and 14 weeks of gestation may be a useful ultrasonographic screening tool for cardiac abnormalities in addition to chromosomal defects. Similarly, Moseli et al.[43] suggested nuchal translucency as a market for the antenatal diagnosis of aortic coarctation.

In a recently published study Hyett et al.[44] examined the utility of measuring nuchal translucency thickness in screening for defects of the heart and great arteries at 10 to 14 weeks of gestation in a population-based cohort study of 29,154 singleton gestations with chromosomally normal fetuses. Of 50 cases with major defects of the heart and great arteries (prevalence of 1.7 per pregnancies), 28 (56%; 95% confidence interval of 42 to 70%) were in the subgroup of 1,822 pregnancies with fetal nuchal translucency thickness above the 95th centile of the normal range. The positive and negative predictive values for this cutoff point were 1.5% and 99.9%, respectively. These authors concluded that measurement of nuchal translucency thickness at 10 to 14 weeks of gestation can identify a large proportion of fetuses with major defects of the heart and great arteries. With these data

in mind, these authors suggested that fetuses with increased nuchal translucency should be considered at high risk.

With regard to possible cardiac dysfunction as a possible cause of nuchal translucency, von Kaisenberg et al.[45] investigated whether there was an alteration in the steady-state levels of expression of genes encoding sarcoplasmic reticulum calcium ATPase (calcium ATPase), known to be downregulated in postnatal cardiac failure. In trisomic fetuses versus controls, there was no significant decrease in calcium ATPase expression, and expression levels of calcium ATPase were not related to increased nuchal translucency. However, the levels expressed in fetuses were already very low, and cardiac dysfunction as a potential etiologic factor could not be excluded with certainty.

Transient Protective Decompression Mechanism

At the time increased nuchal translucency occurs (i.e., late first trimester), bony components, which will subsequently form the posterior fossa and protect the proximal cervical neural tube (occipital bone and cervical vertebrae), are not yet fully developed. Moscoso[46] suggested that this transient "cranio–upper cervical window" may function to protect developing intracranial organs from effects of overperfusion (Fig. 5–17). This theory suggests that overperfusion would

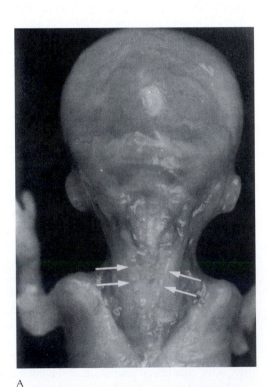
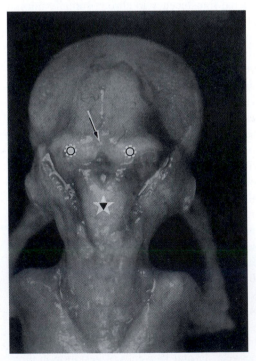

A

B

Figure 5–17. Posterior view of the head and upper cervical region of a human fetus at the end of the 10th week of gestation (foot length: 6 mm). **(A)** Note the "v" shape given by the differentiating vertebral components. **(B)** The neural components of the posterior fossa are not fully differentiated. Developing cerebellum *(dots),* choroid plexus *(long arrow).* The cerebellar vermix is not yet apparent. *(Reproduced with permission from Moscoso G. Ultrasound Obstet Gynecol. 1995;5:5.)*

manifest as a form of "transient physiological edema" at the level of the nuchal fold as a protective decompression mechanism.

Skin Collagen Abnormalities

Interestingly, many of the proteins of the extracellular matrix are encoded on chromosomes 21, 18, or 13.[47] Accordingly, the increased skin thickness in trisomy fetuses may be a consequence of gene-dosage effects. Brand-Saberi et al.[48] reported that alterations in the extracellular matrix of the skin of fetuses with trisomy 21 might explain the morphologic basis for increased nuchal translucency between 10 and 15 weeks of gestation. These authors demonstrated that nuchal translucency represents interstitial edema and correlates with the presence of glycosaminoglycans (especially hyaluronan) and collagen VI, which is partly coded by chromosome 21. Collagen VI (a microfibrillar protein of soft connective tissue) forms a denser mesh in fetal skin with trisomy 21 than in normal fetal skin. The distribution of collagen type VI differs from that of normal fetuses in both nuchal and leg skin. Collagen type VI has been shown to bind to hyaluronan. Interstitial fluid is bound to hyaluronan, which can bind large amounts of fluid because of its negative charge. In this fashion, interstitial fluid may be incorporated directly into the extracellular matrix. The abnormally elevated amounts of hyaluronan can be explained by two genes for collagen type VI, located by the q-terminal region of chromosome 21. It appears that increased cellular synthesis of hyaluronan may be triggered by this binding of hyaluronan to collagen VI, which is overexpressed in trisomy 21 cells.

Brand-Saberi et al.[49] studied the morphology of elevated nuchal skin obtained from fetuses with trisomy 21 and from fetuses with trisomy 18. Dermis samples of fetuses with trisomy 18 appeared to have altered extracellular matrix consisting mainly of collagen type III (reticulin) instead of collagen type I (the major structural protein of soft connective tissue and of tendons and ligaments). In addition to the presence of wide vessels (either veins or lymphatics at the boundary between the dermis and subcutis), nuchal skin from fetuses with trisomy 18 was noted to contain multilocular cavities that were not lined with epithelia. These findings were considered similar to modifications of aging in which distention is attributed to local fluid assembly, reticulin, collagen type V, which do not resist pressure and allow the development of fluid-filled cavities. In contrast, no cavities were noted in nuchal skin of trisomy 21 fetuses. Significantly more hyaluronan was present in the dermis of fetuses with trisomy 21 than in that of fetuses with trisomy 18 and control fetuses. Overall, extracellular matrix changes encountered in fetuses with trisomy 18 were more fundamental than in fetuses with trisomy 21, a finding thought to correlate with the much higher incidence of fetal death in trisomy 18 versus that of trisomy 21.

Von Kaisenberg et al.[47] analyzed human nuchal skin obtained from fetuses with trisomies 21, 18, and 13 and normal control fetuses. In trisomy versus control fetuses, dermal connective tissue was less regular in texture. Using immunohistochemical staining, these authors confirmed that collagen VI is more abundant in fetuses with trisomy 21 than in fetuses with trisomy 18 or 13 or normal karyotype. Similarly, a reduced collagen type I distribution was noted in the skin of fetuses with trisomy 18 compared with normal fetuses and those with trisomies 21 and 13.

In another study, von Kaisenberg et al.[50] determined that the composition of collagen type VI is different from normal in the skin of trisomy 21 fetuses. Immunohistochemistry demonstrated that in trisomy 21 fetuses, collagen type VI formed a dense network extending from the epidermal basement membrane to the subcutis, whereas in normal fetuses dense staining was confined to the upper region of the dermis (Fig. 5–18). Normally, collagen type VI is a triple helix formed of three single chains, $\alpha 1$, $\alpha 2$, and $\alpha 3$. In fetuses with trisomy 21, these authors demonstrated an overexpression of the gene responsible for $\alpha 1$ and $\alpha 2$ chains (COL6A1), which is located on chromosome 21. This overexpression was suggested as an explanation for the retention of interstitial fluid noted in trisomy 21 fetuses.

This theory does not explain the transient appearance of increased nuchal translucency as do the previous two suggested pathophysiologic mechanisms (cardiac and central nervous system decompression mechanisms).

Structural Abnormalities

Increased first-trimester nuchal translucency has been demonstrated in association with structural fetal anomalies other than cardiac. Reported anomalies associated with increased first-trimester nuchal translucency include Smith–Lemli–Opitz syndrome,[51] Fryn's syndrome,[52] and CATCH 22 (cardiac, abnormal facies, thymic hypoplasia, cleft palate, hypocalcemia, and 22 chromosome deletion),[53] and various skeletal dysplasias.[54–56] It is of interest to note that cardiac anomalies similar to those reported in the previous section were noted in a number of these cases: atresia of the aortic arch, truncus arteriosus and subaortal ventricular septal defect in the case of Fryn's syndrome[52]; right ventricular hypoplasia and narrowing of the ductus arteriosus in the case of Smith–Lemli–Opitz syndrome[51]; and large perimembranous ventricular septal defect, interruption of the aortic arch, large patent arterial duct continuous with the descending aorta, and small foramen ovale in the case of the CATCH 22 syndrome.[53] Increased nuchal translucency has also been associated with other congenital (autosomal recessive) disorders such β-thalassemia, as reported by Makrydimas et al.[57]

Souka et al.[58] reported on the prevalence of structural abnormalities and genetic syndromes in 4116 chromosomally normal pregnancies with increased nuchal translucency thickness. Among these fetuses the prevalence of major cardiac defects, diaphragmatic hernia, exomphalos, body stalk anomaly, and fetal akinesia deformation sequence was

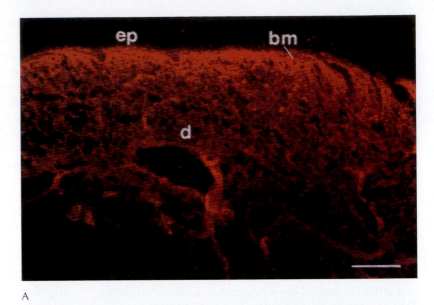

Figure 5–18. Immunofluorescence detection of collagen type VI in a section through nuchal skin of a fetus with trisomy 21 **(A)** and in a normal control fetus **(B),** both at 14 weeks' gestation. In trisomy 21, there is intense staining of the extracellular matrix extending down to the dermis-subcutis junction, whereas in the normal fetus intense staining is restricted to the upper dermis immediately underlying the basement membrane, ep = epidermis; d = dermis; bm = basement membrane. Bar = 0.1 mm. *(Reproduced with permission from von Kaisenberg CS, Brand-Saberi B, Christ B, et al. Obstet Gynecol. 1998;91:319.)*

substantially higher than expected in the normal population. In addition, these authors reported an association between increased nuchal translucency thickness and a wide range of skeletal dysplasias and genetic syndromes that are usually found in fewer than 1 in 10,000 pregnancies. However, the number of affected cases in that study and in previous series of fetuses with increased nuchal translucency thickness is too small for definitive conclusions to be reached. The authors of this extensive study concluded that rates of miscarriage and perinatal death increase, whereas the rates of survival and the prevalence of live births with no obvious abnormalities decrease with increasing nuchal translucency thickness. For a detailed review of first-trimester nuchal translucency screening for fetal structural anomalies in euploid fetuses, the reader is referred to a recent review by Devine and Malone.[59]

MULTIPLE GESTATIONS

Relatively few data regarding increased nuchal translucency in twin gestations have been published.

Aneuploidy

Verdin et al.[60] described an interesting case in which both fetuses in a monozygotic twin gestation exhibited increased nuchal translucency (7 mm and 4.1 mm, respectively). Cytogenic analysis from both amniotic fluid samples revealed trisomy 21, probably resulting from a nondisjunction event in one of the parents.

Pandya et al.[61] retrospectively examined CRL and nuchal translucency of each fetus in eight twin pregnancies in which karyotyping between 10 and 14 weeks of gestation demonstrated that at least one of the fetuses was chromosomally abnormal. Eight fetuses had trisomy 21 and two had trisomy 18. Nuchal translucency was thicker than 2.5 mm in nine (90%) of the trisomic fetuses and in one of the chromosomally normal fetuses. Crown–rump length was below the 5th percentile only in one fetus with trisomy 18.

Sebire et al.[62] assessed the use of nuchal translucency measurement to select a technique of fetal karyotyping in twin gestations. Sixty-seven twin pregnancies in which parents requested fetal karyotyping underwent nuchal translucency measurements. The risk for chromosomal defects in each fetus was calculated from the maternal age and nuchal translucency measurement between 10 and 14 weeks of gestation. In cases where the calculated risk was at least 1 in 50, CVS was the method of choice; if the risk was less than 1 in 50, second-trimester analysis was performed. This selection of technique was determined by the fact that, when chromosomal discordancy exists and selective feticide is considered, the risk of such procedure is significantly higher when performed after 18 to 20 weeks of gestation.[63] Although CVS provides first-trimester cytogenic analysis, it is technically more difficult to ensure that both fetuses have been sampled with this technique, and the procedure-related risk of miscarriage may be higher than with later amniocentesis. Therefore, CVS was considered an option only in pregnancies at high risk for fetal chromosomal abnormalities. In 34 pregnancies the risk was greater than 1 in 50 and indeed 23.5% of these fetuses were found to be chromosomally abnormal. Of the 33 low-risk pregnancies, chromosomally abnormal fetuses were noted in only 1.5% of fetuses. This technique is also prefered when one of the fetuses is found to have a chromosomal abnormality. Documentation of an ultrasonographic marker (in these cases increased nuchal translucency) will assist precise and correct identification of the abnormal twin if selective termination (feticide) is being considered.

Subsequent Twin–Twin Transfusion Syndrome

Sebire et al.[64] studied the possible association between increased nuchal translucency in monochorionic twin gestations and the subsequent development of twin–twin transfusion syndrome (TTS). Among 132 monochorionic gestations, 16 developed severe TTS between 15 and 22 weeks of gestation. In pregnancies that developed severe TTS, the prevalence of nuchal translucency above the 95th centile of the normal range, and the intertwin difference in nuchal translucency and fetal heart rate were significantly higher than in the non-TTS group. No significant differences were noted between the groups in intertwin difference in CRL. For fetal nuchal translucency above the 95th centile, the positive and negative predictive values for the development of TTS were 38% and 91%, respectively. The likelihood ratios of nuchal translucency above or below the 95 centile for the development of severe TTS were 4.7 (between 1.8 and 9.7) and 0.7 (between 0.4 and 0.9), respectively. These findings were thought to demonstrate that underlying hemodynamic changes associated with TTS may manifest as increased nuchal translucency between 10 and 14 weeks of gestation. This association appears to strongly support the cardiac strain pathophysiologic mechanism of first-trimester nuchal translucency, as described earlier.

DOPPLER VELOCIMETRY

Ductus Venosus Flow Velocimetry

Current data regarding Doppler velocimetry and nuchal translucency is also limited. Huisman and Bilardo[41] reported a twin pregnancy discordant for trisomy 18. The affected fetus at 13 weeks of gestation had increased nuchal translucency and reversed end–diastolic ductus venosus flow. At 20 weeks of gestation the nuchal translucency had resolved, and Doppler velocimetry of the central venous system demonstrated normal waveforms.

Montenegro et al.[65] investigated the possible contribution of impaired cardiac function (as depicted by Doppler velocimetry of the ductus venosus) in the pathophysiology of increased nuchal translucency. Of 17 fetuses with nuchal translucency 3 mm or thicker, four had trisomy 21 and one had trisomy 18. All five chromosomally abnormal fetuses with increased nuchal translucency exhibited decreased forward velocity during the atrial contraction phase of less than 2 cm/second. Impaired atrial contraction may implicate cardiac failure or cardiac defects in the pathophysiology of increased nuchal translucency in the first trimester. Further studies are required to confirm these associations.

Matias et al.[66] assessed the role of Doppler ultrasound using ductus venosus flow velocity waveforms in screening for fetal chromosomal abnormalities at 10 to 14 weeks of gestation. In this study, ductus venosus flow velocity waveforms were obtained immediately before fetal karyotyping in 486 consecutive singleton pregnancies at 10 to 14 weeks of gestation. All cases were screened for chromosomal defects by a combination of maternal age and fetal nuchal translucency measurement. Peak systolic and diastolic velocities, the velocity during atrial contraction, and pulsatility index were measured. These authors noted 63 chromosomal defects (38 cases of trisomy 21, 12 cases of trisomy 18, 7 cases of 45,X, and 3 cases of triploidy. In 57 (90.5%) cases, there was reverse or absent flow during the atrial contraction phase of the cardiac cycle. Abnormal ductus venosus flow was observed in 13 (3.1%) of the 423 chromosomally normal fetuses. In the chromosomally abnormal group as opposed to the normal control group, the median systolic and diastolic velocities were significantly lower, and the pulsatility index was significantly higher. However, multivariate regression analysis showed that only the velocity of the atrial wave produced a significant independent contribution in distinguishing between chromosomally normal and abnormal groups. In conclusion, these results suggest that assessment of ductus venosus blood flow in pregnancies considered to be at high risk for chromosomal abnormalities may result in a major reduction in the need for invasive testing with only a small decrease in sensitivity.

These findings also support the hypothesis that one of the mechanisms in the development of increased nuchal translucency is temporary cardiac strain.

Umbilical Artery Flow Velocimetry

Martinez et al.[67] evaluated the performance of the combined use of umbilical artery pulsatility index (PI) and nuchal translucency measurements in first-trimester detection of fetal chromosomal abnormalities. Applying the 95th centile and 3 mm or thicker cutoff points for umbilical artery PI and nuchal translucency, respectively, the detection rate for all chromosomal abnormalities among 553 consecutive women with singleton gestations between 10 and 13 weeks of gestation was 84.2%, with a false-positive rate of 6.6%, positive predictive value of 31.3%, and negative predictive value of 99.4%. Of the 553 women assessed, both ultrasonographic parameters were normal in 502, and of these only three (0.6%) were chromosomally abnormal. In six of eight cases (75%) in whom both parameters were abnormal, a chromosomal abnormality was present. Of the 43 cases in which only one parameter was abnormal, 10 (23.2%) were chromosomally abnormal. These preliminary results suggest that the presence of chromosomal abnormalities may be strongly suspected when an increased nuchal thickness of 3 mm or more is associated with an abnormally high umbilical artery PI between 10 and 13 weeks of gestation.

MATERNAL–FETAL INFECTION

Smulian et al.[68] described a case in which fetal hydrops associated with maternal parvovirus infection during the first trimester of pregnancy sonographically mimicked findings associated with fetal aneuploidy. Transabdominal ultrasonography at 13 weeks of gestation showed a nuchal translucency of 4.5 mm. Transvaginal ultrasonography enhanced visualization of the fetus by demonstrating subcutaneous sonolucency of the fetal scalp, thorax, and abdomen, indicating generalized subcutaneous edema. Two weeks later, fetal demise occurred. Fetal karyotype was normal. These authors suggested that increased first-trimester screening for fetal genetic abnormalities may identify more such fetuses with subcutaneous sonolucencies. Given the potential for first-trimester treatment of fetal hydrops caused by parvovirus with high-dose intravenous γ-globulin therapy, diagnosis of parvovirus infection by serology should be considered in the presence of early sonographic features of fetal hydrops. Sebire et al.[69] investigated the relation between increased fetal nuchal translucency between 10 and 14 weeks of gestation and infection between the mother and the fetus. Four hundred twenty-six chromosomally normal pregnancies with increased nuchal translucency and 63 with "unexplained" second- or third-trimester fetal nuchal edema or hydrops underwent maternal serum infection screening. Patients with positive evidence of recent maternal infection underwent investigation for fetal infection. Evidence of recent maternal infection was present in 6 of the 426 pregnancies (1.4%) with increased fetal nuchal translucency between 10 and 14 weeks of gestation, but in all cases a healthy infant was born with no signs of infection. In contrast, "unexplained" second- or third-trimester fetal hydrops was associated with maternal infection in six of the pregnancies (9.5%) in cases in which there was positive evidence of fetal infection.

LETHALITY AFTER DIAGNOSIS OF NUCHAL TRANSLUCENCY

An increased intrauterine fetal death rate has been observed in association with fetuses with abnormal karyotypes, with an intrauterine demise rate of approximately 40% of such fetuses between 12 weeks of gestation and term.[70] Hyett et al.[71] assessed whether first-trimester nuchal translucency thickness preferentially identifies those fetuses destined to die in utero. The rate of lethality increased with nuchal translucency thickness from 5.3% for those with translucency of 1 to 3 mm to 23.5% for nuchal translucency thicker than 7 mm. Pandya et al.[70] studied six (of 108) fetuses diagnosed with increased nuchal translucency thickness after the first trimester whose parents opted to continue the pregnancy. In five of the six fetuses, the nuchal translucency had resolved, and at the time of the second-trimester scan nuchal thickness was normal. All six trisomy 21 babies were liveborn; these data suggested that increased nuchal translucency does not necessarily identify trisomic fetuses destined to fetal demise. While subsequent demise may occur in some fetuses with first-trimester nuchal translucency, in others this condition may be transient, self-limited, and resolve spontaneously. In such fashion, Rodis et al.[72] reported spontaneous resolution of a cystic hygroma in a fetus with trisomy 21. Spontaneous resolution of other abnormal fluid collections in association with fetal aneuploidy has also been reported. For example, Sherer et al.[5] described spontaneous resolution of a unilateral pleural effusion in a fetus with trisomy 21 at 18 weeks of gestation.

FIRST-TRIMESTER NUCHAL TRANSLUCENCY SCREENING FOR FETAL ANEUPLOIDY

An association between increased first-trimester nuchal translucency and trisomy 21 has been reported by Szabó and Gellen.[73] Subsequently, in the screening process for first-trimester ultrasonographic evidence of abnormal fetal karyotypes, initial studies were performed on populations at increased or high risk (mainly due to advanced maternal age). The true success of screening for fetal chromosomal abnormalities is in screening of general populations, including those at low risk for such disorders. Data consisting of studies, each with 500 patients or more, regarding first-trimester ultrasonographic screening of both these populations are reviewed separately, as are data pertaining to screening for nuchal translucency combined with maternal serum analytes including pregnancy-associated plasma protein-A (PAPP-A) and free beta human chorionic gonadotropin (β-hCG).

Screening of Populations at High Risk

Schulte-Vallentin and Schindler[74] reported on 632 consecutive pregnancies screened sonographically before amniocentesis and chromosome analysis to determine whether increased nuchal translucency could serve as a marker between 10 and 14 weeks of gestation. Eighty-five percent of patients were referred because of advanced maternal age. Of eight patients with "nonechogenic nuchal edema," seven had trisomy 21. These authors used a nuchal translucency between 4 and 7 mm. All seven cases of trisomy 21 were detected by first-trimester nuchal translucency.

Nicolaides et al.[75] examined the significance of fetal translucency between 10 and 14 weeks of gestation in predicting abnormal fetal karyotypes. Of 827 fetuses undergoing amniocentesis or CVS, the incidence of chromosomal defects was 35 (28 of 827). In the 51 (6%) fetuses with nuchal translucency between 3 and 8 mm, the incidence of chromosomal defects was 35% ($n = 18$). Conversely, only 10 of the remaining 776 (1%) fetuses were chromosomally abnormal. These authors concluded that nuchal translucency of 3 mm or thicker is a useful marker for fetal chromosomal abnormalities.

Savodelli et al.[76] assessed 1,400 pregnancies between 10 and 12 weeks of gestation with ultrasonography and then with transabdominal CVS analysis. Of 28 cases of trisomy 21, 15 (54%) exhibited nuchal translucency of between 4 and 7 mm. Similar findings were noted in two of four cases with trisomy 18, in one of two cases of trisomy 13, and in one case of 45,X.

Nicolaides et al.[77] reported 1,273 women with singleton pregnancies undergoing first-trimester karyotyping because of advanced maternal age, parental anxiety, and family history of a chromosomal abnormality in the presence of balanced parental translocation. Nuchal translucency was 3 mm or thicker in 86% of the trisomic and in 4.5% of chromosomally normal fetuses. The observed number of trisomies in the 1185 cases with nuchal translucency thinner than 3 mm was approximately five times less than the number expected on basis of maternal age. In the groups with nuchal translucency of 3 mm ($n = 52$) and thicker than 3 mm ($n = 36$), the observed numbers of trisomies were approximately 5 times and 24 times higher than the respective numbers expected on basis of maternal age. These authors suggested that the risk of fetal trisomy can be derived by combining maternal age

and fetal nuchal translucency between 10 and 13 weeks of gestation. In addition, they predicted that, for a false-positive rate of 5%, the sensitivity of the new screening method must be at least 85%, comparing favorably with the respective 20 to 30% and 50 to 60% of screening based on maternal age alone, or the combination of maternal age and maternal serum analyte screening, respectively.

Brambati et al.[78] assessed nuchal translucency in predicting fetal aneuploidy between 8 and 15 weeks of gestation in 1819 consecutive pregnancies at high risk for chromosomal abnormalities scheduled for CVS analysis. In 43 cases an unbalanced chromosomal abnormality was noted. The incidence of chromosomal aberrations was 18.6% in cases where nuchal translucency was 3 mm and thicker versus 1.7% in cases where nuchal translucency was thinner than 3 mm. Sensitivity, specificity, and relative risk for aneuploidy were 30%, 90%, and 10.83% respectively.

Szabó et al.[79] prospectively screened 3,380 pregnant women, 1,280 of whom were older than 35 years, between 9 and 12 weeks of gestation for nuchal translucency. Women older than 35 years underwent CVS. In women younger than 35 years, CVS was offered only when nuchal translucency was at least 3 mm or in cases of parental chromosomal abnormalities. Overall, 46 chromosomal abnormalities were detected, 43 (93.5%) of which had nuchal translucency by these criteria. The incidence with respect to maternal age was 5.4% ($n = 69$) and 1.28% ($n = 27$) for maternal age older and younger than 35 years, respectively, and the percentage of chromosomal abnormalities was 2.9% and 0.43%, respectively. Risks of trisomies and poor pregnancy outcome were increased with thicker nuchal translucencies. Sensitivity and specificity were 93.5% and 98.4%, respectively.

Pajkrt et al.[80] assessed 2247 women referred for fetal karyotyping with transabdominal ultrasonographic nuchal translucency measurement before invasive prenatal testing. Chromosomal abnormalities were noted in 63 fetuses including 36 with trisomy 21. The likelihood of the presence of chromosomal abnormalities increased with increasing nuchal translucency thickness. Nuchal translucency of 3 mm and thicker identified 25 of 36 (69%) fetuses with trisomy 21, with a false-positive rate of 4.0%. Correction of nuchal translucency measurements for differences due to variation of the measurement with gestational age, by using either a "delta value" or MOMs, did not improve the detection rate.

Pandya et al.[81] reported on 1,015 fetuses undergoing first-trimester karyotyping because of increased nuchal translucency thickness. In that study (of 307 referred cases and 708 routinely scanned patients), the incidence of chromosomal abnormalities increased with both maternal age and nuchal translucency thickness. Observed numbers of trisomies 21, 18, and 13 with nuchal translucencies of 3 mm, 4 mm, 5 mm, and 6 mm thicker were approximately 3 times, 18 times, 28 times, and 36 times higher than the respective numbers expected on the basis of maternal age. In the chromosomally normal group, the incidence of structural defects was 45, which is higher than expected in an unselected population. Rates of fetal loss in the groups with nuchal translucency thickness of 3 mm and 4 mm were 2% and 4%, respectively, similar to the 2.3% rate of fetal loss observed in a group of fetuses with normal nuchal translucency thickness undergoing CVS. For fetal nuchal translucency of 5 mm and thicker, the rate of fetal loss was 13%.

Screening of Populations at Low Risk

After the accumulation of extensive data regarding first-trimester nuchal translucency screening of populations at increased risk, attention has been drawn to populations at low risk. These data are of major importance because these populations represent those in whom the vast majority of pregnancies with fetuses with abnormal chromosomes will occur.

Roberts et al.[82] assessed 1,127 measurements in women attending routine first-trimester (between 8 and 13 weeks of gestation) dating scans, representing the general population. The proportion of fetuses with a nuchal translucency of 3 mm and thicker did not differ with maternal age when divided into 5-year groups. With a cutoff point of 3 mm and thicker, 6% of normal pregnant patients screened positive.

Bewley et al.[83] in the same group of patients reported that among the 1,127 women 70 fetuses (6%) had nuchal translucency of 3 mm and thicker. Of these, five fetuses were karyotypically abnormal (three with trisomy 21 and two with trisomy 18). All aneuploidies occurred in women 39 years and older. Nuchal translucency of 3 mm and thicker was associated with aneuploidy (2.9% vs. 0.28% with nuchal translucency thinner than 3 mm) and specifically with trisomy 21 specifically (1.42% vs. 0.19%). No aneuploidy was identified in women younger than 39 years. The positive predictive value of nuchal translucency in predicting trisomy 21 was lower than previously reported in high-risk groups (1 in 70 vs. 1 in 5), emphasizing that caution should be taken when extrapolating data from high- to low-risk populations. Sensitivity of nuchal translucency 3 mm and thicker in detecting trisomy 21 was also lower (33% vs. 76.9%). As previously reported, increased nuchal translucency was associated with a higher miscarriage rate (2.9% vs. 1.7%).

Hafner et al.[84] prospectively, ultrasonographically assessed 1972 women with singleton pregnancies between 10 and 13 weeks of gestation during initiation of routine antenatal care. Chromosomal abnormalities were found in 11 fetuses. Eight of the 11 chromosomally abnormal fetuses were detected by nuchal translucency thickness of 2.5 mm and greater, suggesting that nuchal translucency screening for aneuploidy is efficient even in unselected populations.

Pajkrt et al.[85] measured nuchal translucency in 1,473 women presenting for routine antenatal care between 10 and 14 weeks of gestation. Trisomy 21 was detected in nine fetuses (0.6%). Screening by maternal age would have diagnosed six of nine fetuses (67%) with trisomy 21, for an invasive testing rate of 24%. Screening for nuchal translucency of 3 mm and thicker identified 67% of fetuses with trisomy 21, with an invasive testing rate of 2.2%. Combining nuchal translucency thickness, corrected for the influence of gestational age by "delta value," and maternal age performed differently according to various chosen cutoff points for adjusted risk. A minimum risk of 1:100 would detect 78% of fetuses with trisomy 21, with a testing rate of 8.1%. Offering karyotyping to all women with a post-test risk of 1:300 would increase the detection rate to 100%, with an invasive testing rate of 19.8%, which is lower than the invasive testing rate of maternal age screening.

Josefsson et al.[86] assessed nuchal translucency as a screening test for chromosomal abnormalities during routine first-trimester ultrasound examination in 1,444 women. Karyotyping was performed with nuchal translucency of 4 mm and thicker. Six fetuses had increased nuchal translucency by this criteria, none of which had any chromosomal abnormality, suggesting further evaluation of this screening modality before widespread use in unselected populations.

Economides et al.[87] assessed 2,256 unselected women (mean maternal age of 30 years, range of 16 to 47 years) with anatomic scanning including nuchal translucency. In the study group, 16 had chromosomal abnormalities (0.7%, 16 of 2,256). Eighty-one percent (13 of 16) of chromosomal abnormalities were diagnosed after routine first-trimester ultrasound because of nuchal translucency in the 99th centile or above for gestational age (sensitivity of 44% and specificity of 99.6%) or the presence of structural anomalies (sensitivity of 38% and specificity of 99.9%).

Theodoropoulos et al.[88] evaluated first-trimester (between 10 and 14 weeks of gestation) nuchal translucency thickness screening for fetal aneuploidy in four fetal medicine units in Greece. Risks for trisomy 21 were calculated by using maternal age and nuchal translucency thickness in 3,550 patients, 277 (7.8%) of whom were older than 37 years. The fetal nuchal translucency thickness increased with CRL, and measurements were above the 95th centile in 101 patients (2.9%). Karyotyping was performed in 360 (10.6%) cases, with the vast majority of invasive procedures performed in patients older than 35 years. The adjusted risk was 1:300 or more in 172 (4.9%) cases, and the high-risk group contained 10 of the 11 (91%) fetuses with trisomy 21 and all 11 fetuses with other chromosomal defects: trisomy 18 ($n = 4$), trisomy 13 ($n = 1$), 47,XXY ($n = 4$), 45,X ($n = 1$), and triploidy ($n = 1$). Therefore, for a false-positive rate of about 5%, the detection rate of trisomy 21 by a combination of maternal age and nuchal translucency thickness is approximately 90%. It is of interest to note that all sonographers participating in this study had received training and appropriate certification from the Fetal Medicine Foundation, London. Training may have resulted in uniformity among participating centers and contributed to the following parameters:

1. the minimum and maximum CRLs were 38 mm and 85 mm, respectively

2. ultrasound was performed transabdominally with curvilinear transducers unless visualization was suboptimal, in which case transvaginal ultrasonography was performed

3. appropriate sagittal views of the fetus were obtained with the fetal image occupying at least 75% of the ultrasound imaging screen

4. maximum translucency was measured with the calipers placed on the fetal skin and on the border of the subcutaneous tissues

Two recent large studies have created major interest in this potential screening tool in unselected populations. Taipale et al.[89] performed transvaginal ultrasonography in 10,010 unselected adolescents and women younger than 40 years with singleton fetuses between 10 and 15.9 weeks of gestation. Nuchal translucency of 3 mm or thicker or cystic hygroma (septated, fluid-filled sacs in the nuchal region) was noted in 76 fetuses (0.8%), 18 (24%) of which had an abnormal karyotype. The sensitivity for detecting trisomies (21, 18, and 13) was 62% (13 of 21 fetuses), and the sensitivity for trisomy 21 alone was 54% (7 of 13 fetuses).

Snijders et al.,[90] by combining maternal age and fetal nuchal translucency at 10 to 14 weeks of gestation, assessed 96,127 women in a multicenter study (22 centers with 306 "appropriately-trained" sonographers). Risk of trisomy 21 was calculated from the maternal age and gestational age-related prevalence, multiplied by a likelihood ratio depending on the deviation from normal nuchal translucency thickness for CRL. The distribution of risks was investigated and the sensitivity of a cutoff risk of 1:300 was calculated. The estimated risk of trisomy 21 from maternal age and nuchal translucency was 1:300 or higher in 7,907 (8.3%) of 95,476 normal pregnancies, in 268 (82.2%) of 326 with trisomy 21, and in 253 (77.9%) of 325 with other chromosomal abnormalities, with a false-positive rate of 8.3%. The 5% of the study population with the highest estimated risk included 77% of the trisomy 21 cases. These authors concluded from this extensive study that selection of the high-risk group for invasive testing by this screening method allows the detection of 80% of affected pregnancies, with approximately 30 invasive tests for identification of one affected fetus. Results of this study have been challenged in that results were based on the estimation that in the absence of screening, 266 full-term live births of infants with Down syndrome would have occurred. This estimation did not account for the well-established increased incidence of intra-uterine demise in up to 40% of pregnancies with Down syndrome between 10 and 14 weeks' gestation. Thus, the true prevalence of Down syndrome would have been 443 fetuses, yielding a lower detection rate of 60% (266 of 443). This more accurate detection rate of Down syndrome does not differ significantly from current detection rates achieved with maternal midtrimester multiple marker screening. Notwithstanding, a beneficial consequence of screening for trisomy 21 by this method is the early

diagnosis of trisomy 18. Among the data presented (multicenter study of 91,091 singleton pregnancies), Sherod et al.[91] described 106 fetuses with trisomy 18, 83% of whom were identified by nuchal translucency screening.

EFFECT OF NUCHAL TRANSLUCENCY ON PERFORMANCE OF SUBSEQUENT MID-TRIMESTER MATERNAL SERUM SCREENING

Kadir and Economides[92] assessed the effect of first-trimester nuchal translucency on second-trimester serum screening for trisomy 21 in 2250 patients. The detection rate of nuchal translucency (above the 99th centile) screening for trisomy 21 was 83% (5 of 6), with a 1.3% false-positive rate, 63.8 likelihood ratio, and positive predictive value of 22.7%. After the introduction of nuchal translucency, the likelihood ratio for a positive result and positive predictive value of second-trimester serum screening decreased from 9.1 to 5 and from 2.7% to 0.45%, respectively. This study demonstrated that nuchal translucency is not only effective in first-trimester screening for trisomy 21 but also has implications on the likelihood ratio and positive predictive values of subsequent second-trimester maternal serum screening. Specifically, a patient positive at mid-trimester serum screening will be less likely to have a fetus with trisomy 21 if first-trimester nuchal translucency was normal.

Similarly, Thilaganathan et al.[93] evaluated the effectiveness of first-trimester nuchal translucency between 10 and 14 weeks of gestation and its effect on subsequent mid-trimester maternal serum screening. A total of 2,290 patients from a general population was assessed. A nuchal translucency-derived risk of 1:200 for an aneuploid pregnancy resulted in a 5% (n = 147) screen positive rate. Using this risk, five of seven (71%) fetuses with trisomy 21 and 14 of 18 (78%) aneuploid fetuses were detected. Second-trimester maternal serum analyte assessment was performed in 1,904 of the patients who had nuchal translucency screening, with a screen positive rate of 7.5% (n = 143). Only one additional case of trisomy 21 would have been detected by mid-trimester maternal serum screening if nuchal translucency screening had been implemented at a risk level of 1:300, suggesting that a first-trimester nuchal translucency screening program will significantly reduce the positive predictive value of subsequent mid-trimester serum screening.

Nuchal Translucency Combined with First-Trimester Maternal Serum Screening

First-trimester maternal serum free β-hCG is higher and PAPP-A is lower in cases of trisomy 21 than in chromosomally normal pregnancies.[94–97] After finding that first-trimester maternal serum analytes including PAPP-A and free β-hCG were truly independent of nuchal translucency, data combining these predictors (ultrasound and serum analytes) were judged scientifically correct and became available. Noble et al.[98] in a study of 2529 pregnancies between 10 and 14 weeks of gestation estimated that inclusion of maternal serum free β-hCG could improve the sensitivity of screening for trisomy 21 by about 5%. For a detailed review of the performance of first-trimester serum biochemical markers in the screening for fetal aneuploidy, the reader is referred to a recent review by Canick and Kellner.[99]

Orlandi et al.[100] assessed 754 singleton pregnancies with first-trimester nuchal translucency measurement and maternal serum free β-hCG and PAPP-A. Nuchal translucency alone detected 57% (8 of 14) of cases of aneuploidy at a 5.8% (42 of 730) false-positive rate. Modeling with age distribution of livebirths, a 5% false-positive rate resulted in detection of trisomy 21 with an efficiency of 61% by maternal serum analyte analysis, 73% by nuchal translucency, and 87% by combining both methods.

Zimmermann et al.[101] retrospectively assessed first-trimester maternal serum free β-hCG and PAPP-A and nuchal translucency in 1151 patients (between 25 and 44 years of age) undergoing CVS, mostly for advanced maternal age. Twenty-three of 1151 women (1:50) had an abnormal fetal karyotype. Nine of the 23 had nuchal translucency of 3 mm and thicker. Logistic regression analysis demonstrated that the detection rate of any chromosomal abnormality (including trisomy 18) was improved if a combination of increased nuchal translucency and maternal serum PAPP-A was used. The detection rate for any chromosomal abnormality for both increased nuchal translucency and decreased PAPP-A level was 39%, with a false-positive rate of 2%. When PAPP-A was less than 0.5 MOM or the nuchal translucency was 3 mm or thicker, 16 of 23 fetuses with an abnormal karyotype could be detected, for an odds ratio of 1:4.6. Addition of maternal serum free β-hCG had only a small impact on the detection rate, and, as expected α-fetoprotein had no effect.

Haddow et al.[102] reported on first-trimester screening for fetal aneuploidy in 4412 women with maternal serum α-fetoprotein, unconjugated estriol, hCG, free β-hCG, PAPP-A, and nuchal translucency thickness. In the study group, 82% of patients were older than 35 years. Fetal chromosomal analysis was performed in all pregnancies. Overall, 61 fetuses with trisomy 21 were documented. A total of 48 pregnancies affected by trisomy 21 and 3169 unaffected pregnancies were identified before 14 weeks of gestation. The rates of detection of fetal trisomy 21 for the five serum markers were as follows: 17% for α-fetoprotein, 4% for unconjugated estriol, 29% for hCG, 25% for free β-hCG, and 42% for PAPP-A, with false-positive rates of 5%. Measurements of serum hCG and free β-hCG were highly correlated. When applied in combination with PAPP-A and maternal age, the detection rate was 63% for hCG (95% confidence interval of 47% to 76%) and 60% for free β-hCG (95% confidence interval of 45% to 4%). Of interest, measurements of nuchal translucency (normal pregnancies, $n = 3991$; trisomy 21 fe-

tuses, $n = 58$) differed considerably across the 16 participating prenatal diagnostic centers and could not be reliably incorporated into calculations of this study. The authors stated that measurements of nuchal translucency adhered to published protocols,[75] but uniformity was not established among all participating centers. The variability among centers in median values and in the ratios of the 95th centiles coupled with their different abilities to obtain the measurements successfully suggest that the performance of nuchal translucency in this study may not accurately reflect its long-term performance at individual centers. For this reason, the nuchal translucency measurements were not included with the results of serum assays in the overall analysis.

De Biasio et al.[103] confirmed the value of combined first-trimester screening for fetal aneuploidy in a group of 1467 women by maternal age, nuchal translucency screening, and maternal serum PAPP-A and free β-hCG between 10 and $13^{6}/7$ weeks of gestation. Among this group of patients with a median maternal age of 31 years 8 months, 704 underwent invasive diagnostic testing due to advanced maternal age. No clinical action was taken on account of first-trimester screening results. Thirteen fetuses had trisomy 21. With a risk cutoff of 1 in 350, 11 affected pregnancies were detected (detection rate of 85%, 95% confidence interval of 56% to 100%), with a 3.3 false-positive rate. The odds of being given a postive result were 1 in 30. Interestingly, only three patients in this study group were younger than 35 years.

These data and results of other studies of smaller populations[104–106] suggest that combined biochemical and ultrasound evaluation for chromosomal abnormalities during the first trimester may yield a detection capability superior to that of current established second-trimester prenatal screening protocols.

Recently, Wald et al. proposed a new screening method in which measurements obtained during both first- and second-trimesters are integrated to provide a single estimate of a woman's risk of having a pregnancy affected by Down's syndrome.[107] To this goal these authors utilized data from previously published studies of various screening methods employed during the first and second trimesters. First-trimester screening consisted of measurement of serum pregnancy-associated plasma protein A in 77 pregnancies affected by Down syndrome and 383 unaffected pregnancies and measurements of nuchal translucency obtained by ultrasonography in 326 affected and 95,476 unaffected pregnancies. The second-trimester tests utilized were various combinations of measurements of serum alpha-fetoprotein, unconjugated estriol, human chorionic gonadotropin, and inhibin A in 77 affected pregnancies. Applying a risk of 1 in 120 or greater as the cutoff to define a positive result on the integrated screening test, the rate of detection of Down's syndrome was 85%, with a false positive rate of 0.9%. To achieve the same rate of detection, current screening tests would have higher false positive rates (5–22%). If the integrated test were to replace the triple test (measurements of serum alpha feto-protein, unconjugated estriol, and human chorionic gonadotropin), currently used with a 5% false positive rate, for screening during the second trimester, the detection rate would be higher (85% versus 69%), with a reduction of four fifths in the number of invasive diagnostic procedures and associated consequent losses of normal fetuses.

Potentially, as a direct result of the lesser need for invasive diagnostic procedures, increasing number of patients may elect to undergo integrated screening for fetal aneuploidy. The reduction in the false positive with the integrated tests is particularly evident for older women. Among women 35 years of age or older, the false positive rate of the integrated test was only 3.35 (with a cutoff of 1 in 120), as compared with 19% for the triple test (with the usual cutoff of 1 in 250), with a gain in detection (92% versus 88%). For every 100,000 women 35 years of age or older who were screened, only 30 unaffected fetuses would be lost because of diagnostic procedures with the integrated test, as compared with 171 with the triple test. Finally, the authors calculated that in the U.S. use of the integrated test instead of the triple test for prenatal screening for Down's syndrome would detect 800 more affected pregnancies and save about 1,400 unaffected fetuses from being lost as a result of amniocentesis or chorionic villus sampling each year, if all women identified as being at high risk underwent definitive, invasive diagnostic tests.

Nuchal Translucency Combined with Fetal Heart Rate

Hyett et al.[108] assessed first-trimester nuchal translucency and fetal heart rate between 10 and 14 weeks of gestation. In 6,903 normal singleton gestations, fetal heart rate decreased from a mean of 171 beats per minute at 10 weeks to 156 beats per minute at 14 weeks. In contrast, in 85 pregnancies with trisomy 21 fetuses, the mean heart rate was significantly higher. No significant association was noted between nuchal translucency and fetal heart rate, leading these authors to suggest calculating the combined risk for trisomy 21 with these two parameters. Of 6,961 pregnancies, it was estimated that inclusion of fetal heart rate with maternal age and nuchal translucency would improve the sensitivity for screening for trisomy 21 by approximately 5%.

THE FUTURE

Questions regarding optimal modalities (or various combinations thereof) in addition to the optimal timing of screening for fetal aneuploidy, whether first or second trimester, remain unanswered. A current prospective multicenter trial in the United States funded by the National Institutes of Health, National Institute of Child Health and Human Development (FASTER, i.e., first- and second-trimester evaluation of risk

of aneuploidy) has been designed and implemented with the following specific aims:

1. to evaluate the success rate of obtaining nuchal translucency measurements and the natural history of increased nuchal thickness
2. to define the detection rate of fetal trisomy 21 and other aneuploidies by using maternal age, nuchal translucency thickness, free β-hCG, and PAPP-A in an unselected population of pregnant patients between $10^{3/7}$ and $13^{6/7}$ weeks of gestation
3. to compare first-trimester screening with nuchal translucency and serum analytes (free β-hCG and PAPP-A) with subsequent second-trimester maternal serum screening (α-fetoprotein, free β-hCG, uE$_3$, and inhibin) in the same patients
4. to assess and compare all currently available noninvasive screening methods for fetal aneuploidy including isolation of fetal cells from maternal blood

Despite unknown factors, it is clear that prenatal diagnosis of most (if not all) fetal aneuploidies is possible. The basic question that remains is, At what expense? or, worded differently, What false-positive rate is acceptable, thereby exposing normal pregnancies to the well-established risks of invasive diagnostic testing?

SUMMARY

Throughout the recent decade, application of first-trimester ultrasonographic measurement of nuchal translucency has clearly been demonstrated to be a useful tool in the early detection of fetal aneuploidy. Studies with large numbers of low-risk patients support first-trimester sonographic screening for fetal aneuploidy, with sensitivities of approximately 80%. Furthermore, recent studies have demonstrated enhanced sensitivity of prenatal screening for fetal chromosomal abnormalities by using protocols combining first-trimester maternal serum analytes with nuchal translucency and maternal age. Large, prospective studies are needed to objectively compare this modality of first- versus second-trimester screening for fetal aneuploidy.

REFERENCES

1. Nyberg DA, Resta RG, Luthy DA, et al. Prenatal sonographic findings of Downs syndrome: Review of 94 cases. *Obstet Gynecol.* 1990;76:370.
2. Benacerraf BR, Miller WA, Frigoletto FD. Sonographic detection of fetuses with trisomy 13 and 18: Accuracy and limitations. *Am J Obstet Gynecol.* 1988;158:404.

3. Nyberg DA, Kramer D, Resta RG, et al. Prenatal sonographic findings of trisomy 18: Review of 47 cases. *J Ultrasound Med.* 1993;12:103.

4. Ginsburg N, Cadkin A, Pergamnet E, et al. Ultrasonographic detection of the second-trimester fetsus with trisomy 18 and trisomy 21. *Am J Obstet Gynecol.* 1990;163:1186.

5. Sherer DM, Abramowicz JS, Sanko SR, et al. Trisomy 21 presented as a transient unilateral pleural effusion at 18 weeks' gestation. *Am J Perinatol.* 1993;10:12.

6. Garden AS, Benzie RJ, Miskin M, et al. Fetal cystic hgyroma colli: Antenatal diagnosis, significance and management. *Am J Obstet Gynecol.* 1986;154:221.

7. Pijpers L, Reuss A, Steward PA, et al. Fetal cystic hygroma: Prenatal diagnosis and management. *Obstet Gynecol.* 1988;72:223.

8. Abramowicz JS, Warsof SL, Lochner Doyle D, et al. Congenital cystic hygroma of the neck diagnosed prenatally: Outcome with normal and abnormal karyotype. *Prenatal Diagn.* 1989;9:321.

9. Rottem S, Bronshtein M, Thaler I, et al. First trimester transvaginal sonographic diagnosis of fetal anomalies. *Lancet.* 1989;1:444.

10. Bronstein M, Rottem S, Yoffe N, et al. First-trimester and early second-trimester diagnosis of nuchal cystic hygroma by transvaginal ultrasonography: Diverse prognosis of the septated lesion. *Am J Obstet Gynecol.* 1989;161:78.

11. van Zalen-Sprock RM, van Vugt JMC, van Geijn HP. First-trimester diagnosis of cystic hygroma—course and outcome. *Am J Obstet Gynecol.* 1992;167:94.

12. Benacerraf BR, Barss V, Laboda LA. A sonographic sign for the detection in the second trimester of the fetus with Down syndrome. *Am J Obstet Gynecol.* 1985;151:1078.

13. Benacerraf BR, Gelman, R, Frigoletto FD. Sonographic identification of second trimester fetuses with Down syndrome. *N Engl J Med.* 1987;317:1371.

14. Benacerraf BR, Frigoletto FD. Soft tissue nuchal fold in the second-trimester fetus: Standards for normal measurements compared with those in Down syndrome. *Am J Obstet Gynecol.* 1987;157:1146.

15. Jones KL. Down syndrome. In: *Smith's Recognizable Patterns of Human Malformation*, 5th ed. Philadelphia: WB Saunders; 1997:8.

16. Johnson MP, Johnson A, Holtzgreve W, et al. First-trimester simple hygroma: Cause and outcome. *Am J Obstet Gynecol.* 1993;168:156.

17. Bonilla-Musoles F, Raga F, Villalobos A, et al. First-trimester neck abnormalities: Three-dimensional evaluation. *J Ultrasound Med.* 1998;17:419.

18. Mahieu-Caputo D, Dommergues M, Morichon-Delvallez N. et al. First-trimester translucency: Aneuploidy, sonographic findings, and maternal age. *Fetal Diagn Ther.* 1996;11:199.

19. Braithwaite JM, Economides DL. The measurement of nuchal translucency with transabdominal and transvaginal sonography success rates, repeatability and levels of agreement. *Br J Radiol.* 1995;68:720.

20. Whitlow BJ, Chatzipapas IK, Economides DL. The effect of fetal neck position on nuchal translucency measurement. *Br J Obstet Gynecol.* 1998;105:872.

21. Schaefer M, Laurichesse-Delmas H, Ville Y. The effect of nuchal cord on nuchal translucency measurement at 10–14 weeks. *Ultrasound Obstet Gynecol.* 1998;11:271.

22. Braithwaite JM, Morris RW, Economides DL. Nuchal translucency measurements: Frequency distribution and changes with gestation in a general population. *Br J Obstet Gynaecol.* 1996;103:1201.

23. Pandya PP, Altman DG, Brizot ML, et al. Repeatability of fetal nuchal translucency thickness. *Ultrasound Obstet Gynecol.* 1995;5:334.

24. Herman A, Maymon R, Dreazen E, et al. Image magnification does not contribute to the repeatability of caliper placement in measuring nuchal translucency thickness. *Ultrasound Obstet Gynecol.* 1998;11:266.

25. Braithwaite JM, Kadir RA, Pepera T, et al. Nuchal translucency measurement: Training of potential examiners. *Ultrasound Obstet Gynecol.* 1996;8:192.

26. Herman A, Maymon R, Dreazen E, et al. Nuchal translucency audit: A novel image-scoring method. *Ultrasound Obstet Gynecol.* 1998;12:398.

27. Pajkrt E, Bilardo CM, van Lith JMM, et al. Nuchal translucency measurement in normal fetuses. *Obstet Gynecol.* 1995;86:994.

28. Pajkrt E, de Graaf IM, Mol BWJ, et al. Weekly nuchal translucency measurements in normal fetuses. *Obstet Gynecol.* 1998;91:208.

29. Yagel S, Anteby EY, Rosen L, et al. Assessment of first-trimester nuchal translucency by daily reference intervals. *Ultrasound Obstet Gynecol.* 1998;11:262.

30. Whitlow BJ, Economides DL. The optimal gestational age to examine fetal anatomy and measure nuchal translucency in the first trimester. *Ultrasound Obstet Gynecol.* 1998;11:258.

31. Schuchter K, Wald N, Hackshaw AK, et al. The distribution of nuchal translucency at 10–13 weeks of pregnancy. *Prenatal Diagn.* 1998;18:281.

32. Thilaganathan B, Khare M, Williams B, et al. Influence of ethnic origin on nuchal screening for Down's syndrome. *Ultrasound Obstet Gynecol.* 1998;12:112.

33. Jackson S, Porter H, Vyas S. Trisomy 18: First-trimester nuchal translucency with pathological correlation. *Ultrasound Obstet Gynecol.* 1995;5:55.

34. Hyett JA, Moscoso G, Nicolaides KH. First-trimester nuchal translucency and cardiac septal defects in fetuses with trisomy 21. *Am J Obstet Gynecol.* 1995;172:1411.

35. Hyett JA, Moscoso G, Nicolaides KH. Cardiac defects in 1st-trimester fetuses with trisomy 18. *Fetal Diagn Ther.* 1995;10:381.

36. Hyett J, Moscoso G, Nicolaides KH. Increased nuchal translucency in trisomy 21 fetuses: Relationship to narrowing of the aortic isthmus. *Hum Reprod.* 1995;10:3049.

37. Hyett JA, Moscoso G, Nicolaides KH. First trimester nuchal translucency and cardiac septal defects in trisomy 21 fetuses. *Am J Obstet Gynecol.* 1995;172:1411.

38. Hyett J, Moscoso G, Papangiotsu G, et al. Abnormalities of the heart and great arteries in chromosomally normal fetuses with increased nuchal translucency thickness at 11–13 weeks' gestation. *Ultrasound Obstet Gynecol.* 1996;7:245.

39. Hyett J, Moscoso G, Nicolaides KH. Abnormalities of the heart and great arteries in first trimester chromosomally abnormal fetuses. *Am J Med Genet.* 1997;69:207.

40. Matias A, Montenegro N, Areias JC, et al. Anomalous fetal

venous return associated with major chromosomopathies in the late first trimester of pregnancy. *Ultrasound Obstet Gynecol.* 1998;11:209.

41. Huisman TWA, Bilardo CM. Transient increase in nuchal translucency thickness and reversed end-diastolic flow in a fetus with trisomy 18. *Ultrasound Obstet Gynecol.* 1997;10:397.

42. Hyett JA, Perdu M, Sharland GK, et al. Increased nuchal translucency at 10–14 weeks of gestation as a marker for major cardiac defects. *Ultrasound Obstet Gynecol.* 1997;10:242.

43. Moseli M, Thilaganathan B. Nuchal translucency: A marker for the antenatal diagnosis of aortic coarctation. *Br J Obstet Gynaecol.* 1996;103:1044.

44. Hyett J, Perdu M, Sharland G, et al. Using fetal nuchal translucency to screen for major congenital cardiac defects at 10–14 weeks gestation: Population based cohort study. *Br Med J.* 1999;318:81.

45. von Kaisenberg CS, Huggon I, Hyett JA, et al. Cardiac expression of sarcoplasmic reticulum calcium ATPase in fetuses with trisomy 21 and trisomy 18 presenting with nuchal translucency. *Fetal Diagn Ther.* 1997;12:270.

46. Moscoso G. Fetal nuchal translucency: A need to understand the physiologic basis. *Ultrasound Obstet Gynecol.* 1995;5:6.

47. von Kaisenberg GS, Krenn V, Ludwig M, et al. Morphological classification of nuchal skin human fetuses trisomy 21, 18, and 13 and at 12–18 weeks and in a trisomy 16 mouse. *Anat Embryol.* 1998;197:105.

48. Brand-Saberi B, Flöel H, Schulte-Vallentin M, et al. Alterations of the fetal extracellular matrix in the nuchal oedema of Down's syndrome. *Ann Anat.* 1994;176:539.

49. Brand-Saberi B, Epperlein HH, Romanos GE, et al. Distribution of extracellular matrix components in nuchal skin from fetuses carrying trisomy 18 and trisomy 21. *Cell Tissue Res.* 1994;277:465.

50. von Kaisenberg CS, Brand-Saberi M, Christ B, et al. Collagen type VI gene expression in the skin of trisomy 21 fetuses. *Obstet Gynecol.* 1998;101:319.

51. Hyett JA, Clayton PT, Moscoso G, et al. Increased first trimester nuchal translucency as a prenatal manifestation of Smith-Lemli-Opitz syndrome. *Am J Med Genet.* 1995;58:374.

52. Hösli JM, Tercanli S, Rehder H, et al. Cystic hygroma as an early first-trimester marker for recurrent Fryn's syndrome. *Ultrasound Obstet Gynecol.* 1997;10:422.

53. Lazanakis MS, Rogers K, Economides L. Increased nuchal translucency and CATCH 22. *Prenatal Diagn.* 1998;18:507.

54. Morton JE, Kilby MD, Rushton I. A new lethal autosomal recessive skeletal dysplasia with associated dysmorphic features. *Clin Dysmorphol.* 1998;7:109.

55. Fisk NM, Vaughan J, Smidt M, et al. Transvaginal ultrasound recognition of nuchal edema in the first-trimester diagnosis of achondrogenesis. *J Clin Ultrasound.* 1991;19:586.

56. Ben Ami M, Perlitz S, Haddad S, et al. Increased nuchal translucency is associated with asphyxiating thoracic dysplasia. *Ultrasound Obstet Gynecol.* 1997;10:297.

57. Makrydimas G, Georgiou I, Syrrou M, et al. Increased nuchal translucency thickness in a fetus at risk for beta-thalassemia. *J Matern Fetal Med.* 1997;6:301.

58. Souka AP, Snijders RJ, Novakov A, et al. Defects and syndromes in chromosomally normal fetuses with increased nuchal translucency thickness at 10–14 weeks of gestation. *Ultrasound Obstet Gynecol.* 1998;11:391.

59. Devine PC, Malone FD. First trimester screening for structural fetal anomalies: Nuchal translucency sonography. *Semin Perinatol.* 1999;23:382.

60. Verdin SM, Braithwaite JM, Spencer K, et al. Prenatal diagnosis of trisomy 21 in monozygotic twins with increased nuchal translucency and abnormal serum. *Fetal Diagn Ther.* 1997;12:153.

61. Pandya PP, Hilbert F, Snijders RJM, et al. Nuchal translucency thickness and crown-rump length in twin pregnancies with chromosomal abnormal fetuses. *J Ultrasound Med.* 1995;14:565.

62. Sebire NJ, Noble PL, Psarra A, et al. Fetal karyotyping in twin pregnancies: Selection of technique by measurement of fetal nuchal translucency. *Br J Obstet Gynaecol.* 1996;103:887.

63. Evans MI, Goldberg JD, Dommergues M, et al. Efficacy of second-trimester selective termination for abnormalities: International collaborative experience among the world's largest centers. *Am J Obstet Gynecol.* 1994;171:90.

64. Sebire NJ, D'Ercole C, Huges K, et al. Increased nuchal translucency at 10–14 weeks of gestation as a predictor of severe twin-to-twin transfusion syndrome. *Ultrasound Obstet Gynecol.* 1997;10:86.

65. Montenegro N, Matias A, Areias JC, et al. Increased nuchal translucency: Possible involvement of early cardiac failure. *Ultrasound Obstet Gynecol.* 1997;10:265.

66. Matias A, Gomes C, Flack N, et al. Screening for chromosomal abnormalities at 10–14 weeks: The role of ductus venosus blood flow. *Ultrasound Obstet Gynecol.* 1998;12:380.

67. Martinez JM, Borrell A, Antolin E, et al. Combining nuchal translucency with umbilical Doppler velocimetry for detecting fetal trisomies in the first trimester of pregnancy. *Br J Obstet Gynaecol.* 1997;104:11.

68. Smulian JC, Egan JF, Rodis JF. Fetal hydrops in the first trimester associated with maternal parvovirus infection. *J Clin Ultrasound.* 1998;26:314.

69. Sebire NJ, Bianco D, Snijders RJ, et al. Increased fetal nuchal translucency thickness at 10–14 weeks: Is screening for maternal–fetal infection necessary? *Br J Obstet Gynaecol.* 1997;104:212.

70. Pandya PP, Snijders RJM, Johnson S, et al. Natural history of trisomy 21 fetuses with fetal nuchal translucency. *Ultrasound Obstet Gynecol.* 1995;5:381.

71. Hyett JA, Sebire NJ, Snijders RJM, et al. Intrauterine lethality of trisomy 21 fetuses with increased nuchal thickness. *Ultrasound Obstet Gynecol.* 1996;7:101.

72. Rodis JF, Vintzileous AM, Campbell WA, et al. Spontaneous resolution of fetal cystic hygroma in Down syndrome. *Obstet Gynecol.* 1988;71:976.

73. Szabó J, Gellen J. Nuchal fluid accumulation in trisomy 21 detected by vaginosonography in the first trimester. *Lancet.* 1990;336:1133.

74. Schulte-Vallentin M, Schindler H. Non-echogenic nuchal oedema as a marker in trisomy 21 screening. *Lancet.* 1992;339:1053.

75. Nicolaides KH, Azar G, Byrne D, et al. Fetal nuchal translucency: Ultrasound screening for chromosomal defects in the first trimester of pregnancy. *Br Med J.* 1992;304:867.

76. Savoldelli G, Binkert G, Achermann J, et al. Ultrasound screening for chromosomal anomalies in the first trimester of pregnancy. *Prenatal Diag.* 1993;13:513.

77. Nicolaides KH, Brizot ML, Snijders RJ. Fetal nuchal translucency: Ultrasound screening for fetal trisomy in the first trimester of pregnancy. *Br J Obstet Gynaecol.* 1994;101:782.

78. Brambati B, Cislaghi C, Tului L, et al. First-trimester Down syndrome screening using nuchal translucency: A prospective study in patients undergoing chorionic villus sampling. *Ultrasound Obstet Gynecol.* 1995;5:9.

79. Szabó J, Gellén J, Szemere G. First-trimester ultrasound screening for fetal aneuploidies in women over 35 and under 35 years of age. *Ultrasound Obstet Gynecol.* 1992;5:161.

80. Pajkrt E, Mol BWJ, van Lith JMM, et al. Screening for Down syndrome by fetal nuchal translucency measurement in a high-risk population. *Ultrasound Obstet Gynecol.* 1998;12:156.

81. Pandya PP, Kondylios A, Hilbert L, et al. Chromosomal defects and outcome in 1,015 fetuses with increased nuchal translucency. *Ultrasound Obstet Gynecol.* 1995;5:15.

82. Roberts LJ, Bewley S, Makinson AM, et al. First trimester fetal nuchal translucency: Problems with screening the general population. 1. *Br J Obstet Gynaecol.* 1995;102:381.

83. Bewley S, Roberts LJ, Mackinson AM, et al. First trimester fetal nuchal translucency: Problems with screening the general population. 2. *Br J Obstet Gynaecol.* 1995;102:386.

84. Hafner E, Schuchter K, Phillip K. Screening for chromosomal abnormalities in an unselected population by fetal nuchal translucency. *Ultrasound Obstet Gynecol.* 1995:6:330.

85. Pajkrt E, van Lith JMM, Mol BWJ, et al. Screening for Down's syndrome by fetal nuchal translucency measurement in a general obstetric population. *Ultrasound Obstet Gynecol.* 1998;12:163.

86. Josefsson A, Molander E, Selbing A. Nuchal translucency as a screening test for chromosomal abnormalities in a routine first trimester ultrasound examination. *Acta Obstet Gynecol.* 1998;77:497.

87. Economides DL, Whitlow BJ, Kadir R, et al. First trimester sonographic detection of chromosomal abnormalities in an unselected population. *Br J Obstet Gynaecol.* 1998;105:58.

88. Theodoropoulus P, Lolis D, Papageorgiou C, et al. Evaluation of first-trimester screening by nuchal translucency and maternal age. *Prenatal Diagn.* 1998;18:133.

89. Taipale P, Hilesmaa V, Salonen R, et al. Increased nuchal translucency as a marker for fetal chromosomal defects. *N Engl J Med.* 1997;337:1654.

90. Snijders RJM, Noble P, Sebire N, et al. UK multicentre project on assessment of risk of trisomy 21 by maternal age and fetal nuchal-translucency thickness at 10–14 weeks of gestation. *Lancet.* 1998;352:343.

91. Sherod C, Sebire NJ, Soares W, et al. Prenatal diagnosis of trisomy 18 at the 10–14 week ultrasound scan. *Ultrasound Obstet Gynecol.* 1997;10:387.

92. Kadir RA, Economides DL. The effect of nuchal translucency measurement on second-trimester biochemical screening for Down's syndrome. *Ultrasound Obstet Gynecol.* 1997;9:244.

93. Thilaganathan B, Slack A, Wathen NC. Effect of first-trimester increased fetal nuchal translucency on second-trimester maternal serum biochemical screening for Down syndrome. *Ultrasound Obstet Gynecol.* 1997;10:261.

94. Macintosh MC, Iles R, Teisner B, et al. Maternal serum human chorionic gonadotropin and pregnancy associated plasma protein A, markers for fetal Down syndrome at 8–14 weeks. *Prenatal Diagn.* 1994;14:203.

95. Brambati B, Macintosh MCM, Teisner B, et al. Low maternal serum level of pregnancy associated plasma protein (PAPP-A) in the first trimester in association with abnormal fetal karyotype. *Br J Obstet Gynaecol.* 1993;100:324.

96. Hurley PA, Ward RHT, Teisner B, et al. Serum PAPP-A measurement in first-trimester screening for Down syndrome. *Prenatal Diagn.* 1993;13:903.

97. Spencer K, Macri JN, Aitken DA, et al. Free-βhCG as first-trimester marker for fetal trisomy. *Lancet.* 1992;339:1480.

98. Noble PL, Abraha HD, Snijders RJM, et al. Screening for fetal trisomy 21 in the first trimester of pregnancy: Maternal serum free-βhCG and fetal nuchal thickness. *Ultrasound Obstet Gynecol.* 1995;6:390.

99. Canick JA, Kellner LH. First trimester screening for aneuploidy: Serum biochemical markers. *Semin Perinatol.* 1999;23:359.

100. Orlandi F, Damiani G, Hallahan TW, et al. First-trimester screening for fetal aneuploidy: Biochemistry. *Ultrasound Obstet Gynecol.* 1997;10:381.

101. Zimmermann R, Hucha A, Savodelli G, et al. Serum parameters and nuchal translucency in first trimester screening for fetal chromosomal abnormalities. *Br J Obstet Gynaecol.* 1996;103:1009.

102. Haddow JE, Palomaki GE, Knight G, et al. Screening of maternal serum for fetal Down's syndrome in the first trimester. *N Engl J Med.* 1998;338:955.

103. De Biasio P, Siccardi M, Volpe G, et al. First-trimester screening for Down syndrome using nuchal translucency measurement with free β-hCG and PAPP-A between 10 and 13 weeks of pregnancy—the combined test. *Prenatal Diagn.* 1999;19:360.

104. Biagiotti R, Brizzi L, Periti E, et al. First trimester screening for Down's syndrome using maternal serum PAPP-A and free β-hCG in combination with fetal nuchal translucency thickness. *Br J Obstet Gynaecol.* 1998;105:917.

105. Scott F, Wheeler D, Sinosich M, et al. First trimester aneuploidy screening using a nuchal translucency, free beta human chorionic gonadotropin and maternal age. *Aust NZ J Obstet Gynaecol.* 1996;36:381.

106. Brizot ML, Snijders RJ, Butler J, et al. Maternal serum hCG and fetal nuchal translucency thickness for the prediction of fetal trisomies in the first trimester of pregnancy. *Br J Obstet Gynaecol.* 1995;102:127.

107. Wald NJ, Watt HC, Hackshaw AK. Integrated screening for Down's syndrome based on tests performed during the first and second trimesters. *N Engl J Med.* 1999;341:461.

108. Hyett JA, Noble PL, Snijders RJM, et al. Fetal heart rate in trisomy 21 and other chromosomal abnormalities at 10–14 weeks of gestation. *Ultrasound Obstet Gynecol.* 1997;7:239.

6

Transvaginal Sonography of Ectopic Pregnancy

Arthur C. Fleischer • *Michael P. Diamond* • *Peter S. Cartwright*

Recent improvements in the sonographic depiction of uterine and adnexal structures with transvaginal sonography and refinements in radioimmunoassay (RIA) of the beta subunit of human chorionic gonadotropin (β-hCG) have markedly enhanced the sonologist's ability to diagnose ectopic pregnancy. Although the sonographic findings in ectopic pregnancy can be subtle, a definitive diagnosis of this entity is possible in most cases when sonographic findings are combined with results of a single or with serial β-hCG assays. Most importantly, sonography is useful in the evaluation of patients with suspected ectopic pregnancy to verify the presence or absence of an intrauterine pregnancy and to identify an ectopic pregnancy in the adnexa.

The possibility that a tube containing an ectopic pregnancy can be "salvaged" by linear salpingostomy is closely related to the stage at which the ectopic pregnancy is detected. Once the tube has ruptured, it usually cannot be salvaged. Therefore, it is most desirable to diagnose an ectopic pregnancy as early as possible.

Early diagnosis is also important in patients undergoing medical treatment of ectopic pregnancy. In addition, transvaginal color Doppler sonography (TV-CDS) may be used to monitor the effectiveness of medical treatment. Transvaginal CDS will have an important role in determining which type of treatment (medical, local methotrexate, or KCl injections) is most appropriate based on the relative vascularity of the choriodecidua within the tube and the presence or absence of embryonic heart motion.

The use of transvaginal sonography (TVS) has greatly enhanced the sonographic evaluation of patients with suspected ectopic pregnancy. Specifically, the presence or absence of an intrauterine gestation can be documented approximately 1 week earlier with TVS than with transabdominal sonography (TAS). In addition, adnexal masses created by ectopic pregnancies can be more frequently detected by TVS.

The additional use of TV-CDS seems to further enhance detection of ectopic pregnancies that might not be apparent on TVS.[1,2] Viable trophoblastic tissue typically produces a vascular ring within the tube that can be recognized by TV-CDS. Application of this technique is discussed further in Chap. 14.

With these modalities and laboratory tests, a very high degree of accuracy (greater than 90%) is possible in establishing the presence or excluding the possibility of ectopic pregnancy.[3]

If left unrecognized, an ectopic pregnancy can result in significant maternal morbidity and mortality. Ectopic pregnancy is responsible for 4 to 10% of all maternal deaths.[4,5] Even though the diagnosis of ectopic pregnancy is often considered in women who present with lower abdominal pain and amenorrhea, it is missed by the initial examining physician in up to 70% of cases.[6] Expeditious and accurate diagnosis of patients who are suspected of having ectopic pregnancy is important so proper management can be instituted. If it is recognized early, before tubal rupture, it may be possible to surgically remove the gestational sac by linear salpingostomy, thereby preserving the tube and future chances of achieving pregnancy. Because salpingectomy is frequently required for advanced ectopic pregnancies, a history of the disorder can be a contributing factor to female infertility. Once a patient has had an ectopic pregnancy, there is a significant chance (about one in four) of recurrence in a future pregnancy.[6]

Another reason for early definitive diagnosis by TVS is the more widespread use of medical treatment of ectopic pregnancies. Color Doppler ultrasound may have a role in the monitoring of the vascularity of the ectopic pregnancy during treatment because with effective treatment blood flow is altered.[7]

INCIDENCE

Several epidemiologic studies have shown that the incidence of ectopic pregnancies is increasing, which may be a reflection of the increased prevalence of salpingitis.[8,9] For example, the age-adjusted incidence of ectopic pregnancy rose from 55.5 to 84.2 per 100,000 women in northern California from 1972 to 1978.[8] Nationwide, the number of ectopic pregnancies has ranged from 17,800 in 1970 to 42,000 in 1978.[9] The death rate, however, decreased by 75% during this period, which is a reflection of an increase in suspicion of ectopic pregnancies by patients and care providers and an improvement in the ability to diagnose this entity in its earliest stages. The incidence of ectopic pregnancies is greatest in patients with salpingitis, previous tubal surgery, or intrauterine device (IUD) use.[10,11]

PATHOGENESIS

The term *ectopic pregnancy* refers to an implantation of the conceptus outside the endometrial cavity. Ninety-five percent of ectopic pregnancies are tubal, and the majority of these occur in the ampullary or isthmic portions of the oviduct. The remaining 5% occur in the abdomen, ovary, cervix, and the retroperitoneal space.

In ampullary ectopic tubal pregnancies, the conceptus implants beneath the epithelium of the fallopian tube to form a fluid-filled gestational sac, which is lined with trophoblastic tissue, in the wall of the tube. Because the fallopian tube has only two thin layers of muscle, the trophoblastic cells that burrow deep into the tubal epithelium distend it and can eventually cause it to rupture. The gestational sac within the tube of a ruptured ectopic pregnancy is usually surrounded by fluid or blood due to erosion of adjacent vessels. In the vast majority of cases, the separation of the decidua from the wall of the tube causes death of the embryo. In rare cases, the embryo may survive an attempt at abortion by reimplantation within the abdomen and reestablishment of the blood supply from the omentum or the mesentery.

Mild uterine enlargement and decidualization of the endometrium are usually present with an ectopic pregnancy and can occasionally be detected clinically. If dilatation and curettage (D&C) is performed on a patient with an ectopic pregnancy, only decidua without chorionic villi will be obtained.

Studies have indicated that up to one-third of all ectopic embryos have an abnormal karyotype, a factor that contributes to their demise and resultant deficient decidual support.[4] Because the ectopic implanted embryo frequently dies before the sixth week of gestation, decidualization may be interrupted and faulty.[12] Other contributing factors to the establishment of an ectopic pregnancy may include endocrine dysfunction, current IUD use, abnormalities of tubal physiology, and previous tubal surgery.[10,11,13]

Another possible etiology of recurrent ectopic pregnancies is the transperitoneal migration of the fertilized egg into the contralateral tube. Predictably, this would result in delayed and faulty implantation of the trophoblasts into the tubal wall. As the relative contributions of those factors to the development of ectopic pregnancy are better understood, measures that can prevent ectopic pregnancy may be determined.

CLINICAL ASPECTS

Proposed explanations for development of ectopic pregnancy include delayed ovulation or delayed transit of the fertilized zygote secondary to fallopian tube malfunction, ovulation from the contralateral ovary with delayed passage of the zygote through the tube, obstruction of zygote passage secondary to intratubal adhesions from pelvic inflammatory disease, and abnormal angulation of the tube relative to the uterine cornu.[4]

Before the use of antibiotics for pelvic inflammatory disease, tubal inflammation resulted in a much higher incidence of complete tubal closure and subsequent sterility. The recent two- to threefold increased incidence of ectopic gestations among previously pregnant patients has been attributed paradoxically to the use of antibiotics for treatment of tubal inflammation.[14] Antibiotics have reduced the incidence of sterility but have resulted in more women with open, but malfunctioning, tubes. The result is an increased incidence of ectopic pregnancy among patients with previous tubal infection. In addition to patients who have a history of pelvic inflammatory disease, patients who have undergone tubal surgery, have a history of infertility, and who have used IUDs have an increased chance of developing an ectopic pregnancy.[10] Ectopic pregnancy is a double-edged sword because it results in both a nonviable pregnancy and the ability to render the patient infertile.[11] Once a patient has had an ectopic pregnancy, there is a one in four chance of recurrence in a future pregnancy.[6]

In the United States, the incidence of ectopic pregnancy is between 1 in 100 and 1 in 400 pregnancies, but in some populations it is as high as 1 in 32 live births.[4,6] Clinically, however, ectopic pregnancy should be considered in the differential diagnosis of any patient presenting with lower abdominal pain[15] because the sometimes massive intraperitoneal bleeding associated with rupture of an ectopic pregnancy is such a serious complication. An analogy can be made between ectopic pregnancy in the 1990s and the great masquerade of pulmonary tuberculosis in the 1930s; its clinical symptoms at presentation differ so much in type and severity.[4] In fact, clinicians are now taught to "think ectopic" for any woman of childbearing age who presents with lower abdominal pain.

The most common presenting symptoms of ectopic pregnancy are pelvic pain, which may be mild and intermittent or persistent and severe, and abnormal vaginal bleeding.[16] The clinical symptomatology and routine laboratory findings in ectopic pregnancy are usually not diagnostic by themselves. Abnormal vaginal bleeding is seen in approximately three-fourths of patients with such pregnancies and can be confused with other causes of first-trimester bleeding, such as threatened or spontaneous abortion. There is, however, no bleeding or menstrual history that is inconsistent with an ectopic gestation. Statistically, vaginal bleeding is more commonly associated with other first-trimester conditions (such as threatened spontaneous abortion, cervical polyp, or infection) than with ectopic pregnancy. Diffuse abdominal pain may be present, as may rebound tenderness from peritoneal irritation resulting from free intraperitoneal bleeding.

The presence of an adnexal mass is not specific for the diagnosis of ectopic pregnancy because a mass can occur in many other conditions, such as corpus luteum cyst, dermoid cyst, or leiomyomata. In our experience, a palpable adnexal mass was noted in less than one-third of cases and did not predict whether or not the gestation had ruptured.[17] Although uncommon, the presence of a palpable adnexal mass (that is, separate from both ovaries and uterine fundus) is highly suggestive of an ectopic pregnancy.

In an emergency setting, culdocentesis (the transvaginal aspiration of fluid from the posterior cul-de-sac) remains an alternative diagnostic aid for evaluating patients suspected of having an ectopic gestation. The aspiration of nonclotting blood indicates the presence of a hemoperitoneum. This finding is not diagnostic of an ectopic pregnancy, however; it may also result from a hemorrhagic corpus luteum, complete or incomplete abortion, ovulation, or previous attempts at culdocentesis. In our experience, 70% of patients with an ectopic pregnancy who underwent this procedure had positive taps; this was one of the key factors resulting in the patient's admission to the hospital.[18] In only 56% of these patients, however, was the tube ruptured; intact tubal pregnancy may produce

several liters of hemoperitoneum by bleeding through the fimbriated end of the tube. A negative culdocentesis usually excludes a ruptured tube.

A recently published study has reported that the sonographic finding of hemoperitoneum is more predictive of ectopic pregnancy than of culdocentesis. They concluded that culdocentesis should not play a role in the evaluation of ectopic pregnancy except in the unusual circumstances in which TVS cannot be performed.[19]

The clinical course of an ectopic pregnancy is related to its site of implantation.[20] The ampullary portion of the tube is the most common location for ectopic implantation. As in other sites, the ectopic pregnancy can expand the tube until it ruptures. Complete or partial tubal abortion may also occur, with the contents of the sac extruded through the fimbriated end of the tube into the peritoneal cavity. If the fimbriated end of the tube is occluded, hematosalpinx will result. Ectopic pregnancies that occur in the narrow isthmic portion of the tube usually distend it eccentrically and, because of the tube's small diameter, rupture early in the pregnancy.

Ectopic pregnancy in the interstitial portion of the tube is uncommon (3 to 4% of all ectopic pregnancies) but it has the most serious potential complications. Because of its location within the muscular portion of the uterus near the major uterine vessels, the pregnancy can survive until 3 to 4 months' gestation. Massive bleeding from the uterine arteries and veins can then result.

Chronic ectopic pregnancies may occur, resulting in hematoma formation in the cul-de-sac.[21] Such patients usually present with recurrent, intermittent low-grade fever associated with a palpable solid mass. On physical examination, there is usually a firm pelvic mass located in the midline and difficult to separate from the uterus. Culdocentesis may be negative because the blood in the cul-de-sac is clotted. In very rare cases, the embryo and products of conception will undergo dehydration in situ with the formation of a lithopedion pregnancy.

Other rare sites of implantation include intra-abdominal, ovarian, cervical, and extraperitoneal. True advanced abdominal ectopic pregnancies may be difficult to differentiate from normal intrauterine pregnancies; the uterus must be defined separately from the amniotic sac and its contents.[22] Abdominal pregnancies are thought to be the result of reimplantation of an aborted fetus after it passes out the fimbriated end of the tube and reimplants on the mesentery or omentum. These pregnancies can progress to term without symptoms, and first present because of difficulty during the initial stages of labor. Extraperitoneal ectopic pregnancies are quite rare and are probably the result of tubal rupture, with expulsion of the fetus between the leaves of the broad ligament. The rupture occurs between the fimbriated end of the tube (where it is not covered by peritoneum) and the site where the two folds of the broad ligament are loosely opposed. The tubal contents may empty into the soft tissue and mesosalpinx and implant in that region.

β-hCG ASSAY

To properly evaluate a patient in whom an ectopic pregnancy is suspected, it is absolutely imperative to correlate the sonographic findings with the results of a pregnancy test. In addition, it is important for the sonographer and sonologist to know the type of pregnancy test used and its relative sensitivity.

The enzyme-linked immunoassays that detect urine human chorionic gonadotropin (hCG) are nonquantitative but very sensitive and may easily be performed in an office or clinic. These tests are useful for determining the presence or absence of a pregnancy and are routinely positive when the serum hCG level is at least 50 mIU/mL (8 to 10 days postconception). They are positive in about 99% of patients with a symptomatic ectopic pregnancy. The enzyme-linked immunoabsorbant assays (ELISA) detecting the beta subunit of the serum hCG molecule are quantitative and most helpful in cases where a problem arises during an early pregnancy, such as suspected ectopic pregnancy or threatened abortion.

All commercially available kits that measure serum β-hCG now use the ELISA technology, and the older radio immuno assays (RIAs) have been replaced. In addition, the earlier confusion over different "international standards" has been resolved, and all kits now use the same standard.

Most of the urine pregnancy tests assay for the whole intact hCG molecule. They may, however, also detect metabolized core fragments of hCG, which contain portions of both the alpha and beta chains of the molecule, but where the beta subunit is "nicked." These "nicked" beta subunit chains may not be detected by a serum β-hCG ELISA, thereby giving the impression of a "false-positive" urine pregnancy test.[23] Clinically, this may be encountered when a patient has a nonviable pregnancy (usually intrauterine) that is in the process of resolving. The trophoblast has ceased producing hCG, has often been expelled, and the serum β-hCG level is very low. Such patients may present with complaints of pain and abnormal bleeding, and an ectopic pregnancy is in the differential diagnosis. Usually, the urine pregnancy test also becomes negative when repeated in 48 h.

The ability to quantitate serum levels of β-hCG allows the clinician to estimate the gestational age of the pregnancy, assuming it is normal. The β-hCG level can then be correlated with the sonographic findings in looking for certain developmental "milestones" (Table 6–1). Transvaginal sonographic features that are expected at the various β-hCG levels are summarized in Figure 6–1. Correlating the serum β-hCG level with the sonographic findings enables the clinician to evaluate the normalcy of the pregnancy in question.

The "milestones" that are helpful include the delineation of a "chorionic sac" at the fifth week, detection of a yolk sac within the gestational sac of approximately 1 cm at 5 to 6 weeks, and an embryo within a sac of approximately 1.5 mm at 6 weeks.

TABLE 6–1. TRANSVAGINAL ULTRASOUND AND EMBRYOLOGIC MILESTONES

Gestational Age (weeks)	Range of Chorionic Sac Mean Dimension (mm)[a]	Embryo Length (mm)[b]	Mean β-hCG mIU/mL[b,c]
4	1.5 × 2.8	0.5	28
5	8–15	1.5–3	300
6	15–40	4–8	3000
7	40–100	9–16	50,000

[a]Data from Davies J. *Human Developmental Anatomy.* New York: Ronald Press; 1962.
[b]Data from Cartwright P, DiPietro D. Beta hCG is a diagnostic and for suspected ectopic pregnancy. *Obstet Gynecol.* 1984;63:76.
[c]Second International Standard.[25]

A *discriminatory zone* for the level of serum β-hCG has been defined for discerning a normal (viable) intrauterine pregnancy from an ectopic pregnancy by means of TVS. This level is between 1500 and 2000 mIU/mL. This means

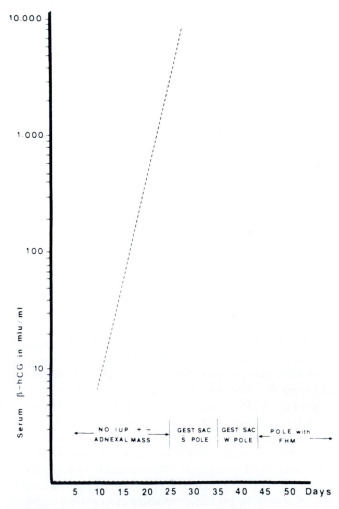

Figure 6–1. β-hCG and TAS milestones.[25] (I.R.P.)

every viable intrauterine pregnancy should be visible sono-graphically by the time the serum β-hCG is 2000 mIU/mL or more. The absence of an intrauterine gestational sac when the serum level is above the discriminatory zone is highly suspicious for an ectopic pregnancy. If no intrauterine gestational sac is seen while the serum β-hCG is below the discriminatory zone, the pregnancy may be either very early intrauterine or ectopic. Even when an adnexal mass is visualized, this may simply be a self-contained hemorrhagic corpus luteum cyst. Measuring the thickness of the endometrial stripe may be of some value. Normal, early intrauterine pregnancies tend to be associated with a thickened endometrium, whereas the stripe is thinner with an ectopic pregnancy. When ambiguity persists, serial β-hCG determinations should be drawn to look for a normal or abnormal progression, and the sonogram should be repeated once the level has risen above the discriminatory zone.

It must be emphasized, however, that these criteria represent guidelines, not absolute endpoints.[24] It is possible for a viable intrauterine pregnancy to demonstrate a low β-hCG level and/or slow progression. Conversely, a normal rise in the β-hCG level may sometimes be associated with an ectopic pregnancy.[24] Also, a multiple gestation or a heterotopic pregnancy may show an uncharacteristically elevated β-hCG level for any given gestational age.

The amount of hCG produced by an ectopic pregnancy is generally less than that by a viable intrauterine pregnancy of the same gestational age,[25] which may be due to an unfavorable location for trophoblast proliferation. This fact is useful, however, only if the date of conception is known. The serum β-hCG level for 192 women with a proven ectopic pregnancy at the time of their initial presentation is shown in Figure 6–2. It is clear that the majority of these patients presented with the serum β-hCG level below the discriminatory zone.

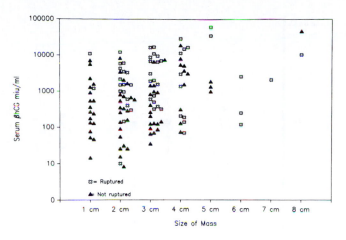

Figure 6–3. β-hCG versus size of mass. (I.R.P.)

The level of serum β-hCG tends to be proportional to the size of a tubal pregnancy (Fig. 6–3). A ruptured tubal pregnancy tends to be associated with a higher level than one that has not ruptured. The range of serum β-hCG levels for any given situation, however, is so broad that this observation has little clinical relevance.

Visualizing an intrauterine sac when the serum β-hCG is below the discriminatory zone may signify an abnormal gestation (Fig. 6–4). An intrauterine "blighted ovum" may appear this way. Also, there is the "pseudogestational sac," which is sometimes associated with an ectopic pregnancy. A pseudogestational sac lacks the "double-sac" sign and is smaller and more irregular than a true gestational sac at a comparable gestational age.

Serial determinations of the serum β-hCG level have proven useful in the clinically stable patient when ambiguity persists even after the sonographic findings have been correlated with a single quantitative β-hCG. Figure 6–5 shows the β-hCG progression in 19 clinically stable patients with an ectopic pregnancy.[25] The first known value is arbitrarily placed on the standard line, and subsequent values are plotted accordingly. It is apparent that most patients showed a plateau or fall in the level during the period of preoperative evaluation. This plateau or fall is diagnostic of a nonviable pregnancy when it occurs at levels below 3000 mIU/mL during at least a 48-hour period. It does not, however, distinguish between a nonviable intrauterine and an ectopic pregnancy. It is also apparent from Figure 6–5 that some ectopic pregnancies may show an initial normal rise in the level of β-hCG. This normal rise, however, is usually short lived, and an abnormal progression soon develops.

Serial β-hCG determinations are also essential after treatment of an ectopic pregnancy by either medical or surgical means. A plateau or rise in the level may be the first indication of a persistent ectopic pregnancy.[26] Furthermore, a negative β-hCG may signify a resolution of the problem before any sonographic findings have resolved.

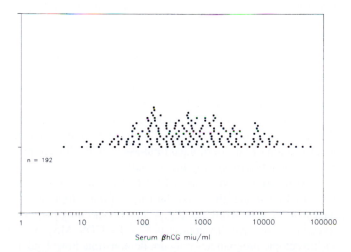

Figure 6–2. β-hCG at time of presentation in 192 surgically proven ectopic pregnancies.[25] (I.R.P.)

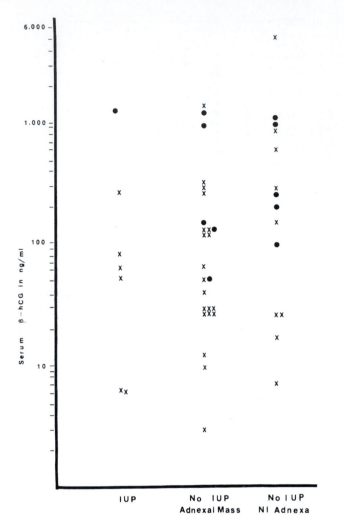

Figure 6–4. β-hCG, ultrasound (TA) findings in 46 proven ectopic pregnancies.[25] ×, Unruptured; ○, ruptured. (I.R.P.)

SONOGRAPHIC EVALUATION

The use of TVS has greatly enhanced the sonographic evaluation of patients with suspected ectopic pregnancy.[27,28] In particular, the presence or absence of an intrauterine gestation can be documented or excluded at an earlier stage (approximately 1 week) than with TAS. In addition, adnexal masses and reliable collections of intraperitoneal fluid created by ectopic pregnancies can more frequently be detected by TVS. The use of TAS and TVS with highly sensitive pregnancy tests has markedly enhanced the ability to detect ectopic pregnancies over techniques and tests available in the recent past. A very high degree of accuracy now exists in the ability to establish the presence or exclude the possibility of an ectopic pregnancy.[27,29]

Transvaginal sonography plays a major role in the evaluation of patients with suspected ectopic pregnancy. Most importantly, vaginal transducer/probes allow accurate and definitive inclusion or exclusion of an intrauterine preg-

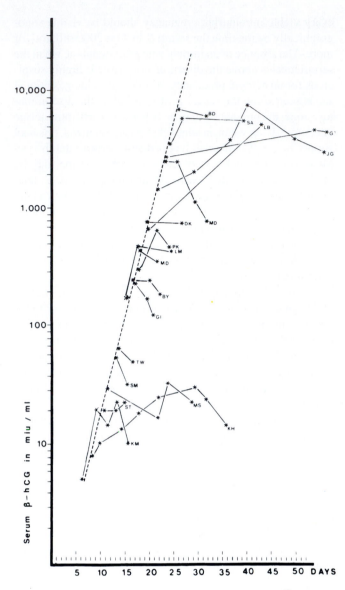

Figure 6–5. Serial β-hCG in 19 clinically stable patients.[25] (I.R.P.)

nancy by demonstration of an intrauterine gestational sac. Transvaginal sonography also can be used to demonstrate an extrauterine gestational sac, corpus luteum, or both. Transabdominal sonography can be used to evaluate these parameters but is, in general, less accurate or definitive. Because the field of view of TVS is limited, TAS can be helpful in the identification of intraperitoneal fluid associated with ectopic pregnancy hemorrhage, rupture, or both.

As mentioned previously, TV-CDS may be a useful adjunct to TVS in that the "vascular ring" of the ectopic pregnancy can be visualized (see Fig. 6–11). Functioning corpora lutea may also have this appearance on TV-CDS. Most nonviable ectopic pregnancies may not demonstrate flow. Under treatment, most ectopic pregnancies demonstrate increased vascularity as defined by the number of colorized pixel elements in the tubal ring.

SCANNING TECHNIQUE

On both TAS and TVS, sonographic examinations should begin by delineation of the uterus in its long axis. One should carefully evaluate the endometrial interfaces for the presence or absence of a gestational sac or decidual thickening. Once the uterus is adequately evaluated, the adnexal region should be carefully examined. If possible, both ovaries should be identified because some ectopic pregnancies are associated with coexisting corpus luteum. On a transverse transvaginal scan, the relative position of the proximal segment of tube can be approximated by recognition of the several anatomic landmarks. These include delineation of the round ligament as it courses directly anterior to the tube near the uterine

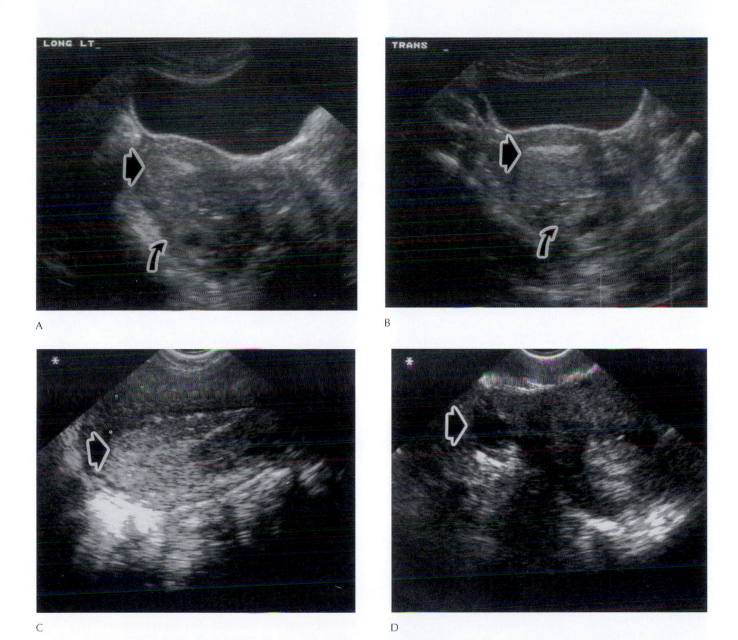

Figure 6–6. Ectopic pregnancy: uterine sonographic findings. **(A)** Longitudinal TA sonogram of unruptured ectopic pregnancy appearing as a complex retrouterine mass posterior to uterus *(curved arrow).* Uterus contains thickened, decidualized endometrium *(arrow).* **(B)** Transverse TAS of **A** showing thickened endometrium *(arrow)* and left adnexal ectopic gestation *(curved arrow).* **(C)** TVS of unruptured ectopic pregnancy. Long axis of uterus shows thickened decidualized endometrium *(arrow).* **(D)** Semiaxial TVS of **C** showing right adnexal mass *(arrow),* which represents an unruptured ectopic pregnancy. A yolk sac is present within gestational sac. *(Figure continued.)*

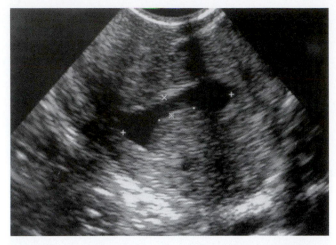

E

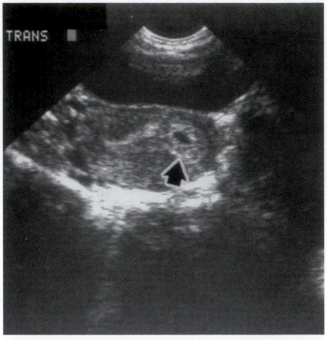

F

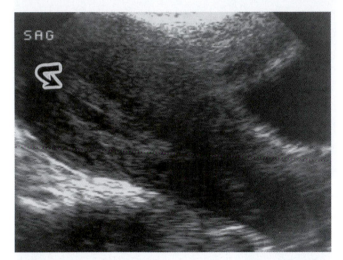

G

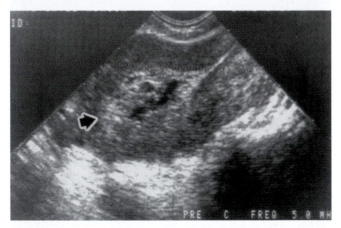

H

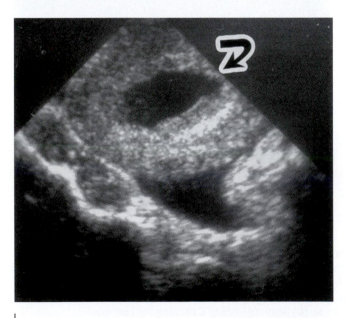

I

Figure 6–6. *(continued)* **(E)** TVS of pseudogestational sac in a patient with proven ectopic pregnancy. The irregular sac *(between +'s)* was mistaken for deformed intrauterine sac. **(F)** Transverse TAS of a 6-week intrauterine pregnancy showing typically eccentric location of gestational sac *(arrow)* within uterine lumen. **(G)** TAS showing irregularly thickened decidualized endometrium *(curved arrow)*. **(H)** TVS of patient in **G,** more clearly showing irregular decidualized endometrium *(arrow)* of proven ectopic pregnancy. **(I)** TVS of decidual cast *(curved arrow)* with blood-distended uterine lumen. Intraperitoneal fluid was also present in cul-de-sac. *(Figure continued.)*

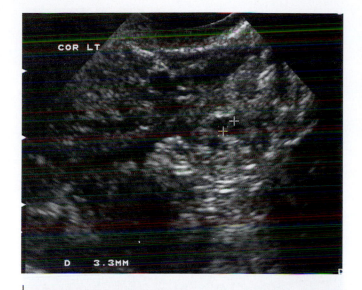

J

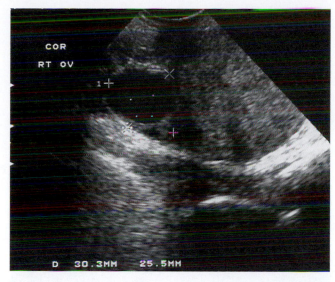

K

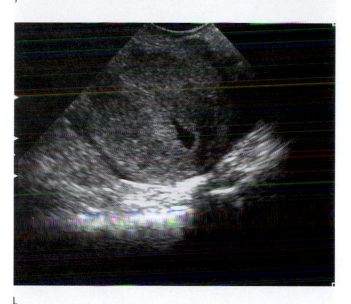

L

Figure 6–6. *(continued)* **(J, K, L)** Unruptured left ectopic pregnancy demonstrating all of the typical sonographic findings. **(J)** TVS of left adnexa showing adnexal "ring." **(K)** TVS of right adnexa showing right corpus luteum. **(L)** TVS of uterus showing decidual thickening and small amount of intraluminal fluid or "pseudosac."

fundus and the location of the interstitial portion of the tube by its proximity to the endometrium, which invaginates into the uterine cornu on a transverse scan in the region of the tubal ostia. If color Doppler is used, the pulse repetition frequency should be low to maximize detection of slow flow.

SONOGRAPHIC FINDINGS

The sonographic findings that are encountered in a patient with ectopic pregnancy differ according to the stage of pregnancy in which the patient is examined and whether or not rupture has occurred. In addition, findings depend on what type of transducer/probe is used. The following discussion is organized into uterine, adnexal, and peritoneal sonographic findings.

Uterine

In most ectopic pregnancies, the uterus demonstrates a thickened endometrial interface due to the decidualization of the endometrium (Fig. 6–6). Particularly with TV scans, the increased fluid content of the decidualized endometrium can be appreciated due to enhanced through transmission distal to this layer. In more advanced ectopic pregnancies, fluid or blood may be present within the decidualized endometrium, simulating the appearance of an early gestational sac. In some cases, before sloughing of the decidua, a hypoechoic interface beneath the decidua can be seen that represents hemorrhage between the necrotic decidua and inner myometrium. In contradistinction to normal intrauterine pregnancies, where the gestational sac is spherical and well defined, the pseudogestational sac created by sloughing decidua found in some advanced ectopic pregnancies is more irregular and angulated.

For a more detailed discussion of the sonographic changes that occur within the uterus in early intrauterine pregnancy, refer to Chap. 5. As opposed to the decidualized endometrium in normal intrauterine pregnancy, the decidualized endometrium of ectopics usually demonstrates little or no diastolic flow on TV-CDS. The myometrium typically shows a poorly vascularized or "cold" pattern. The waveform from the decidualized endometrium of the ectopic pregnancy demonstrates little or no diastolic flow as compared with the decidua of an early intrauterine pregnancy. Tiny (a few millimeters) cysts can be seen within the decidua and they have been reported to correspond to areas of decidual necrosis.[30]

Adnexal

Typically, ectopic pregnancies occur as rounded masses, from 1 to 3 cm in size, which are located in the parauterine region. Masses that result from an ectopic pregnancy typically

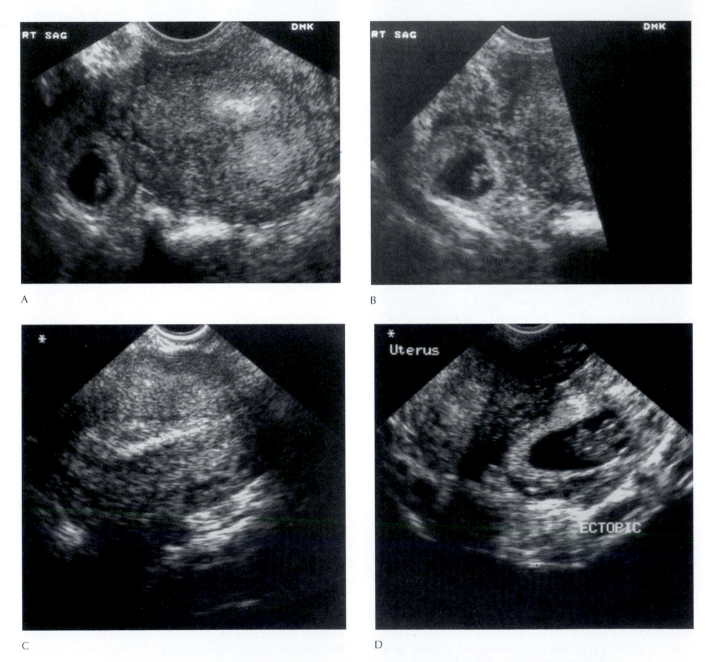

Figure 6–7. Ectopic pregnancy; adnexal findings. **(A)** TV sonogram showing lack of gestational sac within uterus and right adnexal "ring." **(B)** TVS of an unruptured ectopic pregnancy that contains a dead embryo and deflated yolk sac. **(C)** TV sonogram of uterus in long axis and **(D)** left adnexa in advanced (8-week) unruptured ectopic pregnancy. Fetus demonstrated heart activity. *(Figure continued.)*

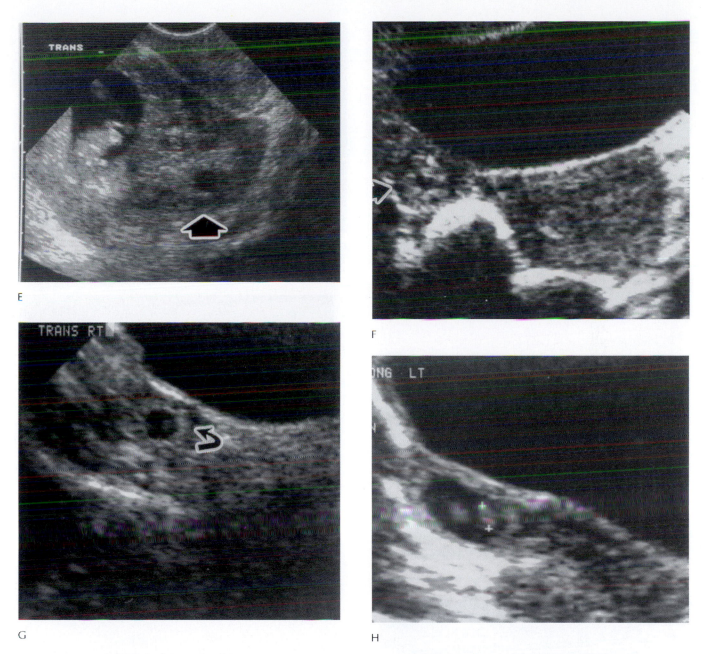

Figure 6–7. *(continued)* **(E)** TV sonogram of advanced (9-week) ruptured ectopic pregnancy. There is clotted blood *(arrow)* within cul-de-sac adjacent to ectopic gestation secondary to rupture of this ectopic pregnancy. Pregnancy had intraluminal fluid as depicted in **E**. **(F)** Magnified transverse TAS of an unruptured right-tubal pregnancy *(arrow)*. *(Courtesy of Gary Thieme, MD.)* **(G)** Transverse TAS of ectopic gestation with embryo within sac *(arrow)*. **(H)** Magnified longitudinal TAS of a 7-week ectopic pregnancy showing embryo *(between + 's)*. *(Courtesy of Philippe Jeanty, MD, PhD.) (Figure continued.)*

consist of a central hypoechoic area surrounded by an echogenic rim of trophoblastic tissue and muscle layer. An embryo can rarely be identified within the gestational sac of an ectopic pregnancy; a yolk sac may be present. In general, a corpus luteum appears as a hypoechoic structure surrounded by a rim of ovarian tissue. Usually, the corpus luteum is more eccentrically located within the ovarian

structure than the more concentric halo representing the rim of trophoblastic tissue and muscle of an ectopic pregnancy. On TV-CDS both viable ectopics and corpora lutea demonstrate a vascular ring surrounding a relatively hypoechoic center.

Transvaginal sonography is particularly helpful in identification of adnexal masses resulting from ectopic gestations

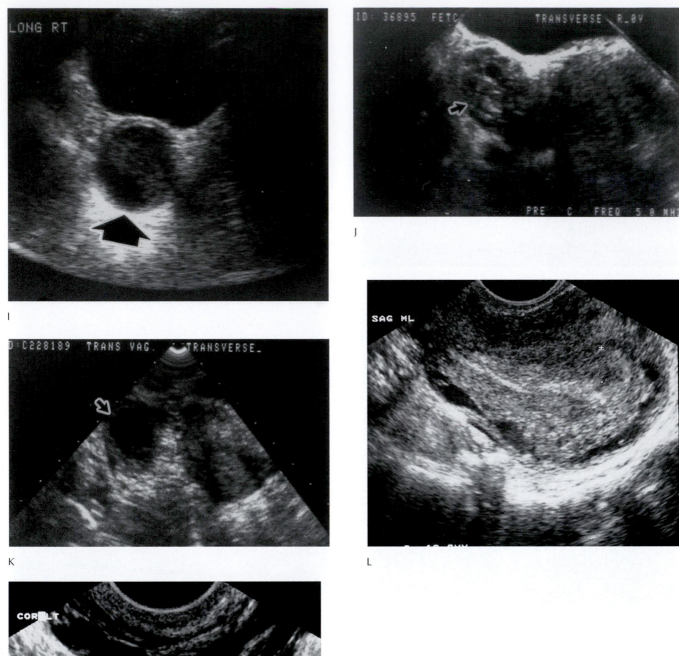

Figure 6–7. *(continued)* **(I)** TAS of hematosalpinx *(arrow)* secondary to ruptured ectopic pregnancy. **(J)** TVS of hematosalpinx *(arrow)* secondary to ruptured ectopic pregnancy. **(K)** TVS of hemorrhagic corpus luteum *(arrow)* that simulated an ovarian ectopic pregnancy **(L, M)** TVS of unruptured ectopic pregnancy showing decidual change in the retroflexed uterus **(L)** and the unruptured ectopic in the left tube **(M)**. A yolk sac is present within the gestational sac.

(Fig. 6–7). In our study, TVS was able to identify adnexal masses in the 1- to 3-cm range that had β-hCGs between 800 and 1000 mIU/mL.[27]

On TV-CDS unruptured ectopic pregnancies with viable trophoblasts demonstrate a vascular ring. This structure can usually be identified as separate from the ipsilateral ovary. The blood flow typically demonstrates low-impedance, high-diastolic flow, but there is a significant range in flow observed in ectopic pregnancies, ranging from low impedance to high impedance with reversed diastolic flow, probably a reflection

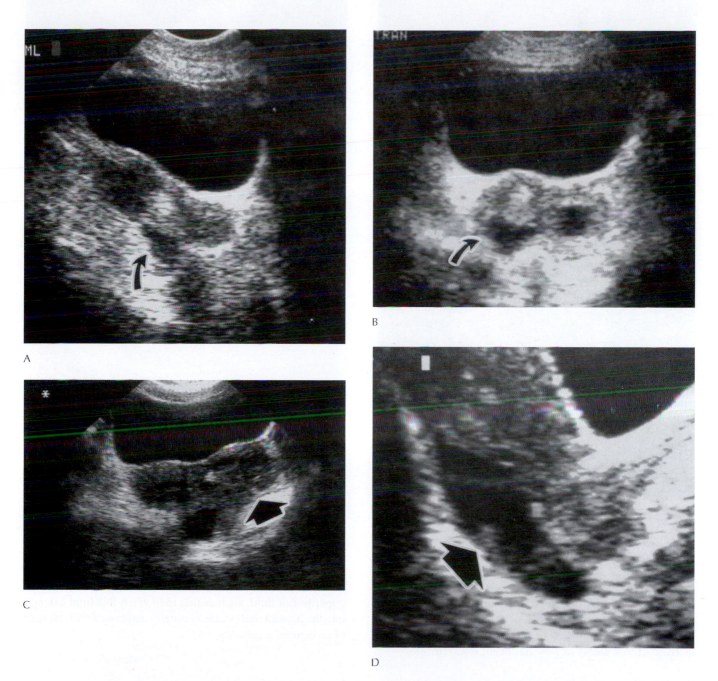

Figure 6–8. Ectopic pregnancy: peritoneal findings. **(A)** Longitudinal and **(B)** transverse sonogram of "leaking" left tubal ectopic pregnancy with unclotted cul-de-sac hemorrhage *(curved arrow).* **(C)** Transverse TAS of clotted hemorrhage secondary to chronic ruptured ectopic pregnancy. Transverse TAS of intraperitoneal hemorrhage associated with ruptured abdominal pregnancy. **(D)** Magnified longitudinal TAS showing partially clotted cul-de-sac hemorrhage *(arrow)* secondary to ruptured ectopic pregnancy. *(Figure continued.)*

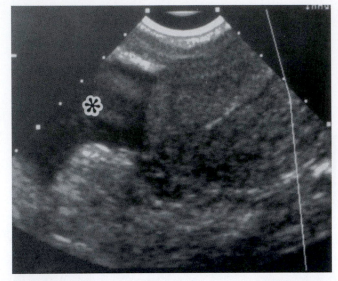

E

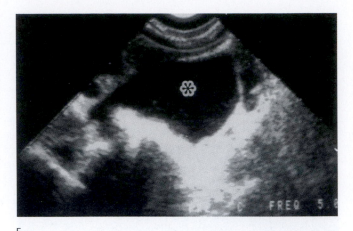

F

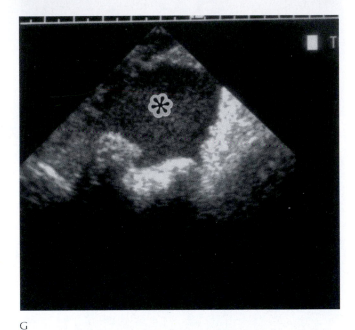

G

Figure 6–8. *(continued)* **(E)** TVS long axis showing clotted blood (⋆) superior to funds. **(F)** TVS showing intraperitoneal free blood (⋆). Low-level echoes were within this partially clotted blood collection in cul-de-sac. **(G)** TVS of free blood (⋆) in cul-de-sac secondary to ruptured ectopic pregnancy. TAS low-level echoes probably were from clotted portions of intraperitoneal blood collection.

of the intactness of the trophoblasts within the muscular layers of the tube.

The vascularity of ectopic pregnancies changes, probably depending on the viability of the trophoblasts as they invade the circular muscle of the tube. With treatment, an increase of vascularity or flow has been observed.[2]

Peritoneal

Along with evaluation of the uterus and adnexa, sonography can detect intraperitoneal fluid that may be associated with hemorrhage, rupture, or both of an ectopic pregnancy (Fig. 6–8). The presence of intraperitoneal fluid does not always correlate with the presence of rupture because there may be

hemorrhage out of the fimbriated ends of tubes in patients with unruptured ectopic pregnancies. Large amounts of intraperitoneal fluid, such as that seen when this fluid extends into the hepatorenal pouch, is usually associated with rupture of an ectopic pregnancy.

RARE TYPES OF ECTOPIC PREGNANCY

Although the majority of ectopic pregnancies (95%) occur within the tube, there are some rare types that can occur within the tube, cervix, ovary, and peritoneal (abdominal) spaces

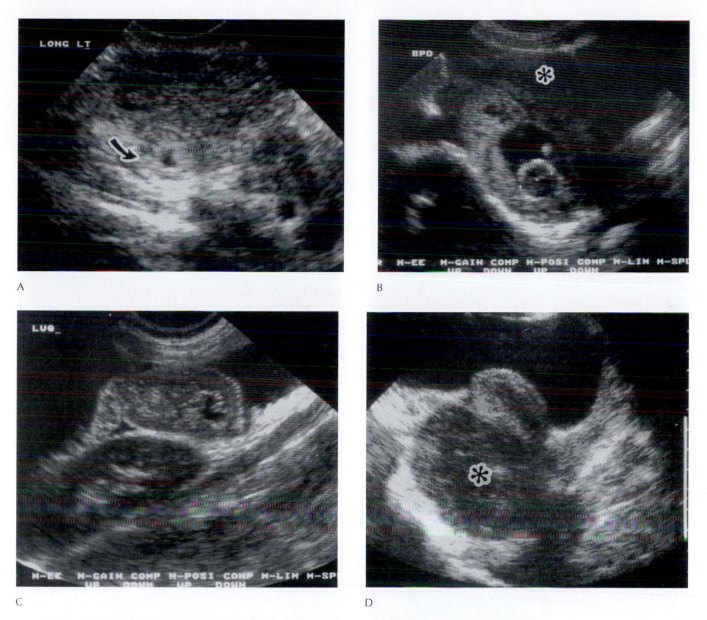

Figure 6–9. Rare types of ectopic pregnancy. **(A)** Semicoronal TVS showing eccentrically located gestational sac *(arrow)* that was found to represent a cornual ectopic pregnancy. **(B)** Longitudinal TAS showing 12-week fetus outside uterus (⋆). **(C)** Same patient as in **B**, showing large amount of intraperitoneal fluid surrounding bowel in this ruptured abdominal ectopic pregnancy. **(D)** Longitudinal TAS showing solid retrouterine mass (⋆) that represented chronic ectopic pregnancy. The β-hCG was negative. *(Figure continued.)*

(Fig. 6–9). Rarely, a patient can present after tubal rupture with a chronic ectopic pregnancy.

Transvaginal sonography is helpful in diagnosing interstitial ectopic pregnancies. One should be aware that the normal intrauterine pregnancy may have a very eccentrically located gestational sac early in development (at approximately 5 to 7 weeks). In interstitial ectopic pregnancies, however, the gestational sac can be identified that is separate from the decidualized endometrium. It may sometimes be difficult to distinguish a cornual ectopic pregnancy that is very eccen-

trically located within the uterus from one located within the isthmic portion of the tube. The myometrium surrounding a cornual ectopic pregnancy is typically abnormally thin (less than 5 mm).

Some have described the "interstitial line" sign as helpful in the sonographic diagnosis of an interstitial pregnancy. This sign describes a linear echogenic interface in the uterine cornu that delineates the cornu. The proximity of the gestational sac relative to this interface establishes the diagnosis of an interstitial ectopic pregnancy.[31]

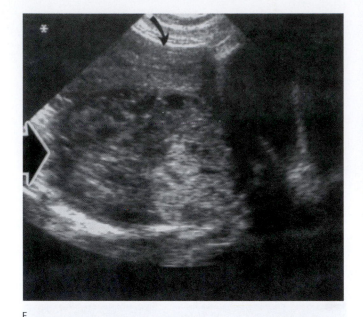

E

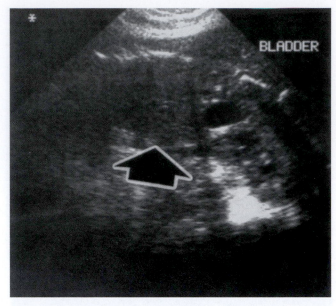

F

G

Figure 6–9. *(continued)* **(E)** Longitudinal TAS showing a hydropic placenta *(large arrow)* posterior to a nongravid uterus *(curved arrow).* **(F)** Fetus in **E** was in right upper quadrant. **(G)** Transverse TAS of 24-week fetus was found to be surrounded by ovarian tissue. Fetal head (★) and cervical spine are shown. *(Figure continued.)*

Another condition that can be confused with an interstitial ectopic pregnancy is an early intrauterine pregnancy in a bicornuate uterus. Transvaginal sonography is particularly helpful in establishing the presence of two endometrial lumina in patients with a bicornuate uterus. Color Doppler sonography can also be helpful in delineating the arcuate vessels within the outer myometrium of the two horns.

Cervical ectopic pregnancies appear as gestational sacs that are abnormally low within the uterus. These can be mimicked by nonviable pregnancies that are in the process of aborting.

Abdominal pregnancies result from abortion or tubal rupture with subsequent fixation of the decidua onto bowel, omentum, or mesentery. These types of ectopic pregnancy

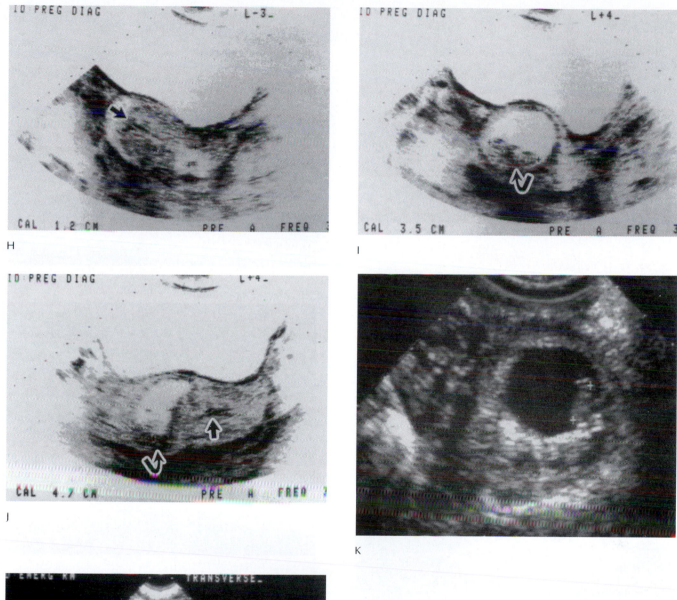

Figure 6–9. *(continued)* **(H, I)** Longitudinal and transverse; **(J)** TAS (black-on-white format) showing an interstitial ectopic pregnancy at 8 weeks. The endometrial lumen *(straight arrow)* is nondistended by the interstitial ectopic gestational sac *(curved arrow). (Courtesy of Grady Stewart, MD.)* **(K)** TVS of left ovarian ectopic pregnancy. An embryo can be identified within the left ovary. **(L)** Transverse TAS of intrauterine pregnancy and ruptured ectopic pregnancy appearing as localized collection of blood in cul-de-sac (⋆). *(Figure continued.)*

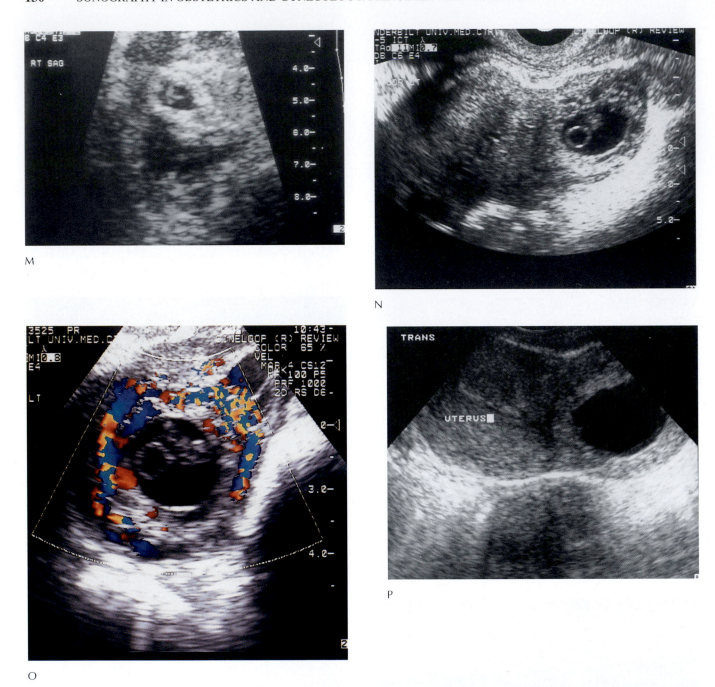

Figure 6–9. *(continued)* **(M)** Cornual ectopic pregnancy showing a large area of subchorionic hemorrhage. **(N)** TVS of what appeared to be an interstitial ectopic pregnancy. At surgery this ectopic pregnancy was within the isthmic portion of the tube. **(O)** TV-CDS of patient in **N** showing vascular ring around the ectopic pregnancy. **(P)** TVS showing cornual ectopic pregnancy. The gestational sac is very eccentrically located. *(Courtesy of G. Sacks, MD.)*

may be difficult to recognize because the uterine wall surrounding some intrauterine pregnancies is so thin. Clues to this disorder include abnormal fetal lie, oligohydramnios, and intraperitoneal fluid. To confirm an intraabdominal pregnancy, one should endeavor to delineate the uterus as a separate structure from the fetus and placenta. In some cases,

magnetic resonance imaging can be useful in assessing the uterus by demonstrating its relation to the cervix and myometrium of the uterus.

Chronic ectopic pregnancies result from rupture of the tube with subsequent hematoma formation. The hematoma may also incite an inflammatory reaction with development

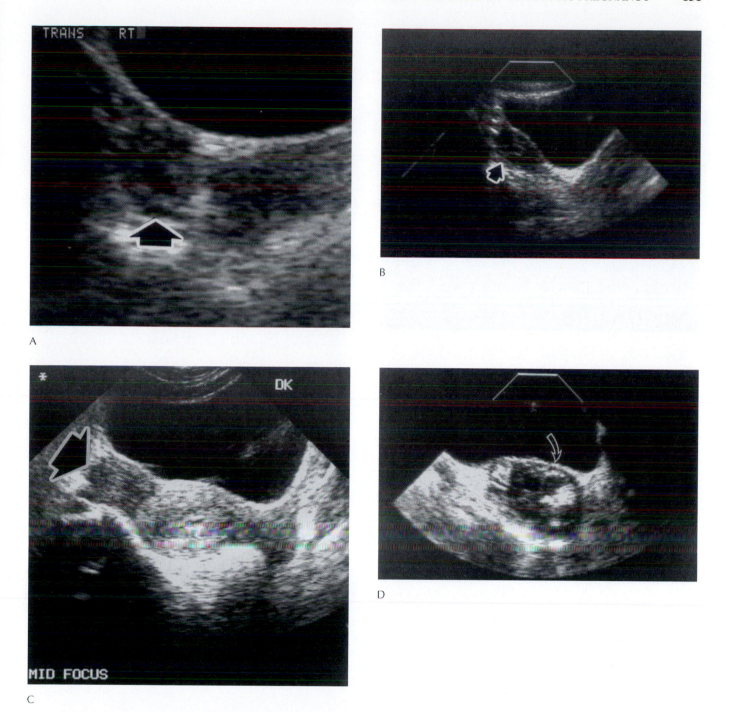

Figure 6–10. Other adnexal masses and conditions. **(A)** Magnified transverse TAS of corpus luteum *(arrow)* within right ovary having similar appearance to ectopic pregnancy. Hypoechoic center is surrounded by echogenic rim of tissue. **(B)** Longitudinal TAS of group of endometriomas *(arrow)* that appear similar to an ectopic pregnancy. **(C)** Longitudinal TAS of pedunculated fibroid *(arrow)* adjacent to uterine fundus, simulating appearance of ectopic pregnancy. Patient's pregnancy test was positive even though intrauterine gestation could not be depicted with TAS. **(D)** Transverse TAS of patient with unruptured ectopic pregnancy adjacent to dermoid cyst. *(Figure continued.)*

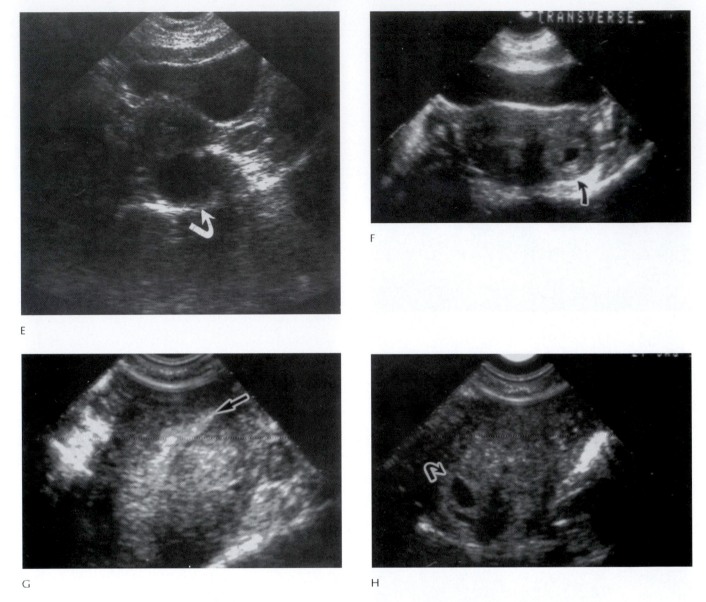

Figure 6–10. *(continued)* **(E)** Transverse TAS of patient with cystic adnexal mass and positive pregnancy test. At surgery, ectopic pregnancy was found next to a cystadenoma of left ovary *(curved arrow)*. **(F)** Transverse TAS showing eccentrically located gestational sac *(curved arrow)*. **(G)** TV sonogram showing thickened endometrium *(arrow)* of nongravid horn of a bicornuate uterus. **(H)** Left horn contained a gestational sac *(curved arrow)*. **E, F, G** of same patient. *(Figure continued.)*

of adhesions. These masses typically appear as rounded solid structures. They can be surrounded by a hydrosalpinx or pyosalpinx. In some cases of chronic ectopic pregnancy, the trophoblasts will be necrotic and the β-hCG low or absent.

Although sonographic documentation of an intrauterine pregnancy virtually excludes the possibility of an ectopic pregnancy, one should not totally disregard the possibility of

the latter, particularly in a patient who has undergone ovulation induction.[32] The incidence of combined intrauterine and extrauterine pregnancy is low and has been reported to be between 1 in 2000 to 1 in 30,000 deliveries.[33] The incidence of heterotopic pregnancy is greatest in women who have been treated with ovulation induction.

Ectopic pregnancy can coexist with other adnexal masses. For example, we have examined patients in whom

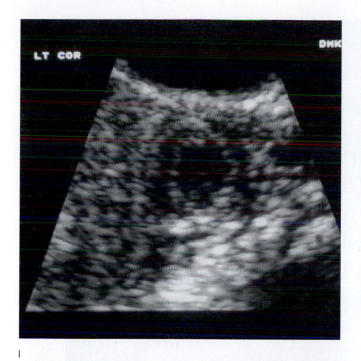

I

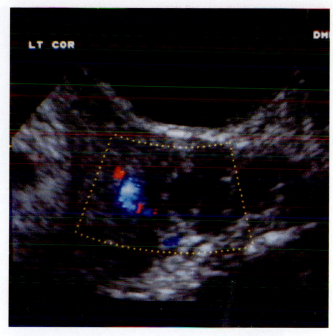

J

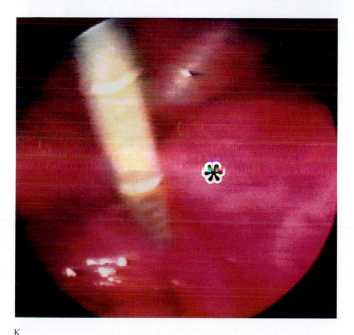

K

Figure 6–10. *(continued)* **(I)** Magnified TVS showing a rounded mass near left cornu. **(J)** TV-CDS of same patient in **J** showing rounded mass near left cornu coexisting with a 6-week intrauterine pregnancy. Only a portion of the intrauterine sac is seen. **(K)** Photograph taken during laparoscopy showing round ligament fibroma (★). *(Courtesy of Barbara Nylander, MD.) (Figure continued.)*

an ectopic pregnancy was found coexisting with a dermoid cyst, ovarian cystadenoma, and fibroids. Whether or not the presence of these masses contributed to the chance of developing an ectopic pregnancy is only speculative. The presence of these masses, however, may alter the angle and course of the tube.

OTHER ADNEXAL MASSES

Transvaginal sonography is particularly helpful in distinguishing corpus luteum that occurs within the ovary from ectopic pregnancies (Fig. 6–10). In general, a corpus luteum appears as a hypoechoic area within the ovary. Corpora lutea

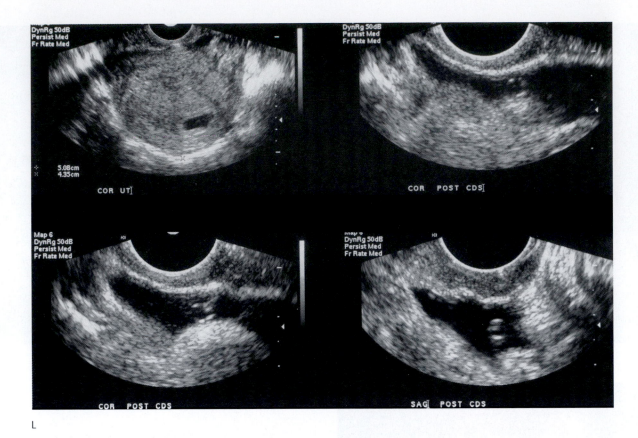

L

Figure 6–10. *(continued)* **(L)** Composite TVS showing fluid in cul-de-sac surrounding a rounded structure. This most likely represented a cyst of Morgangi that arose from the frimbriated end of the tube. The presence of fluid surrounding it allowed its sonographic delineation. Initially, a yolk sac was considered, but a cyst of Morgangi was considered possible although not confirmed at surgery, because the patient had an ongoing pregnancy.

typically tend to be eccentrically located within the ovary, although this is not an absolute criterion for their recognition (Fig. 6–11). On TV-CDS low-impedance, high-diastolic flow is typically seen. A hydrosalpinx can be differentiated from an ectopic pregnancy by delineation of this shape and orientation. It may be difficult in some cases of tubo-ovarian abscess ectopic pregnancy to determine which mass actually represents the ectopic pregnancy.

TREATMENT IMPLICATIONS

Medical treatment of ectopic pregnancies has become standard care in certain patients.[35] A single intramuscular injection of 50 mg of methotrexate has been found to be efficacious in women with an ectopic pregnancy that is smaller than 3 cm, with no embryonic cardiac activity, and less than 50 cc of intraperitoneal fluid.[36]

Patients treated with methotrexate are usually asked to visit the outpatient department for a sonogram and serum hCG level every 2 to 3 days until the hCG levels fall below 10 IU/mL.

In the study by Ylostalo, expectant management was studied in 83 patients, or 26% of all ectopic pregnancies in their clinic. Sixty-nine percent had spontaneous resolution,[37] but 18% required surgical intervention because of worsening clinical symptoms and a rise in hCG.

Color Doppler sonography is useful in determining response to medical treatment. Most responsive ectopic pregnancies demonstrate an increase in size and vascularity with a decrease in β-hCG.[38,39] Others have reported similar findings when the ectopic pregnancy itself was injected under sonographic guidance.[40]

MEDICOLEGAL CONSIDERATIONS

For medicolegal purposes, the sonologist should be aware that in up to 20% of proven ectopic pregnancies the sonographic appearance of uterus and adnexa were normal with

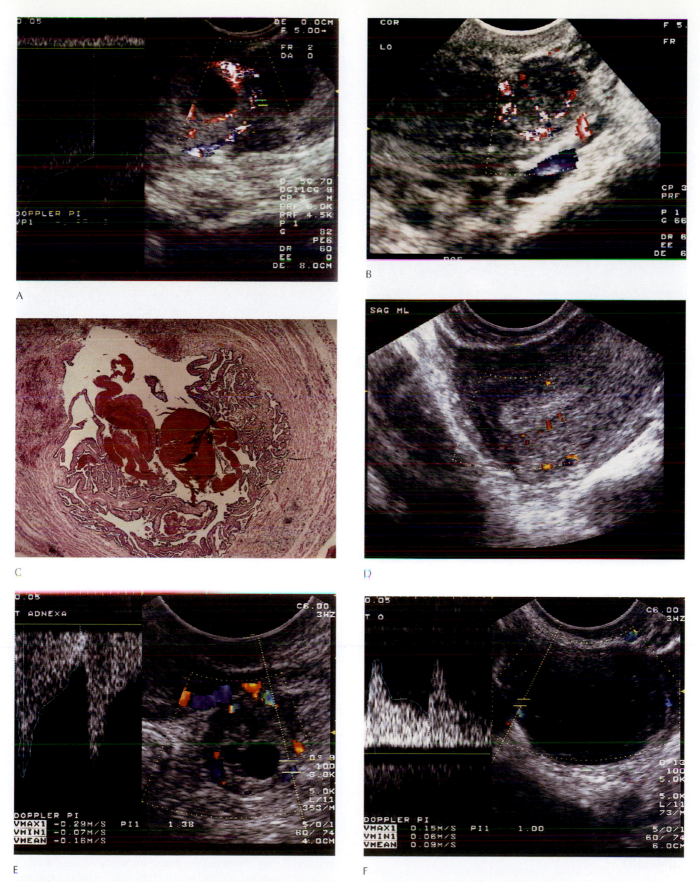

Figure 6–11. TV-CDS of ectopic pregnancy. **(A)** TVS showing no definite adnexal mass. **(B)** TV-CDS of patient in **A** showing two vascular masses, one representing the corpus luteum and the smaller one, an unruptured ectopic pregnancy. **(C)** Low-power photomicrograph of the unruptured ectopic pregnancy in **A** and **B**. Some of the supplying vessels are seen within the tubal muscle layers. **(D)** TVS of unruptured ectopic pregnancy showing "cool" uterine flow. **(E)** Same patient as in **D** showing a vascular right adnexal ring. **(F)** A hemorrhagic corpus luteum. **D, E, F** of same patient. *(Figure continued.)*

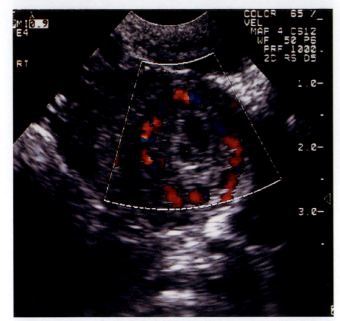

G

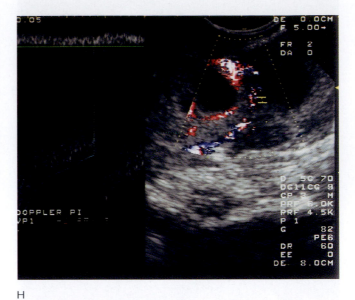

H

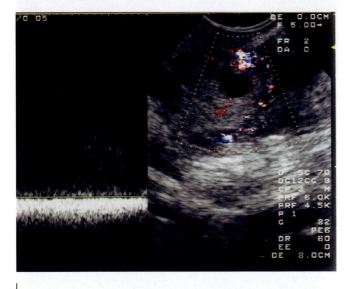

I

Figure 6–11. *(continued)* **(G)** A vascular corpus luteum mimicking the TV-CDS finding of an ectopic pregnancy. **(H, I)** Similarity of corpus luteum and ectopic flow in a patient with two cul-de-sac masses. **H** shows flow within the wall of a corpus luteum. **(I)** Flow in the ectopic pregnancy.

TAS.[34] Even with TVS with or without TV-CDS some cases may not demonstrate definitive findings. Therefore, it may be advisable in some cases where sonographic findings are inconclusive to incorporate a statement in the official report such as the following: "Although the possibility of an ectopic pregnancy is unlikely, it cannot be totally excluded."[41]

SUMMARY

In conclusion, it is believed that the use of TAS or TVS and TV-CDS, or both, with sensitive pregnancy tests can result in a high degree of accuracy in the detection or exclusion of an extrauterine pregnancy. In most cases, it is important to cor-relate the sonographic findings with the β-hCG level. With TVS, most normal intrauterine pregnancies will demonstrate a gestational sac at a level of 800 to 1000 mIU/mL (Second International Standard).[42] In other words, if an intrauterine gestational sac cannot be identified when the β-hCG is above this value, an ectopic pregnancy should be considered to be of increased likelihood.[27] It is anticipated that earlier diagnosis of ectopic pregnancy will result in better clinical outcomes because it may improve the chance for successful medical or surgical treatment. Transvaginal CDS may improve outcome of ectopic pregnancies by tailoring medical or surgical treatment based on the presence or absence of blood flow within the choriodecidua or presence or absence of embryonic or fetal heart motion (Fig. 6–12).

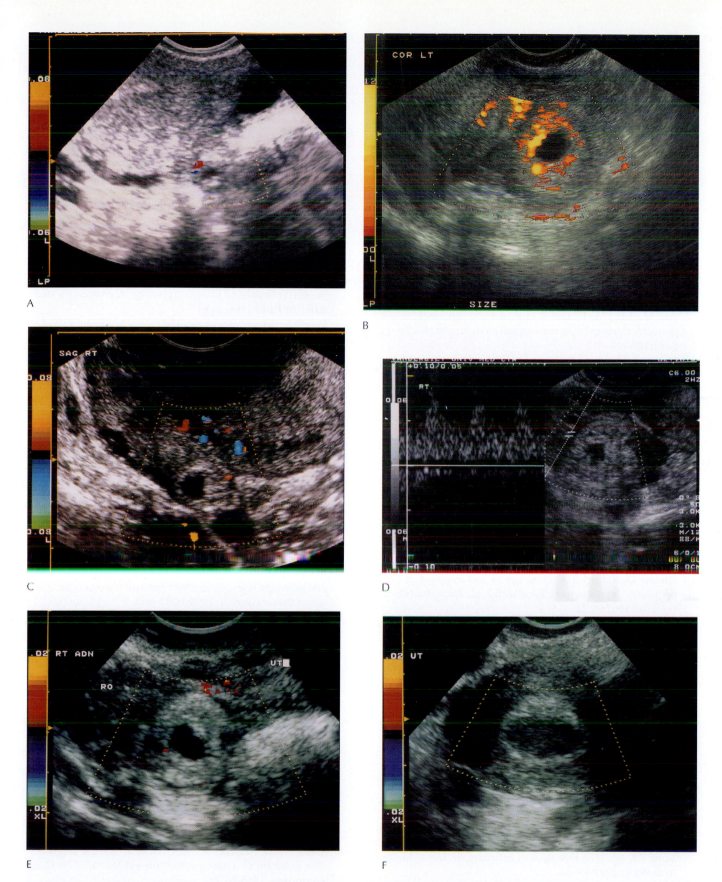

Figure 6–12. TV-CDS depiction of vascularity of ectopic pregnancy. **(A)** Relatively hypovascular ectopic pregnancy showing blood flow as a focal area. **(B)** Hypervascular ectopic pregnancy with flow surrounding the sac. **(C)** Avascular ectopic pregnancy during tubal abortion. **(D)** Hypervascular ectopic pregnancy with low-impedance, high-velocity flow within the tubal wall. **(E, F)** Same patient as in **D** 1 week after methotrexate treatment showing decreased vascularity around the ectopic pregnancy **(E)** and hematometria **(F)**.

REFERENCES

1. Pellerito JS, Taylor KJW, Quedens-Case C, et al. Ectopic pregnancy: Evaluation with endovaginal color flow imaging. *Radiology.* 1992;183:407–411.

2. Emerson DS, Cartier MS, Altieri LA, et al. Diagnostic efficacy of endovaginal color Doppler flow imaging in an ectopic pregnancy screening program. *Radiology.* 1992;183:413–420.

3. Weckstein LN, Boucher AR, Tucker H, et al. Accurate diagnosis of early ectopic pregnancy. *Obstet Gynecol.* 1985;65:393–397.

4. Laing F. Ectopic pregnancy. In: Ferrucci J, ed. *Diagnostic Imaging.* Philadelphia: Lippincott; 1988:1.

5. Tancer M, Delke L, Veridiano N. A fifteen year experience with ectopic pregnancy. *Surg Gynecol Obstet.* 1981;152:179.

6. Breen J. A 21-year survey of 654 ectopic pregnancies. *Am J Obstet Gynecol.* 1970;106:1004.

7. Atri M, Bret PM, Tulandi T, et al. Ectopic pregnancy: Evolution after treatment with transvaginal methotrexate. *Radiology.* 1992;185:749–753.

8. Shiono P, Harlap S. Pellegrin F. Ectopic pregnancies: Rising incidence rates in northern California. *Am J Public Health.* 1983;72:173.

9. Rubin G, Peterson H, Dorfman S, et al. Ectopic pregnancy in the United States 1970 through 1978. *JAMA.* 1983;249:1725.

10. Marchbanks PA, Annegers JF, Coulam CB, et al. Risk factors for ectopic pregnancy: A population-based study. *JAMA.* 1988;259:1823–1827.

11. Taylor RN. Ectopic pregnancy and reproductive technology. *JAMA.* 1988;259:1862–1864.

12. Laing F, Jeffrey R. Ultrasound evaluation of ectopic pregnancy. *Radiol Clin North Am.* 982;20:383.

13. Hershlag A, Diamond MP, DeCherney AH. Tubal physiology: An appraisal. *J Gynecol Surg.* 1989;5:3–25.

14. Kleiner G, Roberts T. Current factors and causation of tubal pregnancy: A prospective clinical pathologic study. *Am J Obstet Gynecol.* 1967;99:21.

15. Doyle MB, DeCherney AH, Diamond MP. Epidemiology and etiology of ectopic pregnancy. *Obstet Gynecol Clin North Am.* 1991;18:1–17.

16. Meyer WR, DeCherney AH, Diamond MP. Tubal ectopic pregnancy: Contemporary diagnosis, treatment, and reproductive potential. *J Gynecol Surg.* 1989;5:343–352.

17. Ackerman R, Deutsch S, Krumholtz B. Levels of human chorionic gonadotropin in unruptured and ruptured ectopic pregnancy. *Obstet Gynecol.* 1982;60:13.

18. Cartwright P, Vaughn W, Tuttle D. Culdocentesis and ectopic pregnancy. *J Reprod Med.* 1984;29:88.

19. Chen PC, Sickler GK, Dubinsky TJ, et al. Sonographic detection of echogenic fluid and correlation with culdocentesis in the evaluation of ectopic pregnancy. *AJR.* 1998;170:1299–1302.

20. Diamond MP. Review of endoscopic surgical procedures in treatment of the infertile woman. In: Mishell DR, Paulsen CA, Lobo RA, eds. *The Year Book of Infertility.* St. Louis: Mosby-Year Book; 1991;45–64.

21. Bedi DG, Fagan CJ, Nocera RM. Chronic ectopic pregnancy. *J Ultrasound Med.* 1984;3:347–352.

22. Stanley R, Horger J, Fagan C, et al. Sonographic findings in abdominal pregnancies. *AJR.* 1986;147:1043.

23. Udoji WC, Victory DF, Cartwright PS, et al. Diagnostic problems with variant forms of human chorionic gonadotropin. *Lab Med.* 1998;29:243–246.

24. Wiser-Estin M, DeCherney AH, Diamond MP. Perils in the differentiation of a viable intrauterine pregnancy (IUP) from an ectopic eccyesis. *Gynecol Endoscopy.* 1993;2:223–226.

25. Cartwright P, DiPietro D. Ectopic pregnancy: Change in serum hCG concentrations. *Obstet Gynecol.* 1984;63:76.

26. Seifer DB, Gutmann JN, Doyle MB, et al. Persistent ectopic pregnancy following laparoscopic linear salpingostomy. *Obstet Gynecol.* 1990;76:1121–1125.

27. Fleischer A, Herbert C, Hill G, et al. Ectopic pregnancy: Features of transvaginal sonography. *Radiology.* 1990;174:375–378.

28. Nyberg DA, Mack LA, Jeffrey RB, et al. Endovaginal sonographic evaluation of ectopic pregnancy: A prospective study. *AJR.* 1987;149:1181–1186.

29. Filly RA: Ectopic pregnancy: The role of sonography. *Radiology.* 1987;162:661–668.

30. Ackerman TE, Levi CS, Lyons EA, et al. Decidual cyst: Endovaginal sonographic sign of ectopic pregnancy. *Radiology.* 1993;189:727–731.

31. Ackerman TE, Levi CS, Dashefsky SM, et al. Interstitial line: Sonographic finding in interstitial (cornual) ectopic pregnancy. *Radiology.* 1993;189:83–87.

32. Yaghoobian J, Pinck RL, Ramanathan K, et al. Sonographic demonstration of simultaneous intrauterine and extrauterine gestation. *J Ultrasound Med.* 1986;5:309–312.

33. Hann LE, Bachmann DL, McArdle CR. Coexistent intrauterine and ectopic pregnancy: A reevaluation. *Radiology.* 1984;152:151.

34. Mahony BS, Filly RA, Nyberg DA, et al. Sonographic evaluation of ectopic pregnancy. *J Ultrasound Med.* 1985;4:221.

35. Cacciatore B, Korhonen J, Stenman UH, et al. Transvaginal sonography and serum hCG in monitoring of presumed ectopic pregnancies selected for expectant management. *Ultrasound Obstet Gynecol.* 1995;5:297–300.

36. Hacket E, Jurkovic E. Ultrasound in the diagnosis and non-surgical management of ectopic pregnancy. In: Jurkovic D, Jauniaux E, eds. *Ultrasound and Early Pregnancy.* London: Parthenon Publishers; 1996;65–80.

37. Ylostalo P, Cacciatore B, Sjoberg J, et al. Expectant management of ectopic pregnancy. *Obstet Gynecol.* 1992;80:345–348.

38. Atri M, Bret PM, Tulandi T, et al. Ectopic pregnancy: Evolution after treatment with transvaginal methotrexate. *Radiology.* 1992;185:749–753.

39. Atri M, Bret PM, Tulandi T. Spontaneous resolution of ectopic pregnancy: Initial appearance and evolution at transvaginal US. *Radiology.* 1993;186:83–86.

40. Tekay A, Martikainen H, Heikkinen H, et al. Disappearance of the trophoblastic blood flow in tubal pregnancy after methotrexate injection. *J Ultrasound Med.* 1993;12:615–618.

41. James AE Jr, Fleischer A, Sacks G, et al. Ectopic pregnancy: The paradigm of a sonographic "missed lesion." *Clin Diagn Ultrasound.* 1986;26:99.

42. Rottem S, Timor-Tritsch IE. Think ectopic. In: Timor-Tritsch IE, Rottem S, eds. *Transvaginal Sonography.* New York: Elsevier; 1988;8:125–141.

7

Fetal Biometry

Philippe Jeanty

IMPORTANCE OF A CRITICAL APPROACH

The literature contains many tables and nomograms that describe the normal growth of various fetal parameters, such as the biparietal diameter, abdominal diameters, femur, and orbits. Some of these tables were established with great care and respect as to basic mathematical principles. Others, however, were prepared in a less careful manner. Deciding which table to use and knowing its limitations are important in everyday practice. For example, using a table whose "confidence limits" were graphically drawn instead of mathematically computed (or worse, a table that does not provide confidence limits) would be difficult to justify should a legal problem arise. The basic principles involved are well established, and the software required for analysis is currently available for most microcomputers. Knowing the basic concepts described in this chapter enables an understanding of the seemingly complicated and esoteric language used in sonographic literature and thereby allows a judgment as to whether or not a study has been performed correctly.

WHY FETAL BIOMETRY?

Before the development of ultrasound, fetal dimensions were measured using radiologic techniques. The development of ultrasound made it possible to measure the bones and soft tissue structures of the fetus faster and more reliably than with x-rays. Fetal growth is so rapid that parameters such as the fetal biparietal diameter (BPD) and femur length change significantly within 1 to 2 weeks. The use of such measurements answers the following questions:

1. What is the age of the fetus?
2. Is the fetus of appropriate size for its age?
3. Are there any malformations?

The first question is crucial in the modern practice of obstetrics and is one of the most frequent reasons for referral in countries where routine scanning is not the practice.

The evaluation of fetal growth and the detection of intrauterine growth retardation are also major concerns because the growth-retarded fetus is at a higher risk of morbidity and mortality.

With the decrease in the traditional causes of perinatal mortality, the detection of congenital malformation has become more important.

PRINCIPLES OF FETAL BIOMETRY

How Are Normal Values Derived?

The normal values (mean, lower, and upper limits of normal) of a given parameter at different gestational ages are defined by measuring that parameter in fetuses of normal patients

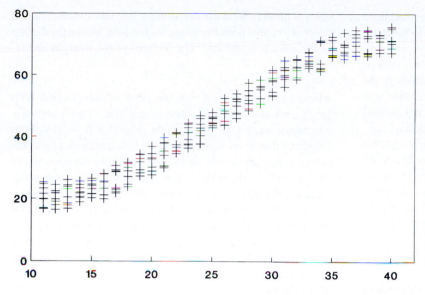

Figure 7–1. Scattergram. Alongside the *X* axis is the independent variable, and alongside the *Y* axis is the dependent variable. Notice that the data are well correlated and well grouped and that an even number of points have been connected for every single gestational age.

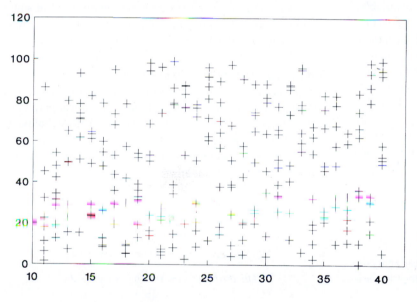

Figure 7–2. In this sample, the data are randomly dispersed. There is no trend, and any value from 0 to 100 can occur at any age. Such a distribution is useless in fetal biometry.

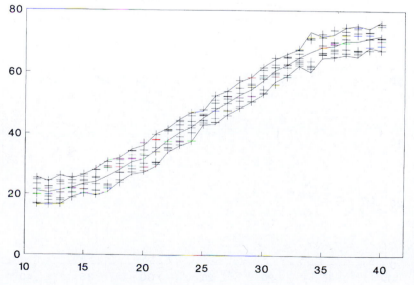

Figure 7–3. The scattergram shown in Figure 7–1 has been further studied, and the mean and confidence limits have been traced. The tracing is irregular and influenced by the variability of the population studied.

sample variability is not taken into account. The procedure that is commonly used consists of fitting a curve to the data.

Curve Fitting. A simple technique to summarize the data of the scattergram is to draw a curve that passes through the mean of the data and to compute the variability around this curve. Curve fitting is done by regression analysis, a statistical tool for evaluating the relation between two variables.

When that relation is known, it is possible to predict values for one variable from the other (e.g., prediction of gestational age from BPD). When two variables are used, one is called the *independent* or *observed variable;* the other is called the *dependent* or *predicted variable.* The independent variable is represented on the *X* axis and the dependent variable is represented on the *Y* axis.

Regression Analysis

The basic principle of regression analysis is to calculate a curve that best describes the relation between two variables (hence, the term *best curve fit*). Although details of the mathematical calculations are beyond the scope of this chapter, it is important to know that the usual procedure to fit a curve is called the *least-squares technique.* That is, a curve is proposed and the vertical distance between each datum point and the curve is measured (Fig. 7–4). The sum of these distances is then taken. (Because some data will be above the curve and some below, taking the simple distances would not be sufficient. The sum of the distances from the "data above" would end up canceling out the sum of the distances from the "data below.") By squaring these distances, their signs are removed. Either a straight or a curved line can be used; accordingly, the regression analysis is called a *linear* or *curvilinear polynomial.*

Linear Regression Analysis. In linear regression analysis, the best straight line that fits the relation between the two variables is plotted. Because the straight line has a mathematical description, it is possible to use its formula for the prediction of the unknown variable. The formula of the straight line is

$$y = a + xb$$

where *a* is the value of *y* at the point of intersection with the *X* axis and *b* is the slope of the line. This curve has one major advantage over all the others: it is so simple to calculate that even some wristwatch calculators can compute a linear regression from a data sample. Linear regression is appropriate in the following situations: (1) for small samples, (2) when the variability of the parameter is large, and (3) when the accuracy of the prediction is not crucial (because it is a preliminary study or because variations from normal are considerably larger than the imprecision of the measurement). Linear regression analysis is not very powerful for accurate prediction because of the tendency to average the raw data.

Although linear regression is frequently used in sonographic literature, most biologic phenomena (e.g., fetal growth) are better described by curvilinear equations.

Curvilinear Polynomial Regression Analysis. When the sample is large (i.e., more than 150 data points obtained over 20 weeks or more), it is possible to fit a curvilinear graph that better describes the evolution of the data. This technique is called *polynomial regression analysis.*

Polynomial regressions are described by mathematical formulas called *polynomial equations.* These are of different orders, depending on the highest power to which the independent variable is raised. For example:

First order: $y = a + bx$

Second order: $y = a + bx + cx^2$

Third order: $y = a + bx + cx^2 + dx^3$

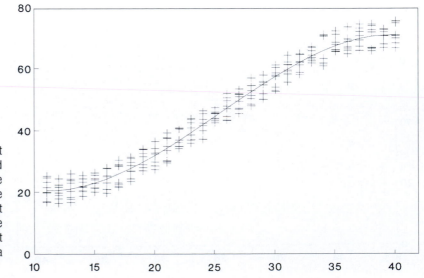

Figure 7–4. A curve has been fitted onto the dataset by calculating the distance between each point and the curve and taking the sum of the square of these distances. Multiple equations can be fitted on the given dataset. The difference among equations is that their fit is more or less appropriate. Some of these equations probably do not fit the earliest or latest portion of the dataset, although they usually have a good representation in the middle portion.

The higher the order of the polynomial equation, the better it describes the data. The ultimate goal of such an approach would be to fit a curve that passes through each point. It can be demonstrated mathematically that such a curve would have an order that is equivalent to the number of points of the sample minus 1. Obviously, such a high-order equation would make computation impractical and would no longer summarize the data.

In practice, the lowest-order polynomial equation that summarizes the data is selected. The selection is made by comparing the coefficients of correlation of the different order polynomial equations for the same data.

Coefficients of Correlation and of Determination. The quality of the fit of the equation is measured by the coefficient of multiple correlation, R, or by the square of this value (the coefficient of determination, R^2). The better the correlation, the closer these coefficients will be to 1. If there is a perfect correlation between the two variables, all the points in the scattergram will be on the regression line. This rarely occurs, however, and it is more likely that some points will be outside the regression line. An R value of 0 indicates that there is no relation between the two variables. Parameters that correlate very well have some R^2 values in the 0.90 to 0.99 range. After the second or third order, the curves will usually demonstrate R^2 values close to each other (Fig. 7–5). Among the curves with a high R value, the most appropriate one is the curve with the lowest order. To discriminate among these curves another test, the F test, is needed.

The F Test. With an increase in the order of polynomial equations, the coefficients (b, c, and d in the above equations) that multiply the independent variable (x in the above equations) become smaller. At high orders, the power by which the in-dependent variable is raised results in values that are very large (40 weeks raised to the third power is 64,000). To compensate, the coefficient must be very small; otherwise, the parameter would be immense. The coefficients may be so small that they are no longer different from 0. In that case, the term does not add precision to the equation and should be eliminated. The F test is a variant of the T test designed to test the hypothesis that the coefficients (b, c, d, ..., n) of the equations are different from 0. This test allows one to ascertain whether or not going to a higher-order equation adds coefficients that are significant without unnecessarily complicating the equation.

Prediction from Equations

The purpose of fetal biometry is to predict information concerning a fetus and then verify how closely that fetus conforms to the predictions. The reference parameter represented on the X axis of graphs, or at the extreme left column of nomograms (e.g., the gestational age), is called the *observed value*. The Y axis value is called the *predicted value*. A common mistake consists of using the predicted value to obtain the observed value. For example, the BPD is measured and read from right to left to the gestational age column to obtain the age. This "two-directional" reading is mathematically incorrect. Among other reasons, the confidence limits will be expressed in the wrong scale (or be impossible to find). It appears a bit confusing that, when data are collected, the relation between the observed variable and the predicted variable is different from that between the predicted variable and the observed variable! One tends to assume that if a BPD of 43 mm corresponds to a gestational age of 19 weeks, then for 19 weeks the mean BPD would be 43 mm. The prediction is, in fact, 46 mm (see Table 7–2) because of the sum-of-squares technique described above.

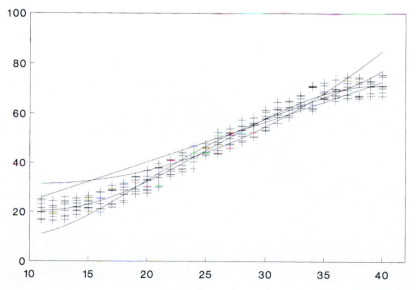

Figure 7–5. Multiple equations can be fitted on the given dataset. The difference among equations is that their fit is more or less appropriate. Some of these equations probably do not fit the earliest or latest portion of the dataset, although they usually have a good representation in the middle portion.

How to Compute the Confidence Limits. Besides being able to describe the mean growth, one must be able to answer the question, How far from the mean can an individual be and still be considered normal? Or, in statistical terms, What is the dispersion around the mean? The statistical parameter that measures this dispersion is the *standard deviation*. The smaller the standard deviation, the less the variability of the sample around the mean. The standard deviation is also used to define the statistical limits of normality. These intervals are called *confidence limits* (Fig. 7–6). Traditionally, the confidence limits are set at the 5th and 95th percentiles (±1.66 standard deviations) or at the 1st and 99th percentiles (±2.38 standard deviations). Two standard deviations correspond to 95% of the population, 2.5% being below the normal limits and 2.5% being above. Outside the lowest and highest percentiles, the parameter is considered abnormal. With the commonly used 5th and 95th percentiles, it is important to remember that 10% of patients tested will be outside normal limits. This does not mean, however, that the patient is abnormal. The predictive value of a given equation is greater if the standard deviation does not change significantly with variations of the observed value. The absence of variation of the standard deviation can be investigated by the Bartlett or Levene test.

Summary

When selecting an equation for your practice, choose one derived from a study based on a large sample of data covering a wide range of values for the independent variable. It should adequately represent the extremes of the curve. If there are many equations that fulfill these criteria, select the curve based on longitudinal rather than on cross-sectional studies. Be careful to check that the study spans the range of gestational age being covered. For example, some studies describe the growth of the femur from 12 to 22 weeks; using these studies outside those limits would be inaccurate.

Do not use the same table to determine gestational age from a parameter and to test the normality of this parameter against the gestational age.

The equations that follow are those of Jeanty and associates except when specified. The rationale for selection of the curve is expressed above. It is beyond the scope of this chapter to discuss all the curves that have been published. The guidelines should help the reader to decide which curves are correct. "Composite" curves, which average excellent curves with less optimal ones, should be avoided.

In all nomograms presented, the observed value is listed in the left column and the predicted value in the right column. A special effort toward standardization has been made. All measurements are expressed in the same units: millimeters, weeks plus days from the first day of the LMP, and grams.

ESTIMATION OF GESTATIONAL AGE

Definition

Different ways of estimating the duration of pregnancy can be used. The conceptual age is calculated from ovulation. The menstrual age is calculated from the first day of the LMP. I use the gestational age, which is calculated from theoretical time of ovulation, plus 2 weeks. This has the advantage over menstrual age of eliminating the problems associated with oligomenorrhea and delayed ovulation.

The weeks are always counted as completed weeks, not as current weeks. A patient whose LMP started on January 1 therefore will be in her fourth week on February 1.

Parameters Proposed for the Assessment of Gestational Age

In all the tables in this section, gestational age is expressed in weeks and days from the (theoretical) onset of the normal

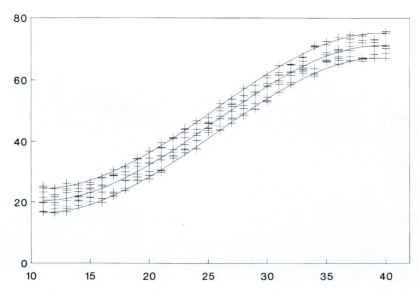

Figure 7–6. The curve and the confidence limit have been placed. Confidence limits are usually selected at the 5th and 95th percentiles.

menstrual period (conception date minus 15 days). Tenths of weeks are not used to avoid difficulties in conversion to days. All measurements are expressed in millimeters instead of centimeters to be consistent with the International System of Units in which secondary units are related to the primary unit by 10 raised to the power of 3 (thousand, million, billion, thousandth, micro, pico, and so forth) and in which the use of centimeters is not recommended.[1]

The parameters proposed to establish gestational age are detailed below.

Crown–Rump Length. The crown–rump length (CRL) (Table 7–1) is the longest demonstrable length of the embryo or fetus, excluding the limbs and yolk sac.[2] The reason for the high accuracy of the CRL is the excellent correlation between length and age in early pregnancy when growth is rapid and minimally affected by pathologic disorders. Even if differences do occur during that time, they are too small to be detected by ultrasound. Although originally described with static scanners, CRL measurement is much faster and just as reliable when obtained in real time. In a scan that demonstrates a longitudinal section of the fetus, the calipers should be placed at the outer edge of the cephalic pole and the outer edge of the fetal rump (Fig. 7–7). The limbs and yolk sac should not be included (Fig. 7–8). The average of three measurements should be used; it is predictive of menstrual age with an error of 3 days (90% confidence limits) from 7 to 10 weeks.

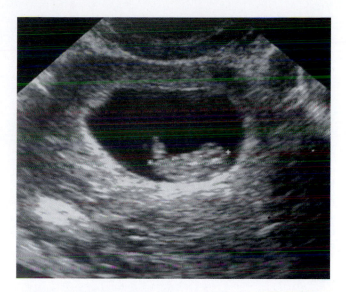

Figure 7–7. Crown–rump length is measured from the top of the head to the outer edge of the fetal rump.

As growth progresses, however, the curvature of the fetus changes and the linear measurements that can be obtained with the calipers are less accurate. The error increases to 5 days between 10 and 14 weeks of gestation.

Biparietal Diameter. Historically, BPD (Table 7–2) was the first parameter used to assess gestational age. Its accuracy is

TABLE 7–1. ASSESSMENT OF THE GESTATIONAL AGE FROM THE CROWN–RUMP LENGTH

	Gestational Age				Gestational Age		
	Percentile				Percentile		
mm	5th	50th	95th	mm	5th	50th	95th
10	6 + 5	7 + 3	8	30	9 + 5	10 + 2	11
11	6 + 6	7 + 4	8 + 2	31	9 + 5	10 + 3	11 + 1
12	7 + 1	7 + 5	8 + 3	32	9 + 6	10 + 4	11 + 2
13	7 + 2	8	8 + 4	33	10	10 + 5	11 + 2
14	7 + 3	8 + 4	8 + 6	34	10 + 1	10 + 6	11 + 3
15	7 + 4	8 + 2	9	35	10 + 2	10 + 6	11 + 4
16	7 + 5	8 + 3	9 + 1	36	10 + 2	11	11 + 5
17	8	8 + 4	9 + 2	37	10 + 3	11 + 1	11 + 6
18	8 + 1	8 + 5	9 + 3	38	10 + 4	11 + 2	11 + 6
19	8 + 2	8 + 6	9 + 4	39	10 + 5	11 + 2	12
20	8 + 3	9	9 + 5	40	10 + 5	11 + 3	12 + 1
21	8 + 4	9 + 1	9 + 6	41	10 + 6	11 + 4	12 + 1
22	8 + 5	9 + 2	10	42	11	11 + 4	12 + 2
23	8 + 6	9 + 3	10 + 1	43	11	11 + 5	12 + 3
24	8 + 6	9 + 4	10 + 2	44	11 + 1	11 + 6	12 + 3
25	9	9 + 5	10 + 3	45	11 + 2	11 + 6	12 + 4
26	9 + 1	9 + 6	10 + 4	46	11 + 2	12	12 + 5
27	9 + 2	10	10 + 5	47	11 + 3	12 + 1	12 + 5
28	9 + 3	10 + 1	10 + 5	48	11 + 4	12 + 1	12 + 6
29	9 + 4	10 + 2	10 + 6	49	11 + 4	12 + 2	13

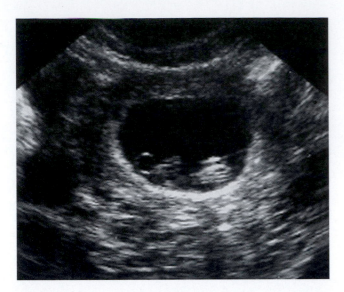

Figure 7–8. One should be careful not to include the yolk sac in the measurement of the crown–rump length.

greatest between 12 and 28 weeks. The consensus that has been reached is to measure the BPD at the level of the thalami (Fig. 7–9). Measurement rostral to the thalami (below the cerebral peduncles) may result in underestimation of the BPD and, consequently, of the gestational age. Biparietal diameter charts are based on measurement from the outer table of the proximal skull to the inner table of the distal skull,[3,4] corresponding to the "leading edge to leading edge" measurement of the A-mode technique. Although the plane of largest BPD may change with the gestational age (and move slightly rostrally), using the same landmark throughout the pregnancy is preferred to avoid unnecessary confusion. It is ill advised to change the plane in late pregnancy because the reference charts were established with the fixed plane described above.

The fetal head can occasionally be flattened and elongated (dolichocephaly) and the BPD thereby artificially decreased (Fig. 7–10). To check for this, the cephalic index (CI) should be obtained. The CI is the ratio of the BPD divided by

TABLE 7–2. ASSESSMENT OF THE GESTATIONAL AGE FROM THE BIPARIETAL DIAMETER

| | Gestational Age | | | | Gestational Age | | | | Gestational Age | | |
| | Percentile | | | | Percentile | | | | Percentile | | |
mm	5th	50th	95th	mm	5th	50th	95th	mm	5th	50th	95th
10	7	10 + 1	13 + 1	40	14 + 2	17 + 3	20 + 3	70	24 + 3	27 + 3	30 + 4
11	7 + 2	10 + 2	13 + 3	41	14 + 4	17 + 5	20 + 5	71	24 + 6	27 + 6	30 + 6
12	7 + 3	10 + 4	13 + 4	42	14 + 6	18	21	72	25 + 1	28 + 2	31 + 2
13	7 + 5	10 + 5	13 + 5	43	15 + 1	18 + 2	21 + 2	73	25 + 4	28 + 5	31 + 5
14	7 + 6	10 + 6	14	44	15 + 3	18 + 4	21 + 4	74	26	29	32 + 1
15	8 + 1	11 + 1	14 + 1	45	15 + 6	18 + 6	21 + 6	75	26 + 3	29 + 3	32 + 4
16	8 + 2	11 + 2	14 + 3	46	16 + 1	19 + 1	22 + 1	76	26 + 6	29 + 6	32 + 6
17	8 + 4	11 + 4	14 + 4	47	16 + 3	19 + 3	22 + 4	77	27 + 1	30 + 2	33 + 2
18	8 + 5	11 + 5	14 + 6	48	16 + 5	19 + 5	22 + 6	78	27 + 4	30 + 5	33 + 5
19	9	12	15	49	17	20 + 1	23 + 1	79	28	31 + 1	34 + 1
20	9 + 1	12 + 2	15 + 2	50	17 + 3	20 + 3	23 + 3	80	28 + 3	31 + 3	34 + 4
21	9 + 3	12 + 3	15 + 3	51	17 + 5	20 + 5	23 + 6	81	28 + 6	31 + 6	35
22	9 + 4	12 + 5	15 + 5	52	18	21	24 + 1	82	29 + 2	32 + 2	35 + 3
23	9 + 6	12 + 6	16	53	18 + 2	21 + 3	24 + 3	83	29 + 5	32 + 5	35 + 6
24	10 + 1	13 + 1	16 + 1	54	18 + 5	21 + 5	24 + 5	84	30 + 1	33 + 1	36 + 2
25	10 + 2	13 + 3	16 + 3	55	19	22	25 + 1	85	30 + 4	33 + 4	36 + 5
26	10 + 4	13 + 4	16 + 5	56	19 + 2	22 + 3	25 + 3	86	31	34	37 + 1
27	10 + 6	13 + 6	17	57	19 + 5	22 + 5	25 + 6	87	31 + 3	34 + 3	37 + 4
28	11	14 + 1	17 + 1	58	20	23 + 1	26 + 1	88	31 + 6	35	38
29	11 + 2	14 + 3	17 + 3	59	20 + 3	23 + 3	26 + 3	89	32 + 2	35 + 3	38 + 3
30	11 + 4	14 + 4	17 + 5	60	20 + 5	23 + 6	26 + 6	90	32 + 5	35 + 6	38 + 6
31	11 + 6	14 + 6	18	61	21 + 1	24 + 1	27 + 1	91	33 + 2	36 + 2	39 + 2
32	12 + 1	15 + 1	18 + 1	62	21 + 3	24 + 4	27 + 4	92	33 + 5	36 + 5	39 + 6
33	12 + 3	15 + 3	18 + 3	63	21 + 6	24 + 6	27 + 6	93	34 + 1	37 + 1	40 + 2
34	12 + 4	15 + 5	18 + 5	64	22 + 1	25 + 2	28 + 2	94	34 + 4	37 + 5	40 + 5
35	12 + 6	16	19	65	22 + 4	25 + 4	28 + 5	95	35	38 + 1	41 + 1
36	13 + 1	16 + 2	19 + 2	66	22 + 6	26	29	96	35 + 4	38 + 4	41 + 4
37	13 + 3	16 + 4	19 + 4	67	23 + 2	26 + 2	29 + 3	97	36	39	42 + 1
38	13 + 5	16 + 6	19 + 6	68	23 + 5	26 + 5	29 + 5	98	36 + 3	39 + 4	42 + 4
39	14	17 + 1	20 + 1	69	24	27 + 1	30 + 1	99	37	40	43

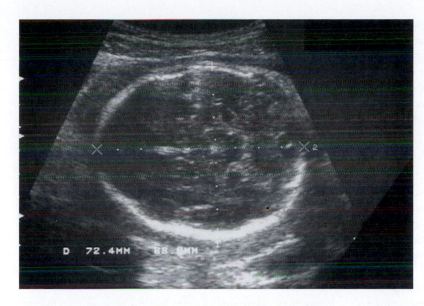

Figure 7–9. Biparietal diameter is measured at the level of the thalamus from the outer to the inner skull.

occipitofrontal diameter (OFD), and its normal range is 0.75 to 0.85. When the CI is close to either end of the confidence limits, the BPD should not be used to assess gestational age.

Doubilet and Greenes correct the BPD when it is deformed.[5] Theirs is a procedure different than the CI. What they have attempted to do is to provide the normal measurement of BPD if the head had not been deformed. They use one of two approaches: either calculate the area of the head and derive the BPD from it or use a circumference correcting the BPD. Although they recommended using the area corrected by BPD, I have been uneasy with that approach because the cross-sectional area of a volume that is compressed is not constant. For example, if you compress a coffee cup between your fingers, the distance between your fingers will decrease, and the cross-sectional area of the cup will decrease; however, the perimeter of the cup remains the same. The same is true of the fetal head. If you press the head side to side, the BPD will decrease, the OFD will increase, and the head area will decrease, but the head perimeter will not change. For these reasons I do not recommend using the error-corrected BPD. If either of these methods is used, the perimeter-corrected BPD would probably be of more value. However, in practice, that would increase the number of calculations needed and would not offer significant advantage over the head perimeter method described below.

Wolfson et al. showed that, in fetuses that have premature rupture of the membranes, the BPD is not very reliable in assessing gestational age.[6] This is no surprise in view of the discussion on dolichocephaly. In fetuses that present for the first time with premature rupture of the membrane, measurement of the femur and humerus should be obtained. An average of these two measurements usually provides the best available assessment.

O'Keeffe et al. conducted a study similar to that of Wolfson et al. O'Keeffe et al. arrived at the same conclusion concerning the use of the BPD and suggested the use of the head perimeter and femur measurements.[7] However, O'Keeffe et al. also suggested the use of the abdomen perimeter. In view of the fact that premature infants are often delayed in growth, the abdomen perimeter should not be used because the abdomen perimeter could be less than expected, resulting in some underestimation of fetal age.

Because shape, growth disturbances, and individual variation affect the size of the head to an increasing degree after 28 weeks of gestation, the BPD should be used with some caution after this point.[8]

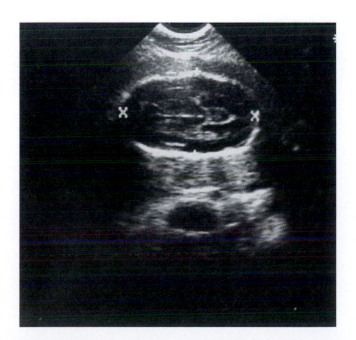

Figure 7–10. Example of dolichocephaly in a fetus that has premature rupture of the membrane.

In the early 1980s, a technique called *growth-adjusted sonographic age* was proposed to correct the gestational age in serially studied fetuses that were suspected of growth disturbances. Although the technique was an excellent idea from a conceptual viewpoint, it was often impractical to use. It has been shown that the technique did not offer any advantage over a single BPD measurement in a population of well-controlled patients.[9]

Head Perimeter. The head perimeter is influenced by growth disorders but to a lesser extent than the BPD. Ott compared the mean error of the head perimeter to the mean error of BPD and found it to be significantly smaller.[10] It is not influenced by dolichocephaly or brachycephaly. The head perimeter is measured in the same plane as the BPD. One should make certain that the longest (anteroposterior) length is obtained, which implies that the cavum pellucidum or the roof of posterior fossa is included in the scan. The head perimeter is either measured with electronic calipers (see Fig. 7–9) or computed by using the formula:

$$\frac{BPD + OFD}{2}\pi \text{ head perimeter} = (BPD + OFD) \times 1.62$$

A nomogram that allows calculation of gestational age from the head perimeter is provided in Table 7–3.

Femur and Humerus Lengths. Femur length (Table 7–4) was originally measured to diagnose limb dwarfism. It was subsequently observed that femur length was an excellent parameter to determine fetal age.[3,11–14] The femur can be measured from 10 weeks onward. The femur is measured from the origin to the distal end of the shaft (Fig. 7–11). The femoral head and distal epiphysis are not included in the measurement. The humerus is measured in the same way (Fig. 7–12). The humerus (Table 7–5) is also commonly measured (see below).

Other Parameters. Crown–rump length, BPD, and femur and humerus lengths are by no means the only parameters useful in estimating gestational age. Among the others that have been proposed are other fetal long bones,[14] binocular distance,[15] head perimeter,[16,17] the abdominal perimeter,[16] clavicle, and the size and shape of the fetal ears.[18] The abdominal perimeter has rapidly been abandoned because it is too sensitive to variations of fetal growth.

Among the other long bones, measurement of the humerus is surely the easiest to obtain and the most reproducible. The tibia comes next; the radius and ulna should be used only when confusing results are obtained from other methods. In practice, the bone-derived gestational ages are averaged and compared with the BPD-derived gestational age. If the difference is greater than 11 days, using the bone-derived gestational age is preferred. Tables 7–5 and 7–6 may

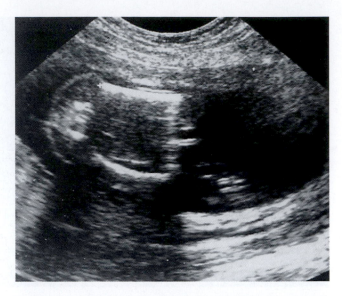

Figure 7–11. Measurement of the femur is obtained from the most proximal portion of the shaft to the distal end. Neither the femoral head nor the distal epiphysis is included. When two femurs are seen in the same section, only the proximal one is measured. Acoustical shadowing from one femur or from other bones can artifactually decrease the length of the other femur.

be used to determine the gestational age from the long bones of the fetus.

The binocular distance is a parameter that has occasionally proven useful. To obtain the right plane, one should start from the conventional section of the BPD and move the transducer caudally until the orbits are visualized. In the correct

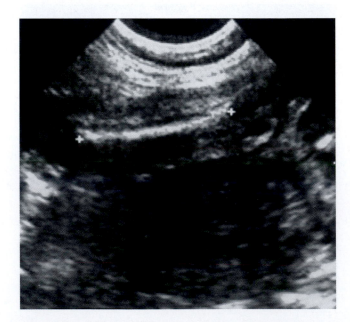

Figure 7–12. Measurement of the humerus is obtained in the same way as measurement of the femur.

TABLE 7–3. ASSESSMENT OF THE GESTATIONAL AGE FROM THE HEAD PERIMETER

mm	Gestational Age Percentile			mm	Gestational Age Percentile			mm	Gestational Age Percentile			mm	Gestational Age Percentile		
	5th	50th	95th		5th	50th	95th		5th	50th	95th		5th	50th	95th
80	10 + 5	12 + 4	14 + 2	160	16 + 5	18 + 3	20 + 1	240	24 + 1	25 + 6	27 + 4	320	33	34 + 6	36 + 4
84	11	12 + 5	14 + 4	164	17	18 + 6	20 + 4	244	24 + 4	26 + 2	28	324	33 + 4	35 + 2	37
88	11 + 2	13	14 + 6	168	17 + 3	19 + 1	20 + 6	248	25	26 + 5	28 + 3	328	34	35 + 5	37 + 4
92	11 + 4	13 + 2	15	172	17 + 5	19 + 3	21 + 2	252	25 + 3	27 + 1	28 + 6	332	34 + 4	36 + 2	38
96	11 + 6	13 + 4	15 + 2	176	18	19 + 6	21 + 4	256	25 + 6	27 + 4	29 + 2	336	35	36 + 5	38 + 4
100	12 + 1	13 + 6	15 + 4	180	18 + 3	20 + 1	21 + 6	260	26 + 1	28	29 + 5	340	35 + 3	37 + 2	39
104	12 + 3	14 + 1	15 + 6	184	18 + 5	20 + 4	22 + 2	264	26 + 4	28 + 3	30 + 1	344	36	37 + 5	39 + 4
108	12 + 5	14 + 3	16 + 1	188	19 + 1	20 + 6	22 + 4	268	27 + 1	28 + 6	30 + 4	348	36 + 4	38 + 2	40
112	13	14 + 5	16 + 3	192	19 + 3	21 + 2	23	272	27 + 4	29 + 2	31	352	37	38 + 5	40 + 4
116	13 + 2	15	16 + 5	196	19 + 6	21 + 4	23 + 3	276	28	29 + 5	31 + 3	356	37 + 4	39 + 2	41
120	13 + 4	15 + 2	17	200	20 + 2	22	23 + 5	280	28 + 3	30 + 1	31 + 6	360	38	39 + 6	41 + 4
124	13 + 6	15 + 4	17 + 2	204	20 + 4	22 + 2	24 + 1	284	28 + 6	30 + 4	32 + 2	364	38 + 4	40 + 2	42 + 1
128	14 + 1	15 + 6	17 + 5	208	21	22 + 5	24 + 3	288	29 + 2	31	32 + 6				
132	14 + 3	16 + 1	18	212	21 + 2	23 + 1	24 + 6	292	29 + 5	31 + 4	33 + 2				
136	14 + 5	16 + 4	18 + 2	216	21 + 5	23 + 3	25 + 2	296	30 + 1	32	33 + 5				
140	15	16 + 6	18 + 4	220	22 + 1	23 + 6	25 + 4	300	30 + 5	32 + 3	34 + 1				
144	15 + 3	17 + 1	18 + 6	224	22 + 4	24 + 2	26	304	31 + 1	32 + 6	34 + 5				
148	15 + 5	17 + 3	19 + 2	228	22 + 6	24 + 5	26 + 3	308	31 + 4	33 + 3	35 + 1				
152	16	17 + 6	19 + 4	232	23 + 2	25	26 + 6	312	32 + 1	33 + 6	35 + 4				
156	16 + 3	18 + 1	19 + 6	236	23 + 5	25 + 3	27 + 2	316	32 + 4	34 + 2	36				

TABLE 7–4. ASSESSMENT OF THE GESTATIONAL AGE FROM THE FEMUR LENGTH

	Gestational Age Percentile				Gestational Age Percentile				Gestational Age Percentile				Gestational Age Percentile		
mm	5th	50th	95th	mm	5th	50th	95th	mm	5th	50th	95th	mm	5th	50th	95th
10	10 + 2	12 + 4	14 + 6	30	17 + 1	19 + 2	21 + 4	50	24 + 5	27	29 + 1	70	33 + 1	35 + 3	37 + 5
11	10 + 4	12 + 6	15 + 1	31	17 + 3	19 + 5	22	51	25 + 1	27 + 2	29 + 4	71	33 + 4	35 + 6	38 + 1
12	11	13 + 1	15 + 3	32	17 + 6	20	22 + 2	52	25 + 4	27 + 5	30	72	34	36 + 2	38 + 4
13	11 + 2	13 + 4	15 + 5	33	18 + 1	20 + 3	22 + 5	53	25 + 6	28 + 1	30 + 3	73	34 + 3	36 + 5	39
14	11 + 4	13 + 6	16 + 1	34	18 + 4	20 + 6	23	54	26 + 2	28 + 4	30 + 6	74	35	37 + 1	39 + 3
15	11 + 6	14 + 1	16 + 3	35	18 + 6	21 + 1	23 + 3	55	26 + 5	29	31 + 2	75	35 + 3	37 + 5	39 + 6
16	12 + 2	14 + 3	16 + 5	36	19 + 2	21 + 4	23 + 5	56	27 + 1	29 + 3	31 + 5	76	35 + 6	38 + 1	40 + 2
17	12 + 4	14 + 6	17 + 1	37	19 + 5	21 + 6	24 + 1	57	27 + 4	29 + 6	32	77	36 + 2	38 + 4	40 + 6
18	12 + 6	15 + 1	17 + 3	38	20	22 + 2	24 + 4	58	28	30 + 2	32 + 3	78	36 + 5	39	41 + 2
19	13 + 2	15 + 4	17 + 5	39	20 + 3	22 + 5	24 + 6	59	28 + 3	30 + 5	32 + 6	79	37 + 2	39 + 3	41 + 5
20	13 + 4	15 + 6	18 + 1	40	20 + 6	23	25 + 2	60	28 + 6	31 + 1	33 + 2	80	37 + 5	40	42 + 1
21	14	16 + 1	18 + 3	41	21 + 1	23 + 3	25 + 5	61	29 + 2	31 + 3	33 + 5				
22	14 + 2	16 + 4	18 + 5	42	21 + 4	23 + 6	26	62	29 + 5	31 + 6	34 + 1				
23	14 + 4	16 + 6	19 + 1	43	22	24 + 1	26 + 3	63	30 + 1	32 + 2	34 + 4				
24	15	17 + 1	19 + 3	44	22 + 2	24 + 4	26 + 6	64	30 + 4	32 + 5	35				
25	15 + 2	17 + 4	19 + 6	45	22 + 5	25	27 + 2	65	31	33 + 1	35 + 3				
26	15 + 5	17 + 6	20 + 1	46	23 + 1	25 + 3	27 + 4	66	31 + 3	33 + 5	35 + 6				
27	16	18 + 2	20 + 4	47	23 + 4	25 + 5	28	67	31 + 6	34 + 1	36 + 2				
28	16 + 3	18 + 4	20 + 6	48	23 + 6	26 + 1	28 + 3	68	32 + 2	34 + 4	36 + 5				
29	16 + 5	19	21 + 2	49	24 + 2	26 + 4	28 + 6	69	32 + 5	35	37 + 1				

TABLE 7–5. ASSESSMENT OF THE GESTATIONAL AGE FROM THE HUMERUS AND ULNA LENGTHS

Humerus

mm	Gestational Age Percentile			mm	Gestational Age Percentile		
	5th	50th	95th		5th	50th	95th
10	9 + 5	12 + 3	15 + 1	40	21 + 3	24 + 2	27
11	10	12 + 5	15 + 4	41	22	24 + 5	27 + 3
12	10 + 2	13 + 1	15 + 6	42	22 + 3	25 + 1	28
13	10 + 5	13 + 3	16 + 1	43	22 + 6	25 + 5	28 + 3
14	11	13 + 5	16 + 4	44	23 + 3	26 + 1	28 + 6
15	11 + 2	14 + 1	16 + 6	45	23 + 6	26 + 5	29 + 3
16	11 + 5	14 + 3	17 + 1	46	24 + 3	27 + 1	29 + 6
17	12	14 + 6	17 + 4	47	24 + 6	27 + 5	30 + 3
18	12 + 3	15 + 1	17 + 6	48	25 + 3	28 + 1	30 + 6
19	12 + 5	15 + 4	18 + 2	49	26	28 + 5	31 + 3
20	13 + 1	15 + 6	18 + 4	50	26 + 3	29 + 1	32
21	13 + 3	16 + 2	19	51	27	29 + 5	32 + 3
22	13 + 6	16 + 4	19 + 2	52	27 + 4	30 + 2	33
23	14 + 2	17	19 + 5	53	28	30 + 6	33 + 4
24	14 + 4	17 + 3	20 + 1	54	28 + 4	31 + 2	34 + 1
25	15	17 + 5	20 + 4	55	29 + 1	31 + 6	34 + 4
26	15 + 3	18 + 1	20 + 6	56	29 + 5	32 + 3	35 + 1
27	15 + 6	18 + 4	21 + 2	57	30 + 2	33	35 + 5
28	16 + 2	19	21 + 5	58	30 + 6	33 + 4	36 + 2
29	16 + 4	19 + 3	22 + 1	59	31 + 3	34 + 1	36 + 6
30	17	19 + 6	22 + 4	60	32	34 + 5	37 + 3
31	17 + 3	20 + 1	23	61	32 + 4	35 + 2	38
32	17 + 6	20 + 4	23 + 3	62	33 + 1	35 + 6	38 + 4
33	18 + 2	21	23 + 6	63	33 + 5	36 + 3	39 + 1
34	18 + 5	21 + 4	24 + 2	64	34 + 2	37	39 + 6
35	19 + 1	22	24 + 5	65	34 + 6	37 + 4	40 + 3
36	19 + 5	22 + 3	25 + 1	66	35 + 3	38 + 1	41
37	20 + 1	22 + 6	25 + 4	67	36 + 1	38 + 6	41 + 4
38	20 + 4	23 + 2	26	68	36 + 5	39 + 3	42 + 2
39	21	23 + 5	26 + 4	69	37 + 2	40 + 1	42 + 6

Ulna

mm	Gestational Age Percentile			mm	Gestational Age Percentile		
	5th	50th	95th		5th	50th	95th
10	10	13 + 1	16 + 1	40	23	26 + 1	29 + 1
11	10 + 3	13 + 3	16 + 4	41	23 + 4	26 + 4	29 + 5
12	10 + 5	13 + 6	16 + 6	42	24 + 1	27 + 1	30 + 1
13	11 + 1	14 + 1	17 + 2	43	24 + 4	27 + 5	30 + 5
14	11 + 3	14 + 4	17 + 4	44	25 + 1	28 + 1	31 + 2
15	11 + 6	14 + 6	18	45	25 + 5	28 + 5	31 + 6
16	12 + 2	15 + 2	18 + 2	46	26 + 2	29 + 2	32 + 3
17	12 + 4	15 + 5	18 + 5	47	26 + 6	29 + 6	32 + 6
18	13	16	19 + 1	48	27 + 3	30 + 3	33 + 3
19	13 + 3	16 + 3	19 + 4	49	28	31	34
20	13 + 6	16 + 6	19 + 6	50	28 + 4	31 + 4	34 + 4
21	14 + 1	17 + 2	20 + 2	51	29 + 1	32 + 1	35 + 1
22	14 + 4	17 + 5	20 + 5	52	29 + 5	32 + 5	35 + 6
23	15	18 + 1	21 + 1	53	30 + 2	33 + 2	36 + 3
24	15 + 3	18 + 4	21 + 4	54	30 + 6	34	37
25	15 + 6	19	22	55	31 + 3	34 + 4	37 + 4
26	16 + 2	19 + 3	22 + 3	56	32 + 1	35 + 1	38 + 1
27	16 + 5	19 + 6	22 + 6	57	32 + 5	35 + 5	38 + 6
28	17 + 1	20 + 2	23 + 2	58	33 + 2	36 + 3	39 + 3
29	17 + 5	20 + 5	23 + 5	59	34	37	40
30	18 + 1	21 + 1	24 + 2	60	34 + 4	37 + 4	40 + 5
31	18 + 4	21 + 5	24 + 5	61	35 + 2	38 + 2	41 + 2
32	19	22 + 1	25 + 1	62	35 + 6	38 + 6	42
33	19 + 4	22 + 4	25 + 5	63	36 + 4	39 + 4	42 + 4
34	20	23 + 1	26 + 1	64	37 + 1	40 + 2	43 + 2
35	20 + 4	23 + 4	26 + 4				
36	21	24	27 + 1				
37	21 + 3	24 + 4	27 + 4				
38	22	25	28 + 1				
39	22 + 4	25 + 4	28 + 4				

151

TABLE 7–6. ASSESSMENT OF THE GESTATIONAL AGE FROM THE TIBIA AND CLAVICLE LENGTHS

Tibia

mm	Gestational Age Percentile		
	5th	50th	95th
10	10 + 3	13 + 2	16 + 1
11	10 + 5	13 + 4	16 + 4
12	11 + 1	14	16 + 6
13	11 + 3	14 + 2	17 + 2
14	11 + 6	14 + 5	17 + 4
15	12 + 1	15	18
16	12 + 4	15 + 3	18 + 2
17	12 + 6	15 + 6	18 + 5
18	13 + 2	16 + 1	19
19	13 + 4	16 + 4	19 + 3
20	14	16 + 6	19 + 6
21	14 + 3	17 + 2	20 + 1
22	14 + 6	17 + 5	20 + 4
23	15 + 1	18 + 1	21
24	15 + 4	18 + 3	21 + 3
25	16	18 + 6	21 + 5
26	16 + 3	19 + 2	22 + 1
27	16 + 5	19 + 5	22 + 4
28	17 + 1	20	23
29	17 + 4	20 + 3	23 + 3
30	18	20 + 6	23 + 6
31	18 + 3	21 + 2	24 + 1
32	18 + 6	21 + 5	24 + 4
33	19 + 2	22 + 1	25
34	19 + 5	22 + 4	25 + 3
35	20 + 1	23	25 + 6
36	20 + 4	23 + 3	26 + 2
37	21	23 + 6	26 + 5
38	21 + 3	24 + 2	27 + 1
39	21 + 6	24 + 5	27 + 5
40	22 + 2	25 + 1	28 + 1
41	22 + 5	25 + 5	28 + 4
42	23 + 1	26 + 1	29
43	23 + 5	26 + 4	29 + 3
44	24 + 1	27	29 + 6
45	24 + 4	27 + 3	30 + 3
46	25	28	30 + 6
47	25 + 4	28 + 3	31 + 2
48	26	28 + 6	31 + 6
49	26 + 3	29 + 3	32 + 2
50	27	29 + 6	32 + 5
51	27 + 3	30 + 2	33 + 2
52	27 + 6	30 + 6	33 + 5
53	28 + 3	31 + 2	34 + 1
54	28 + 6	31 + 6	34 + 5
55	29 + 3	32 + 2	35 + 1
56	29 + 6	32 + 6	35 + 5
57	30 + 3	33 + 2	36 + 1
58	30 + 6	33 + 6	36 + 5
59	31 + 3	34 + 2	37 + 1
60	31 + 6	34 + 6	37 + 5
61	32 + 3	35 + 2	38 + 2
62	33	35 + 6	38 + 5
63	33 + 3	36 + 3	39 + 2
64	34	36 + 6	39 + 6
65	34 + 4	37 + 3	40 + 2
66	35 + 1	38	40 + 6
67	35 + 4	38 + 4	41 + 3
68	36 + 1	39	42
69	36 + 5	39 + 4	42 + 3
70	37 + 2	40 + 1	43

Clavicle

mm	Gestational Age Percentile		
	5th	50th	95th
10	7 + 3	11 + 6	16 + 2
11	8 + 2	12 + 5	17 + 1
12	9 + 1	13 + 4	18
13	10	14 + 3	18 + 6
14	10 + 5	15 + 2	19 + 5
15	11 + 4	16	20 + 3
16	12 + 3	16 + 6	21 + 2
17	13 + 2	17 + 5	22 + 1
18	14 + 1	18 + 4	23
19	14 + 6	19 + 2	23 + 6
20	15 + 5	20 + 1	24 + 4
21	16 + 4	21	25 + 3
22	17 + 3	21 + 6	26 + 2
23	18 + 2	22 + 5	27 + 1
24	19	23 + 3	27 + 6
25	19 + 6	24 + 2	28 + 5
26	20 + 5	25 + 1	29 + 4
27	21 + 4	26	30 + 3
28	22 + 2	26 + 6	31 + 2
29	23 + 1	27 + 4	32
30	24	28 + 3	32 + 6
31	24 + 6	29 + 2	33 + 5
32	25 + 5	30 + 1	34 + 4
33	26 + 3	31	35 + 3
34	27 + 2	31 + 5	36 + 1
35	28 + 1	32 + 4	37
36	29	33 + 3	37 + 6
37	29 + 6	34 + 2	38 + 5
38	30 + 4	35	39 + 4
39	31 + 3	35 + 6	40 + 2
40	32 + 2	36 + 5	41 + 1
41	33 + 1	37 + 4	42
42	34	38 + 3	42 + 6
43	34 + 5	39 + 1	43 + 4
44	35 + 4	40	44 + 3

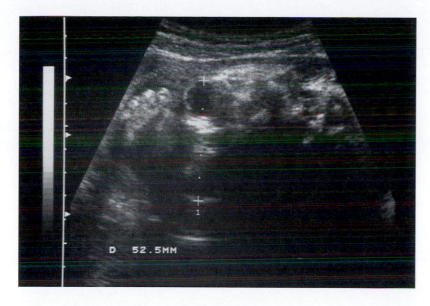

Figure 7–13. Measurement of binocular distance. Both eyes should have the same diameter; the measurement is obtained from the interface between the globe and the orbit on either side.

plane, both eyes should have the same diameter, and the image should be symmetrical (Fig. 7–13). The largest diameter of the eye should be used; the interocular distance should be the smallest. Table 7–7 can be used to derive the gestational age from the binocular distance.

The cerebellar measurement was proposed by Reece et al.[18] who found that the measurement of the cerebellum correlated well with the gestational age and was not much affected by growth retardation (Fig. 7–14). Further, if the measurement is expressed in millimeters, the value is very similar to the gestational age. For instance, if a cerebellum is measured to be 22 mm, the fetus is about 22 weeks in gestational age. This similarity in value makes it easy to use the cerebellum as a rapid check of the gestational age.

The clavicle is also proposed as a measurement to arrive at gestational age. The clavicle has an intramembranous ossification and not an endochondral ossification. This differentiates it from other long bones of the body. The clavicles

TABLE 7–7. ASSESSMENT OF THE GESTATIONAL AGE FROM THE BINOCULAR DISTANCE

| | Gestational Age | | | | Gestational Age | | | | Gestational Age | | |
| | Percentile | | | | Percentile | | | | Percentile | | |
mm	5th	50th	95th	mm	5th	50th	95th	mm	5th	50th	95th
10	7 + 1	7 + 3	7 + 4	30	18 + 1	19 + 2	20 + 3	50	29	31 + 1	33 + 3
11	7 + 5	8	8 + 2	31	18 + 5	19 + 6	21 + 1	51	29 + 4	31 + 5	34
12	8 + 2	8 + 4	8 + 6	32	19 + 1	20 + 3	21 + 5	52	30 + 1	32 + 3	34 + 5
13	8 + 6	9 + 1	9 + 4	33	19 + 5	21 + 1	22 + 3	53	30 + 4	33	35 + 2
14	9 + 3	9 + 5	10 + 1	34	20 + 2	21 + 5	23 + 1	54	31 + 1	33 + 4	36
15	10	10 + 3	10 + 6	35	20 + 6	22 + 2	23 + 5	55	31 + 5	34 + 1	36 + 4
16	10 + 3	11	11 + 3	36	21 + 3	22 + 6	24 + 3	56	32 + 2	34 + 5	37 + 2
17	11	11 + 4	12 + 1	37	21 + 6	23 + 3	25	57	32 + 6	35 + 2	37 + 6
18	11 + 4	12 + 1	12 + 5	38	22 + 3	24	25 + 5	58	33 + 2	36	38 + 4
19	12 + 1	12 + 5	13 + 3	39	23	24 + 5	26 + 2	59	33 + 6	36 + 4	39 + 1
20	12 + 5	13 + 2	14	40	23 + 4	25 + 2	27	60	34 + 3	37 + 1	39 + 6
21	13 + 1	14	14 + 5	41	24 + 1	25 + 6	27 + 4	61	35	37 + 5	40 + 3
22	13 + 5	14 + 4	15 + 2	42	24 + 4	26 + 3	28 + 2	62	35 + 4	38 + 2	41 + 1
23	14 + 2	15 + 1	16	43	25 + 1	27	28 + 6	63	36 + 1	38 + 6	41 + 5
24	14 + 6	15 + 5	16 + 4	44	25 + 5	27 + 4	29 + 4	64	36 + 4	39 + 4	42 + 3
25	15 + 3	16 + 2	17 + 2	45	26 + 2	28 + 2	30 + 1				
26	15 + 6	16 + 6	17 + 6	46	26 + 6	28 + 6	30 + 6				
27	16 + 3	17 + 4	18 + 4	47	27 + 3	29 + 3	31 + 3				
28	17	18 + 1	19 + 1	48	27 + 6	30	32 + 1				
29	17 + 4	18 + 5	19 + 6	49	28 + 3	30 + 4	32 + 5				

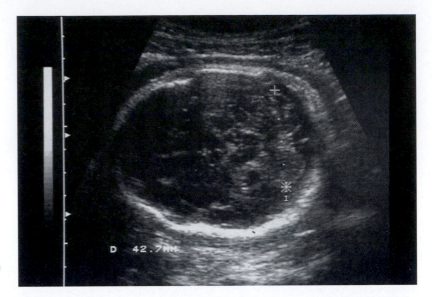

Figure 7–14. Cerebral measurement is one of the longest widths of the cerebellum.

are affected to a very different degree by diseases such as achondroplasia, thanatophoric, dysplasia, and so forth. The clavicle is occasionally useful in such circumstances. Another interesting point is that the length of a clavicle expressed in millimeters is very close to the gestational age expressed in weeks.[19]

Ossification Center. Many investigators have also attempted to determine the gestational age based on identification and measurement of ossification centers such as the distal femoral, proximal tibial, and proximal humeral. This method has been associated with a few problems. The first is that the observation of an ossification center by itself is not sufficiently precise. When only presence of the ossification center is assessed, the fetus can be any age after the age at which the ossification center appears, information of little use in clinical practice.

The measurement of the ossification center is also a problem. What appears as the ossification center on ultrasound is only the interface on the proximal side of the center of the ossification center and not the whole ossification center. The thickness and length are not visible unless the ossification center lies exactly perpendicular to the ultrasound beam. This position is difficult to obtain in clinical practice. The ossification centers are small, and a small error in measurement on any of them is equivalent to a large absolute variation on the assessment of gestational age. Therefore, the use of the ossification center is of little value in clinical practice; even in late gestation, the measurement of the femur and humerus is preferred.[20]

Selection of an Appropriate Table

In view of the large number of different parameters, it is important to know which one to measure and when. Different parameters have different reliability and ease of measurement at different gestational ages. In the list that follows, the parameters are given in decreasing order of preference. This order was established from their reliability, confidence limits, and ease of measurement. It should not be regarded as definitive and can be adapted to specific circumstances.

- From 7 to 10 weeks: CRL
- From 10 to 14 weeks: CRL, BPD, femur length, humerus length
- From 15 to 28 weeks: BPD, femur length, humerus length, head perimeter, binocular distance, other long bone lengths
- After 28 weeks (more accurate for dating): femur length, humerus length, binocular distance, BPD (check that the BPD is correct by evaluating the CI), other long bone lengths, head perimeter

What to Do When Different Parameters Provide Different Estimates

The general rule is that the earlier the estimation of the age, the more accurate it is. If estimate of the fetal age has been made at 15 weeks and a control scan at 27 weeks yields a different estimate, do not change the original estimate: it is more accurate. Ages are more or less equivalent when they are within 11 days of each other (this is an arbitrary limit). Before 20 weeks, parameters should be remeasured when the difference exceeds 1 week.

During a given examination when two similar parameters agree (e.g., two different bones), the average gestational age can be derived from them. When a few parameters provide estimates that are in the same range with only one discordant, recheck that one. If it is still abnormal, do not include it in the final estimate.

How to Report the Results

We are strongly in favor of reporting the lower 5th and the upper 95th confidence limits on the prediction for each measurement.[21] For example, the gestational age should be reported as 35 weeks (between 33 and 37 weeks) because this signifies that there is a 95% chance that the age is within 33 to 37 weeks and that the most likely age is 35 weeks. This is especially important in late gestation and may have legal implications.

The Abdominal Perimeter

The abdominal perimeter is used to assess growth and should not be used to assess gestational age. Otherwise, growth-restricted fetuses would appear younger and not growth restricted. A nomogram of the abdominal perimeter is provided in Table 7–8.

Other Available Nomograms

The following biometric parameters have also been measured, and interested readers are encouraged to obtain the original report if needed. These include the orbit,[22] nose,[23] cheek,[24] chin length and upper lip width,[25] frontal lobe,[26] transcerebellar diameter,[27] thyroid,[28] lungs,[29] heart diameter,[30] liver,[31] sacrum,[32] iliac bone,[33] iliac angle,[34,35] and thigh volume.[36,37] Many more have been published, and the interested reader should do a Medline search to identify the most recent articles.

TABLE 7–8. ABDOMINAL PERIMETER (mm)

Weeks	10th Centile	50th Centile	95th Centile
10	21	43	65
11	31	53	75
12	41	63	85
13	52	74	96
14	63	85	107
15	74	96	118
16	86	108	130
17	97	119	141
18	109	131	153
19	121	143	165
20	133	155	177
21	145	167	189
22	157	179	201
23	169	191	213
24	180	202	224
25	192	214	236
26	204	226	248
27	215	237	259
28	226	248	270
29	237	259	281
30	247	269	291
31	257	279	301
32	267	289	311
33	276	298	320
34	285	307	329
35	293	315	337
36	301	323	345
37	308	330	352
38	314	336	358
39	320	342	364
40	326	348	370

REFERENCES

1. Lippert H, Lehman HP. *SI Units in Medicine: An Introduction to the International System of Units with Conversion Tables and Normal Ranges.* Baltimore: Urban & Schwarzenberg; 1978.
2. Robinson HP, Fleming JEE. A critical evaluation of sonar crown–rump length measurements. *Br J Obstet Gynaecol.* 1975;82:702–710.
3. Hadlock FP, Deter RL, Harrist RB, et al. Fetal biparietal diameter: A critical reevaluation of the relation to menstrual age by means of realtime ultrasound. *J Ultrasound Med.* 1982;1: 97–104.
4. Shepard M, Filly RA. A standardized plane for biparietal diameter measurement. *J Ultrasound Med.* 1982;1:145–150.
5. Doubilet PM, Greenes RA. Improved prediction of gestational age from fetal head measurements. *AJR.* 1984;142: 797–800.
6. Wolfson RN, Zador IE, Halvorsen P, et al. Biparietal diameter in premature rupture of membranes: Errors in estimating gestational age. *J Clin Ultrasound.* 1983;11:371–374.
7. O'Keeffe DF, Garite TJ, Elliott JP, et al. The accuracy of estimated gestational age based on ultrasound measurement of biparietal diameter in preterm premature rupture of the membranes. *Am J Obstet Gynecol.* 1985;151:309–312.
8. Selbing A, Kjessler B. Conceptual dating by ultrasonic measurement of the fetal biparietal diameter in early pregnancy. *Acta Obstet Gynecol Scand.* 1985;64:593–597.
9. Simon NV, Levisky JS, Siegle JC, et al. Evaluation of the dating of gestation via the growth adjusted sonographic age method. *J Clin Ultrasound.* 1984;12:195–199.
10. Ott WJ. The use of ultrasonic fetal head circumference for predicting expected date of confinement. *J Clin Ultrasound.* 1984;12:411–415.
11. Hadlock FP, Harrist RB, Deter RL, et al. Fetal femur length as a predictor of menstrual age: Sonographically measured. *AJR.* 1982;138:875.
12. Hohler CW, Quetel TA. Fetal femur length: Equations for computer calculation of gestational age from ultrasound measurements. *Am J Obstet Gynecol.* 1982;143:479–481.
13. Jeanty P, Romero R. *Obstetrical Ultrasound.* New York: McGraw-Hill; 1984.
14. Jeanty P, Rodesch F, Delbeke D. Estimation of fetal age by long bone measurements. *J Ultrasound Med.* 1984;3:75–79.
15. Jeanty P, Cantraine F, Cousaert E, et al. The binocular distance: A new parameter to estimate fetal age. *J Ultrasound Med.* 1984;3:241–244.
16. Deter RL, Harrist RB, Hadlock FP, et al. Fetal head and abdominal circumferences. II: A critical reevaluation of the relationship to menstrual age. *J Clin Ultrasound.* 1982;10:365–372.
17. Hadlock FP, Deter RL, Harrist RB. Fetal head circumference: Relation to menstrual age. *AJR.* 1982;138:649–653.

18. Reece EA, Goldstein I, Pilu G, et al. Fetal cerebellar growth unaffected by intrauterine growth retardation: A new parameter for prenatal diagnosis. *Am J Obstet Gynecol.* 1987;157:632–638.

19. Yarkoni S, Schmidt W, Jeanty P, et al. Clavicular measurement: A new biometric parameter for fetal evaluation. *J Ultrasound Med.* 1985;4:467–471.

20. Goldstein I, Lockwood C, Belanger K, et al. Ultrasonographic assessment of gestational age with the distal femoral and proximal tibial ossification center in the third trimester. *Am J Obstet Gynecol.* 1988;158:127–130.

21. Jeanty P. A simple reporting system for obstetrical ultrasound examination. *J Ultrasound Med.* 1985;4:591–593.

22. Goldstein I, Tamir A, Zimmer EZ, et al. Growth of the fetal orbit and lens in normal pregnancies. *Ultrasound Obstet Gynecol.* 1998;12:175.

23. Ben Ami M, Weiner E, Perlitz Y, et al. Ultrasound evaluation of the width of the fetal nose. *Prenat Diagn.* 1998;18:1010.

24. Abramowicz JS, Robischon K, et al. Incorporating sonographic cheek-to-cheek diameter, biparietal diameter and abdominal circumference improves weight estimation in the macrosomic fetus. *Ultrasound Obstet Gynecol.* 1997;9:409.

25. Sivan E, Chan L, Mallozzi-Eberle A, et al. Sonographic imaging of the fetal face and the establishment of normative decisions for chin length and upper lip width. *Am J Perinatol.* 1997;14:191.

26. Persutte WH. Microcephaly-no small deal. *Ultrasound Obstet Gynecol.* 1998;11:317.

27. Rotmensch S, Goldstein I, Liberati M, et al. Fetal transcerebellar diameter in Down syndrome. *Obstet Gynecol.* 1997;89:534.

28. Meinel K, Doring K. Growth of the fetal thyroid gland in the 2nd half of pregnancy-biometric ultrasound studies. *Ultraschall Med.* 1997;18:258.

29. Heling KS, Kalache K, Chaoui R, et al. Ultrasound biometry of the fetal lung-measurement planes and reference values. *Zentralbl Gynakol.* 1997;119:625.

30. Hata T, Senoh D, Hata K, et al. Intrauterine sonographic assessments of embryonic heart diameter. *Hum Reprod.* 1997;12:2286.

31. Hata T, Fujiwaki R, Senoh D, et al. Intrauterine sonographic assessments of embryonal liver length. *Hum Reprod.* 1996;11:2758.

32. Pajak J, Heimrath J, Gabrys M, et al. Usefulness of ultrasonographic measurement for fetal sacrum length in assessment of gestational age in physiologic pregnancy. *Ginekol Pol.* 1998;69:563.

33. Zoppi MA, Ibba RM, Floris M, et al. Can fetal iliac bone measurement be used as a marker for Down's syndrome screening? *Ultrasound Obstet Gynecol.* 1998;12:19.

34. Bork MD, Egan JF, Cusick W, et al. Iliac wing angle as a marker for trisomy 21 in the second trimester. *Obstet Gynecol.* 1997;89(5 Pt 1):734.

35. Shipp TD, Bromley B, Lieberman E, et al. The second-trimester fetal iliac angle as a sign of Down's syndrome. *Ultrasound Obstet Gynecol.* 1998;12:15.

36. Lee W, Comstock CH, Kirk JS, et al. Birthweight prediction by three-dimensional ultrasonographic volumes of the fetal thigh and abdomen. *J Ultrasound Med.* 1997;16:799.

37. Chang FM, Liang RI, Ko HC, et al. Three-dimensional ultrasound-assessed fetal thigh volumetry in predicting birth weight. *Obstet Gynecol.* 1997;90:331.

8

Prenatal Diagnosis of Congenital Heart Disease

Gianluigi Pilu • Philippe Jeanty • Antonella Perolo •
Daniela Prandstraller

Abnormalities of the heart and great arteries are the most common congenital abnormalities and occur in about 0.6% of newborns. In general, about half are either lethal or require surgery and half are asymptomatic. The half that is lethal or requires surgery is referred to as *major*. The distribution of anomalies detected in fetuses is different from that in pediatric series because it is strongly biased toward the more severe anomalies. When stillbirths and early fetal deaths are included, the number of anomalies rises. The etiology of heart defects is heterogeneous and probably depends on the interplay of multiple genetic and environmental factors, including maternal diabetes mellitus or collagen disease, exposure to drugs such as lithium, and viral infections such as rubella. Approximately 5% of the defects are associated with chromosomal aberrations in the pediatric population, and the proportion rises to 25% in fetal series.[1] Heart defects are found in more than 99% of fetuses with trisomy 18, in 90% of those with trisomy 13, in 50% of those with trisomy 21, in 40 to 50% of those with deletions or partial trisomies involving a variety of chromosomes, and in 35% of those with 45,X. The risk of recurrence after the birth of one affected child is increased to 2 to 5% and to 10% after the birth of two affected siblings (Table 8–1).[2]

Pioneer studies on the ultrasound investigation of the fetal heart were reported in the early 1970s. Fetal echocardiography has become a well-established technique for the prenatal diagnosis of cardiac heart defects, but the use of this technique is limited at present. However, cardiac defects are one of the most common types of congenital anomalies, and we anticipate that routine sonography will include a basic echocardiographic examination. It is clear that doing so will demand a significant improvement over the present level of expertise and training. The purpose of this chapter is to provide a practical approach to the sonographic prediction of heart disease in the fetus.

SONOGRAPHIC EVALUATION OF FETAL CARDIAC STRUCTURE AND FUNCTION

Real-Time Two-Dimensional Evaluation

Complex cardiac anomalies are frequently associated with an abnormal disposition of the heart and extracardiac viscera. Fetal echocardiography should always include an assessment of the topographic anatomy of the abdomen and chest.

TABLE 8–1. RECURRENCE RISKS OF CONGENITAL HEART DISEASE

Defect	Recurrence Risks (%)		
	One Sibling Affected[a]	Father Affected[b]	Mother Affected[b]
Aortic stenosis	2	3	13–18
Atrial septal defect	2.5	1.5	4–4.5
Atrioventricular canal	2	1	14
Coarctation	2	2	4
Patent ductus arteriosus	3	2.5	3.5–4
Pulmonary stenosis	2	2	4–6.5
Tetralogy of Fallot	2.5	1.5	2.5
Ventricular septal defect	3	2	6–10

[a]Data derived from Nora JJ, Nora AH. *Genetics and counseling in cardiovascular disease.* Springfield, IL; Charles C. Thomas; 1978.
[b]Data derived from Nora JJ, Nora AH. Maternal transmission of congenital heart disease: New recurrence risk figures and the questions of cytoplasmic inheritance and vulnerability to teratogens. *Am J Cardiol.* 1987;59:459.

The left and right sides of the fetus are assessed by determining the relative position of the head and spine. The visceral situs is then assessed by demonstrating the relative position of the stomach, hepatic vessels, abdominal aorta, and inferior vena cava. A transverse section of the fetal chest visualizes the position of the heart (Fig. 8–1).

The heart can be observed in an infinity of planes, but a few sections are the basis on which most of the diagnoses are made.[3] These planes provide views of the four chambers, left and right chambers and great vessels (Fig. 8–2). Although it is convenient to refer to these standardized views for descriptive purposes, in practice it may be difficult to reproduce these exact sections, and the operator should be familiar with small variations of these planes.

The four-chamber view is obtained by making a section that is practically axial to the fetal chest.[4] The important landmarks to identify are the apex of the heart, the base, the interventricular septum, the interatrial septum, the two atrioventricular valves (tricuspid and mitral), and the four cavities delineated by these structures. The thickness of the interventricular septum and of the free ventricular walls is the same. The heart is not midline but shifted to the left side of the chest. The axis of the interventricular septum is about 45 to 20 degrees to the left of the anteroposterior axis of the fetus.[5] The interatrial septum is open at the level of the *foramen ovale.* The foramen ovale flap is visible in the left atrium, beating toward the left side. The insertion of the tricuspid valve along the interventricular septum is more apical than the insertion of the mitral valve. The confluence of the pulmonary veins into the left atrium serves to identify it as such.

By turning the transducer and keeping the left ventricle and the aorta in the same plane, one can obtain views of the left side of the heart, views of the right side of the heart are obtained by moving the transducer toward the cranium and tilting it slightly in the direction of the left shoulder.

Views of the left side of the heart demonstrate important landmarks. The mitral valve is seen between the left atrium and the left ventricle. The posterior leaflet is shorter than the anterior leaflet. The anterior leaflet is in continuity with the posterior wall of the aorta. The anterior wall of the aorta is in continuity with the interventricular septum. The aortic valve can be seen at the base of the aorta.

Views of the right side of the heart demonstrate the right ventricle and the ventricular outflow tract. The main pulmonary artery originates from the anterior ventricle and trifurcates into a large vessel, the ductus going into the descending aorta, and two small vessels, the pulmonary arteries. The pulmonary valve is anterior and cranial to the aortic valve.

There are two *arches* in the fetus and they should be distinguished (Fig. 8–3). The aortic arch is recognized from the ductus, with the following criteria. The brachiocephalic vessels originate from the aortic arch, whereas no vessels emanate from the ductus. The curve of the aortic arch is gentler than that of the ductus, which is slightly more angular. The cavae can be seen in a longitudinal view as they both enter the right atrium.

M-Mode

Because the fetal electrocardiogram is difficult to derive, one uses the M-mode recording to deduce from the mechanical

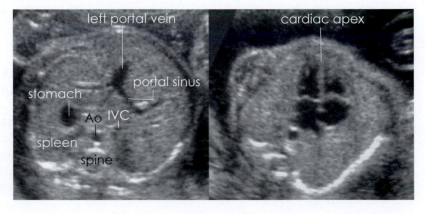

Figure 8–1. Sonographic assessment of the visceral situs. In a transverse scan of the abdomen, the stomach, spleen, and abdominal aorta are seen on the *left;* the portal sinus, gallbladder *(not shown),* and inferior vena cava are seen on the *right.* In a transverse section of the chest, the cardiac apex is seen pointing to the *left.*

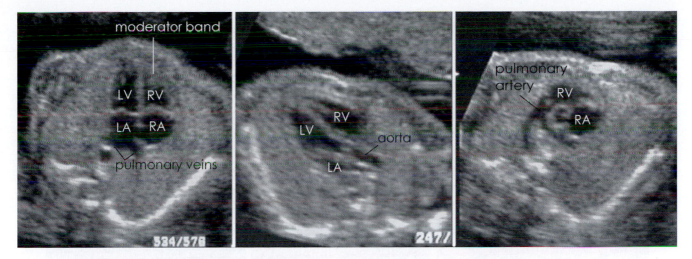

Figure 8–2. Sonographic demonstration of cardiac anatomy in a normal mid-trimester fetus: four-chamber view *(left),* left heart view *(middle),* and right heart view *(right).* LA and LV, left atrium and ventricle, respectively; RA and RV, right atrium and ventricle, respectively.

events the electrical signal that caused them. In M-mode ultrasound, only one line of information is continuously displayed: instead of a two-dimensional scan of the heart, a recording of the variations of echoes along a single line is produced. Thus, M-mode is of little help in the analysis of the morphology of the heart but is useful in assessing motions and rhythms. One simply "drops" an M-mode line over one atrial and ventricular wall and is able to quantitate cardiac frequency and to infer the atrioventricular sequence of contractions.

Color and Pulsed Wave Doppler Sonography

Color and pulsed Doppler sonograms are useful to assess normal anatomy and physiology. Adequate recordings of blood flow through the atrioventricular valves and in the great ves-

sels can be obtained in most cases starting from 14 weeks and even before using vaginal ultrasound (Fig. 8–4). Color and pulsed wave Doppler sonograms are valuable in the assessment of atrioventricular valve regurgitation, which is a major prognostic factor in fetal heart disease[6] (Fig. 8–5). In normal fetuses, the peak velocity in the ascending aorta and pulmonary artery is usually less than 1 m per second. Excessive peak velocities increase the index of suspicion of semilunar valve stenosis that is associated with poststenotic turbulence (Fig. 8–6).

Indications for Fetal Echocardiography

A full cardiac examination is a time-consuming investigation that is not recommended for every patient at present. Unless

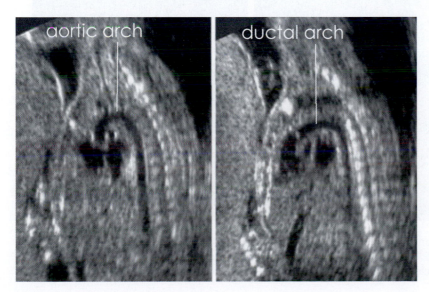

Figure 8–3. Aortic and ductal arch. The long upward course and the presence of the brachiocephalic vessels identify the aortic arch.

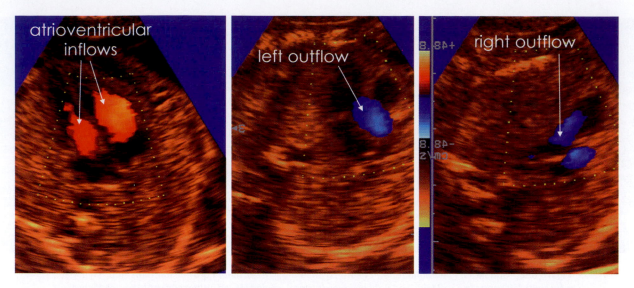

Figure 8–4. Color Doppler echocardiography performed with transvaginal ultrasound in a 15-week fetus.

there is a specific indication for fetal echocardiography, the standard of practice in the United States and in most European countries is to limit the examination to the fetal position, situs, and a four-chamber view. The rest of the investigation concerns the dedicated cardiac examination.[7] Cardiac examinations are easiest to perform between 20 and 24 weeks. However, the use of vaginal sonography allows the diagnosis of a relevant number of anomalies since 10–12 weeks of gestation.[8]

Dedicated examinations (often called *fetal echo* or *echocardiography*) are performed for familial and maternal or fe-

tal reasons (Table 8–2).[9] The result of the examination will affect the prenatal care in several ways. When the examination is normal, the parent can be reassured, with the *caveat* that some anomalies may have been overlooked. Some of the tachyarrhythmias can be treated *in utero*. When the anomaly is treatable, delivery in a tertiary care center with specific expertise in the treatment of congenital heart disease should be encouraged. When a lethal anomaly is discovered, interruption of the pregnancy can be offered; after the legal limit of termination, noninterventional obstetrical care can be offered.

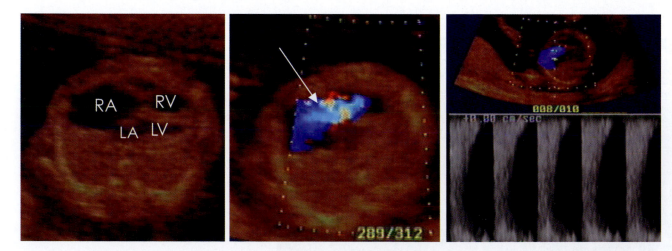

Figure 8–5. Two-dimensional echocardiography shows gross enlargement of the right atrium (RA) in a 17-week fetus. Color and pulsed Doppler sonography demonstrate massive regurgitation of the tricuspid valve, which indicates severe insufficiency of the tricuspid valve. LV, left ventricle; LA, left atrium; RV, right ventricle.

TABLE 8–2. INDICATIONS FOR FETAL ECHOCARDIOGRAPHY

Familial and maternal indications
   Familial history of congenital heart disease
   Maternal disease associated with fetal heart disease (diabetes, autoimmune conditions, etc.)
   Exposure to teratogens
Fetal indications
   Abnormal four-chamber view
   Extracardiac anomalies
   Dysrrhythmias
   Polyhydramnios
   Hydrops

PRENATAL DIAGNOSIS OF CONGENITAL HEART DISEASE

Septal Defects

Atrial Septal Defects. During embryogenesis, the common atrium is first divided by the septum primum into the right and left atria. The septum primum extends from the base of the heart toward the endocardial cushion. The gap between the two is called the *ostium primum*. When the fusion between the septum primum and the endocardial cushion has occurred, the septum primum fenestrates. The resulting communication between the two atria is called the *ostium secundum*. A second septum then extends on the right side of the septum primum and covers part of the ostium secundum. The remaining orifice is the foramen ovale, and the foramen ovale flap is the lower part of the septum primum. Thus, defects that are close to the endocardial cushion are called the *ostium primum*, and defects in the area of the foramen ovale are the *ostium secundum*. Ostium secundum defects are the most common and are

found in 0.07 per 1000 infants.[10] The *primum* atrial septal defect (ASD) is the simplest form of atrioventricular septal defect, which will be considered later on.

Secundum ASDs are most frequently isolated but may be related to other cardiac lesions associated with interatrial shunts (such as mitral, pulmonary, tricuspid or aortic atresia) and are occasionally found as part of syndromes, including Holt–Oram syndrome (ostium secundum defect, hypoplasia of the thumb and radius, triphalangeal thumb, abrachia, and phocomelia).[11]

Although the *in utero* identification of *secundum* ASD has been reported, the diagnosis remains difficult because of the physiologic presence of the foramen ovale. Most likely, only unusually large defects can be recognized with certainty.

Atrial septal defects are not a cause of impairment of cardiac function in utero because a large right-to-left shunt at the level of the atria is a physiologic condition in the fetus. Most affected infants are asymptomatic even in the neonatal period.

Ventricular Septal Defects. Ventricular septal defects (VSDs) are probably the most common congenital cardiac defect.[11] They are classified into perimembranous, inlet, trabecular, or outlet defects depending on their location on the septum. *Perimembranous* defects (80%) are so called because they not only involve the membranous septum below the aortic valve but also extend to variable degrees into the adjacent portion of the septum. The *inlet* defects are on the inflow tract of the right ventricle and thus affect the implantation of the septal chordae of the tricuspid valve. The *trabecular* defects occur in the muscular portion of the septum, and the *outlet* defects are in the infundibular portion of the right ventricle. Trabecular defects (5 to 20%) have not been detected

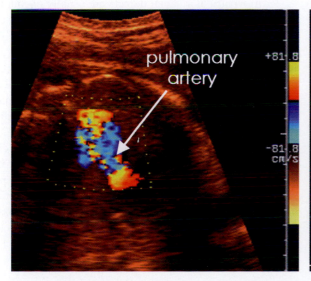
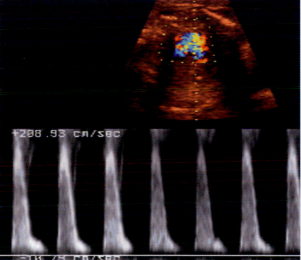

Figure 8–6. In this fetus with a hypertrophic right ventricle, color Doppler sonography shows aliasing of the pulmonary artery, suggestive of poststenotic turbulence. Pulsed Doppler sonography confirms that peak velocity in the main pulmonary trunk exceeds 2 m per second, indicating pulmonary stenosis.

by prenatal ultrasound because they are usually composed of small orifices. Overall, small isolated ventricular septal defects are difficult to detect prenatally, and both false-positive and false-negative diagnoses have been made.

The echocardiographic diagnosis depends on the demonstration of a dropout of echoes in the ventricular septum. Because most ventricular septal defects are perimembranous and subaortic, a detailed view of the left outflow tract is the best way to image them. Defects smaller than 1 to 2 mm will fall beyond the resolution power of current ultrasound equipment and will escape detection. For evaluating the ventricular septum in search of defects, multiple views should be used. Perimembranous defects will be best demonstrated by the four-chamber view. Muscular defects, which are difficult to observe, are best searched for in the short-axis view by trying to demonstrate a connection between the two ventricles.

There is no evidence that VSDs are responsible for hemodynamic compromise in utero. Even a large interventricular communication probably gives rise only to small, bidirectional shunts in the fetus because during intrauterine life the right and left ventricular pressures are believed to be equal. It has been debated as to whether or not shunting across the defects can be detected by the use of color Doppler sonography.

The vast majority of infants are not symptomatic during the neonatal period. Rare exceptions are represented by very large defects, associated with a massive left-to-right shunt that can be associated with congestive heart failure soon after birth. Approximately 25% of small trabecular defects close spontaneously, and a smaller proportion of the membranous defects also occlude.

Atrioventricular Septal Defects. The ontogenesis of the apical portion of the atrial septum, of the basal portion of the interventricular septum, and of the atrioventricular valves depends on the development of mesenchymnal masses defined by endocardial cushions. Abnormal development of these structures is commonly referred to as *endocardial cushion defects, atrioventricular canal defects,* or *atrioventricular septal defects.* In the complete form, called the *persistent common atrioventricular canal,* the tricuspid and mitral valve are fused in a large single atrioventricular valve that opens above and bridges the two ventricles. This valve has an anterior and a posterior leaflet. In the incomplete form, various amounts of tethering of one or both leaflets to the crest of the interventricular septum lead to a connection that creates functional atrial or ventricular septal defects, ventriculoatrial septal defects (a connection between the left ventricle and right atrium), or valvular abnormalities (clefting of the septal leaflet of the mitral valve).

In the complete form of the atrioventricular canal, the common atrioventricular valve may be incompetent, and systolic blood regurgitation from the ventricles to the atria may give rise to congestive heart failure.[12]

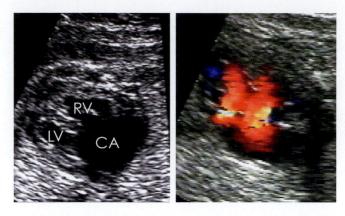

Figure 8–7. Two-dimensional and color Doppler echocardiography shows a common atrium (CA), a large ventricular septal defect, and a common atrioventricular valve, indicating a complete atrioventricular septal defect. LV, left ventricle; RV, right ventricle.

Antenatal echocardiographic diagnosis of complete atrioventricular septal defects is usually easy. An obvious deficiency of the central core structures of the heart is present. Color Doppler ultrasound can be useful in facilitating the visualization of the central opening of the single atrioventricular valve (Fig. 8–7). The atria may be dilated as a consequence of atrioventricular insufficiency. In such cases, color and pulsed Doppler ultrasound allow the physician to identify the regurgitant jet. The incomplete forms are more difficult to recognize. A useful hint is the demonstration of the tricuspid and mitral valve attaching at the same level at the crest of the septum. This apical displacement of the mitral valve elongates the left ventricular outflow tract. The atrial septal defect is of the ostium primum type (because the septum secundum is not affected) and thus is close to the crest of the interventricular septum.

Atrioventricular septal defects are usually encountered either in fetuses with chromosomal aberrations (50% of cases have been associated with aneuploidy, with 60% of these cases being trisomy 21 and 25% being trisomy 18)[13] or in fetuses with cardiosplenic syndromes. In fetuses with chromosomal aberrations, an atrioventricular septal defect is frequently found in association with extracardiac anomalies. In fetuses with cardiosplenic syndromes, multiple cardiac anomalies are almost the rule.

Atrioventricular septal defects do not impair fetal circulation *per se.* However, the presence of atrioventricular valve insufficiency may lead to intrauterine heart failure. The prognosis of atrioventricular septal defects is poor when detected *in utero,* probably because of the high frequency of associated anomalies in antenatal series. Only 4 of 29 (14%) fetuses survived in one series, 2 of whom had trisomy 21 and 1 was inoperable.[14]

Univentricular Heart. According to Becker and Anderson,[15] the term *univentricular heart* defines a group of anomalies characterized by the presence of an atrioventricular junction that is entirely connected to only one chamber in the ventricular mass. With this definition, the univentricular heart includes both those cases in which two atrial chambers are connected, by either two distinct atrioventricular valves or by a common one, to a main ventricular chamber *(classic double-inlet single ventricle)* and those cases in which, because of the absence of one atrioventricular connection (tricuspid or mitral atresia), one of the ventricular chambers is either rudimentary or absent (Fig. 8–8). The main ventricular chamber may be either the left or right type and in some cases may be of indeterminate type. A rudimentary ventricular chamber lacking an atrioventricular connection is a frequent but not constant finding. Antenatal echocardiographic diagnosis is usually easy. The hemodynamics may differ greatly from case to case, depending on the type of ventriculoarterial connection and the sum of the associated cardiac anomalies, which are very frequently seen.

Outflow Obstructions

Aortic Stenosis. Aortic stenosis is commonly divided into supravalvar, valvar, and subaortic forms. Supravalvar aortic stenosis can be due to one of three anatomic defects: a membrane (usually placed above the sinuses of Valsalva), a localized narrowing of the ascending aorta (hourglass deformity), or a diffuse narrowing involving the aortic arch and branching arteries (tubular variety). The valvar form of aortic stenosis can be due to dysplastic, thickened aortic cusps or fusion of the commissure between the cusps. The subaortic forms include a fixed type, representing the consequence of a fibrous or fibromuscular obstruction, and a dynamic type, which is due to a thickened ventricular septum obstructing the outflow tract of the left ventricle. The latter is also known as *asymmetric septal hypertrophy* (ASH) or *idiopathic hypertrophic subaortic stenosis*. A transient form of dynamic obstruction of the left outflow tract is seen in infants of diabetic mothers and is probably the consequence of fetal hyperglycemia and hyperinsulinemia.[16]

Echocardiographic diagnosis of valvar aortic stenosis after birth depends on real-time cross-sectional demonstration of doming of the aortic cusps and Doppler ultrasound identification of post-stenotic turbulence. The left ventricle may have hypertrophic walls or be dilated.[17] Pulsed Doppler ultrasound is valuable for assessing both increased peak velocities in the ascending aorta (Fig. 8–9) and insufficiency of the atrioventricular valves that can accompany the cases with the most severe obstructions.

Asymmetric septal hypertrophy has been identified *in utero*.[18] The only reported case, however, is likely to be an exception because there is evidence indicating that this anomaly usually has an evolutive course, and it is not apparent in the neonatal period.[19] Hypertrophic cardiomyopathy

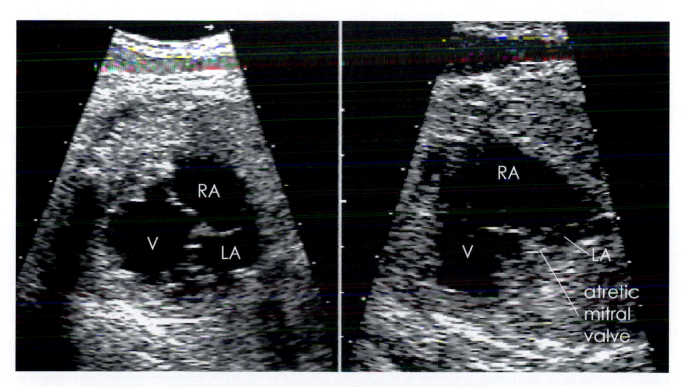

Figure 8–8. Varieties of univentricular heart. *Left:* Two atria with two patent atrioventricular valves are seen emptying into a single ventricular chamber, indicating a double-inlet single ventricle. *Right:* The mitral valve is not patent, the left ventricle is not visualized, and the left atrium is small, indicating mitral valve atresia.

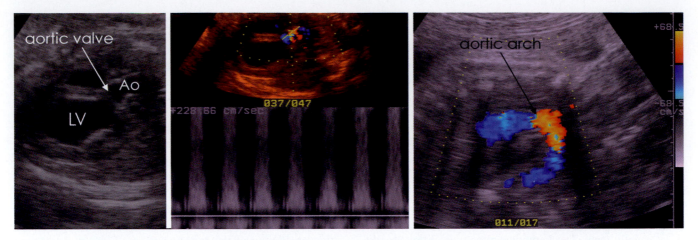

Figure 8–9. The left ventricle (LV) is dilated, with a bright echocardium. The aortic valve is thickened. Color and pulsed Doppler sonograms show axial blood flow within the ascending aorta (Ao), with a peak velocity exceeding 1.5 m per second. Color Doppler sonography demonstrates reverse flow into the aortic arch, indicating critical aortic stenosis, ductal dependent.

in fetuses of diabetic mothers has been reported on several occasions.[20] We are not aware of cases of supravalvular aortic stenosis detected in utero.

Depending on the severity of the aortic stenosis, the association of left ventricular pressure overload and sub-endocardial ischemia due to decrease in coronary perfusion may lead to intrauterine impairment of cardiac function. Although subavalvular and subaortic forms are not generally manifested in the neonatal period, the valvar type can be a cause of congestive heart failure in the newborn and fetus.[21] Aortic stenosis is one of the congenital cardiac defects most frequently found in association with intrauterine growth retardation.[22]

Real-time and pulsed wave Doppler ultrasound allow a precise estimation of the severity of the stenosis. Knowledge of peak velocity allows the prediction of the pressure gradient with reasonable accuracy by using the modified Bernoulli equation. There is concern that cases seen in early gestation may progress in severity. However, in the few cases we had an opportunity to follow throughout gestation, the lesions remained stable.

Coarctation and Tubular Hypoplasia of the Aorta. Coarctation is a localized narrowing of the juxtaductal arch, most commonly between the left subclavian artery and the ductus. A discrete shelf between the isthmus and the descending aorta is the most common finding at anatomic dissection. The pathogenesis of coarctation of the aorta is controversial. Three hypothesis have been suggested. Coarctation may be a true malformation due to an embryogenetic abnormality, or the consequence of aberrant ductal tissue in the aortic wall, resulting in narrowing of the isthmus at the time of closure of the ductus (the so-called *Skodaic theory*), or the anatomic result of an intrauterine hemodynamic perturbance due to an intracardiac anomaly diverting blood flow from the aorta into the pulmonary artery and the ductus arteriosus. There is clinical and pathologic evidence supporting at least the last two hypotheses.

Tubular hypoplasia is a generalized narrowing of the aorta that affects the proximal arch, most commonly the segment between the left common carotid and the left subclavian artery or the isthmus, and may extend in the brachiocephalic vessels.

Cardiac anomalies are present in 90% of cases and include aortic stenosis and insufficiency, ventricular septal defect, atrial septal defect, transposition of the great arteries, truncus, and double-outlet right ventricle. The aortic valve is bicuspid in 25 to 50% of cases. The mitral valve is abnormal in 25 to 50% of cases.[23,24] Complete heart block may coexist.[25]

Noncardiac anomalies include diaphragmatic hernia[26,27] and Turner syndrome but not Noonan syndrome.

The expected finding in coarctation is that of an echogenic shelf poking into the lumen of the aorta. This finding, however, is recognizable in less than half of the fetuses. Coarctation may be a postnatal event, and this limits prenatal diagnosis in many cases. This anomaly, however, has been described in the fetus, although only in late pregnancy.[28]

An enlarged right atrium and right ventricle (when the right ventricle is 1.3 times the size of the left ventricle) with increased tricuspid flow (greater than twice the mitral flow) and an enlarged pulmonary artery have been found in 50% of cases[29,30] (Fig. 8–10). In tubular narrowing, the aorta becomes gracile and loses its caliber. The diagnosis is probably not very reliable due to the difficult access.

Because the blood flow through the isthmus is minimal during intrauterine life, the descending aorta being mainly supplied by the ductus arteriosus, isolated coarctation is not expected to alter hemodynamics significantly. However, cases with tubular hypoplasia of the aortic arch may result in a greater hemodynamic burden, and this could explain the

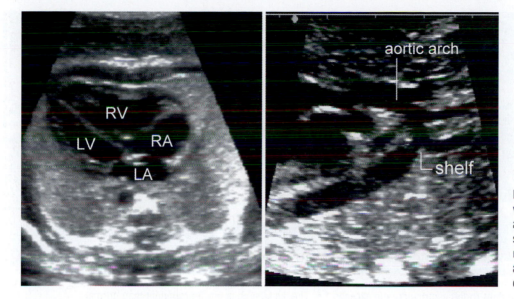

Figure 8–10. The right-to-left ventricular ratio exceeds 1.5, and a close-up of the aortic arch suggests narrowing of the isthmus, with a shelf. These findings are strongly suggestive of aortic coarctation.

dilatation of the right heart that has been documented with echocardiography before birth.

Interrupted Aortic Arch. The interruption can be complete or there may be an atretic fibrous segment between the arch and the descending aorta. The lesion has been considered an extreme form of coarctation.[31] The interruptions are categorized according to their level in relation to the brachiocephalic vessels. In type A (42%), the aorta supplies the three brachiocephalic vessels, and the pulmonary artery supplies the descending aorta via the ductus.[32] In type B (53%), the interruption is proximal to the left subclavian artery. In type C (4%), the interruption is between the right innominate and left common carotid artery. Type C is the most lethal form. A common anomaly (which is still probably beyond prenatal recognition) is the presence of a replaced right subclavian artery that originates from the distal portion of the aorta. Ventricular septal defects are almost always present in type B and occur in 50% of type A cases.

Associated cardiac anomalies include atrial septal defects, subaortic stenosis, hypoplasia of the ascending aorta, bicuspid aortic and/or pulmonic valve, replaced right subclavian artery, and ventricular septal defects. The ventricular septal defect is of the malalignment type with obstruction of the aortic outflow.

Associated extracardiac anomalies include DiGeorge syndrome (association of thymic aplasia, type B interruption, and hypoplastic mandible), holoprosencephaly, cleft lip/palate, esophageal atresia, duplicated stomach, diaphragmatic hernia, horseshoe kidneys, bilateral renal agenesis, oligodactyly, claw hand, and syrenomelia.

The characteristic findings of an *arch* in the higher chest from which no or too few vessels originate should suggest the diagnosis.[33] In a sagittal section, the aorta can be traced into the carotids but cannot be traced into the descending aorta. Another finding is the discrepancy in the size of the ventricles, with a predominance of the right one (Fig. 8–11).

Hypoplastic Left Heart. Hypoplastic left heart syndrome (HLHS) is characterized by a very small left ventricle, with mitral and/or aortic atresia. Blood flow to the head and neck vessels and coronary artery is supplied in a retrograde manner through the ductus arteriosus.

Echocardiographic diagnosis of HLHS in the fetus depends on the demonstration of a diminutive left ventricle and ascending aorta.[34,35] In most cases, the ultrasound appearance is self-explanatory, and the diagnosis an easy one (Fig. 8–12). However, there is a broad spectrum of hypoplasia of the left ventricle. We have seen cases with a ventricular cavity of almost normal size that may represent a diagnostic challenge, particularly in early gestation. Because the four-chamber view is almost normal, these cases certainly may be missed in most routine surveys of fetal anatomy. With closer scrutiny, however, the movement of the mitral valve appears severely impaired to nonexistent, ventricular contractility is obviously decreased, and the ventricle often displays an internal echogenic lining that is probably due to endocardial fibroelastosis. The definitive diagnosis of HLHS depends on demonstration of hypoplasia of the ascending aorta and atresia of the aortic valve. Color flow mapping is an extremely useful adjunct to the real-time examination because it allows the demonstration of retrograde blood flow within the ascending aorta and aortic arch (Fig. 8–13). Doppler sonography is also useful for identifying insufficiency of the atrioventricular valves.

The prognosis for infants with HLHS is extremely poor. This lesion is responsible for 25% of cardiac deaths in the first week of life. Almost all affected infants die within 6 weeks if they are not treated.[36] Palliative procedures have been proposed and long-term survivors have been reported.

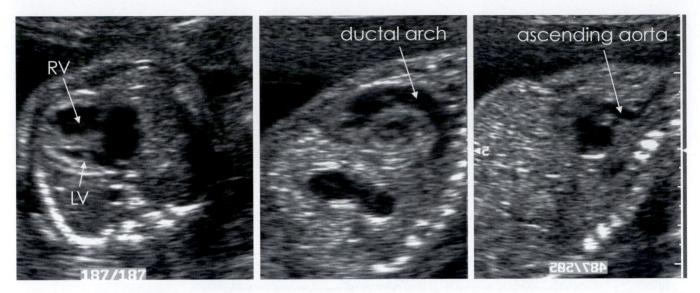

Figure 8–11. The right-to-left ventricular ratio exceeds 1.5. The ductal arch is more prominent than normal. The ascending aorta has a vertical course with no demonstrable connection with the descending aorta. This is an example of an interrupted aortic arch.

Recently, cardiac transplantation in the neonatal period has also been attempted.

Hypoplastic left heart is well tolerated *in utero*. The patency of the ductus arteriosus allows adequate perfusion of the head and neck vessels. Intrauterine growth may be normal, and the onset of symptoms most frequently occurs after birth. Congestive heart failure is seen only in cases with insufficiency of the atrioventricular valves, which represent a distinct minority.

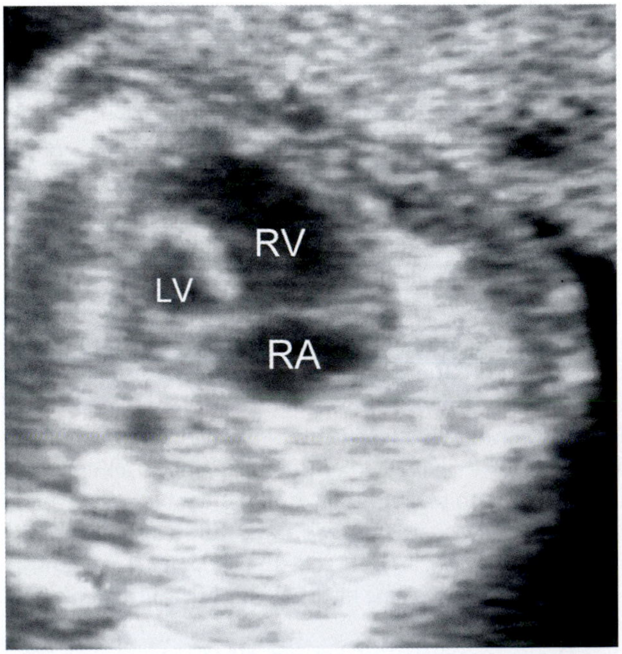

Pulmonary Stenosis. The most common form of pulmonary stenosis is the valvar type, which occurs with the fusion of the pulmonary leaflets. Hemodynamics is altered proportionally to the degree of the stenosis. The work of the right ventricle is increased, as is the pressure, leading to hypertrophy of the ventricular walls. In the most severe cases, right ventricular overload may result in congestive heart failure.

The same considerations formulated for the prenatal diagnosis of aortic stenosis also are valid for pulmonic stenosis. A handful of cases recognized *in utero* have been reported in the literature thus far, mostly severe types with enlargement of the right ventricle and/or poststenotic enlargement or hypoplasia of the pulmonary artery (see Fig. 8–6).

Pulmonary Atresia with Intact Ventricular Septum. Pulmonary atresia with intact ventricular septum (PA:IVS) in infants is usually associated with a hypoplastic right ventricle. However, cases with an enlarged right ventricle and atrium have been described with unusual frequency in prenatal series.[37] Although the prenatal series are small, the discrepancy with the pediatric literature may be due to the very high perinatal loss rate that is found in "dilated" cases. Enlargement of the ventricle and atrium is probably the consequence of tricuspid insufficiency. Prenatal diagnosis of PA:IVS relies on the demonstration of a small pulmonary artery with an atretic pulmonary valve. The considerations previously formulated for the real-time and Doppler diagnosis of HLHS also apply to PA:IVS.

Figure 8–12. A four-chamber view demonstrates a diminutive left ventricle (LV) with a bright and thickened endocardium and no contractility in real-time examination, indicating hypoplastic left heart syndrome.

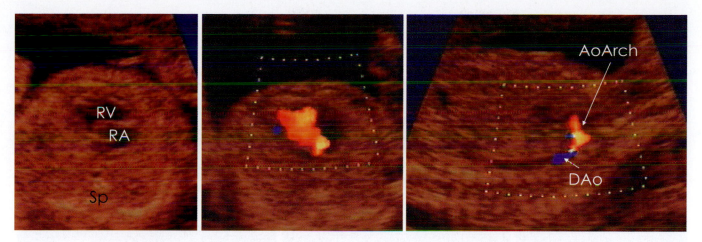

Figure 8–13. The left heart chambers are not visualized. Color Doppler sonography demonstrates only one patent atrioventricular valve and reverse flow within the aortic arch (AoArch), indicating hypoplastic left heart syndrome. Sp, spine; Dao, descending aorta.

Conotruncal Malformations

Conotruncal malformations are a heterogeneous group of defects that involve two different segments of the heart: the conotruncus and the ventricles.

Conotruncal anomalies are relatively frequent. They account for 20% to 30% of all cardiac anomalies[1] and are the leading cause of symptomatic cyanotic heart disease in the first year of life. Prenatal diagnosis is of interest for several reasons. Given the parallel model of fetal circulation, conotruncal anomalies are well tolerated *in utero*. The clinical presentation occurs usually hours to days after delivery and is often severe, representing a true emergency and leading to considerable morbidity and mortality. Nevertheless these malformations have a good prognosis when promptly treated. Two ventricles of adequate size and two great vessels are commonly present, thereby allowing biventricular surgical correction. The outcome is much more favorable than with most of the other cardiac defects that are detected antenatally.

The first reports on prenatal echocardiography of conotruncal malformations date from the beginning of the 1980s. Nevertheless, despite improvement in the technology of diagnostic ultrasound, the recognition of these anomalies remains difficult. The four-chamber view, which many recommend including in the standard sonographic examination of fetal anatomy, is frequently unremarkable in these cases. A specific diagnosis requires meticulous scanning and at times may represent a challenge even for experienced sonologists. Referral centers with special expertise in fetal echocardiography have reported both false-positive[4] and false-negative diagnoses.

Transposition of the Great Arteries. Transposition of the great arteries (TGA) is most commonly found in the complete form, which is characterized by atrioventricular concordance with ventriculoarterial discordance. The aorta arises from the right ventricle and lies anterior to and left of the pulmonary artery, which is connected to the left ventricle and lies posteriorly and medially. The most common form is the so-called D-TGA.

The prevalence is 2 per 10,000 live births.[11] Associated lesions are present in roughly 50% of cases, including ventricular septal defects (which can occur anywhere in the ventricular septum), pulmonary stenosis, unbalanced ventricular size ("complex transpositions"), and anomalies of the mitral valve, which can be straddling or overriding.

According to Becker and Anderson,[15] three types of complete TGA can be distinguished: TGA with intact ventricular septum with or without pulmonary stenosis, TGA with ventricular septal defects, and TGA with ventricular septal defect and pulmonary stenosis.

Complete transposition is probably one of the most difficult cardiac lesions to recognize *in utero*. In most cases, the four-chamber view is normal, and the cardiac cavities and the vessels appear normal. A clue to the diagnosis is the demonstration of the two great vessels not crossing but arising parallel from the base of the heart. The most useful echocardiographic view *in utero* is the equivalent of the subcostal oblique view postnatally,[7] which may demonstrate that the vessel connected to the left ventricle has a posterior course and bifurcates into the two pulmonary arteries. Conversely, the vessel connected to the right ventricle has a long upward couse and gives rise to the brachiocephalic vessels (Fig. 8–14).

Difficulties may arise in the case of a huge, malaligned, ventricular septal defect with overriding of the posterior semilunar root. This combination makes the differentiation from double-outlet right ventricle very difficult.

Corrected TGA is characterized by a double discordance at the atrioventricular and ventriculoarterial levels. The left atrium is connected to the right ventricle, which in turn is

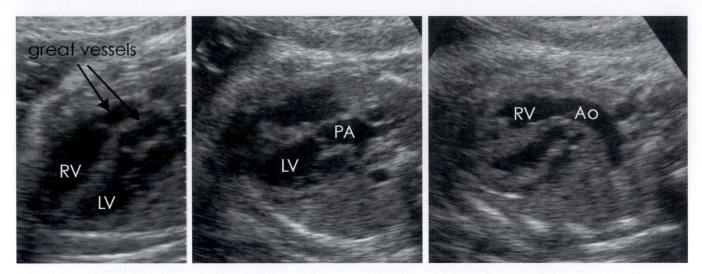

Figure 8–14. Complete transposition of the great vessels. The great vessels arise side by side from the base of the heart. The artery connected with the left ventricle (LV) has a posterior course and bifurcates and thus can be identified with the pulmonary artery (PA). The artery connected with the right ventricle (RV) has a long upward course and gives rise to the brachiocephalic vessels and thus can be identified with the aorta (Ao).

connected to the ascending aorta. Conversely, the right atrium is connected with the right ventricle, which in turn is connected to the ascending aorta. The derangement of the conduction tissue secondary to malalignment of the atrial and ventricular septa may result in dysrrhythmias, namely a complete atrioventricular block.

For diagnostic purposes, the identification of the peculiar difference in ventricular morphology (moderator band, papillary muscles, insertion of the atrioventricular valves) has a preminent role. The appearance of the pulmonary veins connected to an atrium that in turn is connected to a ventricle that has the moderator band at the apex is an important clue, which is identifiable in a simple four-chamber view (Fig. 8–3). Diagnosis requires meticulous scanning to carefully assess all cardiac connections by using the same views as those described for the complete form. The presence of an atrioventricular block increases the index of suspicion.[38]

As anticipated from the parallel model of fetal circulation, complete TGA is uneventful *in utero*. The lack of hemodynamic compromise is indirectly established by the frequency of normal birth weight in these infants. After birth, survival depends on the amount and size of the mixing of the two otherwise independent circulation systems. Patients with TGA and an intact ventricular septum present shortly after birth with cyanosis and tend to deteriorate rapidly. When a large ventricular septal defect is present, cyanosis can be mild. Clinical presentation may be delayed up to 2 to 4 weeks and usually occurs with signs of congestive heart failure. When severe stenosis of the pulmonary artery is associated with a ventricular septal defect, symptoms are similar to those in patients with tetralogy of Fallot.

The time and mode of clinical presentation with corrected TGA depend on the concomitant cardiac defects (ventricular septal defects, pulmonary stenosis, bradycardia, etc.).

Double-Outlet Right Ventricle. In double-outlet ventricle (DORV), most of the aorta and pulmonary valve arise completely or almost completely from the right ventricle. The relation between the two vessels may vary, ranging from a Fallot-like to a TGA-like situation (the Taussig–Bing anomaly). Double ORV is not a single malformation from a pathophysiologic point of view. The term refers only to the position of the great vessels that is found in association with ventricular septal defects, tetralogy of Fallot, transposition, and univentricular hearts.

The prevalence is 0.032 per 1000 live births.[11] Pulmonary stenosis is very common in all types of DORV, but left outflow obstructions, from subaortic stenosis to coarctation, and interruption of the arotic arch can also be seen.

Prenatal diagnosis of DORV can be made reliably in the fetus,[13] but differentiation from other conotruncal anomalies can be very difficult, especially with tetralogy of Fallot and TGA with ventricular septal defect. The main echocardiographic features include (a) alignment of the two vessels totally or predominantly from the right ventricle and (b) the presence in most cases of bilateral coni (subaortic and subpulmonary).

The hemodynamics are dependent on the anatomic type of DORV and the associated anomalies. Because the fetal heart works as a common chamber where the blood is mixed and pumped, the presence of DORV is not expected to be a cause of cardiac failure. Indeed, in our series of 10 cases, we have never seen intrauterine heart failure. As opposed to other conotruncal malformations, we have frequently found extracardiac anomalies and/or chromosomal aberrations associated with fetal DORV.

Tetralogy of Fallot.   The essential features of this malformation are (a) malalignment of the ventricular septal defect with anterior displacement of the infundibular septum associated with subpulmonary narrowing and an overriding aortic root and (b) demonstrable continuity between the right outflow tract and the pulmonary trunk. In about 20% of cases this continuity is lacking, leading to atresia of the pulmonary valve, a condition that is commonly referred to as *pulmonary atresia with ventricular septal defect*. Tetralogy of Fallot can be associated with other specific cardiac malformations that define peculiar entities, including atrioventricular septal defects, found in 4% of cases, and absence of the pulmonary valve, found in fewer than 2%. Hypertrophy of the right ventricle, one of the classic elements of the tetrad, is always absent in the fetus and develops only after birth.

Echocardiographic diagnosis of tetralogy of Fallot relies on the demonstration of a ventricular septal defect in the outlet portion of the septum and an overriding aorta. There is an inverse relation between the size of the ascending aorta and the pulmonary artery, with a disproportion that is often striking (Fig. 8–15). A large aortic root is an important diagnostic clue.[39] Doppler studies provide valuable information. The finding of increased peak velocities in the pulmonary artery corroborates the diagnosis of tetralogy of Fallot by suggesting obstruction of blood flow in the right outflow tract. Conversely, demonstration with color and/or pulsed Doppler that in the pulmonary artery there is neither forward nor reverse flow, allows a diagnosis of pulmonary atresia.

Diagnostic problems arise at the extremes of the spectrum of tetralogy of Fallot. In cases with minor forms of right outflow obstruction and an overriding aorta, differentiation from a simple ventricular septal defect can be difficult. In those cases in which the pulmonary artery is not imaged, a differential diagnosis between pulmonary atresia with ventricular septal defect and truncus arteriosus communis is similarly difficult.

The sonographer should also be alerted to a frequent artifact that resembles overriding of the aorta. Incorrect orientation of the transducer may demonstrate apparent septoaortic discontinuity in a normal fetus. The mechanism of the artifact is probably related to the angle of incidence of the sound beam. Although such an artifact caused the only false-positive finding in our series,[40] our experience since then suggests that careful visualization of the left outflow tract with different insonation angles, the use of color Doppler, and the research of the other elements of the tetralogy should virtually eliminate this problem.

Atrioventricular connections need to be carefully assessed to rule out the possible association with atrioventricular septal defects. Such a combination is associated with an increased risk of concomitant autosomal trisomies, Down syndrome in particular, and results *per se* in a worse prognosis. Abnormal enlargement of the right ventricle, main pulmonary trunk, and artery suggests the absence of a pulmonary valve.[2]

Evaluation of other variables, such as multiple ventricular septal defects and coronary anomalies, would be valuable for a better prediction of surgical timing and operative prognosis. Unfortunately, these findings cannot be recognized with certainty by prenatal echocardiography at present.

Cardiac failure is never seen prenatally or postnatally. Even in cases of tight pulmonary stenosis or atresia, the wide ventricular septal defect provides adequate combined ventricular output, and the pulmonary vascular bed is supplied in a retrograde manner by the ductus. The only exception to this rule is represented by cases with an absent pulmonary valve that may result in massive regurgitation to the right ventricle and atrium.

When severe pulmonic stenosis is present, cyanosis tends to develop immediately after birth. When a lesser degree

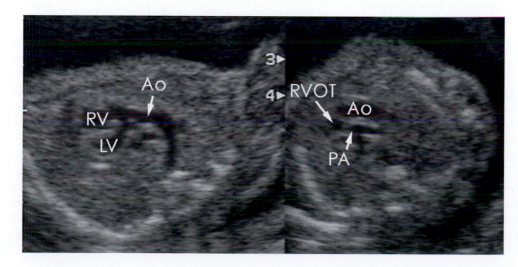

Figure 8–15. Tetralogy of Fallot. The aorta (Ao) overrides the ventricular septum by about 50%. The outflow tract of the right ventricle (RVOT) and the pulmonary artery (PA) are restricted.

of obstruction in pulmonary blood flow is present, the onset of cyanosis may not appear until the first year of life. When there is pulmonary atresia, rapid and severe deterioration follows ductal constriction.

Truncus Arteriosus Communis. Truncus arteriosus is characterized by a single arterial vessel that originates from the heart, overrides the ventricular septum, and supplies the systemic, pulmonary, and coronary circulation systems.

The single arteral trunk is larger than the normal aortic root and is connected predominantly with the right ventricle in roughly 42% of cases, with the left ventricle in 16%, and is equally shared in 42%.[41] The truncal valve may have one, two, or three cusps and is rarely normal. It can be stenotic or, more frequently, insufficient. A malalignment ventricular septal defect, usually wide, is an essential part of the malformation.

Truncus arteriosus can be classified in different ways, according to Collets and Edwards[42] and Van Praagh and Van Praagh.[43] The following situations can be recognized:

- The pulmonary arteries arise from the truncus within a short distance from the valve as a main pulmonary trunk that then bifurcates (type A or I) or without the main pulmonary trunk (type A2 or II and III).
- Less frequently, only one pulmonary artery (usually the right) originates from the truncus, whereas the other is supplied by a systemic collateral vessel from descending aorta (type A3).

Truncus has been associated with interrupted aortic arch (type A4) in 11% of cases. Similar to tetralogy of Fallot and unlike the other conotruncal malformations, truncus is frequently associated with extracardiac malformations in a proportion ranging between 20 and 40%.

Truncus arteriosus can be detected reliably with fetal echocardiography (Fig. 8–16). The main diagnostic criteria are the following:

- a single semilunar valve that overrides the ventricular septal defect
- a direct continuity between one or two pulmonary arteries and the single arterial trunk

The semilunar valve is often thickened and moves abnormally. Doppler ultrasound is of value to assess incompetence of the truncal valve.

A peculiar problem found in prenatal echocardiography is the demonstration of the absence of the pulmonary outflow tract and the concomitant failure to image the pulmonary arteries. In this situation, a differentiation between truncus and pulmonary atresia with ventricular septal defect may be impossible.

Similar to the other conotruncal anomalies, truncus arteriosus is not associated with alteration of fetal hemodynamics. The only remarkable exception is the case with an incompetent truncal valve that may result in massive regurgitation of blood to the ventricles and cause congestive heart

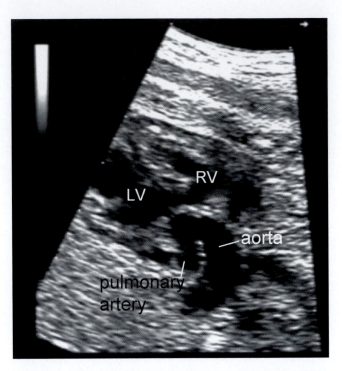

Figure 8–16. Truncus arteriosus type A. A single large vessel is seen arising from the base the heart. The truncal valve is thickened. The aortopulmonary septum is seen dividing the truncus distally into its aortic and pulmonary portions.

failure. This did not occur in our series of five consecutive cases, and we are not aware of any such case reported in the literature. Truncus arteriosus is frequently a neonatal emergency. These patients usually have unobstructed pulmonary blood flow and show signs of progressive congestive heart failure with the postnatal fall in pulmonary resistance. Many patients will present with cardiac failure in the first 1 or 2 weeks of life.

Cardiosplenic Syndromes

In cardiosplenic syndromes, the fetus has either two left or two right sides. Other terms commonly used include *left* or *right isomerism, asplenia,* and *polysplenia.* Unpaired organs (liver, stomach, and spleen) may be absent, mid-line, or duplicated. Because of left atrial isomerism (and thus absence of the right atrium, which is the normal location for the pacemaker) and abnormal atrioventricular junctions, atrioventricular blocks are very common.

Polysplenia. Polysplenia is also called *left isomerism.* The spleens are usually posterior to the stomach but may be variable, which renders their identification even more difficult. As in asplenia, the liver is usually mid-line. The stomach and aorta may be on opposite sides. The cardiac anomalies, although common, are less severe than those affecting asplenia. Cardiac anomalies include:

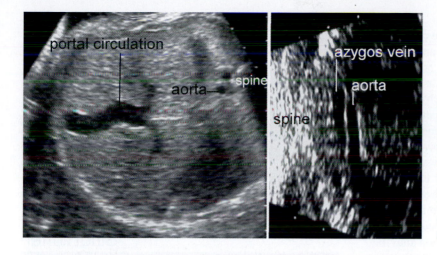

Figure 8–17. Polysplenia. *Left:* Transverse section of the abdomen demonstrates an unusual course of the portal circulation, suggesting a symmetric liver, and an abnormal disposition of the main abdominal vessels: the aorta is found in a central position, anterior to the spine; the inferior vena cava is not identified; and a large venous vessel is seen posterior to the aorta. *Right:* The venous vessel posterior to the aorta is seen reaching the upper thorax and is thus identified as an azygos vein.

- interrupted inferior vena cava with azygos continuation (75%)
- partial anomalous pulmonary venous return; most commonly, the pulmonary vein drains bilaterally to both atria
- bilateral superior vena cava, each entering its own atrium
- rarely, transposition of the great arteries or DORV
- atrial septal defects
- obstructive lesions of the aortic valve
- ventricular septal defect or endocardial cushion defect

Symmetry of the liver can be sonographically recognized *in utero* by the abnormal course of the portal circulation, when a clearly defined portal sinus bending to the right is not displayed. Interruption of the inferior vena cava is also characteristic (Fig. 8–17). In polysplenia, the cava is interrupted and continues into the hemiazygos, which is ipsilateral and posterior to the aorta. The azygos vein drains into the superior vena cava. The hepatic vein does not join the inferior vena cava but crosses over to the left to empty into the azygos continuation or into the nearest atrium (not always the right atrium). Although the spleen can be identified in normal fetuses, its absence is not a reliable finding because the spleen can be difficult to identify or replaced by small splenic nodules.

Associated anomalies include multiple spleens (often too small to be detected), bilateral bilobed lungs, absence of the gallbladder and hypoplastic biliary structures, malrotation of the guts, duodenal atresia preduodenal portal vein, and hydrops.

Asplenia. In asplenia, the fetus has two right sides: one in the normal position, and the other as a mirror image. This is called *right isomerism.* Thus, left-side organs such as the spleen are rudimentary or absent. The liver is generally mid-line, and the stomach is right or left sided. The heart has two "right atria." The cardiac malformations are severe, with a tendency toward a single structure replacing normal paired structures: single atrium, single atrioventricular valve, single ventricle, and single great vessel. The following are typically associated with asplenia:

- bilateral superior vena cava
- DORV or pulmonary atresia
- large atrial septal defect; the interatrial septum is reduced to a fibrous band
- single atrioventricular valve and single ventricle
- total or partial anomalous pulmonary venous return; because there is no "left" atrium, the pulmonary vein connects anomalously; drainage is often either supracardiac or infradiaphragmatic, but even when pulmonary veins enter the atrium, their morphology and connections are abnormal
- large ventricular septal defect
- transposition of the great arteries
- pulmonary restriction (stenosis or atresia)

The condition is more common in male fetuses, and few survive past the first few weeks or months.

Evaluation of the disposition of the abdominal organs is of special value for the sonographic diagnosis of fetal right isomerism. In situs solitus and in situs inversus, the aorta, and vena cava are on contralateral sides of the mid-line, with the cava ipsilateral to the right atrium.[44] In asplenia, the cava is ipsilateral and anterior to the aorta, and the hepatic vein enters the atrium independently from the cava.[45] In the abdomen, the liver is transverse, and the aorta and cava are on the same side (either left or right) of the spine. The spleen cannot be seen,[46] and the stomach is found in close contact with the thoracic wall. The heterogeneous cardiac anomalies found in association with asplenia are usually easily seen, but a detailed diagnosis is usually a challenge. In particular, assessment of connection between the pulmonary veins and the atrium (an element that has a major prognostic influence) can be extremely difficult.

Fetal Dysrhythmias

Irregular patterns of fetal heart rhythms are a frequent finding. Short periods of tachycardia, bradycardia, and ectopic beats are very commonly seen and, in the vast majority of cases, have no clinical significance. A sustained bradycardia of less than 100 beats per minute, a sustained tachycardia of more than 200 beats per minute, and irregular beats occurring more than 1 in 10 should be considered abnormal and require further investigation.[47] The fetal electrocardiogram is of little value in the prenatal diagnosis of dysrhythmias because a satisfactory transabdominal recording can be obtained in a minority of cases. At present, M-mode and pulsed Doppler ultrasound are the best available techniques for the assessment of irregular fetal heart rhythm. The study of the mechanical events of the sequence of contraction may be accomplished in different ways. Simultaneous visualization of atrioventricular valves and ventricular wall motion, aortic valve opening and atrial wall movement with M-mode, and sampling of the ventricular inlet or inferior vena cava with M-mode can be used from time to time. The sequence of excitation can be reasonably inferred by the sequence of contraction (Fig. 8–18).

Premature Atrial and Ventricular Contraction. Premature atrial and ventricular contractions are the most frequent fetal dysrrhythmias.[48] Repeated premature contractions can give rise to complex rhythm patterns. Premature atrial contractions may be either conducted to the ventricles or blocked, depending on the time of the cardiac cycle in which they occur, thus resulting in either an increased or a decreased ventricular rate. Blocked premature atrial contractions should be differentiated from atrioventricular block. Premature atrial and ventricular contractions are considered a benign condition. They probably do not induce any hemodynamic perturbance, do not appear to be associated with an increased risk of structural abnormalities, and usually disappear *in utero* or soon after birth. However, because there is at least a theoretical possibility that in a few cases an ectopic beat may trigger a reentrant tachyarrhythmia, serial monitoring of the fetal heart during pregnancy is suggested. Pulsed Doppler ultrasound evaluation of blood flow in fetuses with premature beats shows that the fetal heart is capable of postextrasystolic popentiation and that the Frank–Starling mechanism is operating since the early stages of fetal development.

Supraventricular Tachyarrhythmias. Supraventricular tachyarrhythmias include supraventricular paroxysmal tachycardia (SVT), atrial flutter, and atrial fibrillation. Supraventricular paroxysmal tachycardia is characterized by an atrial frequency between 200 and 300 beats per minute and a 1:1 atrioventricular conduction rate. It can occur by one of two mechanisms: automaticity and reentry. In the former case, an irritable ectopic focus discharges at high frequency. In the latter case, an electrical impulse reenters the atria, giving rise to repeated electrical activity. Reentry may occur at the level

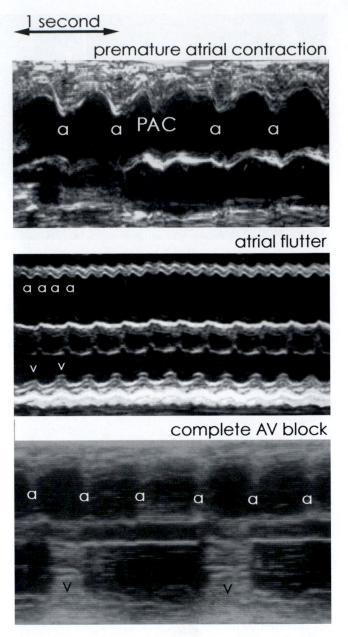

Figure 8–18. Diagnosis of fetal dysrhythmias with M-mode: *a,* atrial contractions; *v,* ventricular contractions. In the *upper* panel, a premature atrial contraction (PAC) is seen. In the *middle* panel, the atria contract rapidly with a frequency of about 440 beats per second, and the ventricles respond with a frequency of 220 beats per second, indicating an atrial flutter with a 2:1 atrioventricular block. In the *lower* panel, the atria contract regularly with a frequency of about 120 beats per second. The ventricles contract with a frequency of about 50 beats per second independent of atrial contractions. This is complete atrioventricular block.

of the sinoatrial node or inside the atrium, the atrioventricular node, and the His Purkinje system. Reentry may also occur along an anomalous atrioventricular connection such as the Kent bundle in Wolff–Parkinson–White syndrome. In atrial flutter, the atrial rate ranges from 300 to 400 beats per minute. Due to variable degrees of atrioventricular block, the ventricular rate ranges between 60 and 200 beats per minute. In atrial fibrillation, the atrial rate is more than 400 beats per minute and the ventricular rate ranges between 120 and 200 beats per minute. Atrial flutter and fibrillation often alternate and are thought to arise from similar mechanisms that include circus movement of the electrical impulse, ectopic formation, multiple reentry, and multifocal impulse formation. Supraventricular paroxysmal tachycardia is by far the most common tachyarrhythmia in children. The most frequent form is the one caused by atrioventricular nodal reentry.

Diagnosis of fetal tachyarrhythmia can be easily accomplished by direct auscultation or continuous Doppler examination. M-mode and/or pulsed Doppler ultrasound can identify the precise heart rate and recognize the atrioventricular sequence of contractions.

The association between fetal tachyarrhythmia and nonimmune hydrops is well established. It has been postulated that a fast ventricular rate results in suboptimal filling of the ventricles, which would lead to decreased cardiac output, right atrial overload, and congestive heart failure. The frequency of nonimmune hydrops is variable. We have seen fetuses with SVT who did well *in utero* and were successfully treated after birth. It can be postulated that, in those cases in which a reentry mechanism is involved, the fetus alternates phases of tachycardia and phases of normal rhythm. Intrauterine pharmacologic cardioversion of fetal tachyarrhythmia by maternal administration of drugs has been successful in many cases. Transplacental passage of anti-arrhythmic drugs is limited when fetal hydrops is present, and under these conditions a direct administration by ultrasound-guided funipuncture has been proposed. The optimal approach to the treatment of this condition is still uncertain. Digoxin, verapamil, propranolol, quinidine, procainamide, flecainide, and amiodarone have all been used. The interested reader is referred to specific works in this subject. Independently from the therapeutic regimen employed, the largest available series suggest a survival rate in the range of approximately 90%.[49–51]

Atrioventricular Block. Atrioventricular (AV) block can result from immaturity of the conduction system, absence of connection to the AV node, or abnormal anatomic position of the AV node. Atrioventricular block is commonly classified into three types. First-degree AV block corresponds to a simple conduction delay that is associated to a prolongation of the PR interval on the electrocardiogram. Second-degree AV block is subdivided into Mobitz types I and II. Mobitz type I consists of a progressive prolongation of the PR interval that finally leads to the block of one atrial impulse (Luciani–Wenckebach phenomenon). In Mobitz type II, the ventricular rate is a submultiple of the atrial rate (e.g., 2:1, 3:1). In third-degree or complete AV block, there is a complete dissociation of atria and ventricles, usually with independent and slow activation of the ventricles. Third-degree AV block has been associated with more than half of the cases of cardiac structural anomalies, mostly with atrioventricular discordance.[52] In cases without structural cardiac diseases, the etiology of AV block mostly depends on the presence of maternal antibodies against SSA and SSB antigens. Transplacental passage of these antibodies would lead to inflammation and damage of the conduction system. Anti-SSA antibodies have been reported in more than 80% of mothers who delivered infants with AV block, although only 30% had clinical evidence of connective tissue disease, mostly lupus erythematosus.[53–56]

First- and second-degree AV block are not usually associated with any significant hemodynamic perturbance. Third-degree AV block may lead to bradycardia that causes a decreased cardiac output and congestive heart failure *in utero*. In the largest available antenatal series that included 55 cases diagnosed *in utero*, the adverse prognostic factors included the presence of structural cardiac disease, hydrops, and a ventricular rate of fewer than 55 beats per minute.[57]

Intrauterine ventricular pacing was attempted in one case. A lead was inserted through the maternal abdominal and uterine wall and the fetal thorax and placed inside the right ventricle. Although a regular ventricular frequency was obtained, fetal death ensued a few hours later.[58] Plasmapheresis to reduce the transplacental passage of anibodies has been employed with limited success. The use of maternal steroids to limit the inflammatory response in the fetal cardiac conducting system has been reported with successful results. The use of immunosuppressive agents has also been advocated.[59]

EARLY DIAGNOSIS OF FETAL HEART DISEASE WITH TRANSVAGINAL SONOGRAPHY

Transvaginal high-frequency, high-resolution ultrasound probes allow a very detailed evaluation of embryonic and fetal anatomy very early in gestation. A four-chamber view of the fetal heart after 12 weeks of gestation is usually possible with this equipment. A detailed examination of cardiac connection is frequently possible by 14 weeks. The capability of transvaginal sonography to predict fetal malformation very early in gestation is currently under investigation (Fig. 8–19). Reports from different institutions suggest that the diagnosis of several types of cardiac anomalies is feasible in the interval between the late first trimester and the early second trimester.[60–62]

Several investigators have suggested that, in pregnancies at risk for fetal heart disease, an echocardiographic examination should be performed at approximately 14 weeks with a transvaginal probe. However, experience suggests that several lesions will not be diagnosed until the mid-trimester. Thus, it seems prudent that in these cases a second examination be scheduled at approximately 20 weeks for a definitive echocardiographic examination.

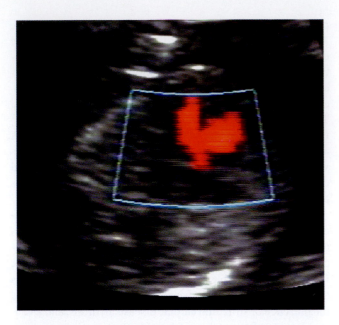

Figure 8–19. In a 13-week fetus with increased nuchal translucency, color Doppler transvaginal echocardiography demonstrates a complete atrioventricular septal defect. Chorionic villus sampling was performed and revealed trisomy 21.

DIAGNOSTIC ACCURACY OF FETAL ECHOCARDIOGRAPHY

Fetal echocardiography allows the antenatal diagnosis of congenital heart disease, but the accuracy of this technique has been difficult to establish. Prenatal echocardiography has a tendency to detect the more severe anomalies (univentricular heart, severe outflow obstructions, and endocardial cushion defects) and miss the more benign lesions. Defects that have commonly been missed include ventricular septal defect (membranous and muscular), secundum atrial septal defect, coarctation, supravalvar aortic stenosis, and tetralogy of Fallot.[63] Lesions that affect the four-chamber view are detected more often than conotruncal lesions. Further, the natural evolution of some anomalies may be such that they only appear in the third trimester. Examples of these anomalies include premature occlusion of the foramen ovale,[64] pulmonary stenosis with intact ventricular septum,[65] and cardiac tumors.[66]

Studies in which a detailed fetal echocardiogram was performed reported sensitivities in the range of 70 to 85%.[67–70]

A standard sonographic examination of fetal anatomy in the mid-trimester should always include a four-chamber view. The sensitivity of this approach in detecting congenital heart disease is, however, controversial. Some studies have found a sensitivity of as high as 80%, whereas others have reported disappointing results, with sensitivities of 5 to 15%.[71,72]

Recent evidence suggests that a high detection rate of cardiac lesions (more than 50%) can be achieved by referral to a specialist in echocardiography for patients with increased nuchal translucency at 10 to 14 weeks.[73,74]

REFERENCES

1. Allan LD. Fetal echocardiography. *Clin Obstet Gynecol.* 1998;31:61.
2. Allan LD, Crawford DC, Chita SK, et al. Familial recurrence of congenital heart disease in a prospective series of mothers referred for fetal echocardiography. *Am J Cardiol.* 1986;58:334.
3. Cyr DR, Guntheroth WG, Mack LA, et al. A systematic approach to fetal echocardiography using real time/two dimensional sonography. *J Ultrasound Med.* 1986;5:343.
4. Klinkenbijl J, Wenink AC. Morphology of sections through the fetal heart. *Int J Cardiol.* 1988;20:87.
5. Comstock CH. Normal fetal heart axis and position. *Obstet Gynecol.* 1987;70:255.
6. Silverman NH, Kleinman CS, Rudolph AM, et al. Fetal atrioventricular valve insufficiency associated with nonimmune hydrops: A two dimensional echocardiographic and pulsed Doppler ultrasound study. *Circulation.* 1985;72:825.
7. Cyr DR, Guntheroth WG, Mack LA, et al. A systematic approach to fetal echocardiography using real time/two dimensional sonography. *J Ultrasound Med.* 1986;5:343.
8. Gembruch U, Knopfle G, Bald R, et al. Early diagnosis of congential heart disease by transvaginal echocardiography. *Ultrasound Obstet Gynecol.* 1993;3:310.
9. Kleinman CS, Santulli TV Jr. Ultrasonic evaluation of the fetal human heart. *Semin Perinatol.* 1983;7:90.
10. Fyler DC, Buckley LP, Hellenbrand WE, et al. Report of the New England Regional Cardiac Program. *Pediatrics.* 1980;65(suppl):375.
11. Brons JT, van Geijn HP, Wladimiroff JW, et al. Prenatal ultrasound diagnosis of the Holt Oram syndrome. *Prenat Diagn.* 1988;8:175.
12. Kleinman CS, Donnerstein RL, DeVore GR, et al. Fetal echocardiography for evaluation of *in utero* congestive heart failure: A technique for study of nonimmune fetal hydrops. *N Engl J Med.* 1982;306:568.
13. Machado MV, Crawford DC, Anderson RH, et al. Atrioventricular septal defect in prenatal life. *Br Heart J.* 1988;59:352.
14. Machado MV, Crawford DC, Anderson RH, et al. Atrioventricular septal defect in prenatal life. *Br Heart J.* 1988;59:352.
15. Becker AE, Anderson RH. *Pathology of Congenital Heart Disease.* London: Butterworths; 1981.
16. Walther FJ, Siassi B, King J, et al. Cardiac output in infants of insulin-dependent diabetic mothers. *J Pediatr.* 1985;107:109.
17. Huhta JC, Carpenter RJ, Moise KJ, et al. Prenatal diagnosis and postnatal management of critical aortic stenosis. *Circulation.* 1987;75:573.
18. Stewart PA, Buis-Liem T, Verwey RA, et al. Prenatal ultrasonic diagnosis of familial asymmetric septal hypertrophy. *Prenat Diagn.* 1986;6:249.
19. Wright GB, Keane JF, Nadas AS, et al. Fixed subaortic stenosis in the young. Medical and surgical course in 83 patients. *Am J Cardiol.* 1983;52:830.
20. Rizzo G, Arduni D, Romanini C. Accelerated cardiac growth

and abnormal cardiac flows in fetuses of type I diabetic mothers. *Obstet Gynecol.* 1992;80:369.

21. Allan LD, Little D, Campbell S, et al. Fetal ascites associated with congenital heart disease. Case report. *Br J Obstet Gynaecol.* 1981;88:453.

22. Reynolds JL. Intrauterine growth retardation in children with congenital heart disease. Its relation to aortic stenosis. *Birth Defects Orig Art Ser.* 1972;8:143.

23. Becker AE, Becker MJ, Edwards JE. Anomalies associated with coarctation of the aorta. *Circulation.* 1970;41:1067.

24. Rosenquist GC. Congenital mitral valve disease associated with coarctation of the aorta. *Circulation.* 1974;49:985.

25. Machado MV, Tynan MJ, et al. Fetal complete heart block. *Br Heart J.* 1988;60:512.

26. Crawford DC, Drake DP, Kwaitkowski D, et al. Prenatal diagnosis of reversible cardiac hypoplasia associated with congenital diaphragmatic hernia: Implications for postnatal management. *JCU.* 1986;14:718.

27. Siebert JR, Hass JE, Beckwith JB. Left ventricular hypoplasia in congenital diaphragmatic hernia. *J Pediatr Surg.* 1984;19:567.

28. Allan LD, Crawford DC, Tynan MI. Evolution of coarctation of the aorta in intrauterine life. *Br Heart J.* 1984;52:471.

29. Allan LD, Chita SK, Anderson RH, et al. Coarctation of the aorta in prenatal life: An echocardiographic, anatomical, and functional study. *Br Heart J.* 1988;59:356.

30. Benacerraf BR, Saltzman DH, Sanders SP. Sonographic sign suggesting the prenatal diagnosis of coarctation of the aorta. *J Ultrasound Med.* 1989;8:65.

31. Van Mierop L, Kutsche LM. Interruption of the aortic arch and coarctation of the aorta: Pathogenetic relations. *Am J Cardiol.* 1971;54:829.

32. Van Praagh R, Bernhard W, Rosenthal A, et al. Interrupted aortic arch: Surgical treatment. *Am J Cardiol.* 1971;27:200.

33. Marasini M, Pongiglione G, Lituania M, et al. Aortic arch interruption: Two dimensional echocardiographic recognition in utero. *Pediatr Cardiol.* 1985;6:147.

34. Sahn DJ, Shenker L, Reed KL, et al. Prenatal ultrasound diagnosis of hypoplastic left heart syndrome in utero associated with hydrops fetalis. *Am Heart J.* 1982;104:1368.

35. Silverman NH, Enderlein MA, Golbus MS. Ultrasonic recognition of aortic valve atresia *in utero. Am J Cardiol.* 1984;53:391.

36. Doty DB. Aortic atresia. *J Thorac Cardiovasc Surg.* 1980; 79:462.

37. Allan LD, Crawford DC, Tynan MJ. Pulmonary atresia in prenatal life. *J Am Coll Cardiol.* 1986;8:1131.

38. Schmidt KG, Ulmer HE, Silverman NH, et al. Perinatal outcome of fetal complete atrioventricular block: A multicenter experience. *JACC* 1991;17:1360.

39. De Vore GR, Siassi B, Platt LD. Fetal echocardiography VIII. Aortic root dilatation—a marker for tetralogy of Fallot. *Am J Obstet Gynecol.* 1988;159:129.

40. Pilu G, Baccarani G. Prenatal diagnosis of cardiac structural abnormalities. *Fetal Ther.* 1986;1:86.

41. Hernanz-Schulman M, Fellows KE. Persistent truncus arteriosus: Pathologic, diagnostic and therapeutical considerations. *Semin Roentgenol.* 1985;20:121.

42. Collett RW, Edwards JE. Persistent truncus arteriosus. A classification according to anatomic types. *Surg Clin North Am.* 1949;29:1245.

43. Van Praagh R, Van Praagh S. The anatomy of common aorticopulmonary trunk (truncus arteriosus communis) and its embryologic implications. A study of 57 necropsy cases. *Am J Cardiol.* 1965;16:406.

44. Huhta JC, Smallhorn JF, Macartney FJ. Cross-sectional echocardiographic diagnosis of situs. *Br Heart J.* 1982.

45. Stewart PA, Becker AE, Wladimiroff JW, et al. Left atrial isomerism associated with asplenia: Prenatal echocardiographic detection of complex congenital cardiac malformations. *J Am Coll Cardiol.* 1984;4:1015.

46. Chitayat D, Lao A, Wilson RD, et al. Prenatal diagnosis of asplenia/polysplenia syndrome. *Am J Obstet Gynecol.* 1988; 158:1085.

47. Allan LD, Anderson RH, Sullivan ID, et al. Evaluation of fetal arrhythmias by echocardiography. *Br Heart J.* 1983;50:240.

48. Kleinman CS, Donnerstein RL, Jaffe CC, et al. Fetal echocardiography. A tool for evaluation of *in utero* cardiac arrhythmias and monitoring of *in utero* therapy: Analysis of 71 patients. *Am J Cardiol.* 1983;51:237.

49. Kleinman CS, Copel JA, Weinstein EM, et al. *In utero* diagnosis and treatment of fetal supraventricular tachycardia. *Semin Perinatol.* 1985;9:113.

50. Maxwell DJ, Crawford DC, Curry PVM, et al. Obstetric importance, diagnosis and management of fetal tachycardias. *Br Med J.* 1988;297:107.

51. Hansmann M, Gembruch U, Bald R, et al. Fetal tachyarrhythmias: Transplacental and direct treatment of the fetus. A report of 60 cases. *Ultrasound Obstet Gynecol.* 1991;1:162.

52. Griffiths SP. Congenital complete heart block. *Circulation.* 1971;43:615.

53. Chameides L, Truex RC, Vetter V, et al. Association of maternal systemic lupus erythematosus with congenital complete heart block. *N Engl J Med* 1977;297:1204.

54. McCue CM, Mantakas ME, Tingelstad JB, et al. Congenital heart block in newborns of mothers with connective tissue disease. *Circulation.* 1977;56:82.

55. Scott JS, Maddison PJ, Taylor PV, et al. Connective tissue disease, antibodies to ribonucleoprotein and congenital heart block. *N Engl J Med.* 1983;309:209.

56. Singsen BH, Akthar JE, Weinstein MM, et al. Congenital complete heart block and SSA antibodies. Obstetric implications. *Am J Obstet Gynecol.* 1985;152:655.

57. Schmidt KG, Ulmer HE, Silverman NH, et al. Perinatal outcome of fetal complete atrioventricular block: A multicenter experience. *J Am Coll Cardiol.* 1991;17:1360.

58. Carpenter RJ, Strasburger JF, Garson A, et al. Fetal ventricular pacing for hydrops secondary to complete atrioventricular block. *J Am Coll Cardiol.* 1986;8:1434.

59. Olah KS, Gee H. Fetal heart block associated with maternal anti-Ro (SS-A) antibody. Current management. A review. *Br J Obstet Gynaecol.* 1991;98:751.

60. Gembruch U, Knolpfe G, Chatterjee M, et al. First trimester diagnosis of fetal congenital heart disease by transvaginal two-dimensional and Doppler echocardiography. *Obstet Gynecol.* 1990;75:496.

61. Bronshtein M, Zimmer EZ, Milo S, et al. Fetal cardiac abnormalities detected by transvaginal sonography at 12–16 weeks' gestation. *Obstet Gynecol.* 1991;78:374.

62. Johnson P, Sharland G, Maxwell D, et al. The role of transvaginal sonography in the early detection of congenital heart disease. *Ultrasound Obstet Gynecol.* 1992;2:248.

63. Allan LD, Crawford DC, Tynan M. Evolution of coarctation of the aorta in intrauterine life. *Br Heart J.* 1984;52:471.

64. Pesonen E, Haavisto H, Ammala P, et al. Intrauterine hydrops caused by premature closure of the foramen ovale. *Arch Dis Child.* 1983;58:1015.

65. Todros T, Presbitero P, Gaglioti P, et al. Pulmonary stenosis with intact ventricular septum: Documentation of development of the lesion echographically during fetal life. *Int J Cardiol.* 1988;19:355.

66. Weber HS, Kleinman CS, Hellenbrand WE, et al. Development of a benign intrapericardial tumor between 20 and 40 weeks of gestation. *Pediatr Cardiol.* 1988;9:153.

67. Achiron R, Glaser J, Gelernter I, et al. Extended fetal echocardiographic examination for detecting cardiac malformations in low risk pregnancies. *Br Med J.* 1992;304:671.

68. Bromley B, Estroff JA, Sanders SP, et al. Fetal echocardiography: Accuracy and limitations in a population at high risk and low risk for heart defects. *Am J Obstet Gynecol.* 1992;166:1473.

69. Davis GK, Farquhar CM, Allan LD, et al. Structural cardiac abnormalities in the fetus: Reliability of prenatal diagnosis and outcome. *Br J Obstet Gynaecol.* 1990;97:27.

70. Stumpflen I, Stumpflen A, Wimmer M, et al. Effect of detailed fetal echocardiography as part of routine antenatal ultrasonographic screening on detection of congenital heart disease. *Lancet.* 1996;348:854.

71. Tegnander E, Eik-Nes SH, Johansen OJ, et al. Prenatal detection of heart defects at the routine fetal examination at 18 weeks in a non-selected population. *Ultrasound Obstet Gynecol.* 1995;5:372.

72. Todros T, Faggiano F, Chiappa E, et al. Accuracy of routine ultrasonography in screening heart disease prenatally. *Prenat Diagn.* 1997;17:901.

73. Hyett J, Perdu M, Sharland G, et al. Using fetal nuchal translucency to screen for major congenital cardiac defects at 10–14 weeks of gestation: Population based cohort study. *Br Med J.* 1999;318:81.

74. Zosmer N, Souter VL, Chan CS, et al. Early diagnosis of major cardiac defects in chromosomally normal fetuses with increased nuchal translucency. *Br J Obstet Gynaecol.* 1999;106:829.

9

Fetal Functional Echocardiography

Giuseppe Rizzo • Alessandra Capponi • Carlo Romanini

In adults, blood circulates sequentially through the systemic and pulmonary vasculature, and there is essentially no mixture of oxygenated blood and deoxygenated blood. Fetal cardiac hemodynamic differs from that of the postnatal period. During fetal life, blood is oxygenated in the placenta and returns to the fetal body through the umbilical vein. Studies on chronically instrumented fetal lambs have shown that in physiologic conditions approximately 55% of umbilical vein blood bypasses the hepatic circulation, entering directly in the inferior vena cava through the ductus venosus.[1] From the inferior vena cava, this highly oxygenated blood preferentially streams through the foramen ovale into the left atrium, left ventricle, and descending aorta.[2] Poorly oxygenated blood from the hepatic and superior vena cava circulations enters the right atrium and is almost completely directed through the tricuspid valve into the right ventricle and pulmonary artery.[2] Because fetal blood is not oxygenated in the lungs, an additional shunt (i.e., the ductus arteriosus) operates to bypass the pulmonary circulation, preferentially directing the right ventricle output to the descending aorta. As a consequence, both ventricles eject blood into the systemic circulation in parallel. The output of the left ventricle is directed through the ascending aorta to upper body, thus making available the most highly oxygenated blood to the heart and the brain. The right ventricle ejects less oxygenated blood through the patent ductus arteriosus and the descending aorta to the lower body and placenta.

These features of the fetal circulation raise interesting and important questions concerning the mechanisms responsible for providing oxygen and substrates to the different organs in normal and pathologic pregnancies. However there are limitations to the study of these mechanisms in the human fetus, and much of the understanding and present knowledge of fetal hemodynamics are derived from animal studies. However, recently technologic advances in ultrasound have made possible studying the human fetal heart. In particular, the advent of pulsed and color Doppler techniques have allowed examination of the fetal cardiovascular system, thus enabling hemodynamic studies on fetuses under both normal and abnormal conditions.

This chapter outlines the principles of fetal Doppler echocardiography and its practical uses, and it discusses its current and possible future applications.

TECHNIQUE

General Principles

The parameters used to describe fetal cardiac velocity waveforms differ from those used in fetal peripheral vessels. In peripheral circulation, indices such as the pulsatility index, resistance index, or systolic/diastolic (S/D) ratio are used. These indices are derived from relative ratios of systolic, diastolic, and mean velocity and thus are independent from the absolute blood velocity values and the angle of insonation of the Doppler beam.[3]

In contrast, in cardiac Doppler, all measurements represent absolute values. Measurements of absolute flow velocities require knowledge of the angle of insonation, which may be difficult to obtain with accuracy. The error in the estimation of the absolute velocity resulting from the uncertainty of angle measurement is strongly dependent on the magnitude in the angle itself. For angles smaller than about 20 degrees, the error will be reduced to an insignificant level. For larger angles, the cosine term in the Doppler equation changes the small uncertainty in the measurement of the angle to a large error in velocity estimation.[3] As a consequence, recordings should be always obtained with the Doppler beam as parallel as possible to the bloodstream, and all recordings with an estimated angle greater than 20 degrees should be rejected.

Color Doppler may help by demonstrating the flow direction in real time, thus allowing the sonographer to properly align the Doppler beam in the direction of the blood flow. To record velocity waveforms, pulsed Doppler is generally preferred to continuous-wave Doppler because of its range resolution. During recordings, the sample volume is placed immediately distal to the locations of investigation (e.g., distal to the aortic semilunar valves to record the left ventricle outflow). However, under conditions of particularly high velocities (e.g., in the ductus arteriosus), continuous Doppler may be useful because this modality is not affected aliasing.

Parameters Measured

The parameters most commonly used to describe the cardiac velocity waveforms are[4]

- the *peak velocity* (PV), expressed as the maximum velocity at a given moment (e.g., systole, diastole) on the Doppler spectrum
- the *time to peak velocity* (TPV), or acceleration time, expressed by the time interval between the onset of the waveform and its peak
- the *time-velocity integral* (TVI), calculated by measuring the area underneath the Doppler spectral waveform

It is possible also to calculate *absolute cardiac flow* from both atrioventricular valves and outflow tracts by multiplying the TVI by the valve area and the fetal heart rate (HR). These measurements are prone to errors mainly due to inaccuracies in estimating the valve area. Area is derived from the valve diameter, which is near the limits of ultrasound resolution. This parameter is then halved and squared in the calculation, thus amplifying potential errors. However, they can be used in longitudinal studies with short intervals between examinations in which the valve dimensions are assumed to remain relatively constant. Furthermore, it is also possible to accurately calculate the relative ratio between the right and left cardiac output (RCO/LCO); avoiding the measurements of the cardiac valve because the relative dimensions of aortic and pulmonary valves remain constant throughout gestation in the absence of cardiac structural diseases.[5]

The evaluation of *ventricular ejection force* (VEF) has also been recently used to assess fetal cardiac function.[6,7] VEF is a Doppler index based on Newton's law that estimates the energy transferred from right and left ventricular myocardial shortening to work done by accelerating blood into the pulmonary and systemic circulations, respectively.[8] This index appears to be less affected by changes in preload and afterload than other Doppler indices.[8] Results seem to be more accurate than those obtained with other Doppler variables such as peak velocities (used in the assessment of ventricular function in adults with chronic congestive heart failure).

VEF is calculated according to Newton's second law of motion. The force developed by the ventricular contraction accelerates a column of blood into the aorta or pulmonary artery and represents transfer of energy of myocardial shortening to work done on the pulmonary and systemic circulation. Newton's second law estimates the force as the product of mass and acceleration. The mass component in this model is the mass of blood accelerated into the outflow tract over a particular interval and may be calculated as the product of the density of blood (1.055), the valve area, and the flow velocity time integral during acceleration (FVI$_{AT}$), which is the area under the Doppler spectrum envelope up to the time of peak velocity. The acceleration component of the equation is estimated as the PV divided by the TPV. Thus, VEF is calculated with the following equation.[6]

$$VEF = (1.055 \times valve\ area \times FVI_{AT}) \times (PV/TPV).$$

Doppler Depiction of Fetal Cardiac Circulation

In the human fetus, velocity waveforms can be recorded at any point including venous return, foramen ovale, atrioventricular valves, outflow tracts, pulmonary arteries, and ductus arteriosus. Various factors affect the morphology of the velocity waveforms from different districts. Among these are preload,[9,10] afterload,[10,11] myocardiac contractility,[12] ventricular compliance,[13] and fetal HR.[14] The impossibility in obtaining simultaneous recordings of pressure and volume does not fully describe the contribution of these factors to the human fetal hemodynamics. However, because each parameter and site of recording are more specifically affected by one of these factors, it is possible to indirectly elucidate the underlying pathophysiology by performing measurements at different sites.

Venous Circulation. Blood flow velocity waveforms may be recorded from the superior and inferior vena cava, ductus venosus, hepatic veins, pulmonary veins, and umbilical vein. The vascular areas studied more frequently are the inferior vena cava (IVC) and the ductus venosus (DV).

The IVC velocity waveforms, recorded from the segment of the vessel just distal to the entrance of the ductus venosus,[15] are characterized by a triphasic profile with a first forward wave concomitant with ventricular systole, a

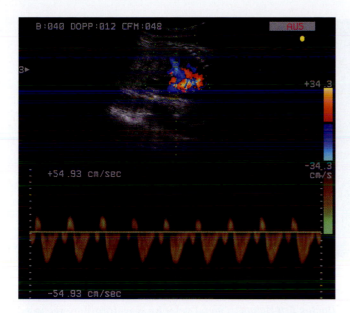

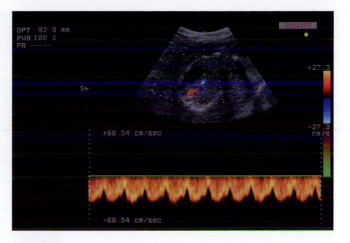

Figure 9–2. Blood flow velocity waveforms from the ductus venosus in a normal fetus at 34 weeks of gestation. The systolic-to-atrial contraction ratio is 0.48.

Figure 9–1. Velocity waveforms from the inferior vena cava in a normal fetus at 32 weeks of gestation depict the systolic (S) and diastolic (D) waves (bottom) and the reverse flow during atrial contraction (top). The preload index is 0.46.

second forward wave of smaller dimensions occurring with early diastole, and a third wave with reverse flow during atrial contraction[16,17] (Fig. 9–1). Several indices have been suggested to analyze IVC waveforms, but we have recently demonstated that the preload index (PLI) is more efficient than the others described in literature in predicting fetal compromise.[18] This index, expressed by the ratio between the PV during atrial contraction and the PV during systole (PLI = A/S),[19] is related to the pressure gradient between the right atrium and the right ventricle during end diastole, which is a function of both ventricular compliance and ventricular end diastolic pressure.[20]

The ductus venosus may be seen in a transverse section of the upper fetal abdomen at the level of its origin from the umbilical vein. Color is then superimposed, and the pulsed Doppler sample volume is placed just above its inlet (close to the umbilical vein) at the point of maximum flow velocity identified by color brightness. Ductus venosus flow velocity waveforms exhibit a biphasic pattern with a first peak concomitant with systole (S), a second peak concomitant with diastole (D), and a nadir during atrial contraction (A) (Fig. 9–2). Among the indices suggested to quantify velocity waveforms from DV, the ratio between S-peak velocity to A-peak velocity (S/A) proved to be a angle-independent parameter that efficiently describes DV hemodynamics.[18,21]

The morphology of the velocity waveforms from the hepatic veins is similar to that of IVC. There is a scarcity of reports on the use of these vessels in the human fetus, and from the data available it may be argued that the analysis of these vessels may have the same significance as IVC.

Pulmonary veins velocity waveforms may be recorded at the level of their entrance in the right atrium. Their morphology also is characterized by forward velocities during atrial contraction[22] (Fig. 9–3). The striking differences in the velocity waveform morphology of the IVC and the pulmonary vein is of interest and may reflect the different hemodynamic conditions occurring in the systemic and pulmonary venous circulation during fetal life.[23]

Umbilical venous blood flow is usually continuous (Fig. 9–4). However, in the presence of a reverse flow during atrial contraction in the IVC, pulsations in umbilical venous flows do occur. In normal pregnancies these pulsations occur only before the 12th week of gestation, and they are secondary to the stiffness of the ventricles at this gestational age, causing a high percentage of reverse flow in the IVC.[24] Later in gestation the presence of pulsations in the umbilical vein suggest severe cardiac compromise.

Atrioventricular Valves. Flow velocity waveforms at the level of mitral and tricuspid valves are recorded from the apical four-chamber view of the fetal heart and are characterized by two diastolic peaks corresponding to early ventricular filling (E wave) and to active ventricular filling during atrial contraction (A wave) (Fig. 9–5). The ratio between the E and A waves (E/A) is a widely accepted index of ventricular diastolic function, and it is an expression of both the cardiac compliance and preload conditions.[4,9,25]

Outflow Tracts. Flow velocity waveform from the aorta and pulmonary artery are recorded from the five-chamber and short-axis views of the fetal heart, respectively (Figs. 9–6 and 9–7). Peak velocity and TPV are the most commonly used indices. The former is influenced by several factors including valve size, myocardial contractility, and afterload[4,10,11]

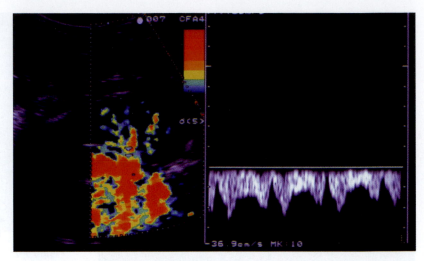

Figure 9–3. Velocity waveform from a pulmonary vein in a normal fetus at 30 weeks of gestation. Note the presence of forward flow during atrial contraction.

and the latter is believed to be affected by the mean arterial pressure.[26]

Coronary Blood Flow. Coronary blood flow may be visualized with the use of high-resolution ultrasound equipment and color Doppler echocardiography. In normal fetuses both right and left coronary arteries may be identified after 31 weeks of gestation under optimal conditions.[27] In compromised fetuses these vessels may be identified at a earlier gestational age, probably because of increased coronary blood flow.[27]

Pulmonary Vessels. Velocity waveforms may be recorded from the right and left pulmonary arteries or from peripheral vessels within the lung.[28–31] The morphology of the waveforms is different according to the site of sampling, and there is a progressive increase in the diastolic component in the more distal vessels[30,31] (Fig. 9–8). Analysis of the vessels may be used to study the normal development of lung circulation.

Ductus Arteriosus. Ductal velocity waveforms are recorded from a short-axis view showing the ductal arch and are characterized by a continuous forward flow through the entire cardiac cycle[32] (Fig. 9–9). The parameter most commonly analyzed is the PV during systole or, similarly to peripheral vessels, the pulsatility index (PI = [systolic velocity − diastolic velocity]/mean velocity).[32,33]

Reproducibility

A major concern in obtaining absolute measurements of velocities or flow is reproducibility. To obtain reliable recordings, it is important to minimize the angle of insonation, to verify in real time and color flow imaging the correct position of the sample volume before and after each Doppler recording, and to limit the recordings to periods of fetal rest and apnea because behavioral states greatly influence

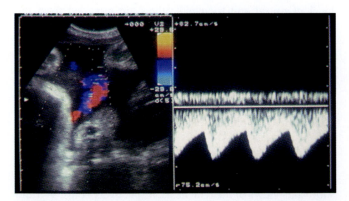

Figure 9–4. Blood flow velocity waveforms from the umbilical artery *(bottom)* and vein *(top)* in a normal fetus at 34 weeks of gestation. Note the continous flow pattern in the umbilical vein.

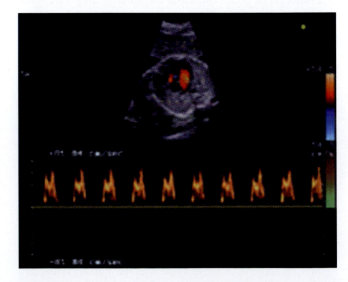

Figure 9–5. Velocity waveform from the mitral valve at 35 weeks of gestation. The early-to-active ventricular filling ratio is 0.83.

< 10%[38]). Further, the use of angle-independent indices from the venous circulation may further improve reproducibility.

NORMAL RANGES OF DOPPLER ECHOCARDIOGRAPHIC INDICES

The advent of transvaginal color Doppler equipment has allowed sonographers to record cardiac flow velocity waveforms from 8 weeks of gestation onward.[39,40] Particularly marked changes occur at all cardiac levels from this gestational age up to 20 weeks. In particular, the PLI in the IVC decreases significantly[39,41] (see Fig. 9–9), the E/A ratios of both atrioventricular levels increases dramatically[39,40] (Fig. 9–10) and PV and TVI values in outflow tracts increase, which is particularly evident in the pulmonary valve.[39] These changes suggest a rapid development of ventricular compliance that may explain the decrease of IVC PLI, the increase of E/A, and a shift of cardiac output toward the right ventricle, probably secondary to the decreased right ventricle afterload related to a fall in placental resistances.

After 20 weeks of gestation there is another, but less evident, decrease of IVC PLI[18] associated with a significant decrease of the S/A ratio of the DV[21] (Table 9–1).

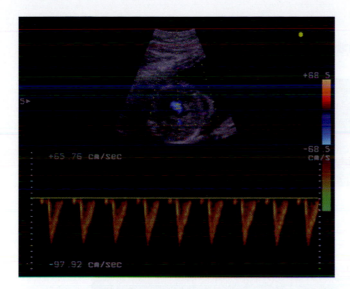

Figure 9–6. Velocity waveform from the ascending aorta in a normal fetus at 33 weeks of gestation. The peak velocity is 74 cm/s, and the time to peak velocity is 38 ms.

the recordings.[34,35] Under these conditions it is necessary to select a series (at least five) of consecutive velocity waveforms characterized by uniform morphology and high signal-to-noise ratio before performing the measurements. By using this technique of recording and analysis, we managed to obtain a coefficient of variation below 10% for all the echocardiographic indices with the exception of those requiring measurement of valve dimensions. These results are in agreement with those reported by other centers (coefficient of variation < 7%,[36] coefficient of variation < 7.6%,[37] maximal variation

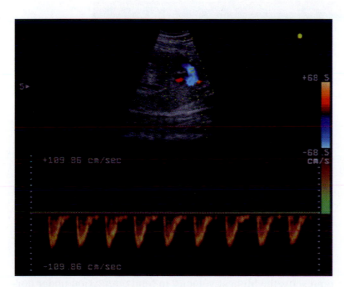

Figure 9–7. Velocity waveform from the pulmonary artery in a normal fetus at 33 weeks of gestation. The peak velocity is 66 cm/s and the time to peak velocity is 28 ms.

TABLE 9–1. NORMAL REFERENCE LIMITS (5TH, 50TH, AND 95TH CENTILES) OF THE PRELOAD INDEX (PLI) FROM THE INFERIOR VENA CAVA AND THE ATRIAL-TO-SYSTOLIC RATIO (A/S) IN THE DUCTUS VENOSUS

	PLI				A/S		
Weeks	5th	50th	95th	Weeks	5th	50th	95th
18	0.24	0.39	0.75	18	1.81	2.75	4.18
19	0.23	0.38	0.72	19	1.76	2.68	4.08
20	0.22	0.36	0.70	20	1.72	2.61	3.97
21	0.21	0.35	0.67	21	1.67	2.55	3.88
22	0.21	0.34	0.65	22	1.63	2.48	3.78
23	0.20	0.33	0.62	23	1.59	2.42	3.68
24	0.19	0.31	0.60	24	1.55	2.36	3.59
25	0.18	0.30	0.58	25	1.51	2.30	3.50
26	0.18	0.29	0.56	26	1.47	2.24	3.41
27	0.17	0.28	0.54	27	1.44	2.19	3.33
28	0.17	0.27	0.52	28	1.40	2.13	3.25
29	0.16	0.26	0.50	29	1.37	2.08	3.16
30	0.15	0.25	0.48	30	1.33	2.03	3.09
31	0.15	0.24	0.46	31	1.30	1.98	3.01
32	0.14	0.23	0.45	32	1.27	1.93	2.93
33	0.14	0.23	0.43	33	1.24	1.88	2.86
34	0.13	0.22	0.42	34	1.20	1.83	2.79
35	0.13	0.21	0.40	35	1.17	1.79	2.72
36	0.12	0.20	0.39	36	1.14	1.74	2.65
37	0.12	0.20	0.39	37	1.12	1.70	2.58
38	0.11	0.20	0.39	38	1.09	1.66	2.52
39	0.11	0.20	0.39	39	1.06	1.61	2.46
40	0.11	0.20	0.39	40	1.03	1.57	2.39

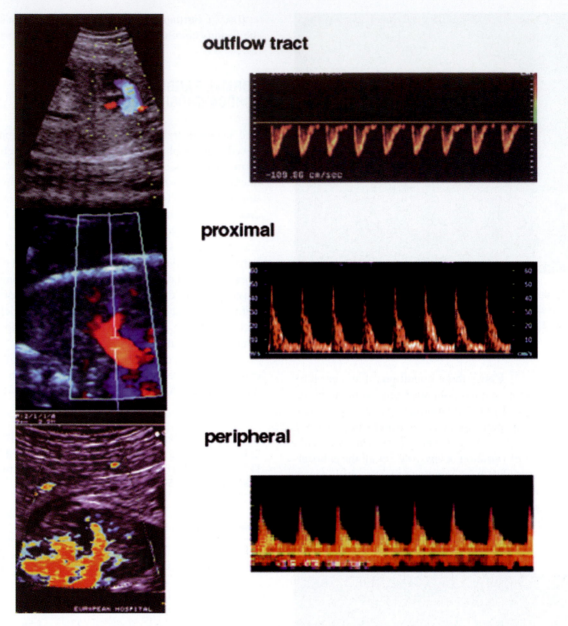

Figure 9–8. Velocity waveforms from the fetal lung circulation. Note the different morphology of blood flow velocity waveforms from the outflow tract to the peripheral vessels.

At the level of the atrioventricular valves, the E/A ratios increase[42,43] (Table 9–2), and PV values linearly increase at the level of both pulmonary and aortic valves (44) (Tables 9–3 and 9–4). Small changes are present in TPV values during gestation.[45] TPV values at the level of pulmonary valve are lower than those at the aortic level, suggesting a slightly higher blood pressure in the pulmonary artery than in the ascending aorta[46] (Tables 9–3 and 9–4). Quantitative measurements have shown that the right cardiac output (RCO) is higher than the left cardiac output (LCO) and that from 20 weeks onward the RCO/LCO ratio remains constant, with a mean value of 1.3[47,48] (Table 9–5). This value is lower than that reported in fetal sheep (RCO/LCO = 1.8), and this difference may be explained by the higher brain weight in humans.[49]

In normal fetuses VEF exponentially increases with advancing gestation at the level of both right and left ventricles.[6] No significant differences are present between right and left VEF values, and the ratio between right and left VEF values remains stable during gestation (mean value = 1.09).[7]

Ductal PV increases linearly with gestation, and its value represents the highest velocity in fetal circulation under normal conditions. The PI values are constant.[32,33] Values of systolic velocity above 140 cm/s in conjuction with a diastolic

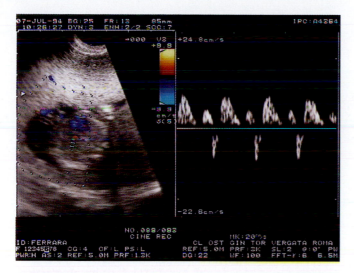

Figure 9–9. Blood flow velocity waveforms from the inferior vena cava in a normal fetus at 11 weeks of gestation. Note the high amount of reverse flow during atrial contraction.

velocity greater than 35 cm/s or a PI of less than 1.9 are considered expressions of ductal constriction.[32]

CARDIAC DOPPLER FINDINGS IN ABNORMAL GESTATION

Growth-Retarded Fetuses

Intrauterine growth-retarded (IUGR) fetuses with uteroplacental insufficiency have characteristic changes of peripheral vascular resistances (i.e., the so-called brain-sparing effect)

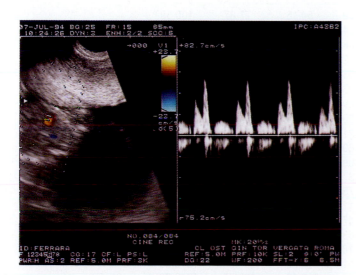

Figure 9–10. Blood flow velocity waveforms from the tricuspid valve in a normal fetus at 13 weeks of gestation. Note the low early-to-active ventricular filling ratio value (0.40).

TABLE 9–2. NORMAL REFERENCE LIMITS (5TH, 50TH, AND 95TH PERCENTILES) OF E/A RATIOS FROM MITRAL AND TRICUSPID VALVES

	Mitral Valve			Tricuspid Valve		
Weeks	5th	50th	95th	5th	50th	95th
20	0.400	0.592	0.783	0.47	0.65	0.84
21	0.419	0.609	0.798	0.49	0.67	0.85
22	0.437	0.625	0.813	0.50	0.68	0.87
23	0.454	0.640	0.827	0.51	0.70	0.88
24	0.469	0.655	0.841	0.53	0.71	0.89
25	0.484	0.670	0.855	0.54	0.72	0.90
26	0.498	0.683	0.869	0.55	0.73	0.91
27	0.511	0.696	0.882	0.56	0.74	0.92
28	0.524	0.709	0.894	0.57	0.75	0.93
29	0.536	0.721	0.906	0.57	0.76	0.94
30	0.547	0.732	0.917	0.58	0.76	0.95
31	0.558	0.743	0.927	0.59	0.77	0.95
32	0.568	0.753	0.937	0.59	0.77	0.96
33	0.577	0.762	0.947	0.59	0.78	0.96
34	0.586	0.771	0.955	0.60	0.78	0.96
35	0.594	0.779	0.963	0.60	0.78	0.97
36	0.602	0.786	0.971	0.60	0.78	0.97
37	0.608	0.793	0.978	0.60	0.78	0.97
38	0.613	0.799	0.985	0.60	0.78	0.97
39	0.618	0.805	0.992	0.60	0.78	0.97
40	0.621	0.810	0.999	0.60	0.78	0.96

E/A, ratio of early ventricular filling to active ventricular filling.

TABLE 9–3. NORMAL REFERENCE LIMITS (5TH, 50TH, AND 95TH PERCENTILES) OF PV (CM/S) AND TPV (MS) FROM AORTIC VALVE

	PV			TPV		
Weeks	5th	50th	95th	5th	50th	95th
20	44.29	62.29	80.29	28.13	41.93	55.73
21	45.59	63.59	81.59	28.46	42.26	56.06
22	46.90	64.90	82.90	28.79	42.59	56.39
23	48.20	66.20	84.20	29.12	42.92	56.72
24	49.50	67.50	85.50	29.45	43.25	57.05
25	50.81	68.81	86.81	29.78	43.58	57.38
26	52.11	70.11	88.11	30.11	43.91	57.71
27	53.41	71.41	89.41	30.44	44.24	58.04
28	54.72	72.72	90.72	30.77	44.57	58.37
29	56.03	74.03	92.03	31.10	44.90	58.70
30	57.33	75.33	93.33	31.43	45.23	59.03
31	58.63	76.63	94.63	31.76	45.56	59.36
32	59.94	77.94	95.94	32.09	45.89	59.69
33	61.24	79.24	97.24	32.42	46.22	60.02
34	62.55	80.55	98.55	32.75	46.55	60.35
35	63.85	81.85	99.85	33.08	46.88	60.68
36	65.15	83.15	101.15	33.41	47.21	61.01
37	66.46	84.46	102.46	33.74	47.54	61.34
38	67.76	85.76	103.76	34.07	47.87	61.67
39	69.07	87.07	105.07	34.40	48.20	62.00
40	70.37	88.37	106.37	34.73	48.53	62.33

PV, Peak velocity; TPV, time to peak velocity.

TABLE 9–4. NORMAL REFERENCE LIMITS (5TH, 50TH, AND 95TH PERCENTILES) OF PV (CM/S) AND TPV (MS) FROM PULMONARY ARTERY

	PV			TPV		
Weeks	5th	50th	95th	5th	50th	95th
20	32.30	51.80	71.30	25.26	38.06	50.86
21	33.50	53.00	72.50	24.93	37.73	50.53
22	34.69	54.19	73.69	24.60	37.40	50.20
23	35.89	55.39	74.89	24.27	37.07	49.87
24	37.08	56.58	76.08	23.94	36.74	49.54
25	38.28	57.78	77.28	23.61	36.41	49.21
26	39.47	58.97	78.47	23.28	36.08	48.88
27	40.67	60.17	79.67	22.95	35.75	48.55
28	41.86	61.36	80.86	22.62	35.42	48.22
29	43.06	62.56	82.06	22.29	35.09	47.89
30	44.25	63.75	83.25	21.96	34.76	47.56
31	45.45	64.95	84.45	21.63	34.43	47.23
32	46.64	66.14	85.64	21.30	34.10	46.90
33	47.84	67.34	86.84	20.97	33.77	46.57
34	49.03	68.53	88.03	20.64	33.44	46.24
35	50.23	69.73	89.23	20.31	33.11	45.91
36	51.43	70.93	90.43	19.98	32.78	45.58
37	52.62	72.12	91.62	19.65	32.45	45.25
38	53.82	73.32	92.82	19.32	32.12	44.92
39	55.01	74.51	94.01	18.99	31.79	44.59
40	56.21	75.71	95.21	18.66	31.46	44.26

PV, Peak velocity; TPV, time to peak velocity.

that affect cardiac hemodynamics.[50] Secondary to the brain-sparing, selective modifications occur in cardiac afterload; decreased left ventricle afterload due to the cerebral vasodilation and increased right ventricle afterload due to the systemic and pulmonary vasoconstriction.[4,30] Furthermore, hypoxemia may impair myocardial contractility, whereas polycythemia, usually present, may alter blood viscosity and therefore preload.[4]

As a consequence, IUGR fetuses show impaired ventricular filling properties, with a lower E/A ratio at the level of atrioventricular valves,[43] lower PV in aorta and pulmonary arteries[51] (Figs. 9–11 and 9–12), increased aortic and decreased pulmonary TPV,[45] and a relative increase of LCO associated with decreased RCO.[37] These hemodynamic intracardiac changes are compatible with a preferential shift of cardiac output in favor of the left ventricle, leading to improved perfusion to the brain. Thus, in the first stages of the disease, the supply of substrates and oxygen can be maintained at near normal levels despite any reduction of placental transfer.

Longitudinal studies of IUGR fetuses have elucidated the natural history of these hemodynamic modifications during uteroplacental insufficiency.[52–54] Such studies have shown that both TPV in the aorta and pulmonary arteries and the ratios between right and left ventricle outputs remain stable during serial recordings. These findings are consistent

TABLE 9–5. NORMAL REFERENCE LIMITS (5TH, 50TH, AND 95TH PERCENTILES) OF LCO (ML/MIN) AND RCO (ML/MIN) CALCULATED AT THE LEVEL OF OUTFLOW TRACT

	LCO			RCO		
Weeks	5th	50th	95th	5th	50th	95th
20	42.42	60.61	78.79	54.16	77.37	100.59
21	48.59	69.42	90.24	68.25	97.49	126.74
22	57.98	82.83	107.68	71.87	102.67	133.47
23	70.60	100.86	131.12	86.04	122.91	159.78
24	86.45	123.50	160.55	103.75	148.21	192.67
25	105.53	150.75	195.98	125.00	178.57	232.14
26	127.83	182.61	237.39	149.79	213.99	278.18
27	153.36	219.08	284.80	178.13	254.47	330.81
28	182.11	260.16	338.21	210.00	300.01	390.01
29	214.09	305.85	397.60	245.42	350.61	455.79
30	249.30	356.15	462.99	284.38	406.26	528.14
31	287.74	411.06	534.37	326.89	466.98	607.08
32	329.40	470.57	611.75	372.93	532.76	692.59
33	374.29	534.70	695.11	422.52	603.60	784.68
34	422.41	603.44	784.47	475.65	679.50	883.35
35	473.75	676.79	879.83	532.32	760.46	988.60
36	528.33	754.75	981.18	592.53	846.48	1100.42
37	586.12	837.32	1088.51	656.29	937.56	1218.82
38	647.15	924.50	1201.85	723.59	1033.70	1343.80
39	711.40	1016.29	1321.17	794.43	1134.90	1475.36
40	778.88	1112.69	1446.49	868.81	1241.15	1613.50

LCO, Left cardiac output; RCO, right cardiac output.

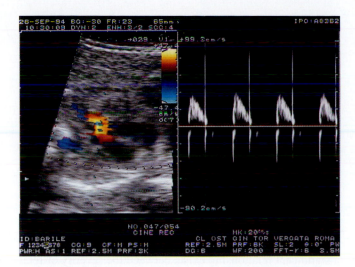

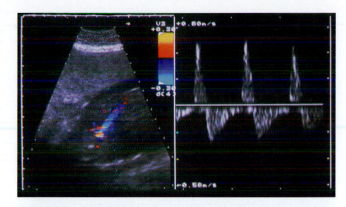

Figure 9–13. Inferior vena cava velocity waveforms in a fetus with intrauterine growth retardation at 29 weeks of gestation. Note the marked increase of the A wave.

Figure 9–11. Blood flow velocity waveforms from the ascending aorta at 28 weeks of gestation in a fetus with intrauterine growth retardation. Peak velocity is 42 cm/s (normal mean value for gestation = 72 cm/s).

with the absence of other significant changes in outflow resistances (a parameter inversely related to TPV values) and with cardiac output redistribution after the establishment of the brain-sparing mechanism.[52] However, in deteriorating IUGR fetuses, PV and cardiac output gradually decline, suggesting a progressive deterioration of cardiac function.[52] As a consequence, cardiac filling is also impaired. Studies of the fetal venous circulation[53,54] have demonstrated that an increase of IVC reverse flow during atrial contraction occurs with progressive fetal deterioration, suggesting a higher pressure gradient in the right atrium (Fig. 9–13). The next step

of the disease is the extension of the abnormal reversal of blood velocities in the IVC to the DV, resulting in an increase of the S/A ratio, mainly due to a reduction of the A component in the velocity waveforms[21,54] (Fig. 9–14). High venous pressure leads to a reduction of velocity at end diastole in the umbilical vein, causing typical diastolic pulsations[55] (Fig. 9–15). The development of these pulsations is close to the onset of fetal HR anomalies and is frequently associated with acidemia and fetal endocrine changes.[55–57] At this stage, coronary blood flow may be visualized; if fetuses are not delivered, intrauterine death may occur after a median of 3.5 days.[27]

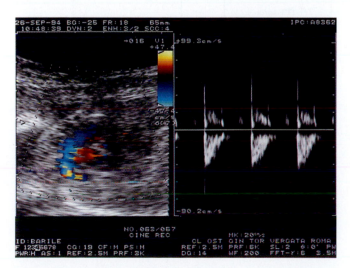

Figure 9–12. Blood flow velocity waveforms from the pulmonary artery in the same fetus shown in Figure 9–11. Peak velocity is 35 cm/s (normal mean value for gestation = 61 cm/s).

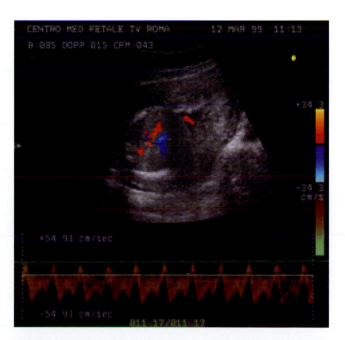

Figure 9–14. Ductus venosus velocity waveforms in a fetus with intrauterine growth retardation at 28 weeks of gestation. The A wave is reversed.

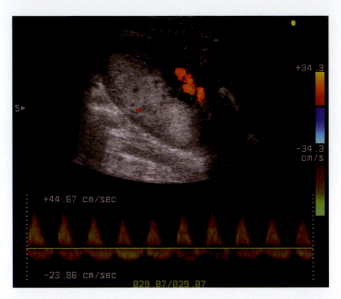

Figure 9–15. Umbilical artery and vein velocity waveforms in a severely growth retarded fetus at 27 weeks of gestation. Note the absence of end diastolic velocities in the artery and the presence of pulsations in the vein.

Studies of VEF in IUGR have demonstrated that it is significantly and symmetrically decreased in both ventricles.[6] The presence of a symmetrical decrease of VEF from both ventricles, despite the dramatically different hemodynamic conditions present in the vascular district of ejection of the two ventricles (i.e., reduced cerebral resistances for the left ventricle and increased splachnic and placental resistances for the right ventricle), supports a pivotal role for intrinsic myocardial function as a compensatory mechanism of the IUGR fetus after the establishment of the brain-sparing effect. Indeed, in fetuses followed longitudinally until either intrauterine death or the onset of abnormal fetal HR patterns requiring early delivery, VEF dramatically decreases over a short time interval (i.e., 1 week), showing an impairment of ventricular force close to that of fetal distress.[6] Furthermore, a significant relationship exists between the severity of fetal acidosis at cordocentesis and VEF values.[6] This confirms the pivotal role of the fetal heart dysfunction in progressive fetal compromise.

A schematic description of these hemodynamic changes and suggested pathophysiologic significance is shown in Figure 9–16. We speculate that the fall in cardiac output and

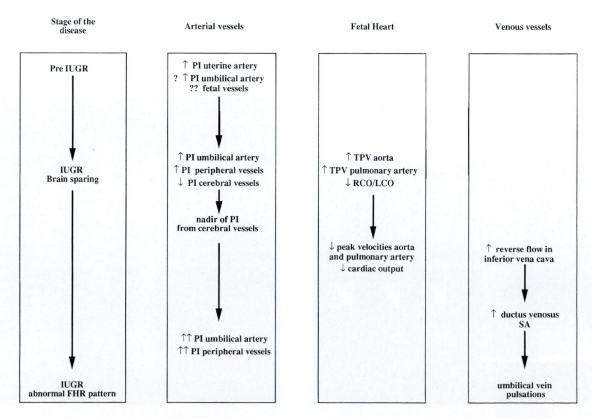

Figure 9–16. Suggested pathophysiologic steps and corresponding hemodynamic changes in deteriorating fetuses with intrauterine growth retardation.

VEF may reflect decompensation of a normally protective mechanism responsible for the brain-sparing effect. According to this model, the fetal heart adapts to placental insufficiency to maximize brain substrate and oxygen delivery. With progressive deterioration of the fetal condition, this protective mechanism is overwhelmed by the fall in cardiac output, and fetal distress occurs.

Fetuses of Diabetic Mothers

Infants of diabetic mothers are at risk for developing hypertrophic cardiomyopathy.[58] This disease is characterized by a thickening of the interventricular septum and ventricular free walls, as well as systolic and diastolic dysfunction of the neonatal heart, which may result in congestive heart failure in the immediate postnatal period.[59] Echocardiography studies of the fetal heart have demonstrated that hypertrophic cardiomyopathy is present prenatally and may worsen *in utero*.

M-mode studies in fetuses of insulin-dependent diabetic mothers have shown an increased thickness of ventricular walls that is particularly evident at the level of interventricular septum[60–62] (Fig. 9–17). The increased cardiac size does not merely reflect the larger size of fetuses of diabetic mothers (i.e., macrosomia) but represents a selective organomegaly. Controlling cardiac size for fetal abdominal circumference or biparietal diameter (biometric parameters closely related to fetal weight) showed an increased wall thickness irrespective of fetal size.[60,61]

Longitudinal echocardiographic studies have elucidated the natural history of fetal hypertrophic cardiomyopathy. Fetuses of diabetic mothers showed an accelerated increase of cardiac size, and the growth curves differ from those of

normal fetuses.[62] Although the cardiac walls are already thicker than in normal fetuses at 20 weeks of gestation, the accelerated increase of cardiac size is more marked during the late second trimester.[62] The cause of the greater fetal growth rate during the late second trimester is unclear. Because no differences were present in the metabolic control, it has been speculated that a different degree of sensitivity of fetal myocardium occur during gestation to factors accelerating its growth. This hypothesis is supported by the data of Thorsson and Hintz[63] who showed a reduction from fetus to adult in the number and affinity of insulin receptors.

Echocardiographic studies[60,62] have shown that the increase in cardiac wall thickness affects fetal cardiac function.

Fetuses of diabetic mothers show lower E/A ratios at the level of both atrioventricular valves when compared with normal fetuses[62] (Fig. 9–18). Longitudinal studies have shown that these changes are already present in early gestation and that a delayed development of diastolic function occurs, with a slower rate of change in E/A ratios during gestation.[63] Transvaginal echocardiography has demonstrated differences in cardiac functional development as early as 12 weeks of gestation, and these differences seem to be particularly evident in cases with poor metabolic control.[64]

The low E/A values might be explained by an impaired development of ventricular compliance in fetuses of diabetic mothers secondary to cardiac wall thickening. This is consistent with the significant relationship between interventricular septum and lateral ventricular wall thickness and the severity of the impairment of E/A ratios.[62]

The E/A ratio is also influenced by the preload. Polycythemia is frequently present at birth in infants of

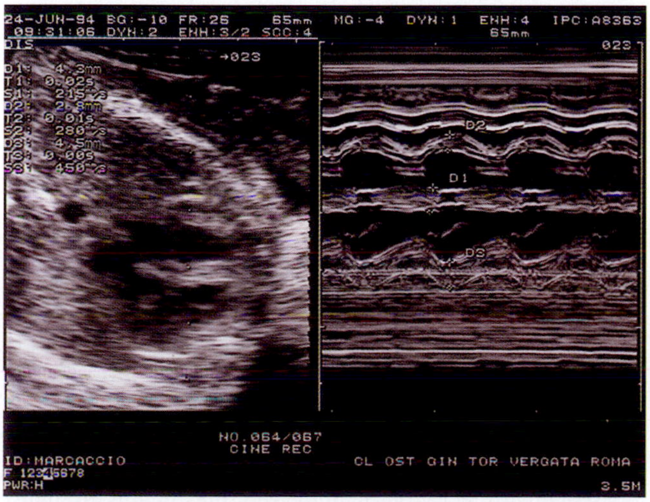

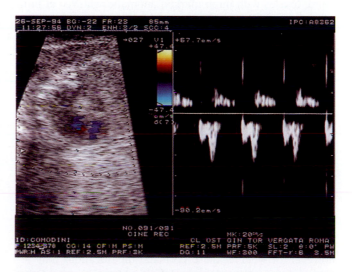

Figure 9–17. Real-time and M-mode tracing at the level of the fetal heart in a 24-week fetus with a diabetic mother. The intraventricular wall septal thickness is 4.3 mm (expected mean for biparietal diameter = 2.2 mm).

Figure 9–18. Blood flow velocity waveforms at the level of tricuspid valve in a fetus of insulin-dependent diabetic mother at 32 weeks of gestation. The early-to-active ventricular filling ratio is 0.48 (expected mean for gestation = 0.77).

diabetic mothers.[65] This condition increases blood viscosity, which may reduce preload and thus potentially affect the E/A ratio during intrauterine life. This hypothesis is supported by recent data showing a significant relation between fetal hematocrit and E/A values after controlling for cardiac thickness and fetal HR,[66] suggesting a significant role of fetal blood viscosity on cardiac diastolic function.

Peak velocities at the level of aortic and pulmonary outflow tracts are significantly higher in fetuses of diabetic mothers than in normal fetuses.[60] Increased PVs may be secondary to reduced outflow tract dimensions, decreased afterload, increased cardiac contractility, or increased volume flow. Differentiation between these factors is difficult in the human fetus. An obstruction of the left ventricle outflow tract due to the hypertrophy of the septal musculature, resulting in an increase of aortic PVs, has been described in infants of diabetic mothers.[67] However, in this condition the obstruction is usually limited to the left ventricle outflow tract and does not affect the right ventricle and thus does not explain the presence of a concomitant increase of pulmonary PVs. Similarly, a decrease in afterload seems unlikely on the basis of the lack of differences in TPVs between control fetuses and fetuses of diabetic mothers. An increased contractility is compatible with postnatal studies showing a systolic ventricular contractile function above normal in infants of diabetic mothers.[68] The higher values of PVs may be explained on the basis of an increased intracardiac volume flow secondary to the relative larger size of such fetuses since cardiac output is also a function of fetal weight.

These abnormalities in cardiac hemodynamics also impair venous circulation. We have recently shown that the PLI in the IVC is increased in fetuses of diabetic mothers. Furthermore, fetuses with more marked anomalies showed at birth a lower pH in the umbilical artery, an increased hematocrit, and higher morbidity. In addition, no changes were noted in fetal peripheral vessels.

On this basis we speculated that the mechanisms inducing fetal distress are different in fetuses of diabetic mothers than in those with IUGR. In the former group, the development of hyperthrophic cardiomyopathy plays a pivotal role in the genesis of fetal distress; in the latter group the changes in cardiac function are secondary to modification in peripheral resistance. A diagram of the suggested pathophysiology occurring in fetuses of diabetic mother is shown in Figure 9–19.

After birth, the hypertrophic changes of the myocardium regress to normal over a period of several months and are usually not present at 1 year of age.[58,68] There is no account, however, of whether these perinatal modifications may affect cardiac function during adult life. Moreover, significant changes occur during the transitional circulation. In normal infants, the E/A ratios at the level of both atrioventricular valves significantly increase during the first days of life and the E wave is usually higher than the A wave, resulting in

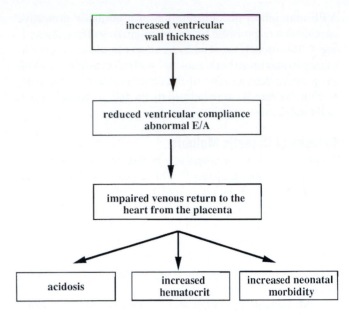

Figure 9–19. Suggested pathophysiologic steps of perinatal distress in fetuses of insulin-dependent diabetic mothers.

an E/A higher than 1.[69] In newborns of diabetic mothers, no changes of E/A ratios occur during the first 5 days of life, and their value remains lower than 1.[69] These changes may explain the relatively high incidence of transient tachypnea and pulmonary edema.[58]

Fetal Anemia

Red cell isommunization results in a progressive destruction of fetal red blood cells leading to fetal anemia. Intravascular fetal blood transfusions by cordocentesis are the standard treatment of fetal anemia, and this procedure leads to rapid injection of large amounts of blood into the fetal circulatory space.

Doppler echocardiography has elucidated the hemodynamic response of the human fetus to anemia and its rapid correction by transfusion.[70,71]

In anemia, the LCO and RCO are significantly higher than normal, and there is a significant relationship between the severity of the fetal anemia and cardiac output.[70,71] As a consequence of the high volume flow, PVs at outflow tracts are increased.[70] Furthermore, the E/A at both atrioventricular valves is increased[71] (Fig. 9–20). Venous flow is similarly affected, with an increase of PV in DV and a loss of pulsatility.[72,73]

Fetal cardiac output is increased, presumably to maintain adequate oxygen delivery to organs. Although the mechanisms responsible for the increase of cardiac output are still unclear, two main factors have been implicated[74]: first, decreased blood viscosity leading to increased venous return and cardiac preload; and second, peripheral vasodilatation

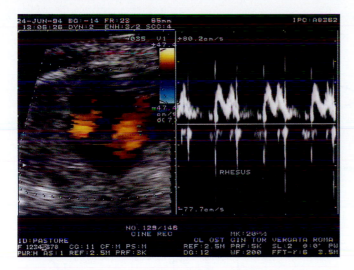

Figure 9–20. Blood flow velocity waveforms from the tricuspid valve in an anemic fetus at 28 weeks of gestation. The early-to-active ventricular filling ratio is 0.97 (expected mean for gestation = 0.77) and fetal hemoglobin is 7.4 g/dL.

due to a fall in blood oxygen content and therefore reduced cardiac afterload. The role of the first mechanism is supported by the high E/A ratio in anemic fetuses.

There is no evidence to support redistribution of cardiac output similar to that described in the hypoxic IUGR fetus (brain-sparing effect) because the RCO/LCO ratio is normal in anemic fetuses.[71] This is in agreement with the normal PI present in fetal peripheral vessels in anemic fetuses.[74] These findings suggest that in red cell isoimmunization, the changes in fetal cardiac function are related mainly to low blood viscosity, leading to a hyperdynamic state. After intravascular transfusion, there is a significant temporary fall in RCO and LCO[70,71] associated with an increased E/A ratio.[71] The latter changes are probably due to the increased preload secondary to the relatively large amount of blood transfused.

The decreased cardiac output may be secondary to four different factors (HR, preload, myocardial contractility, or afterload). The first factor may be excluded because cardiac output decreases in the absence of any significant changes in fetal HR.[70] Preload should be decreased to support the decrease in cardiac output, but the high E/A values suggest an increase rather than a decrease of preload.[71] Similarly, impaired myocardial contractility seems unlikely to play a role on the basis of the velocity waveforms of the aorta and pulmonary artery.[70] Therefore, an increase in cardiac afterload seems to be the best explanation for the decrease in cardiac output after a transfusion.[71]

It is noteworthy that the fall in cardiac output in the human fetus is proportional to the expansion of the fetoplacental volume.[71] Moreover, within 2 hours of transfusion, all the echocardiographic parameters return toward the normal range, suggesting a rapid recovery of the fetal cardiac function.[71]

Discordant Twins

Twin pregnancies have a high rate of perinatal complications that are particularly evident in pairs with discordant growth.[76] Studies limited to the umbilical artery have provided conflicting results in twins as to whether discordant size is associated with discordant Doppler indices.[77–80] These discrepancies may be explained on the basis of the following classification criteria.

We evaluated two groups of twin pregnancies with discordant growth secondary to different etiologies.[81] In the first group, the etiology was malnutrition of one twin due to placental insufficiency limited to one placenta. Criteria of inclusion were the presence of dichorionic placentas, thus virtually excluding the possibility of blood shunts between fetuses; the absence of chromosomal and structural anomalies, excluding intrinsic causes of the growth defect; and delivery based on the presence of late decelerations, suggestive of fetal hypoxemia of the smaller twin. In the larger twin, serial studies showed the absence of any differences from normal singleton pregnancies in all the vessels investigated, thus suggesting normal placental and fetal hemodynamics. In contrast, the smaller twin showed progressive changes of Doppler indices similar to those described for singleton growth-retarded fetuses associated with placental insufficiency. Therefore, the absolute values of the Doppler indices in the smaller twin, or the delta values between the smaller and the larger twin, may be a tool for fetal surveillance or prediction of fetal distress similar as in singleton pregnancies. This finding confirms that of previous studies showing how a high delta value in the umbilical artery can predict low birthweight and adverse perinatal outcome in twin pregnancies.[77,78] The combined study of several vascular areas may improve the diagnostic efficacy of Doppler ultrasonography.

The second group of twin pregnancies studied were those affected by twin-to-twin transfusion syndrome. The classic pathophysiologic background of this syndrome is a shift of blood volume from the donor twin to the recipient twin.[82] As a result of the transfusion, the donor twin becomes anemic, decreases its growth rate, and develops oligohydramnios. The recipient twin becomes polycythemic and plethoric and, as consequence of the volume overload, may develop polyhydramnios, cardiomegaly, mitral and tricuspid regurgitation, cardiac insufficiency, and hydrops.[82–84] However, this concept has been recently questioned by data obtained at cordocentesis showing only small differences in fetal hemoglobin between fetuses with classic signs of twin-to-twin transfusion syndrome.[85] These observations suggest that the mechanism responsible for this syndrome is more complex than mere shifts of blood volume that probably become massive only at a late stage in the disease. Serial studies obtained in this second group of twin fetuses support this concept by showing changes of Doppler indices only at the time of the last recording, close to the delivery (associated with fetal distress in most of the cases).

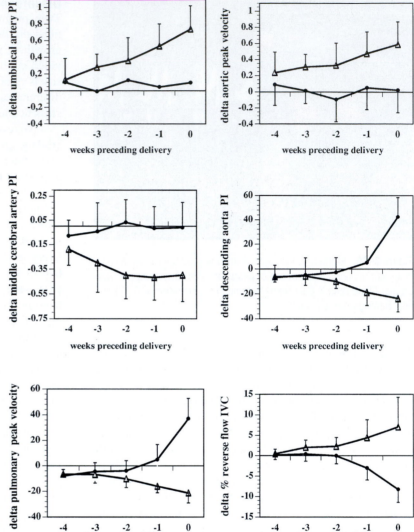

Figure 9–21. Serial changes in delta value (difference between the Doppler indices between the smaller and larger twin) in pregnancies complicated by placental insufficiency of one twin (triangles) or twin-to-twin transfusion syndrome (circles). (*Reproduced with permission from Rizzo G, Arduini D, Romanini C.* Am J Obstet Gynecol. *1994;170:1321–1327.*)

These changes are present at the cardiac and venous levels and are consistent with anemia (increased PV at outflow tract and decreased pulsatility in IVC) in the smaller twin and of massive blood transfusion (decreased PV at outflow tract, increased pulsatility in IVC, and umbilical vein pulsations) in the larger twin (Fig. 9–21). These Doppler patterns are similar to those described before and immediately after intravascular blood transfusion of anemic fetuses. The absence of differences in PI values in the peripheral circulation close to delivery is not surprising because these indices are minimally affected by fetal anemia or polycythemia[75] and confirms previous studies focusing on the umbilical artery.[80]

In summary, Doppler ultrasound in twins may be useful in the presence of a discordant growth. In the presence of placental insufficiency, Doppler echocardiography can help identify those fetuses at high risk for increased perinatal mortality and morbidity. In the management of twin-to-twin

transfusion syndrome, Doppler echocardiography appears to be a useful tool to improve the perinatal management of this condition.

REFERENCES

1. Edelstone DI, Rudolph AM. Preferential streaming of ductus venosus blood to the brain and heart in fetal lambs. *Am J Physiol.* 1979;237:H724–H729.
2. Rudolph AM. Distribution and regulation of blood flow in the fetal and neonatal lamb. *Circ Res.* 1985;57:811–821.
3. Burns PN. Doppler flow estimations in the fetal and maternal circulations: Principles, techniques and some limitations. In: Maulik D, McNellis D, eds. *Doppler Ultrasound Measurement of Maternal–Fetal Hemodynamics.* Ithaca, NY: Perinatology Press; 1987;43–78.
4. Rizzo G, Arduini D, Romanini C. Doppler echocardiographic

assessment of fetal cardiac function. *Ultrasound Obstet Gynecol.* 1992;2:434–445.

5. Comstock CH, Riggs T, Lee W, Kirk J. Pulmonary to aorta diameter ratio in the normal and abnormal fetal heart. *Am J Obstet Gynecol.* 1991;165:1038–1043.

6. St John Sutton M, Gill T, Plappert T, et al. Assessment of right and left ventricular function in term of force development with gestational age in the normal human fetus. *Br Heart J.* 1991;61:285–289.

7. Rizzo G, Capponi A, Rinaldo D, et al. Ventricular ejection force in growth retarded fetuses. *Ultrasound Obstet Gynecol.* 1995;5:247–252.

8. Isaaz K, Ethevenot G, Admant P, et al. A new Doppler method of assessing left ventricular ejection force in chronic congestive heart failure. *Am J Cardiol.* 1989;64:81–87.

9. Stottard MF, Pearson AC, Kern MJ, et al. Influence of alteration in preload of left ventricular diastolic filling as assessed by Doppler echocardiography in humans. *Circulation.* 1989;79:1226–1236.

10. Gardin JM. Doppler measurements of aortic blood velocity and acceleration: Load-independent indexes of left ventricular performance. *Am J Cardiol.* 1989;64:935–936.

11. Bedotto JB, Eichorn EJ, Grayburn PA. Effects of left ventricular preload and afterload on ascendic aortic blood velocity and acceleration in coronaric artery disease. *Am J Cardiol.* 1989;64:856–859.

12. Brownwall E, Ross J, Sonnenblick EH. *Mechanism of Contraction in the Normal and Failing Heart.* 2nd ed. Boston: Little Brown; 1976:92–129.

13. Takaneka K, Dabestani A, Gardin JM, et al. Left ventricular filling in hypertrophic cardiomyopathy: A pulsed Doppler echocardiographic study. *J Am Coll Cardiol.* 1986;7:1263–1271.

14. Kenny J, Plappert T, Doubilet P, et al. Effects of heart rate on ventricular size, stroke volume and output in the normal human fetus: A prospective Doppler echocardiographic study. *Circulation.* 1987;76:52–58.

15. Rizzo G, Caforio L, Arduini D, Romanini C. Effects of sampling site on inferior vena cava flow velocity waveforms. *J Mater Fetal Invest.* 1992;2:153–156.

16. Reed KL, Appleton CP, Anderson CF, et al. Doppler studies of vena cava flows in human fetuses—Insights into normal and abnormal cardiac physiology. *Circulation.* 1990;81:498–505.

17. Appleton CP, Hatle LK, Popp RL. Superior vena cava and hepatic vein Doppler echocardiography in healthy adults. *J Am Coll Cardiol.* 1987;10:1032–1039.

18. Rizzo G, Capponi A, Talone PE, et al. Doppler indices from inferior vena cava and ductus venosus in predicting pH and oxygen tension in umbilical blood at cordocentesis in growth retarded fetuses. *Ultrasound Obstet Gynecol.* 1996;7:401–410.

19. Kanzaki T, Chiba Y. Evaluation of preload condition of the fetus by inferior vena cava blood flow pattern. *Fetal Diagn Ther.* 1990;5:168–174.

20. Okamura K, Murotsuki J, Kobajashi M, et al. Umbilical venous pressure and Doppler flow patterns of inferior vena cava in the fetus. *Am J Perinatol.* 1994;11:255–259.

21. Rizzo G, Capponi A, Arduini D, Romanini C. Ductus venosus velocity waveforms in appropriate and small for gestational age fetuses. *Early Hum Dev.* 1994;39:15–26.

22. Better DJ, Kaufman S, Allan LD. The normal pattern of pulmonary venous flow on pulsed Doppler examination of the human fetus. *J Am Soc Echocardiogr.* 1996;9:281–285.

23. Rizzo G, Capponi A, Pasquini L, et al. Abnormal fetal pulmonary venous blood flow velocity waveforms in the presence of complete transposition of the great arteries. *Ultrasound Obstet Gynecol.* 1996;7:299–300.

24. Rizzo G, Arduini D, Romanini C. Pulsations in umbilical vein: A physiological finding in early pregnancy. *Am J Obstet Gynecol.* 1992;167:675–677.

25. Labovitz AJ, Pearson C. Evaluation of left ventricular diastolic function: Clinical relevance and recent Doppler echocardiographic insights. *Am Heart J.* 1987;114:836–851.

26. Kitabatake A, Inoue M, Asao M, et al. Noninvasive evaluation of pulmonary hypertension by a pulsed Doppler technique. *Circulation.* 1983;68:302–309.

27. Baschat AA, Gembruch U, Reiss I, et al. Demonstration of fetal coronary blood flow by Doppler ultrasound in relation to arterial and venous flow velocity waveforms and perinatal outcome. The heart sparing effect. *Ultrasound Obstet Gynecol.* 1997;9:162–172.

28. Laudy JAM, De Riddler MA, Wladimiroff J. Doppler velocimetry in branch pulmonary arteries of normal human fetuses during the second half of pregnancy. *Pediatr Res.* 1997;41:897–901.

29. Rasanen J, Hutha JC, Weiner S, et al. Fetal branch pulmonary arterial vascular impedance during the second half of pregnancy. *Am J Obstet Gynecol.* 1996;174:1441–1449.

30. Rizzo G, Capponi A, Chaoui R, et al. Blood flow velocity waveforms from peripheral pulmonary arteries in normally grown and growth-retarded fetuses. *Ultrasound Obstet Gynecol.* 1996;8:87–92.

31. Chaoui R, Taddei F, Rizzo G, et al. Doppler echocardiography of the main stems of the pulmonary arteries in the normal human fetus. *Ultrasound Obstet Gynecol.* 1998;11:173–179.

32. Huhta JC, Moise KJ, Fisher DJ, et al. Detection and quantitation of constriction of the fetal ductus arteriosus by Doppler echocardiography. *Circulation.* 1987;75:406–412.

33. Van de Mooren K, Barendregt LG, Waladimiroff J. Flow velocity waveforms in the human fetal ductus arteriosus during the normal second trimester of pregnancy. *Pediatr Res.* 1991;30:487–490.

34. Rizzo G, Arduini D, Valensise H, Romanini C. Effects of behavioural states on cardiac output in the healthy human fetus at 36–38 weeks of gestation. *Early Hum Dev.* 1990;23:109–115.

35. Huisman TW, Brezinka C, Stewart PA, et al. Ductus venosus flow velocity waveforms in relation to fetal behavioural states. *Br J Obstet Gynaecol.* 1994;101:220–224.

36. Groenenberg IAL, Hop WCJ, Wladimiroff JW. Doppler flow velocity waveforms in the fetal cardiac outflow tract; reproducibility of waveform recording and analysis. *Ultrasound Med Biol.* 1991;17:583–587.

37. Al-Ghazali W, Chita SK, Chapman MG, Allan LD. Evidence of redistribution of cardiac output in asymmetrical growth retardation. *Br J Obstet Gynaecol.* 1989;96:697–704.

38. Reed KL, Meijboom EJ, Sahn DJ, et al. Cardiac Doppler flow velocities in human fetuses. *Circulation.* 1986;73:41–56.

39. Rizzo G, Arduini D, Romanini C. Fetal cardiac and extracardiac circulation in early gestation. *J Mater Fetal Invest.* 1991;1:73–78.

40. van Splunder P, Stijnen T, Wladimiroff JW. Fetal atrioventricular flow-velocity waveforms and their relationship to arterial and venous flow velocity waveforms at 8 to 20 weeks of gestation. *Circulation.* 1996;94:1372–1378.

41. Wladimiroff JW, Huisman TWA, Stewart PA, Stijnen T. Normal fetal Doppler inferior vena cava, transtricuspid and umbilical artery flow velocity waveforms between 11 and 16 weeks' gestation. *Am J Obstet Gynecol.* 1992;166:46–49.

42. Reed KL, Sahn DJ, Scagnelli S, et al. Doppler echocardiographic studies of diastolic function in the human fetal heart: Changes during gestation. *J Am Coll Cardiol.* 1986;8:391–395.

43. Rizzo G, Arduini D, Romanini C, Mancuso S. Doppler echocardiographic assessment of atrioventricular velocity waveforms in normal and small for gestational age fetuses. *Br J Obstet Gynaecol.* 1988;95:65–69.

44. Kenny JF, Plappert T, Saltzman DH, et al. Changes in intracardiac blood flow velocities and right and left ventricular stroke volumes with gestational age in the normal human fetus: A prospective Doppler echocardiographic study. *Circulation.* 1986;74:1208–1216.

45. Rizzo G, Arduini D, Romanini C, Mancuso S. Doppler echocardiographic evaluation of time to peak velocity in the aorta and pulmonary artery of small for gestational age fetuses. *Br J Obstet Gynaecol.* 1990;97:603–607.

46. Machado MVL, Chita SC, Allan LD. Acceleration time in the aorta and pulmonary artery measured by Doppler echocardiography in the midtrimester normal human fetus. *Br Heart J.* 1987;58:15–18.

47. Allan LD, Chita SK, Al-Ghazali W, et al. Doppler echocardiographic evaluation of the normal human fetal heart. *Br Heart J.* 1987;57:528–533.

48. De Smedt MCH, Visser GHA, Meijboom EJ. Fetal cardiac output estimated by Doppler echocardiography during mid- and late gestation. *Am J Cardiol.* 1987;60:338–342.

49. Rizzo G, Arduini D. Cardiac output in anencephalic fetuses. *Gynecol Obstet Invest.* 1991;32:33–35.

50. Peeters LLH, Sheldon RF, Jones MD, et al. Blood flow to fetal organ as a function of arterial oxygen content. *Am J Obstet Gynecol.* 1979;135:637–646.

51. Rizzo G, Arduini D. Fetal cardiac function in intrauterine growth retardation. *Am J Obstet Gynecol.* 1991;165:876–882.

52. Rizzo G, Arduini D, Romanini C. Inferior vena cava flow velocity waveforms in appropriate and small for gestational age fetuses. *Am J Obstet Gynecol.* 1992;166:1271–1280.

53. Hecker K, Hackeloer BJ. Cardiotocogram compared to Doppler investigation of the fetal circulation in the premature growth-retarded fetus: Longitudinal observations. *Ultrasound Obstet Gynecol.* 1997;9:152–161.

54. Rizzo G, Capponi A, Soregaroli M, et al. Umbilical vein pulsations and acid base status at cordocentesis in growth retarded fetuses with absent end diastolic velocity in umbilical artery. *Biol Neonate.* 1995;68:163–168.

55. Gudmundusson S, Tulzer G, Hutha JC, Marsal K. Venous Doppler in the fetus with absent end diastolic flow in umbilical artery. *Ultrasound Obstet Gynecol.* 1996;7:262–267.

56. Capponi A, Rizzo G, De Angelis C, et al. Atrial natriuretic peptide levels in fetal blood in relation to inferior vena cava velocity waveforms. *Obstet Gynecol.* 1997;89:242–247.

57. Gutgesell HP, Speer ME, Rosenberg HS. Characterization of the cardiomyopathy in infants of diabetic mothers. *Circulation.* 1980;61:441–450.

58. Reller MD, Kaplan S. Hypertrophic cardiomyopathy in infants of diabetic mothers: An update. *Am J Perinatol.* 1988;5:353–358.

59. Weber HS, Copel JA, Reece A, et al. Cardiac growth in fetuses of diabetic mothers with good metabolic control. *J Pediatr.* 1991;118:103–107.

60. Rizzo G, Arduini D, Romanini C. Cardiac function in fetuses of type I diabetic mothers. *Am J Obstet Gynecol.* 1991;164:837–843.

61. Vielle JC, Sivekoff M, Hanson R, Fanaroff AA. Interventricular septal thickness in fetuses of diabetic mothers. *Obstet Gynecol.* 1992;79:51–54.

62. Rizzo G, Arduini D, Romanini C. Accelerated cardiac growth and abnormal cardiac flows in fetuses of type I diabetic mothers. *Obstet Gynecol.* 1992;80:369–376.

63. Thorsson AV, Hintz RL. Insulin receptors in the newborn: Increase in receptor affinity and number. *N Engl J Med.* 1977;297:908–912.

64. Rizzo G, Arduini D, Capponi A, Romanini C. Cardiac and venous flows in fetuses of insulin dependent diabetic mothers: Evidence of abnormal hemodynamics in early gestation. *Am J Obstet Gynecol.* 1995;173:1775–1781.

65. Widness J, Susa J, Garcia J. Increased erytropoiesis and elevated erytropoietin levels in infants born to diabetic mothers and in hyperinsulinemic rhesus fetuses. *J Clin Invest.* 1981;67:637–641.

66. Rizzo G, Pietropolli A, Capponi A, et al. Analysis of factors affecting ventricular filling in fetuses of type I diabetic mothers. *J Perinat Med.* 1994;22:125–132.

67. Gutgesell HP, Mullins CE, Gillette PC, et al. Transient hypertrophic subaortic stenosis in infants of diabetic mothers. *J Pediatr.* 1976;89:120–125.

68. Mace S, Hirschfeld SS, Riggs T, et al. Echocardiographic abnormalities in infants of diabetic mothers. *J Pediatr.* 1979;95:1013–1019.

69. Condoluci C, Rizzo G, Arduini D, Romanini C. Transitional circulation in infants of diabetic mothers. In: *6th Fetal Cardiology Symposium. Abstract Book* 23. Rome; 1991.

70. Moise KJ, Mari G, Fisher DJ, et al. Acute fetal hemodynamic alterations after intrauterine transfusion for treatment of severe red blood cell alloimmunization. *Am J Obstet Gynecol.* 1990;163:776–784.

71. Rizzo G, Nicolaides KH, Arduini D, Campbell S. Effects of intravascular fetal blood transfusion on fetal intracardiac Doppler velocity waveforms. *Am J Obstet Gynecol.* 1990;163:1231–1238.

72. Oepkes D, Vandenbussche FP, Van Bel F, Kanhai HHH. Fetal ductus venosus blood flow velocities before and after transfusion in red-cell alloimmunized pregnancies. *Obstet Gynecol.* 1993;82:237–241.

73. Hecker K, Snijders R, Campbell S, Nicolaides K. Fetal venous, arterial and intracardiac blood flows in red blood cell isoimmunization. *Obstet Gynecol.* 1995;85:122–128.

74. Fumia FD, Edelstone DI, Holzman IR. Blood flow and oxygen delivery as functions of fetal hematocrit. *Am J Obstet Gynecol.* 1984;150:274–282.

75. Bilardo CM, Nicolaides KH, Campbell S. Doppler studies in red cell isoimmunization. *Clin Obstet Gynecol.* 1989;32:719–727.

76. Ho SK, Wu PK. Perinatal factors and neonatal morbidity in twin pregnancy. *Am J Obstet Gynecol.* 1975;122: 979–987.

77. Farmakides G, Schulman H, Saldana LR, et al. Surveillance of twin pregnancies with umbilical artery velocity waveforms. *Am J Obstet Gynecol.* 1986;153;789–792.

78. Giles WB, Trudinger BJ, Cook CM. Fetal umbilical artery velocity waveforms in twin pregnancies. *Br J Obstet Gynaecol.* 1985;92:490–497.

79. Pretorius DH, Machester D, Barkin S, et al. Doppler ultrasound of twin–twin transfusion syndrome. *J Ultrasound Med.* 1988;7: 117–124.

80. Giles WB, Trudinger BJ, Cook CM, Connelly AJ. Doppler umbilical artery Doppler studies in the twin–twin transfusion syndrome. *Obstet Gynecol.* 1990;76:1097–1099.

81. Rizzo G, Arduini D, Romanini C. Cardiac and extra-cardiac flows in discordant twins. *Am J Obstet Gynecol.* 1994;170: 1321–1327.

82. Blickstein I. The twin–twin transfusion syndrome. *Obstet Gynecol.* 1990;76:714–721.

83. Weiner CP, Ludormisky A. Diagnosis, pathophysiology and treatment of chronic twin-to-twin transfusion. *Fetal Diagn Ther.* 1994;9:283–290.

84. Hecker K, Ville Y, Snijders RJM, Nicolaides K. Doppler studies of the fetal circulation in twin–twin transfusion syndrome. *Ultrasound Obstet Gynecol.* 1995;5:318–324.

85. Saunders NJ, Snijders RJM, Nicolaides KH. Twin–twin transfusion syndrome during the 2nd trimester is associated with small intertwin hemoglobin differences. *Fetal Diagn Ther.* 1991;6:34–36.

Sonography of the Placenta

Beverly A. Spirt • Lawrence P. Gordon

The placenta provides the essential connection between the mother and the developing fetus. Many clinical problems are attributed to the placenta despite the fact that they cannot always be explained after pathologic examination; the term *placental insufficiency* has long been used to explain delayed fetal growth and development, despite the fact that there are no anatomic or histologic explanations of this condition. With the increasing use of Doppler ultrasound to study abnormalities of the maternal vasculature and uteroplacental circulation, however, a practical definition of *placental insufficiency* may evolve.

A thorough understanding of the anatomy of the normal placenta and its variations, as well as the pathologic conditions that are known to occur, is necessary to correctly interpret the sonographic appearance of this short-lived organ. This chapter focuses on the sonographic anatomy of the normal and abnormal placenta, with anatomic and pathologic correlation.

DEVELOPMENT OF THE PLACENTA

The early gestational sac is covered by chorionic villi, which are visible at transvaginal sonography as a hyperechoic rim at about 4 to $4^1/_2$ weeks menstrual age (Fig. 10–1A). At about 5 weeks, the villi opposite the implantation site begin to regress, producing a smooth, relatively avascular membrane (chorion laeve). Continued proliferation of the remaining villi

forms the early placenta (Fig. 10–1B). By 9 to 10 weeks, the diffuse granular echotexture of the placenta is clearly apparent at sonography. This texture is produced by echoes emanating from the villous tree, which is bathed in maternal blood (Fig. 10–1C). The placenta retains this general sonographic appearance throughout the pregnancy, with the notable exception of calcium deposition.

Placental Calcification

Placental calcium deposition is a normal physiologic process that occurs throughout pregnancy.[1] During the first 6 months, the calcification is microscopic; macroscopic plaques appear in the third trimester, most commonly after 33 weeks.[2,3] The calcium is deposited primarily in the basal plate and septa but is also found in the perivillous and subchorionic spaces. Plaques of calcium are readily detected at sonography as echogenic foci that do not produce significant acoustic shadows (Fig. 10–2). The circular configuration seen in heavily calcified placentas results from septal calcifications.

Placental calcification has been studied by histologic,[4,5] chemical,[6] radiographic,[2] and sonographic[3] techniques with the following conclusions. The incidence of placental calcification increases exponentially with increasing gestational age, beginning at about 29 weeks[2–4,6] (Fig. 10–3). More than 50% of placentas show some degree of calcification after 33 weeks.[3] There is no increased calcification in postmature placentas.[4,6] Placental calcification is more common in women of lower parity[2–4] and is probably related to maternal

A

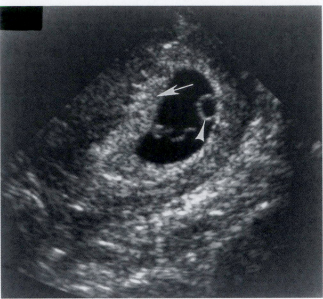

B

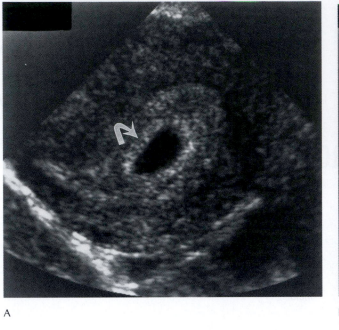

C

Figure 10–1. Normal placental development. **(A)** Transvaginal scan at 5.5 weeks showing gestational sac with hyperechoic rim *(curved arrow)* representing chorionic villi. **(B)** Transvaginal scan at 9 weeks showing early placenta *(arrow)*. Arrowhead, yolk sac. **(C)** Transabdominal scan at 15.7 weeks showing typical diffuse granular echotexture of the placenta (P). Note relatively hypoechoic myometrium (M). F, Fetus.

serum calcium levels.[1,7] Placental calcification is also more common in late summer and early fall deliveries, when maternal serum calcium levels are highest.[5,7] There is no proof that placental calcification has any pathologic or clinical significance.[1,8,9]

MACROSCOPIC LESIONS OF THE PLACENTA: NORMAL

Maternal blood pooling in the perivillous and subchorionic space is a normal occurrence and is visualized at sonogra-

phy as anechoic or hypoechoic areas within the placenta. Slow flow can be demonstrated in these spaces with the use of a high-frequency transducer. Eventually, fibrin deposition occurs. Table 10–1 lists the common, normal macroscopic lesions of the placentas (Fig. 10–4). Of these, subchorionic fibrin deposition, intervillous thrombosis, perivillous fibrin deposition, and septal cysts have been diagnosed sonographically.

Subchorionic Fibrin Deposition

Subchorionic anechoic or hypoechoic areas are visualized in approximately 15% of obstetric sonograms (Fig. 10–5). These correspond to areas of subchorionic fibrin deposition

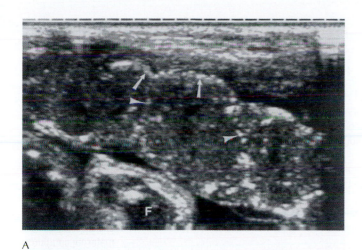

A

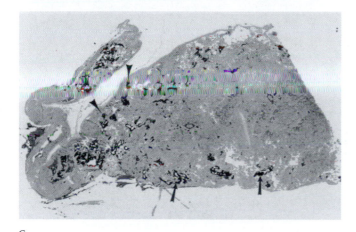

B

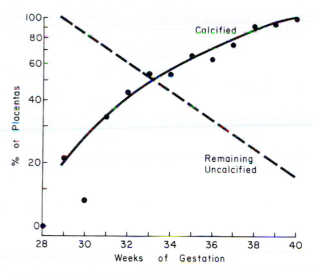

Figure 10–3. Placental calcification versus gestational age. *(Reprinted with permission from Spirt BA, Cohen WN, Weinstein HM. The incidence of placental calcification in normal pregnancies. Radiology. 1982;142:707.)*

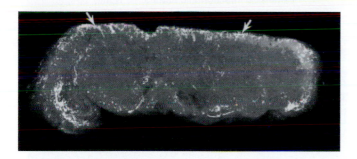

C

Figure 10–2. Placental calcification. **(A)** Anterior placenta at 39 weeks contains prominent calcifications, especially in basal plate *(arrows)* and septa *(arrowheads)*. F, Fetus. **(B)** Radiograph of tissue slice confirms presence of calcification. *(Arrows indicate basal plate.)* **(C)** Photomicrograph of tissue stained for calcium shows deposits along the basal plate *(arrows)*, in subchorionic area *(arrowheads)*, and in perivillous space *(open arrows)*.

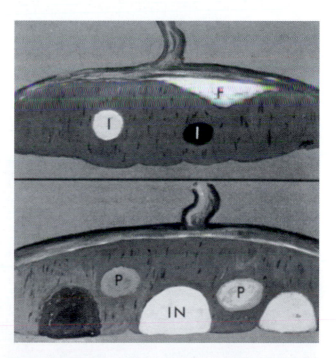

Figure 10–4. Common macroscopic lesions of the placenta. Subchorionic fibrin deposition (F) appears as laminated yellow–white plaques, sometimes associated with fresh blood. Intervillous thrombosis (I) appears as round to oval lesions varying from red to laminated white, depending on age. Perivillous fibrin deposition (P) is seen as nonlaminated plaques varying from brown to white depending on age. True infarcts (IN) appear as dark red to white nonlaminated lesions adjacent to basal plate.

TABLE 10–1. COMMON MACROSCOPIC LESIONS OF THE PLACENTA

	Incidence (Full-Term Uncomplicated Pregnancies, %)[1]	Etiology	Microscopic Description	Clinical Significance
Intervillous thrombosis	36	Bleeding from fetal vessels	Laminated fibrin and red cells surrounded by villi	Fetal–maternal hemorrhage
(Massive) perivillous fibrin deposition	22	Pooling and stasis of blood in intervillous space	Fibrosed villi entrapped in fibrin	None
Septal cyst	19	Obstruction of septal venous drainage by edematous villi	Small cyst (5–10 mm) within septum containing acellular fluid	None
Infarct	25	Disorder of maternal vessels; retroplacental hemorrhage	Coagulation necrosis of villi	Depends on extent and associated maternal condition
Subchorionic fibrin deposition	20	Pooling and stasis of blood in subchorionic space	Laminated subchorionic fibrin without villi; secondary cyst formation may occur	None

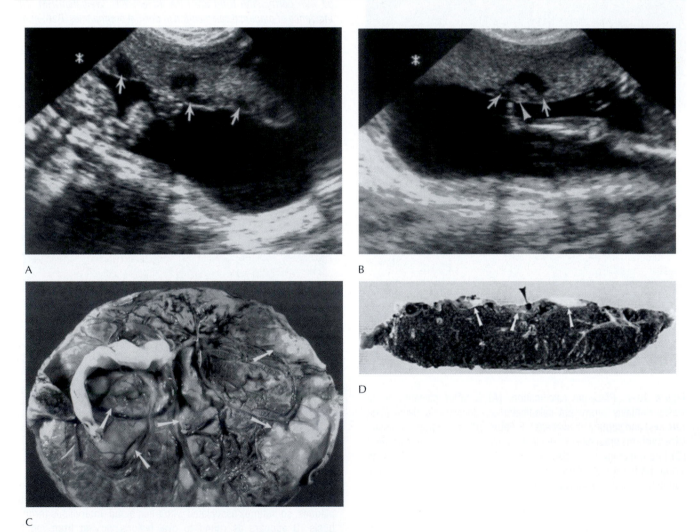

Figure 10–5. Subchorionic fibrin deposition. **(A)** Sagittal scan at 21.5 weeks shows multiple subchorionic anechoic/hypoechoic lesions *(arrows)*. **(B)** Transverse scan 90 degrees to central lesion in **A** showing subchorionic lesion *(arrows)* with vessel overlying it *(arrowhead)*. **(C)** Gross photograph of placenta showing multiple deposits of subchorionic fibrin corresponding to lesions seen at sonography *(arrows)*. **(D)** Section of placenta showing laminated subchorionic fibrin deposition *(arrows)* corresponding to lesions in **A**. Note vessel *(arrowhead)* overlying central lesion (see **B**).

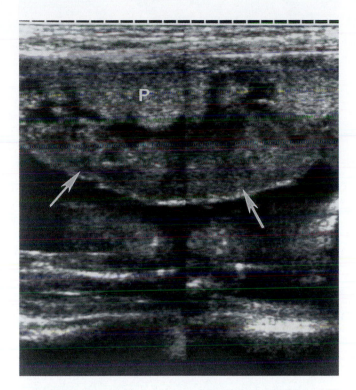

Figure 10–6. Subchorionic fibrin deposition. Anterior placenta (P) with prominent subchorionic blood pooling *(arrows)* at 21 weeks. The complex low-level echo pattern was seen in real time to represent slow flow.

in the term placenta[10] and have no clinical significance.[1] *Subchorionic fibrin* refers to a laminated collection of fibrin between the chorionic plate and placental villi. It is a result of pooling and stasis of maternal blood in the intervillous space beneath the chorion, which leads to thrombosis and secondary fibrin deposition. Slow flow is often visible with real-time sonography (Fig. 10–6). Subchorionic blood pooling and fibrin deposition may be quite prominent at sonography (Fig. 10–7); it is important to recognize this entity so as not to confuse it with a chorioangioma.

Intervillous Thrombosis

Intervillous thromboses are intraplacental areas of hemorrhage with a variable gross appearance that depends on the age of the lesion. Fresh lesions are dark red but, with aging, change to brown, yellow, and finally white. Usually, there are visible laminations that microscopically consist of layers of fibrin. Both fetal and maternal red blood cells are present, suggesting that a leakage of fetal cells from a villous tear stimulates maternal coagulation.[11] Intervillous thromboses have been found in up to 36% of term placentas from uncomplicated pregnancies.[1]

At sonography, intervillous thromboses appear as anechoic or hypoechoic intraplacental lesions that vary in size from a few millimeters to several centimeters[12,13] (Fig. 10–8). They may extend to the subchorionic space or the basal plate. These lesions have been documented sonographically as early

as 19 weeks.[13] The incidence of intervillous thrombosis is increased in cases of Rh isoimmunization,[1,12,14,15] suggesting that the presence of intervillous thrombosis might lead to sensitization.

Some authors have suggested that intraplacental lesions may be associated with elevated maternal serum α-fetoprotein (MSAFP) levels in patients with normal-appearing fetuses;[16–18] however, with the exception of a case report documenting an intervillous thrombosis in a patient with elevated MSAFP,[19] these studies do not provide pathologic documentation regarding the lesions seen at antenatal sonography. If the correlation is valid, it should be true only in the case of intervillous thromboses, because these are the only macroscopic placental lesions that are known to contain fetal blood.

Perivillous Fibrin Deposition

Perivillous fibrin deposition results from pooling and stasis of blood in the intervillous space. The lesions consist of nonlaminated plaques, varying in color from brown to white depending on age. Sonographically, they appear as intraplacental anechoic or hypoechoic lesions (Fig. 10–9). Almost all full-term placentas contain some degree of perivillous fibrin deposition; in approximately 22%, the plaques are large enough to be seen macroscopically.[1] Perivillous fibrin deposition is of no clinical significance.[8]

Maternal Lakes

"Maternal lakes" are anechoic lesions in the placenta that correspond to blood filled spaces at delivery. This entity is not described in the pathology literature. We believe that maternal lakes represent an early stage of intervillous thrombosis and/or perivillous fibrin deposition before the fibrin is laid down. Flow can be demonstrated in some of these lesions at real-time sonography and color flow Doppler examination (Fig. 10–10). It is likely that in those lesions with particularly active flow, less fibrin is deposited so that the lesion is "empty" on gross inspection at delivery (Fig. 10–11). Aberrant blood flow to the placenta may result in an increased number of maternal lakes, as has been described in cases of placenta creta (see later discussion).

Infarcts

As with other organs, placental infarcts result from a disruption in the maternal vascular supply leading to coagulation necrosis of villi. Infarcts occur most commonly at the base of the placenta and vary in size from a few millimeters to many centimeters. Although small infarcts are found in 25% of placentas of uncomplicated pregnancies, they occur with increased frequency in pregnancies complicated by preeclampsia and essential hypertension. Small infarcts have no clinical significance;[1] however, extensive infarction, involving more than 10% of the placental parenchyma, is a reflection of maternal vascular disease.[8]

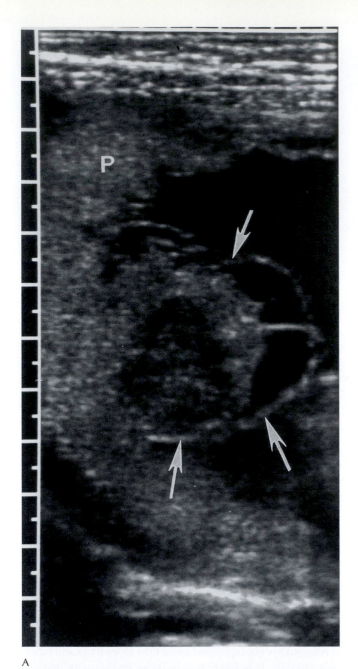

A

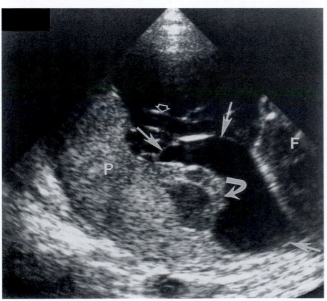

B

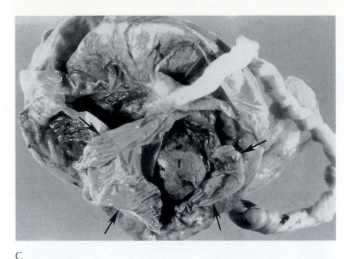

C

D

E

Figure 10–7. Subchorionic fibrin deposition. **(A)** At 21 weeks, a prominent complex subchorionic lesion with a large cystic component is seen *(arrows)*. No flow was demonstrated within. P, Placenta. **(B)** At 25 weeks, the solid component was smaller *(curved arrow)*. *Arrows,* overlying cyst; *open arrow,* umbilical cord; F, Fetus. Gross photographs of fetal surface **(C)** and cross section **(D)** of term placenta show opened cyst *(arrows)* adjacent to cord insertion. The cyst was formed by the chorion and contained clear fluid and fibrin (f). **(E)** Photomicrograph confirms that the cyst wall is made up of chorion *(arrow)*. f, Fibrin; P, Placenta.

200

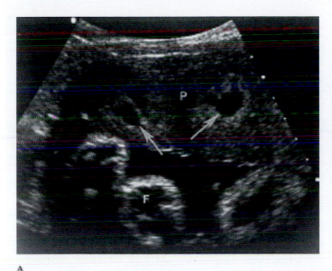
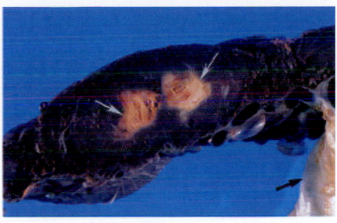

A   B

Figure 10–8. Intervillous thrombosis. **(A)** Two irregular-shaped intraplacental hypoechoic lesions *(arrows)* are seen in this anterior placenta at 33 weeks; several similar lesions were noted in this placenta. **(B)** Laminated fibrin, characteristic of intervillous thrombosis, is demonstrated in two adjacent lesions *(arrows)* after delivery. P, Placenta; F, Fetus; *black arrow,* umbilical cord.

Placental infarcts cannot be documented at sonography unless they are complicated by hemorrhage.[20] This likely reflects the fact that infarcts are composed of necrotic villi, whereas those macroscopic lesions that are visible at sonography contain fluid and/or fibrin.

MACROSCOPIC LESIONS OF THE PLACENTA: ABNORMAL (TABLE 10–2)

Gestational Trophoblastic Disease

The gestational trophoblast contributes to the formation of placental villi. Neoplasms of the gestational trophoblast may be divided into those with villi (complete and partial hydatidiform moles) and those without villi (persistent trophoblastic neoplasia, including choriocarcinoma, invasive mole, and placental site trophoblastic tumor).

The complete hydatidiform mole is characterized by replacement of the placenta with enlarged, hydropic villi and the lack of an embryo. It is believed to result from abnormal fertilization of an empty ovum by either a single sperm with duplication of the paternal haploid set of chromosomes (46,XX) or two spermatozoa (dispermy), resulting in a heterozygous karyotype (46,XY or 46,XX).[21,22] The incidence of hydatidiform mole in the United States and Europe is 1 in 1500 pregnancies, with a higher incidence of 1 in 522 pregnancies in Japan.[23]

TABLE 10–2. ABNORMAL MACROSCOPIC LESIONS OF THE PLACENTA

	Incidence (Full-Term Uncomplicated Pregnancies, %)[1]	Etiology	Microscopic Description	Clinical Significance
Hydatidiform mole		1. Complete mole	Generalized swelling of all villi	May develop persistent trophoblastic neoplasia
		2. Tripoidy; partial mole	Mild to moderate swelling of some villi	Associated with symptoms of preeclampsia
Chorioangioma	1	Vascular malformation	Multiple capillaries in a loose stroma	Usually none, dependent on size
Teratoma	Rare	?	Tissue elements of three embryonic germ layers	None
Metastatic lesions	Rare	Melanoma, carcinoma of breast and carcinoma of the lung are most frequent		
Abscess	Rare	Listeriosis, staphylococcus, streptococcus, tuberculosis	Necrotic villi, with intravillous and intervillous inflammation	Neonatal sepsis; listeriosis is associated with premature labor

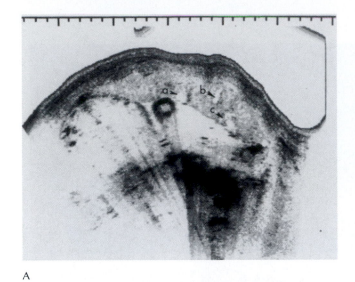

A

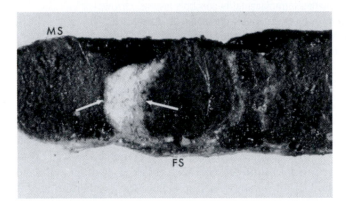

B

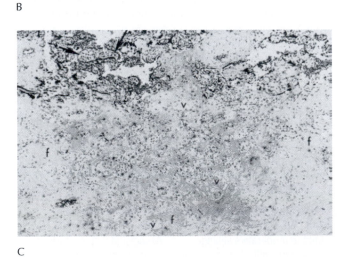

C

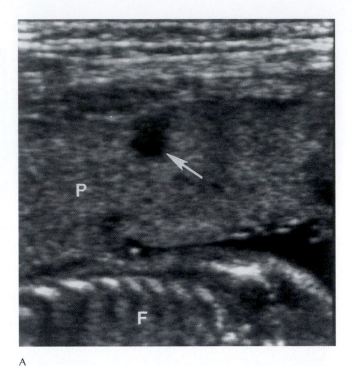

A

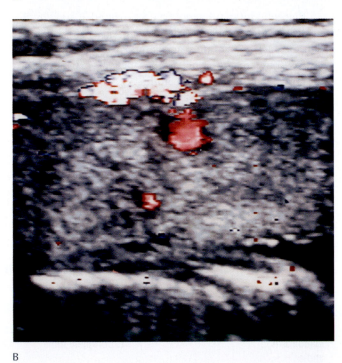

B

Figure 10–9. Perivillous fibrin deposition. **(A)** Transverse scan at 31 weeks shows three intraplacental anechoic lesions (a, b, c). **(B)** This placenta contained multiple areas of perivillous fibrin deposition. Gross specimen at right angle to lesion "a" in **A** shows irregular, nonlaminated collection of perivillous fibrin *(arrows)*. FS, Fetal surface; MS, Maternal surface. **(C)** Fibrin (f) separates villi (v) and obliterates intervillous space. Normal villi surrounded by maternal red cells are present at the periphery *(arrows)*. (H & E × 55.)

Figure 10–10. Maternal lake. **(A)** Anterior placenta at 21 weeks contains hypoechoic intraplacental lesion *(arrow)*. **(B)** Flow is demonstrated with color flow Doppler. P, Placenta; F, Fetus.

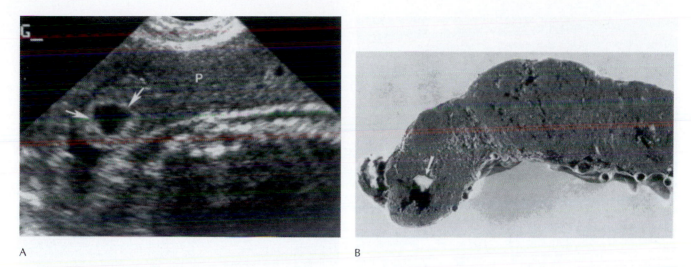

A   B

Figure 10–11. Maternal lake. **(A)** Sector scan at 35 weeks showing anechoic intraplacental lesion *(arrows).*
(B) At delivery, lesion *(arrow)* contained blood that fell out upon sectioning.

At sonography, the uterus is filled with echogenic material containing multiple anechoic vesicles of different sizes (Fig. 10–12). The vesicles enlarge with advancing gestational age. Early in pregnancy, transvaginal sonography is helpful in diagnosing hydatidiform mole (Fig. 10–13). A viable fetus may coexist with a complete mole in the case of a multiple pregnancy with one empty ovum (Fig. 10–14). Elevated serum β-human chorionic gonadotropin (β-hCG) levels are found with hydatidiform mole. Persistent trophoblastic neoplasia occurs in up to 20% of patients with complete hydatidiform mole.[22] Thus, serum β-hCG levels must be closely followed to ensure that they decrease to zero after evacuation of the mole.

Partial hydatidiform mole refers to a placenta containing areas of molar change alternating with normal villi. The fetus is usually abnormal. Most partial moles are triploid

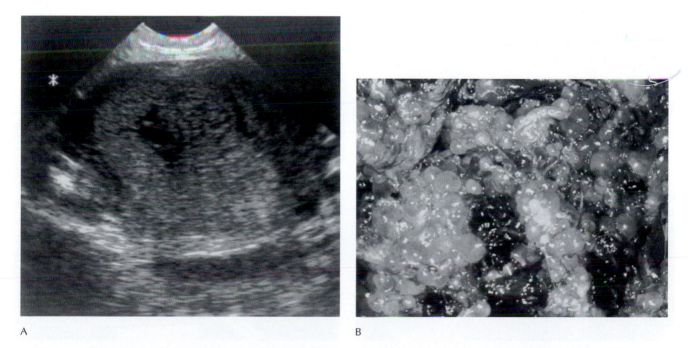

A   B

Figure 10–12. Hydatidiform mole. **(A)** Sagittal scan of the uterus shows a diffuse vesicular echo pattern.
(B) Gross specimen demonstrates multiple grapelike cysts. (**B,** *Courtesy of Dr. David Jones, Department of Pathology, SUNY Health Science Center at Syracuse, New York. Reprinted with permission from Spirt BA, Kagan EH, Rozanski RM. Sonolucent areas in the placenta: Sonographic and pathologic correlation. AJR. 1978;131:961.)*

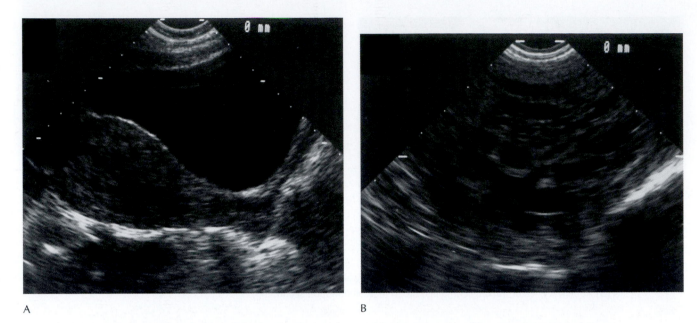

A   B

Figure 10–13. Early hydatidiform mole. **(A)** Transabdominal sagittal scan of the uterus at 10 to 12 weeks amenorrhea shows inhomogeneous uterine echotexture. **(B)** Transvaginal scan shows typical vesicular pattern of hydatidiform mole. *(Courtesy of Medical Imaging Department, Crouse Hospital, Syracuse, New York. Reprinted with permission from Spirt BA, Gordon LP. Sonographic evaluation of the placenta. In: Rumack C, Charbonneau W, Wilson S, eds.* Diagnostic Ultrasonography. *Chicago: Year Book Medical Publishers; 1991.)*

(69 chromosomes). At sonography, a large placenta with diffuse anechoic intraplacental lesions is seen (Fig. 10–15). Triploid pregnancies have a high incidence of first-trimester spontaneous abortion. In the second trimester, partial moles may present with early onset of preeclampsia. Persistent trophoblastic neoplasia occurs in a small percentage of patients with triploid partial moles, necessitating close monitoring of chorionic gonadotropin levels in all cases of partial hydatidiform moles as well as complete moles.[21,22,26–30]

Primary Neoplasm

There are two nontrophoblastic primary tumors of the placenta: the relatively common chorioangioma and the rare

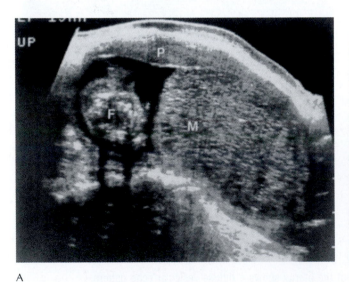

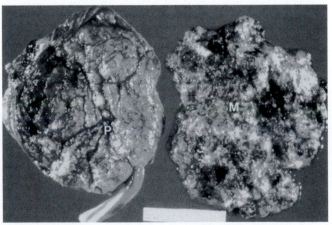

A   B

Figure 10–14. Coexistent fetus and mole. **(A)** Sagittal scan at 26 weeks shows anterior placenta (P) and fetus (F) with coexisting mole (M). **(B)** At delivery, the hydatidiform mole and the placenta were separate. *(Reprinted with permission from Spirt BA, Gordon LP, Oliphant M. Prenatal Ultrasound: A Color Atlas with Anatomic and Pathologic Correlation. New York: Churchill Livingstone; 1987.)*

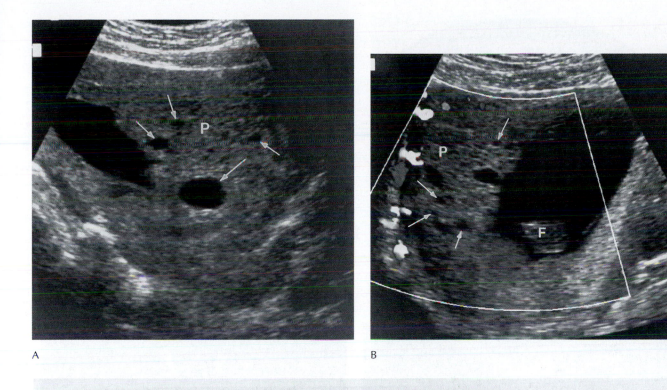

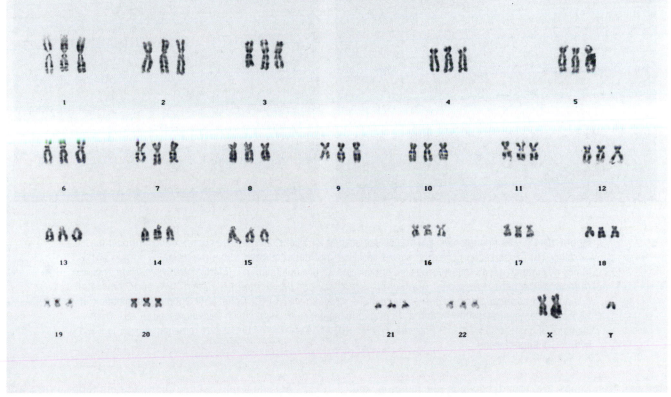

Figure 10–15. Partial hydatidiform mole. **(A, B)** Transabdominal scans at 10 weeks of amenorrhea show large placenta (P) with multiple anechoic lesions of different sizes *(arrows),* and fetal demise. F, Fetus. **(C)** Chromosomal analysis confirmed triploidy.

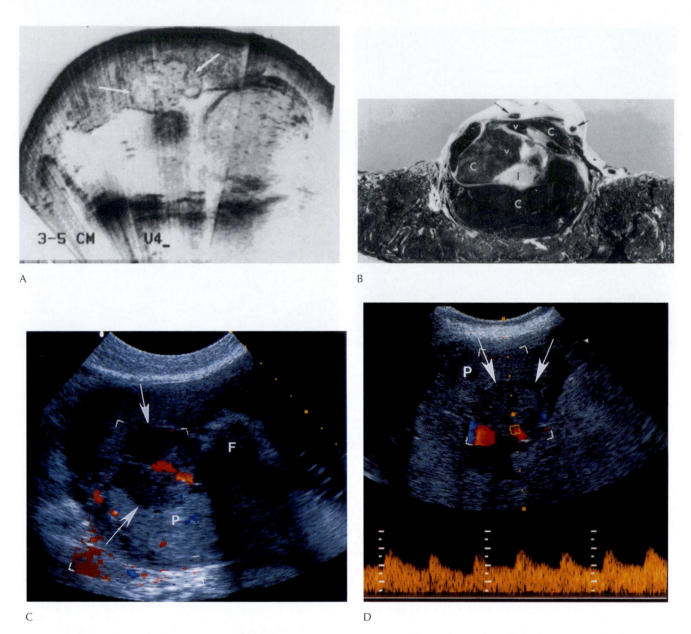

Figure 10–16. Chorioangiomas. **(A)** Transverse scan at 24 weeks shows large complex subchorionic mass *(arrows)*. **(B)** Cross-section of tumor shows vessels (v) of different sizes within the lesion. A portion of the tumor had infarcted, and fetal hydrops did not develop. C, Chorioangioma; I, Infarct. *(Arrows indicate vessels from umbilical cord.) (Reprinted with permission from Spirt BA, Gordon LP, Cohen, WN, et al. Antenatal diagnosis of chorioangioma of the placenta. AJR. 1980;135:1273.)* **(C)** Color flow Doppler examination at 29 weeks demonstrates flow within a 4-cm chorioangioma *(arrows),* which had increased in size from a diameter of 3 cm at 25 weeks. P, Placenta; F, Fetus. **(D)** At 34 weeks, the tumor size remained the same. Fetal hydrops did not develop.

teratoma. Teratomas are found between the amnion and the chorion and are of no clinical significance.[1] The chorioangioma is a vascular malformation seen in approximately 1% of carefully studied placentas.[1] Small tumors occur within the placenta, whereas large tumors may protrude from the fetal surface. The microscopic appearance is that of proliferating capillaries present in a loose fibrous stroma.

At sonography, a large chorioangioma appears as a well-circumscribed solid intraplacental mass lesion within which vessels may be seen[31] (Fig. 10–16). Doppler examination is useful to demonstrate the vascularity of these lesions. Large chorioangiomas (larger than 5 cm) are associated with fetal hydrops, cardiomegaly and congestive heart failure, low birth weight, premature labor, or fetal demise.[32–34] Small lesions usually have no associated problems.

Secondary Neoplasms

Neoplasms that may metastasize to the placenta include melanoma, carcinoma of the breast, and carcinoma of the lung.

Abscess

Macroabscesses of the placenta are unusual. Staphylococcus, β-hemolytic streptococcus, *Mycobacterium tuberculosis*, and *Listeria monocytogenes* are among those organisms known to involve the placenta by either ascending infection or hematogenous spread.[1] Although listeriosis usually results in microabscesses, macroabscesses have been reported.[35]

THE RETROPLACENTAL AREA

The placenta should be easily distinguished from the retroplacental myometrium and decidua basalis, which appear relatively hypoechoic when compared to the placenta (Fig. 10–17). Maternal blood flows to the placenta via the spiral arterioles. These terminate at the base of the placenta and supply blood to the intervillous space. Blood drains from the placenta through endometrial veins, which are present all along the base of the placenta,[36–38] and in the septa (Fig. 10–18). These veins are often visible at sonography (Fig. 10–19).

During the third month of gestation, placental septa develop. These are composed of decidua and trophoblasts and

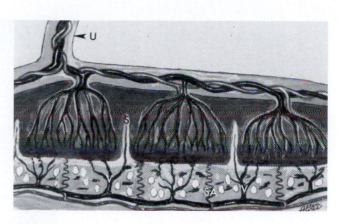

Figure 10–18. Diagram of placental circulation. U, Umbilical Cord; SA, Spiral Arterioles; V, Draining Veins; S, Septum. *(Reprinted with permission from Spirt BA, Kagan EH. Sonography of the placenta. Semin Ultrasound. 1980;1:293.)*

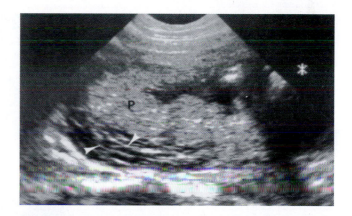

A

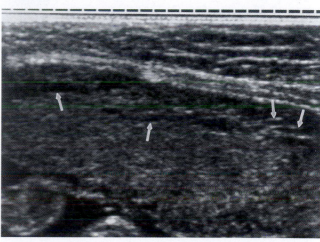

B

Figure 10–19. Retroplacental veins. **(A)** Sector scan at 20 weeks demonstrates venous drainage *(arrowheads)* of posterior placenta. P, Placenta. **(B)** Anterior placenta at 25 weeks. Note retroplacental veins *(arrows)*.

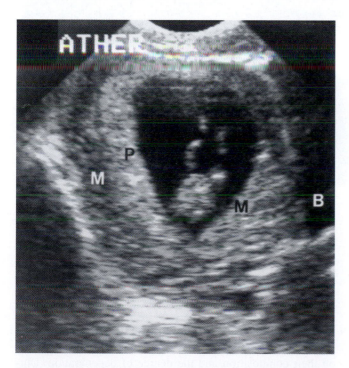

Figure 10–17. The placenta and myometrium. Sagittal sector scan at 11.5 weeks clearly shows the posterior placenta (P). The retroplacental myometrium (M) appears relatively hypoechoic, whereas the myometrium (M) at the inferior aspect of the uterus appears more echogenic. B, Maternal Bladder.

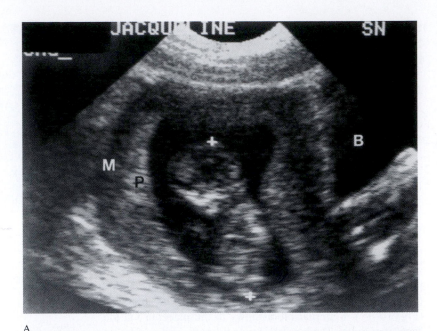

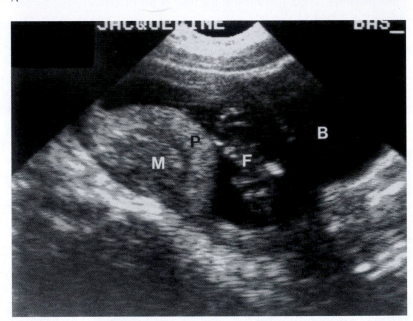

Figure 10–20. Contraction. **(A)** Sagittal sector scan at 12 weeks shows the posterior placenta (P). **(B)** Scan in the same location 20 mins later shows a contraction involving the placenta (P) and myometrium (M). F, Fetus; B, Maternal Bladder.

extend from the basal plate toward the fetal surface. They divide the maternal surface into 15 to 20 lobes that have no physiologic significance.[1]

Contractions

Transient myometrial thickening results from normal uterine contractions (Braxton Hicks), which are imperceptible to the mother. These contractions most commonly occur in the second trimester, but can be seen earlier (Figs. 10–20 and 10–21). A contraction may mimic placenta previa and should be followed over time to exclude that diagnosis (Fig. 10–22); usually, rescanning the patient approximately 30 minutes after the initial examination will suffice. A con-

traction should also be distinguished from a leiomyoma, which would not change over a relatively short period of time (Fig. 10–23).

Leiomyomas

Leiomyomas have a variable sonographic appearance ranging from hypoechoic to hyperechoic and complex, depending on their composition and the degree of degeneration. During the course of pregnancy, they may change in size and echotexture. Retroplacental leiomyomas are distinguishable from contractions at sonography by their stable appearance over time; the presence of multiple leiomyomas helps in the diagnosis.

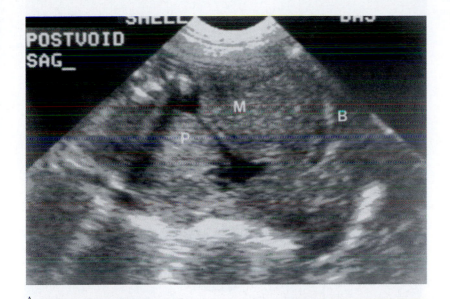

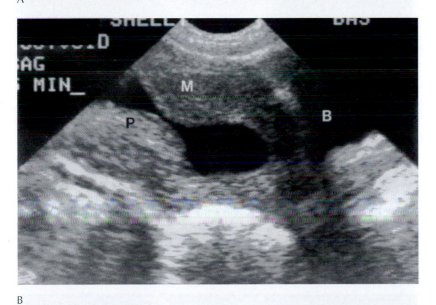

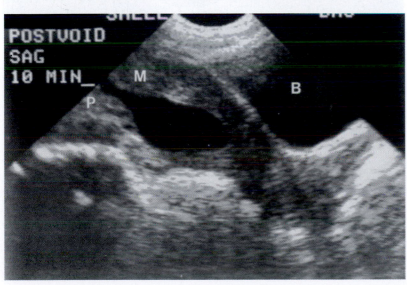

Figure 10–21. Contraction. **(A)** Sagittal sector scan at 15 weeks shows a contraction involving the posterior placenta (P) and anterior myometrium (M) in the lower segment of the uterus. B, Maternal Bladder. **(B)** Five mins later, the contraction is less pronounced. **(C)** Ten mins later, the placenta and anterior myometrium appear smooth.

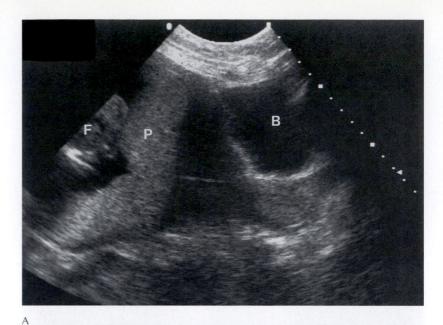

A

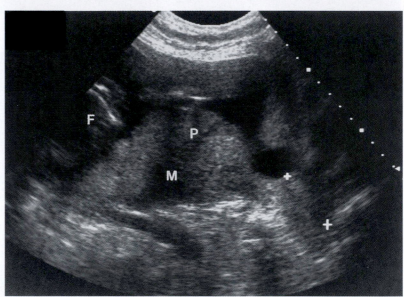

B

Figure 10–22. Contraction mimicking placenta previa.
(A) Sagittal midline scan at 23 weeks shows apparent placenta previa. **(B)** Twenty-five mins later, midline sagittal scan shows posterior placenta, well away from the cervix *(cursors)*. The contraction (M) is now posterior. **(C)** Transverse image shows that the placenta is left sided, with anterior and posterior extensions. B, Maternal Bladder; F, Fetus; P, Placenta.

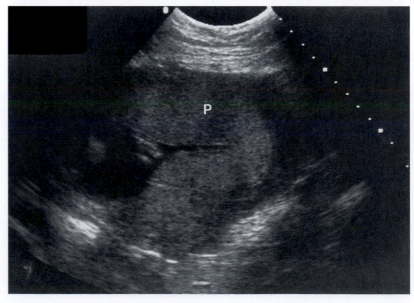

C

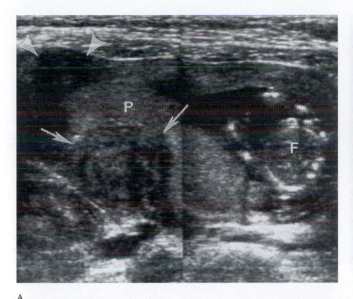

A

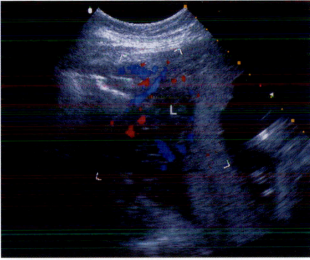

B

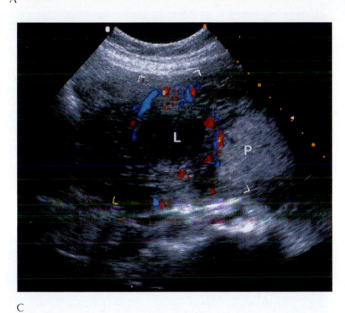

C

Figure 10–23. Myomas. **(A)** At 16 weeks, small anterior fibroid *(arrowheads)* and prominent posterior, retroplacental fibroid *(arrows)* are demonstrated. P, Placenta; F, Fetus. Right transverse **(B)** and sagittal **(C)** color flow Doppler images of a retroplacental fibroid at 27 weeks show that the retroplacental vessels are maintained. P, Placenta; L, Leiomyoma.

Placenta Creta

Placenta creta, thought to be due to a focal or diffuse deficiency of the decidua basalis,[1] occurs in varying degrees: placenta accreta vera, in which the villi attach to but do not invade the myometrium; placenta increta, wherein the myometrium is invaded; and placenta percreta, in which the villi fully penetrate the myometrium. Placenta creta is more frequent in patients with previous cesarean section, increased parity, prior manual removal of a placenta, and uterine scars. In an unscarred uterus with placenta previa, the risk of placenta creta is 5%. In the case of placenta previa after one cesarian section, the risk of placenta creta is 24%. After four or more cesarean sections, the risk of placenta creta in the case of placenta previa is 67%.[39]

Placenta creta results in severe hemorrhage, usually necessitating hysterectomy. Rupture of the uterus occurs in ap-

proximately 14% of cases.[22] Villous invasion into adjacent structures such as the bladder may also occur.

At sonography, placenta creta should be suspected if the usual retroplacental hypoechoic zone of decidua/myometrium is absent (Fig. 10–24).[40–42] These placentas are also characterized by an increased number of large intervillous spaces (lakes)[43,44] in which turbulent flow may be seen with color flow and spectral Doppler sonography.[45–47]

In the case of a posterior placenta, magnetic resonance imaging has been useful to diagnose placenta creta.[48]

THE MEMBRANES

The amnion is seen as a separate membrane (Fig. 10–25) until the end of the first trimester, when the amnion and chorion

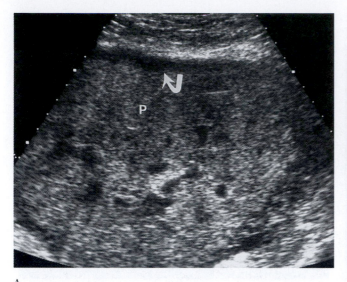

A

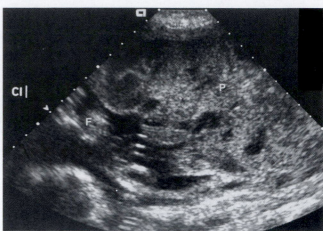

B

Figure 10–24. Placenta creta. **(A)** Placenta accreta. Sagittal scan at 30 weeks shows anterior placenta (P) with multiple lakes. The retroplacental stripe *(curved arrow)* is visible. Premature rupture of the membranes had occurred. The patient delivered 4 days after this scan, and focal placenta accreta was noted at pathology. Hysterectomy was performed for severe postpartum bleeding and retained placenta 1 week later. Placenta accreta was confirmed at pathology. *(Courtesy of Medical Imaging Department, Crouse Hospital, Syracuse, New York.)* **(B, C)** Placenta percreta in a patient with placenta previa and three prior cesarean sections. **(B)** Sagittal scan at 27 weeks shows multiple placental lakes *(arrows)*. *(Courtesy of Medical Imaging Department, Crouse Hospital, Syracuse, New York.)* **(C)** Midline sagittal scan at 35 weeks shows complete placenta previa, with placental tissue extending to the maternal bladder (B). Irregularity of the bladder wall *(arrows)* suggests invasion. After cesarean section, a hysterectomy was performed. The placenta had invaded the bladder wall. *(Courtesy of Dr. Robert Silverman, Perinatal Center, SUNY Upstate Medical University, Syracuse, New York.)* P, Placenta; F, Fetus; C, Cervix.

C

fuse to form an avascular membrane surrounding the amniotic cavity. In rare cases, the membranes remain separate throughout the pregnancy (Fig. 10–26).

The calcified yolk sac remnant, which is located between the amnion and the chorion, may be seen at sonography on the fetal surface of the placenta (Fig. 10–27).

Placenta Extrachorialis

A placenta in which the fetal membranes do not extend to the edge, so that the chorionic plate is smaller than the basal plate, is called *placenta extrachorialis*. The attachment of the fetal membranes to the chorionic plate forms a ring that may be flat (circummarginate) or folded (circumvallate) (Fig. 10–28). This ring may be partly or totally circumferential. The fold of

membranes can be seen at sonography (Fig. 10–29) through the second trimester. The circummarginate placenta has no clinical significance, whereas a complete circumvallate placenta may be associated with a higher incidence of premature labor, threatened abortion, perinatal mortality, and marginal hemorrhage.[1,49,50]

The Umbilical Cord Insertion

The umbilical cord inserts on the fetal surface of the placenta, usually in an eccentric location. A placenta with a marginally inserted cord is often referred to as a *battledore placenta* (Fig. 10–30). This occurs in fewer than 6% of cases and is of no clinical significance. An important variation of umbilical cord attachment is the rare velamentous insertion,

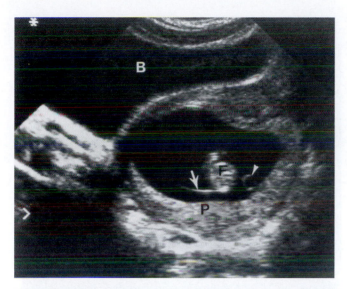

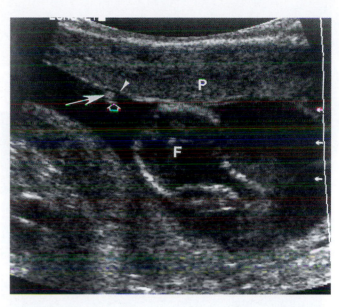

Figure 10–25. The amniotic membrane. Transverse sector scan at 10.8 weeks shows the amniotic membrane *(arrow)*. The yolk sac *(arrowhead)* is seen between the amnion and the placenta.

Figure 10–27. Yolk sac remnant. At 14 weeks, the yolk sac remnant *(arrow)* is seen between amnion *(open arrow)* and chorion *(arrowhead)*. P, Placenta; F, Fetus.

where the fetal vessels attach to the membranes at a variable distance from the fetal surface (Fig. 10–31). This occurs in fewer than 2% of cases.[1,51] Velamentous insertion is potentially hazardous because the fetal vessels are less protected and may be damaged during labor. In addition, fetal vessels running intramembranously across the internal os (vasa previa) (Fig. 10–32) may tear, leading to fetal blood loss. Color flow Doppler examination is helpful to accurately assess an abnormal umbilical cord insertion.[52] As with placenta previa, vasa previa is an indication for cesarean section.

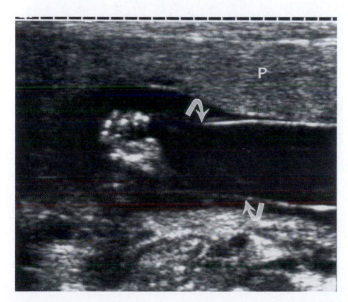

Figure 10–26. Persistent nonfusion of the chorion and amnion. At 21.5 weeks, a membrane *(curved arrows)* is seen surrounding the fetus. At term, the amnion and chorion were unfused. P, Placenta.

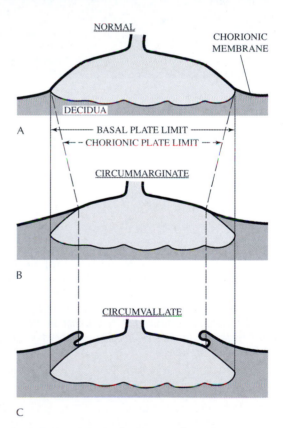

Figure 10–28. Cross-sectional diagram comparing extrachorial placentas with normal placenta. **(A)** Normal placenta, showing the transition of membranous to villous chorion at the placental edge. **(B)** Circummarginate placenta: the transition from membranous to villous chorion occurs at a distance from the placental edge. **(C)** Circumvallate placenta, similar to **B** except for a fold in the chorioamniotic membrane. *(Reprinted with permission from Spirt BA, Kagan EH. Sonography of the placenta. Semin Ultrasound. 1980;1:293).*

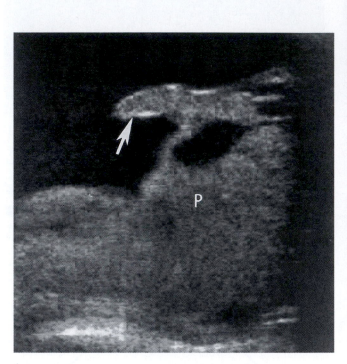

A

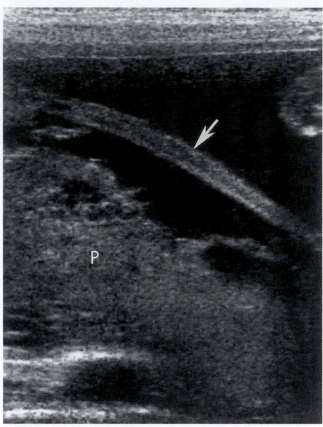

B

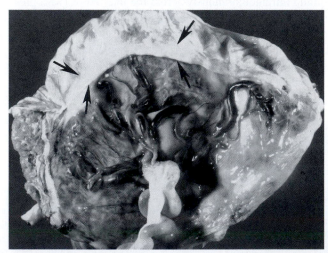

C

Figure 10–29. Extrachorial placenta. Transverse **(A)** and oblique **(B)** scans at 26.5 weeks show a thick membrane fold *(arrow)* involving a portion of the placenta (P). **(C)** At delivery, a partial circumvallate placenta was confirmed *(arrows)*. *(Reprinted with permission from Spirt BA, Gordon LP. Imaging of the placenta. In: Traveras JM, Ferrucci JT. Radiology: Diagnosis—Imaging—Intervention. Philadelphia: JB Lippincott Co; 1992.)*

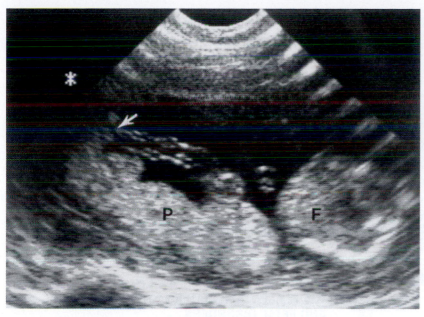

A

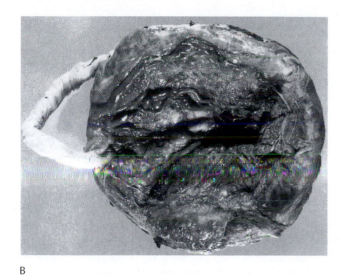

B

Figure 10–30. Battledore placenta. **(A)** Transverse scan at 20 weeks shows a posterior placenta (P) with a marginal cord insertion *(arrow),* confirmed at delivery **(B)**. F, Fetus.

VARIATIONS IN SHAPE

At the end of the fourth month, the placenta has attained its final thickness and shape; however, circumferential enlargement continues into the third trimester. The appearance of the placenta and myometrium may change with contractions (see earlier discussion). It may also change with different degrees of bladder filling; this effect occurs most commonly in the second trimester. The full bladder compresses the anterior portion of the lower uterine segment against the posterior wall, artificially elongating the cervix. It may be necessary to repeat the examination after voiding to exclude the presence of a placenta previa (Fig. 10–33).

Succenturiate Lobes

In up to 8% of placentas, succenturiate (accessory) lobes are present.[1,53–55] These consist of separate masses of chorionic villi connected to the main placenta by vessels within the membrane (Fig. 10–34). It is important to make the diagnosis antenatally because of the following complications: a succenturiate lobe may be retained in utero, resulting in

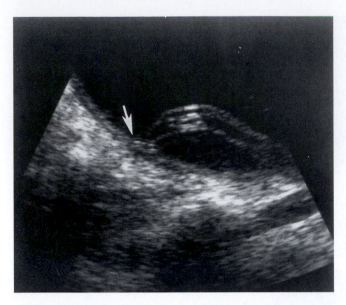

Figure 10–31. Velamentous insertion. Sector scan at 25 weeks shows the umbilical cord inserting into the membranes *(arrow)*. Note polyhydramnios.

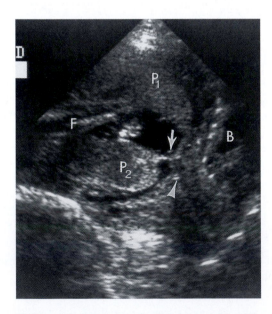

Figure 10–32. Vasa previa. Longitudinal scan at 25 weeks shows a vessel *(arrow)* overlying the internal cervical os *(arrowhead)*. The placenta was on the left, with anterior (P₁) and posterior (P₂) extensions. B, Maternal Bladder. Vasa previa was confirmed at cesarean section. *(Reprinted with permission from Spirt BA, Gordon LP. Sonographic evaluation of the placenta. In: Rumack C, Charbonneau W, Wilson S. eds.* Diagnostic Ultrasound. *Chicago: Year Book Medical Publishers; 1991;935–953.)*

postpartum hemorrhage; it may overlie the internal cervical os; or the vessels that connect it to the main placental mass may traverse the internal os (vasa previa) and rupture during labor, resulting in fetal blood loss.

Placenta Membranacea

Other variations of placental shape that are of clinical significance include placenta membranacea and a variant of that condition, the annular or ring-shaped placenta. Both are associated with antepartum and postpartum hemorrhage. These conditions result from failure of regression of the chorionic villi in the first trimester, so that it covers most or all of the surface of the amniotic sac.[1] Placenta membranacea may be diagnosed at sonography if placental tissue is seen to extend over most of the uterine cavity.[56]

THE PLACENTA IN MATERNAL AND FETAL DISORDERS

The placenta can lose up to 30% of its surface area and still maintain its function;[1,8] however, maternal vascular problems may induce a placental response to the anoxia that results from decreased uteroplacental blood flow. It is the decreased uteroplacental circulation that is believed to play a role in intrauterine growth restriction (IUGR).[8] Prior to Doppler sonography, uteroplacental blood flow could not be studied noninvasively. As more data are obtained, Doppler evaluation of the uteroplacental circulation will likely provide useful information for the detection and management of some cases of IUGR.

The most consistent placental abnormality in cases of Rh incompatibility, diabetes, anemia, and preeclampsia is variation in size. Visual assessment is usually sufficient to judge whether a placenta is too large or too small.

The placenta may be markedly enlarged in cases of hemolytic disease of the newborn. This appears to be secondary to both villous edema and hyperplasia of the villous tree.[1] The amount of villous edema may vary in different areas of the same placenta. Sonographic examination shows a large placenta with an echo pattern that is similar to that of normal placentas (Fig. 10–35). Septal cysts are frequent, due to mechanical obstruction of septal venous drainage by the villous edema.[1]

Placentas of diabetic mothers are often large due to villous edema.[1,53] Septal cysts are more frequent in these placentas as well. Placentas of mothers who are severely anemic also tend to be large but histologically normal.[1]

Placentas from preeclamptic mothers tend to be slightly smaller than the norm.[1] There is a high incidence of placental infarction in such patients, ranging from 33% of mild cases to 60% of severely affected patients. There is an increased incidence of retroplacental hematomas with preeclampsia,[1] which undoubtedly accounts in part for the increased

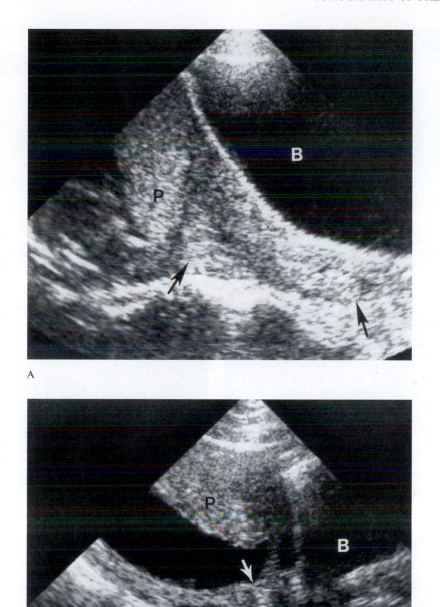

Figure 10–33. Bladder effect. **(A)** Sagittal sector scan at 18.5 weeks shows an elongated cervix *(arrows)* with the anterior placenta (P) covering the area of the cervix. **(B)** Postvoid scan shows the placenta (P) to be well away from the internal os *(arrow)* of the cervix. B, Maternal Bladder.

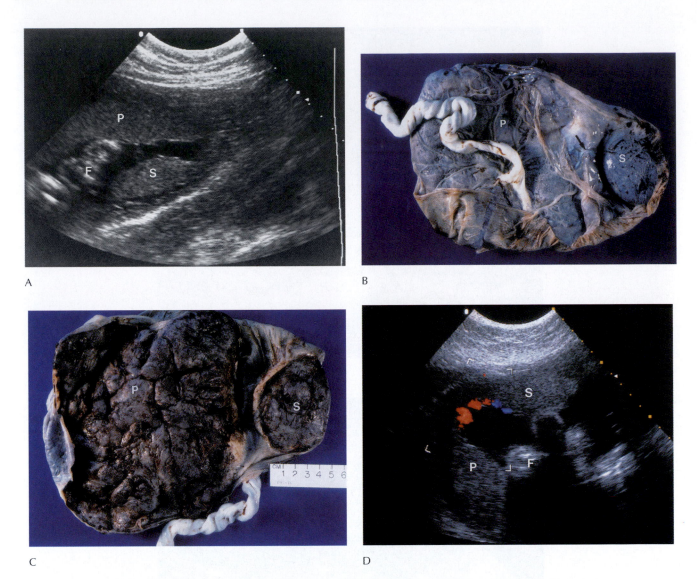

Figure 10–34. Succenturiate lobes. **(A)** Sagittal scan at 28.5 weeks shows anterior placenta (P) with posterior succenturiate lobe (S). F, Fetus. Succenturiate lobe (S) was confirmed at delivery. **(B)** Fetal surface. Arrow, vessel connecting succenturiate lobe (S) with main placenta (P). **(C)** Maternal surface. **(D)** Color flow Doppler image at 31 weeks shows vessels connecting anterior succenturiate lobe (S) to posterior placenta (P). F, Fetus.

incidence of infarction in these patients. Small placentas are also found in association with chromosomal abnormalities, severe maternal diabetes, and chronic infection.[53]

ANTEPARTUM HEMORRHAGE

Bleeding from placenta previa and abruptio placentae usually occurs at or close to term, whereas retroplacental or marginal hemorrhage may occur as early as the first trimester.

Retroplacental/Submembranous Hematoma
Retroplacental hemorrhage may manifest itself in three ways: (1) external bleeding without formation of a significant in-

trauterine hematoma; (2) formation of a retroplacental or marginal hematoma with or without external bleeding; and (3) formation of a submembranous hematoma at a distance from the placenta, with or without external bleeding. Sonographic examination in cases of antepartum bleeding may be negative if most of the bleeding is external.

A retroplacental or submembranous hematoma will appear as a hypoechoic or complex collection at sonography[57–59] (Figs. 10–36 and 10–37). At least one follow-up examination should be performed to ensure that the hematoma has decreased in size. Even if follow-up study indicates that the lesion has disappeared, careful examination of the placenta following delivery will show a thin layer of organized hematoma or fibrin along the membranes.

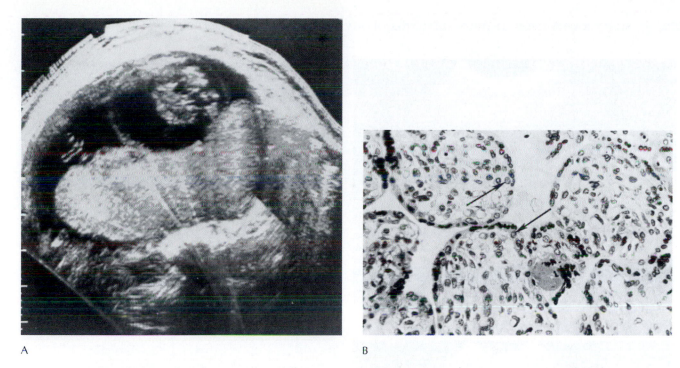

A

B

Figure 10–35. Maternal–fetal Rh incompatibility. **(A)** Transverse scan at 28 weeks shows a grossly enlarged placenta. Note the marked fetal ascites. *(Courtesy of Dr. Edward Bell, Syracuse, New York.)* **(B)** Microscopically, the villi are hypercellular with persistence of cytotrophoblasts *(arrows).* Mild edema is present. (H & E × 100.)

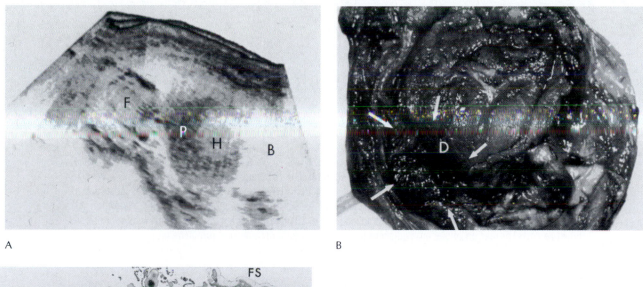

A

B

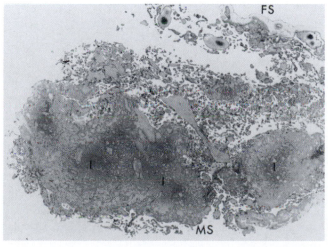

C

Figure 10–36. Retroplacental hematoma. **(A)** Midline sagittal scan at 18 weeks shows a 3.5-cm retroplacental mass (H). P, Placenta; B, Maternal Bladder; F, Fetus. **(B)** Hysterotomy was performed due to severe disseminated intravascular coagulation. A hematoma was present with a corresponding depression in the placenta (D, *arrows*). **(C)** Microscopic section through area D shows infarcts (I) based on the maternal surface (MS) at the site of the hematoma. FS, Fetal Surface. *(Reprinted with permission from Spirt BA, Kagan EH, Aubry RH. Clinically silent retroplacental hematoma. Sonographic and pathologic correlation. J Clin Ultrasound. 1981;9:203.)*

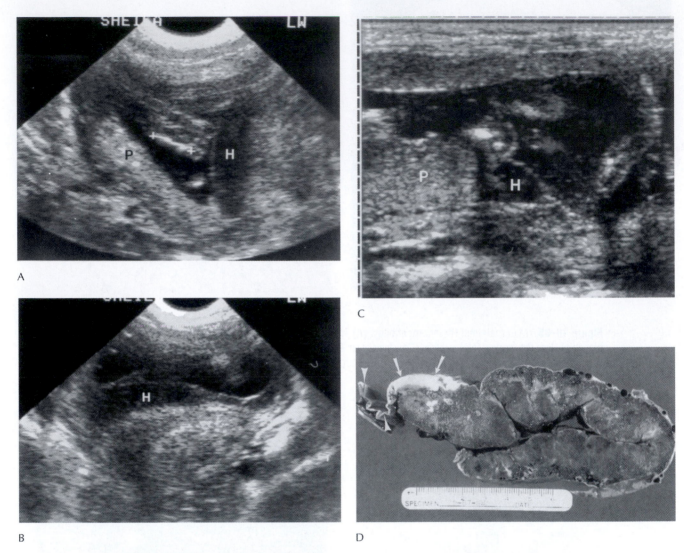

Figure 10–37. Submembranous hematoma. **(A)** Sagittal and **(B)** transverse sector scans at 13 weeks in patient with vaginal bleeding show subchorionic collection (H) containing low-level echoes adjacent to posterior placenta (P) **(C)** Follow-up sagittal scan at 21 weeks shows anechoic subchorionic collection (H) adjacent to placenta (P). Collection has decreased in size. **(D)** Section of term placenta shows subchorionic fibrin *(arrows)* at margin of placenta adjacent to insertion of fetal membranes *(arrowheads)*.

In early pregnancy, subchorionic hematoma may be distinguished from a nonfused amnion by evaluating the thickness of the membrane. The membrane above a subchorionic hematoma is thicker than the amnion (Fig. 10–38).

The clinical significance of retroplacental hemorrhage depends on the size and extent of the lesions. Small hematomas of less than 60 cc are not associated with an increased risk of miscarriage.[60–62] Disseminated intravascular coagulation may occur in cases of large, chronic retroplacental hematomas as a result of tissue breakdown.[57]

Abruptio Placentae

The term *abruptio placentae* is usually reserved for the clinical syndrome of acute separation of the placenta, accompanied by severe bleeding, pain, and hypovolemic shock. In most cases, immediate cesarean section is necessary. In those patients sufficiently stable to be examined before delivery, a poorly defined echogenic retroplacental collection causing apparent thickening of the placenta is seen at sonography (Fig. 10–39). Traditionally, abruptio placentae has been associated with maternal hypertension. Increased vascular

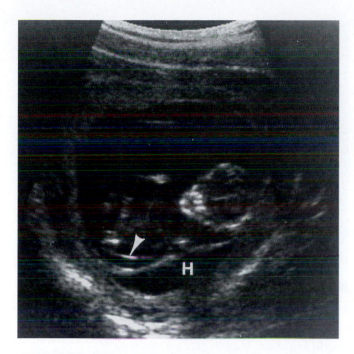

Figure 10–38. Submembranous hematoma. Sector scan at 12 weeks in a patient with vaginal bleeding shows a subchorionic hematoma (H). Note the thin, unfused amnion *(arrowhead).*

resistance in the uteroplacental arteries has been documented in association with abruptio placenta in hypertensive patients.[63,64] Placental abruption has also been reported in association with cocaine abuse, which is known to have hypertensive and vasoconstrictive effects.[65]

Placenta Previa

Placenta previa, in which the placenta covers part or all of the internal cervical os, is a common cause of bleeding in the third trimester, although it occurs in fewer than 1% of deliveries[66] (Fig. 10–40). Placenta previa is often overdiagnosed in the first two trimesters, because it is commonly mimicked by two conditions: overfilling of the urinary bladder and contractions (see earlier discussion).[67] Thus, if placenta previa is suspected, it is important to reexamine the patient after voiding and/or after approximately half an hour has passed. After 20 weeks, it is usually difficult to visualize the internal os of the cervix using the transabdominal approach, because of shadowing by the fetal calvaria. Translabial sonography provides a useful means of diagnosing placenta previa in that situation (see Fig. 10–40B).[68]

Placenta previa may be asymmetric, with the edge of an anterior or posterior placenta extending over the internal os of

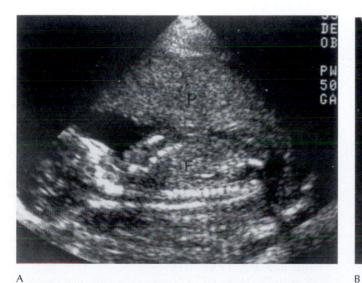

A

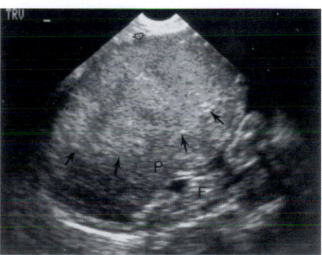

B

Figure 10–39. Abruptio placentae. **(A)** Real-time sector scan at 17 weeks shows an anterior placenta (P). **(B)** At 35 weeks, the patient presented with vaginal bleeding and hypotension. An inhomogeneous hyperechoic collection *(arrows)* is present between the placenta (P) and myometrium *(open arrow).* F, Fetus. At cesarean section, a 75% abruption was found. *(Courtesy of Dr. Michael Oliphant, Crouse Hospital, Syracuse, New York).*

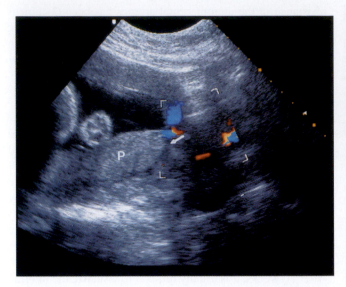
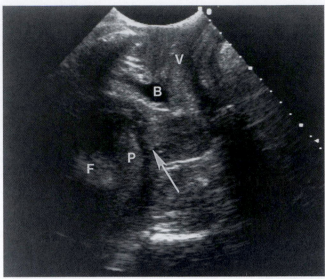

A   B

Figure 10–40. Asymmetric placenta previa. **(A)** Color Doppler image at 27 weeks shows edge of posterior placenta (P) overlying the internal os of the cervix *(arrow)*. **(B)** Asymmetric placenta previa is confirmed on transperineal scan at 32 weeks. B, Maternal Bladder; V, Vagina; arrow, internal os of cervix; P, Placenta.

the cervix, or central, with an inferior placenta symmetrically located over the cervix. In either case, cesarean section is indicated.

REFERENCES

1. Fox H. *Pathology of the Placenta.* Philadelphia: Saunders; 1978.
2. Tindall VR, Scott JS. Placental calcification. A study of 3,025 singleton and multiple pregnancies. *J Obstet Gynaecol Br Commonw.* 1965;72:356.
3. Spirt BA, Cohen WN, Weinstein HM. The incidence of placental calcification in normal pregnancies. *Radiology.* 1982;142:707.
4. Wentworth P. Macroscopic placental calcification and its clinical significance. *J Obstet Gynaecol Br Commonw.* 1965; 72:215.
5. Fujikura D. Placental calcification and seasonal difference. *Am J Obstet Gynecol.* 1963;87:46.
6. Jeacock MK. Calcium content of the human placenta. *Am J Obstet Gynecol.* 1963;87:34.
7. Mull JW, Bill AH. Variations in serum calcium and phosphorus during pregnancy. *Am J Obstet Gynecol.* 1934;27:510.
8. Fox H. Pathology of the placenta. *Clin Obstet Gynecol.* 1986;13:501.
9. Spirt BA, Gordon LP. The placenta as an indicator of fetal maturity—Fact and fancy. *Semin Ultrasound.* 1984;5:290.
10. Spirt BA, Kagan EH, Rozanski RM. Sonolucent areas in the placenta: Sonographic and pathologic correlation. *AJR.* 1978;131:961.
11. Kaplan C, Blanc WA, Elias J. Identification of erythrocytes in intervillous thrombi: A study using immunoperoxidase identification of hemoglobins. *Hum Pathol.* 1982;13:554.
12. Hoogland HJ, de Haan J, Vooys GP. Ultrasonographic diagno-

sis of intervillous thrombosis related to Rh isoimmunization. *Gynecol Obstet Invest.* 1979;10:237.
13. Spirt BA, Gordon LP, Kagan EH. Intervillous thrombosis: Sonographic and pathologic correlation. *Radiology.* 1983;147:197.
14. Javert CT, Reiss C. The origin and significance of macroscopic intervillous coagulation hematomas (red infarcts) of the human placenta. *Surg Gynecol Obstet.* 1952;94:257.
15. Devi B, Jennison RF, Langley FA. Significance of placental pathology in transplacental hemorrhage. *J Clin Pathol.* 1968;21:322.
16. Perkes EA, Baim RS, Goodman KJ. Second-trimester placental changes associated with elevated maternal serum fetoprotein. *Am J Obstet Gynecol.* 1982;144:935.
17. Fleischer AC, Kurtz AB, Wapner RJ, et al. Elevated alphafetoprotein and a normal fetal sonogram: Association with placental abnormalities. *AJR.* 1988;150:881.
18. Bernstein IM, Barth RA, Miller R. Elevated maternal serum alpha-fetoprotein: Association with placental sonolucencies, fetomaternal hemorrhage, vaginal bleeding, and pregnancy outcome in the absence of fetal anomalies. *Obstet Gynecol.* 1992;79:71.
19. Jauniaux E, Gibb D, Moscoso G. Ultrasonographic diagnosis of a large placental intervillous thrombosis associated with elevated maternal serum α-fetoprotein level. *Am J Obstet Gynecol.* 1990;163:1558.
20. Harris RD, Simpson WA, Pet LR, et al. Placental hypoechoic/anechoic areas and infarction: Sonographic-pathologic correlation. *Radiology.* 1990;176:75.
21. Roberts DJ, Mutter GL. Advances in the molecular biology of gestational trophoblastic disease. *J Reprod Med.* 1994;39:201.
22. Wolf NG, Lage JM. Genetic analysis of gestational trophoblastic disease: A review. *Semin Oncol.* 1995;22:113.
23. Fox H. General pathology of the placenta. In: Fox H, ed. *Haines*

and Taylor Obstetrical and Gynaecological Pathology. 3rd ed. Edinburgh: Churchill-Livingstone; 1987:972.

24. Szulman AE, Surti U. The syndromes of hydatidiform mole. I: Cytogenetic and morphologic correlations. *Am J Obstet Gynecol.* 1978;131:655.

25. Szulman AE, Philippe E, Boue JG, et al. Human triploidy: Association with partial hydatidiform moles and nonmolar conceptuses. *Hum Pathol.* 1981;12:1016.

26. Redline RW, Hassold T, Zaragoza MV. Prevalence of the partial molar phenotype in triploidy of maternal and paternal origin. *Hum Pathol.* 1998;29:505.

27. Szulman AE, Surti U. The syndromes of hydatidiform mole. II: Morphologic evolution of the complete and partial mole. *Am J Obstet Gynecol.* 1978;132:20.

28. Szulman AE, Wong LC, Hsu C. Residual trophoblastic disease in association with partial hydatidiform mole. *Obstet Gynecol.* 1981;57:392.

29. Heifetz SA, Czaja J. In situ choriocarcinoma arising in a partial hydatidiform mole: Implications for the risk of persistent trophoblastic disease. *Pediatr Pathol.* 1992;12:601.

30. Gardner HA, Lage JM. Choriocarcinoma following a partial hydatidiform mole: A case report. *Hum Pathol.* 1992;23:468.

31. Spirt BA, Gordon LP, Cohen WN, et al. Antenatal diagnosis of chorioangioma of the placenta. *AJR.* 1980;135:1273.

32. Battaglia MC, Woolever CA. Fetal and neonatal complications associated with recurrent chorioangiomas. *Pediatrics.* 1967;41:62.

33. Wallenburg HCS. Chorioangioma of the placenta. *Obstet Gynecol Surg.* 1971;26:411.

34. Fox H. Non-trophoblastic tumours of the placenta. In: Fox H, ed. *Haines and Taylor Obstetrical and Gynaecological Pathology.* 3rd ed. Edinburgh: Churchill-Livingstone; 1987;1030.

35. Topalovski M, Yang SS, Boonpasat Y. Listeriosis of the placenta: Clinicopathologic study of seven cases. *Am J Obstet Gynecol.* 1993;169:616.

36. Ramsey EM, Corner CW, Donner MW. Serial and cineradioangiographic visualization of maternal circulation in the primate (hemochorial) placenta. *Am J Obstet Gynecol.* 1963;86:213.

37. Ramsey EM. Circulation in the maternal placenta of the rhesus monkey and man with observations on the marginal lakes. *Am J Anat.* 1956;98:159.

38. Ramsey EM. Development and anatomy of the placenta. In: Fox H, ed. *Haines and Taylor Obstetrical and Gynaecological Pathology.* 3rd ed. Edinburgh: Churchill-Livingstone; 1987:959.

39. Clark SL, Koonings PP, Phelan JP. Placenta previa/accreta and prior cesarian section. *Obstet Gynecol.* 1985;66:89.

40. Pasto ME, Kurtz AB, Rifkin MD, et al. Ultrasonographic findings in placenta increta. *J Ultrasound Med.* 1983;2:155.

41. deMendonca LK. Sonographic diagnosis of placenta accreta: Presentation of six cases. *J Ultrasound Med.* 1988;7:211.

42. Finberg HJ, Williams JW. Placenta accreta: Prospective sonographic diagnosis in patients with placenta previa and prior cesarian section. *J Ultrasound Med.* 1992;11:333.

43. Guy GP, Peisner DB, Timor-Tritsch IE. Ultrasonographic evaluation of uteroplacental blood flow patterns of abnormally located and adherent placentas. *Am J Obstet Gynecol.* 1990;163:723.

44. Hoffman-Tretin JC, Koenigsberg M, Rabin A. Placenta accreta:

45. Lerner JP, Deane S, Timor-Tritsch IE. Characterization of placenta accreta using transvaginal sonography and color Doppler imaging. *Ultrasound Obstet Gynecol.* 1995;5:198.

46. Chou MM, Ho ESC. Prenatal diagnosis of placenta previa accreta with power amplitude ultrasonic angiography. *Am J Obstet Gynecol.* 1997;177:1523.

47. Kirkinen P, Helin-Martikainen H-L, Vanninen R, et al. Placenta accreta: Imaging by gray-scale and contrast-enhanced color Doppler sonography and magnetic resonance imaging. *J Clin Ultrasound.* 1998;26:90.

48. Levine D, Hulka CA, Ludmir J, et al. Placenta accreta: Evaluation with color Doppler US, power Doppler US, and MR imaging. *Radiology.* 1997;205:773.

49. Scott JS. Placenta extrachorialis (placenta marginata and placenta circumvallate): A factor in antepartum hemorrhage. *J Obstet Gynaecol Br Commonw.* 1960;67:904.

50. Naftolin F, Khudr G, Benirschke K, et al. The syndrome of chronic abruptio placentae, hydrorrhea, and circumvallate placentae. *Am J Obstet Gynecol.* 1973;116:347.

51. Kohler HG. Pathology of the umbilical cord and fetal membranes. In: Fox H, ed. *Haines and Taylor Obstetrical and Gynaecological Pathology.* 3rd ed. Edinburgh: Churchill-Livingstone; 1987:1079.

52. DiSalvo DN, Benson CB, Laing FC, et al. Sonographic evaluation of the placental cord insertion site. *AJR.* 1998;170:1295.

53. Perrin EVDK, Sander CH. Introduction: How to examine the placenta and why. In: Perrin EVDK, ed. *Pathology of the Placenta.* New York: Churchill Livingstone; 1984.

54. Earn AA. Placental anomalies. *Can Med Assoc J.* 1951;65:118.

55. Torpin R, Hart BF, Placenta bilobata. *Am J Obstet Gynecol.* 1941;42:38.

56. Molloy CE, McDowell W, Armour R, et al. Ultrasonic diagnosis of placenta membranacea in utero. *J Ultrasound Med.* 1983;2:377.

57. Spirt BA, Kagan EH, Aubry RH. Clinically silent retroplacental hematoma: Sonographic and pathologic correlation. *J Clin Ultrasound.* 1981;9:203.

58. Nyberg DA, Cyr DR, Mack LA, et al. Sonographic spectrum of placental abruption. *AJR.* 1987;148:161.

59. Spirt BA, Kagan EH, Rozanski RM. Abruptio placenta: Sonographic and pathologic correlation. *AJR.* 1979;133:877.

60. Nyberg DA, Mack LA, Benedetti TJ, et al. Placental abruption and placental hemorrhage: Correlation of sonographic findings with fetal outcome. *Radiology.* 1987;164:357.

61. Pedersen JF, Mantoni M. Prevalence and significance of subchorionic hemorrhage in threatened abortion: A sonographic study. *AJR.* 1990;154:535.

62. Stabile I, Campbell S, Grudzinskas JG. Threatened miscarriage and intrauterine hematomas: Sonographic and biochemical studies. *J Ultrasound Med.* 1989;8:289.

63. Morrow RJ, Knox Ritchie JW. Uteroplacental and umbilical artery blood velocity waveforms in placental abruption assessed by Doppler ultrasound. Case report. *Br J Obstet Gynaecol.* 1988;95:723.

64. Oosterhof H, Aarnoudse JG. Placental abruption preceded by abnormal flow velocity waveforms in the uterine arteries. Case report. *Br J Obstet Gynaecol.* 1993;98:225.

65. Townsend RR, Laing FC, Jeffrey RB. Placental abruption associated with cocaine abuse. *AJR.* 1988;150:1339.
66. Iyasu S, Saftlas AK, Rowley DL, et al. The epidemiology of placenta previa in the United States, 1979 through 1987. *Am J Obstet Gynecol.* 1993;168:1424.
67. Artis AA, Bowie JD, Rosenberg ER, et al. The fallacy of placental migration: Effect of sonographic techniques. *AJR.* 1985;144:799.
68. Hertzberg BS, Bowie JD, Carroll BA, et al. Diagnosis of placenta previa during the third trimester: Role of transperineal sonography. *AJR.* 1992;159:83.

Sonography of the Umbilical Cord and Intrauterine Membranes

Arthur C. Fleischer

The umbilical cord and membranes share similar developmental origins, and both are considered in this chapter. This chapter also discusses and illustrates the sonographic depiction of the umbilical cord, with emphasis on normal and abnormal morphology.

With the increased use of percutaneous umbilical cord blood sampling and Doppler studies, there has been renewed interest in the sonographic evaluation of the umbilical cord. Transvaginal sonography (TVS) has also demonstrated developmental anomalies of the cord in early pregnancy. Improved visualization of the cord enables the diagnosis of conditions such as nuchal cord and cord entanglement in twins.

Intrauterine membranes can be delineated with sonography in patients who have bleeding episodes and in some uncomplicated pregnancies. Their assessment is clinically important in multifetal pregnancies. Because determination of zygosity and chorionicity may suggest certain potential complications, such as potential twin-to-twin transfusion, this aspect of multifetal pregnancies is discussed in detail in Chapter 26. This chapter will discuss the sonographic distinction between intrauterine membranes that can be associated with poor pregnancy outcome and those that usually are not.

Sonographic delineation of the umbilical cord and its fetal and placental insertion has important clinical implications. Eccentric, membranous, and velamentous placental cord insertions can be recognized antenatally, requiring close follow-up for pregnancy complications.[1] Similarly, anatomic depiction of the umbilical cord is required for meaningful Doppler assessment of flow in the umbilical arteries and vein. The Doppler values obtained from the cord differ according to where the structure is sampled. Highest impedance in the umbilical arteries is typically present at the placental insertion and the lowest at the fetal insertion. Thus, most studies measure the impedance in a loop of free cord between the two insertion sites. Abnormally high values have been correlated to a reduced number of tertiary chorionic villi arteries and/or maldevelopment of the placental terminal villous tree.[2,3]

FORMATION OF THE UMBILICAL CORD

The umbilical cord is formed in the early weeks of embryogenesis from the body stalk (which contains the umbilical arteries, umbilical veins, and allantois) and the yolk stalk (which contains the omphalomesenteric stalk and remnant of the original yolk sac attachment). During this process, one of the umbilical veins involutes to form a single vein, and the omphalomesenteric vessels are obliterated. The result is an umbilical cord, covered by amnion and containing a single umbilical vein, and two umbilical arteries supported in

Wharton's jelly, a gelatinous substance that consists mainly of collagen. Although the walls of the umbilical vessels have a large proportion of muscle, they lack collagen and elastin and so are able to change configuration with changes in osmotic pressure in the amniotic fluid.

STRUCTURE AND FUNCTION OF THE UMBILICAL CORD

The umbilical cord is quite variable in length and normally contains two umbilical arteries and a single large umbilical vein surrounded by a clear gelatinous Wharton's jelly. The Wharton's jelly that surrounds the vessels apparently has the function of protecting the vessels from undue torsion and compression.[1] A layer of amnion covers the umbilical cord except near the fetal insertion, where an epithelial covering is substituted. The arteries wind around the umbilical vein in a spiral fashion, and because the vessels are longer than the cord itself, there may be a number of foldings and tortuosities producing protrusions or false knots on the cord surface. Both the helical pattern (coiling) at the cord vessels and the presence of Wharton's jelly confer turgor to the cord, which helps prevent kinking and cord prolapse. Cord length and helical coiling are related to fetal movement. Compromised fetuses tend to have less tightly coiled cord than ones with active movement.

Oxygenated blood flows in the umbilical vein from the placenta to the fetus and, on reaching the fetal abdominal wall, passes through the liver posteriorly and cephalad to terminate at the portal sinus (the main left portal vein). Deoxygenated

blood from the fetal aorta passes to the hypogastric arteries, which wind superiorly and medially along the superolateral margin of the bladder, to enter the cord as the umbilical arteries, which carry blood back to the placenta.

SONOGRAPHIC ANATOMY OF THE NORMAL CORD

The umbilical stalk and the yolk sac are seen as early as 7 weeks adjacent to the anterior abdominal wall of the developing fetus (Fig. 11–1). In the second and third trimesters, the umbilical cord is readily visualized. As imaged in long axis, the cord may be seen as a series of parallel lines and shorter angled linear interfaces arising from the umbilical arteries that wrap around the central vein (Fig. 11–1H). In short axis, the arteries and umbilical vein may be seen as three separately circular lucencies (Fig. 11–1F). Pulsations of the cord, occurring at the same rate as fetal heart rate, may be seen in real time.

Because there are different directions of flow in the umbilical cord, color Doppler image will demonstrate one color in the vein and another in the arteries (Fig. 11–1H).

When there is oligohydramnios, some segments of the cord may be difficult to visualize. Color Doppler sonography (CDS) may allow better tracing of the cord in these cases.

The placental insertion site of the cord may appear as a V- or U-shaped sonolucent area arising from the chorionic plate. The placental site of cord insertion into the placenta is variable, often into the central portion of the placenta, but with eccentric cord insertion occurring in 48% to 75% of cases.[4,5]

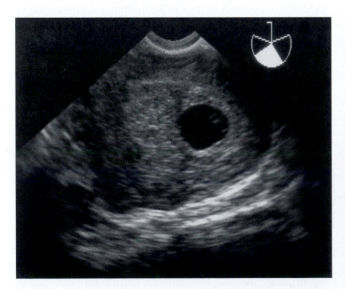

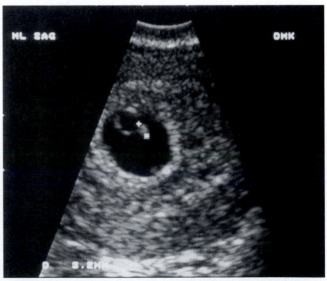

A

B

Figure 11–1. Development of the umbilical cord. **(A)** Transvaginal sonogram at 5 weeks shows "double bleb" corresponding to the amnion and yolk sac on either side of the embryo. **(B)** Same as **A** 5 days later. The yolk sac/embryo complex is depicted clearly. The embryo measures 3 mm in length. *(Figure continued.)*

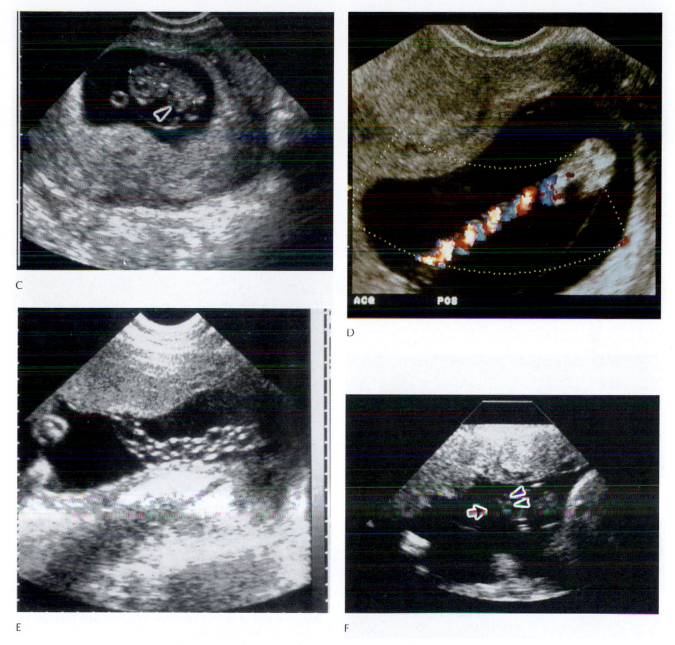

Figure 11–1. *(continued)* (C) Developing umbilical cord at 8 weeks. There is a suggestion of bowel herniating into the base of the cord *(arrowhead)*. The yolk sac is extraamniotic. **(D)** Color Doppler sonogram shows the umbilical cord at 10 weeks. **(E)** Long axis of the umbilical cord in a 20-week pregnancy demonstrates the spiral course of umbilical arteries. **(F)** Sonographic image of normal umbilical cord depicted in true short axis shows two arteries *(arrowheads)* adjacent to the single umbilical vein *(large arrow)*. *(Figure continued.)*

CORD ABNORMALITIES

Eccentric cord insertions include marginal, where the cord inserts from the placental edge, or velamentous or membranous, where the cord forms from the individual chorionic surface vessels that run beneath the chorionic membrane for some variable distance beyond the margin of the placenta before the cord forms as a distinct structure. In 5% to 6% of pregnancies, marginal or velamentous insertion of the cord may occur.[6] These conditions, abnormal placental cord insertions and vasa previa, can be explained by the concept of *placental trophotropism. Trophotropism* describes a process of focal enlargement or atrophy of the placenta probably dependent on several factors that determine relative myometrial perfusion.

Vasa previa is defined as blood vessels of the fetal circulation passing across the internal os of the cervix. This condition is associated with an increased risk of rupture of the

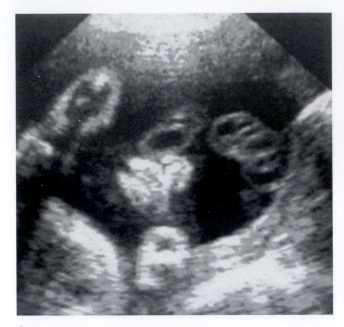

G

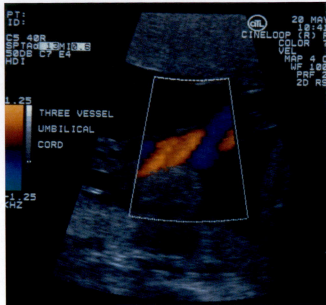

H

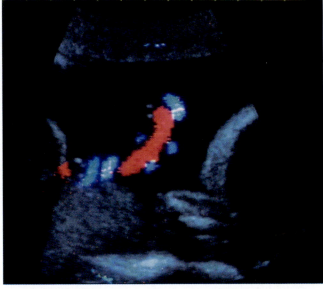

I

Figure 11–1. *(continued)* **(G)** Normal umbilical cord adjacent to the fetal face demonstrates the vein and two arteries in oblique section. **(H)** Normal umbilical cord has two arteries (in red) coiling around the central single vein as depicted with amplitude CDS. **(I)** Color Doppler image of normal umbilical cord, with vein depicted as red and arteries depicted as blue.

vessel and fetal exsanguinations and, if definitely diagnosed, an absolute indication for operative delivery. Vasa previa is caused by the presence of either a velamentous cord or a succenturiate lobe.

At the insertion of the cord into the anterior abdominal wall of the fetus (fetal insertion), the origins of the umbilical vein and hypogastric arteries may be seen (Fig. 11–1C). Weakness in the anterior abdominal wall of the involuted right umbilical vein is the site for gastrochesis, an eccentric herniation of bowel. A replaced right umbilical vein may be associated with fetal anomalies.[7]

Abnormalities of Cord Length

Although the average cord length is 55 cm, a normal range of cord length of 30 to 120 cm may be seen. Extremes of cord length may occur from apparently no cord (acordia)[8] to lengths of up to 300 cm.[9] Excessively long cords may predispose to vascular occlusion by thrombi and by true knots and also to cord prolapse during labor. Rarely, excessively short umbilical cords may be responsible for abruptio placentae, uterine inversion, or intrafunicular hemorrhage.[3] Sonographic delineation of the umbilical cord with color Doppler sonography may be helpful in a qualification

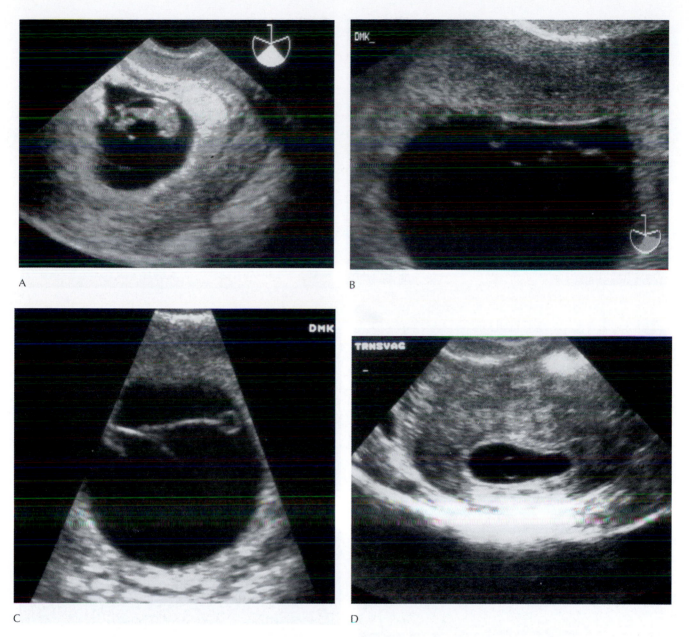

Figure 11–2. Umbilical cord and related malformations. **(A)** Allantoic cyst arising within the umbilical cord. **(B)** Omphalomesenteric cyst arising from the cord at 7 weeks. **(C)** Vitelline duct and shrunken yolk sac seen at 8 weeks associated with embryonic demise. **(D)** Enlarged yolk sac (larger than 6 mm) associated with embryonic demise. *(Figure continued.)*

assessment of cord length. Thus, a subjective assessment of cord length is possible (Fig. 11–2). An absent or excessively short cord is also seen in body stalk anomaly.

Abnormalities of Cord Position

Loops of umbilical cord usually lie anterior to the fetal abdominal wall and adjacent to the limbs. In a number of instances, however, there may be loopings of the cord around the fetal neck or limbs, or loops of cord may lie between the fetal presenting part and the lower uterine segment

(funic presentation). The most important umbilical cord malpositions include prolapses, knots, and neck, body, and shoulder loopings. Kamina and DeTourris in a series of 1750 deliveries, found 4 prolapses, 232 neck loopings, 45 shoulder loopings, and 13 cord knots.[10] Walker and Pye found an incidence of nuchal cord of 17% at delivery.[11] Other studies have reported a nuchal cord (around the back of the head and neck) to be present in one of four pregnancies, but the cord did not seem to have a negative impact on pregnancy outcome (Fig. 11–3).[8,10–15] Multiple loops are

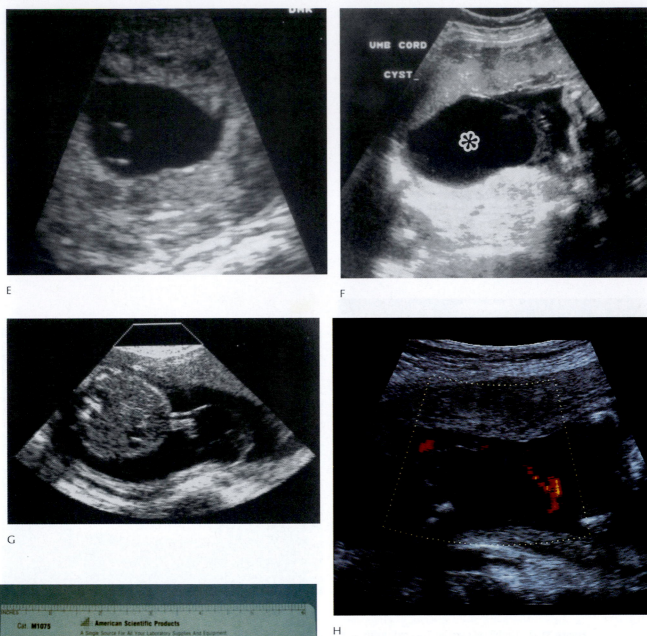

Figure 11–2. *(continued)* **(E)** Shrunken yolk sac adjacent to the amnion in embryonic demise. **(F)** Large cystic structure (∗) within the umbilical cord represents an allantoic cyst. **(G)** Multiple loculated cysts within the umbilical cord represent an allantoic cyst. **(H)** Cystic degeneration of Wharton's jelly as imaged with CDS. *(Courtesy of Lin Dincon, MD.)* **(I)** Specimen of **H** showing an area of cystic degeneration.

seen in only 2% of pregnancies. Therefore, it is important to recognize but not react to the presence of a nuchal cord unless there are concomitant signs of compromise of the fetal condition such as decreased fetal movement or suppressed fetal condition (low biophysical score, abnormal umbilical Doppler).

If suspected on initial scans, the presence of a nuchal cord should be definitively documented as a cord that completely encircles the fetal neck. Color Doppler imaging is useful in establishing the number of cords because it shows the number of veins and arteries in a loop of cord, thereby distinguishing it from multiple loops.

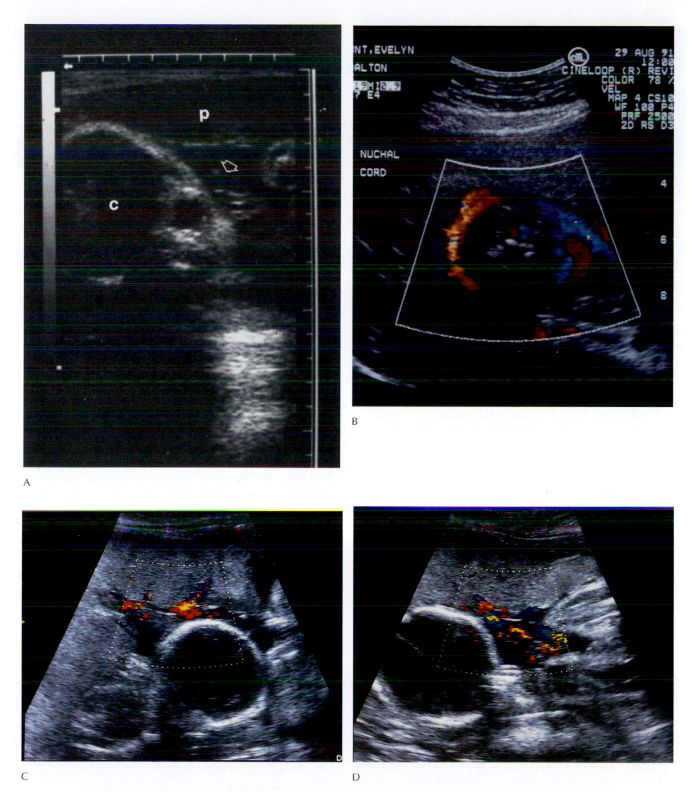

Figure 11–3. Nuchal cord. **(A)** In this third-trimester fetus with demonstrated variable decelerations on a nonstress test, there is sonographic evidence of a loop of cord *(arrow)* wrapped around the fetal neck. C, fetal cranium; p, placenta. **(B)** Short axis through the neck shows tightly wrapped nuchal cord. The nuchal cord is demonstrated by one loop completely encircling the neck of the fetus. **(C)** Tangled cords in monoamniotic twin pregnancy. **(D)** Origins of the umbilical cord in an image of a placenta belonging to the left fetus. *(Figure continued.)*

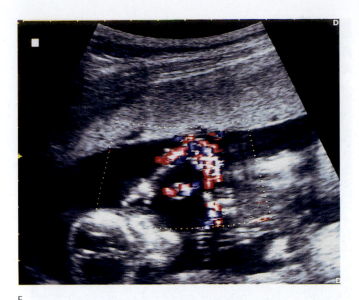

E

Figure 11–3. (continued) (E) Tangled cords in monoamniotic twin pregnancy as shown on CDS. (Courtesy of Philippe Jeanty, MD, PhD.)

Cord morphology, which includes number and arrangement of vessels, is becoming incorporated into routine obstetric sonograms because of the association with structural fetal anomalies, and it is anticipated that the presence of nuchal cords will be encountered more frequently. Controversy remains as to whether or not to report the presence of a nuchal cord, because it is so common and is usually not associated with fetal compromise. However, it is felt that if a nuchal cord is seen and definitively documented, it should be reported and the obstetrician notified. Such findings may result in more frequent antenatal testing. Detection of a nuchal cord in a critical case of a compromised fetus makes it an important entity to recognize antenatally with sonography.

Coiling of the cord around the neck is an uncommon cause of fetal death in singletons and most multiple gestations. A significant portion of the high perinatal mortality rate in monoamniotic twins is attributable to umbilical cord accidents, most frequently because of the entanglement or true knotting of the two cords, leading to occlusion and asphyxia of one or both fetuses.[9]

Occasionally, loops of the cord may be seen lying between the fetal presenting part of the lower segment, referred to as *cord* or *funic presentation*. It is important to recognize this because such a position predisposes to cord prolapse and possible fetal death at the time of rupture of the membranes. Funic presentation is more common with malpresentations, such as breech or transverse lie. The condition, especially before 32 weeks, may often be transient and clinically insignificant; however, one should look for causes that may produce a persistent cord presentation and the risk of cord prolapse. These causes include a marginal cord insertion from the caudal margin of low-lying placenta, uterine structural anomalies such as fibroids or uterine adhesions, or congenital malformations that may prevent the fetus from engaging well into the lower uterine segment.

Single Umbilical Artery

Although the normal umbilical cord contains two umbilical arteries, a single umbilical artery (SUA) may be seen in approximately 1% of all singleton births, 5% of twins, and 2.5% of abortuses (Figs. 11–4 and 11–5).[16] The absent artery forms but becomes atrophic. There is a higher association of fetal anomaly with absent left than with right umbilical arteries is a mnemonic (H. Finberg, personal communication, 1999). Bernischke and Driscoll were the first to describe a relation between SUA and fetal malformations by showing an increased incidence of genitourinary tract anomalies.[17] More recent studies have shown structural anomalies of the fetus in one-third of pregnancies with an SUA, in particular cardiac malformations.[18,19] Malformations of other organ systems may also be associated with SUA (Table 11–1). The incidence of SUA has been found to be increased in pregnancies subsequently ending in abortion, because of trisomy 21, in offspring of diabetic mothers and in black patients. It is also important to note that there is a 7% incidence of fetal anomalies in apparently normal fetuses on sonography that appear to have an isolated single umbilical artery.[19] Therefore, it is advisable to consider karyotypic abnormality when an SUA is detected.

There is a fourfold increase in perinatal mortality in pregnancies with SUA.[19] Many of these deaths are secondary to the major congenital malformations associated with SUA, but others remain unexplained. In following infants with SUA, Froehlich and Fujihura[20,21] found a high mortality (14%) rate, but in those who survived infancy, serious anomalies were no more common than in a control group. Conversely, Bryan and Kohler,[22] who followed up on 98 infants, found that previously unrecognized malformations became apparent in 10.

Prenatal sonographic diagnosis of SUA in two fetuses at 34 and at 36 weeks was first reported by Jassani and Brennan.[18] The first infant subsequently died in utero, and

TABLE 11–1. SINGLE UMBILICAL ARTERY

Single Umbilical Artery: Associated Conditions[a]	
IUGR	42%
MS anomalies	32%
GU anomalies	20%
GI anomalies	11%
Skin anomalies	9%
CV anomalies	8%
Resp. anomalies	6%
Misc. anomalies	3%

n = 80.
[a]Excerpted from reference #15 and 16.

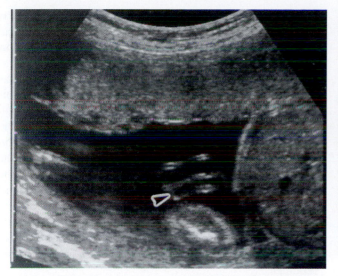

A

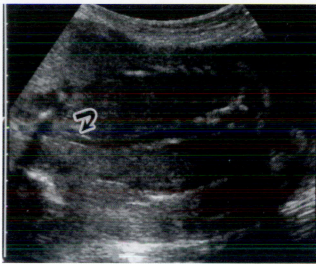

B

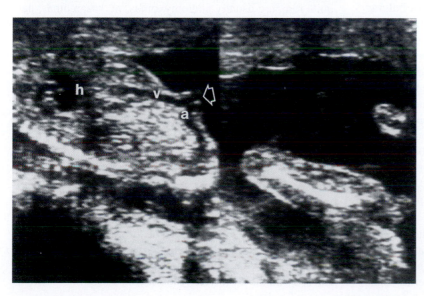

C

Figure 11–4. Single umbilical artery. **(A)** Long axis of the cord demonstrates the umbilical vein and single umbilical artery *(arrowhead)*. **(B)** Long-axis image of iliac vessels demonstrate unilateral agenesis of the left hypogastric artery with preservation of the right artery *(arrow)*. *(Courtesy of Philippe Jeanty, MD, PhD.)* **(C)** Color Doppler sonography shows a single artery within the umbilical cord. *(Courtesy of ATL, Inc.)*

Figure 11–5. Insertion of the cord into the fetal abdomen. Sagittal section of mid-trimester fetus shows insertion of the cord *(arrow)* into the anterior abdominal wall. Division into the umbilical vein (v) and hypogastric artery (a) is shown. h, Heart.

the second showed evidence of mild left hydronephrosis. In a study involving 30 fetuses with SUA, additional anomalies were found in 15, with 12 of these having a major anomaly, including cardiac, cranial, skeletal, and diaphragmatic anomalies. In a more recent study of 118 fetuses with an SUA, 3% had structural defects seen at delivery. Eighty-four percent of all anomalies in these fetuses were prospectively recognized on sonography, with a 7% false-negative rate for obstetric sonography.

In a recent report by Chow, the most common anomalies that were associated with SUA were the heart (51%) and gastrointestinal tract (38%).[19] Thus, it is important to perform a detailed anatomic survey for fetal anomalies when an SUA is detected.

To summarize the discussion of SUA, the following points are made:

1. There is a strong association of fetal anomalies with SUA involving any organ system.
2. If SUA is associated with a detected fetal anomaly, there is a high risk of aneuploidy. Therefore, amniocentesis or chordocentesis is advised.
3. A fetus with SUA and no detectible anomaly is still at risk (although small) for a clinical abnormality, and clinical judgment needs to guide decisions as to whether or not to karyotype.

Other Disorders of the Umbilical Cord

Knots. Umbilical cord knots are very common. Despite reports of 6% mortality, clinical opinion is that knots causing death are rare. Benign knots are rarely reported in birth statistics, resulting in an underdetermination of true incidence. True knot of the cord has been reported as being diagnosed prenatally by serial umbilical cord Doppler images that showed the development of reversed diastolic flow.

False knots, which clinically have no importance, essentially represent a varix, or a redundancy, of the umbilical vessels and are recognized grossly as a focal eccentric bulging of the cord. Sonographically, they may be recognized by irregular vascular protrusions from the cord.

True knots are thought to be caused by excessive fetal movement and, if they become tight, may lead to cord knots. Once formed, these knots may or may not cause fetal compromise. Their physiologic impact on the fetus needs to be assessed with cord Doppler interrogation.[2,3] If there is absent or reversed diastolic low, a compromised fetal condition may be present and may be associated with the cord abnormality.

Umbilical cord entanglement can be seen in monoamniotic twin pregnancies. The mass created by the entangled cords can be verified with color Doppler sonography.

Umbilical Cord Hematoma. Hematoma of the umbilical cord is a rare occurrence. It generally occurs late in pregnancy[20,21,24] and has been reported in a comprehensive review[25] to have an incidence of 1 in 5505 deliveries. Such hematomas most often result from rupture of the wall of the umbilical vein and may develop secondary to mechanical trauma between fetal and maternal tissues, traction on a short cord or on loops of cord around the fetus, or a rare congenital weakness in a vessel wall.[24] Umbilical cord hematomas can also be iatrogenic and caused by percutaneous umbilical cord sampling. These hematomas are associated with a very high perinatal loss; in Dippel's series,[25] 47% of the infants were stillborn. One mechanism of in utero fetal demise may be compression of the umbilical vessels by the increased pressure of blood filling the Wharton's jelly in the substance of the cord.[26] Prenatal diagnosis of umbilical cord hematoma has been reported by Ruvinsky and Wiley in a patient referred at 32 weeks of gestation with in utero fetal demise.[27] The ultrasound examination showed a 6 × 8 cm sonolucent, septated intrauterine mass adjacent to the fetal abdomen.

True Cord Cysts. True cord cysts may be due to allantoic or omphalomesenteric duct remnants, whereas false cysts result from focal liquefaction of Wharton's jelly, often occurring within a regional zone of thickening of the jelly. All are very uncommon in the second and third trimesters. Cysts can be seen a bit more frequently, although they are still uncommon in the first trimester with TVS. Most spontaneously resolve by the end of the first trimester. Such cysts, even when large, usually do not jeopardize fetal circulation, but isolated case reports of cord accidents from cysts and other focal cord lesions indicate the need for ongoing monitoring studies for fetuses who have any cord lesion. Sachs et al.[26] reported the prenatal diagnosis of a 5-cm cystic mass within the umbilical cord, several centimeters from the abdominal wall, at 21 weeks of gestation. Visualization of vessels in the lateral wall of the mass and an intact anterior abdominal wall allowed exclusion of other pathologies.

Neoplasms. Neoplasms of the umbilical cord, which are quite rare, are usually angiomyxomas, myxosarcomas, dermoids, and teratomas, the most common of which is the angiomyxoma.[28] These more commonly occur in a location near the placental margin. Hemangioma of the cord has been reported as a cause of increased amniotic fluid or fetoprotein.[29] Hemangiomas of the umbilical cord are rare but may appear as echogenic masses related to the cord.[30] They may be associated with elevated α-fetoprotein values and, in severe cases, with congestive heart failure of the fetus.

Umbilical Hernia. Umbilical hernia, which is one of the most commonly encountered abnormalities in early infancy,[31] is especially common in black and low-birth-weight infants.[32–34] Umbilical hernias are usually not significant clinically and close spontaneously in the first 3 years of life. Umbilical hernia has been reported as being more common in trisomy 21, congenital hypothyroidism, mucopolysaccharidoses, and the Beckwith syndrome.[31]

Sonographically, umbilical hernia may be recognized as a protrusion from the anterior abdominal wall, with a normal insertion of the umbilical vessels.

Omphalocele and Gastroschisis. Omphalocele and gastroschisis represent abnormalities of closure of the anterior abdominal wall. With omphalocele there is a mid-line umbilical defect with protrusion of abdominal structures, such as bowel and liver, into the base of the umbilical cord (Fig. 11–6), producing a sonographic appearance of a mass adjacent to the anterior abdominal wall, covered with a membrane, and into the apex of which the umbilical cord appears to insert. There is a high incidence of other anomalies (e.g., intestinal, cardiac, and renal anomalies). Recent studies have shown a difference in the risk of aneuploidy in fetuses with small omphaloceles that tend to contain bowel only, whereas large ones contain both bowel and liver.

With gastroschisis, a right paraumbilical abdominal wall defect results in protrusion of bowel and other intraabdominal contents into the amniotic fluid. The cord normally inserts just to the left of the defect; therefore, the gastroschisis will appear as a complex mass adjacent to the base of the cord. The exteriorized bowel loops are not covered by a membrane and therefore are directly exposed to amniotic fluid. A more detailed discussion of the entities can be found in Chapter 18 on sonography of fetal gastrointestinal tract anomalies.

Recent studies have suggested that fetuses with a non-coiled umbilical cord are at greater risk for karyotypic and poor fetal conditions when compared with controls.[35] The detection of a coiled cord can be enhanced with the use of color Doppler sonography to show the "pitch" (number of coils per unit length) of umbilical arteries as they course around the umbilical vein.

INTRAUTERINE MEMBRANES

Development of Amnion and Chorion

Differentiation of the trophoblastic cells from the embryo precursors occurs at approximately 5 days after conception. The trophoblast is further differentiated into two components: the cytotrophoblast and the syncytiotrophoblast. The former is mononuclear, and the latter is multinuclear. The syncytiotrophoblast secretes human chorionic gonadotropin and is responsible for proteolytic invasion into the decidua.

The chorion results from the fusion of the trophoblast and extraembryonic mesenchyme and is organized into chorionic villi, which comprise the major functioning units of the placenta. Atrophy of the villi associated with the decidua capsularis results in the chorion laeve, which eventually becomes the chorionic membrane. The remaining villi establish the chorion frondosum, the fetal component of the placenta. The maternal component of the placenta arises from the decidua basalis. The chorion frondosum can be recognized sonographically in the first trimester as a thickened

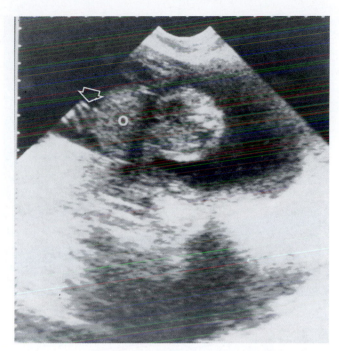

A

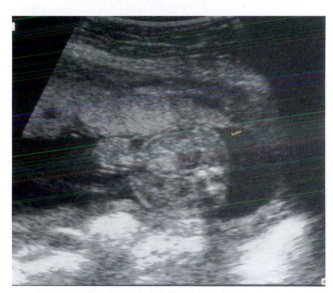

B

Figure 11–6. Omphalocele. **(A)** Transverse section of the fetal trunk shows a large omphalocele (o). The umbilical cord *(arrow)* is implanted at the apex of the omphalocele. **(B)** Omphalocele in a 20-week fetus with displaced cord vessel.

region of echogenic tissue bordering a portion of the gestational sac, indicating the site of the developing placenta. The chorionic membrane is continuous with the fetal surface of the placenta and is firmly adherent to it. This observation is helpful in guiding chorionic villus sampling.

The blastocyst implants into the decidualized endometrium approximately 1 week after fertilization. A layer of

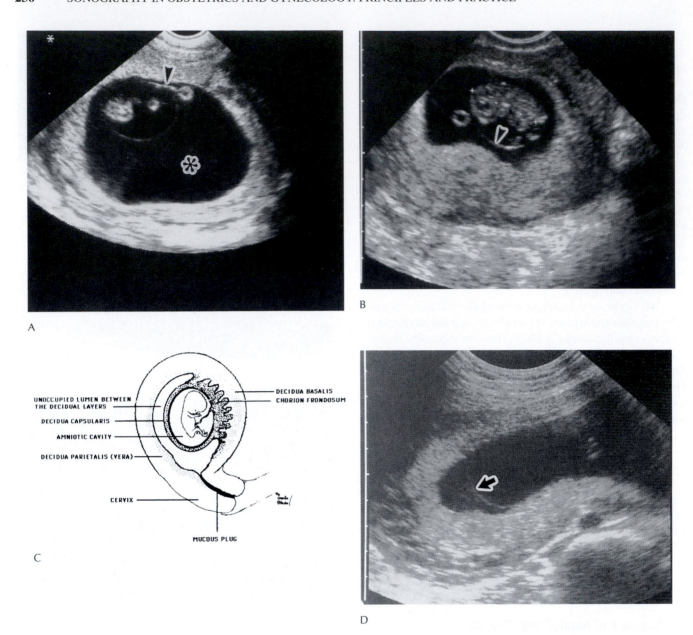

Figure 11–7. Development of amnion and chorion. **(A)** Transgavinal sonogram demonstrates the amnion and yolk sac with the yolk stalk *(arrowhead)*. Fluid in the extracoelomic space (∗) is more echogenic than that within the amniotic cavity. **(B)** Transvaginal sonogram of 9-week intrauterine pregnancy demonstrates the amnion *(arrowhead)*. **(C)** Diagram shows the relation of the amniotic cavity to decidua and chorion before fusion. *(Drawn by Charles Odwin, RT, RDMS, and printed with permission.)* **(D)** Unfused chorioamnion *(arrow)* at 14 weeks.

cells then separates, forming the extracoelomic membrane and creating the primary yolk sac. Simultaneously, the amniotic cavity forms. The embryonic disk lies between the yolk sac and the amniotic sac, allowing real-time visualization of embryonic cardiac pulsation even before demonstration of the embryo. With development of the secondary yolk sac, the primary yolk sac shrinks. The yolk sac and amnion form to separate, opposite surfaces of the embryo. The embryo rotates as the amnion grows, with the amnion

incorporating the embryo and body stalk within it. The amnion ends up adjacent to, but not incorporating, the secondary yolk sac.

The primary and then secondary yolk sacs form along the embryonic surface, facing the chorion frondosum, and attaches to the gestational sac wall along a region that becomes the body stalk and eventually the umbilical cord. The amnion develops along the opposite embryonic surface, growing out to fill the extraembryonic coelom. As it does so, the embryo

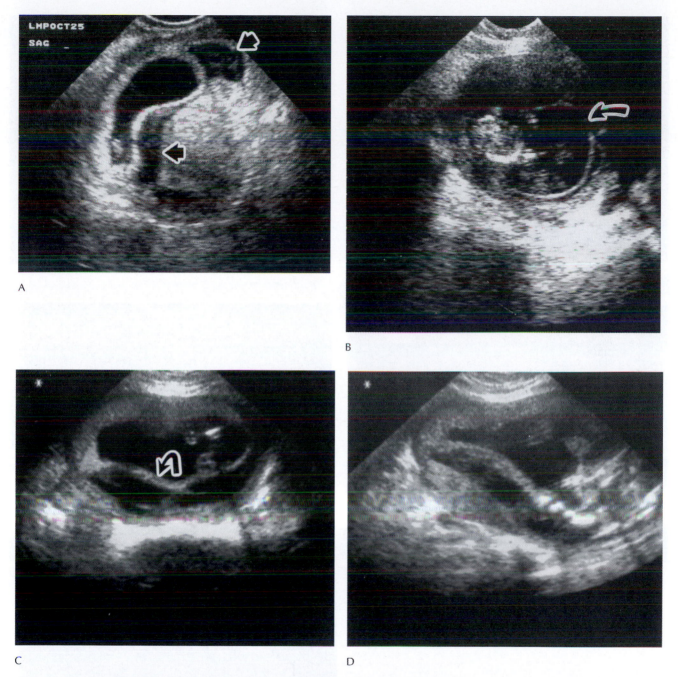

Figure 11–8. Retrochorionic hemorrhage. **(A)** Transvaginal sonogram of elevated chorion with two areas of retrochorionic hemorrhage at 8 weeks. **(B)** Extensive elevation of the chorion *(curved arrow)* and separation from the surrounding decidualized endometrium at 12 weeks associated with fetal demise. **(C)** Transverse transabdominal sonogram of a 20-week pregnancy demonstrates an elevated chorion *(arrow)* with retrochorionic hemorrhage. **(D)** Long-axis image of **C** demonstrates elevated chorion with retrochorionic hemorrhage. The elevated chorion interface is thicker than the amnion. Subchorionic collections stop at the placental edge, whereas subamniotic ones can strip from the chorion over the placenta and may extend to the cord attachment. *(Figure continued.)*

rotates, with the amnion gradually enveloping the fetus and the cord. The secondary yolk sac remains extraamniotic, progressively presses against the chorion, and eventually involutes by 12 weeks.

The amnion progressively expands, completely filling the chorionic cavity (or extraembryonic coelom), by 12 to 14 weeks. This coelom may persist as a potential space for several additional weeks. The amnion generally becomes

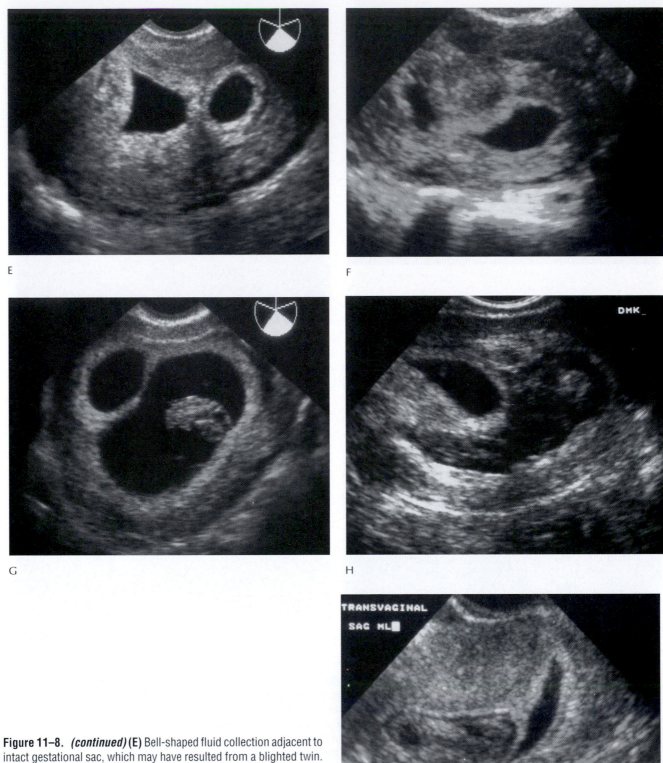

Figure 11–8. *(continued)* **(E)** Bell-shaped fluid collection adjacent to intact gestational sac, which may have resulted from a blighted twin. **(F)** Contractions simulating retrochorionic hemorrhage adjacent to normal gestational sac. **(G)** Second fluid collection adjacent to normal 8-week pregnancy, which may have resulted from a "vanishing twin." **(H)** Extensive retrochorionic hemorrhage associated with separation of decidua basalis. **(I)** This retrochorionic hemorrhage was associated with spontaneous abortion.

adherent to the chorion by 15 to 16 weeks. Amniocentesis done between 12 and 15 weeks may be technically difficult because of this primary amniotic–chorionic separation. The needle may not pierce the amnion but simply indent it, carrying the amnion ahead of it, thus preventing successful amniotic fluid sampling.

The superior resolution afforded by the higher frequency, near-field focused transvaginal approach has significantly altered the sonographic "milestones" of normal early intrauterine pregnancies. The first milestone, the chorionic mass, appears as a 2- to 3-mm hypoechoic complex with the thickened decidualized endometrium. This complex may be seen as early as 5 weeks 4 days since the first day of the last menstrual period. The secondary yolk sac is consistently

demonstrated in a normal intrauterine pregnancy at 5 to 5½ weeks (Fig. 11–7). The thin amniotic membrane is delineated from 7 to 16 weeks (Fig. 11–7B through D). The embryo/fetus is seen to lie within the amniotic sac; the yolk sac is extraamniotic.

Retrochorionic Hemorrhage

The presence of an intrauterine membrane or interface can be detected in patients with a history of vaginal bleeding or as an incidental finding on an obstetric sonogram. An intrauterine membrane arising from the unfused amnion is a normal finding for up to 16 weeks of gestation, at which time it should fuse with the chorion. In patients who experience bleeding in the late first and early second trimester, it is not uncommon

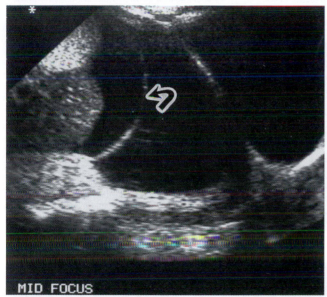

A

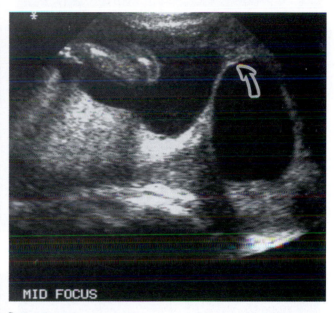

B

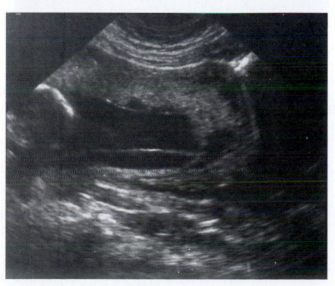

C

Figure 11–9. Abnormal amnion. **(A)** Thin intrauterine interface *(arrow)* corresponds to an amniotic band not involving a fetal part. **(B)** Amniotic sheet probably draped over an intrauterine synechia *(curved arrow)*. **(C)** Thin elevated amnion in an area of amniotic hemorrhage.

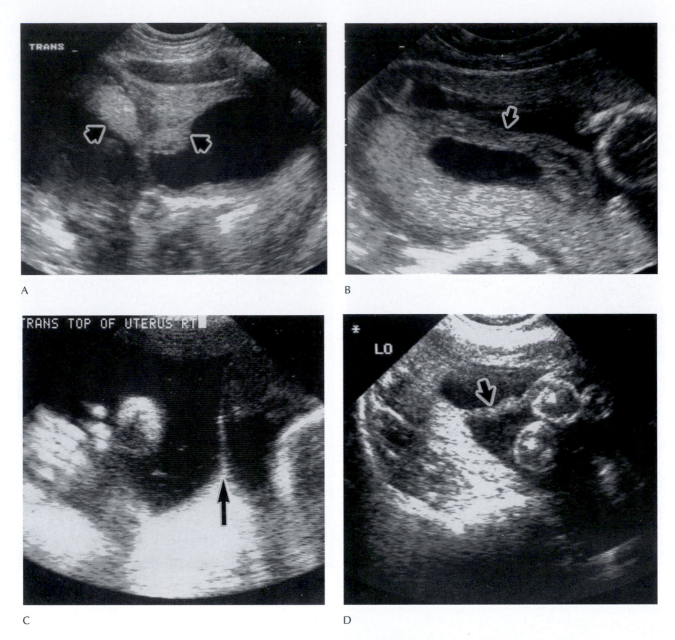

Figure 11–10. Uterine septa. **(A)** Transverse sonogram of 12-week pregnancy with intrauterine septum. The placenta *(arrow)* has implanted on both sides of the septum. **(B)** Long axis of the edge of the septum *(arrow)* coursing in a more horizontal plane than that shown in **A**. **(C)** Transverse sonogram demonstrates thin intrauterine septum *(arrow)* in a near-term pregnancy. The placenta and fetal head are on the left side of the septum; the fetal extremities are on the right. **(D)** Uterine septum *(arrow)* with fetal extremities in the lower part. *(Courtesy of Carl Zimmerman, MD.)*

to find areas of elevated chorion representing areas of hemorrhage. The hypoechoic space may extend to the area of the cervix, allowing for passage of blood vaginally. Areas of elevated chorion are usually thicker than areas of disrupted amnion, which tend to be more centrally located within the amniotic cavity. Typically, patients with retrochorionic hemorrhage have episodes of bleeding, but if the hemorrhage does not extend behind the placenta to involve the basal plate, these areas may regress as the pregnancy progresses.

The fact that choriomyometrial separation can be associated with vaginal bleeding between 10 and 20 weeks has become more apparent with the increased use of sonography.[36,37] The sonographic features associated with retrochorionic hemorrhage include an elevated layer of chorion with an extrachorionic crescent-shaped fluid collection, which may appear purely cystic or complex if organized hemorrhage is present (Fig. 11–8). The prognosis of such abnormalities relates to the size of the hemorrhage,

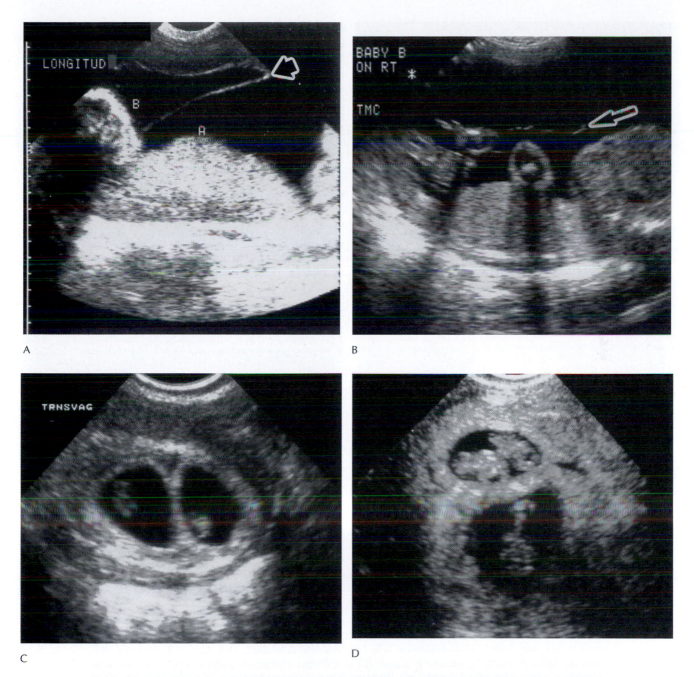

Figure 11–11. Membranes in a multifetal pregnancy. **(A)** Diamniotic, dichorionic, thick membrane *(arrow)*. **(B)** Thin, diamniotic, monochorionic membrane *(arrow)*. **(C)** Transvaginal sonogram shows dichorionic, diamniotic twin pregnancy at 7 weeks. Note the cleavage within the two sets of chorion/amnion. **(D)** Triplet pregnancy with two embryos within the same amnion; one is separate. *(Figure continued.)*

particularly as it compares to the size of the gestational sac. Those patients with small hemorrhages have an excellent chance of a favorable outcome, but those patients with a hemorrhage exceeding 60 cc or greater than 40% of the gestational sac have a less favorable outcome, even if embryonic viability is demonstrated at the initial exam.[38] Prognosis is also probably related to whether the hemorrhage accumulates or is expelled. If it has been expelled,

sonography may not recognize the true extent of the affected area.

It may be difficult definitively to distinguish sonographically between a retrochorionic hemorrhage and a "vanishing" twin in the first trimester. An empty sac or one associated with embryonic demise is usually rounder than the typical crescent-shaped area of retrochorionic hemorrhage.

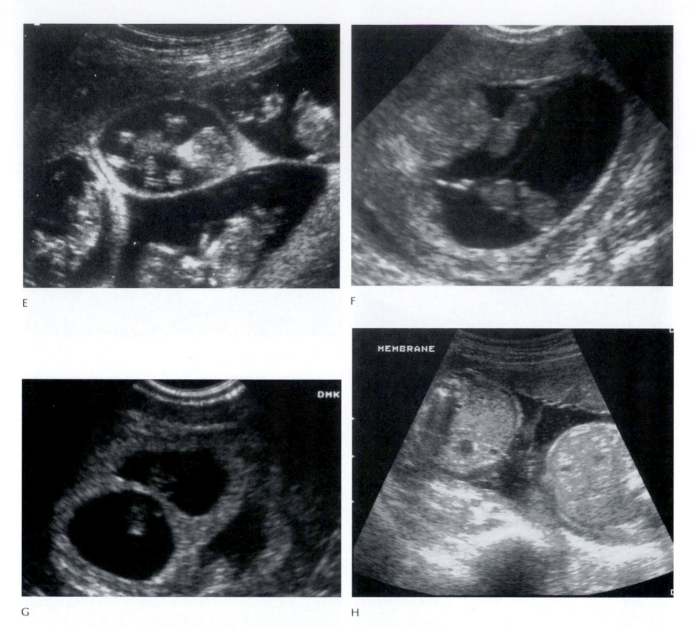

Figure 11–11. *(continued)* **(E)** Quadruplet pregnancy at 9 weeks 5 days, with each fetus within its own amnion. **(F)** Twin 8-week 3-day pregnancy, with one fetus having no cord. This represents the body stalk anomaly associated with the absence of a cord. **(G)** Twin 8-week intrauterine pregnancy with retrochorionic hemorrhage simulating a third deflated sac. **(H)** Monochorionic twin pregnancy at 24 weeks. Note the lack of a placental tissue invaginating between the membranes of the fetuses, which suggests nonchorionicity.

Abnormal Conditions Associated With Membranes, Septa, or Synechiae

Amniotic band syndrome is thought to be a sequela of rupture of the amnion, with formation of fibrous bands that may cross fetal parts and cause significant maldevelopment (Fig. 11–9A).[39] The entrapped fetal part typically is entangled within the area of the membrane. Amniotic band syndrome has been associated with craniospinal malformations and with gastroschisis and limb and finger amputation.[40,41]

Therefore, it is important to document the integrity of only the fetal part that lies in proximity to the disrupted amnion.

A thin interface within the uterus may be encountered in patients in whom the amniotic membrane is draped over a uterine synechia. This uterine malformation has been termed an *amniotic sheet* and has not been associated with an increased incidence of fetal malformation (Fig. 11–9B).[42,43] Amniotic sheets are composed of four layers, two amniotic and two chorion. Their average thickness is 2.4 mm

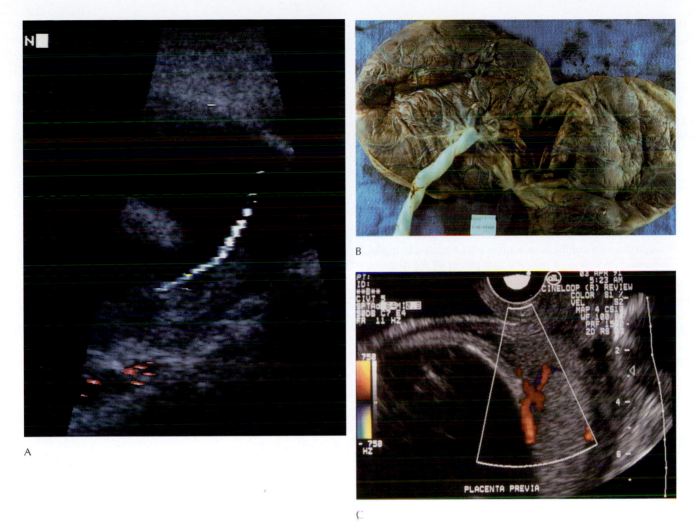

Figure 11–12. Color Doppler sonogram of vasa privia. **(A)** Arterial vessel overlying the chorionic plate in area of the internal cervical os. **(B)** Delivered placenta of patient shown in **A** showing transected vessel crossing an area of the internal cervical os. *(Courtesy of Richard Rosemond, MD.)* **(C)** Transvaginal color Doppler sonogram shows placental vessel in the area of the internal cervical os. *(Courtesy of ATL, Inc.)*

in the mid-portion and 4.5 mm at the free edge. Mothers with amniotic sheets have an increased incidence of previous spontaneous or therapeutic abortion.[44–46] Uterine synechia seems to be associated with a higher incidence of bleeding episodes.[44–46]

Uterine septa tend to be thicker than the interfaces created by amnion and chorion (Fig. 11–10). The septae may consist of myometrium, a fibrous septation, or both, which typically have a (mid) sagittal orientation within the uterus. Implantation can occur on the septum and probably accounts for the high incidence of spontaneous abortion.[47] Placentation on a septum also predisposes to abruption and possibly growth retardation of the fetus. There does not seem to be any increased incidence of complications in patients in whom the placental insertion is on the amniotic sheet.[48]

Twin Pregnancies

It is important to document the presence of a membrane between fetuses of a multifetal pregnancy. The thickness of the membrane can be used to discriminate a monochorionic, diamniotic, or dichorionic twin pregnancy. Dichorionic membranes are typically well defined and have a definite measurable width (usually greater than 2 mm) (Fig. 11–11).[49,50] Monochorionic membranes tend to be thin or hairlike and are visualized in short segments. Errors in assessment of membrane thickness may be related to technical factors, such as a thin membrane appearing thick because of its specular reflection or a thick membrane appearing thin because of physiologic thinning that occurs in late pregnancy.[51] The amnion and chorion of dichorionic twin pregnancies tend to form a triangular configuration that projects into the amnion, termed a *twin peak*.[52] Prenatal sonographic determination of the makeup of the membrane is important because dichorionic diamniotic gestations have the best prognosis, and monochorionic monoamniotic gestations have the poorest. However, sonographic demonstration of either a single placental site or the inability to show membrane may occur in any of the types of twinning.[53] Intertwining of umbilical cords, conjoined twins, or more than three vessels in the umbilical cord occurs only with monochorionic monoamniotic twinning.

SUMMARY

This chapter has described the sonographic depiction of the umbilical cord and intrauterine membranes (Fig. 11–12). Although disorders of these structures occur relatively rarely, sonographic depiction of the type and extent of the disorder can aid management in these complicated pregnancies.

ACKNOWLEDGMENT

The author thanks Dr. Harris Finberg for his helpful remarks concerning this chapter and Dr. David Graham for his initial contribution to this chapter in previous editions.

REFERENCES

1. Di Slavo DN, Benson CB, Laing FE, et al. Sonographic evaluation of the placental cord insertion site. *AJR.* 1998;170:1295.
2. Krebs C, Marcara LM, Leiser R, et al. Intrauterine growth restriction with absent end-diastolic flow velocity in the umbilical artery is associated with maldevelopment of the placental terminal villous tree. *Am J Obstet Gynecol.* 1996;175:1534.
3. Kingdom JCP, Burrell SJ, Kaufmann P. Pathology and clinical implications of abnormal umbilical artery Doppler waveforms. *Ultrasound Obstet Gynecol.* 1997;9:271.
4. Kohorn EI, Walker RMS, et al. Placental localization. *Am J Obstet Gynecol.* 1969;103:868.
5. Purola E. The length and insertion of the umbilical cord. *Ann Chir Gynecol.* 1968;573:621.
6. Fox H. *Pathology of the Placenta.* Philadelphia: Saunders; 1978:426.
7. Jeanatry P. Persistent right umbilical vein: An ominous prenatal finding? *Radiology.* 1990;177:735.
8. Browne FJ. On the abnormalities of the umbilical cord which may cause antenatal death. *J Obstet Gynaecol Br Emp.* 1925;32:17.
9. Pritchard JA, MacDonald PC. *Williams Obstetrics,* 16th ed. New York: Appleton-Century-Crofts; 1980.
10. Kamina P, DeTourris H. The diagnosis of umbilical cord complications with the help of ultrasonic tomography. *Electromedica.* 1977;7:50.
11. Walker CW, Pye BG. The length of the human umbilical cord: A statistical report. *Br Med J.* 1960;1:546.
12. Spellacy WN, Gravem H, et al. The umbilical cord complications of true knots, nuchal coils and cords around the body. *Am J Obstet Gynecol.* 1966;94:1136.
13. Vintzileos AM, Nochimson DJ, et al. Ultrasonic diagnosis of funic presentation. *J Clin Ultrasound.* 1983;11:516.
14. Jouppila P, Kirkinen P. Ultrasonic diagnosis of nuchal encirclement by the umbilical cord. A case and methodological report. *J Clin Ultrasound.* 1982;10:59.
15. Miser WF. Outcome of infants born with nuchal cords. *J Fam Pract.* 1992;34:441.
16. Nyberg D, Mahoney B, Luthy D. Single umbilical artery; prenatal detection of concurrent anomalies. *J Ultrasound Med.* 1991;10:247.
17. Bernischke K, Driscoll SG. *The Pathology of the Human Placenta.* New York: Springer; 1967.
18. Jassani MN, Brennan JR, et al. Prenatal diagnosis of single umbilical artery by ultrasound. *J Clin Ultrasound.* 1980;8:447.
19. Chow J, Benson C, Doubilet P. Frequency and nature of structural anomalies in fetuses with single umbilical arteries. *J Ultrasound Med.* 1998;17:765.
20. Froehlich LA, Fujikura T. Significance of a single umbilical artery. *Am J Obstet Gynecol.* 1966;94:274.
21. Froehlich L, Fujikura T. Follow-up of infants with single umbilical artery. *Pediatrics.* 1973;52:6.
22. Bryan Em, Kohler HG. The missing umbilical artery. II: Pediatric follow-up. *Arch Dis Child.* 1975;50:714.
23. Nyberg DA, Mahony BS, Luthy D. Single umbilical artery prenatal detection of concurrent anomalies. *J Ultrasound Med.* 1991;10:247.
24. Peckham CH, Yerushalmy J. Applasia of one umbilical artery: Incidence by race and certain obstetric factors. *Obstet Gynecol.* 1965;26:359.
25. Dipple AL. Hematomas of the umbilical cord. *Surg Gynecol Obstet.* 1940;70:51.
26. Sachs L, Fourcroy JL, et al. Prenatal detection of umbilical cord allantoic cyst. *Radiology.* 1982;45:445.
27. Ruvinsky ED, Wiley TL, et al. In utero diagnosis of umbilical cord hematoma by ultrasonography. *Am J Obstet Gynecol.* 1981;140:833.
28. Novak ER, Woodruff JD. *Novak's Gynecologic and Obstetric Pathology.* Philadelphia: Sanders; 1967.
29. Barnson AJ, Donnai P, et al. Hemangioma of the cord: Further cause of raised maternal serum and liquor alphafetoprotein. *Br Med J.* 1980;281:1251.
30. Pollack M, Boind L. Hemangioma of the umbilical cord: Sonographic appearance. *J Ultrasound Med.* 1989;8:163.
31. Bello MJ. Umbilical and other abdominal wall hernias. In: Holder TM, Ashcroft KW, eds. *Pediatric Surgery.* Philadelphia: Saunders; 1980.
32. Crump EP. Umbilical hernia. I: Occurrence of the infantile type in negro infants and children. *J Pediatr.* 1952;40:214.
33. Evans A. The comparative incidence of umbilical hernias in colored and white infants. *JAMA.* 1941;33:158.
34. Jackson DJ, Moglen LH. Umbilical hernia: A retrospective study. *Calif Med.* 1970;113:8.
35. Strong TH, Elliott JP, Radin TG. Non-coiled umbilical blood vessel: A new marker for the fetus at risk. *Obstet Gynecol.* 1993;81:409.
36. Kaufman AJ, Fleischer AC, Thieme GA, et al. Separated

chorioamnion and elevated chorion: Sonographic features and clinical significance. *J Ultrasound Med.* 1985;4:119.

37. Burrows PE, Lyons EA, Phillips HJ. Intrauterine membranes: Sonographic findings and clinical significance. *J Clin Ultrasound.* 1982;10:1.

38. Sauerbrei EE, Phan DH. Placental abruption and subchorionic hemorrhage in the first half of pregnancy: US appearance and clinical outcome. *Radiology.* 1986;160:109.

39. Torpin R. *Fetal Malformations Caused by Amnion Rupture During Gestation.* Springfield, IL: Charles C. Thomas; 1986:6.

40. Worthen NJ, Lawrence D, Bustillo M. Amniotic band syndrome: Antepartum ultrasonic diagnosis of discordant anencephaly. *J Clin Ultrasound.* 1980;8:453.

41. Hill LM, Kislak S, Jones N. Prenatal ultrasound diagnosis of a forearm constriction band. *J Ultrasound Med.* 1988;7:293.

42. Randel SB, Filly RA, Callen PW, et al. Amniotic sheets. *Radiology.* 1988;166:633.

43. Stamm E, Waldstein G, Thickman D, et al. Amniotic sheets: Natural history and histology. *J Ultrasound Med.* 1991;10:501.

44. Finberg HJ. Uterine synechia in pregnancy: Expanded criteria for recognition and clinical significance in 28 cases. *J Ultrasound Med.* 1991;10:547.

45. Ball R, Buchmedi S, Longnecker M. Clinical significance of sonographically detached uterine synechia in pregnant patients. *J Ultrasound Med.* 1997;16:465.

46. Finberg H. Uterine synechia in pregnancy: Expanded criteria for recognition and clinical significance in 28 cases. *J Ultrasound Med.* 1991;10:547.

47. Fedele L, Dorta M, Brioschi D, et al. Pregnancies in septate uteri: Outcome in relation to site of uterine implantation as determined by sonography. *AJR.* 1989;152:781.

48. Korbin CD, Benson CB, Doubilet PM. Placenta implantation on the amniotic sheet: Effect on pregnancy outcome. *Radiology.* 1998;206:773.

49. Mahony BS, Filly RA, Callen PW. Amnionicity and chorionicity in twin pregnancies: Prediction using ultrasound. *Radiology.* 1985;155:205.

50. Hertzberg BS, Kurtz AB, Choi HY, et al. Significance of membrane thickness in the sonographic evaluation of twin gestations. *AJR.* 1987;148:151.

51. Townsend RR, Simpson GF, Filly RA. Membrane thickness in ultrasound prediction of chorionicity of twin gestations. *Ultrasound Med.* 1988;8:327.

52. Finberg HJ. The "twin peak" sign. Reliable evidence of dichorionic twinning. *J Ultrasound Med.* 1992;11:571.

53. Filly RA, Goldstein RB, Callen PW. Monochorionic twinning. Sonographic assessment. *AJR.* 1990;154:459.

Doppler Ultrasound: Application to Fetal Medicine

Giancarlo Mari • Laura Detti

Several studies have demonstrated that Doppler ultrasound represents an important diagnostic tool in modern obstetrics.[1,2] Indeed, the American College of Obstetrics and Gynecology has endorsed the use of Doppler ultrasound of the umbilical artery in high-risk pregnancies.[3]

Information obtained with Doppler ultrasound helps obstetricians in managing patients in the following situations: 1) pregnancies complicated by intrauterine growth restriction (IUGR), 2) pregnancies in which the fetus is at risk for anemia because of red blood cell alloimmunization, 3) multiple gestations, and 4) pregnancies treated with prostaglandin inhibitors to monitor the ductus arteriosus.

This chapter has been divided into five sections that follow a brief introduction of Doppler blood flow velocity waveforms (FVWs). The first section discusses Doppler blood FVWs of the umbilical artery (UA) and middle cerebral artery (MCA) in appropriate-for-gestational-age (AGA) fetuses. The second section discusses blood FVWs of the UA and MCA in fetuses and presents clinical cases. Blood FVWs of AGA and IUGR fetuses in other cardiovascular districts also are presented. The third section discusses the use of Doppler ultrasound in pregnancies complicated by red blood cell alloimmunization. The fourth section discusses the use of Doppler ultrasound in multiple gestations. The fifth section discusses the effects of indomethacin on fetal ductus arteriosus blood FVWs.

FLOW VELOCITY WAVEFORMS: GENERAL PRINCIPLES

Blood flow velocity of the fetal vascular system can be either pulsatile or continuous. The arteries always have a pulsatile pattern, whereas the veins have either a pulsatile or a continuous pattern. Figure 12–1 shows a typical Doppler arterial blood FVW. Figure 12–2 shows FVW of an umbilical artery and vein.

The Angle Between the Ultrasound Beam and Blood Flow Is Not Known

Flow velocity waveforms reflect blood velocity and vascular impedance. The *conditio sine qua non* for the assessment of the true velocity is dependent upon the angle between the ultrasound beam and the direction of the blood flow, which needs to be as close as possible to 0 degrees. As the incident angle increases, blood velocity is progressively underestimated. Therefore, indices that are angle independent are used. These indices are:

1. Systolic-to-diastolic (S/D) ratio.[4]
2. Resistance index (RI).[5]
3. Pulsatility index (PI).[6]

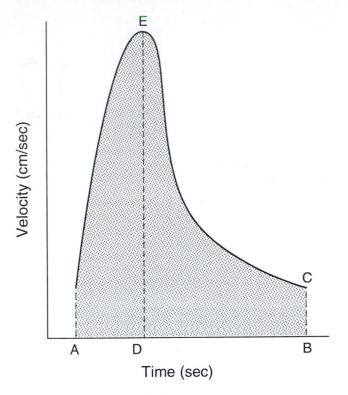

Figure 12–1. Typical Doppler flow velocity waveform of a fetal artery. A represents the beginning of the waveform that coincides with the beginning of the cardiac systole. DE is the peak systolic velocity. CB is the end-diastolic velocity. Velocity is shown on the *y* axis. Note that the velocity is the true blood velocity only if the angle between the ultrasound beam and the blood flow is close to 0 degrees.

The S/D ratio and the RI are easy to calculate (see Figs. 12–1 and 12–2). The PI is more complex because it requires the calculation of the mean velocity, but modern Doppler ultrasound equipment provides those values in real time. In practice, for the UA, the cerebral artery and the uterine arteries, none of the indices is superior to the others and any index may be used.

The three indices provide information on vascular impedance,[7] which is not the same as vascular resistance. In fact, impedance has a more extensive meaning than resistance because it depends on the vascular resistance, preload, heart rate, and cardiac contractility. The term *vascular resistance*, however, has been extensively used in the literature and it is commonly accepted. Our presumption is that by calculating one of these indices and, therefore, estimating the vascular resistance, we may obtain information on the amount of blood flow. One example will clarify this concept. If we assess the PI (or the RI or S/D ratio) at the level of the MCA in AGA fetuses and IUGR fetuses at the same gestational age, the IUGR fetuses will have a lower PI value at the MCA than the AGA fetuses.[8] Our interpretation of these results is that in IUGR fetuses there is a lower vascular resistance at the MCA than in AGA fetuses. This suggests an increased blood flow to the brain. However, we do not know the real value of the vascular resistance and the real amount of cerebral blood flow.

The Angle Between the Ultrasound Beam and Blood Flow Is Close to 0 Degrees

When the angle between the ultrasound beam and the blood flow is close to 0 degrees, a value close to the true value

Figure 12–2. Flow velocity waveforms (FVWs) of the umbilical artery and umbilical vein. The umbilical vein (UV) has a constant velocity, whereas the umbilical artery is pulsatile because it reflects the systole and the diastole of the cardiac cycle. In this specific case, the umbilical vein blood flow was directed toward the transducer and, therefore, the waveform is represented above the baseline, and the umbilical artery blood flow was directed away from the transducer and, therefore, FVWs are represented below the baseline. PV, Peak systolic velocity; EDV, end-diastolic velocity; MV, mean velocity (the mean velocity is equal to the ratio between the area under the curve and the period [time between one cardiac cycle and the next]). Systolic/diastolic (S/D) ratio = PV/ED. Resistance index: (RI) = (PV − EDV)/PV. Pulsatility index: (PI) = (PV − EDV)/MV.

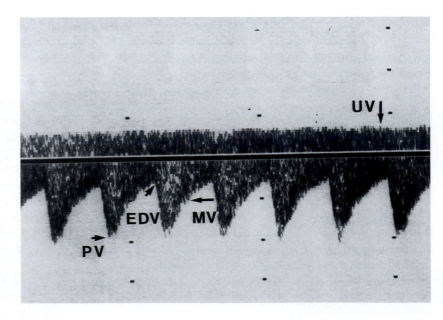

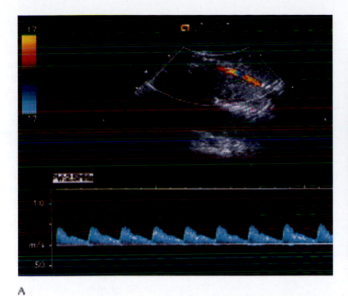
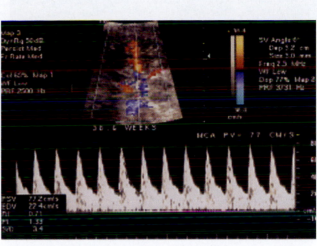

A   B

Figure 12–3. (A) Flow velocity waveforms of the descending aorta. The angle between the ultrasound beam and the blood velocity is greater than 30 degrees; therefore the velocity reported on the *y* axis is not the true velocity (it is underestimated). **(B)** Flow velocity waveforms of the middle cerebral artery. The angle between the ultrasound beam and the blood flow is close to 0 degrees; therefore, the peak systolic velocity of 77 cm per second is very close to the true velocity of the blood flow.

of the blood velocity is obtained. An example is shown in Fig. 12–3A and B. In Fig. 12–3A the angle between the ultrasound beam and the blood flow is greater than 30 degrees, whereas in Fig. 12–3B the angle is close to 0 degrees. In Fig. 12–3A the velocity is underestimated; in Fig. 12–3B the value of the velocity is close to the true value of the blood velocity.

APPROPRIATE-FOR-GESTATIONAL AGE FETUSES

Umbilical Blood Flow Velocity Waveforms

Placental blood FVW are assessed by studying the UA. This artery may be easily studied with any Doppler system. Flow velocity waveforms of the UA are slightly different at the abdominal wall and at the placental insertion,[9] with the indices higher at the fetal abdominal wall than at the placental insertion (Fig. 12–4A and B). The difference, however, is minimal and, therefore, in practice it is not important to obtain the waveforms always at the same level. Any Doppler instrument and any index (PI, RI, and S/D ratio) may be used to assess the UA FVWs.

Flow velocity waveforms of the UA change with advancing gestation (Fig. 12–5).[4,10] End-diastolic velocity (EDV) is often absent in the first trimester[11] and the diastolic component increases with advancing gestation (see Fig. 12–5). The PI, RI, and S/D ratio decrease with advancing gestation, probably due to a decrease in placental vascular resistance (Fig. 12–6).[11–13]

Flow velocity waveforms must always be obtained during periods of fetal apnea because fetal breathing affects the waveforms (Fig. 12–7).

Cerebral Blood Flow Velocity Waveforms

The circle of Willis is composed anteriorly of the anterior cerebral arteries (branches of the internal carotid artery that are interconnected by the anterior communicating artery) and posteriorly of the two posterior cerebral arteries (branches of the basilar artery that are interconnected on either side with the internal carotid artery by the posterior communicating artery). These two trunks and the MCA, another branch of the internal carotid artery, supply the cerebral hemispheres on each side. These arteries have different FVWs (Fig. 12–8)[14]; therefore, it is important to know which artery is under study.

The MCA is the vessel of choice to assess the fetal cerebral circulation because it is easy to identify, is highly reproducible, and provides information on the brain-sparing effect.[8] In addition, it can be studied easily with an angle of 0 degrees between the ultrasound beam and the direction of blood flow (Figs. 12–9 and 12–10); therefore, information on the true velocity of the blood flow may be obtained.[15]

The reference values of the MCA FVWs and PI during gestation are shown in Figs. 12–11 and 12–12 and Table 12–1. The lower PI values early and late in gestation may be due to the increased metabolic requirements of the brain during these periods.[16]

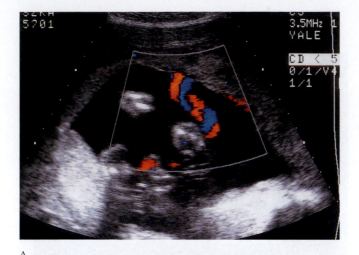

A

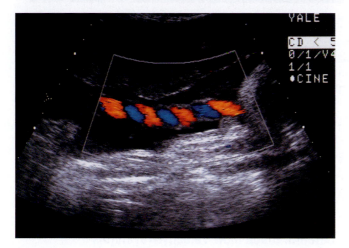

B

Figure 12–4. (A) Umbilical cord at the placental insertion. **(B)** Umbilical cord at the abdominal wall insertion. The umbilical artery waveforms in **A** have a slightly lower index (pulsatility index, systolic/diastolic ratio, resistance index) than in **B**. In practice, however, it is not important to differentiate between the waveforms obtained at these two sites.

Several conditions are associated with an increase or a decrease of the MCA PI when compared to normal values (Tables 12–2 and 12–3).

INTRAUTERINE GROWTH-RESTRICTED FETUS

The IUGR fetus is a fetus that does not reach its potential growth. Environmental factors responsible may be maternal systemic disease (diabetes, hypertension, chronic renal disease, collagen vascular disease, or preeclampsia), smoking, drug use, or impaired uteroplacental perfusion.

Abnormality in the establishment and maintenance of adequate uteroplacental perfusion is probably the single most

TABLE 12–1. MIDDLE CEREBRAL ARTERY PULSATILITY INDEX

Gestational Age (wk)	Normal Values		
	Lower Limit[a]	Predicted Value	Upper Limit[b]
15	0.99	1.57	2.14
16	1.08	1.71	2.33
17	1.16	1.83	2.51
18	1.23	1.95	2.67
19	1.30	2.05	2.81
20	1.35	2.14	2.93
21	1.40	2.22	3.04
22	1.44	2.29	3.13
23	1.48	2.34	3.20
24	1.51	2.38	3.26
25	1.52	2.41	3.30
26	1.54	2.43	3.32
27	1.54	2.44	3.33
28	1.54	2.43	3.32
29	1.52	2.41	3.30
30	1.50	2.38	3.26
31	1.48	2.34	3.20
32	1.44	2.28	3.12
33	1.40	2.21	3.03
34	1.35	2.13	2.92
35	1.29	2.04	2.79
36	1.22	1.94	2.65
37	1.15	1.82	2.49
38	1.07	1.69	2.32
39	0.98	1.56	2.13
40	0.89	1.40	1.92
41	0.78	1.24	1.70
42	0.67	1.06	1.45

PI, Pulsatility index; GA, gestational age. PI $= -1.9763 + (0.32737\ GA) + (-0.00611\ GA^2)$.
[a]Predicted value $- (2 \times 0.184 \times$ predicted value).
[b]Predicted value $+ (2 \times 0.184 \times$ predicted value).
Reproduced with permission from Mari G, Deter RL. Am J Obstet Gynecol. 1992;166:1262–1270.

common cause of IUGR. However, in patients without risk factors we do not know the *primum movens* responsible for the placental insufficiency.[17–21]

In most of the cases IUGR does not recur in the subsequent pregnancy. However, in some cases, it recurs in all subsequent pregnancies (hydiopathic recurrent IUGR).

TABLE 12–2. FACTORS ASSOCIATED WITH A LOW MIDDLE CEREBRAL ARTERY PULSATILITY INDEX

Brain growth spurt
Postuterine contractions
High fetal heart rate
Severe anemia
Post-transfusion
Therapeutic amniocentesis
Ductal constriction and tricuspid insufficiency
Hypoxemia and acidemia

TABLE 12–3. FACTORS ASSOCIATED WITH A HIGH MIDDLE CEREBRAL ARTERY PULSATILITY INDEX

Uterine contractions
Low heart rate
Oligohydramnios
Fetal head compression
Sustained hypoxemia with acidemia
Hydranencephaly
Indomethacin

The IUGR fetus is at greater risk for adverse perinatal outcome when compared with normal fetuses and fetuses that are constitutionally small. Doppler ultrasound can help identify those fetuses that are small because of uteroplacental insufficiency.

In our experience, the two vessels that should be assessed with Doppler ultrasound when an IUGR fetus is suspected are the UA and MCA. In the future, it may be possible to use the ductus venosus FVWs.

Umbilical Blood Flow Velocity Waveforms

In the presence of placental insufficiency, there is greater placental resistance, which is reflected in a decreased diastolic component of the UA waveforms.[17-21] An abnormal UA waveform has a PI value (or RI or S/D ratio) above the normal range. As the placental insufficiency worsens, the diastolic velocity decreases, then becomes absent, and later is reversed

(Fig. 12–13). Some fetuses have decreased diastolic velocity that remains constant with advancing gestation and never becomes absent or reversed, which may be due to a milder form of placental insufficiency.

Cerebral Blood Flow Velocity Waveforms

Animal and human experiments have shown that in the IUGR fetus there is an increase of blood flow to the brain.[22-24] This increase of blood flow can be demonstrated by Doppler ultrasound of the MCA.[8] This effect has been called the *brain sparing effect* (BSE) and is demonstrated by a lower value of the PI (see Fig. 12–12). It is important to emphasize that the MCA PI changes with advancing gestational age. Figure 12–14 shows two sets of waveforms obtained in one IUGR fetus at 24 weeks and in one AGA fetus at term. The two waveforms are similar; however, the MCA PI is abnormal at 24 weeks (BSE) but normal at 39.2 weeks. In IUGR fetuses with a PI below the normal range, there is a greater incidence of adverse perinatal outcome.[8] The BSE may be transient, as has been reported during prolonged hypoxemia in animal experiments,[25] and the overstressed human fetus can also lose the BSE (Fig. 12–15).[26] It has been reported that the MCA PI is below the normal range when PO_2 is reduced.[27] Maximum reduction in PI is reached when the fetal PO_2 is 2 to 4 standard deviations below normal for gestation. When the oxygen deficit is greater, there is a tendency for the PI to rise; this presumably reflects the development of brain edema.

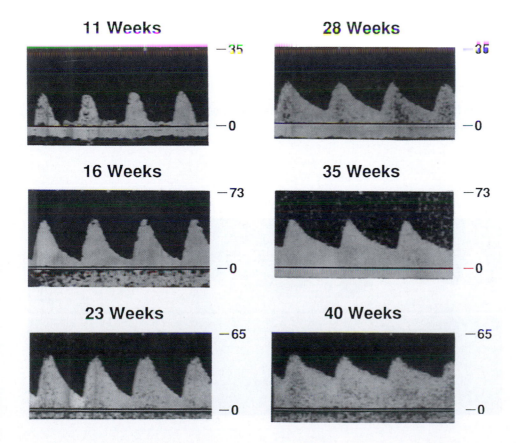

11 Weeks — 35 — 0

28 Weeks — 35 — 0

16 Weeks — 73 — 0

35 Weeks — 73 — 0

23 Weeks — 65 — 0

40 Weeks — 65 — 0

Figure 12–5. Flow velocity waveforms of the umbilical artery with advancing gestation. Note that the end-diastolic velocity increases more than the peak velocity with advancing gestation and this is quantified by a decreased pulsatility index, systolic/diastolic ratio, or resistance index, or all of these, with advancing gestation.

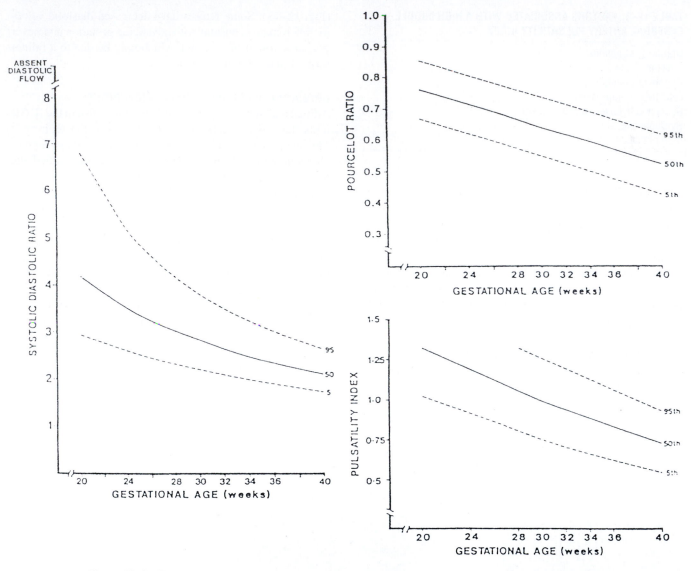

Figure 12–6. The normal values for the umbilical artery. *(Reproduced with permission from Thompson RS, Trudinger BJ, Cook CM.* Br J Obstet Gynaecol. *1988;95:589–591.)*

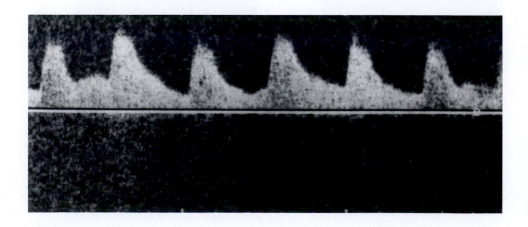

Figure 12–7. Flow velocity waveforms of the umbilical artery during fetal breathing. Note that the waveforms are different from each other.

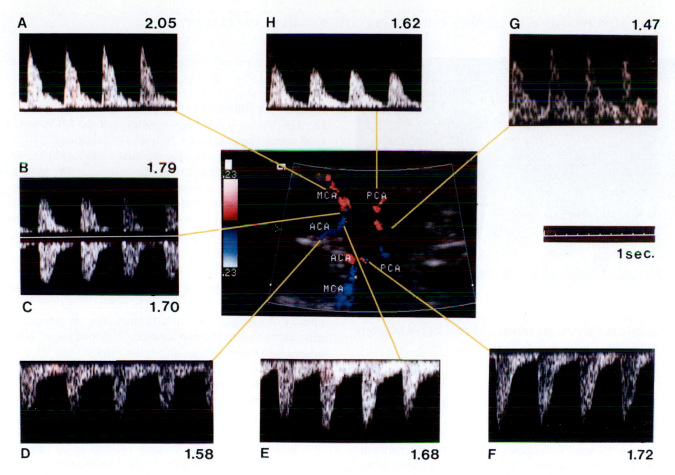

Figure 12–8. Circle of Willis. Note that different cerebral arteries have a different value of pulsatility index. MCA, middle cerebral artery; ACA, anterior cerebral artery; PCA, posterior cerebral artery.

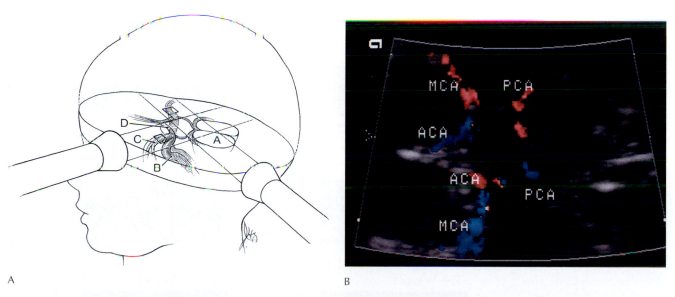

Figure 12–9. (A) Drawing showing the plane used in Doppler ultrasonography studies of the middle cerebral artery. A, pons; B, internal carotid artery; C, middle cerebral artery; D, anterior cerebral artery. *(Reproduced with permission from Mari G, Moise JK, Deter RL, et al. Am J Obstet Gynecol. 1989;160:698–703.)* **(B)** Circle of Willis in a fetus at 20 weeks' gestation. The posterior communicating artery that connects the internal carotid artery and the posterior cerebral artery is not well represented because the angle between the ultrasound beam and the direction of blood flow in this artery is approximately 90 degrees and, therefore, no Doppler signal is recorded. MCA, middle cerebral artery; ACA, anterior cerebral artery; PCA, posterior cerebral artery. *(Reproduced with permission from Mari G. J Ultrasound Med. 1994;13:343–346.)*

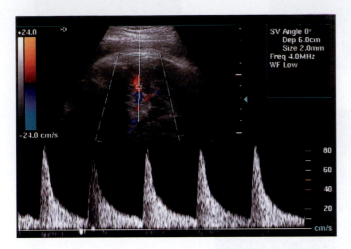

Figure 12–10. Flow velocity waveforms of the middle cerebral artery (MCA). Note that the MCA may be studied with an angle close to 0 degrees and, therefore, the velocity is close to the real velocity of the blood flow.

In IUGR fetuses, the disappearance of the BSE and/or the presence of reversed flow of the MCA is a critical event for the fetus and appears to precede fetal death.[26,28–30] This has been confirmed in fetuses when obstetric interventions were refused by the parents. Unfortunately, to demonstrate this concept, it is necessary to perform a longitudinal study on severely IUGR fetuses up to the point of fetal demise. Reversed flow of the MCA velocity waveforms can be observed with head compression in normal pregnancies (Fig. 12–16). [31]

Ratio of the Cerebral to the Umbilical Artery

In AGA fetuses it has been reported that the MCA-to-UA ratio remains constant after 30 weeks of gestation.[32]

Bahado-Singh et al. have reported a statistically significant increase in perinatal morbidity and mortality in cases with an abnormal cerebroplacental ratio.[33] This ratio appeared to improve the prediction of perinatal outcome compared with umbilical artery velocimetry alone. The cerebroplacental ratio did not appear to correlate significantly with outcome in fetuses at more than 34 weeks of gestation.

Diagnosis of Fetuses with Intrauterine Growth Restriction Before 24 Weeks of Gestation. The substrate for the development of uteroplacental insufficiency may be detected as early as the time of the implantation.[34,35] However, no effect is seen on Doppler ultrasound or on growth until 20 to 24 weeks of gestation. In fact, these fetuses do show signs of growth restriction or abnormal Doppler ultrasound before this period. Rarely is an IUGR fetus diagnosed before 20 weeks of gestation (see IUGR case 5). When this occurs, the possibility of delivering a viable infant is unlikely.

In our experience, admitting patients to the hospital based only on the diagnosis of IUGR fetus before 24 weeks of gestation, when the fetal weight is below 500 g, does not improve pregnancy outcome and the prognosis is poor if delivery occurs at this time.

Figure 12–11. Flow velocity waveforms of the fetal middle cerebral artery at different gestational ages. *(Reproduced with permission from Mari G, Deter RL. Am J Obstet Gynecol. 1992;166: 1262–1270.)*

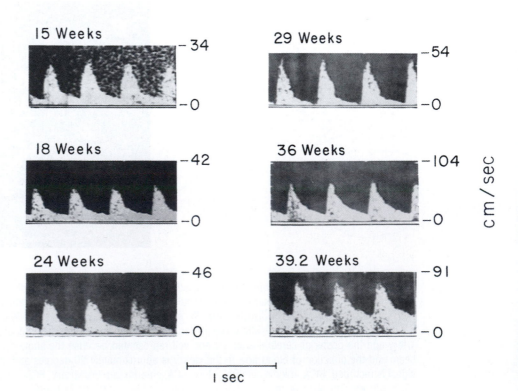

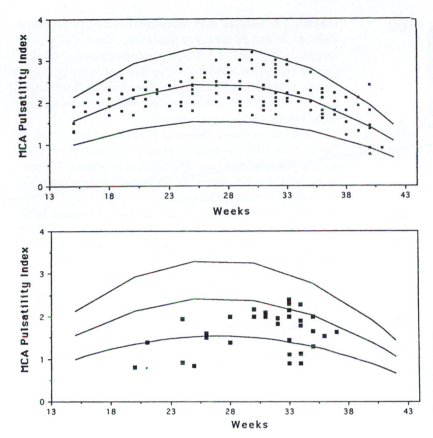

Figure 12–12. Reference range of middle cerebral artery pulsatility index (PI) as a function of gestational age *(top)*. Middle cerebral artery PI in small-for-gestational-age fetuses *(large squares)* plotted on reference range *(bottom)*. *(Reproduced with permission from Mari G, Deter RL. Am J Obstet Gynecol. 1992;166:1262–1270.)*

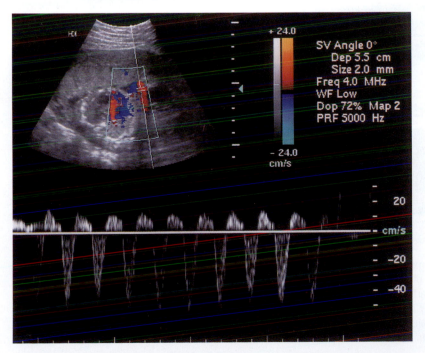

Figure 12–13. Case 1. Flow velocity waveforms of the umbilical artery show reverse flow during diastole.

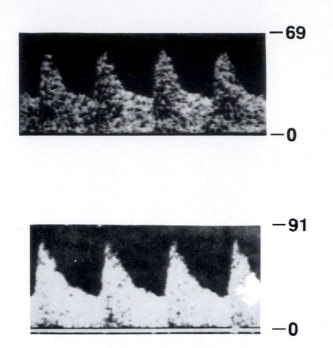

Figure 12–14. Middle cerebral artery flow velocity waveforms in an intrauterine growth-retarded fetus at 24 weeks and in an appropriate-for-gestational-age fetus at 39.2 weeks.

Diagnosis of Fetuses with Intrauterine Growth Restriction Between 24 and 28 Weeks of Gestation. The UA may have an abnormal PI (RI or S/D ratio) values; however, EDV is present both at the abdominal insertion and at the placental insertion. The MCA PI is normal. The amniotic fluid is normal. In these cases we manage the patient as an outpatient with Doppler ultrasound every week.

The UA may have abnormal PI (RI or S/D ratio) value; however, the EDV is present at both the abdominal insertion and the placental insertion. The MCA is abnormal. The amniotic fluid is either normal or abnormal. In these cases we admit the patient to the hospital.

If the UA FVWs have either absent or reversed EDV, we admit the patient to the hospital. After admission, steroid therapy for the fetal lung maturity, bed rest, and oxygen therapy may be useful. However, if the UA and the MCA have an abnormal value at this early gestational age, very likely the process will deteriorate and the chances of a delivery close to term are very low.

In our experience, most of the fetuses admitted to the hospital with absent/reversed EDV of the UA and abnormal MCA are delivered within 4 weeks. Reasons for

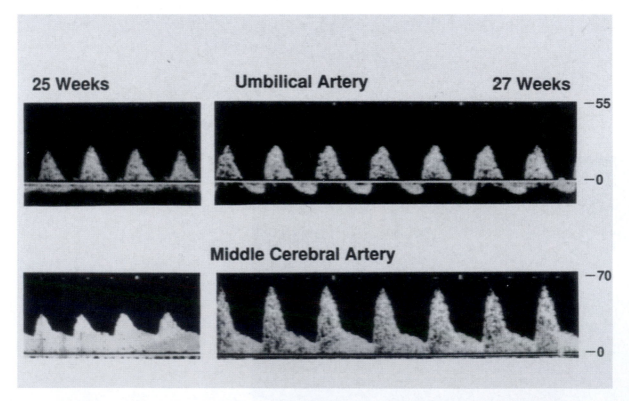

Figure 12–15. Flow velocity waveforms of the umbilical artery and middle cerebral artery (MCA) at 25 and 27 weeks of gestation in a case of a severely growth-retarded fetus. At 25 weeks there was absent end-diastolic velocity of the umbilical artery flow velocity waveforms (FVW), pulsation of the umbilical vein, and the brain-sparing effect (shown by high diastole of the MCA). At 27 weeks there was reverse diastolic FVW of the umbilical artery, and the brain-sparing effect was not present. The fetus died 24 h after this study. *(Reproduced with permission from Mari G, Wasserstrum N.* Am J Obstet Gynecol. *1991;164:776–778.)*

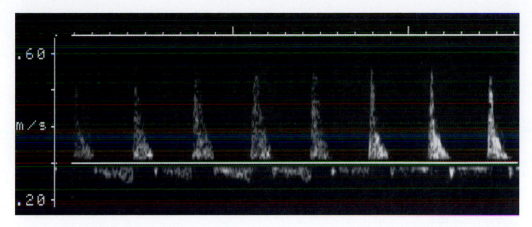

Figure 12–16. Flow velocity waveforms of the middle cerebral artery in a appropriate-for-gestational-age fetus. The reverse flow was transient.

delivery are 1) lack of fetal growth (we expect that fetal abdominal circumference increases by at least 1 cm per week and/or fetal weight increases by 100 g per week); 2) development of HELLP (hemolysis, elevated liver enzymes, low platelets) syndrome, or 3) nonreassuring fetal testing. Interestingly enough, these IUGR fetuses are at lower risk for the development of intraventricular hemorrhage. In fact, it has been reported that IUGR fetuses with BSE are less likely to develop intraventricular hemorrhage.[36] The reason is not completely understood. However, the stress secondary to IUGR may play an important role in this process.

If the fetus is not delivered, the process of uteroplacental insufficiency continues. Tricuspid regurgitation may appear; umbilical vein pulsation,[37] and intermittent ductus venosus reverse flow initially may be present (see IUGR case 1) and later it may be continuous. The biophysical profile (BPP) becomes abnormal. The fetus starts to lose the BSE, and fetal demise occurs. Oligohydramnios may appear at any stage of this process. The time interval between the above events is variable (from 6 to 12 h to several weeks). This scenario applies to a specific, common IUGR and not to the fetuses who have a different underlying pathology such as abruption or toxic drug exposure.

Diagnosis of Fetus with Intrauterine Growth Restriction After 28 Weeks of Gestation.

It is our experience that between 28 and 34 weeks of gestation, in the presence of abnormal UA and MCA, but normal fetal heart rate monitoring and BPP conservative management is a good option.[38] After 34 weeks we perform an amniocentesis, and if the L/S (lecithin/sphingomyelin) ratio is greater than 2.5 with positive PG (phosphatidylglycerol) we ripen the cervix and initiate induction of labor.

Management of Fetuses with Intrauterine Growth Restriction (Cases Reports)

Tables 12–4 and 12–5 present clinical data of 10 small fetuses in whom Doppler ultrasound was helpful in clinical decision making.

Case 1 (Figs. 12–13, 12–17, and 12–18). The patient was admitted to the hospital at 28 weeks because of severe IUGR, oligohydramnios, and abnormal Doppler image of the UA, MCA, and reverse flow of the ductus venosus. The nonstress test was nonreactive with presence of long-term variability, and occasional decelerations. The biophysical profile showed persistent fetal breathing, good movements, and tone. The fetus remained stable for 2 weeks. In this period, the ductus venosus showed intermittent reverse FVWs. Two weeks after admission to the hospital a cesarean delivery was performed because of lack of growth. The fetus presented as breech. The infant initially did well. Later there was progressive deterioration in lung function. Total parenteral nutrition was started. Glucose control was difficult to maintain, with many episodes of hypoglycemia. On day 22 of life there was an episode of pulmonary hemorrhage followed by cardiac arrest. The infant was resuscitated; the electroencephalogram was flat and the baby unresponsive. Head ultrasound was still relatively normal at this stage, with mild ventricular dilation. Abdominal ultrasound showed ascites, but liver and kidneys appeared normal. The infant died on day 24.

Case 2. The patient was admitted to the hospital because of IUGR, oligohydramios, absent EDV of the UA, and presence of BSE. The fetus was delivered 2 weeks later because of lack of growth.

Case 3. The patient was admitted to the hospital because of IUGR and reversed flow of the UA and presence of BSE. At the admission, fetal breathing, movements, and tone were

TABLE 12–4. DATA OF 10 PREGNANCIES COMPLICATED BY FETUSES SMALL FOR GESTATIONAL AGE OR INTRAUTERINE GROWTH RESTRICTION

No.	MA	Pathology	G	P	Reason for Ultrasound	GA at Diagnosis	EFW	AF	UA FVW	MCA FVW	DV FVW	Breathing	Movements	Tone	FHR	GA at Delivery	Reason	Sex
1	28	None	2	0	S < D	28.3	1%	Oligo	RF	BSE	RF	+	+	+	LTV	30.3	Lack of growth	M
2	20	Sickle cell anemia	1	0	S < D	23.1	1%	Oligo	AEDV	BSE	NL	+	+	+	LTV	25.2	Lack of growth	M
3	25	None	3	2	S < D	31.5	1%	NL	AEDV	BSE	NL	+	+	+	LTV/VD	31.5	NRFT	M
4	35	Cocaine use	5	3	Cocaine use	25	3%	NL	AEDV	BSE	NL	+	+	+	LTV	28	NRFT	F
5	35	H/O IUGR	6	2	H/O IUGR	17	<1%	NL	RF	BSE	RF	absent	+	+	present	19	IUFD	F
6	24	CHTN Prev-FD	3	1	CHTN Prev-FD	24	>10%	NL	Abnl	NL	NL	+	+	+	LTV	25.5	NRFT	F
7	31	None	1	0	S < D	29.4	1%	NL	AEDV	BSE	NL	+	+	+	+acc	29.4	NRFT	F
8	20	Crohn's disease	1	0	Crohn's disease	32	5%	NL	NL	NL	NL	+	+	+	+acc	39.2	NL SVD	F
9	33	None	3	2	S < D	24	5%	Oligo	NL	NL	NL	–	+	+	LTV	39.1	NL SVD	M
10	36	None	4	2	S < D	24.1	>10%	NL	NL	NL	NL	+	+	+	LTV	30.2	HELLP	M

MA, maternal age; GA, gestational age; EFW, estimated fetal weight; AF, amniotic fluid; UA, umbilical artery; MCA, middle cerebral artery; DV, ductus venosus; FVW, flow velocity waveform; FHR, fetal heart rate; S < D, size less than dates; AEDV, absent end-diastolic velocity; BSE, brain-sparing effect; NL, normal; LTV, long-term variability; NRFT, non-reassuring fetal testing; H/O, history of; IUGR, intrauterine growth restriction; IUFD, intrauterine fetal demise; CHTN, chronic hypertension; Prev-FD, previous fetal demise; HELLP, hemolysis, elevated liver enzymes low platelets.

TABLE 12–5. NEONATAL DATA OF THE 10 FETUSES WITH INTRAUTERINE GROWTH RESTRICTION

No.	Apgars 1, 5*	Arterial pH (BE)	Venous pH (BE)	Weight (g)	RDS	BPD	IVH	Hospital Stay (Days)	Outcome
1	8, 8	7.17 (−14)	7.27 (−9)	475	Y	Y	N	24	Died on day 24
2	5, 7	7.21 (−9)	7.23 (−8)	520	Y	Y	N	115	Discharged home
3	4, 7	6.93 (−18)	6.97 (−17)	840	Y	N	N	41	Discharged home
4	0, 2	6.92 (−17)	7.14 (−15)	614	Y		?	4	Died on day 4
5	0, 0	—	—	—	—	—	—	—	IUFD at 19 weeks
6	7, 8	7.16 (−9)	—	665	Y	Y	N	89	Discharged home
7	2, 5	7.03	7.07	890	Y	N	N	56	Discharged home
8	9, 9	—	—	2020	N	N	N	2	Discharged home
9	9, 9	—	—	2900	N	N	N	2	Discharged home
10	6, 7	7.21 (−5)	7.29 (−4)	1150	N	N	N	42	Discharged home

*1, 5, score at 1 min and 5 min after birth.
BE, base excess; RDS, respiratory distress syndrome; BPD, bronchopulmonary dysplasia; IVH, intraventricular hemorrhage; Y, yes; N, no.

present. Seven hours after admission the fetus was delivered because of nonreassuring fetal testing (NRFT). The fetus was acidotic at birth.

Case 4. The patient had the first ultrasound at 25 weeks. The amniotic fluid was normal, and there was fetal breathing, movements, and tone. End-diastolic velocity of the UA was absent and BSE was present. Based on these findings and previous history of stillbirth, it was decided to admit the patient to the hospital, but the patient declined. At 28 weeks of gestation she presented to the clinic and was admitted. Cesarean delivery (CD) was performed because of NRFT. The fetus died on day 5.

Case 5. This is a case of a hydiopathic recurrent IUGR fetus. The patient's first two pregnancies ended in miscarriage in the first trimester. The third pregnancy was complicated by an IUGR fetus that was delivered at 34 weeks of gestation. The fifth pregnancy was complicated by an IUGR fetus diagnosed at 19 weeks of gestation. However, it was established that the fetus had a skeletal dysplasia and no Doppler ultrasound was performed. Her current pregnancy was complicated by IUGR diagnosed at 17 weeks of gestation. The diagnosis was once again skeletal dysplasia. No Doppler ultrasound was performed. The patient was referred to our unit for an ultrasound. At 17.1 weeks of gestation, the fetal biometry was consistent with 15 weeks. Doppler ultrasound showed absent EDV of the UA and presence of BSE. The patient was counseled and the diagnosis was changed to hydiopathic recurrent IUGR. The prognosis for her fetus was poor and she declined intervention. At 19 weeks of gestation she presented because of absence of fetal movements. There was no presence of fetal heart rate. The work-up for recurrent pregnancy loss and recurrent IUGR was negative. In this patient, Doppler ultrasound was an important clue for the diagnosis.

Case 6. This patient with chronic hypertension had a history of previous fetal demise in the third trimester. During her current pregnancy she was seen every 2 weeks in our clinic. Ultrasound to assess fetal growth was performed every 4 weeks starting at 16 weeks of gestation. At 24 weeks

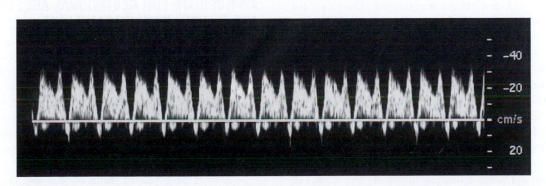

Figure 12–17. Case 1. Flow velocity waveforms of the ductus venosus at admission to the hospital show reverse flow in diastole.

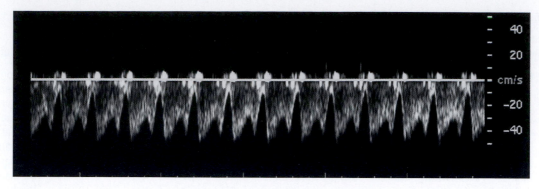

Figure 12–18. Case 1. Flow velocity waveforms of the ductus venosus 2 days after admission to the hospital.

of gestation, the estimated fetal weight was greater than the 10th percentile. However, the UA PI was slightly abnormal and the MCA PI was normal. The amniotic fluid was normal. Fetal movements, breathing, and tone were present. It was decided to repeat the Doppler study in 1 week. When the patient returned to the clinic, there was absent EDV of the UA and presence of BSE. The patient was admitted to the hospital. Three days later there was reversed flow of the UA. Two days later a CD was performed because of NRFT.

Case 7. The patient was referred because of size-less-than-date findings (S < D). The ultrasound showed a small fetus. The amniotic fluid was normal. There was presence of fetal breathing, movements, and tone. Doppler ultrasound showed absence of EDV of the UA and presence of BSE. The patient was admitted because of IUGR and abnormal Doppler of the UA and MCA. The patient started to contract and the evening of the admission to the hospital a CD was performed because of NRFT. Placental abruption was diagnosed at the time of the cesarean delivery.

Case 8. The patient was referred because of S < D. The EFW was below the 10th percentile. The amniotic fluid was normal, and there was presence of breathing, movements, and tone. Doppler of the UA and MCAs was normal. Therefore, the patient was managed as an outpatient. She delivered a healthy infant at 39.2 weeks of gestation.

Case 9. This case is similar to the previous one with the difference that there was decreased amniotic fluid (amniotic fluid index of 5.0). Doppler of the UA and MCA was normal. The patient was admitted to the hospital and remained for 3 weeks. In this period, the fluid increased and growth improved. Doppler of the UA and MCA remained normal. The patient was discharged home. She was then managed as outpatient and delivered a healthy infant at 39.1 weeks of gestation.

Case 10. The patient was referred at 24.1 weeks of gestation because of S < D. The EFW was at the lower limit of normal. The amniotic fluid was normal. Doppler of the UA and MCA was normal. The patient was managed as an outpatient until 29 weeks of gestation when Doppler of the UA and MCA appeared abnormal. The amniotic fluid was normal. The patient was admitted to the hospital. Doppler of the UA improved, whereas the BSE remained present. Nine days after admission the patient developed HELLP syndrome and a CD was performed because of noninducible cervix.

In summary, it is important to emphasize that the imaging results of the UA and MCA alone do not indicate when to deliver the fetus; however, they need to be interpreted with other diagnostic tools, such as the biophysical profile and the assessment of fetal growth.[39–42] The clinical value of the umbilical and cerebral Doppler studies is in determing which fetuses require admission to the hospital and further intensive surveillance.

OTHER FLOW VELOCITY WAVEFORMS OF THE CARDIOVASCULAR SYSTEM IN APPROPRIATE-FOR-GESTATIONAL-AGE FETUSES AND FETUSES WITH INTRAUTERINE GROWTH RESTRICTION

Many other fetal arteries and veins have been studied in AGA and IUGR fetuses. Their study has increased our understanding of fetal physiology and pathophysiology in AGA and IUGR fetuses. However, in our experience, the study of these vessels, as currently performed, does not add new information to the study of the UA and MCA in the management of IUGR fetuses.

A brief overview of these vessels and Doppler of the fetal heart follows.

Descending Aorta

Flow velocity waveforms from the fetal descending aorta are usually recorded at the level of the diaphragm. In fact, FVWs at the level of the diaphragm and distally to the origin of the renal arteries are different (Fig. 12–19A and B).[43,44] The PI of the fetal descending aorta is 1.96 ± 0.30 (SD) at the diaphragm and 1.68 ± 0.28 (SD) after the origin of the renal arteries.[43] The PI is the preferred measure in the descending aorta because end-diastolic flow may be absent in normal fetuses. Flow velocity waveforms in the descending aorta represent the summation of flow to the kidneys, bowel, placenta, and lower extremities. The PI of the fetal descending aorta remains relatively constant throughout gestation because placental and renal resistance decrease with advancing gestation, while lower extremity vascular resistance increases.[45] In severe IUGR fetuses there is reversed flow of the descending aorta.

Celiac Trunk

The celiac trunk arises from the aorta (Fig. 12–20) between the crura of the diaphragm at the level of the 12th thoracica

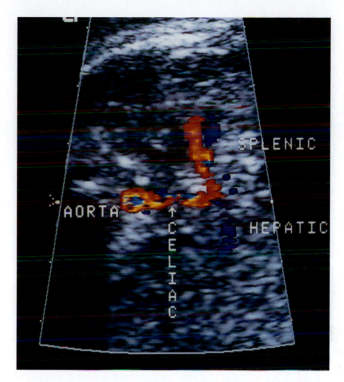

Figure 12–20. Transverse section of the fetal abdomen at the level of the descending aorta, celiac trunk, splenic artery, and hepatic artery. *(Reproduced with permission from Mari G, Abuhamad AZ, Uerpairkoit B, et al.* Ultrasound Obstet Gynecol. *1995;172:820–825.)*

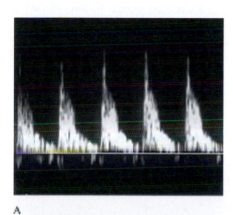

A

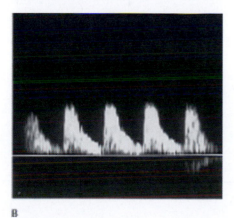

B

Figure 12–19. Flow velocity waveforms of the descending aorta **(A)** at the level of the diaphragm and **(B)** distally to the origin of the renal arteries.

vertebra. It has three main branches: the splenic, common hepatic, and left gastric arteries. The splenic artery supplies the spleen, a great part of the stomach, and the pancreas. The superior mesenteric artery arises anteriorly from the abdominal aorta just below the celiac artery at the level of the two renal arteries (Fig. 12–21). It supplies the distal part of the duodenum, jejunum, cecum, appendix, ascending colon, and most of the transverse colon.

Splenic Artery

Splenic artery PI values are presented in Figure 12–22. Any index may be used to assess the splenic artery. Abuhamad et al.[46] found that IUGR fetuses have a lower splenic artery PI value. This suggests that in cases of chronic hypoxia there is increased blood flow to the spleen because of increased erythropoiesis.[47,48]

Superior Mesenteric Artery

Superior mesenteric artery FVWs are shown in Figure 12–23. With advancing gestation, PI values increase.[49] This may reflect increased bowel resistance because of increased bowel length with advancing gestation. The superior mesenteric artery FVWs does not seem to be useful in evaluating IUGR fetuses.[50]

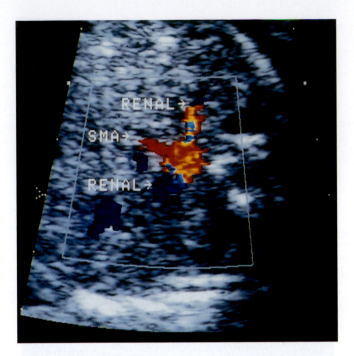

Figure 12–21. Transverse section of the fetal abdomen at the level of the kidneys with the two renal arteries and the superior mesenteric artery at their origin from the descending aorta. *(Reproduced with permission from Mari G, Abuhamad AZ, Uerpairkoit B, et al. Ultrasound Obstet Gynecol. 1995;172:820–825.)*

Adrenal Artery

Figures 12–24 and 12–25 show the abdominal section where the adrenal artery is sampled. Fetal adrenal artery FVWs are shown in Fig. 12–26. In IUGR fetuses there is a lower adrenal artery PI, suggesting an "adrenal stress response" as reported in animal studies (Fig. 12–27).[51]

Renal Artery

The renal artery can be studied in a coronal section of descending aorta and after its origin from the descending aorta in the kidneys (Figs. 12–28 and 12–29). Doppler waveforms of the renal artery and vein are displayed on either side of the baseline (Figs. 12–30 and 12–31).

The PI must be used to assess the renal artery because the EDV is often absent in the second trimester and early third trimester.[52,53] The normal values of the renal artery PI are shown in Figure 12–32. In fetuses with severe IUGR, the renal artery PI is above the reference range.

Femoral, Internal Iliac, and External Iliac Arteries

The femoral artery FVWs are obtained soon after its origin (Figs. 12–33 to 12–35). The normal values of the femoral artery PI and FVWs are shown in Fig. 12–36. There is no difference between the femoral artery PI and the external iliac artery PI.[45]

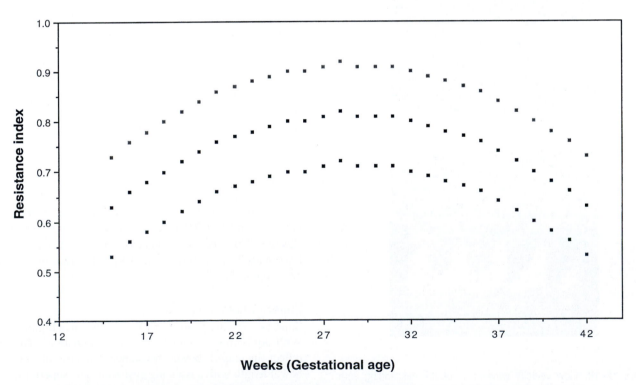

Figure 12–22. Reference range (mean +/− 2 SE) of splenic artery resistance index with gestation. Resistance index = 0.057 (weeks) − 0.001 (weeks)^2: R = 0.53. *(Reproduced with permission from Abuhamad AZ, Mari G, Evans M. Am J Obstet Gynecol. 1995;172:820–825.)*

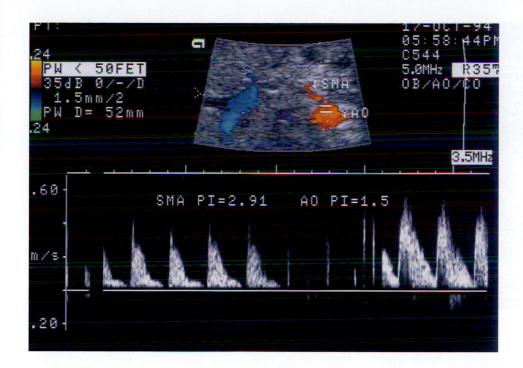

Figure 12–23. Flow velocity waveforms of the superior mesenteric artery (SMA) and descending aorta (AO). The sample volume was initially placed on the SMA and then moved to the AO. PI = Pulsality index.

The internal iliac artery is the intraabdominal continuation of the UA and, therefore, reflects the UA FVWs.

Superior Cerebellar Artery

The superior cerebellar artery arises from the basilar artery before this artery divides into the two posterior cerebral arteries (Fig. 12–37). The PI of the superior cerebellar artery is similar to that of the MCA. Uerpairkoit et al.[54] found that the PI of the superior cerebeller artery is lower than normal in IUGR fetuses, whereas it is in the normal range in small-for-gestational-age fetuses (Fig. 12–38A and B).

Coronary Sinus

Coronary blood flow by color Doppler imaging is possible in the human fetus. However, pulsed wave Doppler measurements are infrequently obtained, making this unfeasible for routine assessment of myocardial blood flow.[55]

Fetal Venous System in Appropriate-for-Gestational-Age Fetuses

Most of the studies on the fetal venous blood flow have been performed on the blood flow coming from the placenta. Recently, the venous circulation on the fetal brain has been

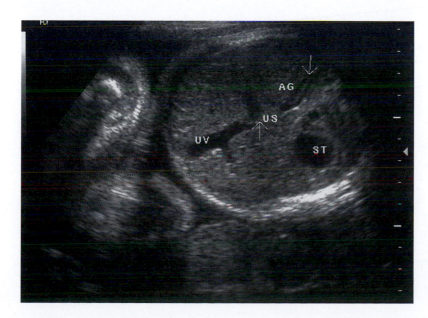

Figure 12–24. Axial section of the fetal abdomen at the level of the adrenal artery. UV, umbilical vein; US, umbilical sinus; AG, adrenal gland; ST, stomach. *(Reproduced with permission from Mari G, Uerpairojkit B, Abuhamad A, et al. Ultrasound Obstet Gynecol. 1996;8:82–86.)*

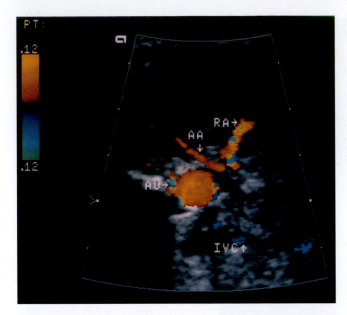

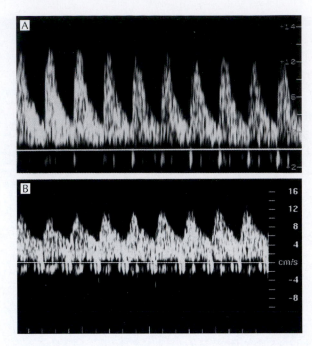

Figure 12–25. Axial section of the fetal abdomen showing the adrenal artery (AA), the descending aorta (AO), the renal artery (RA), and the inferior vena cava (IVC). *(Reproduced with permission from Mari G, Uerpairojkit B, Abuhamad A, et al. Ultrasound Obstet Gynecol. 1996;8:82–86.)*

Figure 12–26. Flow velocity waveforms of the adrenal artery in an appropriate-for-gestational-age fetus **(A)** and in a fetus with intrauterine growth restriction **(B)**. *(Reproduced with permission from Mari G, Uerpairojkit B, Abuhamad A, et al. Ultrasound Obstet Gynecol. 1996;8:82–86.)*

elucidated.[56] In addition, it has been suggested that the study of the pulmonary circulation can be useful in the diagnosis of pulmonary hypoplasia.[57]

Blood flow coming from the placenta returns to the heart through the umbilical vein, ductus venosus, and inferior vena

cava (Figs. 12–39 to 12–41). Approximately 50% of the blood flow from the umbilical vein goes to the liver and 50% to the ductus venosus.[58,59] The umbilical vein has continuous flow that becomes pulsatile at the portal sinus (Fig. 12–42). [60,61]

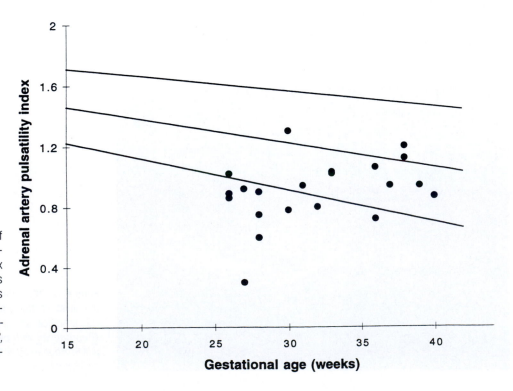

Figure 12–27. Reference range of values for the adrenal artery obtained with the pulsatility index (5th and 95th percentiles). Dots represent the values in fetuses with intrauterine growth restriction. *(Reproduced with permission from Mari G, Uerpairojkit B, Abuhamad A, et al. Ultrasound Obstet Gynecol. 1996;8:82–86.)*

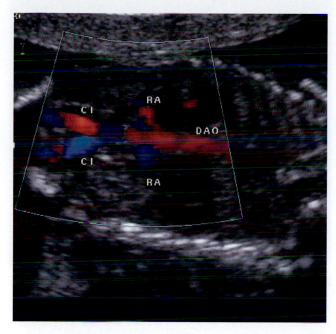

Figure 12–28. Coronal section of the fetal descending aorta (DAO). RA, renal artery at the origin from the aorta; CI, common iliac artery.

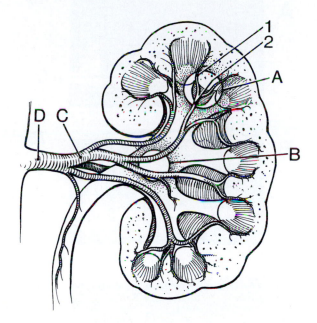

Figure 12–29. Drawing of the fetal kidney. The letters indicate where the waveforms in Fig. 12–30 were obtained.

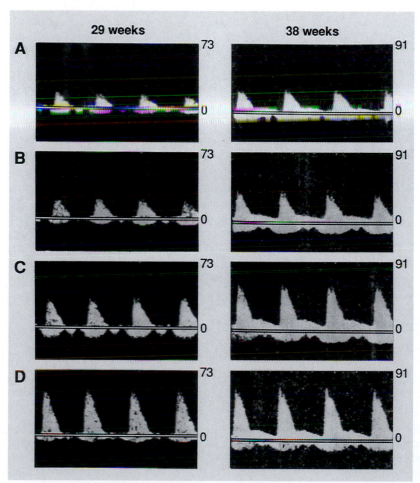

Figure 12–30. Flow velocity waveforms of the renal artery obtained at different levels (see Fig. 12–29).

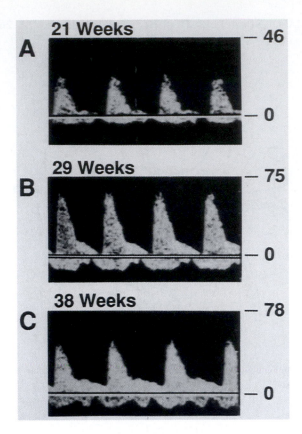

Figure 12–31. Flow velocity waveforms of the renal artery at different gestational ages.

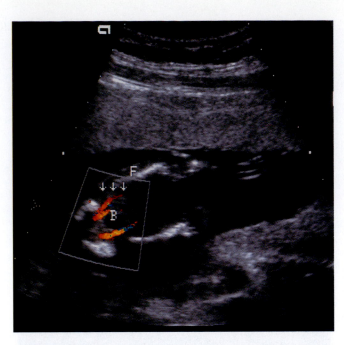

Figure 12–33. Axial section of bladder (B) and thigh showing the two umbilical arteries around the bladder and the femoral artery (three *arrows*). F, femur.

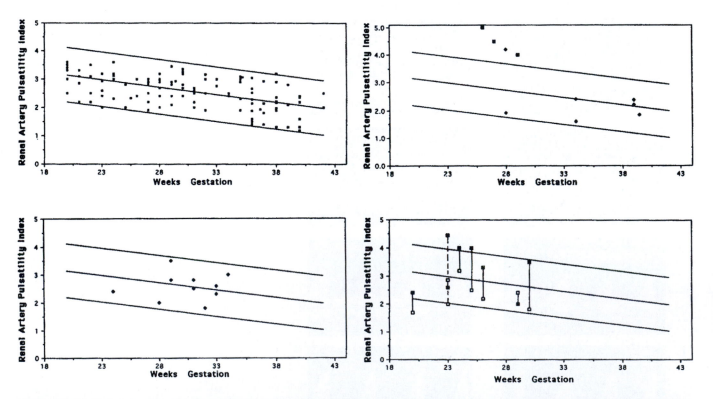

Figure 12–32. Reference range for the renal artery pulsatility index (mean ± 2 SE) *(top left)*. The pulsatility index is reported in intrauterine growth-retarded fetuses with oligohydramnios *(top right);* the three fetuses represented by the three squares died. On the *bottom left,* the renal artery pulsatility index is reported in fetuses with polyhydramnios. On the *bottom right* the renal artery pulsatility index is reported in twins with polyhydramnios–oligohydramnios (the *open squares* represent the twins with polyhydramnios, whereas the *dark squares* represent the twins with oligohydramnios). *(Reproduced with permission from Mari G, Kirshon B, Abuhamad A. Obstet Gynecol. 1993;81:560–564.)*

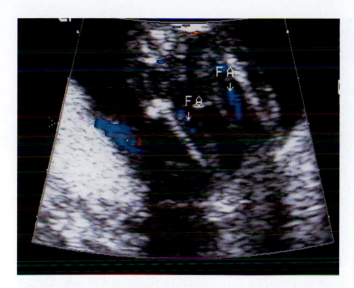

Figure 12–34. The two femoral arteries (FAs).

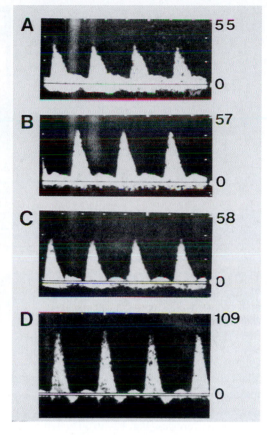

Figure 12–35. Flow velocity waveforms of the femoral artery at 18 **(A)**, 24 **(B)**, 30 **(C)**, and 39 weeks of gestation **(D)** with forward diastolic flow in **A**, presence of a notch in **B** and **C**, and reverse flow in **D**. *(Reproduced with permission from Mari G. Am J Obstet Gynecol. 1991;165:143–151.)*

The blood flow through the ductus venosus goes to the inferior vena cava.

The inferior vena cava, before its entrance into the right atrium, has a triphasic pulsatile pattern (Fig. 12–43).[62,63] The first forward wave begins to increase with atrial relaxation, reaches a peak during ventricular systole, and then falls to a nadir at the end of ventricular systole. The second forward wave occurs during early diastole, and the third wave, characterized by a reverse flow, is present in late diastole with atrial contractions. In healthy fetuses a significant decrease of reverse flow during atrial contraction is present with advancing gestation (Fig. 12–44).[63] These changes are considered to be related to improved ventricular compliance and to the reduction of right ventricular afterload, due to the fall in placental resistance occuring with advancing gestation.

The ductus venosus transports oxygenated blood from the umbilical vein to the left atrium and ventricle, and then to the myocardium and brain. The ductus venosus blood FVW has a biphasic pattern (Fig. 12–45).[64] The two peaks reflect the two peaks of the inferior vena cava; blood flow slows at the time of atrial contraction. In the first trimester it is possible to have reversed blood flow that may be due to the immaturity of the sphincter of the ductus venosus and may

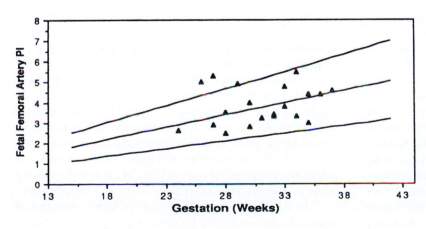

Figure 12–36. Reference range (mean $\pm$ 2 SD) of femoral artery pulsatility index with gestation constructed from a study of 12 appropriate-for-gestational-age fetuses followed up longitudinally. *Triangles* represent pulsatility index values of 20 fetuses with intrauterine growth retardation. *(Reproduced with permission from Mari G. Am J Obstet Gynecol. 1991;165:143–151.)*

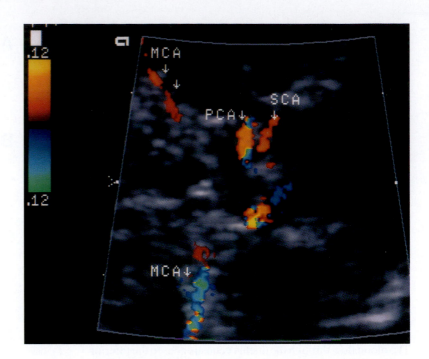

Figure 12–37. Axial section of fetal brain. SCA, superior cerebellar artery; PCA, posterior cerebral artery; MCA, middle cerebral artery.

also explain the umbilical vein pulsatile pattern seen in the first trimester.[65]

A common error is the sampling of the left hepatic vein rather than ductus venosus (Fig. 12–46). The left hepatic vein FVW is similar to the IVC FVW and it has reverse flow in AGA fetuses.

Fetal Venous System in Intrauterine Growth Restriction

The umbilical vein velocities become pulsatile in the severely IUGR fetus[37,66] Fetuses with pulsation in the umbilical vein in the second and third trimesters have a higher morbidity and mortality, even in the setting of normal UA blood flow.

In IUGR fetuses the inferior vena cava is characterized by increased reverse flow during atrial contraction.[63] The mechanism of this increase is attributed to abnormal ventricular filling characteristics, an abnormal ventricular chamber or wall compliance, or abnormal end-diastolic pressure.

The presence of reverse flow at the ductus venosus (Fig. 12–47) has been observed in IUGR fetuses, in cardiac abnormalities, and in cord complications.[67–69] In IUGR fetuses it is an ominous sign. Goncalves et al.[67] observed five fetuses with reverse FVWs at the ductus venosus and in each case died *in utero*. In 18 fetuses with abnormal UA and MCA, with a ratio greater than 1 and no reverse flow in the ductus venosus, none of the fetuses died. A more recent study in IUGR fetuses reported that abnormal ductus venosus FVWs, defined by the presence of reversed flow in diastole, was the only significant parameter associated with perinatal death.[68] Another study reported that an abnormal ductus venosus velocimetry recorded in high-risk pregnancies is a poor indicator of adverse perinatal outcome.[70] Therefore,

more studies are necessary on ductus venosus FVWs to assess whether their study will add more information to the study of the UA and MCA.

Fetal Cardiac Flow Velocity Waveforms in Appropriate-for-Gestational-Age Fetuses and Fetuses with Intrauterine Growth Restriction

Atrioventricular Valves. Atrioventricular (AV) valve velocities can be obtained from a four-chamber view (Fig. 12–48) by placing the sample volume just distal to the valve leaflets. Usually, two peaks are present in the AV valve signal (Fig. 12–49, left): the first peak reflects passive ventricular filling in early diastole (E) and the second peak reflects the atrial contraction in late diastole (A). Early in gestation, A is much higher than E (Fig. 12–50A), indicating that the atrial contraction is important in the fetus. With advancing gestation, E increases and reaches A (Fig. 12–50B), suggesting that the atrial systole becomes less important with maturation of the ventricular myocardium.[71–75] At birth and after birth, E becomes higher than A (Fig. 12–50C), suggesting a less important role for atrial contraction.

The index used most to quantify these waveforms is the E/A ratio. When the AV valve velocity waveforms are studied at a low incident angle, the blood velocity obtained is close to the true velocity. The increase of E/A ratio with advancing gestation has been considered a sign of progressive improvement in myocardial compliance. Of note is that with advancing gestation the peak velocity of the A wave does not change, whereas the peak velocity of the E wave increases.

In IUGR fetuses the E/A ratio is higher than that of normal fetuses controlled for gestational age. These changes

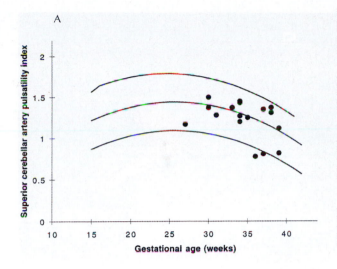

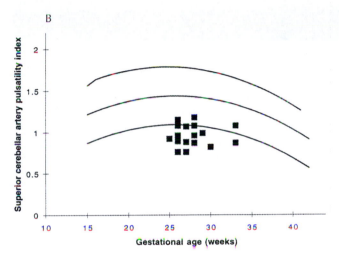

Figure 12–38. Reference range of the fetal superior cerebellar artery values obtained from the pulsatility index (5th and 95th percentiles) during gestation. In **A** and **B** are reported P_1 values in fetuses with small *(circles)* and appropriate *(squared dots)* cerebellum measurements. *(Reproduced with permission from Uerpairojkit B, Chan L, Reece AE, et al.* Obstet Gynecol. *1996;87:995–999.)*

are attributed to changes in preload without impairment in fetal myocardial diastolic function.

Aortic and Pulmonary Valve Flow Velocity Waveforms in Appropriate-for-Gestational-Age Fetuses. Aortic valve (AoV) and pulmonary valve (PuV) velocities are studied at the levels of their respective outflow tracts. The following are the indices that have been used to quantify these waveforms.

Peak Velocity, Acceleration Time, Ejection Time, and Time Velocity Integral

Peak velocity (PV) of both valves increase with advancing gestation.[76] In IUGR fetuses the AoV and PuV have been noted to decrease,[77] which may be secondary to increased placental resistance.

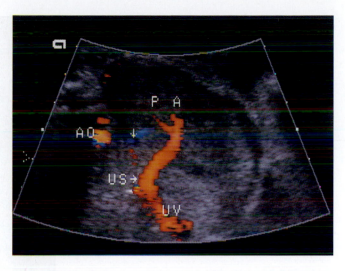

Figure 12–39. Oblique section of the fetal abdomen. The *arrow* indicates the inferior vena cava. UV, umbilical vein; US, umbilical sinus; A, anterior division of the portal vein; P, posterior division of the portal vein; AO, descending aorta.

The acceleration time (AT) is the time from the beginning of the systole to the highest velocity in systole (Fig. 12–51). In the fetus, the AT of the PuV is shorter than the AT of the AoV.[78] After birth and closure of the ductus arteriosus, the AT of the AoV becomes shorter than the AT of the PuV (Mari and Huhta, unpublished data). These data suggest that the decreased pulmonary vascular resistance and increased systemic vascular resistance play an important role in these changes. These findings confirm the data in adults;

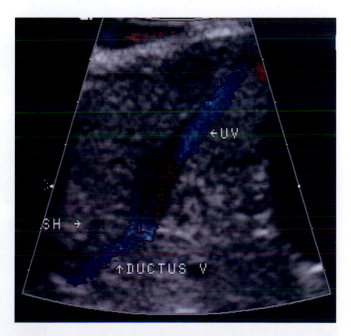

Figure 12–40. Sagittal section of the fetal body. UV, umbilical vein; Ductus V, ductus venosus; SH indicates the left hepatic vein.

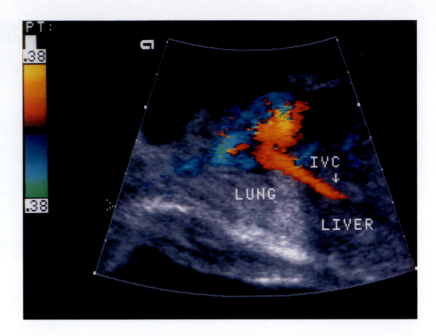

Figure 12–41. Midsagittal section of the fetal body. IVC, inferior vena cava.

that the AT of the PuV and AoV are significantly related to the blood pressure in the systemic and pulmonary circulation, respectively.[79]

Measurement of Fetal Cardiac Output with Doppler Ultrasound

Many investigators have attempted volumetric studies at the level of the fetal heart[76–81] based on the following formula:

$$Q = TVI \times HR \times A$$

where Q is absolute flow per minute, TVI is the time velocity integral, HR is fetal heart rate, and A is the area of the valve.

The velocity of blood passing through a valve is not constant but changes with the cardiac cycle; therefore, the TVI, integral to the velocity waveforms over the entire cardiac cycle, is considered to be a measure of the length of the column of blood.

The main problem in the calculation of absolute flow per minute (Q) is the measurement of the valve area. We can assume that the blood flow at the level of the valvular area is close to laminar and that the Doppler spectrum

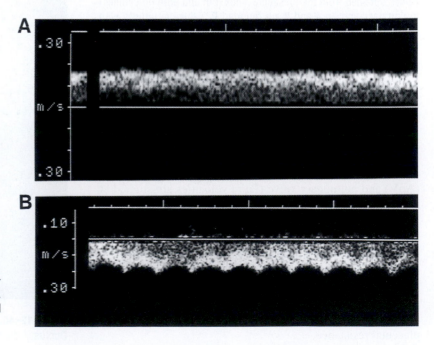

Figure 12–42. Flow velocity waveforms of the umbilical vein **(A)** and umbilical sinus **(B)** in the normal fetus. Note that the flow becomes pulsatile at the umbilical sinus.

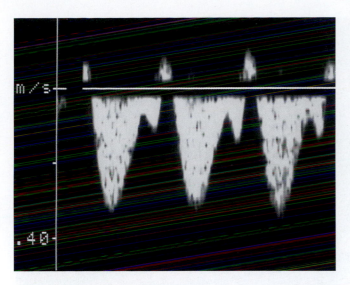

Figure 12–43. Flow velocity waveforms of the inferior vena cava with its typical triphasic pattern.

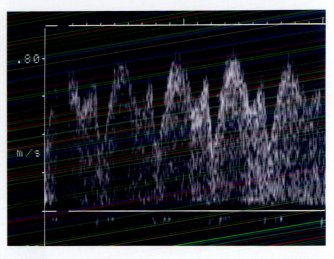

Figure 12–45. Flow velocity waveforms of the ductus venosus in the normal human fetus at 27 weeks of gestation.

reflects all velocities inside the valve. Newer spectral analyzers in many ultrasound machines can provide true-intensity-weighted mean flow measurements that take spectral broadening into account. In addition, we can obtain Doppler waveforms with an angle close to 0 degrees (less than 20 degrees) between the ultrasound beam and the blood flow. A small error in the calculation of the area, which is determined on the basis of one-half of the diameter squared, however, may deeply affect the measurement. For example, a 0.5-mm error in the measurement of a 4-mm valve will produce a 25% variation in the flow calculation.

Animal studies have demonstrated that the calculation of the blood flow may be reliable.[82] The study of the human fetus, however, is different from the "ideal" situation of animal research. An alternative approach can be used to measure the cardiac output (CO) indirectly if the valve diameter remains constant. For example, if measurements are taken in a short interval, valvular area does not change and an intervention

that changes flow will be detected from changes in TVI, HR, or both. The product of TVI and HR was measured at the AoV and PuV before and after two doses of nifedipine.[83] No difference was noted in the two sets of measurements. Although the true value of CO could not be evaluated because the valve diameter was not measured, these results suggested that there were no changes in CO after nifedipine. Subsequently, the effect of fetal transfusion on CO was determined by using the same formula.[84,85] More recently, Gonzalez et al.[86] used the same formula to assess the effects of nitroglycerin on the fetal CO.

Fetal Cardiac Output in Fetuses with Intrauterine Growth Restriction

In IUGR fetuses, there is, presumably, a redistribution of the blood flow from the right to the left ventricle and an increase of blood flow to the brain. It has been reported that, under

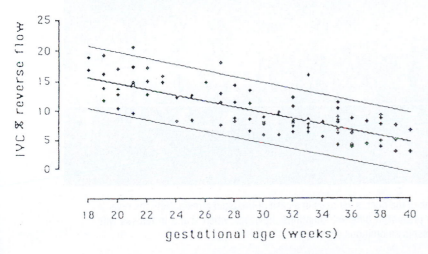

Figure 12–44. Reference range (mean and linear regression of individual 95% confidence intervals) with gestation of inferior vena cava percentage of reverse flow during atrial contractions. *(Reproduced with permission from Rizzo G, Arduini D, Romanini C. Am J Obstet Gynecol. 1992;166:1271–1280.)*

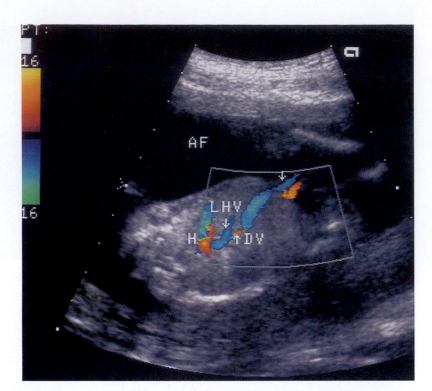

Figure 12–46. Sagittal section of the fetal body. Note that both the ductus venosus (DV) and the left hepatic vein (LHV) empty into the inferior vena cava. H, heart; AF, amniotic fluid.

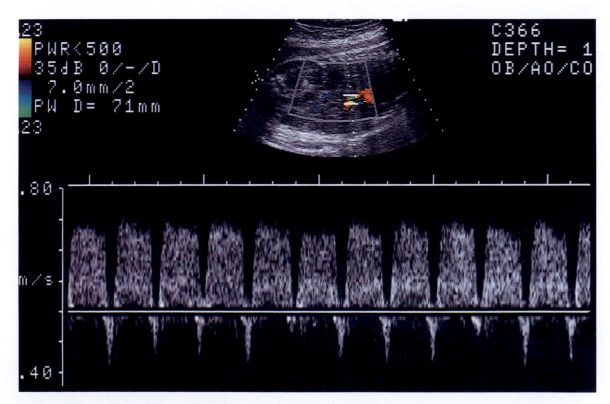

Figure 12–47. Flow velocity waveforms of the ductus venosus in a case of tricuspid atresia. Note the reverse flow in diastole. Reverse flow may be present in different situations; however, when found in fetuses with intrauterine growth restriction, it represents an ominous sign.

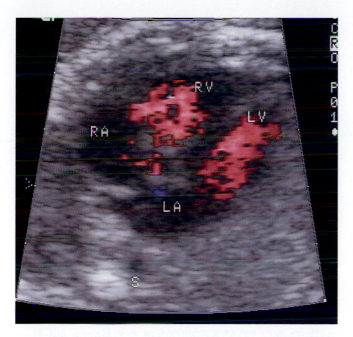

Figure 12–48. Four-chamber view of the heart. The color red indicates that the blood is flowing from the two atria to the two ventricles. RA, right atrium; LA, left atrium; RV, right ventricle; LV, left ventricle.

these conditions, Doppler ultrasound may show this redistribution by calculating the amount of blood flow through the two ventricles.[77]

RED CELL ALLOIMMUNIZATION

We previously studied the effects of intravascular transfusion (IVT) on the circulation of the anemic fetus.[87–89] The PI of eight fetal vessels were studied before, within 2 h, and the day after IVT. A significant decrease in the PI of all the vessels

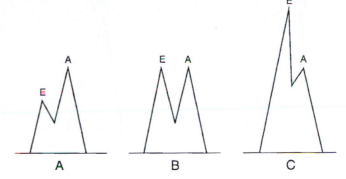

Figure 12–50. Drawing showing the AV valve early in gestation (**A**), late in gestation (**B**), and following birth (**C**).

was noted soon after transfusion, with a return to baseline the day after IVT. More recently, the effects of fetal anemia have been described on the portal venous system.[90]

The CO before and immediately after IVT has been calculated by using the formula

$$Q = TVI \times HR$$

Right-side CO was reduced by 22% and left-side CO was reduced by 19%. No alterations in heart rate were noted after IVT, leading us to deduce that stroke volume was transiently depressed.[84] These findings were confirmed by a subsequent investigation.[85]

Prediction of Fetal Hematocrit

The fetal hematocrit increases with advancing gestation. Fetal anemia is diagnosed when the hematocrit is below 2 standard deviations of the mean for gestational age.

The PI of several fetal vessels and the fetal CO are not good parameters to diagnose fetal anemia.[91,92] We have noted that the PI of the cerebral arteries can become abnormal when

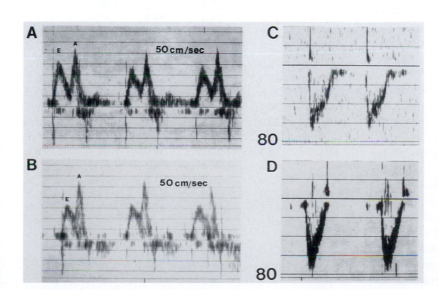

Figure 12–49. Flow velocity waveforms of the mitral (**A**), tricuspid (**B**), pulmonary (**C**), and aortic (**D**) valves. The time between two consecutive waveforms at the AV valves represents the systole, whereas the time between two consecutive waveforms at the pulmonary and aortic valves represents the diastole. There is no waveform in systole at the AV valve and no waveforms in diastole at the aortic and pulmonary valves in the normal heart.

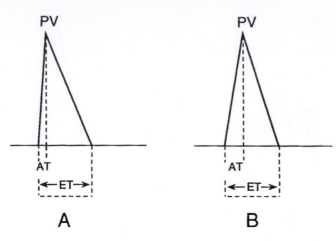

Figure 12–51. Drawing showing the acceleration time (AT) at the pulmonary valve **(A)** and at the aortic valve **(B)**. In the human fetus, the AT is shorter at the pulmonary valve. PV, peak systolic velocity; ET, ejection time.

the hematocrit is close to 10%. Under this condition, the PI of the MCA decreases, suggesting hypoxemia in the severely anemic fetus. The MCA PI in 101 cases of fetal anemia was below 2 standard deviations in seven anemic fetuses (unpublished data). In these fetuses, the hematocrit was below 15%. When anemia is severe, there is an increase of blood flow to the brain, which is reflected by a low MCA PI. However, this redistribution of blood flow does not occur in all the severely anemic fetuses and it allows recognition of only a small number of anemic fetuses.

Peak Velocity of the Middle Cerebral Artery and Fetal Anemia

In anemia the blood viscosity decreases and the blood velocity increases.[93] A correction of fetal anemia decreases fetal blood velocity. The MCA can be studied with a 0 degree angle between the ultrasound beam and the direction of blood flow. This allows the calculation of the true blood velocity at the level of the MCA. In Table 12–6 and Fig. 12–52, the normal values of the MCA peak velocity with advancing gestation are reported.

In 1990, we reported the first study that showed at the MCA, the peak systolic velocity (PSV) is a better predictor of anemia than the PI.[94] In 1993, we reported that in anemic fetuses, the MCA PSV had a sensitivity of 100% in detecting anemia secondary to red blood cell alloimmunization.[95] In 1995, we confirmed these results in a prospective study.[15] In 1997, we reported that the trend of the MCA was at least as effective as the delta optical density at 450 nanometers (ΔOD_{450}) to predict fetal anemia.[96] However, the assessment of the MCA PSV was less expensive and less invasive than amniocentesis. Figure 12–53 shows a graph that we have used since 1997 to follow fetuses at risk of anemia because of red blood cell alloimmunization. We have found this graph useful

and therefore, we do not perform amniocenteses in patients at risk for fetal anemia due to red blood cell alloimmunization. We perform a cordocentesis based only in the presence of the high velocity of the MCA PSV.

To successfully apply this model, the following steps are essential.

1. The fetus should be at risk for anemia.
2. Experienced operator.
3. Soon after the orientation of the fetus *in utero,* magnify the area of the MCA.
4. The MCA PSV has to be determined at an incident angle between the ultrasound beam and the vessel close to 0 degrees. The highest PV should be recorded (see Fig. 12–3B).

TABLE 12–6. VALUES OF THE MIDDLE CEREBRAL ARTERY PEAK VELOCITY (MCA PV) AS A FUNCTION OF GESTATIONAL AGE AT DIFFERENT MULTIPLES OF THE STANDARD ERROR OF ESTIMATION (MSEE)[a] OF THE MEAN

	MSEE				
Weeks	−2	−0.5	0	0.8	2
15	14.2	18.5	20.2	23.2	28.6
16	14.9	19.4	21.1	24.3	30.0
17	15.6	20.3	22.1	25.5	31.4
18	16.4	21.3	23.2	26.7	32.9
19	17.1	22.3	24.3	27.9	34.5
20	17.9	23.3	25.5	29.3	36.1
21	18.8	24.4	26.7	30.7	37.8
22	19.7	25.6	27.9	32.1	39.6
23	20.6	26.8	29.3	33.6	41.5
24	21.2	28.1	30.6	35.2	43.5
25	22.6	29.4	32.1	36.9	45.5
26	23.7	30.8	33.6	38.7	47.7
27	24.8	32.3	35.2	40.5	50.0
28	26.0	33.8	36.9	42.4	52.3
29	27.2	35.4	38.9	44.5	54.8
30	28.5	37.1	40.5	46.6	57.4
31	29.9	38.9	42.4	48.8	60.2
32	31.3	40.7	44.4	51.1	63.0
33	32.8	42.6	46.5	53.5	66.0
34	34.4	44.7	48.7	56.1	69.1
35	36.0	46.8	51.1	58.7	72.4
36	37.7	49.0	53.5	61.5	75.9
37	39.5	51.3	56.0	64.4	79.5
38	41.4	53.8	58.7	67.5	83.2
39	43.3	56.3	61.5	70.7	87.2
40	45.4	59.0	64.4	74.1	91.3
41	47.5	61.8	67.4	78.6	95.7
42	49.8	64.7	70.7	81.3	100

[a] MCA PV (MSEE) = [Ln MCA PV − 2.30921 − 0.0463954 × age (wks)]/ 0.174782.

Reproduced with permission from Mari G, Adrignolo A, Abuhamad AZ, et al. Ultrasound Obstet Gynecol. 1995;5:400–405.

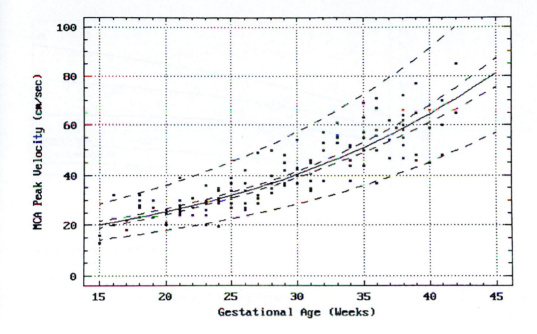

Figure 12–52. Reference range of middle cerebral artery peak velocity (MCA PV) as a function of gestational age constructed from a study of 135 normal fetuses. The *inner dotted lines* represent 95% confidence intervals and the *outer dotted lines* represent 95% prediction intervals. The values of the MCA PV are in centimeters per second. MCA PV (MSEE) = [Ln MCA PV − 2.30921 − 0.0463954 × age (wk)] 0.174782. (R^2 = 78.7). Standard error of estimation = 0.174782. MSEE, multiples of standard error of estimation. *(Reproduced with permission from Mari G, Adrignolo A, Abuhamad AZ, et al. Ultrasound Obstet Gynecol. 1995;400–405.)*

5. Sample the MCA soon after its origin from the internal carotid artery.
6. Repeat 3–5 times.

A multicenter study determined that 70% of invasive procedures (amniocentesis and cordocentesis) used to assess a fetus at risk for anemia because of maternal red blood cell alloimmunization are unnecessary (Fig. 12–54A).[97] The sensitivity of an increased peak velocity of systolic blood flow in the middle cerebral artery for the prediction of moderate or severe anemia was 100% either in the presence or absence of hydrops (95% confidence interval, 86 to 100%), with a

false positive rate of 12% (Fig. 12–54B).[97] A preliminary prospective study has confirmed these results.[98]

Similar results may be obtained while studying the splenic artery.[99] However, we have selected the MCA PV because it is easy to obtain an angle of 0 degrees between the ultrasound beam and this blood vessel and the values are highly reproducible.

Two interesting clinical cases follow.

One patient was a 26-year-old gravida 2, para 1 woman seen at 32 weeks of gestation. The pregnancy was complicated by fetal demise of one twin. The co-twin had been followed to assess growth which was normal. The UA

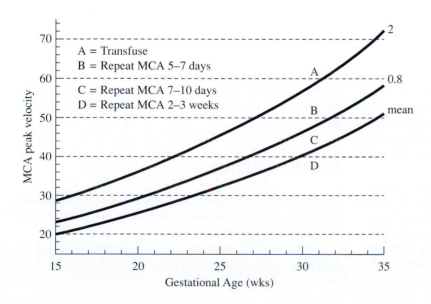

Figure 12–53. Risks zone of fetal anemia; 0.8 and 2 represent values of multiple standard error from the mean. *(Modified with permission from Mari G, Adrignolo A, Abuhamad AZ, et al. Ultrasound Obstet Gynecol. 1995;5:400–405.)*

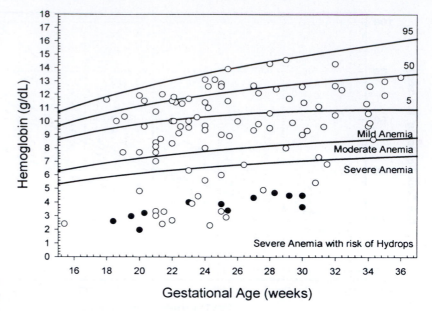

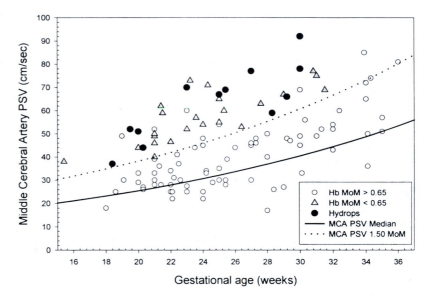

Figure 12–54. (A) Hemoglobin concentrations in 111 fetuses that underwent cordocentesis because they were at risk of anemia. The reference range in the normal fetuses was between 0.84 and 1.16 times the median (corresponding to the 5th and 95th percentiles). Values for the 111 fetuses that underwent cordocentesis are plotted individually. *Solid circles* indicate fetuses with hydrops. *(Reproduced with permission from Mari G et al. N Engl J Med. 2000;343:66–68).* **(B)** Peak velocity of systolic blood flow in the middle cerebral artery in 111 fetuses at risk for anemia due to maternal red-cell alloimmunization. *Open circles* indicate fetuses with either no anemia or mild anemia (≥0.65 multiples of the median hemoglobin concentration). *Triangles* indicate fetuses with moderate or severe anemia (<0.65 multiples of the median hemoglobin concentration). The *solid circles* indicate the fetuses with hydrops. The *solid curve* indicates the median peak systolic velocity in the middle cerebral artery, and the dotted curve indicates 1.5 multiples of the median. *(Reproduced with permission from Mari G et al. N Engl J Med. 2000;342:9–14).*

velocimetry was normal. The MCA PSV (116 cm per second) was above the normal range. The patient was RH negative and had received RhoGAM. In few days, the fetus developed ascites. At delivery the fetal hematocrit was 12%. The diagnosis was Rh alloimmunization. The infant was transfused and did well.

The second patient had an uncomplicated pregnancy until 36 weeks of gestation, when she presented to the labor floor because of decreased fetal movement. A nonstress test showed a sinusoidal pattern. The ultrasound was normal. The UA PI was normal. The MCA had a velocity value of 111 cm per second. A cesarean delivery was performed and

a female infant was delivered. The hematocrit was 7%. The diagnosis was fetal-to-maternal transfusion. The infant did well.

MULTIPLE GESTATION

For the study of the UA in twins, pulsed Doppler ultrasound is required because continuous Doppler does not distinguish between the UAs of the twins.

Giles et al.[100] reported that the S/D ratio of the UA in twin pregnancies, where both twins are AGA, showed close

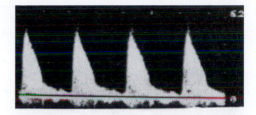

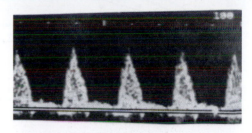

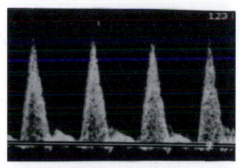

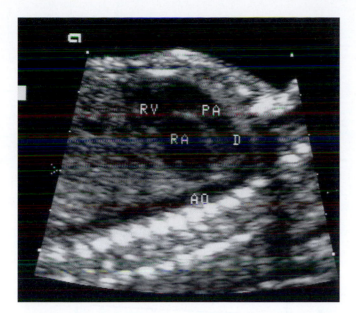

Figure 12–55. Sagittal section of fetal body. PA, pulmonary artery; D, ductus arteriosus; AO, descending aorta; RA, right atrium; RV, right ventricle.

agreement with the singleton pregnancy results in the third trimester.

Umbilical Artery Flow Velocity Waveforms and Perinatal Outcome in Twins

Gaziano et al.[101] reported that twins with an abnormal UA FVW tended to be born 3 to 4 weeks earlier and exhibited a greater number of stillbirths and structural malformations and greater morbidity when compared with fetuses without abnormal Doppler results.

Giles et al.[100] studied 272 twin pregnancies. When information from Doppler ultrasound of the UA was made available to the referring obstetricians, thereby influencing clinical management, they noted a decrease in perinatal mortality and a reduction in the number of infants requiring admission to the intensive care nursery.

Umbilical Artery Flow Velocity Waveforms in Discordant Twins

Discordant growth in twin gestation can result from placental crowding, twin-to-twin-transfusion syndrome, a poor placental implantation site, or chromosomal anomalies. This condition is associated with a significant increase in perinatal morbidity and mortality.

The diagnosis of discordant twins is made mainly with ultrasound. Divon et al.[102] compared intertwin differences in ultrasonographically derived fetal weight, biparietal diameter, abdominal circumference, femur length, and UA S/D ratio. They reported that the best predictor for diagnosis of

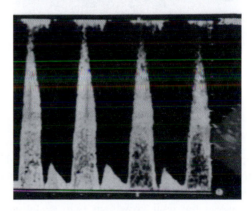

Figure 12–56. Flow velocity waveforms of the ductus arteriosus from 15 weeks of gestation *(top)* to term *(bottom). (Reproduced with permission from Mari G, Deter RL, Uerpairojkit B.* J Clin Ultrasound. *1996;24:185–196.)*

discordant twins appeared to be the presence of either a difference in S/D ratio greater than 15% or a different estimated fetal weight greater than 15%. They correctly identified 14 of the 18 discordant twins.

Degani et al.[103] reported that changes in the Doppler of the internal carotid artery and UA preceded sonographic diagnosis of small-for-gestational-age fetuses by a mean interval of 3.7 weeks and demonstrated better sensitivity and specificity.

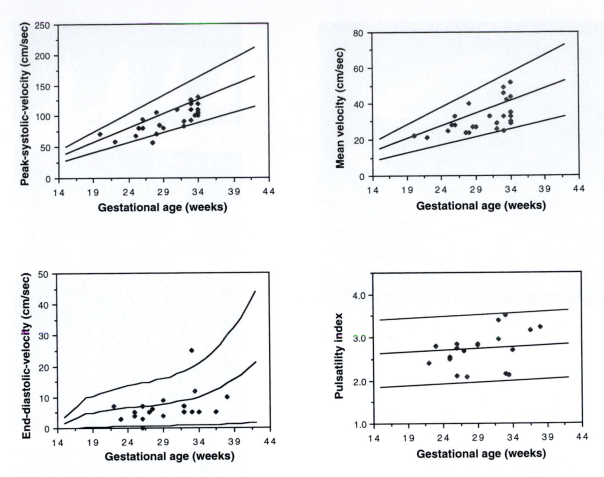

Figure 12–57. Reference of the fetal ductus arteriosus velocity waveforms (5th and 95th percentiles) during gestation. The dots indicate values in IUGR fetuses. *(Reproduced with permission from Mari G, Deter RL, Uerpairojkit B.* J Clin Ultrasound. *1996;24:185–196.)*

Recently, it has been reported that abnormal UA velocimetry can be observed in small twins more often in monochorionic than dichorionic twins.[104]

We assess the fetal growth in twin gestations every 4 weeks. We also assess the UA in twin gestation because, in case of an abnormal UA, we intensify fetal surveillance.

Doppler Ultrasound in Twin-to-Twin Transfusion Syndrome

Several fetal vessels have been studied in pregnancies complicated by twin-to-twin transfusion syndrome.[105,106] Doppler ultrasound of the UA in either twin is associated with poor perinatal outcome.[107]

It appears that the study of the UA FVW in twin gestations may be useful to diagnose discordant twins, decrease perinatal mortality, reduce the number of infants requiring newborn special care unit admission, and predict the out-come in pregnancies complicated twin-to-twin transfusion syndrome.

DUCTUS ARTERIOSUS

The fetal ductus arteriosus is a muscular tube connecting the main pulmonary artery to the descending aorta immediately distal to the left subclavian artery (Fig. 12–55). It has an important role during fetal life when 60 to 65% of the combined CO passes through the ductus arteriosus.[108] and it normally closes shortly after birth. The ductal arch is usually visualized in sagittal scans and the entire arch can be examined with either pulsed Doppler, with a sample volume of at least 5 mm, or continuous wave Doppler because the velocity at different parts of the ductus are different and the area of interest is generally that portion with the highest velocity. Velocity at the ductus is usually the highest obtained in fetal circulation.

In the normal human fetus, ductal velocity increases with advancing gestation (Fig. 12–56) and the study of ductus arteriosus FVWs is not useful in IUGR fetuses (Fig. 12–57).[109]

Indomethacin and Ductus Arteriosus

Indomethacin, a prostaglandin synthetase inhibitor, has been used in the management of preterm labor and polyhydramnios. Additional use of this medication has been limited, mainly over concern of its possible constricitive effect on the fetal ductus arteriosus. *In utero* closure of the ductus arteriosus causes increased pulmonary blood flow and may result in neonatal pulmonary hypertension, shunting of blood through the foramen ovale, and ultimately persistent circulation after birth.

It has been shown that indomethacin causes constriction of the ductus arteriosus and tricuspid insufficiency in the human fetus.[110,111] This effect is readily reversible. In our experience, 50% of the fetuses exposed to indomethacin do not have any effect on the ductus arteriosus. In these fetuses, however, the human fetal pulmonary arterial vascular impedance is increased by maternal indomethacin therapy even without ductal constriction.[112]

We propose the following classification to define ductal constriction (Figs. 12–58 and 12–59).

Mild Constriction (20% of Patients Treated with Indomethacin). The PV of the ductus arteriosus increases with respect to baseline value. The EDV remains constant.

Moderate Constriction (20% of Patients Treated with Indomethacin). The PV and EDV of the ductus arteriosus increase above baseline values. There is absence of tricuspid insufficiency.

Severe Constriction (10% of Patients Treated with Indomethacin). In our experience, after indomethacin therapy, there is at first an increase of the ductus PSV, which is followed by an increase of EDV. Of note is the following observation: when the EDV is greater than 100 to 120 cm per second, tricuspid insufficiency is often present (Fig. 12–59).

In our experience with more than 100 fetuses treated with indomethacin, the discontinuation of the drug is followed by a return to normal of the Doppler ductal parameters in the next 36 hours.

The reason why only 50% of the fetuses develop ductal constriction may be due to different sensitivities to indomethacin. In addition, gestational age plays an important role. For example, we have never seen severe ductal constriction before 22 weeks of gestation. The interaction between ductal constriction and the other neonatal complications of fetal indomethacin exposure requires further investigation.

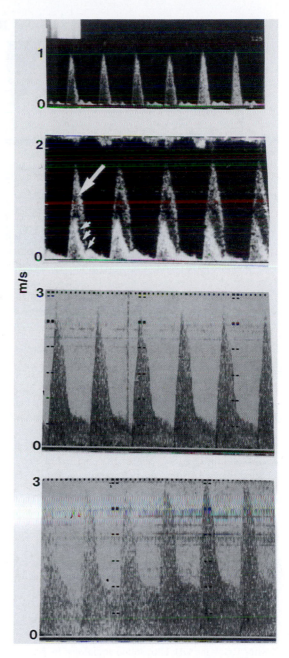

Figure 12–58. Flow velocity of the fetal ductus arteriosus before *(top)* and after indomethacin (see text). The *large arrow* points to the waveform of the ductus arteriosus, whereas the three *small arrows* point to the waveform of the pulmonary artery. This may be obtained either with a continuous Doppler or by enlarging the sample volume. On the *y* axis, the velocity is indicated in meters per second.

m/s

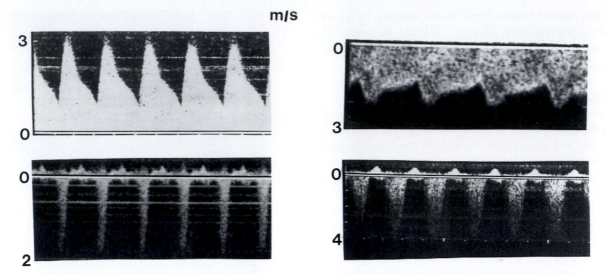

Figure 12–59. Flow velocity waveforms of the ductus arteriosus *(top)* and presence of tricuspid regurgitation *(bottom)*. The velocity is indicated in meters per second.

REFERENCES

1. Allfirevic Z, Neilson JP. Doppler ultrasonography in high risk pregnancies: Systematic review with meta-analysis. *Am J Obstet Gynecol.* 1995;172:1379–1387.

2. Almstrom H, Axelsson O, Cnattingius S, et al. Comparison of umbilical artery velocimetry and cardiotocography for surveillance of small for gestational age fetuses. *Lancet.* 1992;340:936–940.

3. American College of Obstetrics and Gynecology (ACOG). Utility of antepartum umbilical artery Doppler velocimetry in intrauterine growth retardation. Committee Opinion No. 188, ACOG, November 1997.

4. Stuart B, Drumm J, FitzGerald DE, et al. Fetal blood velocity waveforms in normal pregnancy. *Br J Obstet Gynaecol.* 1980;87:780–785.

5. Pourcelot L. Application cliniques de l'examen Doppler transcutane. In: Perronneau P, ed. *Velocimetrie ultrasonoré Doppler.* Paris: Seminaire INSERM; 1974:213–240.

6. Gosling RG, King DH. Ultrasound angiology. In: Marcus AW, Adamson L, eds. *Arteries and Veins.* New York: Churchill-Livingstone; 1975:61–98.

7. Milnor WR, Pulsatile blood flow. *N Engl J Med.* 1972;287:27–34.

8. Mari G, Deter RL. Middle cerebral artery flow velocity waveforms in normal and small for gestational age fetuses. *Am J Obstet Gynecol.* 1992;166:1262–1270.

9. Maulik D, Yarlagadda AP, Youngblood JP, et al. Components of variability of umbilical arterial Doppler velocimetry: A prospective analysis. *Am J Obstet Gynecol.* 1989;160:1406–1412.

10. FitzGerald DE, Drumm J. Noninvasive measurements of human fetal circulation using ultrasound: A new method. *Br Med J.* 1977;ii:1450–1451.

11. Thompson RS, Trudinger BJ, Cook CM. Doppler ultrasound waveform indices: AB ratio, pulsatility index and Pourcelot ratio. *Br J Obstet Gynaecol.* 1988;95:589–591.

12. Trudinger BJ, Stevens D, Connelly A, et al. Umbilical artery flow velocity waveforms and placental resistance: The effects of embolization of the umbilical circulation. *Am J Obstet Gynecol.* 1987;157:1443–1449.

13. Trudinger BJ, Giles WB, Cook CM, et al. Fetal umbilical artery flow velocity waveforms and placental resistance: Clinical significance. *Br J Obstet Gynaecol.* 1985;92:23–30.

14. Mari G, Moise JK, Deter RL, et al. Doppler assessment of the pulsatility index in the cerebral circulation of the human fetus. *Am J Obstet Gynecol.* 1989;160:698–703.

15. Mari G, Adrignolo A, Abuhamad AZ, et al. The diagnosis of fetal anemia with Doppler ultrasound in the pregnancy complicated by Rhesus-isoimmunization. *Ultrasound Obstet Gynecol.* 1995;5:400–405.

16. Dobbing J, Sands J. Timing of neuroblast multiplication in developing human brain. *Nature.* 1970;226:639–640.

17. Fleischer A, Schulman H, Farmakides G, et al. Umbilical velocity wave ratios in intrauterine growth retardation. *Am J Obstet Gynecol.* 1985;151:502–506.

18. Devoe LD, Gardner P, Dear C, et al. The significance of increasing umbilical artery systolic-diastolic ratios in third-trimester pregnancy. *Obstet Gynecol.* 1992;80:684–687.

19. Rochelson BL, Schulman H, Fleischer A, et al. The clinical significance of Doppler umbilical artery velocimetry in the small for gestational age fetus. *Am J Obstet Gynecol.* 1987;156:1223–1226.

20. Trudinger BJ, Cook CM, Giles WB. Fetal umbilical artery velocity waveforms and subsequent neonatal outcome. *Br J Obstet Gynaecol.* 1991;98:378–384.

21. Gudmundsson S, Marsal K. Umbilical and uteroplacental blood flow velocity waveforms in pregnancies with fetal growth retardation. *Eur J Obstet Gynecol Reprod Biol.* 1988;27:187–196.

22. Cohn HE, Sacks EJ, Heymann MA, et al. Cardiovascular responses to hypoxemia and acidemia in fetal lambs. *Am J Obstet Gynecol.* 1974;120:817–814.

23. Marsal K, Lingman G, Giles W. Evaluation of the carotid, aortic and umbilical blood velocity (abstract C33). In: *Proceedings of the Eleventh Annual Conference of the Society for the Study of Fetal Physiology.* Oxford: 1984.

24. Wladimiroff JW, Tonge HM, Stewart PA. Doppler ultrasound assessment of the cerebral blood flow in the human fetus. *Br J Obstet Gynecol.* 1986;93:471–475.

25. Richardson BS, Rurak D, Patrick JE, et al. Cerebral oxidative metabolism during sustained hypoxemia in fetal sheep. *J Dev Physiol.* 1989;11:37–43.

26. Mari G, Wasserstrum N. Flow velocity waveforms of the fetal circulation preceedings fetal demise in a case of lupus anticoagulant. *Am J Obstet Gynecol.* 1991;164:776–778.

27. Vyas S, Nicolaides KH, Bower S, et al. Middle cerebral artery flow velocity waveforms in fetal hypoxemia. *Br J Obstet Gynaecol.* 1990;97:797–803.

28. Sepulveda W, Peek MJ. Reverse end-diastolic flow in the middle cerebral artery: An agonal pattern in the human fetus. *Am J Obstet Gynecol.* 1996;174:1645–1647.

29. Chandran R, Serra Serra V, Sellers SM, et al. Fetal middle cerebral artery flow velocity wavefroms—A terminal pattern. Case report. *Br J Obstet Gynaecol.* 1991;98:937–938.

30. Respondek M, Woch A, Kaczmarek P, et al. Reversal of diastolic flow in the middle cerebral artery of the fetus during the second half of the pregnancy. *Ultrasound Obstet Gynecol.* 1997;9:324–329.

31. Vyas S, Campbell S, Bower S, et al. Maternal abdominal pressure alters fetal cerebral blood flow. *Br J Obstet Gynaecol.* 1990;97:740–747.

32. Gramellini D, Folli MC, Raboni S, et al. Cerebral–umbilical Doppler ratio as a predictor of adverse perinatal outcome. *Obstet Gynecol.* 1992;79:416–420.

33. Bahado-Singh R, Kovanci E, Jeffres A, Oz U, et al. The Doppler cerebroplacental ratio and perinatal outcome in intrauterine growth restriction. *Am J Obstet Gynecol.* 1999;180: 750–756.

34. Brosens I, Robertson WB, Dixon HG. The role of the spiral arteries in the pathogenesis of preeclampsia. *Obstet Gynecol Ann.* 1972;1:177–191.

35. Brosens I, Dixon HG, Robertson WB. Fetal growth retardation and the arteries of the placental bed. *Br J Obstet Gynecol.* 1977;84:656–663.

36. Mari G, Abuhamad AZ, Keller M, et al. Is the fetal brain sparing effect a risk factor for the development of IVH in the premature infant? *Ultrasound Obstet Gynecol.* 1996;8:329–332.

37. Gudmundsson S, Tulzer G, Huhta JC, et al. Venous Doppler in the fetus with absent end-diastolic flow in the umbilical artery. *Ultrasound Obstet Gynecol.* 1996;7:262–267.

38. Kurkinen-Raty M, Kivela A, Jouppila P. The clinical significance of an absent end-diastolic velocity in the umbilical artery detected before the 34th week of pregnancy. *Acta Obstet Gynecol Scand.* 1997;76:398–404.

39. Marsal K, Persson PH. Ultrasonic measurement of fetal blood velocity wave form as a secondary diagnostic test in screening for intrauterine growth retardation. *J Clin Ultrasound.* 1988;16:239–244.

40. Yoon BH, Romero R, Roh CR, et al. Relationship between the fetal biophysical profile score, umbilical artery Doppler velocimetry, and fetal bleed acid–base status determined by cordocentesis. *Am J Obstet Gynecol.* 1993;169:1586–1594.

41. Hecher K, Hackeloer BJ. Cardiotocogram compared to Doppler investigation of the fetal circulation in the premature growth-restricted fetus: Longitudinal observation. *Ultrasound Obstet Gynecol.* 1997;9:152–161.

42. Hata T, Manabe A, Hata K, et al. Fetal circulatory system in growth-retarded fetus with late decelerations and oligohydramnios. *Gynecol Obstet Invest.* 1994;37:96–98.

43. Lingman G, Marsal K. Fetal central blood circulation in the third trimester of normal pregnancy: A longitudinal study: I. Aortic and umbilical blood flow. *Early Hum Dev.* 1986;13: 137–150.

44. Eik-Nes SH, Brubaak AO, Ulstein MK. Measurement of human fetal blood flow. *Br Med J.* 1980;280:283–284.

45. Mari G. Arterial blood flow velocity waveforms of the pelvis and lower extremities in normal and growth-retarded fetuses. *Am J Obstet Gynecol.* 1991;165:143–151.

46. Abuhamad AZ, Mari G, Bogdan D, et al. Splenic artery flow velocity waveforms in appropriate and small-for-gestational-age fetuses. *Am J Obstet Gynecol.* 1995;172:820–825.

47. Finne PH, Halvorsen S. Regulation of erythropoiesis in the fetus and newborn. *Arch Dis Child.* 1972;47:683–687.

48. Fischer JW. Control of erythropoietin production. *Proc Soc Exp Biol Med.* 1984;173:289–305.

49. Abuhamad A, Mari G, Cortina R, et al. Superior mesenteric artery Doppler velocimetry and ultrasonographic assessment of fetal bowel in gastroschisis: A prospective longitudinal study. *Am J Obstet Gynecol.* 1997;176:985–990.

50. Rhee E, Detti L, Mari G. Superior mesenteric artery flow velocity waveforms in small for gestational age fetuses. *J Matern Fetal Med.* 1998;7:120–123.

51. Mari G, Uerpairojkit B, Abuhamad A, et al. Adrenal artery velocity waveforms in the appropriate and small-for-gestational-age fetus. *Ultrasound Obstet Gynecol.* 1996;8:82–86.

52. Vyas S, Nicolaides KH, Campbell S. Renal flow-velocity waveforms in normal and hypoxemic fetuses. *Am J Obstet Gynecol.* 1989;161:168–172.

53. Mari G, Kirshon B, Abuhamad A. Fetal renal artery flow velocity waveforms in normal pregnancies and pregnancies complicated by polyhydramnios and oligohydramnios. *Obstet Gynecol.* 1993;81:560–564.

54. Uerpairojkit B, Chan L, Reece AE, et al. Cerebellar Doppler velocimetry in the appropriate and small-for-gestational-age fetus. *Obstet Gynecol.* 1996;87:995–999.

55. Baschat AA, Gembruch U. Examination of fetal coronary sinus blood flow by Doppler ultrasound. *Ultrasound Obstet Gynecol.* 1998;11:410–414.

56. Laurichesse-Delmas H, Grimaud O, Moscoso G, et al. Color Doppler study of the venous circulation in the fetal brain and hemodynamic study of the cerebral transverse sinus. *Ultrasound Obstet Gynecol.* 1999;13:34–42.

57. Yoshimura S, Masuzaki H, Miura K, et al. Diagnosis of fetal pulmonary hypoplasia by measurement of blood flow velocity waveforms of pulmonary arteries with Doppler ultrasonography. *Am J Obstet Gynecol.* 1999;180:441–446.

58. Rudolph A. Distribution and regulation of blood flow in the fetal and neonatal circulation. *Circ Res.* 1985;57:811–821.

59. Edelstone DI, Rudolph AM, Heymann MA. Liver and ductus venosus blood flows in fetal lamb in utero. *Circ Res.* 1977;42: 426–433.

60. Splunder IP, Huisman TWA, Stijnen T, et al. Presence of

pulsations and reproducibility of waveform recording in the umbilical and left portal vein in normal pregnancies. *Ultrasound Obstet Gynecol.* 1994;4:49–53.

61. Mari G, Uerpairojkit B, Copel JA. Abdominal venous system of the normal fetus. *Obstet Gynecol.* 1995;86:729–733.

62. Reed KL, Appleton CP, Anderson CF, et al. Doppler studies of vena cava flows in human fetuses. *Circulation.* 1990;81:498–505.

63. Rizzo G, Arduini D, Romanini C. Inferior vena cava flow velocity waveforms in appropriate-and small-for-gestational-age fetuses. *Am J Obstet Gynecol.* 1992;166:1271–1280.

64. Kiserud T, Eik-Nes SH, Blaas H-GK, et al. Ultrasonographic velocimetry of the fetal ductus venosus. *Lancet.* 1991;338:1412–1414.

65. Rizzo G, Arduini D, Romanini C. Umbilical vein pulsations: A physiologic finding in early gestation. *Am J Obstet Gynecol.* 1992;167:675–677.

66. Nakai Y, Miyazaki Y, Matsuoka Y. Pulsatile umbilical venous flow and its clinical significance. *Br J Obstet Gynecol.* 1992;99:977–980.

67. Goncalves LF, Romero R, Silva M, et al. Reverse flow in the ductus venosus: An ominous sign (abstract 33). *Am J Obstet Gynecol.* 1995;172:266.

68. Ozcan T, Sbracia M, Levi-d'Ancona R, et al. Arterial and venous Doppler velocimetry in the severely growth restricted fetus and associations with adverse perinatal outcome. *Ultrasound Obstet Gynecol.* 1998;12:39–44.

69. Baz E, Zikulnig L, Hackleloer BJ, et al. Abnormal ductus venosus blood flow: A clue to umbilical cord complication. *Ultrasound Obstet Gynecol.* 1999;13:204–206.

70. Hofstaetter C, Gudmundsson S, Dubiel M, et al. Ductus venosus velocimetry in high-risk pregnancies. *Eur J Obstet Gynecol Reprod Biol.* 1996;70:135–140.

71. Reed KL, Anderson CF, Shenker L. Changes in intracardiac Doppler blood flow velocities in fetuses with absent umbilical artery diastolic flow. *Am J Obstet Gynecol.* 1987;157:774–779.

72. Rizzo G, Arduini D, Romanini C, et al. Doppler echocardiographic assessment of atrioventricular velocity waveforms in normal and small-for-gestational-age fetuses. *Br J Obstet Gynaecol.* 1988;95:65–69.

73. Shapiro I, Degani S, Leibowitz Z, et al. Fetal cardiac measurements derived by transvaginal and transabdominal cross-sectional echocardiography from 14 weeks of gestation to term. *Ultrasound Obstet Gynecol.* 1998;12:404–418.

74. Fouron JC, Carceller AM. Determinants of the Doppler flow velocity profile through the mitral valve of the human fetus. *Br Heart J.* 1993;70:457–460.

75. Hata T, Hata K, Takamiya O, et al. Fetal ventricular relaxation assessed by Doppler echocardiography. *J Cardiovasc Ultrasonogr.* 1988;7:207–213.

76. Kenny JP, Plappert T, Doubilet P, et al. Changes in intracardiac blood flow velocities and right and left ventricular stroke volumes with gestational age in the normal human fetus: A prospective Doppler echocardiographic study. *Circulation.* 1986;74:1208–1216.

77. Al-Ghazali W, Chita SK, Chapman MG, et al. Evidence of redistribution of cardiac output in asymmetrical growth retardation. *Br J Obstet Gynaecol.* 1989;96:697–704.

78. Machado MVL, Chita SC, Allan LD. Acceleration time in the aorta and pulmonary artery measured by Doppler echocardiog-

raphy in the midtrimester normal human fetus. *Br Heart J.* 1987;58:15–18.

79. Kitabatake A, Inoue M, Asao M, et al. Non-invasive evaluation of pulmonary hypertension by pulsed Doppler technique. *Circulation.* 1983;68:302–309.

80. DeSmedt MCH, Visser GHA, Meijboom EJ. Fetal cardiac output estimated by Dopler echocardiography during mid- and late gestation. *Am J Cardiol.* 1987;87:338–342.

81. Allan LD, Chita SK, Al-Ghazali W, et al. Doppler echocardiograpic evaluation of the normal human fetal heart. *Br Heart J.* 1987;57:528–533.

82. Shiraishi H, Silverman NH, Rudolph AM. Accuracy of right ventricular output estimated by Doppler echocardiography in the sheep fetus. *Am J Obstet Gynecol.* 1993;168:947–953.

83. Mari G, Kirshon B, Moise KJ, et al. Doppler assessment of the fetal and uteroplacental circulation during nifedipine therapy for preterm labor. *Am J Obstet Gynecol.* 1989;161:1514–1518.

84. Moise JK, Mari G, Fisher DJ, et al. Acute fetal hemodynamic alterations after intrauterine transfusion for severe red cell alloimmunization. *Am J Obstet Gynecol.* 1990;163:776–784.

85. Rizzo G, Nicolaides KH, Arduini D, et al. Effects of intravascular fetal blood transfusion on fetal intracardiac Doppler velocity waveforms. *Am J Obstet Gynecol.* 1990;163:1231–1238.

86. Gonzalez R, Medina L, Arriagada P, et al. Transdermal administration of a nitric oxide donor is not associated with changes in major fetal cardiac and systemic hemodynamic parameters. *Am J Obstet Gynecol.* 1999;180:S3.

87. Mari G, Moise KJ, Deter RL, et al. Flow velocity waveforms of the umbilical and cerebral arteries before and after intravascular transfusion. *Obstet Gynecol.* 1990;75:584–589.

88. Mari G, Moise KJ, Deter RL, et al. Flow velocity waveforms of the vascular system in the anemic fetus before and after intravascular transfusion for severe red cell alloimmunization. *Am J Obstet Gynecol.* 1990;162:1060–1064.

89. Mari G, Moise KJ, Deter RL, et al. Doppler ultrasound assessment of the renal blood flow velocity waveforms in the anemic fetus before and after intravascular transfusion for severe red cell alloimmunization. *J Clin Ultrasound.* 1991;19:15–19.

90. Levi-d'Ancona R, Rahman F, Ozcan T, et al. The effect of intravascular blood transfusion on the flow velocity waveforms of the portal venous system of the anemic fetus. *Ultrasound Obstet Gynecol.* 1997;10:333–337.

91. Copel JA, Grannum PA, Green JJ, et al. Fetal cardiac output in the isoimmunized pregnancy: A pulsed Doppler-echocardiographic study of patients undergoing intravascular intrauterine transfusion. *Am J Obstet Gynecol.* 1989;161:361–365.

92. Nicolaides KH, Bilardo CM, Campbell S. Prediction of fetal anemia by measurement of the mean blood velocity in the fetal aorta. *Am J Obstet Gynecol.* 1990;162:209–212.

93. Mari G, Rahman F, Oloffson et al. Increase of fetal hematocrit decreases the middle cerebral artery peak systolic velocity in pregnancies complicated by rhesus alloimmunization. *J Matern Fetal Med.* 1997;6:206–208.

94. Mari G, Moise JK, Kirshon B, et al. Middle cerebral artery pulsatility index and maximal velocity as indicators of fetal anemia. Proceedings of the Society for Gynecologic Investigation, St. Louis, March 1990.

95. Mari G, Adrignolo A, Abuhamad A, et al. Doppler ultrasound in the management of the pregnancy complicated by fetal anemia. *Am J Obstet Gynecol.* 1993;168:318.

96. Mari G, Penso C, Sbracia M, et al. Delta OD 450 and Doppler velocimetry of the middle cerebral artery peak velocity in the evaluation for fetal alloimmune hemolytic disease. Which is the best? *Am J Obstet Gynecol.* 1997;176:S18.

97. Mari G. For the Collaborative group for Doppler assessment of the blood velocity in anemic fetuses. Noninvasive diagnosis by Doppler ultrasonography of fetal anemia due to maternal red-cell alloimmunization. *N Engl J Med.* 2000;342:9–14.

98. Mari G. For the Collaborative group for Doppler assessment of the blood velocity in anemic fetuses. Noninvasive multinational alternative to cordocentesis for detection of fetal anemia—A prospective trial. Proceedings, Society of Maternal-Fetal Medicine. Miami, January 2000. *Am J Obstet Gynecol.* 2000;182:S21.

99. Bahado-Singh R, Oz U, Kovanchi E, et al. Main splenic artery peak systolic velocity (PSV): A strong predictor of severe fetal anemia due to Rh-alloimmunization. *Am J Obstet Gynecol.* 1999;180:S20.

100. Giles WB, Trudinger BJ, Cook CM, et al. Umbilical artery flow velocity waveforms and twin pregnancy outcome. *Obstet Gynecol.* 1988;72:894–897.

101. Gaziano EP, Knox H, Ferrera B, et al. Is it time to reassess the risk for the growth-retarded fetus with normal Doppler velocimetry of the umbilical artery? *Am J Obstet Gynecol.* 1994;170:1734–1743.

102. Divon MY, Girz BA, Sklar A, et al. Discordant twins: A prospective study of the diagnostic value of real-time ultrasonography combined with umbilical artery velocimetry. *Am J Obstet Gynecol.* 1989;161:757–760.

103. Degani S, Gonen R, Shapiro I, et al. Doppler flow velocity waveforms in fetal surveillance of twins: A prospective longitudinal study. *J Ultrasound Med.* 1992;11:537–541.

104. Gaziano E, Gaziano C, Brandt D. Doppler velocimetry determined redistribution of fetal blood flow: Correlation with growth restriction in diamniotic monochorionic and dizygotic twins. *Am J Obstet Gynecol.* 1998;178:1359–1367.

105. Mari G, Abuhamad A, Soper R, et al. Doppler ultrasound in the pregnancy complicated by polyhydramnios–oligohydramnios twins (abstract 470). *Am J Obstet Gynecol.* 1994;170:405.

106. Hecher K, Ville Y, Nicolaides KH. Fetal arterial Doppler studies in twin–twin transfusion syndrome. *J Ultrasound Med.* 1995;14:101–108.

107. Mari G. Amnioreduction in twin–twin transfusion syndrome—A multicenter registry, evaluation of 579 procedures. *Am J Obstet Gynecol.* 1998;178:S65.

108. Rudolph AM, Heymann MA. Circulatory changes during growth in the fetal lamb. *Circ Res.* 1970;26:289–299.

109. Mari G, Deter RL, Uerpairojkit B. Flow velocity waveforms of the ductus arteriosus in appropriate and small-for-gestational-age fetuses. *J Clin Ultrasound.* 1996;24:185–196.

110. Huhta JC, Moise JK, Fisher DJ, et al. Detection and quantification of constricition of the fetal ductus arteriosus by Doppler echocardiography. *Circulation.* 1987;75:406–412.

111. Mari G, Moise KJ, Deter RL, et al. Doppler assessment of the pulsatility index of the middle cerebral artery during constriction of the fetal ductus arteriosus following indomethacin therapy. *Am J Obstet Gynecol.* 1989;161:1528–1531.

112. Rasanem J, Debbs RH, Wood DC, et al. The effects of maternal indomethacin therapy on human fetal branch pulmonary arterial vascular impedance. *Ultrasound Obstet Gynecol.* 1999;13:112–116.

13

Doppler Velocimetry of the Uteroplacental Circulation

Luís F. Gonçalves • Roberto Romero • Maria-Teresa Gervasi • Eli Maymon • Percy Pacora • Gianluigi Pilu

Doppler velocimetry of the uteroplacental circulation has been proposed as a screening test to identify women at high risk for the development of preeclampsia and small-for-gestational-age (SGA) fetuses. Prophylaxis of preeclampsia with aspirin and/or nitric oxide (NO) donors to high-risk patients identified on the basis of abnormal uterine artery Doppler flow velocity waveforms (FVWs) has been attempted with varying degrees of success. In this chapter, we review the anatomy and development of the uteroplacental circulation, the pathologic changes associated with placental implantation failure, the rationale for using Doppler velocimetry to detect these changes, and the studies proposing the use of prophylactic agents to prevent preeclampsia and abnormal perinatal outcome in patients with abnormal uterine artery Doppler FVWs.

ANATOMY AND DEVELOPMENT OF THE UTEROPLACENTAL CIRCULATION

Blood supply to the uterus is provided by the uterine and ovarian arteries. The uterine arteries are branches of the internal iliac artery. Upon reaching the isthmic portion of the uterus, they ascend through the lateral wall before anastomosing with the ovarian arteries at the cornu of the uterus (Fig. 13–1).[1] Blood supply to the anterior and posterior walls is provided by the arcuate arteries, which run circumferentially around the uterus. Radial branches extend from the arcuate arteries at right angles toward the endometrium, where they divide into two or more spiral arteries (Fig. 13–2).[2–6]

During pregnancy, approximately 100 spiral arteries connect the maternal circulation to the intervillous space.[2] These vessels undergo important physiologic modifications to accommodate the 10-fold increase in blood flow necessary to meet the metabolic requirements of the fetus and placenta. During the first trimester, a first wave of endovascular trophoblast invades the walls of the spiral arteries in the decidua, stopping at the decidual–myometrial junction at about 15 weeks. During the second trimester, a second wave of endovascular trophoblast invades the myometrial segment of the spiral arteries, interacts with terminal segment of the radial arteries, and replaces their musculoelastic wall tissue with a mixture of fibrinoid and fibrous tissue.[3] The conversion of small muscular spiral arteries into large vascular channels transforms the uteroplacental

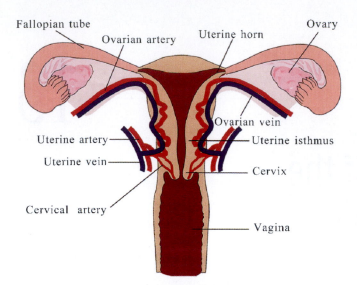

Figure 13–1. Blood supply to the uterus. *(Reproduced with permission from Cuningham FG, MacDonald PC, Gant NF, et al. In: Cuningham FG, MacDonald PC, Leveno K, Gilstrap LC II, eds. Williams Obstetrics. Norwalk, CT: Appleton & Lange; 1993:57–79.)*

circulation from a high resistance into a low resistance vascular system.

In pregnancies complicated by preeclampsia and/or SGA fetuses, trophoblastic invasion is almost completely restricted to the decidual segment of the spiral arteries, with little or no evidence of invasion beyond the decidual–myometrial junction. Failure of normal trophoblastic invasion beyond 24 to 26 weeks results in high impedance to blood flow in the uteroplacental circulation and is associated with the development of preeclampsia later in pregnancy. Doppler velocimetry of the uterine arteries has the potential to detect high impedance to blood flow and, thus, to identify patients at risk for the development of preeclampsia and SGA.[4-10]

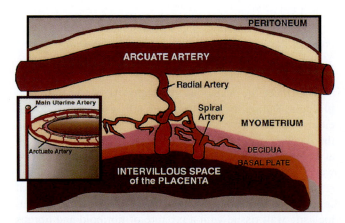

Figure 13–2. Blood supply to the endometrium. *(Reproduced with permission from Brosens I, Robertson WB, Dixon HG. J Obstet Gynecol Br Commonw. 1966;73:357–63.)*

INSTRUMENTATION AND EXAMINATION TECHNIQUE

Both continuous-wave (CW) and pulsed-wave (PW) Doppler have been employed in the study of the uteroplacental circulation. Continuous-wave Doppler has the advantage of being less expensive, but it does not allow visualization of the vessels being sampled. Therefore, the waveform must be identified by pattern recognition, also known as "audio *vessel signature*," raising concerns about the reproducibility of the method. This issue has been addressed in a study of 35 normal pregnancies between 20 and 40 weeks, in which the right uterine artery was evaluated with CW and PW Doppler by the same investigator, to reduce inter-observed variation.[11] No difference was observed between systolic-to-diastolic (S/D) ratios obtained with either CW or PW Doppler (2.03 ± 0.67 versus 2.03 ± 0.46, respectively; $p > 0.10$). The correlation between the two methods, although low, was statistically significant ($r = 0.58$, $p < 0.01$). However, when S/D ratios were elevated (>3.0) the indices obtained with CW Doppler were significantly higher than those obtained with PW Doppler, suggesting that pattern recognition may be less reliable when the uterine artery S/D ratio is elevated. In this circumstance, the waveform may appear similar to, and be confused with that of the iliac artery signal.

Color Doppler imaging (CDI) allows accurate mapping of the uterine arteries as they cross the external iliac arteries in real time, proper placement of the pulsed Doppler gate, and is the preferred technique for performing uterine artery Doppler velocimetry.[12] When the examination is conducted during the second trimester, a general obstetric ultrasound is performed before the examination and placental location is determined. The transducer is then directed toward the iliac fossa, the external iliac artery is imaged in a longitudinal section, and the uterine artery mapped with CDI as it crosses the external iliac artery (Fig. 13–3). This procedure allows precise positioning of the pulsed Doppler gate within the vessel lumen and acquisition of appropriate waveforms for spectral analysis (Fig. 13–4). Transvaginal ultrasound is used for studies performed during the first trimester. Close proximity to the pelvic structures, the use of high-frequency transducers, and a low angle of insonation improve image quality and Doppler signals.

The waveform obtained is subjectively inspected for the presence of an early diastolic notch (Fig. 13–5), which is associated with the subsequent development of preeclampsia.[13-17] Measurements obtained from the Doppler velocity waveform envelope allow the calculation of angle-independent Doppler indices [systolic/diastolic ratio (S/D or A/B), resistance index (RI), and pulsatility index (PI)] that reflect the degree of resistance to blood flow downstream of the interrogation site. Abnormality has been defined as either an absolute cutoff (for example, RI > 0.58) or a measurement greater than a particular centile of the reference range. Studies using receiver operator characteristic (ROC) curves have shown a PI greater than 1.5,[18] an RI greater than 0.68,[19] or an RI in the

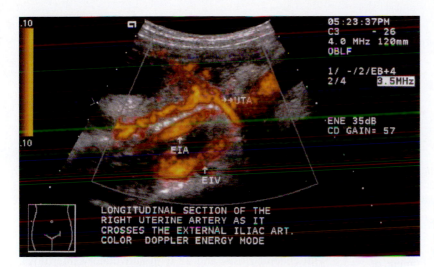

Figure 13–3. Color Doppler energy picture showing the uterine artery at its apparent cross with the external iliac artery. This is the preferred site to obtain a waveform.

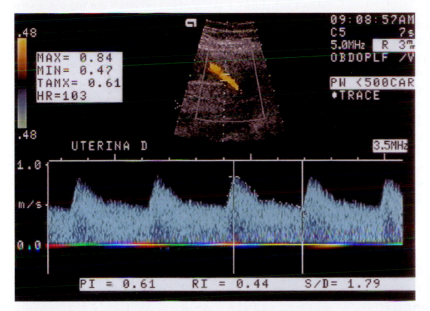

Figure 13–4. Normal uterine artery velocity waveform. Note the high velocities during diastole.

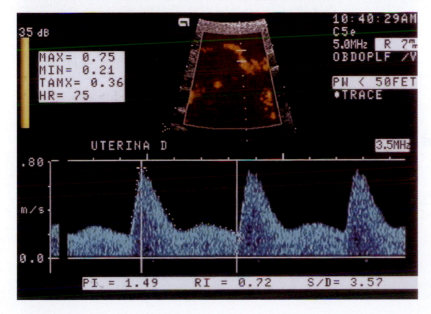

Figure 13–5. Abnormal uterine artery velocity waveform. The waveform is characterized by low-diastolic velocities, increased resistance index, pulsatile index, and systole-to-diastole ratios and persistent diastolic notch (arrows).

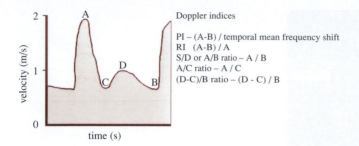

Figure 13–6. Doppler indices used to evaluate resistance to blood flow on flow velocity waveforms obtained from the uterine arteries. A, peak systolic velocity; B, end diastolic velocity; C, early diastolic velocity; D, maximum diastolic velocity.

region of the 90th centile[20] to predict the development of preeclampsia and SGA.

Although good inter-observer agreement has been demonstrated for the subjective assessment of diastolic notching among experienced operators,[15,21] newer Doppler indices have been proposed to objectively assess the shape of the uterine artery waveform, in particular the presence and intensity of the early diastolic notch.[18,22,23] These indices are the peak systolic over protodiastolic ratio (A/C)[18,22,23] and the maximum diastolic velocity minus protodiastolic velocity over end-diastolic velocity ratio [(D − C)/B][18] (Fig. 13–6). Irion et al.[23] reported that an A/C ratio equal to or greater than 2.5 had a sensitivity of 88% and a specificity of 86% to detect a notch. In a subsequent study comparing objective and subjective assessments of 50 abnormal uterine artery Doppler waveforms, Bower et al.[18] found that a (D − C)/B ratio greater than 0.15 reached the closest agreement with the subjective diagnosis of a diastolic notch.

DOPPLER VELOCITY WAVEFORMS OF THE NORMAL UTEROPLACENTAL CIRCULATION

The Nonpregnant Uterus

Uterine artery waveforms obtained from the nonpregnant uterus are characterized by high impedance to blood flow.

Doppler indices (S/D ratio, PI, and RI) change according to the phase of the menstrual cycle.[24] Absent end-diastolic velocities and early diastolic notches are more pronounced during the follicular phase.[25,26] In a study of 150 normal women, Kurjak et al.[27] reported the average uterine artery RI during the proliferative phase to be 0.88 ± 0.04 (2 SE). The RI started to drop one day before ovulation, reached a nadir of 0.84 ± 0.04 (2 SE) on day 18, and remained at this level for the rest of the cycle.

A high resistance to flow during the midluteal phase of the cycle (day 21) has been associated with infertility.[28,29] Steer et al.[29] studied a group of 23 women having artificial insemination with donor sperm because their partners were azoospermic and 161 women receiving treatment for infertility (35 unexplained infertility; 91 with tubal disease, 8 with endometriosis, and 22 with anovulatory infertility). Table 13–1 shows a comparison between the uterine artery pulsatility indices obtained during the midluteal phase of the menstrual cycle for each group. Regardless of specific etiology, the PI was higher in women with infertility.

Likewise, in women undergoing *in vitro* fertilization (IVF), those with a higher PI on the day of follicular aspiration have a lower probability of successful pregnancy.[30,31] Steer et al.[32] demonstrated that a mean PI greater than 3.0 before embryonic transfer predicted up to 35% of inplantation/pregnancy failures. The findings suggest a potential value for uterine artery Doppler velocimetry in identifying endometrial receptivity before *in vitro* fertilization. It seems that in cycles with a high uterine impedance, embryos could be cryopreserved until the uterus becomes more receptive.

First Trimester

In human pregnancies, the intervillous maternal circulation is only fully established at approximately 11 to 12 weeks.[33,34] Before 12 weeks, the intervillous space of the definitive placenta is separated from the uterine circulation by a trophoblastic shell, and trophoblastic plugs obliterate the tip of the uteroplacental arteries. Thus, a very limited amount of maternal blood reaches the intervillous space during the first trimester, and color Doppler signals are usually not seen on the placental substance (Fig. 13–7).[35–40] This is consistent with the

TABLE 13–1. MIDLUTEAL UTERINE ARTERY PULSATILITY INDEX OF NORMAL AND SUBFERTILE WOMEN

Clinical Condition	No. of Women	Age in Years (Range)	Years of Infertility	Pulsatility Index (Range)	p
Normal	23	31 (25–35)		1.9 (0.8–2.7)	
Unexplained infertility	35	34.1 (25–40)	4.2	2.45 (1.0–7.0)	0.036
Tubal damage	92	34.5 (24–41)	4.6	2.65 (1.3–8.0)	0.003
Endometriosis	8	33 (21–40)	3.1	2.32 (2.1–5.7)	0.041
Anovulatory infertility	22	32 (21–40)	3.0	3.03 (1.6–7.0)	0.004

Reproduced with permission from Steer CV, Tan SL, Mason BA, et al. Fertil Steril. 1994;61:53.

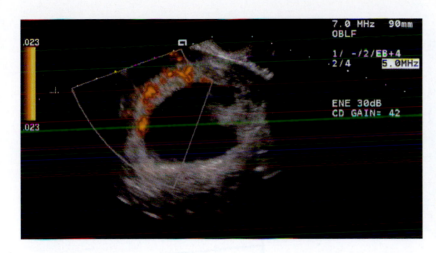

Figure 13–7. Abnormal placenta at 8 weeks. Blood flow is detected within the placental mass by color Doppler energy at this very early stage. This finding is associated with higher pregnancy loss rates.

clinical observation that chorionic villus samples obtained before 12 weeks are rarely tinted by blood in comparison with samples obtained in the second trimester or later.[33] Detection of blood flow in the intervillous space during the first trimester is associated with higher pregnancy loss rates (Fig. 13–8).[41,42] After 12 weeks, blood flow can be systematically detected by CDI of the placental substance.[35–40]

In contrast, FVWs can be obtained from the implantation site as early as 5 weeks after the last menstrual period and are characterized by low impedance to blood flow. A prominent diastolic component is observed, with the mean RI ranging from 0.41 ± 0.10 (SD) to 0.48 ± 0.08 (SD).[35,43,44] The RI gradually decreases from 6 to 12 weeks.[45] Flow velocity waveforms obtained from the uterine arteries are characterized by elevated S/D ratios, reduced end-diastolic velocities, and the presence of a notch in the systolic deceleration slope.[45] The vascular resistance decreases as gestation progresses into the second trimester (Fig. 13–9).[45–49]

Coppens et al.[40] conducted a longitudinal study of uteroplacental blood flow in 37 normal early human pregnancies.

Uterine artery blood flow was characterized by a high systolic component and low end diastolic flow pattern, associated with a prominent early diastolic notch, consistently present from 8 to 14 weeks of gestation. Waveforms from the arcuate arteries also showed a diastolic notch but had higher diastolic velocities in comparison with the uterine arteries. The spiral arteries showed the lowest resistance, with high diastolic blood flow and a small diastolic notch that disappeared in about half of the cases by 10 weeks and in all cases by 13 weeks. In 62% of the cases, the diastolic notch of the arcuate arteries disappeared the week after the disappearance of the notch in the spiral arteries. Normal values for PI in uterine, arcuate, and spiral arteries, from 8 to 14 weeks, are presented in Table 13–2.

Second and Third Trimesters

The second trimester is characterized by a progressive enlargement of the cross-sectional area of the main uterine artery,[47,50] increase in peak velocity and volume flow rates,[47–49,51–53] and a progressive fall in impedance to blood

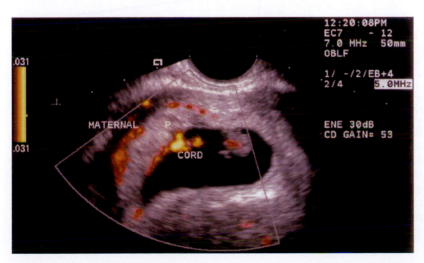

Figure 13–8. The placenta of a normal 8-week pregnancy with superimposed color Doppler energy. Even with settings to detect extremely low-velocity blood flow, no signals are obtained from the placental substance.

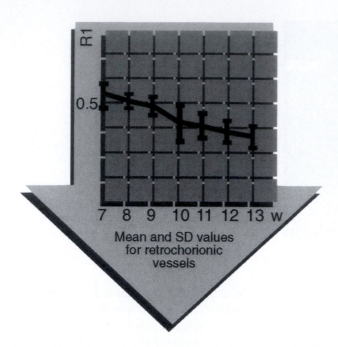

Figure 13–9. Uterine artery resistance index during the first trimester and throughout gestation. *(Reproduced with permission from Mercé LT, Barco MJ, de la Fuente F. Acta Obstet Gynecol Scand. 1989;68:603.)*

flow.[45,46,49,51,54–56] The diastolic notch and the difference between S/D ratios of placental versus nonplacental sites should disappear after 24 to 26 weeks of gestation.[46,47,49,51,57,58] Normal values for the RI of the uterine and arcuate arteries are shown in Figures 13–10 and 13–11.

Puerperium

Profound modifications in uterine perfusion occur within a few hours after delivery. In the first 24 hours postpartum, the blood flow falls considerably, the S/D ratio increases, and the blood velocity remains high. By the second day

TABLE 13–2. MEAN VALUES (±2 SD) FOR PULSATILITY INDEX IN UTERINE, ARCUATE, SPIRAL, AND UMBILICAL ARTERIES IN NORMAL EARLY GESTATION (8–14 WEEKS)

Gestational Age (Weeks)	Spiral Artery	Arcuate Artery	Uterine Artery
	Pulsatility Index		
8	0.85 ± 0.34	1.76 ± 0.36	2.95 ± 0.78
9	0.77 ± 0.24	1.63 ± 0.44	2.65 ± 0.99
10	0.73 ± 0.26	1.33 ± 0.50	2.43 ± 0.64
11	0.67 ± 0.22	1.17 ± 0.38	2.18 ± 0.60
12	0.61 ± 0.26	0.97 ± 0.26	1.92 ± 0.44
13	0.54 ± 0.18	0.91 ± 0.31	1.77 ± 0.42
14	0.54 ± 0.20	0.85 ± 0.33	1.76 ± 0.50

Reproduced with permission from Coppens M, Loquet P, Kollen M, et al. Ultrasound Obstet Gynecol. 1996;7:114.

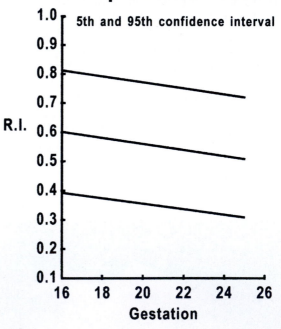

Figure 13–10. Uterine artery resistance index throughout gestation. **(A)** Placental site. **(B)** Nonplacental site. *(Reproduced with permission from Bewley S, Campbell S, Cooper D. Br J Obstet Gynaecol. 1989;96:1040.)*

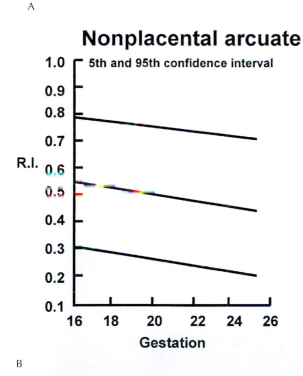

A

B

Figure 13–11. Arcuate artery resistance index throughout gestation. **(A)** Placental site. **(B)** Nonplacental site. *(Reproduced with permission from Bewley S, Campbell S, Cooper D. Br J Obstet Gynaecol. 1989;96:1040.)*

postpartum, both the S/D ratio and PI increase considerably and the diastolic notch reappears. After an initial rise in impedance to blood flow, no further changes are noted until the 6th puerperal week, when the RIs start to rise again, lasting until the third month of puerperium.[48,54]

Influence of Sampling Site and Placental Implantation on Flow Velocity Waveforms

Choosing the appropriate vessel to obtain the Doppler sample is important. Figure 13–12 shows sampling sites used by different investigators to obtain uteroplacental Doppler FVWs. These sites include the main uterine arteries,[59] the arcuate arteries along the lateral uterine wall,[60] and the subplacental vessels.[56,61] Much controversy has been generated by comparing studies using different sampling sites.[62] Studies evaluating the arcuate, radial, and spiral arteries during the second trimester are subject to sampling bias and are difficult to reproduce. Furthermore, waveforms obtained from these sites do not necessarily reflect the status of the whole uteroplacental circulation, because only a small section is examined. Waveforms from the main uterine arteries provide a more accurate picture of perfusion status, reflecting the sum of resistances in the uteroplacental vascular bed.[63–65] As mentioned before, CDI allows easy identification of the main uterine artery as it crosses the external iliac artery, thus improving reproducibility (see Figs. 13–3 to 13–5). Waveforms obtained from this site are comparable to waveforms obtained from the main uterine artery near its origin from the internal iliac artery.[64]

The combination of RIs from four different locations (right and left uterine and arcuate arteries) into an averaged index has been proposed as a means to overcome methodologic problems when comparing studies of Doppler waveforms sampled at different sites.[66] However, the predictive values for abnormal pregnancy and perinatal outcomes were lower than those reported by studies using the uterine or arcuate arteries alone. Therefore, that approach is not justified and does not warrant their substitution for this method.

Sampling both uterine arteries is also important.[67] The RI, PI and S/D ratios are lower in the ipsilateral site of placental implantation.[28,46,68] This difference is more pronounced during the first half of the pregnancy and should gradually disappear as the pregnancy approaches the third trimester (see Figs. 13–10 and 13–11).[28,46,64] In a study of 71 pregnancies, Schulman et al.[59] demonstrated that persistence of a difference between the S/D ratios of left and right uterine arteries after 26 weeks of gestation ($\Delta \geq 1$) was associated with an increased risk for the development of preeclampsia [50% (14 of 28) versus 14% (6 of 43); relative risk (RR) = 2.55, 95% confidence interval (CI) = 1.5 to 4.3] and SGA [39% (11 of 28) versus 5% (2 of 43), RR = 2.88, 95% CI = 1.8 to 4.6].

Elevated Doppler Indices in the Uterine Arteries as a Measure of Impedance to Blood Flow in the Uteroplacental Circulation. Evidence that elevated PI, RI, and S/D ratios and the presence of a diastolic notch in the uterine artery FVW reflect increased impedance to blood flow in the placental circulation comes from three sources: computer models of the uteroplacental circulation,[69,70] embolization of the uteroplacental circulation in animal models,[71,72] and studies

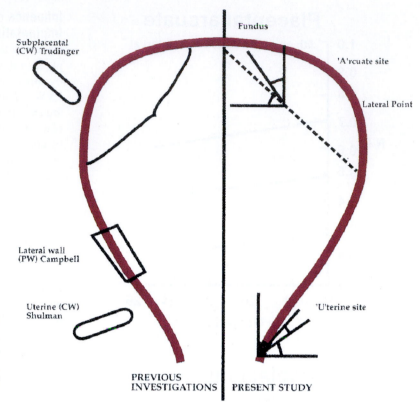

Figure 13–12. Sampling sites used in the studies of Doppler velocimetry of the uteroplacental circulation. *(Reproduced with permission from Bower SJ, Campbell S. In: Chervenak FA, Isaacson GC, Campbell S, eds. Ultrasound Obstet Gynecol. Boston: Little & Brown; 1993: 579–586.)*

comparing histologic evaluation of placental bed biopsies with Doppler velocimetry of the uterine arteries.[73,74]

Computer Models of the Uteroplacental Circulation. The uterine artery FVW has two components: a pulsatile and a steady flow component. The pulsatile component is formed by the interaction of an outgoing and a reflected wave, which bounces back to the maternal heart upon reaching the uteroplacental vascular bed.

Adamson et al.[69] developed a computer model to evaluate the effect of placental resistance, arterial diameter, and blood pressure on the shape of the uterine artery velocity waveform. Their model was designed to simulate resistance to flow, vessel compliance, and main uterine artery blood inertia, as well as the physical properties of all the vessels branching from the main uterine artery to form the distal vascular bed (arcuate, radial, and spiral arteries). The variables analyzed [uteroplacental vascular resistance, uterine artery radius, and mean arterial blood pressure (MAP)] were altered over realistic ranges, either independently or in combination, to examine their effects on the uterine artery FVW. When the resistance of the distal vascular bed was increased six-fold while keeping constant the uterine artery radius and MAP (Fig. 13–13), the following observations were made: 1) decreased mean velocity and blood flow; 2) elevated PI and S/D ratios; and 3) development of a notch in the early diastolic portion of the FVW, caused by destructive interaction

between outgoing and reflected waves. A reduction in the uterine artery radius resulted in an increase in mean velocity, elevated PI and S/D ratios, but no diastolic notch. An increase in the MAP caused elevation in mean blood

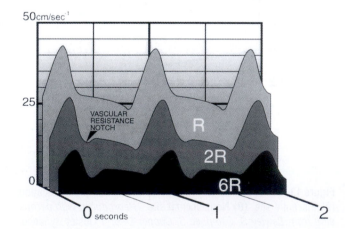

Figure 13–13. Effect of a sixfold increase in the resistance of the distal vascular be in the uterine artery waveform. Interactions between outgoing and reflected waves produce a notch in the early diastolic component of the waveform. This effect is not observed when the radius of the uterine artery or the mean arterial pressure is modified without an increase in the peripheral vascular resistance. *(Reproduced with permission from Adamson SL, Morrow RJ, Bascom PAJ, et al. In: Mo LYL, Ritchie WK, eds. Ultrasound Med Biol. 1989;5:437.)*

velocity without changing the RIs, or generating a diastolic notch. These observations suggest that the changes in uterine artery Doppler velocimetry observed in preeclampsia are not mediated by high blood pressure, but rather are the consequence of an abnormally elevated uteroplacental vascular resistance, expressed by elevations in Doppler indices and the presence of a diastolic notch.

Talbert[70] proposed another model to study uteroplacental blood flow. The model used resistance and capacitance elements in all components of the uteroplacental circulation, making it possible to simulate various physiologic situations and observe changes in the Doppler FVWs. Uteroplacental blood flow parameters were changed within physiologic limits for a 1000-g human fetus at 28 weeks of gestation. The first experiment described was a 33% reduction in blood flow, achieved by raising the resistance to flow in the transcotyledonary region and spiral arteries. The results were increased uterine artery PI and RI, but no diastolic notch. In the second experiment, intervillous obstruction was modeled by increasing central cotyledon pressure by nearly doubling transcotyledonal resistance, which caused distention and reduction of flow resistance of the spiral and radial arteries. The uterine artery PI and RI increased, but no diastolic notch was produced. When placental resistances were kept within normal limits and the distensibilities of uterine and arcuate artery walls were raised, a diastolic notch was produced, with normal uterine artery PI and RI. The typical FVW observed *in vivo* in abnormal uterine artery Doppler studies (increased PI, RI, and the presence of a diastolic notch) was produced by a combination of increased placental resistance and distensibility of the uterine and arcuate artery walls.

Embolization of the Uteroplacental Circulation of Pregnant Ewes.
Ochi et al.[71,72] embolized the uterine spiral arteries of pregnant ewes at 16 to 17 weeks of gestation through the stepwise injection of gelfoam microbeads into the uterine arteries and analyzed the associated Doppler velocimetric changes. Embolization of the uteroplacental circulation resulted in a dose-dependent decrease in blood flow, an increase in uterine vascular resistance, a dose-dependent attenuation of the pregnancy-related physiologic elevation in the diastolic flow velocity, an increase in PI,[71] and the appearance of a diastolic notch.[72] The findings suggest that elevated PI and the presence of a diastolic notch in the uterine artery velocity waveform indicate increased vascular resistance of the uteroplacental circulation.

Correlation of Placental Bed Biopsies and Uterine Artery Doppler Velocity Waveforms.
Olofsson et al.[73] and Lin et al.[74] compared histologic findings of placental bed biopsies obtained at the time of cesarean section with uterine artery waveforms. They studied placental bed biopsies taken at cesarean section in 26 complicated (study group) and 29 uncomplicated (control group) pregnancies after performing Doppler velocimetry of the uterine arteries. Physiologic changes were absent in 77% (20 of 26) of the complicated pregnancies and present in all controls. Patients with abnormal placental bed biopsies were more likely to have elevated uterine artery PIs and abnormal pregnancy outcomes [pregnancy-induced hypertension (PIH) and SGA]. Similar conclusions were reached by Lin et al.[74] who studied 43 patients who had Doppler examination of the uterine arteries within 7 days of delivery and found that 92% (12 of 13) of the patients with a uterine artery S/D ratio greater than or equal to 2.5 failed to show trophoblast migration into the myometrium. Patients with impaired trophoblast migration into the myometrium delivered more prematurely (33.1 ± 2.7 versus 36.1 ± 2.2 weeks, $p < 0.02$) and had a higher rate of SGA fetuses (1290.2 ± 319.1 versus 1870.5 ± 523.1 g, $p < 0.02$).

Prediction of Preeclampsia and SGA Fetuses.
Abnormal uterine artery Doppler FVWs are characterized by elevated RI, PI, or S/D ratios and the presence of a diastolic notch (see Fig. 13–5). As discussed before, pregnancies complicated by preeclampsia and, to a lesser extent, SGA fetuses, show evidence of impaired trophoblastic invasion of the myometrial portion of the spiral arteries.

Several investigators have studied the potential role of uteroplacental Doppler to identify patients at risk for preeclampsia, SGA, preterm delivery, or adverse perinatal outcomes. Tables 13–3 to 13–6 summarize the results of such studies for high-risk[19,75–78] or unselected populations.[17,22,66,78–89] In 14 studies,[17,19,75,77–79,81–83,85–89] Doppler was considered effective in identifying a high-risk population for the development of preeclampsia and/or SGA; in three,[22,66,76] the results were inconclusive; and in three,[80,83,88] the results did not support a role for uteroplacental Doppler velocimetry as a screening test in pregnancy. Divergence among the studies is attributed to differences in patient selection and gestational age for screening, type of equipment used (CW, PW, or color Doppler), multiple definitions of abnormal FVWs, different vessels examined, and heterogeneous outcome criteria.[19,90] Sensitivities for the detection of preeclampsia ranged from 25 to 100%. The sensitivity improved as gestational age approached 26 weeks, when the main uterine arteries were the vessels interrogated (rather than other vessels, such as arcuate arteries) and when a persistent diastolic notch was one of the criteria used for analysis.[83] Positive predictive values ranged from 2% to 50% in low-risk populations (see Table 13–5) and increased from 17% to 70% in high-risk populations (see Table 13–3). Bower et al.[86] proposed a two-stage screening protocol for preeclampsia with uterine artery Doppler velocimetry performed at 18–22 weeks and 24 weeks. In their study of 2,058 low-risk patients, 16% (329 of 2,058) had a diastolic notch in either uterine artery at 18–22 weeks. Persistence of an abnormal waveform increased the RR for moderate and severe preeclampsia by 24-fold. SGA babies with abnormal waveforms during

TABLE 13–3. PREDICTIVE VALUES FOR THE DEVELOPMENT OF PIH IN HIGH-RISK POPULATIONS

Author Year	Vessel	Gestational Age (Weeks)	Population With Complete Follow-up	Abnormal Result	Prevalence	Sensitivity	Specificity	PPV	NPV	Outcome Measure
Arduini[75] 1987	Arcuate	18–20	60 pregnancies at risk for PIH	RI > 0.57	37%	64%	84%	70%	80%	PIH 1
Jacobson[76] 1990	Arcuate	24	91 pregnancies at risk for PIH	RI ≥ 0.58	29%	44%	73%	33%	81%	PIH 2
Jacobson[76] 1990	Arcuate	24	91 pregnancies at risk for PIH	RI ≥ 0.58	10%	67%	63%	17%	95%	PIH 3
Montenegro[77] 1992	Uterine	26	71 pregnancies at high risk*	Persistent diastolic notch	37%	100%	82%	76%	100%	PIH 4
Zimmermann[19] 1997	Uterine	21–24	175 pregnancies at high risk for PIH	Bilateral notch	18%	22%	90%	39%	88%	PIH 5
Zimmermann[19] 1997	Uterine	21–24	175 pregnancies at high risk for PIH	RI ≥ 0.68	18%	23%	84%	29%	79%	PIH 5
Zimmermann[19] 1997	Radial/spiral	21–24	175 pregnancies at high risk for PIH	RI ≥ 0.38	18%	45%	50%	21%	75%	PIH 5
Zimmermann[19] 1997	Radial/spiral	21–24	175 pregnancies at high risk for PIH	Bilateral notch	18%	32%	90%	48%	82%	PIH 6 or SGA < 10th centile
Zimmermann[19] 1997	Uterine	21–24	175 pregnancies at high risk for PIH	RI ≥ 0.68	18%	56%	84%	51%	87%	PIH 6 or SGA < 10th centile
Zimmermann[19] 1997	Radial/spiral	21–24	175 pregnancies at high risk for PIH	RI ≥ 0.38	18%	76%	50%	30%	88%	PIH 6 or SGA < 10th centile
Caforio[78] 1999	Uterine	18–20	335 high risk†	RI ≥ 90th centile	9%	94%	69%	23%	99%	PIH 4
Caforio[78] 1999	Uterine	22–24	335 high risk†	RI ≥ 90th centile	12%	97%	71%	31%	99%	PIH 4

*Defined as nulliparous, chronic hypertension or previous history of preeclampsia.
†Defined as chronic hypertension, type 1 diabetes, autoimmune disease, systemic lupus erythematosus, renal disease, previous obstetric history of stillbirths, intrauterine growth retardation, or stillbirths and habitual abortions.
NPV, negative predictive value; PIH 1, blood pressure ≥ 140/90 on two occasions at least 4 h apart; PIH 2, blood pressure of at least 90 mmHg with a rise of 25 mmHg from booking or a rise of 15 mmHg if the booking diastolic pressure was already 90 mmHg; PIH 3, blood pressure of at least 90 mmHg with a rise of 25 mmHg from booking or a rise of 15 mmHg if the booking diastolic pressure was already 90 mmHg + 500 mg/24 h of proteinuria; PIH 4, blood pressure ≥ 140/90 mmHg on two occasions at least 4 h apart + 300 mg/24 h of proteinuria; PIH 5, blood pressure > 145/85 mmHg (two occasions > 24 h apart); PIH 6, blood pressure > 145/85 mmHg (two occasions > 24 h apart) and proteinuria (>+ on dipstick testing on more than two occasions more than 24 h apart); PPV, positive predictive value; RI, resistance index; SGA, small for gestational age.

TABLE 13–4. PREDICTIVE VALUES FOR THE DEVELOPMENT OF SGA IN HIGH-RISK POPULATIONS

Author Year	Vessel	Gestational Age (Weeks)	Population With Complete Follow-up	Abnormal Result	Prevalence	Sensitivity	Specificity	PPV	NPV	Outcome Measure
Jacobson[76] 1990	Arcuate	24	91	RI ≥ 0.58	18%	71%	68%	28%	91%	SGA < 10th centile

NPV, negative predictive value; PPV, positive predictive value.

pregnancy were also more likely to be admitted to the neonatal intensive care unit (NICU) than those with normal uterine artery FVWs. When patients were re-examined at 24 weeks, 59% (193 of 329) showed normal uterine artery Doppler waveforms.[15] Persistent notch in the early diastolic component of the waveform improved the predictive value of the test (from 4.3 to 28%) and was associated with a 68-fold risk for the development of preeclampsia. Harrington et al.[89] examined the possibility of predicting preeclampsia and SGA at 12 to 16 weeks with transvaginal uterine and umbilical artery Doppler velocimetry. The parameters evaluated included the presence or absence of an early diastolic notch, vessel diameter, RI, PI, time averaged mean velocity (TAV), maximum systolic velocity, and volume flow in the uterine arteries and RI and PI in the umbilical arteries. The main outcome measures of the study were intrauterine death, birth weight, preeclampsia, and antepartum hemorrhage. Women who subsequently developed preeclampsia had significantly lower mean uterine artery TAV, lower volume flow, and elevated RI. The odds ratio (OR) for the development of preeclampsia in women with bilateral notches was 43.54 (95% CI = 5.84 to 324.73). These patients were also more likely to have SGA babies (OR = 8.61, 95% CI = 4.0 to 20.0) or deliver prematurely (OR = 2.38, 95% CI = 1.19 to 4.75).

A large study conducted by Irion et al.[88] in low-risk populations, with similar inclusion criteria, Doppler examination technique, and outcome variables as the study of Bower et al.,[15] was not able to reproduce the results. The likelihood ratio for the development of preeclampsia in patients with a notch in the uterine arteries examined at 26 weeks was only 1.94 (95% CI = 1.14 to 3.31). The authors concluded that Doppler of the uteroplacental circulation "does not fulfill the requirements for a screening test in unselected populations." However, they acknowledged that the likelihood ratios for the abnormal test justify the interest in the technique in patients at higher risk of obstetric or perinatal complications [i.e., those with risk factors for preeclampsia identified by medical history, increased second-trimester arterial blood pressure, risk factors for intrauterine growth retardation (IUGR) and prematurity or those with abnormal biological tests]. Among the other studies that failed to show a benefit of uterine artery Doppler velocimetry as a screening test in pregnancy, the study by Newnham et al.[83] evaluated only the presence of SGA as an outcome variable. In the study of Harrenty et al.,[61] PIs obtained from subplacental vessels (ra-

dial or spiral arteries) were compared between a group of 32 normal pregnancies and a group of 32 pregnancies complicated by preeclampsia. All examinations were performed during the third trimester, and the waveforms with lowest resistance to flow were selected for analysis. No differences in PI were detected between the two groups. Because of a sampling bias, these results are not surprising. Placental bed biopsies from patients with preeclampsia show areas lacking trophoblastic invasion scattered among areas with normal physiologic change.[6] By selecting only those areas with the lowest resistance to flow, the possibility of sampling vessels with normal trophoblastic invasion but with abnormal placentation is increased.

One point that has been frequently overlooked when evaluating uterine artery Doppler studies is the high negative predictive value of the test.[87,90] Most recent studies in unselected populations have reported negative values ranging from 96 to 99%[17,22,66,78,82,83,85,86,89] and a substantial reduction in the risk of developing preeclampsia or delivering an SGA baby. Thus, it has been proposed that a normal uterine artery Doppler study at 24 weeks could serve to organize prenatal care by identifying a group of low-risk women who would be ideal candidates for community care during pregnancy.[87,90] Kurdi et al.[87] performed uterine artery Doppler velocimetry in 946 low-risk women at 20 weeks to test this hypothesis and found that 99% of the women with normal uterine artery Doppler FVWs did not develop preeclampsia and 96% did not deliver an SGA baby (birth weight below the 5th centile). Moreover, no women with normal Doppler studies required delivery before 37 weeks for preeclampsia or an SGA fetus. Indeed, in women with normal uterine artery Doppler, the OR for developing any complication during pregnancy (defined as preeclampsia, placental abruption, delivery of an SGA baby below the 10th centile, or a pregnancy that resulted in stillbirth or a neonatal death) was 0.24 (95% CI = 0.17 to 0.34). The authors concluded that these women form a "truly low-risk group, who should be suitable for community-led care, thereby enabling obstetricians to concentrate more time and energy on high-risk pregnancies."

Prediction of Superimposed Preeclampsia in Patients With Chronic Hypertension. The incidence of superimposed preeclampsia in pregnancies complicated by chronic hypertension ranges from 4.7 to 52%, depending on the severity of hypertension at the onset of pregnancy and on the diagnostic

TABLE 13–5. PREDICTIVE VALUES FOR THE DEVELOPMENT OF PIH IN LOW-RISK POPULATIONS

Author Year	Vessel	Gestational Age (Weeks)	Population With Complete Follow-up	Abnormal Result	Prevalence	Sensitivity	Specificity	PPV	NPV	Outcome Measure
Campbell[79] 1986	Arcuate	16–18	126	RI > 0.58	12%	67%	64%	20%	93%	PIH 9
Hanretty[80] 1989	Arcuate	26–30	291	S/D ratio > 2.07	24%	7%	94%	26%	76%	PIH 7
Hanretty[80] 1989	Arcuate	34–36	318	S/D ratio > 2.00	26%	5%	98%	44%	74%	PIH 7
Schulman[81] 1989	Uterine	26	255	Mean RI > 0.62	—	—	—	33%	—	PIH (not defined)
Steel[82] 1990	Uterine	16–22	1123	RI > 0.58	3%	79%	91%	23%	99%	PIH 4
Bewley[66] 1991	2 uterine, 2 arcuate	16–24	925	Mean RI > 95th centile	5%	24%	95%	20%	96%	PIH 8
Harrington[83] 1992	Uterine	20	2437	RI > 95th centile or notch	2%	76%	86%	13%	99%	PIH 2
Harrington[83] 1992	Uterine	24	2437	RI > 95th centile or notch	2%	76%	96%	35%	99%	PIH 2
Harrington[83] 1992	Uterine	26	2437	RI > 95th centile or notch	2%	74%	97%	44%	99%	PIH 2
Valensise[85] 1993	Uterine	22	272	RI > 0.58	3%	88%	93%	30%	99%	PIH 4
Bower[86] 1993	Uterine	18–22	2058	RI > 95th centile or notch	2%	82%	86%	11%	99%	PIH 4
North[22] 1994	Uterine	19–24	458	RI > 0.56 on placental side	3%	27%	89%	8%	97%	PIH 4
North[22] 1994	Uterine	19–24	458	Elevated A/C ratio	3%	53%	88%	14%	98%	PIH 4
Harrington[17] 1996	Uterine	24	1204	Bilateral notch	4%	55%	98%	50%	98%	PIH 4
Harrington[89] 1997	Uterine	12–16	626	Bilateral notch	4.7%	90%	46%	8%	99%	PIH 4
Harrington[89] 1997	Uterine	12–16	626	Any notch	4.7%	97%	46%	8%	99.6%	PIH 4
Irion[88] 1998	Uterine	26	1159	Notch	4%	26%	87%	7%	—	PIH 4
Irion[88] 1998	Uterine	26	1159	A/C ratio ≥ 2.5	4%	34%	85%	8%	—	PIH 4
Irion[88] 1998	Uterine	22–24	530	RI ≥ 90th centile	0.5%	100%	75%	2%	100%	PIH 4

A/C, peak systolic/protodiastolic ratio; NPV, negative predictive value; PIH 1, blood pressure ≥ 140/90 on two occasions at least 4 h apart; PIH 2, blood pressure of at least 90 mmHg with a rise of 25 mmHg from booking or a rise of 15 mmHg if the booking diastolic pressure was already 90 mmHg; PIH 3, blood pressure of at least 90 mmHg with a rise of 25 mmHg from booking or a rise of 15 mmHg if the booking diastolic pressure was already 90 mmHg + 500 mg/24 h of proteinuria; PIH 4, blood pressure > 140/90 mmHg (two occasions 4 h apart) and proteinuria (>300 mg/24 h or > ++ on dipstick testing); PIH 5, blood pressure > 145/85 mmHg (two occasions > 24 h apart) and proteinuria (>+ on dipstick testing on more than two occasions more than 24 h apart); PIH 7, blood pressure > 140/90 mmHg, requiring further investigation or treatment; PIH 8, blood pressure > 140/90 mmHg (two occasions 4 h apart) and proteinuria (>150 mg/24 h or > ++ on dipstick testing); PIH 9, blood pressure rise (systolic > 30 mmHg or diastolic > 15 mmHg) with proteinuria or generalized edema; PPV, positive predictive value; RI, resistance index; S/D, systolic/diastolic ratio.

TABLE 13–6. PREDICTIVE VALUES FOR THE DEVELOPMENT OF SGA IN LOW-RISK POPULATIONS

Author Year	Vessel	Gestational Age (Weeks)	Population With Complete Follow-up	Abnormal Result	Prevalence	Sensitivity	Specificity	PPV	NPV	Outcome Measure
Campbell[79] 1986	Arcuate	16–18	126	RI > 0.53	14%	67%	65%	24%	92%	SGA < 10th centile
Hanretty[80] 1989	Arcuate	26–30	291	S/D ratio > 2.07	6%	7%	94%	5%	95%	SGA < 5th centile
Hanretty[80] 1989	Arcuate	34–36	318	S/D ratio > 2.00	5%	0	97%	0	95%	SGA < 5th centile
Schulman[81] 1989	Uterine	26	255	Mean RI > 0.62	9%	17%	97%	44%	92%	SGA not defined
Newnham[83] 1990	Subplacental	24	253	RI > 0.50	7%	6%	92%	5%	93%	SGA < 10th centile
Steel[82] 1990	Uterine	16–22	1123	RI > 0.58	5%	43%	91%	23%	99%	SGA < 5th centile
Bewley[66] 1991	2 uterine, 2 arcuate	16–24	925	Mean RI > 95th centile	6%	19%	95%	19%	96%	SGA < 5th centile
Valensise[85] 1993	Uterine	22	272	RI > 0.58	8%	67%	95%	54%	97%	SGA < 10th centile
Bower[86] 1993	Uterine	18–22	2058	RI > 95th centile or notch	5%	46%	86%	15%	97%	SGA < 5th centile
North[22] 1994	Uterine	19–24	458	RI > 0.56 on placental side	7%	50%	90%	27%	91%	SGA < 10th centile
North[22] 1994	Uterine	19–24	458	Elevated A/C ratio (objective assessment of diastolic notch)	7%	87%	49%	23%	96%	SGA < 10th centile
Harrington[17] 1996	Uterine	24	1204	Bilateral notch	11%	22%	98%	50%	91%	SGA < 10th centile
Irion[88] 1998	Uterine	26	1159	Notch	11%	30%	88%	24%	—	SGA < 10th centile
Irion[88] 1998	Uterine	26	1159	A/C ratio ≥ 2.5	11%	29%	86%	21%	—	PIH 4
Irion[88] 1998	Uterine	26	1159	S/D (A/B) ratio > 90th centile	11%	26%	92%	28%	—	PIH 4
Irion[88] 1998	Uterine	26	1159	RI ≥ 0.58	11%	29%	89%	25%	—	PIH 4

A/B and S/D, systolic/diastolic ratio; PIH 4, blood pressure > 140/90 mmHg (two occasions 4 h apart) and proteinuria (>300 mg/24 h or >++ on dipstick testing); RI, resistance index; SGA, small for gestational age.

criteria used.[91] Superimposed preeclampsia is strongly associated with a worse perinatal outcome in this group of patients. [91]

Uterine artery Doppler velocimetry has been investigated as a test to predict, among patients with chronic hypertension, those who could develop superimposed preeclampsia.[92,93] Caruso et al.[92] studied 42 women with chronic hypertension with uterine artery Doppler velocimetry at 23 to 24 weeks. The prevalence of superimposed preeclampsia was 21%, and the lowest uterine artery waveform RI above the 90th centile predicted this outcome with a sensitivity of 100%, specificity of 88%, positive predictive value (PPV) of 69%, and negative predictive value (NPV) of 100%. Patients with abnormal uterine artery Doppler velocimetry were more likely to deliver a premature (30.5 ± 3.3 versus 38.3 ± 1.8 weeks, $p = 0.0005$) or low-birth-weight baby (1140 ± 651 versus 3034 ± 532 g, $p = 0.0005$), have a cesarean section for fetal distress [46% (6 of 13) versus (0 of 29), $p = 0.0005$], deliver a newborn with an Apgar score below 7 at 5 minutes [(61.5% (8 of 13) versus (0 of 29), $p = 0.0005$], or have their baby admitted to the NICU [69.2% (9 of 13) versus 13.8% (4 of 29), $p = 0.0005$]. Perinatal mortality rate was also higher for patients with abnormal uterine artery Doppler velocimetry [53.8% (7 of 13) versus (0 of 29), $p = 0.0005$]. In another study of 78 chronic hypertensive patients, Frusca et al.[93] found that the presence of bilateral diastolic notches in the uterine arteries was significantly more prevalent among patients who developed superimposed preeclampsia [23% (3 of 13) versus 0% (0 of 65), $p < 0.001$] or delivered SGA babies [85% (11 of 13) versus 3% (2 of 65), $p < 0.001$]. Of interest was the low prevalence of superimposed preeclampsia (only 3.8%). The authors commented that, although this may be due to the small number of patients, it could also reflect a benefit of low-dose aspirin therapy (50 mg/day), which was prescribed to all patients from the 12th week until delivery.

UTERINE ARTERY DOPPLER IN PREGNANCIES COMPLICATED BY PREECLAMPSIA

Doppler of the uterine arteries has also been evaluated as a test to identify, among pregnancies complicated by preeclampsia, those with a higher maternal and fetal risk. Van Asselt et al.[94] evaluated 28 women with severe preeclampsia [systolic blood pressure ≥ 160 mmHg and diastolic ≥ 110 mmHg and/or proteinuria of +3 (≥3.0 g/L)] and 28 with mild preeclampsia [systolic blood pressure = 145–155 mmHg and diastolic = 90–105 mmHg and proteinuria +1 or +2 (>0.3 and <3.0 g/L)]. Uterine artery Doppler waveforms were obtained with CDI, and a mean PI of both uterine arteries above 1.20 was considered abnormal. Umbilical artery FVWs were also obtained during the examination; an abnormal umbilical artery FVW was defined as a PI higher than two standard de-

viations above the mean for gestational age. The results of the last examination before delivery were correlated to perinatal outcome, mean maternal blood pressure, and degree of proteinuria. Uterine artery PI was positively correlated with the degree of proteinuria. Patients with abnormal uterine and umbilical artery FVWs were more likely to deliver prematurely (38.6 ± 2.5 weeks for normal uterine and umbilical artery waveforms; 36.5 ± 2.5 weeks for abnormal uterine and normal umbilical artery waveforms; 36.6 ± 3.3 weeks for normal uterine and abnormal umbilical artery waveforms; 37.7 ± 5.1 weeks for abnormal uterine and umbilical artery waveforms; $p = 0.0005$); deliver more SGA fetuses [5.3% (4 of 76) for normal uterine and umbilical artery waveforms; 33.3% (5 of 15) for normal uterine and abnormal umbilical artery waveforms; 25% (2 of 8) for normal uterine and abnormal umbilical artery waveforms; 77.8% (7 of 9) abnormal uterine and umbilical artery waveforms; $p = 0.0001$], and have more NICU admissions [15.8% (12 of 76) for normal uterine and umbilical artery waveforms; 53.3% (8 of 15) for abnormal uterine and normal umbilical artery waveforms; 62.5% (5 of 8) for normal uterine and abnormal umbilical artery waveforms; 88.9% (8 of 9) for abnormal uterine and umbilical artery waveforms; $p = 0.0001$]. Women with an unilateral notch in the uterine arteries were 8 times more likely to deliver an SGA newborn [37% (10 of 27) versus 6.5% (4 of 62), OR = 8.5, 95% CI = 2.7 to 27] and 10 times more likely to do so when bilateral notches were present [42.1% (8 of 19) versus 6.5% (4 of 62), OR = 10.6, 95% CI = 3.2 to 35.2]. When bilateral notches were present, there was also a 4 to 5 times increased risk for a cesarean section [68.4% (13 of 19) versus 33.9% (21 of 62), OR = 4.2, 95% CI = 1.5 to 12.2] and admission to the NICU [52.6% (10 of 19) versus 19.4% (12 of 62), OR = 4.6, 95% CI = 1.6 to 13.3]. Similar findings were reported by Joern and Rath,[95] who examined 142 pregnancies complicated by preeclampsia/HELLP syndrome and/or SGA, and by Hofstaetter et al.,[96] who studied a heterogeneous group of 421 high-risk pregnancies (SGA, preeclampsia, PIH, diabetes mellitus, prolonged pregnancy, third-trimester hemorrhage, premature rupture of membranes, decreased fetal movements, bad obstetric history, poly- or oligohydramnios, fetal heart arrhythmia, and abnormal cardiotocogram). When both uterine and umbilical arteries were abnormal, outcome was poorer, with a higher rate of preterm delivery and lower birth weight. Outcome was not significantly affected when only the umbilical arteries were pathologic.

RANDOMIZED CONTROLLED TRIALS

Two randomized controlled trials assessed the value of screening with the uterine and umbilical arteries. Newnham et al.[97] randomized women in the third trimester and, therefore, did not assess the effect of screening early in pregnancy. Also, the development of preeclampsia and SGA were not evaluated as outcomes in that study. Davies et al.[98] randomized 2600 unselected women to Doppler or control groups at 19 to 20 weeks of gestation. Women in the Doppler group had the uterine arteries examined at 19 to 20 weeks, followed by a second scan at 24 weeks if the results of the first examination were abnormal. Low-risk women had umbilical artery Doppler performed at 32 weeks. High-risk women (defined as those with hypertension, diabetes, previous SGA livebirth, previous stillbirth or neonatal death, hypertension in a previous pregnancy or at booking, smoking more than 10 cigarettes per day) or women who screened positive at the 24-week uterine artery Doppler study had ultrasound examinations every month. Hypertension developed in fewer women in the Doppler group [7.9% (98 of 1246) versus 11.3% (139 of 1229), RR = 0.70, 95% CI = 0.54 to 0.89]. No improvement in perinatal outcome was demonstrated in pregnancies allocated to the Doppler group. The authors speculated that, although the reduction of hypertension in the Doppler group could have been the result of an action taken in response to the abnormal uterine artery examinations in the second trimester, it could have also been a chance finding, because there was no defined intervention instituted.

COMBINATION OF UTERINE ARTERY DOPPLER VELOCIMETRY WITH OTHER TESTS

The combination of uterine artery Doppler with other methods to evaluate maternal adaptation to pregnancy has been proposed to overcome the low positive predictive value of the test.[99] Other tests include 24-h automated maternal blood pressure[100] or biochemical markers such as α-fetoprotein,[101–103] β-human chorionic gonadotropin (β-hCG),[104] a combination of maternal serum α-fetoprotein, β-hCG, and uric acid levels,[105] the N-terminal peptide of proatrial natriuretic peptide,[106] and urinary kallicrein: creatinine ratios.[107]

Uterine Artery Doppler Velocimetry Combined With 24-h Automated Blood Pressure Monitoring

Benedetto et al.[100] conducted a case-control study to evaluate the value of adding 24-h automated blood pressure (BP) monitoring to uterine artery Doppler screening in detecting a combination of PIH, preeclampsia, and SGA. Ninety women with singleton pregnancies at high risk for PIH, preeclampsia, or SGA and abnormal uterine artery Doppler FVWs at 20 to 22 weeks (mean RI > 0.58, diastolic notches) were compared with a control group ($n = 90$) with the same risk factors but normal uterine artery Doppler. Women selected for the control group were those examined immediately after each patient with an abnormal Doppler. All patients underwent 24-h BP monitoring with a portable automated device

immediately after recruitment. The primary endpoints of the study were the development of PIH or preeclampsia and SGA. The overall incidence of PIH or preeclampsia with or without SGA, or of SGA alone, was significantly higher in the abnormal Doppler than in the control group [42% (38 of 90) versus 17% (15 of 90), $p < 0.05$]. The highest incidence of PIH and preeclampsia, with or without SGA, occurred in the group with abnormal uterine Doppler associated with a systolic midline estimating statistic of rhythm (MESOR) of at least 111 mmHg or a diastolic MESOR at least 68 mmHg [51.1% (23 of 45) versus 2.2% (1 of 45), $p < 0.0001$]. This difference, although less marked, was also observed in the normal uterine Doppler group [31.6% (6 of 19) versus 4.2% (3 of 71), $p < 0.01$]. Abnormal uterine artery Doppler alone predicted PIH/preeclampsia with or without SGA, with a 73% sensitivity, 55% specificity, 27% PPV, and 90% NPV. The predictive value of the test improved two-fold with the addition of a diastolic MESOR greater than or equal to 0.68: 64% sensitivity, 91% specificity, 62% PPV, and 92% NPV. The results suggest that screening pregnant women with a two-stage test (uterine artery Doppler plus 24-h BP monitoring) may significantly increase the performance of uterine artery Doppler screening in identifying pregnancies at high risk for PIH and preeclampsia.

Uteroplacental Doppler Velocimetry in Patients With Elevated Maternal Serum α-Fetoprotein

In addition to the well-established association between elevated levels of maternal serum α-fetoprotein (MSAFP) and neural tube defects, this marker has been linked to an increased risk of perinatal death, preterm delivery, and SGA. Three studies[101–103] have shown that fetuses with idiopathic elevation of MSAFP above 2.5 multiples of the median (MOM) and abnormal uterine artery Doppler velocimetry are at increased risk for abnormal perinatal outcome, including PIH, SGA, and preterm birth.

In the first study, uterine artery Doppler velocimetry was performed at 18 to 22 weeks and again at 24 to 26 weeks in a group of 98 pregnancies with elevated MSAFP and normal fetal anatomy by ultrasound.[101] Fourteen percent of the fetuses (14 of 98) died in the perinatal period, 21.4% (21 of 98) were delivered prematurely, and 17.3% (17 of 98) were SGA. A persistent diastolic notch after 24 to 26 weeks predicted 79% of the perinatal deaths. These findings were confirmed in the study by Bromley et al.[102] who reported poor outcome in 47% of 199 second-trimester pregnancies with elevated MSAFP levels and severe early uterine artery diastolic notch at 18 to 19 weeks. Similarly, Konachak et al.,[103] in a study of 103 patients with unexplained elevated MSAFP levels, found that abnormal uterine artery Doppler velocimetry performed at 17 to 22 weeks was associated with an increased risk of PIH, low birth weight, and preterm delivery.

Uterine Artery Doppler in Pregnancies With Elevated Free β-hCG

In a retrospective study of 329 consecutive women with elevated maternal serum-free β-hCG levels during Down's syndrome screening, Palacio et al.[104] reported values greater than or equal to 5.0 MOM were associated with a high incidence of PIH, SGA, or intrauterine fetal death (RR = 2.3, 95% CI = 1.3 to 3.9). Twenty-six women were selected for a prospective study based on a free β-hCG value greater than or equal to 5.0 MOM at 15 to 18 weeks and normal fetal karyotype. Patients had uterine and umbilical artery Doppler velocimetry performed at 20 weeks and every month thereafter. Abnormal outcome, in this group was observed in 8 fetuses (30.8%) and included isolated fetal growth restriction ($n = 3$), PIH ($n = 3$; two with associated SGA), and intrauterine fetal demise (IUFD) with SGA ($n = 2$). The presence of a diastolic notch at 24 weeks predicted adverse perinatal outcome with a sensitivity of 88%, specificity of 94.4%, PPV of 87.5%, and NPV of 94.4%.

Combination of MSAFP, Maternal Serum hCG (MShCG), and Uric Acid Levels

Jauniaux et al.[105] studied 41 singleton pregnancies selected because of bilateral diastolic notches in the FVWs and/or an increased PI above the 95th centile between 20 and 24 weeks of gestation. MSAFP, MShCG, and uric acid levels were measured and results compared with pregnancy outcome. All women were followed monthly until delivery. Among 20 patients with normal outcome, 19 had normal uterine artery Doppler velocimetry at their second visit. Twenty-one pregnancies had abnormal outcomes: severe proteinuric PIH with SGA (8 of 21), isolated SGA (8 of 21), mild PIH with normal fetal growth (3 of 21), and placental abruption (2 of 21). MSAFP, MShCG, and uric acid levels were increased in the first visit among pregnancies with adverse perinatal outcomes (MSAFP: 2.9 $\pm$ 0.8 versus 1.7 $\pm$0.9 MOM, $p < 0.01$; MShCG: 2.8 $\pm$ 1.1 versus 1.4 $\pm$0.9 MOM, $p < 0.05$; uric acid: 3.9 $\pm$ 1.1 versus 2.9 $\pm$ 0.7, $p < 0.01$). MSAFP and MShCG dropped by the second visit, whereas uric acid levels kept increasing in complicated pregnancies until delivery. Sixty-four percent (7 of 11) of the patients with PIH presented with a combination of high MSAFP and MShCG at the first visit; no patients with normal outcome presented with elevation of both markers ($p < 0.01$).

STRATEGIES TO PREVENT THE DEVELOPMENT OF PREECLAMPSIA IN PATIENTS WITH ABNORMAL UTEROPLACENTAL DOPPLER WAVEFORMS

A good screening test is only useful when preventive measures or treatment for the condition under investigation are available. Calcium supplementation, fish oils and linoleic acid, low-dose aspirin, NO donors, and antioxidants (vitamins C and E) have been proposed as prophylactic agents for preeclampsia. In the following paragraphs, we review the effect of these aspects on the prevention of preeclampsia, with emphasis on high-risk patients selected by uterine artery Doppler velocimetry screening.

Calcium

Several studies have suggested a role for calcium supplementation in the reduction of preeclampsia.[108,109] Intracellular calcium stimulates smooth muscle contraction, whereas extracellular calcium has the opposite effect. Extracellular calcium activates membrane phospholipase to produce prostaglandins and may increase the prostacyclin-to-thromboxane ratio.

A meta-analysis conducted in 1994[108] showed an overall reduction in the incidence of hypertension (0.44; 95% CI = 0.33 to 0.59), preeclampsia (0.34; 95% CI = 0.22 to 0.54), and preterm delivery (0.66; 95% CI = 0.45 to 0.97) in women recruited between 20 and 32 weeks and who took 1.5 to 2.0 g of calcium daily. Levine et al.[108] in a larger randomized controlled trial was not able to reproduce these results. In their study, 4589 healthy nulliparous women at 13 to 21 weeks were assigned to receive 2 g of either elemental calcium or placebo for the remainder of their pregnancies. The rate of preeclampsia was not different between the treatment and control groups [6.9% (158 of 2295) versus 7.3% (168 of 2294), RR = 0.94, 95% CI = 0.76 to 1.16].

Herrera et al.,[110] in a small placebo controlled study (43 women in each arm), showed a substantial reduction in the incidence of preeclampsia [9.3% (4 of 43) versus 37.2% (16 of 43), RR = 0.25, 95% CI = 0.09 to 0.069, $p < 0.001$] in high-risk women receiving a combination of 600 mg calcium and 450 mg linoleic acid.

No trials have been conducted exploring the possibility of supplementing calcium to women with abnormal uterine artery Doppler FVWs.

Fish Oils and Linoleic Acid

Before the development of the disease, women with preeclampsia have a depletion of high-density lipoprotein (HDL) and excess low-density lipoproteins (LDLs), very-low-density lipoproteins (VLDLs), and trygliceride. The combination of elevated fatty acids and increased production of cytokines [tumor necrosis factor (TNF), interleukin-1 (IL-1), and IL-6] is associated with release of reactive free radicals. Reactive free radicals cause platelet activation and enhanced thromboxane release, inhibition of prostacyclin production, increased endothelin release (a vasoconstrictor), inactivation of NO (a vasodilator), white cell activation, and direct endothelium damage.

Fish oils reduce the load of potentially harmful LDLs and are preferentially metabolized to prostacyclin rather than to thromboxane. It was expected that diet supplementation with these compounds could have a protective effect on the endothelium by decreasing the overproduction of reactive free radicals observed in patients with preeclampsia. Two studies[111,112] failed to show a beneficial effect of fish oil in pregnancy, although, as described above, a small trial combining calcium and fish oil supplementation[110] did show a substantial reduction in the incidence of preeclampsia in treated patients.

Aspirin

Low-dose aspirin (50 to 150 mg/day) has been extensively investigated as a prophylactic agent for women at risk of uteroplacental or umbilical placental vascular thrombosis and insufficiency. An imbalance favoring the production of thromboxane A_2 (TxA_2) over prostacyclin (PGI_2), two prostanoids derived from the arachdonic acid metabolism, is thought to play an important role in the pathogenesis of preeclampsia and at least some cases of SGA.[113] Low-dose aspirin irreversibly inhibits almost all platelet cyclo-oxygenase activity, thereby blocking the production of TxA_2, a potent vasoconstrictor and platelet aggregating agent, and has been proposed as a prophylactic agent to prevent the development of preeclampsia.[114]

Although some trials have suggested a significant reduction in the rates of preeclampsia and SGA when women at high risk are selected for treatment,[115–123] a beneficial effect of universal prophylaxis with low-dose aspirin has not been confirmed by several large randomized clinical trials in unselected or low-risk populations.[124–131] One small[132] and two large[133,134] recent randomized clinical trials also failed to show any benefit of aspirin prophylaxis in high-risk pregnancies. The Collaborative Low-Dose Aspirin Study in Pregnancy (CLASP) trial[133] recruited 9364 women between 12 and 32 weeks of gestation, in 16 countries, and randomized them to either 60 mg aspirin/day or placebo. Women were eligible to enter the study if, "in the opinion of the responsible clinician, were at sufficient risk of preeclampsia or IUGR for the use of low-dose aspirin to be contemplated, but without clear indications for or against its use." Follow-up was available for 9309 patients: 4659 allocated to aspirin and 4650 allocated to placebo. No differences in the rates of preeclampsia [6.7% (313 of 4659) versus 7.6% (352 of 4650), odds reduction 12%, not significant (NS)], SGA [6.6% (317 of 4810) versus 8.3% (401 of 4821)], and perinatal death [2.7% (129 of 4810) versus 2.8% (136 of 4821), odds reduction 5%, NS] were detected between patients receiving aspirin or placebo. However, aspirin reduced the likelihood of delivery before 37 weeks [19.7% (920 of 4659) versus 22.2% (1033 of 4650), odds reduction 14%, 95% CI = 22 to 5%, $p = 0.003$], and this effect was stronger among women delivering preterm because of proteinuric preeclampsia [3% versus 4.1%, odds reduction 28%, 95% CI = 46 to 4% reduction, $p = 0.003$]. Caritis et al,[134] in a subsequent study, enrolled 2539 pregnant women at high risk for preeclampsia between 13 and 26 weeks [insulin-treated diabetes ($n = 471$), chronic hypertension ($n = 774$), multifetal gestations ($n = 688$), or a previous history of preeclampsia ($n = 606$)] and allocated them to receive either aspirin (60 mg/day) or placebo. No differences were observed between treatment and control groups in the rates of preeclampsia (18% versus 20%, RR = 0.9, 95% CI = 0.8 to 1.1), SGA fetuses (10% versus 9%, RR = 1.2, 95% CI = 0.9 to 1.5), preterm delivery (40% versus 43%, RR = 0.9, 95% CI = 0.8 to 1.1), and perinatal deaths (3% versus 5%, RR = 0.8, 95% CI = 0.5 to 1.1).

Aspirin Prophylaxis in Patients With Abnormal Uterine Artery Flow Velocity Waveforms.

Among the studies that selected women for aspirin prophylaxis on the basis of abnormal uterine artery Doppler velocimetry, three showed a reduction in the rate of preeclampsia[135–139] and one did not.[140] The results of these studies are summarized in Table 13–7 and discussed in more detail below.

Montenegro et al.[135,136] studied 104 women at risk for the development of preeclampsia (primiparity, chronic hypertension, or preeclampsia in previous pregnancies). Uterine artery Doppler velocimetry was performed at 26 weeks in all patients and considered abnormal if an early diastolic notch was visualized in at least one of the uterine arteries. Sixty-seven women had a persistently abnormal waveform and were randomized to receive either aspirin (50 mg/day until delivery, $n = 33$) or placebo ($n = 34$). The proportion of women who did not develop preeclampsia was significantly lower in the group treated with aspirin than in the control group [9% (3 of 33) versus 76% (26 of 34), $p < 0.001$]. Twenty-one of the patients with a persistent diastolic notch had a placental bed biopsy performed after birth. Ninety-five percent of the patients (20 of 21) had evidence of abnormal placentation as there was no evidence of trophoblastic invasion of the myometrial portion of the spiral arteries. No patients with a normal uterine artery Doppler velocimetry developed preeclampsia. After excluding the patients treated with aspirin, the predictive value of a diastolic notch in the uterine artery waveform after 26 weeks for preeclampsia was: sensitivity of 100% (26 of 26), specificity of 82.2% (37 of 45), PPV of 76% (26 of 34), and NPV of 100% (37 of 37).

As part of a French trial on the use of aspirin for the prevention of preeclampsia and IUGR (EPREDA),[125] 90 high-risk multipara (previous history of preeclampsia or IUGR) were randomized at 14 weeks and received either aspirin (150 mg/day, $n = 60$) or placebo ($n = 30$) from 17 weeks of gestation onward.[137] According to results of uterine artery Doppler velocimetry at 24 weeks, patients were further subdivided in two groups: 1) normal Doppler velocimetry [$n = 74$ (82.2%); 32.4% (24 of 74) in the placebo group and 67.6% (50 of 74) in the treatment group] and 2) abnormal Doppler velocimetry [$n = 16$ (17.8%); 37.5% (6 of 16) in the placebo group and 62.5% (10 of 16) in the treatment group]. The prevalence of SGA (defined as birth weight below the 5th centile for age) was significantly higher in the group with abnormal uterine

TABLE 13–7. RANDOMIZED CLINICAL TRIALS OF LOW-DOSE ASPIRIN WITH AN ABNORMAL UTERINE ARTERY DOPPLER VELOCIMETRY

Author Year	Population	Randomization Criteria	Aspirin Dose (mg/day)	Treatment	Placebo	Preeclampsia			SGA			Severe Preeclampsia Requiring Delivery Before 37 Weeks		
						Treatment	Placebo	p	Treatment	Placebo	p	Treatment	Placebo	p
Montenegro[135] 1990	Nulliparous, chronic hypertension, preeclampsia in previous pregnancies	Persistent notch after 26 weeks	50	33	34	9% (3/33)	76% (26/34)	<0.001	—	—	—	—	—	—
Uzan[137] 1990	Preeclampsia or SGA in previous pregnancies	Abnormal D/S ratio; persistent notch after 24 weeks	150	10	6	10% (1/10)	50% (3/6)	<0.05	20% (2/10)	66% (4/6)	<0.05	—	—	—
Bower[139] 1996	High-risk women enrolled in the CLASP trial[133]	Elevated RI; persistent notch after 24 weeks	60	31	29	29% (9/31)	41% (12/29)	0.32	26% (8/31)	41% (12/29)	0.20	3% (1/31)	24% (7/29)	0.02
Morris[140] 1996	Nulliparous women	Elevated RI; persistent notch at 18 weeks	100	52	50	8% (4/52)	14% (7/50)	NS	15% (8/52)	20% (10/50)	NS	—	—	—

D/S, diastolic/systolic ratio; NS, not significant; RI, resistance index; SGA, small for gestational age.

302

artery velocimetry [37.5% (6 of 16) versus 13.5% (10 of 74), $p < 0.05$]. Among these patients, those who received low-dose aspirin had a significantly better pregnancy outcome as measured by a lower incidence of SGA [20% (2 of 10) versus 66.7% (4 of 6), $p < 0.05$] and preeclampsia [10% (1 of 10) versus 50% (3 of 6), $p < 0.05$].

Bower et al.[139] analyzed a subset of women recruited for the CLASP trial[133] because of abnormal uterine artery Doppler velocimetry at 24 weeks of gestation (presence of a diastolic notch or an RI > 95th centile for gestational age). Women were randomized to receive aspirin (60 mg/day) or placebo. Over a period of 2 years, 63 women agreed to participate, 55 of whom complied with the treatment; 3 were lost to follow-up. Results were analyzed on an intention-to-treat basis. Thirty-one patients were allocated to the treatment group and 29 to the placebo group. Twenty-nine percent (9 of 31) of the patients developed preeclampsia in the aspirin group versus 41% (12 of 29) in the placebo group (OR = 0.58, 95% CI = 0.20 to 1.69, $p = 0.32$). However, there was a significant reduction on the incidence of severe preeclampsia [12.9% (4 of 31) versus 37.9% (11 of 29), OR = 0.24, 95% CI = 0.07 to 0.88, $p = 0.03$], preeclampsia requiring delivery before 37 weeks [3% (1 of 31) versus 24% (7 of 29), OR = 0.10, 95% CI = 0.01 to 0.91, $p = 0.02$], and preeclampsia requiring delivery before 34 weeks [0 of 31 versus 5 of 29 (17%), $p = 0.02$] in patients treated with aspirin.

Morris et al.[140] screened women during the 18-week routine ultrasound scan with uterine artery Doppler velocimetry. Those with an S/D ratio above 3.3 or, with an early diastolic notch, an S/D ratio above 3.0 were offered to participate in a randomized, double-blind, placebo-controlled trial of low-dose aspirin (100 mg/day). Nineteen percent of the women screened had an abnormal uterine artery FVWs at 18 weeks (186 of 955), and 102 (54.8%) agreed to be randomized. Patients allocated to receive aspirin had a tendency to develop less preeclampsia, but the difference was not statistically significant [8% (4 of 52) versus 14% (7 of 50), RR = 0.55, 95% CI = 0.17 to 1.76]. There were no differences in the rates of PIH [15% (8 of 52) versus 14% (7 of 50), RR = 1.09, 95% CI = 0.43 to 2.80], preterm delivery [6% (3 of 52) versus 10% (5 of 50), RR = 0.58, 95% CI = 0.14 to 2.29], SGA [15% (8 of 52) versus 20% (10 of 50), RR = 0.78, 95% CI = 0.34 to 1.80], or any adverse outcome [56% (29 of 52) versus 56% (28 of 50), RR = 0.99, 95% CI = 0.70 to 1.40]. The authors commented that failure to confirm a potential benefit of Doppler screening in the reduction of preeclampsia for patients treated with aspirin, from 14 to 8% in this study, could be due to an inadequate sample site.

These studies show a tendency toward a lower incidence of preeclampsia for patients with abnormal Doppler velocimetry treated with aspirin, but larger trials are needed to see whether the results can be reproduced.

A possible explanation for the overall aspirin failure in preventing preeclampsia has been recently suggested by a study of prostacyclin and thromboxane changes in pregnant women recruited early in pregnancy for the Calcium for Preeclampsia Prevention Trial (CPEP).[108] Excretion of urinary metabolites of PGI_2 (PGI-M) and TxA_2 (Tx-M) were measured from timed urine collections obtained prospectively from pregnant women enrolled in the CPEP trial. Urine samples were collected before 22 weeks, between 26 and 29 weeks, and at 36 weeks of gestation. Rates of PGI-M and TxA_2 were compared between women who developed preeclampsia ($n = 134$) and controls ($n = 139$).[141] The results of the study demonstrate that the imbalance favoring TxA_2 or PGI_2 in patients with preeclampsia is actually due to significantly lower levels of PGI_2 starting early in pregnancy (17% lower than controls, 95% CI = 6 to 27%, $p = 0.005$). The TxA_2 levels were not significantly higher overall (9% higher than controls, 95% CI = −3 to 23%, $p = 0.14$). Therefore, aspirin trials may have failed because an increase in thromboxane production is not the initial abnormality and future interventions should probably be designed to correct the relative prostacyclin deficiency.

Nitric Oxide Donors

Although the imbalance in PGI_2 to TxA_2 allows for an explanation of the many clinical features of preeclampsia (vasoconstriction, platelet destruction, and reduced uteroplacental blood flow), it does not clarify the whole spectrum of pathophysiologic changes associated with the disease. Glomerular endotheliosis and ultrastructural changes observed in the placental bed, and other parts of the circulation are evidence that global endothelium dysfunction contributes substantially to the pathogenesis of preeclampsia.[142,143]

Nitric oxide,[144] also known as endothelium-derived relaxing factor (EDRF),[145] is a highly unstable mediator produced by the vascular endothelium in response to the action of a family of enzymes known as NO synthases. The biological precursor of the gas is L-arginine[146] and the byproduct, L-citrulline, can be measured in tissue as a marker of NO synthase activity. Nitric oxide causes smooth muscle relaxation by acting on the intracellular enzyme guanylate cyclase, stimulating the production of cyclic guanosine monophosphate (cGMP) from guanosine triphosphate (GTP), and dephosphorylation of myosin light chains. It also inhibits platelet aggregation and, therefore, has antithrombotic properties.[147] Nitric oxide is produced by the endothelium at a background rate and is released in response to acethylcoline, bradykinin, and nitrovasodilators.[148] If necessary, larger amounts of NO can be produced over a short period by macrophages, vascular smooth muscle, and trophoblastic tissue in response to cytokines and inflammation.[149] Nitric oxide activity is potentiated by superoxide dismutase[150] and L-arginine.[146] The relaxation effect is abolished by destruction of the endothelium, inhibited by oxyhemoglobin and L-nitro-arginine methyl ester, and inactivated by superoxide anions.[146]

There is evidence linking defective NO synthesis or metabolism to preeclampsia:

- the endothelium is focally disrupted by the trophoblast in preeclampsia;[146]
- administration of L-nitro-arginine methyl ester (a NO activity inhibitor) causes a dose-dependent increase in blood pressure and proteinuria in rats,[151] a dose-dependent reduction in birth weight and increased mortality of rat pups,[153] and reverses the pregnancy-induced refractoriness to vasopressor agents;[151]
- circulating levels of the NO metabolite, nitrite, are decreased in patients with preeclampsia;[152]
- inhibition of NO synthesis in pregnant rats produces signs similar to those of preeclampsia;[153]
- there is a drastic reduction of NO release from the endothelium of umbilical cord vessels from patients with PIH and increased perfusion pressure of both artery and vein;[154]
- in preeclampsia, there is evidence of platelet activation and they also have an exaggerated intracellular response to NO.[155]

This evidence raised interest in using NO donors either to ameliorate the course of established preeclampsia or to prevent it. The NO donors tested to date were nitroglycerin or glyceryl trinitrate (GTN), isosorbide dinitrate, and S-nitrosoglutathione.

Preliminary Studies With GTN. Ramsey et al.[156] studied the effect of GTN and PGI$_2$ on uterine artery Doppler FVWs during the first and second trimesters of normal pregnancy. Ten patients at 8 to 10 weeks of gestation received an intravenous infusion of GTN before pregnancy termination. The drug caused a significant drop in the uterine artery RI and reduction of diastolic notching in 8 women, mimicking the physiologic alterations observed normally during the second trimester. A second group, consisting of 15 women with abnormal uterine artery FVWs (mean RI > 6.0 and bilateral diastolic notches) at 24 to 26 weeks of gestation, also received a GTN infusion. In this group, there was a dose-dependent reduction in the uterine artery Doppler RI, but no changes in maternal blood pressure, pulse rate, carotid artery RI, or fetal umbilical artery FVWs. Interestingly, the same effect could not be reproduced by infusing PGI$_2$ in the same patients after a 30-minute GTN washout period.

Giles[157] reported improved umbilical artery S/D ratios in pregnancies complicated by impaired fetal growth after administering 300 μg of sublingual nitroglycerin.

Grunewald et al.[158] infused incremental doses of GTN in 12 women with severe preeclampsia: 0.25 μg/min every 5 to 10 mins until a reduction in diastolic BP to 100 mmHg occurred or a maximum dose of 5.0 μg was reached. They observed a significant reduction in maternal BP and umbilical

artery PI, without significant interference with fetal heart rate or uterine artery PI.

Luzi et al.[159] compared the sublingual administration of 0.3 mg of GTN in two groups of high-risk pregnancies: 10 patients with mild preeclampsia and 10 patients with threatened preterm labor near 30 weeks. Maternal BP and the PI of uterine, umbilical, and middle cerebral arteries dropped in both groups after administration of sublingual GTN; however, changes were significantly more pronounced in pregnancies complicated by preeclampsia. These results suggest that the hemodynamic responses to sublingual administration of 0.3 mg of GTN are different in preeclamptic pregnancies and in patients with preterm labor. The increased effect of NO donors, in this setting, may be attributed to NO release by the drug, which would offset the decreased production of NO postulated to contribute to the pathogenesis of preeclampsia.

Preliminary Studies With Isosorbide Dinitrate. Sublingual administration of isosorbide dinitrate (5 mg) to 16 low-risk patients before pregnancy termination for nonmedical indications, between 17 and 24 weeks, caused a fall in maternal BP and an increase in heart rate.[160] Uterine artery resistance fell to a lesser degree than did umbilical artery Doppler resistance. Maximum changes in maternal BP and heart rate occurred 6 mins after isosorbide dinitrate administration. Maximum uterine artery RI changes were observed at 10 mins and returned to baseline values within 30 mins of the experiment. In a similar study design,[161] the same investigators administered 5 mg of isosorbide dinitrate to 11 women at 8 to 10 weeks before pregnancy termination. They also observed a fall in maternal BP associated with a concomitant increase in heart rate and a decreased resistance in the uterine artery, with maximum effect achieved after 10 mins.

Preliminary Studies With S-nitrosoglutathione. S-nitrosoglutathione is a NO donor unavailable for clinical use at the present time which has[162] a preferential effect on platelet activation over vascular relaxation.[163]

However, administration of S-nitrosoglutathione to a patient with reduced synthesis of endogenous NO (such as in preeclampsia) is associated with an exaggerated vasodilatory response. Intravenous infusion of S-nitrosoglutathione (50 to 250 μg/min over 60 to 90 min) to 10 women with severe preeclampsia or preeclampsia with severe fetal compromise, at 21 to 33 weeks of gestation, resulted in a dose-dependent fall in BP, uterine artery resistance, and effective inhibition of platelet activation. However, there were no significant changes in the umbilical artery, fetal thoracic aorta, or middle cerebral artery PI, suggesting absence of adverse effects in the fetal circulation.[162]

Randomized Controlled Trials. Two randomized controlled trials have examined the effect of NO donors in pregnancies complicated by preeclampsia. The first trial was designed to determine whether a prophylactic GTN, in women with high-resistance waveforms, could reduce the risk of preeclampsia.[164] Forty consecutive patients at 24 to 26 weeks, with bilateral notches and mean uterine artery Doppler RI greater than 0.58 were enrolled in a double-blind, randomized trial. Patients with preexisting hypertension, SGA fetuses (abdominal circumference less than the 5th centile for gestational age), and fetal anomalies were excluded. Patients taking antihypertensive or cardiovascular medications were also excluded, as were those with evidence of diabetes mellitus or chronic renal disease or proteinuria above 0.3 g/L. Patients were randomly allocated to receive 5 mg/day of active transdermal Deponit 5 GTN ($n = 21$) or placebo patches ($n = 19$) and were followed up every 2 to 3 weeks until delivery. The main outcome measures were: 1) gestational age at development of preeclampsia; 2) gestational age at development of SGA (abdominal circumference below the 5th centile for gestational age, or gestation at delivery of a baby weighing less than the 10th centile); 3) gestation at delivery (if less than 37 weeks); 4) maternal systolic and diastolic BPs; 5) mean uterine RI; and 6) fetal umbilical artery PI and middle cerebral artery PI. No significant changes were observed for systolic BP, diastolic BP, mean uterine RI, umbilical artery RI, and MCA PI over time in both groups. No significant differences between the two groups were observed for gestational age at delivery (GTN: 38.5 ± 3.0 weeks versus 37.3 ± 3.1 weeks), birth weight (GTN: 2782 ± 638 versus 2565 ± 684 g), development of preeclampsia [GTN: 24% (5 of 21) versus 21% (4 of 19)], delivery before 37 weeks [GTN: 10% (2 of 21) versus 32% (6 of 19)], or diagnosis of SGA [GTN: 29% (6 of 21) versus 37% (7 of 19)]. However, when the Kaplan–Meier estimate of the survivor function was used to compare the adverse events between GTN and placebo groups, 71% (15 of 21) of the patients in the GTN group left the trial with no adverse events (i.e., full-term birth of a normally grown baby without evidence of pre-eclampsia) versus 26% (5 of 19) in the placebo group. The hazard ratio was 0.267 (95% CI = 0.102 to 0.701), equating to a reduction in hazard of 73%. Further studies are required to address this issue.

In the second trial, Thaler et al.[165] studied the effect of sublingual isosorbide dinitrate in 23 women with PIH (defined as at least two recordings of diastolic BP $\geq$ 90 mmHg, 4 h apart, at any stage after 20 weeks of gestation; daily protein excretion did not exceed 300 mg in any patient). Twelve patients received a sublingual tablet of isosorbide dinitrate (5 mg) and had maternal heart rate, BP, uterine artery, and umbilical artery velocity waveforms recorded 2 mins before and every 2 mins after the medication for 20 mins. Ten patients received placebo. Significant changes in maternal BP, heart rate, uterine artery S/D ratio, and umbilical artery S/D ratio were observed in patients receiving isosorbide dinitrate but not in those receiving placebo. Mean maternal BP dropped from 103 ± 1.8 mmHg to 90.5 ± 2.9 mmHg at 14 mins ($p < 0.0001$), the heart rate increased from 97.3 ± 3.8 beats per minute to

115 ± 3.5 beats per minute at 12 mins ($p < 0.0001$), the mean S/D ratio in the umbilical artery fell from 3.07 ± 0.33 to 2.58 ± 0.23 at 8 mins ($p < 0.0007$) and the mean uterine artery S/D ratio dropped from 3.27 ± 0.6 to 2.38 ± 0.28 at 10 mins ($p < 0.0001$).

Combining Aspirin and NO Donors. The combination of low-dose aspirin and NO donors has been suggested as a novel approach to manage fetuses at high risk for placental insufficiency.[166] Low-dose aspirin and NO donors have different, but possibly synergic, mechanisms of action. Low-dose aspirin increases the endothelial and platelet prostacyclin-to-thromboxane ratio. Nitric oxide donors, release NO in the circulation, with direct action on the vascular endothelium, causing relaxation.

Oyelese et al.[166] used a combination of aspirin (75 mg/day) and GTN patches (5 mg/day) in two cases with poor obstetric histories attributed to severe placental insufficiency. The first patient had a previous fetal loss because of placental infarction at 27 weeks, and the second patient had a previous pregnancy complicated by severe preeclampsia requiring delivery at 32 weeks. Both had severe bilateral diastolic notches at 20 and 24 weeks in the index pregnancy. In the first case, a 1600-g fetus was electively delivered at 32 weeks because of oligohydramnios and fetal redistribution of flow. In the second case, the fetus was delivered because of preterm labor and weighed 1650 g.

Antioxidants

There is compelling evidence suggesting that the normal protective role of the maternal vascular endothelium is severely compromised in women with preeclampsia. Decreased endothelial prostacyclin synthesis, decreased bioavailability of NO, greater cell permeability, and increased endothelial expression of cell adhesion molecules and increased availability of prothrombotic factors are consistent with endothelial cell activation. Free radicals have emerged as likely mediators of maternal vascular malfunction. Superoxide anions and markers of lipid activation (e.g., malondyaldehyde[167] and 8 epiprostaglandin-F2α[168]) are increased in the plasma of women with preeclampsia. Plasminogen-activator inhibitor 1 (PAI-1) is synthesized predominantly by endothelial cells and is thought to be a marker of endothelial-cell activation. PAI-2 is synthesized by the placenta.[169] The ratio of PAI-1 to PAI-2 decreases in normal pregnancy but is high in preeclampsia suggesting endothelial cell activation and placental insufficiency.[170]

Randomized Controlled Trial of Antioxidants (Vitamins C and E) to Prevent Preeclampsia. Chappel et al.[171] conducted a randomized controlled trial to evaluate the potential benefit of antioxidant supplementation (vitamins C and E) on markers of endothelial and placental function and the rates of preeclampsia in high-risk pregnancies. Two hundred eighty-three women were identified as high risk for preeclampsia because of abnormal two-stage uterine artery Doppler velocimetry at 20 and 24 weeks[15] or previous maternal history. Patients were randomly allocated to receive 1000 mg vitamin C and 400 IU natural-source vitamin E daily ($n = 142$) or placebo ($n = 141$) throughout pregnancy. The primary outcome measure was the ratio of PAI-1 to PAI-2, and the secondary outcome was the frequency of preeclampsia. One hundred sixty women completed the study: 81 in the placebo group (14 did not attend and 34 had normal velocimetry at 24 weeks; 13 withdrew from the study) and 79 in the study group (10 did not attend and 38 had normal velocimetry at 24 weeks; 14 withdrew from the study). Vitamin supplementation was associated with a 21% reduction (95% CI = 4 to 35%; $p = 0.015$) in the ratio of PAI-1 to PAI-2 over gestation compared with the placebo group. Women who received vitamin C and E supplementation developed preeclampsia significantly less often than those who received placebo. Among patients who finished the trial, only 8% (6 of 79) of those treated with vitamin supplementation developed preeclampsia versus 26% (21 of 81) in the placebo group (adjusted OR = 0.24; 95% CI = 0.08 to 0.7; $p = 0.002$). The results remained unchanged when the analysis was performed on an intention-to-treat basis [vitamin group, 8% (11 of 141), versus placebo group, 17% (24 of 142); adjusted OR = 0.39; 95% CI = 0.17 to 0.90]. The authors speculated that the potential benefit of vitamins C and E in this group could be due to inhibition of reactive oxygen species: vitamin C is a potent scavenger of superoxide radicals[172] and may have helped preserve NO; it also maintains intracellular glutathione concentrations;[173] both vitamin C and E decrease LDL oxidation.[173,174]

PRETERM LABOR

Uterine artery Doppler velocimetry, performed at admission for preterm labor, has been shown to correlate significantly with failed tocolysis, a short interval between admission and delivery and abnormal perinatal outcome. Brar et al.[175] studied the uterine and umbilical artery FVWs of 60 patients in preterm labor receiving either ritodrine ($n = 20$) or magnesium sulfate tocolysis ($n = 40$). A uterine artery S/D ratio greater than 2.6 or the presence of a diastolic notch was considered abnormal. Fifty-eight percent (7 of 12) of the patients with abnormal uterine artery velocimetry failed tocolysis and delivered within 48 h of the examination, as compared with 14.6% (7 of 48) of the patients with a normal waveform ($p < 0.01$). In a subsequent study, 92 patients had uterine and umbilical artery FVWs determined at admission.[176] The outcome variables were preterm delivery (before 37 weeks), SGA rate, rate of cesarean section for fetal distress, number of days in the NICU, and neonatal death rate. An abnor-

mal uterine artery Doppler waveform had a PPV of 78.6% and an NPV of 69.2% for preterm delivery. The PPV and NPV for abnormal perinatal outcome were 64.3% and 82.1%, respectively.[177] These results were confirmed in a case-control study of 55 patients in preterm labor who were compared with 30 control patients not in labor.[178] No difference in uterine artery impedance to flow was observed between the study and control groups. However, 90.1% (10 of 11) of the patients with a pathologic uterine artery velocity waveform (PI > 0.90) delivered preterm, whereas only 36% (16 of 44) of the patients with a normal PI did so ($p < 0.05$). The PPV and NPV for preterm delivery in this series were 90.9% and 63.6%, respectively.[178]

The effect of different tocolytic agents on uteroplacental blood flow has also been investigated. Tocolysis with either beta-adrenergic drugs or magnesium sulfate is associated with a reduction in the impedance to blood flow in the uteroplacental circulation.[177,179] In the case of beta-adrenergic drugs, the reduction in impedance to flow may be caused by a reduction in peripheral resistance.[177] In the case of magnesium sulfate, it is likely that the decreased impedance to flow is a result of a reduction in peripheral uterine vasculature resistance.[179,180] Short-term tocolysis with nifedipine does not appear to have an influence on either the fetal or the uteroplacental circulations when evaluated by Doppler velocimetry.[181]

Rizzo et al.[182] studied multiple vessels (uterine, umbilical, fetal thoracic descending aorta, renal artery, and middle cerebral artery) with Doppler velocimetry in patients with preterm labor. Patients in preterm labor had higher uterine RI values when compared with normal reference values for gestational age, but no difference was found between those who delivered within 48 h or after 48 h of admission (0.75 ± 0.95 versus 0.85 ± 76, $p = 0.681$). However, PI values from the MCA were significantly lower in the group of fetuses who delivered within 48 h (1.80 ± 1.32 versus −0.39 ± 1.19, $p \le 0.001$).

DIABETES MELLITUS

Hyperglycemia may impair placental development and hence predispose the pregnancy to adverse perinatal outcome. Few studies have assessed uteroplacental perfusion with Doppler.[183–189]

It has been demonstrated that insulin-dependent diabetic pregnancies do not show the normal decline in uterine artery PIs during the third trimester.[188] Absolute PI values, however, remain within normal limits and do not help predict perinatal outcome. In contrast, increased discordance in the uterine artery S/D ratios during the third trimester (≥ 0.6) may be of value in identifying patients at risk for fetal distress.[189] A compilation of data from five other studies, including 217 diabetic patients (68 class A, 73 class B, 46 class C, 11 class D, 8 class F, and 11 class R according to White's classification[190]) who had serial Doppler velocimetry studies of the uterine arteries performed throughout the pregnancy, showed the test to be within normal limits, regardless of the diabetic class except in diabetic pregnancies complicated by preeclampsia.

SUMMARY

Most studies of uterine artery Doppler velocimetry have shown that an abnormal test increases the likelihood of pre-eclampsia. The presence of a diastolic notch, a PI greater than 1.5, or an RI greater than 0.68, especially when bilateral, are probably the best parameters for considering the test abnormal in the second trimester.

Aspirin prophylaxis remains a controversial subject. Most randomized trials that have used abnormal uterine artery FVWs to randomize patients into aspirin or placebo therapy show a benefit of aspirin in reducing the incidence of preeclampsia or preeclampsia requiring delivery before 37 weeks. Novel approaches to prophylaxis based on uterine artery Doppler screening are encouraging, namely the use of NO donors, NO donors plus aspirin, or antioxidants (vitamins C and E). Results of larger trials are awaited with interest.

Until now, the best screening strategy has been to scan patients at 20 weeks and rescan those with abnormal Doppler velocimetry at 24 weeks to minimize the false-positive tests. It has been demonstrated that a diastolic MESOR equal to or greater than 0.68, in 24-h automated BP monitoring, for patients with abnormal uterine artery Doppler at 24 weeks, increases the PPV of the test by two-fold.

Ultrasound is facing a new era. Widespread nuchal trans-lucency screening at 11 to 14 weeks, better equipment resolution, and improved knowledge are bringing prenatal diagnosis into the first trimester.[191] It is possible that the ideal time for the initial evaluation of the uterine circulation would be the ultrasound scan performed at 13 to 14 weeks, when fetal anatomy can be evaluated in detail with the transvaginal probe[192] and nuchal translucency assessed. Data from Harrington et al.[89] have shown that the absence of a diastolic notch between 12 and 16 weeks has a high NPV for the development of preeclampsia or delivery of an SGA fetus. Patients with normal nuchal translucency, normal fetal anatomy, and normal uterine artery Doppler velocimetry at the 13-week scan would constitute a truly low-risk group. Conversely, patients with uterine artery notches at this stage would be the ideal candidates for larger trials, to test the possible prophylactic regimens for the prevention of preeclampsia. A second-stage exam could be performed at 23 to 24 weeks to minimize the false-positive results, reassess fetal anatomy, and measure cervical length. Only those patients with a persistently abnormal uteroplacental circulation would remain

in prophylactic regimens, thereby maximizing the chances of preventing adverse perinatal outcome and minimizing the risks of unnecessary treatment.

ADDENDUM

Since submission of this chapter, a randomized management trial of low-dose, slow-release aspirin given to women with abnormal uterine artery Doppler studies at 20 weeks of gestation has been published.[193] In this trial, women were considered screen positive if there were bilateral notches with a mean RI > 0.55 (>50th centile), or a unilateral notch and a mean RI > 0.65 (>90th centile), or a mean RI > 0.70 (>95th centile) in the absence of notches. Screen-positive women were allocated to a control or a treatment group, the latter receiving 100 mg slow-release aspirin from 20 to 37 weeks. Doppler studies were repeated at 24 weeks and treatment discontinued in case of normal waveforms. The four main outcome variables were: gestational age at delivery, development of preeclampsia, occurrence of antepartum hemorrhage, or delivery of an SGA baby. The final analysis was performed in 940 women: 107 in the treatment group, 103 in the control group, and 730 with normal Doppler waveforms. No differences between control and treatment groups were observed for the main outcome variables: gestational age at delivery (38.3 ± 3.9 weeks versus 38.1 ± 3.3 weeks, NS), development of preeclampsia [8.4% (9 of 103) versus 6.5% (7 of 107), NS], occurrence of antepartum hemorrhage [0% (0 of 103) versus 0.9% (1 of 107), NS] or delivery of an SGA baby [33.9% (35 of 103) versus 29.9% (32 of 107), NS]. However, a significantly lower incidence of any complication [51.4% versus 71.8%, OR = 0.41 (CI = 0.35 to 0.45), $p < 0.01$] or severe complications [15% versus 29.1%, OR = 0.43 (CI = 0.22 to 0.84), $p < 0.05$] was observed in patients allocated to aspirin. Severe complications were defined as any case with preeclampsia requiring delivery before 34 weeks, placental abruption, delivery of an SGA baby below the third percentile, an Apgar score below 7 at 5 mins, admission to NICU, or a pregnancy that resulted in a stillbirth or neonatal death. "Any" complication included: any severe complication, all cases of preeclampsia delivered after 34 weeks, and SGA babies below the 10th percentile.

REFERENCES

1. Cuningham FG, MacDonald PC, Gant NF, et al. Anatomy of the reproductive tract of women. In: Cuningham FG, MacDonald PC, Leveno K, Gilstrap LC II, eds. *Williams Obstetrics*. Norwalk, CT: Appleton & Lange; 1993:57.
2. Brosens I, Robertson WB, Dixon HG. Anatomy of the maternal side of the placenta. *J Obstet Gynecol Br Commonw*. 1966;73:357.

3. Brosens I, Robertson WB, Dixon HG. The physiological response of the vessels of the placental bed to normal pregnancy. *J Pathol Bacteriol.* 1967;93:569.

4. Brosens I, Robertson WB, Dixon HG. The role of the spiral arteries in the pathogenesis of preeclampsia. *Obstet Gynecol Annu.* 1972;1:177.

5. Brosens I, Dixon HG, Robertson WB. Fetal growth retardation and the arteries of the placental bed. *Br J Obstet Gynecol.* 1977;84:656.

6. Khong TY, De Wolf R, Robertson WB, Brosens I. Inadequate maternal vascular response to placentation in pregnancies complicated by preeclampsia and by small-for-gestational age infants. *Br J Obstet Gynecol.* 1986;93:1049.

7. Robertson WB, Brosens I, Dixon G. Uteroplacental vascular pathology. *Eur J Obstet Gynecol Reprod Biol.* 1975;5:47.

8. Sheppard BL, Bonnar L. The ultrastructure of the arterial supply of the human placenta pregnancies complicated by growth retardation. *J Obstet Gynecol Br Commonw.* 1976;83:948.

9. Garretsen G, Huisjes HJ, Elema JD. Morphological changes of the spiral arteries in the placental bed in relation to preeclampsia and fetal growth retardation. *Br J Obstet Gynecol.* 1981;88:876.

10. Hustin J, Foidart JM, Lambotte R. Maternal vascular lesions in preeclampsia and intrauterine growth retardation: Light microscopy and immunofluorescence. *Placenta.* 1983;4:489.

11. Mehalek KE, Berkowitz GS, Chitkara U, et al. Comparison of continuous-wave and pulsed Doppler S/D ratios of umbilical and uterine arteries. *Obstet Gynecol.* 1988;72:603.

12. Arduini D, Rizzo G, Boccolini MR, et al. Functional assessment of uteroplacental and fetal circulations by means of color Doppler ultrasonography. *J Ultrasound Med.* 1990;9:249.

13. Fleischer A, Schulman H, Farmakides G, et al. Uterine artery Doppler velocimetry in pregnant women with hypertension. *Am J Obstet Gynecol.* 1986;154:806.

14. Thaler I, Weiner Z, Itskovitz J. Systolic or diastolic notch in uterine artery blood flow velocity waveforms in hypertensive patients: Relationship to outcome. *Obstet Gynecol.* 1992;80:806.

15. Bower S, Bewley S, Campbell S. Improved prediction of preeclampsia by two-stage screening of uterine arteries using the early diastolic notch and color Doppler imaging. *Obstet Gynecol.* 1993;82:78.

16. Chan FY, Pun TC, Lam C, et al. Pregnancy screening by uterine artery Doppler velocimetry—Which criterion performs best? *Obstet Gynecol.* 1995;85:596.

17. Harrington K, Cooper D, Lees C, et al. Doppler ultrasound of the uterine arteries: Importance of bilateral notching in the prediction of preeclampsia, placental abruption or delivery of a small for gestational age baby. *Ultrasound Obstet Gynecol.* 1996;7:182.

18. Bower S, Kingdom J, Campbell S. Objective and subjective assessment of abnormal uterine artery Doppler flow velocity waveforms. *Ultrasound Obstet Gynecol.* 1998;12:260.

19. Zimmermann P, Eiriö V, Koskinen J, et al. Doppler assessment of the uterine and uteroplacental circulation in the second trimester in pregnancies at high risk for preeclampsia and/or intrauterine growth retardation: Comparison and correlation between different Doppler parameters. *Ultrasound Obstet Gynecol.* 1997;9:330.

20. Joern H, Klein A, Kuehlwein H, Rath W. Critical comparison of indices and threshold values for assessing placenta performance using Doppler ultrasound. *Ultrasound Med Biol.* 1997;23:1179.

21. Farrel T, Chien PFW, Mires GJ. The reliability of the detection of an early diastolic notch with uterine artery Doppler velocimetry. *Br J Obstet Gynaecol.* 1998;105:1308.

22. North, RA, Ferrier C, Long D, et al. Uterine artery Doppler flow velocity waveforms in the second trimester for the prediction of preeclampsia and fetal growth retardation. *Obstet Gynecol.* 1994;83:378.

23. Irion O, Masse J, Forest J-C, Moutquin J-M. Peak systolic over protodiastolic ratio as an objective substitute for the uterine artery notch. *Br J Obstet Gynecol.* 1996.7:182.

24. Santolaya-Forgas J. Physiology of the menstrual cycle by ultrasonography. *J Ultrasound Med.* 1992;11:139.

25. Goswamy RK, Steptoe PC. Doppler ultrasound studies of the uterine artery in spontaneous ovarian cycles. *Hum Reprod.* 1988;3:721.

26. Scholtes MC, Wladimiroff JW, van Rijen HJ, Hop WC. Uterine and ovarian flow velocity waveforms in the normal menstrual cycle: A transvaginal Doppler study. *Fertil Steril.* 1989;52:981.

27. Kurjak A, Kupesic-Urek S, Schulman H, Zalud I. Transvaginal color flow Doppler in the assessment of ovarian and uterine blood flow in infertile women. *Fertil Steril.* 1991;56:870.

28. Deutinger J, Rudelstorfer R, Bernaschek G. Vaginosonographic Doppler velocimetry in both uterine arteries: Elevated left-right differences and relationship to fetal haemodynamics and outcome. *Early Hum Dev.* 1991;25:187.

29. Steer CV, Tan SL, Mason BA, Campbell S. Midluteal-phase vaginal color Doppler assessment of uterine artery impedance in a subfertile population. *Fertil Steril.* 1994;61:53.

30. Goswamy RK, Williams G, Steptoe PC. Decreased uterine perfusion—A cause of infertility. *Hum Reprod.* 1988;3:955.

31. Sterzik K, Grab D, Sasse V, et al. Doppler sonographic findings and their correlation with implantation in an in vitro fertilization program. *Fertil Steril.* 1989;52:825.

32. Steer CV, Campbell S, Tan SL, Crayford T. The use of transvaginal color flow imaging after in vitro fertilization to identify optimum uterine conditions before embryo transfer. *Fertil Steril.* 1992;57:372.

33. Hustin J, Schaaps JP. Echographic and anatomic studies of the maternotrophoblastic border during the first trimester of pregnancy. *Am J Obstet Gynecol.* 1987;157:162.

34. Hustin J, Schaaps JP, Lambotte R. Anatomical studies of the utero-placental vascularization in the first trimester of pregnancy. *Troph Res.* 1988;3:49.

35. Jaffe R, Warsof SL. Transvaginal color Doppler imaging in the assessment of uteroplacental blood flow in the normal first trimester pregnancy. *Am J Obstet Gynecol.* 1991.164:781.

36. Jauniaux E, Jurkovic D, Campbell S. In vivo investigations of anatomy and physiology of early human placental circulations. *Ultrasound Obstet Gynecol.* 1991;1:435.

37. Jauniaux E, Jurkovic D, Campbell S, Justin J. Doppler ultrasound features of the developing placental circulations: Correlation with anatomic findings. *Am J Obstet Gynecol.* 1992;166:585.

38. Jaffe R, Woods JF. Color Doppler imaging and in vivo assessment of the anatomy and physiology of the early uteroplacental circulations: Correlation with anatomic findings. *Am J Obstet Gynecol.* 1992;166:585.

39. Jauniaux E, Johson MR, Jurkovic D, et al. The role of relaxin in the development of the uteroplacental circulation in early pregnancy. *Obstet Gynecol.* 1994;85:338.

40. Coppens M, Loquet P, Klollen F, et al. Longitudinal evaluation of uteroplacental and umbilical blood flow changes in normal early pregnancy. *Ultrasound Obstet Gynecol.* 1996;7:114.

41. Khong TY, Liddel HS, Robertson WB. Defective haemochorial placentation as a cause of miscarriage: A preliminary study. *Br J Obstet Gynaecol.* 1987;94:649.

42. Hustin J, Jauniaux E, Schaaps JP. Histological study of the maternoembryonic interface in spontaneous abortion. *Placenta.* 1990;11:477.

43. Alfirevic Z, Kurjak A. Transvaginal color Doppler ultrasound in normal and abnormal early pregnancy. *J Perinat Med.* 1990;18:173.

44. Dillon E, Case CQ, Ramos IM, et al. Endovaginal pulsed and color Doppler in first-trimester pregnancy. *Ultrasound Med Biol.* 1993;19:517.

45. Mercé LT, Barco MJ, de la Fuente F. Doppler velocimetry measured in retrochorionic space and uterine arteries during early human pregnancy. *Acta Obstet Gynecol Scand.* 1989;68:603.

46. Deutinger J, Rudelstorfer, Bernaschek G. Vaginosonographic velocimetry of both main uterine arteries by visual vessel recognition and pulsed Doppler method during pregnancy. *Am J Obstet Gynecol.* 1988;159:1072.

47. Thaler I, Manor D, Itskovitz J, et al. Changes in uterine blood flow during pregnancy. *Am J Obstet Gynecol.* 1990;162:121.

48. Kofinas AD, Espeland MA, Penry M, et al. Uteroplacental Doppler flow velocity waveform indices in normal pregnancy: A statistical exercise and development of appropriate reference values. *Am J Perinatol.* 1992;9:94.

49. van Zalen-Sprock MM, van Gut JMG, Colenbrander GJ, van Geijin HP. First-trimester uteroplacental and fetal blood flow velocity waveforms in normally developing fetuses: A longitudinal study. *Ultrasound Obstet Gynecol.* 1994;4:284.

50. Thoresen M, Jarlis W. Doppler measurements of changes in human mammary and uterine blood flow during pregnancy and lactation. *Acta Obstet Gynecol Scand.* 1988;67:741.

51. den Ouden M, Cohen-Overbeek TE, Wladimiroff JW. Uterine and fetal umbilical artery flow velocity waveforms in normal first trimester pregnancies. *Br J Obstet Gynecol.* 1990;97:716.

52. Jurkovic D, Jauniaux E, Hustin J, et al. Transvaginal color Doppler assessment of the uteroplacental circulation in early pregnancy. *Obstet Gynecol.* 1991;77:365.

53. Palmer SK, Zamudio S, Coffin C, et al. Quantitative estimation of human uterine artery blood flow and pelvic blood flow redistribution in pregnancy. *Obstet Gynecol.* 1992;80:1000.

54. Cohen-Overbeek T, Pearce M, Campbell S. The antenatal assessment of utero-placental and feto-placental blood flow using Doppler ultrasound. *Ultrasound Med Biol.* 1985;2:329.

55. McCowan LM, Ritchie K, Mo LY, et al. Uterine artery flow velocity waveforms in normal and growth-retarded pregnancies. *Am J Obstet Gynecol.* 1988;158:499.

56. Trudinger BJ, Giles WB, Cook CM. Flow velocity waveforms in the maternal uteroplacental and fetal umbilical placental circulations. *Am J Obstet Gynecol.* 1985;152:155.

57. Tekay A, Jouppila P. A longitudinal Doppler ultrasonographic assessment of the alterations in peripheral vascular resistance of uterine arteries and ultrasonographic findings of the involuting uterus during the puerperium. *Am J Obstet Gynecol.* 1993;168:190.

58. Kofinas AD, Penry M, Swain M, Hatjis CG. Effect of placental laterality on uterine artery resistance and development of preeclampsia and intrauterine growth retardation. *Am J Obstet Gynecol.* 1989;161:1536.

59. Schulman H, Ducey J, Farmakides G, et al. Uterine artery Doppler velocimetry: The significance of divergent systolic/diastolic ratios. *Am J Obstet Gynecol.* 1987;157:1539.

60. Campbell S, Griffin DR, Pearce JM, et al. New Doppler technique for assessing uteroplacental blood flow. *Lancet.* 1983;i:675.

61. Hanretty KP, Whittle MJ, Rubin PC. Doppler uteroplacental waveforms in pregnancy-induced hypertension: A reappraisal. *Lancet.* 1988;1(8590):850.

62. Bewley S, Campbell S, Cooper D. Uteroplacental Doppler flow velocity waveforms in the second trimester: A complex circulation. *Br J Obstet Gynaecol.* 1989;96:1040.

63. Bower SJ, Campbell S. Doppler velocimetry of the uterine artery as a screening test in pregnancy. In: Chervenak FA, Isaacson GC, Campbell S, eds. *Ultrasound in Obstetrics and Gynecology.* Boston: Little & Brown; 1993:579.

64. Oosterhof H, Aarnoudse JG. Ultrasound pulsed Doppler studies of the uteroplacental circulation: The influence of sampling site and placental implantation. *Gynecol Obstet Invest.* 1992;33:75.

65. Pearce JM, Campbell S, Cohen-Overbeek T, et al. Reference ranges and sources of variation for indices of pulsed Doppler flow velocity waveforms from the uteroplacental and fetal circulation. *Br J Obstet Gynecol.* 1988;95:248.

66. Bewley S, Cooper D, Campbell S. Doppler investigation of uteroplacental blood flow resistance in the second trimester: A screening study for preeclampsia and intra-uterine growth retardation. *Br J Obstet Gynecol.* 1991;98:871.

67. Kofinas AD, Penry M, Simon NV, Swain M. Interrelationship and clinical significance of increased resistance in the uterine arteries in patients with hypertension or preeclampsia or both. *Am J Obstet Gynecol.* 1992;166:601.

68. Kofinas AD, Penry M, Greiss GC, et al. The effect of placental location on uterine artery flow velocity waveforms. *Am J Obstet Gynecol.* 1988;159:1504.

69. Adamson SL, Morrow RJ, Bascom PAJ, et al. Effect of placental resistance, arterial diameter, and blood pressure on the uterine arterial velocity waveform. A computer modeling approach. *Ultrasound Med Biol.* 1989;5:437.

70. Talbert DG. Uterine flow velocity waveform shape as an indicator of maternal and placental development failure mechanisms: A model-based synthesizing approach. *Ultrasound Obstet Gynaecol.* 1995;6:261.

71. Ochi H, Suginami H, Matsubara K, et al. Micro-bead embolization of the spiral arteries and changes in uterine artery flow velocity waveforms in the pregnant ewe. *Ultrasound Obstet Gynecol.* 1995;6:272.

72. Ochi H, Matsubara K, Kusanagi Y, et al. Significance of a diastolic notch in the uterine artery flow velocity waveform induced by uterine embolisation in the pregnant ewe. *Br J Obstet Gynecol.* 1998;105:1118.

73. Olofsson P, Laurini RN, Marsal K. A high uterine artery pulsatility index reflects a defective development of placental bed spiral arteries in pregnancies complicated by hypertension

and fetal growth retardation. *Eur J Obstet Reprod Biol.* 1993;49:161.

74. Lin S, Shimizu I, Suehara N, et al. Uterine artery Doppler velocimetry in relation to trophoblast migration into the myometrium of the placental bed. *Obstet Gynecol.* 1995;85:760.

75. Arduini D, Rizzo G, Romanini C, Mancuso S. Utero-placental blood flow velocity waveforms as predictors of pregnancy-induced hypertension. *Eur J Obstet Gynecol Reprod Biol.* 1987;26:335.

76. Jacobson S, Imhof R, Manning N, et al. The value of Doppler assessment of the uteroplacental circulation in predicting preeclampsia or intrauterine growth retardation. *Am J Obstet Gynecol.* 1990;162:110.

77. Montenegro CAB, Perim SMC, Rezende-Filho J, et al. Uterine artery Doppler screening at 26 weeks gestation in the prediction of preeclampsia. Abstract 097 presented at the 8th World Congress on Hypertension in Pregnancy, Buenos Aires, Argentina, November 8–12, 1992.

78. Caforio L, Testa AC, Mastromarino C, et al. Predictive value of uterine artery velocimetry at midgestation in low and high-risk populations: A new perspective. *Fetal Diagn Ther.* 1999;14:201.

79. Campbell S, Pearce JM, Hackett G, et al. Qualitative assessment of uteroplacental blood flow: Early screening test for high-risk pregnancies. *Obstet Gynecol.* 1986;68:649.

80. Hanretty KP, Primrose MH, Neilson JP, Whittle MJ. Pregnancy screening by Doppler uteroplacental and umbilical artery waveforms. *Br J Obstet Gynaecol.* 1989;96:1163.

81. Schulman H, Winter D, Farmakides G, et al. Pregnancy surveillance with Doppler velocimetry of uterine and umbilical arteries. *Am J Obstet Gynecol.* 1989;160:192.

82. Steel SA, Pearce JM, McParland P, Chamberlain GVP. Early Doppler ultrasound screening in prediction of hypertensive disorders of pregnancy. *Lancet.* 1990;335:1548.

83. Newnham JP, Patterson LL, James IR, et al. An evaluation of the efficacy of Doppler flow velocity waveform analysis as a screening test in pregnancy. *Am J Obstet Gynecol.* 1990;162:403.

84. Harrington KF, Campbell S, Bewley S, Bower S. Doppler velocimetry studies of the uterine artery in the early prediction of preeclampsia and intra-uterine growth retardation. *Eur J Obstet Gynecol Reprod Biol.* 1991;42:S14.

85. Valensise H, Bezzeccheri V, Rizzo G, et al. Doppler velocimetry of the uterine artery as a screening test for gestational hypertension. *Ultrasound Obstet Gynecol.* 1993;3:18.

86. Bower S, Schuchter K, Campbell S. Doppler ultrasound screening as part of routine antenatal scanning: Prediction of preeclampsia and intrauterine growth retardation. *Br J Obstet Gynecol.* 1993;100:989.

87. Kurdi W, Campbell S, Aquilina J, et al. The role of color Doppler imaging of the uterine arteries at 20 weeks' gestation in stratifying prenatal care. *Ultrasound Obstet Gynecol.* 1998;12:339.

88. Irion O, Massé J, Forest JC, Moutquin JM. Prediction of preeclampsia, low birth weigth for gestation and prematurity by uterine artery blood flow velocity waveforms analysis in low risk nulliparous women. *Br J Obstet Gynaecol.* 1998; 105:422.

89. Harrington K, Goldfrad C, Carpenter RG, Campbell S. Transvaginal uterine and umbilical artery Doppler examination of 12–16 weeks and the subsequent development of preeclampsia and intrauterine growth retardation. *Ultrasound Obstet Gynecol.* 1997;9:94.

90. Aquilina J, Harrington K. Pregnancy hypertension and uterine artery Doppler ultrasound. *Curr Opin Obstet Gynecol.* 1996; 8:435.

91. Sibai BM. Hypertension and pregnancy. Chronic hypertension in pregnancy. *Clin Perinatol.* 1991;18:833.

92. Caruso A, Caforio L, Testa AC, et al. Chronic hypertension in pregnancy: Color Doppler investigation of uterine arteries as a predictive test for superimposed preeclampsia and adverse perinatal outcome. *J Perinat Med.* 1996;24:141.

93. Frusca T, Soregaroli M, Zanelli S, et al. Role of uterine artery Doppler investigation in pregnant women with chronic hypertension. *Eur J Obstet Gynecol Reprod Biol.* 1998;29:47.

94. van Asselt K, Gudmundsson S, Lindqvist P, Marsal K. Uterine and umbilical artery velocimetry in preeclampsia. *Acta Obstet Gynecol Scand.* 1998;77:614.

95. Joern H, Rath W. Comparison of Doppler sonographic examinations of the umbilical and uterine arteries in high-risk pregnancies. *Fetal Diagn Ther.* 1998;13:150.

96. Hofstaetter C, Dubiel M, Gudmundsson S, Marsal K. Uterine artery Doppler assisted velocimetry and perinatal outcome. *Acta Obstet Gynecol Scand.* 1996;75:612.

97. Newnham JP, O'Dea MRA, Reid KP, Diepeveen DA. Doppler flow velocity waveform analysis in high risk pregnancies: A randomised controlled trial. *Br J Obstet Gynaecol.* 1991;98:956.

98. Davies JA, Gallivan S, Spencer JAD. Randomised controlled trial of Doppler ultrasound screening of placental perfusion during pregnancy. *Lancet.* 1992;340:1299.

99. Valensise H. Uterine artery Doppler velocimetry as a screening test: Where we are and where we go. *Ultrasound Obstet Gynecol.* 1998;12:81.

100. Benedetto C, Valensise H, Marozio L, et al. A two-stage screening test for pregnancy-induced hypertension and preeclampsia. *Obstet Gynecol.* 1998;92:1005.

101. Aristidou A, Van Den Hof M, Campbell S, Nicolaides K. Uterine artery Doppler in the investigation of pregnancies with raised maternal serum alpha-fetoprotein. *Br J Obstet Gynecol.* 1990;97:431.

102. Bromley B, Frigoletto FD, Harlow BL, et al. The role of Doppler velocimetry in the structurally normal second-trimester fetus with elevated levels of maternal serum α-fetoprotein. *Ultrasound Obstet Gynecol.* 1994;4:377.

103. Konachak PS, Bernstein IM, Capeless MD. Uterine artery Doppler velocimetry in the detection of adverse obstetric outcomes in women with unexplained elevated maternal serum α-fetoprotein levels. *Am J Obstet Gynecol.* 1995; 173:1115.

104. Palacio M, Jauniaux E, Kingdom J, et al. Perinatal outcome in pregnancies with a positive serum screening for Down's syndrome due to elevated levels of free beta-human chorionic gonadotropin. *Ultrasound Obstet Gynecol.* 1999;13:58.

105. Jauniaux E, Gulbist B, Tunkel S, et al. Maternal serum testing for alpha-fetoprotein and human chorionic gonadotropin in high-risk pregnancies. *Prenat Diagn.* 1996;16:1129.

106. Pouta AM, Vuolteenaho OJ, Laatikainen TJ. An increase of the plasma N-terminal peptide of proatrial natriuretic peptide in preeclampsia. *Obstet Gynecol.* 1997;89:747.

107. Millar JG, Campbell SK, Albano JDM, et al. Early prediction of preeclampsia by measurement of kallikrein and creatinine on a random urine sample. *Br J Obstet Gynecol*. 199;103:421.

108. Carroli G, Duley L, Belizan JM, Villar J. Calcium supplementation during pregnancy: A systematic review of randomized controlled trials. *Br J Obstet Gynecol*. 1994;101:753.

109. Levine RJ, Hauth JC, Curet LB, et al. Trial of calcium to prevent preeclampsia. *N Engl J Med*. 1997;337:69.

110. Herrera JA, Arevalo-Herrera M, Herrera S. Prevention of preeclampsia by linoleic acid and calcium supplementation: A randomized controlled trial. *Obstet Gynecol*. 1998;91:585.

111. Olsen SF, Sorensen JD, Secher NJ, et al. Randomized controlled trial of fish-oil supplementation on pregnancy duration. *Lancet*. 1992;339:1003.

112. Sorensen JD, Olsen SF, Pedersen AK, et al. Effects of fish oil supplementation in the third trimester of pregnancy on prostacyclin and thromboxane production. *Am J Obstet Gynecol*. 1993;168:915.

113. Walsh SW. Preeclampsia: An imbalance in placental prostacyclin and thromboxane production. *Am J Obstet Gynecol*. 1985:152:335.

114. Goodlin RC, Haesslein HO, Fleming J. Aspirin for the treatment of recurrent toxaemia. *Lancet*. 1978;ii:51.

115. Wallenburg HCS, Dekker GA, Makovitz JW, et al. Low-dose aspirin prevents pregnancy-induced hypertension and preeclampsia in angiotensin-sensitive primigravidae. *Lancet*. 1986;1(8471):1.

116. Michael CA, Seville P, Walters BNJ. Randomized double-blind placebo controlled trial of aspirin in the prevention of preeclampsia. In: Proceedings of the VIIth World Congress of Hypertension in Pregnancy, Perugia, Italy. 1990:73.

117. Schiff E, Peleg E, Goldenberg M, et al. The use of aspirin to prevent pregnancy-induced hypertension and lower the ratio of thromboxane A2 to prostacyclin in relatively high risk pregnancies. *N Engl J Med*. 1989;321:351.

118. McParland P, Pearce JM, Chamberlain GVP. Doppler ultrasound and aspirin in recognition and prevention of pregnancy-induced hypertension. *Lancet*. 1990;335:1552.

119. Uzan S, Beaufils S, Breart G, et al. Prevention of fetal growth retardation with low-dose aspirin: Findings of the EPREDA trial. *Lancet*. 1991;337:1427.

120. Davies NJ, Farguharson RG, Wakinshaw SA. Low-dose aspirin and nulliparae. *Lancet*. 1991;338:324.

121. Porreco RP, Hickok DE, Williams MA, et al. Low-dose aspirin and hypertension in pregnancy. *Lancet*. 1993;341:312.

122. Uzan M, Uzan S, Bréart G, et al. Can uterine artery velocimetry be a predictor for IUGR and be an indication for ASA treatment. *Fetal Diagn Ther*. 1992;7:204.

123. Uzan M, Haddad B, Bréart G, Uzan S. Uteroplacental Doppler and aspirin therapy in the prediction and prevention of pregnancy complications. *Ultrasound Obstet Gynecol*. 1994;4:342.

124. Beaufils M, Donsimoni R, Uzan S, et al. Prevention of preeclampsia by early antiplatelet therapy. *Lancet*. 1985;1:840.

125. Uzan S, Beaufils M, Breart G, et al. Prevention of fetal growth retardation with low-dose aspiring: Findings of the EPREDA trial. *Lancet*. 1978;337:1427.

126. Italian Study of Aspirin in Pregnancy. Low-dose aspirin in prevention and treatment of intrauterine growth retardation and pregnancy-induced hypertension. *Lancet*. 1993;341:396.

127. Hauth JC, Goldenberg RL, Parker JR, et al. Low-dose aspirin therapy to prevent preeclampsia. *Am J Obstet Gynecol*. 1993;168:1083.

128. Sibai BM, Caritis SN, Thron E, et al. Prevention of preeclampsia with low-dose aspirin in health, nulliparous, pregnant women. *N Engl J Med*. 1993;329:1213.

129. ECPPA. Randomized trial of low-dose aspirin for prevention of maternal and fetal complications in high risk pregnant women in Brazil. *Br J Obstet Gynaecol*. 1996;103:39.

130. Rotchel YE, Cruickshank JK, Gay MP, et al. Barbados Low Dose Aspirin Study in Pregnancy (BLASP): A randomised trial for the prevention of preeclampsia and its complications. *Br J Obstet Gynaecol*. 1998;105:286.

131. Golding J. Jamaica Low Dose Aspirin Study Group. A randomised trial of low dose aspirin for primiparae in pregnancy. *Br J Obstet Gynaecol*. 1998;105:293.

132. Vinikka L, Hartikainen-Sorri A-L, Lumme R, et al. Low dose aspirin in hypertensive pregnant women: Effect on pregnancy outcome and prostacyclin-thromboxane balance in mother and newborn. *Br J Obstet Gynaecol*. 1993;100:809.

133. CLASP: a randomised trial of low-dose aspirin for prevention and treatment of preeclampsia among 9364 pregnant women. *Lancet*. 1994;343:619.

134. Caritis S, Sibai B, Hauth J, et al. NICHD Maternal-Fetal Medicine Units. Low-dose aspirin to prevent preeclampsia in women at high risk. *N Engl J Med*. 1998:338:701.

135. Montenegro CAB, Perim SMC, Rezende-Filho J, et al. The value of uterine artery Doppler ultrasound and aspirin in the prediction and prevention of preeclampsia. Abstract 096, Presented at VIIIth World Congress on Hypertension in Pregnancy, Buenos Aires, Argentina, November 8–12, 1992.

136. Perim SMC. Valor do ácido acetil-salicílico na prevenção da toxemia gravídica (thesis). Rio de Janeiro, Brazil: School of Medicine, Federal University of Rio de Janeiro; 1991.

137. Uzan M, Uzan S, Bréart G, et al. Can uterine artery velocimetry be a predictor for IUGR and be an indication for ASA treatment. *Fetal Diagn Ther*. 1992;7:204.

138. Uzan M, Haddad B, Bréart G, Uzan S. Uteroplacental Doppler and aspirin therapy in the prediction and prevention of pregnancy complications. *Ultrasound Obstet Gynecol*. 1994;4:342.

139. Bower SJ, Harrington KF, Schuchter K, et al. Prediction of preeclampsia by abnormal uterine Doppler ultrasound and modification by aspirin. *Br J Obstet Gynaecol*. 1996;103:625.

140. Morris JM, Fay RA, Ellwood DA, et al. A randomized controlled trial of aspirin in patients with abnormal uterine artery blood flow. *Obstet Gynecol*. 1996;87:74.

141. Mills JL, DerSimonian R, Raymond E, et al. Prostacyclin and thromboxane changes predating clinical onset of preeclampsia: A multicenter prospective study. *JAMA*. 1999;282:356.

142. Shanklin DR, Sibai BM. Ultrastructural aspects of preeclampsia. I. Placental bed and uterine boundary vessels. *Am J Obstet Gynecol*. 1989;161:735.

143. Barton JR, Hiett AK, O'Connor WN, et al. Endomyocardial ultrastructural findings in preeclampsia. *Am J Obstet Gynecol*. 1991;165:389.

144. Radomski MW, Palmer RM, Moncada S. Endogenous nitric oxide inhibits human platelet adhesion to vascular endothelium. *Lancet*. 1987;2:1057.

145. Palmer RMJ, Ferrige AG, Moncada S. Release of nitric oxide accounts for the biological activity of endothelium-derived relaxing factor. *Nature*. 1987;327:524.

146. Palmer RMJ, Rees DD, Aston DS, Moncada S. L-arginine is the physiological precursor for the formation of nitric oxide in endothelium-dependent relaxation. *Biochem Biophys Res Commun*. 1988;153:1251.

147. Bhordwaj R, Page CP, May GR, Moore PK. Endothelium-derived relaxing factor inhibits platelet aggregation in human whole blood in vitro and in the rat in vivo. *Eur J Pharmacol*. 1988;157:83.

148. Furchgott RF. The role of endothelium in the response of vascular smooth muscle to drugs. *Annu Rev Pharmacol Toxicol*. 1984;24:175.

149. Nathan C. Nitric oxide as a secretory product of mammalian cells. *FASEB J*. 1992;6:3051.

150. Gryglewski RJ, Palmer RMJ, Moncada S. Superoxide anion is involved in the breakdown of endothelium-derived vascular relaxing factor. *Nature*. 1986;320:454.

151. Gant NF, Whalley PJ, Everett RB, et al. Control of vascular reactivity in pregnancy. *Am J Kidney Dis*. 1987;9:303.

152. Seligman SP, Buyon JP, Clancy RM, et al. The role of nitric oxide in the pathogenesis of preeclampsia. *Am J Obstet Gynecol*. 1994;171:944.

153. Yallampalli C, Garfield RE. Inhibition of nitric oxide synthesis in rats during pregnancy produces signs similar to those of preeclampsia. *Am J Obstet Gynecol*. 1993;169:1316.

154. Pinto A, Sorrentino R, Sorrentino P, et al. Endothelial-derived relaxing factor released by endothelial cells of human umbilical vessels and its impairment in pregnancy-induced hypertension. *Am J Obstet Gynecol*. 1994;164:507.

155. Janes SL, Goodall AH. Flow cytometric detection of circulating activated platelets and platelet hyper-responsiveness in pre-eclampsia and pregnancy. *Clin Sci*. 1994;86:731.

156. Ramsay B, De Belder A, Campbell S, et al. A nitric oxide donor improves uterine artery diastolic blood flow in normal early pregnancy and in women at high risk of pre-eclampsia. *Eur J Clin Invest*. 1994;24:76.

157. Giles W. Reduction in human fetal umbilical-placental vascular resistance by glyceryl trinitrate (letter). *Lancet*. 1992;342:242.

158. Grunewald C, Kublickas M, Carlström L, et al. Effects of nitroglycerin on the uterine and umbilical circulation in severe preeclampsia. *Obstet Gynecol*. 1995;86:600.

159. Luzi G, Caserta G, Iammarino G, et al. Nitric oxide donors in pregnancy: Fetomaternal hemodynamic effects induced in mild preeclampsia and threatened preterm labor. *Ultrasound Obstet Gynecol*. 1999;14:101.

160. Thaler I, Amit A, Jakobi P, Itskovitz-Eldor J. The effect of isosorbide dinitrate on uterine artery and umbilical artery flow velocity waveforms at mid-pregnancy. *Obstet Gynecol*. 1996;88:838.

161. Amit A, Thaler I, Paz Y, Itskovitz-Eldor J. The effect of a nitric oxide donor on Doppler flow velocity waveforms in the uterine artery during the first trimester of pregnancy. *Ultrasound Obstet Gynecol*. 1998;11:94.

162. Lees C, Langford E, Brown AS, et al. The effects of S-nitrosoglutathione on platelet activation, hypertension, and uterine and fetal Doppler in severe preeclampsia. *Obstet Gynecol*. 1996;88:14.

163. de Belder AJ, MacAllister R, Radomski MW, et al. Effects of S-nitroso-glutathione in the human forearm circulation: Evidence for selective inhibition of platelet activation. *Cardiovasc Res*. 1994;28:691.

164. Lees C, Valensise H, Black R, et al. The efficacy and fetal-maternal cardiovascular effects of transdermal glyceryl trinitrate in the prophylaxis of pre-eclampsia and its complications: A randomized double-blind placebo-controlled trial. *Ultrasound Obstet Gynecol*. 1998;12:334.

165. Thaler I, Amit A, Kamil D, Itskovitz-Eldor J. The effect of isosorbide dinitrate on placental blood flow and maternal blood pressure in women with pregnancy induced hypertension. *Am J Hypertens*. 1999;12:341.

166. Oyelese KO, Black RS, Lees CC, Campbell S. A novel approach to the management of pregnancies complicated by uteroplacental insufficiency and previous stillbirth. *Aust NZ J Obstet Gynecol*. 1998;38:391.

167. Hubel CA, McLaughlin MK, Evans RW, et al. Fasting serum triglycerides, free fatty acids, and malondialdehyde are increased in preeclampsia, are positively correlated and decrease within 28 hours postpartum. *Am J Obstet Gynecol*. 1996;174:975.

168. Barden A, Beilin LJ, Ritchie J, et al. Plasma and urinary 8-isoprostane as an indicator of lipid peroxidation in pre-eclampsia and normal pregnancy. *Clin Sci*. 1996;91:711.

169. Halligan A, Bonnar J, Sheppard B, et al. Haemostatic, fibrinolytic and endothelial variables in normal pregnancies and preeclampsia. *Br J Obstet Gynaecol*. 1994;101:488.

170. Reith A, Booth NA, Moore NR, et al. Plasminogen activator inhibitors (PAI-1 and PAI-2) in normal pregnancies, pre-eclampsia and hydatidiform mole. *Br J Obstet Gynaecol*. 1993;100:370.

171. Chappell LC, Seed PT, Briley AL, et al. Effect of antioxidants on the occurrence of pre-eclampsia in women at increased risk: A randomised trial. *Lancet*. 1999;354:810.

172. Nishikimi M. Oxidation of ascorbic acid with superoxide anion generated by the xanthine–xanthine oxidase system. *Biochem Biophys Res Commun*. 1975;63:463.

173. Fuller CJ, Grundy SM, Norkus EP, Jialal I. Effect of ascorbate supplementation on low density lipoprotein oxidation in smokers. *Atherosclerosis*. 1996;119:139.

174. Jialal I, Grundy SM. Effect of dietary supplementation with alphatocopherol on the oxidative modification of low density lipoprotein. *J Lipid Res*. 1992;33:899.

175. Brar HS, Medearis AL, Greggory R, et al. Maternal and fetal blood flow velocity waveforms in patients with preterm labor. Prediction of successful tocolysis. *Am J Obstet Gynecol*. 1988;159:947.

176. Brar HS, Medearis AL, Greggory R, et al. Maternal and fetal blood flow velocity waveforms in patients with preterm labor. Relationship to outcome. *Am J Obstet Gynecol*. 1989;161:1519.

177. Brar HS, Medearis AL, Greggory R, et al. Maternal and fetal blood flow velocity waveforms in patients with preterm labor: Effect of tocolytics. *Obstet Gynecol*. 1988;72:209.

178. Robel R, Ruckhaberle KE, Faber R, et al. Doppler sonographic examinations of uteroplacental, fetoplacental, and fetal hemodynamics and their prognostic value in preterm labor. *J Perinat Med*. 1991;19:341.

179. Keely MM, Wade RV, Laurent SL, et al. Alterations in maternal fetal Doppler flow velocity waveforms in preterm labor

patients undergoing magnesium sulfate tocolysis. *Obstet Gynecol.* 1993;81:191.

180. Thagarajah S, Harbert G Jr, Bourgeois FJ. Magnesium sulfate and ritodrine hydrochloride: Systemic and uterine hemodynamic effects. *Am J Obstet Gynecol.* 1985;153:666.

181. Mari G, Kirshon B, Moise KJ Jr, et al. Doppler assessment of the fetal and uteroplacental circulation during nifedipine therapy for preterm labor. *Am J Obstet Gynecol.* 1989; 161:1514.

182. Rizzo G, Capponi A, Arduini D, et al. Uterine and fetal blood flows in pregnancies complicated by preterm labor. *Gynecol Obstet Invest.* 1996;42:163.

183. Bracero LA, Jovanovic L, Rochelson B, et al. Significance of umbilical and uterine artery velocimetry in the well-controlled pregnant diabetic. *J Reprod Med.* 1989;34:273.

184. Bracero LA, Schulman H. Doppler studies of the uteroplacental circulation in pregnancies complicated by diabetes. *Ultrasound Obstet Gynecol.* 1991;1:391.

185. Salvesen DR, Higueras MT, Brudenell M, et al. Doppler velocimetry and fetal heart rate studies in nephropathic diabetics. *Am J Obstet Gynecol.* 1992;167:1297.

186. Salvesen DR, Higueras MT, Mansur CA, et al. Placental and fetal Doppler velocimetry in pregnancies complicated by maternal diabetes mellitus. *Am J Obstet Gynecol.* 1993;168:845.

187. Kofinas AD, Penry M, Swain M. Uteroplacental Doppler flow velocity waveform analysis correlates poorly with glycemic control in diabetic pregnant women. *Am J Obstet Gynecol.* 1991;8:273.

188. Grunewald C, Divon M, Lunell N. Doppler velocimetry in last trimester pregnancy complicated by insulin-dependent diabetes mellitus. *Acta Obstet Gynecol Scand.* 1996;75:804.

189. Bracero LA, Evanco J, Byrne D. Doppler velocimetry discordance of the uterine arteries in pregnancies complicated by diabetes. *J Ultrasound Med.* 1997;16:387.

190. White P. Classification of obstetric diabetes. *Am J Obstet Gynecol.* 1978;130;228.

191. Snijders RJ, Noble P, Sebire N, et al. UK multicentre project on assessment of risk of trisomy 21 by maternal age and fetal nuchal-translucency thickness at 10–14 weeks of gestation. Fetal Medicine Foundation First Trimester Screening Group. *Lancet.* 1998;352:343.

192. Whitlow BJ, Economides DL. The optimal gestational age to examine fetal anatomy and measure nuchal translucency in the first trimester. *Ultrasound Obstet Gynecol.* 1998;11:258.

193. Harrington K, Kurdi W, Aquilina J, et al. A prospective management study of slow-release aspirin in the palliation of uteroplacental insufficiency predicted by uterine artery Doppler at 20 weeks. *Ultrasound Obstet Gynecol.* 2000;15:13.

14

Color Doppler Sonography in Obstetrics

Donald S. Emerson

Whether or not sonographers and sonologists thought color Doppler sonography for obstetric imaging was needed, their exposure to it makes it virtually impossible to return to practicing without it. The introduction of color Doppler sonography into obstetric imaging continues a trend that began with the transition from static to real-time sonographic imaging. Real-time sonography made possible an imaging philosophy that places physiologic insight at the core of uterine and fetal assessment (i.e., that uterine and fetal structural abnormalities are best understood within the context of physiology). Color Doppler sonography adds yet a new layer of dynamic anatomy with new physiologic insights. Thoughtful application of this philosophy can often greatly enhance ultrasound's diagnostic and prognostic capacity, which is especially important in the current health care reform environment when the clinical usefulness of medical procedures is subjected to greater scrutiny.

PRINCIPLES OF USE

Color Doppler ultrasound effectively enriches obstetric imaging with physiologic information when it is used in a targeted manner. In other words, color Doppler (with pulsed Doppler) sonography should be used as an adjunct to conventional sonography, as an additional imaging tool to clarify specific functional questions left unanswered by or possibly raised by real-time ultrasound. These questions can be classified broadly into the following categories.

1. What is the metabolic status of the imaged tissue? Color Doppler sonography provides a gross indication of an organ's metabolic activity because it reveals otherwise unobservable blood flow patterns and because overall tissue vascularity and specific arterial time–velocity waveforms provide a rough measure of metabolic activity. Greater spatial density of vessels, higher systolic velocities, and higher diastolic-to-systolic velocity ratios are all approximate indicators of diminished vascular bed resistance in the supplied tissues, implying increased metabolic activity. This is particularly useful in the evaluation of intrauterine flow patterns in very early normal and complicated pregnancies when conventional sonography is blandly unrevealing regarding uterine and adnexal physiologic status[1] (see Fig. 14–5). This type of information also provides the fundamental basis for intrauterine growth retardation–related Doppler interrogations.[2]

2. Are there hemodynamic aberrations that can explain the structural and functional abnormalities seen with conventional sonography? There are local and global flow states that may be the cause of, or at least be closely associated with, abnormal findings in the fetal sonographic structural survey.

For instance, the cause of fetal hydrops with faulty cardiac structural development may remain obscure until color Doppler sonography reveals tricuspid regurgitation.[3] In another condition, the abundant high-velocity, low-resistance arteriovenous flow around the head and neck seen with color Doppler ultrasound directly identifies the cause of high-output failure in the fetus with aneurysm of the vein of Galen[4,5] (see Fig. 14–29). Or, for instance, demonstration of reversed flow in the fetal aortic arch is a very powerful confirmation of severe aortic stenosis or atresia.[6] Color and pulsed Doppler sonography also can be used to examine the temporal relations of intracardiac events to clarify the nature of fetal arrhythmias.[7,8]

3. Can a unique feeding vessel be detected to clarify the nature of the tissue it supplies? Certain abnormal maternal adnexal tissues or fetal structures may be recognized, although not specifically classified, with conventional sonography. Color Doppler sonography, however, may discover the supplying or, possibly, draining vessel, thereby revealing the identity of the structure in question. A notable example is cystic adenomatoid malformation (CAM) of the lung, which can be identical in appearance in the fetus to bronchopulmonary sequestration. Demonstration of a supplying systemic artery identifies the mass as sequestration, whereas a supplying artery branching from the pulmonary artery indicates the presence of CAM[9,10] (see Fig. 14–26). Furthermore, demonstration of a draining vein joining the pulmonary veins indicates a high likelihood of intralobar sequestration. Alternatively, a solid, otherwise nondescript adnexal mass is almost certainly identified as the ectopic pregnancy mass when a certain form of ectopic pregnancy blood flow (bizarre type) is recognized with color and pulsed Doppler sonography[1] (see Fig. 14–10).

4. Is there important vascular anatomy present to which conventional sonography is partly or totally blind but that is demonstrable with color Doppler sonography? At times, even with advanced equipment, certain fetal vascular structures are not clearly visible or even visible at all, possibly due to maternal size and fetal positioning. This problem, a particularly difficult one in the case of the fetal outflow tracts in health and disease, can be obviated with color Doppler sonography, which often proves effective in revealing aortic and pulmonary artery outflow tracts (and their spatial relationship) when conventional sonography fails.[11,12] At other times, vessels may be visible with gray-scale imaging, but the use of color Doppler readily tracks their connections, as in azygos continuation of interrupted inferior vena cava, in anomalous pulmonary venous return, or in abdominal heterotaxy.[13,14]

TECHNIQUE

Extraction of useful information from color Doppler sonography depends on attention to proper technique. This includes knowledge of vascular anatomy, insight into hemodynamic physiology, awareness of specific diagnostic goals, appreciation of exposure and safety issues, understanding of practical physical principles of Doppler sonography, and familiarity with the controls and display output of the equipment. When integrated, these components of proper technique will help construct an intelligent and information-rich Doppler interrogation. Some additional important points of technique follow.

1. Color Doppler sonography is an additional layer on top of conventional sonography. Color Doppler sonography should be used only after thorough high-quality conventional ultrasound imaging. The Doppler investigation should then be guided by attention to the particular question or set of questions to be answered with this modality. During the course of the Doppler investigation, the vascular findings should be compared with the findings of conventional real-time ultrasound to determine whether the conclusions are discordant or in agreement. This comparison will often provide new insights into the nature of a pathologic condition (see Fig. 14–17).

2. Color and pulsed Doppler sonographies are complementary. Although the color Doppler map is capable of directly conveying vascular information, it is more frequently used as a sensitive means for identifying vessels for pulsed Doppler interrogation. Color Doppler sonography does provide independent information regarding general vascularity of tissue or presence or direction of flow within vascular channels. Nevertheless, complementary use of pulsed Doppler serves as a reality check, confirming or disproving the color flow findings and exposing the confounding effects of artifacts. Furthermore, compared with the color flow map, the time–velocity blood flow waveforms demonstrated with pulsed Doppler sonography contain much more complete and quantifiable data describing the nature of the flow.[15,16] Nevertheless, color Doppler guidance can be critical to the performance of rapid and consistently accurate pulsed Doppler investigations, because it clearly identifies proper interrogation sites and facilitates proper Doppler angle correction.[15,17,18]

3. A multitiered strategy should be employed to limit exposure levels to Doppler. Fears regarding fetal exposure to Doppler ultrasound are based on experimental models demonstrating primarily thermal effects with the potential for teratogenicity rather than on direct evidence of damage due to typical diagnostic-level exposures in human fetuses.[19,20] Nevertheless, because Doppler sonography is more capable of tissue-heating effects than conventional sonography, it is prudent to employ a multitiered strategy to limit embryonic and fetal exposure to Doppler. A well-reasoned indication for use of Doppler is the first step in this strategy because it will discourage nonindicated examinations and, significantly, can often lead to a briefer indicated examination. Next, the examiner should maintain careful awareness of the elapsed time of examination and keep in perspective the clinical importance of the sought-after vascular information. The examination can be shortened further through the liberal use of the cine loop function and of videotape review. Doppler transmit power should be set at the lowest level compatible with a satisfactory examination. Use of a narrow color box will limit generalized fetal exposure.

4. Attention to proper settings and appropriate use of equipment yield enhanced Doppler sensitivity with fewer artifacts. Both pulse repetition frequency (PRF) and transducer frequency directly affect sensitivity to low-velocity blood flow and susceptibility to aliasing from high-velocity flow. A higher frequency transducer and a lower PRF should be chosen for enhanced detection of low-velocity flow, whereas a lower frequency transducer and a higher PRF are better suited to handle high-velocity signals (see Fig. 14–14). Frame rates tend to be lower for color Doppler than for conventional sonography and may introduce timing artifacts because of relatively high fetal heart rates. For instance, inadequate frame rates will cause diastolic and systolic events to be spuriously overlapped (see Fig. 14–12). Possibly the most important factor, but also the most difficult to control in a fetal examination, is the angle between the long axis of flow and the Doppler beam. At an angle of 90 degrees, almost no signal is recorded; and between 60 and 90 degrees, even though flow is detected on the color map and the spectral tracing, accuracy of blood velocity measurement is unacceptably low. A common but neglected artifact is misinterpretation of the Doppler data.[15] For example, the color Doppler map relates only to mean and not peak Doppler shift (or velocity) per pixel, and frequency shift or blood velocity that is measured is only for that component of flow oriented directly toward or away from the transducer.

EARLY PREGNANCY

Although there is much to be learned about the physiology of early pregnancy through the use of color Doppler sonography,[21] the list of clinical indications for its use in very early gestation in very brief: (1) to diagnose or exclude ectopic pregnancy and (2) to diagnose molar pregnancy (and, in particular, to diagnose myometrial invasion). Potential clinical indications in early pregnancy include early diagnosis of intrauterine pregnancy failure and diagnosis of associated ovarian torsion. Safety concerns regarding potential harmful effects in the developing embryo should convince users to minimize Doppler exposure in the early first trimester. Thus, it should be reserved for clinically indicated uses and research protocols and, even then, the time of examination and power levels should be kept as low as possible.

Ectopic Pregnancy: Rationale for Use of Color Doppler Sonography

The well-recognized overlap in sonographic findings of very early normal and failed intrauterine pregnancy and of ectopic pregnancy often leads to a diagnostic impasse that must

then be resolved through additional laboratory tests, follow-up ultrasound examinations, and, possibly, surgery. This extra workup leads to delays in diagnosis, to higher cost of care, and to possible invasive management. The overall management of ectopic pregnancy, both diagnostic and therapeutic, however, has been moving steadily toward less invasive and noninvasive approaches, and transvaginal and color Doppler sonography have played significant roles in this transformation.[22] The argument in favor of diagnostic surgery for ectopic pregnancy, that therapeutic surgery is a necessity in any case and, therefore, diagnosis can be accomplished during the same surgical procedure, is less compelling today given the availability of medical therapy with a single systemic injection of methotrexate.[23] Thus, as diagnostic ultrasound becomes more sensitive and specific in the diagnosis of ectopic pregnancy, delays in diagnosis and dependence on surgery for diagnosis should lessen. Transvaginal sonography has improved the diagnostic yield of ultrasound in ectopic pregnancy; the addition of color Doppler sonography enhances the diagnostic yield even more.[1,24]

The empty uterus sign, one of the most common sonographic signs of ectopic pregnancy, is not very specific. It is present in early normal and failed pregnancy before the appearance of the gestational sac, in failed pregnancy after loss of the gestational sac, and, of course, in ectopic pregnancy. Specificity of this sign improves when compared with a concurrent serum human chorionic gonadotropin (hCG) level, especially when compared with the discriminatory zone, the serum hCG level above which all normal intrauterine pregnancies should be sonographically detectable.[25,26] Nevertheless, there are limitations to the use of the discriminatory zone and the empty uterus sign. Although there is a heightened probability of ectopic pregnancy when an empty uterus is associated with an hCG level above the discriminatory zone, there remains also a significant possibility of failed intrauterine pregnancy,[27] a condition for which one would like not to offer methotrexate or surgery. Also, the empty uterus is completely indeterminate at serum hCG levels *below* the discriminatory zone. Color Doppler sonography, however, is capable of identifying vascular signs of early intrauterine pregnancy, both normal and failed, in a sonographically empty uterus, at hCG levels above or below the discriminatory zone.

Very small intrauterine fluid sacs, before the appearance of the double decidual sac sign and before the appearance of a yolk sac or embryo, are also sonographically diagnostically indeterminate. Although the majority of these small sacs represent normal intrauterine pregnancies, they may also represent failed or failing intrauterine pregnancies or, more ominously, pseudogestational sacs reported to be associated with 8 to 29% of cases of ectopic pregnancy.[25,28–30] Furthermore, larger abnormal intrauterine fluid sacs that are commonly identified as failed intrauterine pregnancies may also actually represent pseudogestational sacs.[22] Color Doppler sonography is capable, however, of distinguishing between these diagnoses by virtue of the vascular information it identifies.

Thus, in a patient in whom there is some suspicion of ectopic pregnancy, demonstration of an indeterminate or an unusual anembryonic intrauterine sac with transvaginal sonography should be followed up with a color Doppler investigation for greater diagnostic specificity.[1]

Detection of a live embryo in the adnexa is the most specific sonographic sign of ectopic pregnancy; however, there are other adnexal masses that are less specific, although decidedly more frequent (and thus sensitive) signs of ectopic pregnancy, such as cystic masses, termed *adnexal* or *tubal rings,* and solid and complex masses.[22] By detecting characteristic vascular flow patterns within ectopic pregnancy masses, color Doppler sonography enhances confidence in the noninvasive diagnosis of ectopic pregnancy. Furthermore, because the location of ectopic masses tends to follow the laterality of the corpus luteum, demonstration of a corpus luteum can assist the sonographer in finding the ectopic mass.[24,31] Color Doppler sonography detects characteristic luteal flow around the corpus luteum, even when the corpus luteum is barely seen or not detectable at all with conventional transvaginal sonography due to internal hemorrhage.

In summary, the role of color Doppler sonography in the workup of a possible ectopic pregnancy encompasses the following four points:

1. Differentiation of the empty uterus sign into either intrauterine pregnancy (normal and abnormal) or no intrauterine pregnancy (with a greatly increased chance of ectopic pregnancy).
2. Differentiation of pseudogestational sacs (of ectopic pregnancy) and true intrauterine gestational scas (of normal and failing pregnancy).
3. Assistance in the detection, and confirmation of the nature, of adnexal ectopic masses.
4. Identification of the site of the corpus luteum.

Ectopic Pregnancy: Color Doppler Technique

Transvaginal sonography is the ultrasound method of choice for evaluation of normal and failing early intrauterine pregnancy and for the workup of possible ectopic pregnancy. Color Doppler sonography is recruited only after thorough transvaginal two-dimensional real-time imaging if the ultrasound results are indecisive or to improve confidence in the noninvasive diagnosis of ectopic pregnancy prior to treatment. Color Doppler sonography is performed using the transvaginal probe to achieve as high a Doppler sensitivity as possible by virtue of the higher frequency transducer and the shorter distance to the imaging target. As stressed earlier, color and pulsed Doppler methods are complementary. Diagnostic errors will result from use of color Doppler sonography without pulsed Doppler interrogation.

Potential embryonic Doppler exposure is minimized by resorting to uterine Doppler only when necessary, by maintaining power levels as low as possible, by using a very small color box, by limiting the time of the examination, and by using cine loop review.

Color Doppler sonography of the uterus is used both for the information on the color flow map and for its guidance of pulsed Doppler interrogation. The major color map information is the overall vascularity of the inner portion of the uterus. To compare the relative uterine vascularity of different patients in a standard manner, the most sensitive color scale (or PRF) setting is used to produce the color flow map (we use scale values from -3.0 to $+3.0$ cm per second). A highly magnified field of view of the expected area of vascularity is then selected, and color Doppler is used to search for a focal site of highest velocity flow likely to contain characteristic vascularity for sampling with pulsed Doppler ultrasound.

Color Doppler sonography of the ovaries and adnexa also follows after thorough transvaginal imaging. On occasion, higher Doppler power levels than those used in the uterus are needed to demonstrate ovarian flow. It should be stressed that color Doppler sonography in general cannot differentiate between a corpus luteum and an ectopic mass because their flow patterns are usually nearly identical. The important differentiation between these two types of masses must be accomplished first on the basis of conventional sonographic signs. Only then should color and pulsed Doppler be used for confirmation. Color and pulsed Doppler may actually identify a previously unseen ectopic mass.[1,24,32]

Color Doppler Ectopic Pregnancy Workup: Intrauterine Pregnancy Findings

Color and pulsed Doppler sonographies can trace the major branching of the uterine vasculature, from the main uterine arteries to the arcuate arteries, to the radial arteries, and ultimately to the spiral arteries deep in the endometrium. Each of the vessels is recognized by its particular location within the uterus and its characteristic waveform. Spiral arteries undergo a structural alteration in early pregnancy, resulting in a characteristic waveform that is termed *peritrophoblastic flow.* Peritrophoblastic flow is associated only with intrauterine pregnancy, whether normal or failing, and is found close to the gestational sac (if present) and within or just outside the endometrium (Figs. 14–1 and 14–2). Compared with nongravid radial and spiral artery flow, peritrophoblastic flow is characterized by higher peak systolic velocity and higher diastolic flow, indicating lower impedance. Peak systolic velocity increases with increasing sac size, yielding a range of velocities appropriate for normal early pregnancy[33] (Table 14–1). Overall uterine vascularity is not increased in normal early pregnancy, however, and is very similar to that seen in a nongravid uterus (cold or warm). Occasional periendometrial veins are seen in normal pregnancy.[34]

There are at least two situations in which findings of intrauterine pregnancy are falsely positive. Intrauterine leiomyomata can induce increased intrauterine vascularity on the color flow map and increased venous flow and low-impedance

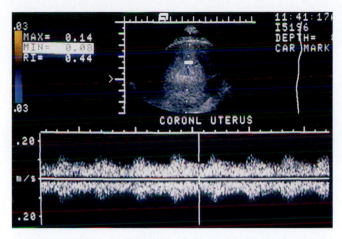

Figure 14–1. Intrauterine peritrophoblastic flow indicates early intrauterine pregnancy (IUP) despite absence of gestational sac. Notice that the pulsed Doppler sampling site is over a focus of color adjacent to the thickened endometrium. Overall uterine vascularity is rather cool and peak systolic velocity is 14 cm/s, appropriate for a very early IUP. Subsequent scan demonstrated normally developing gestational sac and embryo. *(Reproduced with permission from Emerson DS, Cartier MS, Altieri LA, et al.* Radiology. *1992;183:413–420.)*

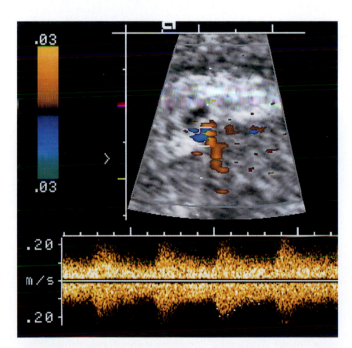

Figure 14–2. Indeterminate intrauterine gestational sac (3 mm) with color and pulsed Doppler demonstration of focal peritrophoblastic flow. Overall uterine vascularity is cool, and peak systolic velocity of the peritrophoblastic flow is 22 cm/s, both indicating a normal early intrauterine pregnancy. *(Reproduced with permission from Emerson D, Felker R. Early Intrauterine Pregnancy. In: Color Doppler Sonography in Obstetrics and Gynecology, Fleischer A, Emerson D, eds. New York: Churchill Livingstone; 1993:169–192.)*

TABLE 14–1. DIAGNOSTIC CRITERIA FOR ENDOVAGINAL SONOGRAPHY WITH TRANSVAGINAL COLOR AND PULSED DOPPLER

Viable IUP

1. Intrauterine sac 0–5 mm: Cool or warm color Doppler uterine appearance
2. Intrauterine sac >5 mm: Warm color Doppler uterine appearance
3. Focally increased intrauterine color with peritrophoblastic flow (near endometrium or small gestational sac):
   a. peak systolic velocity 8–30 cm/s with no intrauterine sac
   b. peak systolic velocity 10–30 cm/s at 4 wk (sac 1–5 mm)
   c. peak systolic velocity 10–60 cm/s at 5 wk (sac 6–10 mm)
4. Minimal or absent intrauterine venous flow
5. CL flow in one or both ovaries (peak systolic velocity >10 cm/s)

Failed IUP

1. Completed AB:
   a. No CL flow
   b. No intrauterine sac
   c. Cold to warm uterus
   d. Intrauterine peritrophoblastic flow absent or extremely low (peak systolic velocity <6 cm/s)
   e. Minimal or absent intrauterine venous flow
2. Incomplete AB:
   a. CL flow may be seen in one or both ovaries
   b. Warm or hot uterus (diffuse uterine vascularity) with color Doppler
   c. Geographically increased intrauterine color with color Doppler
   d. Increased intrauterine venous flow
   e. Peritrophoblastic flow present (peak systolic velocities generally above the normal IUP range, but can be normal or low)

Ectopic Pregnancy

1. Cold or warm color Doppler uterine appearance
2. No or small amount of intrauterine venous flow
3. No intrauterine peritrophoblastic flow
4. CL flow in one or both ovaries
5. Peritrophoblastic-like flow or other bizarre arterial flow in adnexal mass (absence of flow in adnexal mass may be seen)

Indeterminate Diagnosis (Consistent with All of the Above Diagnoses)

Pattern I

1. Cold or warm uterus with color Doppler
2. No peritrophoblastic flow in uterus
3. Minimal or increased intrauterine venous flow
4. No adnexal mass or adnexal peritrophoblastic-like flow
5. CL flow in one or both ovaries

Pattern II

1. Warm uterus or intrauterine low velocity peritrophoblastic-like flow with fibroids present or within 4 days after dilatation and curettage
2. No definitive intrauterine gestational sac or adnexal mass

AB, spontaneous abortion; CL, corpus luteal; IUP, Intrauterine pregnancy.
Reproduced with permission from Emerson DS, Cartier MS, Altieri LA, et al. Radiology. *1992;183:413–420.*

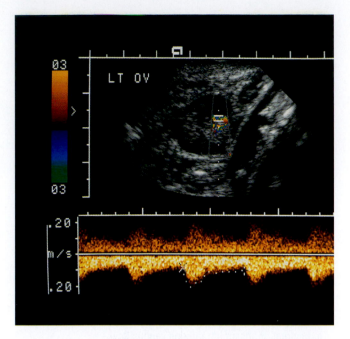

Figure 14–3. Corpus luteal flow in an ovary associated with a normal early intrauterine pregnancy. This form of flow is seen in at least one ovary in early pregnancy even without sonographic demonstration of a classic corpus luteum. Peak systolic velocity is approximately 20 cm/s.

arterial waveforms indistinguishable from peritrophoblastic flow on the pulsed Doppler tracing. Dilatation and curettage can also stimulate uterine vascularity in a similar manner. Fibroids and recent dilatation and curettage thus can simulate the color and pulsed Doppler vascular findings of normal and failed intrauterine pregnancy.

Beginning shortly after ovulation and continuing into early pregnancy, increased ovarian metabolic activity associated with the corpus luteum is reflected by a change in the ovarian artery waveform from a high-resistance (low-diastolic flow) waveform to a low-resistance pattern, called *corpus luteum arterial flow*. This is detectable with color and pulsed Doppler ultrasound in virtually all first-trimester pregnant patients in at least one ovary[1] (Fig. 14–3). (Although we have detected the changes of low-impedance arterial flow in both ovaries in up to 25% of cases of early pregnancy, one ovary typically has higher velocity flow.[1] This ovary defines the likely side of the ectopic pregnancy.)

Color Doppler Ectopic Pregnancy Workup: Failed Intrauterine Pregnancy Findings

Two major patterns of uterine flow are recognized with early failed intrauterine pregnancy, one with incomplete spontaneous abortion and one with complete spontaneous abortion (see Table 14–1). In incomplete spontaneous abortion, overall

uterine vascularity is increased over what would be seen in normal early pregnancy (warm or hot vascularity). Peritrophoblastic arterial flow is identified, typically with systolic velocities above the normal range for intrauterine pregnancy. Periendometrial venous flow is also increased, both in spatial density and in velocity. Corpus luteal flow is found in one or both ovaries. These Doppler findings may be associated with an empty uterus, a small indeterminate sac, or a larger abnormal sac on transvaginal conventional sonography (Figs. 14–4 and 14–5). The incomplete spontaneous abortion pattern of vascular flow is sufficient for definitive diagnosis even in the absence of characteristic conventional sonographic signs.

In complete spontaneous abortion, uterine vascularity is cold or warm, there is no intrauterine peritrophoblastic flow, and intrauterine venous flow is minimal or absent. This pattern is associated with an empty uterus on conventional transvaginal ultrasound imaging. Unfortunately, the pattern is largely indeterminate because it could occur in the setting of an ectopic pregnancy or, possibly, an extremely early intrauterine pregnancy. The one vascular characteristic that may serve to differentiate the pattern of complete spontaneous abortion from both ectopic pregnancy and intrauterine pregnancy is the absence of corpus luteal flow in the ovaries in many, but not all, cases of complete spontaneous abortion.

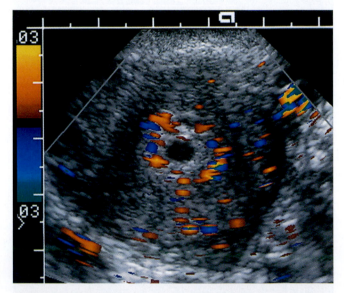

Figure 14–4. Failed intrauterine pregnancy imaged by transvaginal color Doppler sonography. Conventional sonography demonstrates a small sac with a yolk sac, appropriate for a normal early pregnancy. Color Doppler map, however, reveals hot uterine vascularity. Pulsed Doppler interrogation *(not shown)* identified abnormally high-velocity peritrophoblastic flow and increased venous flow. These findings are all indicative of failed intrauterine pregnancy. *(Reproduced with permission from Emerson D, Felker R. Early Intrauterine Pregnancy. In: Color Doppler Sonography in Obstetrics and Gynecology, Fleischer A, Emerson D, eds. New York: Churchill Livingstone; 1993:169–192.)*

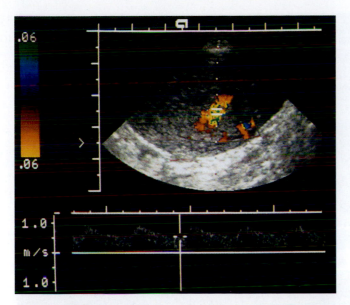

Figure 14–5. Failed intrauterine pregnancy by transvaginal color Doppler sonography. Conventional sonography revealed an empty uterus, consistent with a failed intrauterine pregnancy, very early intrauterine pregnancy, and an ectopic pregnancy. Color Doppler map reveals hot uterine vascularity with a broad geographic focus of color. Pulsed Doppler interrogation within this region of increased vascularity identified peritrophoblastic flow with a peak systolic velocity above the normal range for early normal pregnancy with or without a sac. *(Reproduced with permission from Emerson DS, Cartier MS, Altieri LA, et al. Radiology. 1992;183:413–420.)*

Color Doppler Ectopic Pregnancy Workup: Ectopic Pregnancy Findings

In an ectopic pregnancy, uterine vascularity is cold or warm, no intrauterine peritrophoblastic flow is identified, periendometrial venous flow is minimal, and corpus luteal flow is identified in one or both ovaries. Even in the presence of a pseudogestational sac, there is no intrauterine peritrophoblastic flow (Fig. 14–6). There is no difference in corpus luteal flow parameters between intrauterine pregnancy and ectopic pregnancy.[31] Corpus luteal flow is found ipsilateral to the ectopic pregnancy in 95% of cases and thus can function as a guide to finding the ectopic mass.[31]

When an adnexal ectopic mass is identified, typical peritrophoblastic flow is found within it in 79% of masses, no flow is seen in 6% of masses, and bizarre flow is found in 15% of masses[1] (Figs. 14–7 and 14–8). Peritrophoblastic flow (PTB) does not guarantee that an ectopic mass is the ectopic pregnancy mass because this flow pattern is very similar to corpus luteal flow (CL), although in Kurjak and associates' series ectopic peritrophoblastic flow had a lower resistance index (RI) than did corpus luteal flow (ectopic pregnancy PTB RI < 0.4 < CL RI).[32] Furthermore, although there is a general belief that the color flow map sign of a surrounding ring of vascularity is characteristic of an ectopic pregnancy mass, this same finding is regularly identified around the corpus luteum. Presence of a ring of vascularity and peritrophoblastic flow are helpful only after conventional transvaginal sonography clarifies the location of the mass as being outside the ovary and thus not likely to be a corpus luteum (Fig. 14–9).

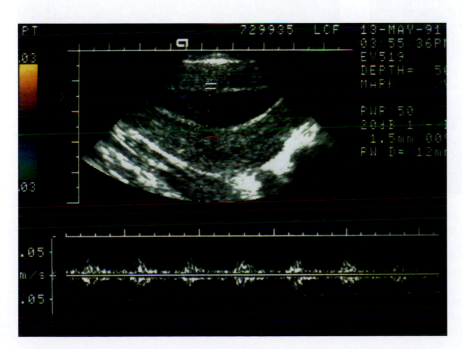

Figure 14–6. Large pseudogestational sac in a patient with an ectopic pregnancy. Transvaginal sonography could not differentiate between a failed intrauterine pregnancy and a pseudogestational sac. A failed intrauterine sac of this size should be associated with warm or hot uterine vascularity and with the presence of peritrophoblastic flow. Cool uterine vascularity and absence of intrauterine peritrophoblastic flow, however, resulted in a specific diagnosis of pseudogestational sac. Arterial waveform is characteristic of a spiral artery in a nongravid uterus. *(Reproduced with permission from Emerson DS, Cartier MS, Altieri LA, et al. Radiology. 1992;183:413–420.)*

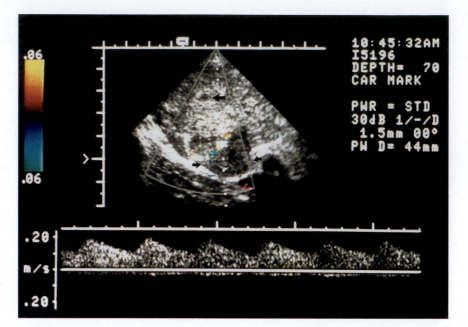

Figure 14–7. Ectopic pregnancy. Transvaginal color Doppler sonography reveals cool uterine vascularity and absent peritrophoblastic flow despite presence of a small endometrial fluid sac *(large arrow)*. This indicates that the sac is a pseudogestational sac. Distal to the uterus is a 2-cm solid mass with characteristic peritrophoblastic flow, the ectopic pregnancy mass. *(Reproduced with permission from Emerson DS, Cartier MS, Altieri LA, et al. Radiology. 1992;183:413–420.)*

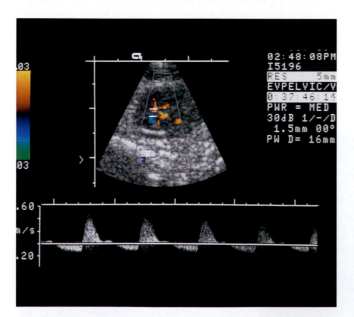

Figure 14–8. Ectopic pregnancy with bizarre arterial waveform. Transvaginal color Doppler sonography identifies central vascularity within this 1-cm solid adnexal mass. Pulsed Doppler waveform is unusual in that it had a high peak systolic velocity (43 cm/s) and retrograde diastolic flow. This waveform and other similar bizarre waveforms are associated with only a small percentage of ectopic pregnancy cases, but when identified, indicate that the mass is truly an ectopic pregnancy. *(Reproduced with permission from Emerson DS, Cartier MS, Altieri LA, et al. Radiology. 1992;183:413–420.)*

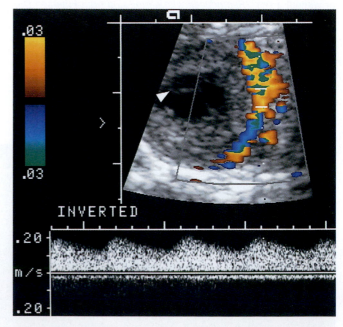

Figure 14–9. Corpus luteum masquerading as an ectopic pregnancy. Conventional sonography demonstrates a thick-walled adnexal cyst with an internal linear echo suggesting a yolk sac *(arrowhead)*. Color and pulsed Doppler reveal a ring of vascularity and a low-impedance waveform. Similar Doppler findings are associated with both ectopic masses and corpora luteum. *(Reproduced with permission from Emerson D, Felker R. Ectopic Pregnancy. In: Color Doppler Sonography in Obstetrics and Gynecology, Fleischer A, Emerson D, eds. New York: Churchill Livingstone; 1993:193–216.)*

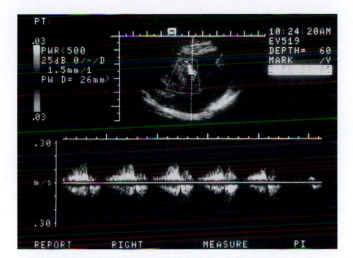

Figure 14–10. Bizarre arterial waveform in this nonspecific adnexal mass is responsible for diagnosis of heterotopic pregnancy in a patient with a 9-week intrauterine pregnancy. Patient was asymptomatic, and there was no clinical suspicion of concurrent ectopic pregnancy. Nevertheless, because we have seen this bizarre waveform only in ectopic pregnancy, the possibility of heterotopic pregnancy was strongly suggested. Diagnosis was confirmed at surgery *(Courtesy of Lisa A. Altieri, MD, Nashville, TN; reproduced with permission from Emerson D, Felker R. Ectopic Pregnancy. In: Color Doppler Sonography in Obstetrics and Gynecology, Fleischer A, Emerson D, eds. New York: Churchill Livingstone; 1993:193–216.)*

We have not seen bizarre flow in any other pelvic structures except for ectopic pregnancy masses and thus believe it to be a signature waveform. Presence of this type of waveform may, in fact, take diagnostic precedence over conventional imaging signs (Fig. 14–10).

There is a relation between serum hCG levels and the presence of ectopic peritrophoblastic flow and an inverse relation between serum hCG and RIs of this flow.[32,35,36] Differences in vascularity between different ectopic masses have generated the hope that color and pulsed Doppler findings

could help direct patients into appropriate treatment regimens, ranging from surgery to medical therapy to conservative follow-up. Nevertheless, we have found no relation between ectopic pregnancy pretreatment vascularity (peak velocity, RI) and the time to resolution during systemic methotrexate thereapy.[37]

Color Doppler Ectopic Pregnancy Workup: Indeterminate Findings

Despite the enhanced diagnostic yield of color Doppler sonography in the workup of potential ectopic pregnancy, some vascular patterns are diagnostically indeterminate. In particular, presence of corpus luteal flow despite absence of an intrauterine gestational sac, of intrauterine peritrophoblastic flow, and of an adnexal mass can indicate extremely early intrauterine pregnancy, failed intrauterine pregnancy, or ectopic pregnancy. Thus, after vigilantly but unsuccessfully searching for an ectopic mass in a patient with this sonographic and vascular pattern, the study should be called indeterminate and the possibility of ectopic pregnancy should continue to be considered.

Color Doppler Ectopic Pregnancy Workup: Benefits

The actual clinical benefit accrued by adding the color Doppler examination to transvaginal sonography in patients at risk for ectopic pregnancy is variable, depending on patient population characteristics and how the test results are used. We evaluated the use of color Doppler sonography for ectopic pregnancy workup at our medical center within the context of an emergency room serum progesterone screening program and an outpatient noninvasive ectopic pregnancy management program[23,38] (Table 14–2). We found that the benefits of transvaginal color Doppler sonography went beyond the actual increase in diagnostic sensitivity for ectopic pregnancy itself (71% diagnostic sensitivity for transvaginal sonography versus 87% for transvaginal color Doppler sonography).[1] (Pellerito's series yielded an even greater difference in sensitivity between transvaginal sonography and

TABLE 14–2. DIAGNOSTIC BENEFIT OF COLOR DOPPLER SONOGRAPHY IN PATIENTS AT RISK FOR ECTOPIC PREGNANCY[a]

	TVS		TVS + CDS	
	% Sensitivity	% Specificity	% Sensitivity	% Specificity
All Dx	62	—	82	—
EP	71	98	87	99
IUP	90	97	99	99
Failed IUP	24	100	59	100

[a]Based on 304 patients. To count as a correct definitive diagnosis, ultrasound had to be correct at the time of the first ultrasound examination.
TVS, Transvaginal sonography; CDS, color Doppler sonography; Dx, Diagnoses; EP, ectopic pregnancy; IUP, normal intrauterine pregnancy; failed IUP, incomplete and completed spontaneous abortion.
Reproduced with permission from Emerson DS, Cartier MS, Altieri LA, et al. Radiology. 1992; 183:413–420.

color Doppler sonography, 54 versus 95%, secondary, in part, to more stringent conventional sonographic criteria for ectopic pregnancy.[24]) Of even greater benefit was the ability of color Doppler to exclude ectopic pregnancy in other patients by diagnosing normal and failed intrauterine pregnancy despite indeterminate transvaginal sonography. Otherwise, these patients may have undergone additional further testing and, possibly, diagnostic surgery. A significant additional benefit of color Doppler sonography was the confirmatory evidence that sonographically demonstrated adnexal masses were truly ectopic pregnancy masses, by demonstrating ectopic pregnancy vascularity within the masses and negative vascular signs of intrauterine pregnancy. This increased diagnostic confidence is an important element in a noninvasive ectopic pregnancy management program.

Molar Pregnancy

Although an unequivocal abundance of high-flow vascularity might be expected to be found within molar pregnancies, the literature shows no consensus on flow levels within uncomplicated tumor masses.[39–42] The experience at our laboratory points to only mild increases in vascularity and typically no flow within the characteristic vesicles. Most of the vascularity is noted at the border of the uterine wall and mass, consisting of pertitrophoblastic-type flow and venous flow. Kurjak and coworkers noted very low-impedance flow with RI levels below normal and failed intrauterine pregnancy.[43] Invasive moles, however, demonstrate rather dramatic increases in vascularity on the color flow map and the pulsed Doppler spectrum.[40,43,44] Very high-velocity flow is seen within areas of tumor invasion into the uterine wall, whether in sonographically normal myometrium or abnormal hypoechoic sinuses (Fig. 14–11). Color Doppler sonography has demonstrated perforation of the uterine wall by the invading tumor.[45] Impedance is extremely low, yielding an arteriovenous shunt type of waveform.[44] Uterine wall hypervascularity recedes with regression of the tumor.[40] The implication of these findings is that, whereas color Doppler sonography may not prove diagnostically useful for nonin-

vasive moles, it is likely to be very helpful for diagnosis of myometrial invasion and for follow-up of response to therapy.

Theca lutein cysts are not as commonly seen today with earlier diagnosis of molar pregnancy; however, when present, there is increased vascularity within the cyst walls, with both low-impedance arterial flow and venous flow.

FETAL VASCULAR ANATOMY

Color Doppler sonography has demonstrated for the first time the fetal vascular tree in great detail in noninstrumented normal live human fetuses. Although the heart and great vessels continue to be the primary objects of color Doppler investigation, other organ systems are beginning to be evaluated.

Color Doppler demonstrates fetal organ blood flow from the first trimester, although it conveys more detailed anatomic content from the second trimester as the fetus grows.[46,47] Flow is demonstrated from the umbilical vein to the ductus venosus and then into the inferior vena cava to the right atrium.[48–50] The umbilical vein has been evaluated from the standpoint of both the normal absence or abnormal presence of modulations in the venous waveform and the more technically challenging calculation of flow volumes.[51–54] Ductus venosus flow patterns have been studied in normal fetuses and have shown high-velocity venous type flow with prominent troughs due to changing intra-atrial pressures and with a direct trajectory into the left atrium.[50,52,55,56] A mean of only 24% (range of 0 to 50%) of umbilical venous flow is normally shunted past the liver in the ductus venosus to the inferior vena cava.[52] Inferior vena cava waveforms have been evaluated for the degree of or percentage of time with reversed flow.[49,57]

Intracardiac flow reveals not only the definitive postnatal currents (Figs. 14–12 and 14–13) but also the fetal right-to-left shunting across the foramen ovale. Doppler studies of flow within the heart and its connecting veins and arteries have established norms for fetal life.[58–60] Flow can be traced with color Doppler sonography out from the great vessels and into the lungs[61] (see Figs. 14–23 and 14–24), into the

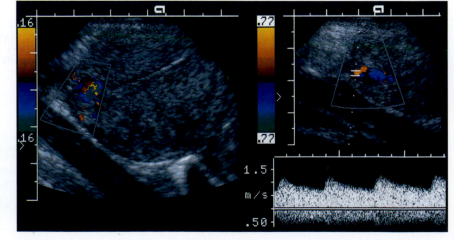

Figure 14–11. Invasive mole. Patient returned with rising serum hCG levels after initial treatment. Color Doppler map reveals very focal areas of increased vascularity within the myometrium. Pulsed Doppler interrogation of this area identified low-resistance, turbulent, high peak velocity (120 cm/s) arterial flow. Abnormal vascularity receded with subsequent therapy.

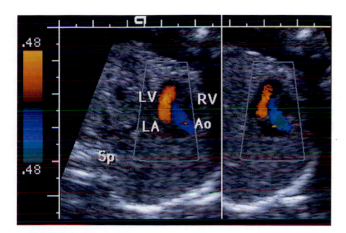

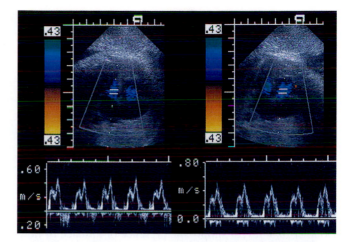

Figure 14–12. Color Doppler sonography of left ventricular outflow view demonstrates flow into the left ventricle *(coded red)* and flow out into the aorta *(coded blue)* in these images selected from a cine loop. The slow frame rate (relative to fetal cardiac rate) artifactually blends systolic *and* diastolic events. Review of individual frames of the cine loop helps to establish the proper timing of events: the *left* image emphasizes diastolic features (velocity and volume of ventricular inflow are greater than outflow), and the *right* image emphasizes systolic features. It is also possible to increase the color Doppler frame rate by changing imaging parameters. *(Reproduced with permission from Emerson D, Cartier M. The Fetus: Scanning Technique and Normal Anatomy. In: Color Doppler Sonography in Obstetrics and Gynecology, Fleischer A, Emerson D, eds. New York: Churchill Livingstone; 1993:217–252.)*

Figure 14–13. Color and pulsed Doppler sonographies effectively demonstrate flow across the atrioventricular valves (*left* image, mitral valve; *right* image, tricuspid valve). Color map provides an overview of intracardiac blood flow currents for a rapid global assessment. It also guides placement of the pulsed Doppler range gate. Spectral tracing reveals the normal M-shaped waveform across these valves, graphically depicting atrial and ventricular events over time. The first peak, the "E" point, occurs in early diastole when blood flows rapidly and passively into the ventricle following ventricular relaxation. The second peak, the "A" point, occurs during active atrial contraction or the atrial kick. Mitral and tricuspid waveforms are quite similar in utero. *(Reproduced with permission from Emerson D, Cartier M. The Fetus: Scanning Technique and Normal Anatomy. In: Color Doppler Sonography in Obstetrics and Gynecology, Fleischer A, Emerson D, eds. New York: Churchill Livingstone; 1993:217–252.)*

ductus arteriosus to the descending aorta, and into the head and neck vessels. Flow is easily seen within the head with color Doppler sonography, making it a practical endeavor to obtain pulsed Doppler waveforms of the middle, anterior, and posterior cerebral arteries and in the vertebral and intracerebellar arteries[62–66] (Fig. 14–14).

The color flow map reveals flow and guides pulsed Doppler interrogation in the descending aorta and in many of its branches, including the celiac axis, superior mesenteric artery, renal arteries, adrenal arteries, and the iliac bifurcation.[67] There is a measurable forward diastolic component in the descending aortic waveform from the midtrimester on, reflecting the effects of not only the high-resistance branches to visceral organs and skeletal muscles but also of the low-resistance placental bed.[68,69] Quantitative study of renal blood flow is made significantly easier to perform using color Doppler sonography.[70,71]

ABNORMAL FETAL ANATOMY

As discussed in the introduction to this chapter, color Doppler sonography provides an extra layer of anatomy and physiology with which to understand and evaluate fetal abnormalities and malformations. It is not a screening tool. Rather, it functions as a problem-solving tool, answering questions not

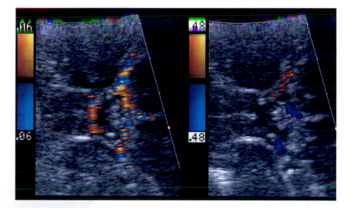

Figure 14–14. Color Doppler flow map of the circle of Willis. It is often necessary to image with different scale settings (due to specific pulse repetition frequencies) to gather complete vascular information. The image on the *left* was acquired with a low-velocity scale (−6.0 to +6.0 cm/s) for enhanced low-flow sensitivity. Although this caused some aliasing (artifactually reversed color coding), it also revealed nearly the entire vascular circle. The image on the *left,* obtained with a higher velocity scale (−48.0 to +48.0 cm/s), more accurately represented flow in the middle cerebral and anterior cerebral arteries but was insensitive to flow through much of the rest of the vascular circle. *(Reproduced with permission from Emerson D, Cartier M. The Fetus: Scanning Technique and Normal Anatomy. In: Color Doppler Sonography in Obstetrics and Gynecology, Fleischer A, Emerson D, eds. New York: Churchill Livingstone; 1993:217–252.)*

answered by, or possibly raised by, the real-time gray-scale ultrasound examination.[72] Thus, although there are large numbers of fetal structural abnormalities, color Doppler sonography has a recognized clinical role in only a limited subset of these cases. The role of Doppler in intrauterine growth retardation and placental insufficiency is covered in Chapters 12 and 15.

Cardiac and Great Vessel Abnormalities

Anomalies of the heart and great vessels represent the overwhelming majority of cases for which color Doppler sonography has additional clinically important information to add to the fetal examination.[73] At the most basic level, color Doppler may reveal simply the presence or absence of flow across an atrioventricular valve or within the aorta or pulmonary artery. At the next level, the color flow map would inform the examiner about the direction of flow, for example, identifying retrograde flow across the tricuspid valve during systole or retrograde flow across the ductus arteriosus in pulmonary atresia. At the next level, one would use the color map to trace the flow of blood into the heart, between the chambers, and out of the heart into the appropriate vessels. At the next level, color Doppler would be used to direct the pulsed Doppler interrogation, to confirm impressions from the color flow map, to identify previously unseen vessels and flow conduits, to analyze the time–velocity waveform for characteristic and unique features and to measure quantifiable parameters, such as peak systolic velocity, end-diastolic velocity, and pulsatility index.

Color Doppler sonography is particularly useful in defining the following structures and flow parameters of the fetal heart and great vessels[11,74,75]:

1. Atrioventricular valve stenosis or regurgitation.
2. Aortic and pulmonary valve stenosis or atresia (with retrograde aortic or ductus arteriosus flow).
3. Demonstration of great vessel relationship and ventricular connections.
4. Direction of flow across ventricular septal defects.

Color Doppler does not necessarily change the diagnoses derived from conventional sonography, but it will often add additional information for a more complete appreciation of all the defects and of the altered physiology.[76] Most color Doppler studies report on findings from after 16 weeks' menstrual age. However, even though color Doppler sonography suffers from poorer spatial resolution and lower frame rates than conventional sonography, there appears to be an expanding role for color Doppler in first-trimester cardiac evaluation using transvaginal sonography.[60,77]

Color Doppler sonography effectively confirms the presence of a ventricular septal defect (VSD) detected with conventional sonography. Even more significant, however, is the capacity of color Doppler sonography to determine the direction of flow across the defect. In an isolated VSD the flow is bidirectional, right to left in systole and reversed in diastole.[74,78] In association with abnormalities of the cardiac outflow tracts or atrioventricular valves, flow becomes more consistently unidirectional or the normal bidirectionality is reversed, thereby providing a clue to other structural defects[74,78] (Fig. 14–15). Color Doppler sonography can confirm a conventional sonographic diagnosis of atrioventricular septal defect (endocardial cushion defect) (Fig. 14–16), although a more significant contribution lies in its ability to detect associated valvular regurgitation.[3,11]

Color Doppler sonography confirms or detects critical valvular stenosis and atresia in a number of ways. In the case of the atrioventricular valves, the absence of flow or the presence of minimal flow across the valve into the ventricle is an obvious deviation from the normal flow pattern seen with color and pulsed Doppler. A confirmatory secondary color Doppler sign would be flow across a VSD *into* the affected ventricle if the outflow tract is unobstructed. When, in addition, only minimal or no flow into a diminutive ventricle is seen, the diagnosis of hypoplastic left or right heart syndrome is made (Fig. 14–17). A secondary color Doppler sign of mitral stenosis would be preferential left-to-right flow

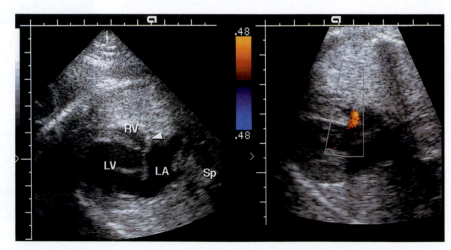

Figure 14–15. Ventricular septal defect (VSD) with unidirectional flow *(red)*. VSD flow occurs only from the enlarged left ventricle (LV) into the diminutive right ventricle (RV) due to a combination of tricuspid atresia *(arrowhead)* and patent right ventricular outflow tract. Color Doppler almost invariably provides additional important anatomic and pathophysiologic information in the case of complex congenital cardiac disease. LA, left atrium; Sp, spine.

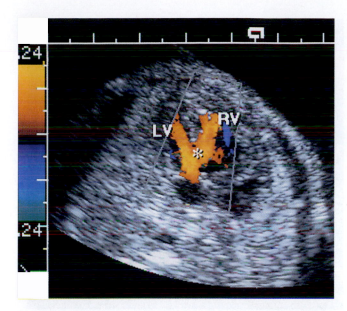

Figure 14–16. Color Doppler sonographic depiction of abnormal flow currents confirming diagnosis of atrioventricular septal defect. The common current of inflow into both ventricles (∗) is due to the defect in the inflow septum. LV, left ventricle; RV, right ventricle.

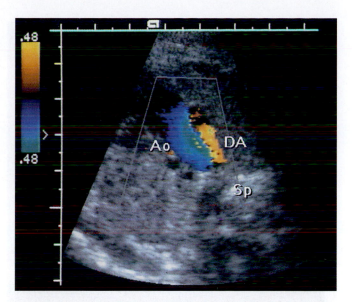

Figure 14–18. Transverse view of fetal chest at the level of the posterior sweep of the aortic (Ao) and ductus arteriosus (DA) arches. Normally the two vessels are of a similar diameter with flow directed in a similar direction, namely from the ventricular outflow tracts posteriorly to the descending aorta. Here, the aorta is significantly larger than the ductus arteriosus, and there is reversed flow in the ductus arteriosus *(yellow)*. This is a case of tetralogy of Fallot with proximal pulmonary artery atresia in which blood flow reaches the left and right pulmonary arteries via retrograde flow in the ductus arteriosus. Sp, spine. *(Reproduced with permission from Emerson D, Cartier M. Fetal Abnormalities and Malformations. In: Color Doppler Sonography in Obstetrics and Gynecology, Fleischer A, Emerson D, eds. New York: Churchill Livingstone; 1993:253–286.)*

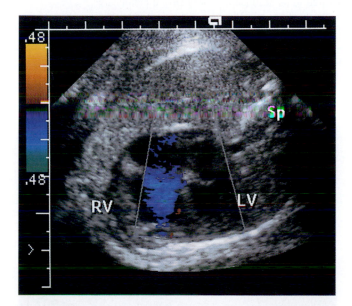

Figure 14–17. Inflow into right ventricle (RV) only and not into left ventricle (LV) despite a relatively normal four-chamber view. Real-time imaging, however, revealed almost no motion of the mitral valve and no sign of left ventricular myocardial shortening. Furthermore, the aortic valve was severely stenotic. It is likely that this was an early phase of hypoplastic left heart syndrome (HLHS) in evolution. Subsequent ultrasound examinations revealed progressive further narrowing of the ascending aorta and increasing discrepancy between the normal right ventricle and the small right ventricle, ultimately appearing as classic HLHS. Sp, spine. *(Reproduced with permission from Emerson D, Cartier M. Fetal Abnormalities and Malformations. In: Color Doppler Sonography in Obstetrics and Gynecology, Fleischer A, Emerson D, eds. New York: Churchill Livingstone; 1993:253–286.)*

across the foramen ovale into the right atrium.[11] In critical aortic stenosis or aortic atresia, in addition to demonstrating no flow across the valve, color Doppler demonstrates retrograde flow in the aortic arch.[6] The color flow map shows no flow across the pulmonary valve in valvular atresia or critical stenosis. The diagnosis is confirmed (and better understood) with color Doppler demonstration of retrograde ductus arteriosus flow feeding the central pulmonary artery (Fig. 14–18).

Color Doppler sonography is particularly useful for the demonstration of valvular regurgitation because this might not be seen or even suspected with conventional sonography. Pulsed Doppler sonography can be used to grade the severity of the regurgitant flow but can partly or entirely miss the abnormal current without the use of color Doppler guidance. Color Doppler, however, not only guides pulsed Doppler interrogation but also can provide a direct visual assessment of the size of the regurgitant jet (Fig. 14–19A and B). The tricuspid valve is the primary valve affected in this manner in fetal life, usually due to valve dysplasia but also due to pulmonary stenosis or atresia, indomethacin-induced ductus arteriosus constriction, atrioventricular septal defect, and supraventricular tachycardia.[74] It has been suggested that the duration of atrioventricular valve regurgitation is a

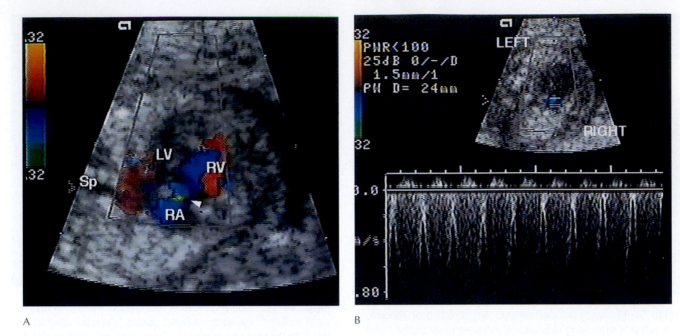

A   B

Figure 14–19. Transvaginal color Doppler demonstration of tricuspid regurgitation in a 14-week fetus with complex congenital cardiac disease. **(A)** Color Doppler map of four-chamber view reveals a large current of blood flow *(blue)* coursing back from the right ventricle (RV) across the tricuspid valve *(arrowhead)* into and filling the right atrium (RA). On real-time color Doppler sonography, regurgitant flow appeared nearly consistently throughout the cardiac cycle. This appeared to be secondary to very severe pulmonary regurgitation. LV, left ventricle; Sp, spine. **(B)** Pulse Doppler interrogation of the tricuspid regurgitant jet reveals the characteristic high-velocity turbulent waveform that, in this case, encompasses the entire cardiac cycle.

consistently measurable indicator of the degree of cardiac dysfunction in supraventricular tachycardia and in atrioventricular septal defects, and it can be used to effectively monitor response to therapy.[3,79] Mitral valve regurgitation may occur due to aortic atresia or critical stenosis.[80]

Malpositioned great vessels are readily diagnosed with conventional sonography when views of the outflow tracts are incorporated into the fetal cardiac survey. Color Doppler provides excellent assistance in this diagnosis because the vessels are often clearly visible on the color flow map even when conventional imaging is limited due to overlying shadowing from ribs. Double-outlet right ventricle, transposition of the great vessels, interrupted aortic arch, truncus arteriosus, and tetralogy of Fallot are identifiable by color Doppler sonography both directly, through the demonstration of the great vessels, and indirectly, through the demonstration of associated cardiac defects[11,74,81] (Figs. 14–20 to 14–22).

Investigations into the type of fetal arrhythmia using M-mode tracings are often limited by fetal positioning and difficulties in the demonstration of atrial contractions and in timing intracardiac events. Color and pulsed Doppler sonographies can be used to measure atrioventricular valve flow waveforms, but, unless inflow and outflow tract flows can be measured simultaneously or M-mode and color flow tracings can be superimposed, the method may not always provide the answer. A novel solution, first proposed by Chan

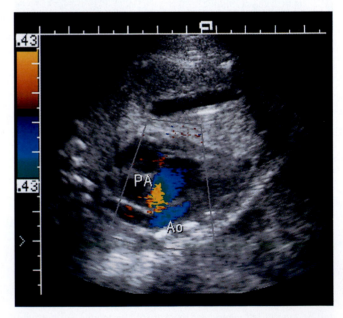

Figure 14–20. Transposition of the great vessels (TOGV). Color Doppler simplifies the task of identifying the outflow vessels and tracing blood flow within them. In this oblique transverse view (left side up), the pulmonary artery (PA) was followed out of the left ventricle and the aorta (Ao) was followed out of the right ventricle. Note the parallel course of the great vessels, characteristic of this abnormality. Also notice the discrepancy in size of the vessels. TOGV is often associated with other abnormalities, including valvular stenoses (as in this case).

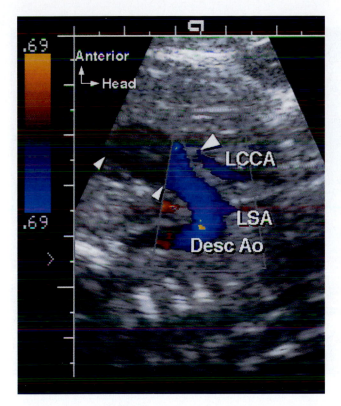

Figure 14–21. Longitudinal scan of 29-week fetus with interrupted aortic arch. The dilated main pulmonary artery *(between the two small arrowheads)* continues into the large ductus arteriosus and then into the descending aorta (Desc Ao). The left subclavian artery (LSA) is shown arising from the very proximal descending aorta. The ascending aorta, most of which is out of the plane of this image, terminates *(large arrowhead)* in the right innominate artery *(not shown)* and the left common carotid artery (LCCA). The aortic arch is interrupted between the take-off of the LCCA and the LSA. These relationships were greatly clarified through the use of the color flow maps.

and associates, is to use color and pulsed Doppler to obtain a simultaneous spectral tracing of inferior vena cava and aortic flows as a tool to determine the relative timing of atrial and ventricular events.[7] De Vore and Horenstein introduced a variant of this technique in which color and pulsed Doppler methods are used to simultaneously record waveforms of the pulmonary artery and vein.[8] This technique has an advantage in that intrapulmonary waveforms are relatively easy to obtain and are not as dependent on fetal positioning as in the aortic–inferior vena cava Doppler interrogation (Fig. 14–23).

Pulmonary Flow

Conventional real-time ultrasound clearly delineates the proximal and distal limbs of the pulmonary circulation. Color Doppler sonography, however, reveals the pulmonary circulation to a much fuller extent than does gray-scale sonography[82] (Fig. 14–24). Color Doppler quickly identifies vessels for pulsed Doppler interrogation and accurately guides Doppler angle adjustment. The unique pulsed Doppler waveform of the fetal pulmonary arterial bed is characterized by an extremely rapid initial flow acceleration followed by a very early and rapid deceleration phase producing a unique needle-like systolic peak.[61] Further deceleration occurs fairly rapidly during diastole (see Fig. 14–23).

Color and pulsed Doppler sonographies provide qualitative diagnostic information in the workup of fetal pulmonary abnormalities. The following list indicates some general situations in which the additional vascular information contributes to a fuller understanding of the pathology.[12]

1. An abnormal pulmonary arterial or venous flow pattern indicates presence of an additional cardiac abnormality in a fetus with a previously recognized cardiac malformation. This has helped

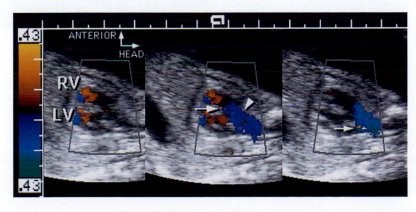

Figure 14–22. Composite of three frames from a color Doppler sonogram revealing truncus arteriosus in a fetus at 21 weeks. The fetus is imaged in a longitudinal plane yielding a short axis view of both ventricles (RV, LV). *Left* image (diastole): Each ventricle is shown in the filling phase. *Middle* image (early systole): Outflow from both ventricles *(coded blue)* join at the ventricular septal defect *(arrow)* into a single current and continue on into the single outflow vessel, the truncus *(arrowhead)*. *Right* image (systole): A small posterior branch, the main pulmonary artery *(small arrow)*, is seen during the time of highest flow velocity in the truncus. The pulmonary artery could not be identified with gray scale sonography. Without clear demonstration of the pulmonary artery, the final prenatal diagnosis would have been less specific and would have included not only ductus arteriosus but also tetralogy of Fallot with pulmonary atresia.

Figure 14–23. Color and pulsed Doppler sonographies of the pulmonary artery (PA, *red*) and vein (PV, *blue*) for diagnosis of fetal cardiac arrhythmia. Simultaneous spectral tracing of the unique fetal pulmonary arterial waveform above the baseline and the pulmonary venous waveform below the baseline makes it possible to correlate ventricular and atrial events. The *small arrow* marks a large trough in venous flow produced by a normal atrial contraction. This is followed by a normal ventricular contraction, represented by the sharp peak above the baseline. The next normal atrial contraction, farther to the right, is again followed by a normal ventricular contraction. An extra venous trough then appears during systole *(large arrow)* due to a premature atrial contraction (PAC). Occurring too early to be conducted (there is no extra ventricular contraction), the PAC is responsible for a delay in the next ventricular contraction (a pause) as the atrial pacemaker is reset. The next normal atrial contraction *(arrowhead)* occurs an appropriate interval after the PAC and is followed by a greater than normal ventricular contraction.

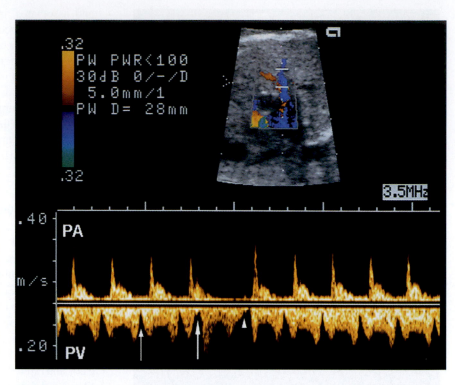

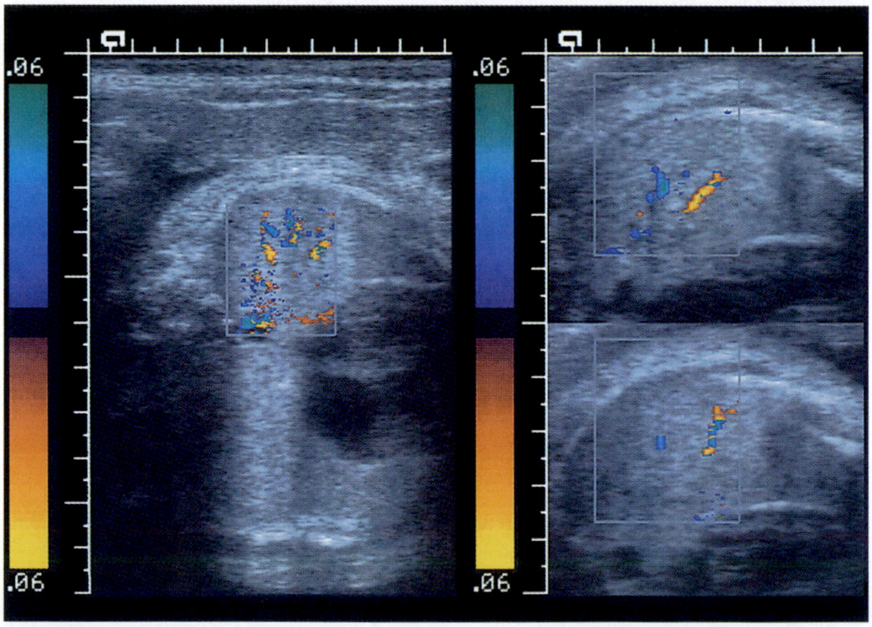

Figure 14–24. Color Doppler maps of flow within parenchymal branches of the pulmonary arteries and veins. These are not seen with conventional gray-scale sonography. Arteries *(coded blue)* and veins *(coded yellow)* can be followed out to the distal aspects of the lungs, making it significantly easier to interrogate specific vessels. *(Reproduced with permission from Emerson D, Cartier M. The Fetus: Scanning Technique and Normal Anatomy. In: Color Doppler Sonography in Obstetrics and Gynecology, Fleischer A, Emerson D, eds. New York: Churchill Livingstone; 1993:217–252.)*

us to identify an unsuspected constricted foramen ovale in a fetus with hypoplastic left heart.

2. Doppler demonstration of normal pulmonary bed arterial flow in a fetus with no demonstrable pulmonary valve or trunk indicates that the main or branch pulmonary arteries must be supplied by retrograde ductus arteriosus flow or by a truncus arteriosus (see Figs. 14–18 and 14–22). This has encouraged us to continue searching for the supplying vessel even when it was initially not readily visible.

3. Color Doppler enhances the mapping of anomalous pulmonary venous return connections. It is performed much more rapidly, with

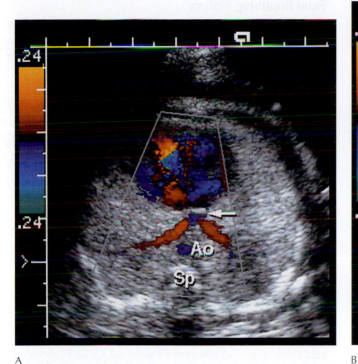

A

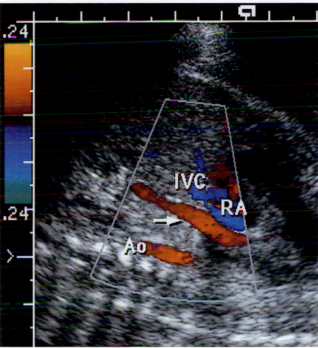

B

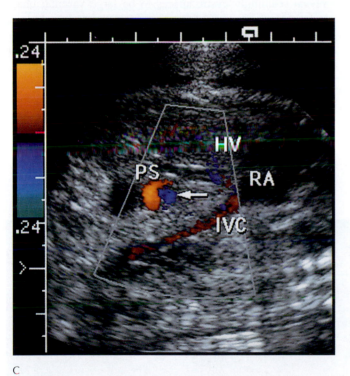

C

Figure 14–25. Total anomalous venous return with infradiaphragmatic drainage in a 30-week fetus. **(A)** Transverse view of the pulmonary veins *(red)* converging to a common pulmonary vein *(blue)* behind the heart. The common pulmonary vein does not enter the left atrium. Instead, it passes behind the heart down into the abdomen. Ao, aorta; Sp, spine. **(B)** Longitudinal image of chest and abdomen. The anomalous common pulmonary vein *(arrow)* is coded red because it courses in a caudal direction into the upper abdomen. The aorta (Ao) is similarly coded red. The inferior vena cava (IVC) is coded blue because it flows in an opposite direction. RA, right atrium. **(C)** Longitudinal view of the lower chest and upper abdomen reveals distal segment of the anomalous common pulmonary vein *(arrow, blue)* draining into the portal sinus (PS, *red*). The inferior vena cava (IVC) is coded red and a hepatic vein (HV) is coded blue. RA, right atrium. *(Reproduced with permission from Emerson D, Becker J, Felker R, et al. Fetus. 1993;3:7474-1–7474-6.)*

more complete and accurate information[14] (Fig. 14–25A through C).

4. Pulmonary arterial and venous flow can be demonstrated with color and pulsed Doppler to be dampened, either locally or globally, due to an intrathoracic mass. Doppler manifestations of this include poor visualization of the pulmonary vasculature on the color map and very low velocities on recordable vascular waveforms.

5. Color Doppler permits monitoring results of therapeutic reduction of an intrathoracic mass by demonstrating rebounding pulmonary arterial flow. The marked increase in vascularity on the color flow map and the rise in peak systolic

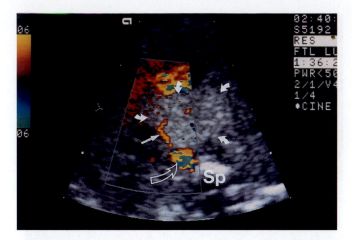

Figure 14–26. Pulmonary sequestration in a 28-week fetus. Color Doppler sonography identifies the systemic artery *(straight arrow)* coursing from the aorta *(open arrow)* to supply the echogenic lung mass *(small curved arrows)* located in the posteromedial right lung base behind the heart. The conventional sonographic image was consistent with sequestration and cystic adenomatoid malformation. The additional vascular information yielded a more specific diagnosis. Sp, spine.

velocity of the arterial waveform probably occur due to a significant fall in resistance to blood flow as lung compression is relieved.

6. Color Doppler identifies supplying arteries and draining veins of intrathoracic masses. We have found this to be particularly effective in improving the specific diagnosis of cystic adenomatoid malformation of the lung and bronchopulmonary sequestration (Fig. 14–26). Color Doppler has been used to identify a herniated liver in a case of diaphragmatic hernia.[83]

Fetal Breathing Motion

Color Doppler sonography is well suited to reveal not only blood flow but also the inward and outward flow of amniotic fluid in the respiratory tract secondary to fetal breathing motion. Placement of the color box and the pulsed Doppler range gate near the fetal nose, mouth, pharynx, or larynx detects the presence of breathing motion more sensitively than by observing abdominal motion[84–86] (Fig. 14–27). Furthermore, this technique graphically depicts patterns of inspiration and expiration that may be altered during fetal distress.[85] In a preliminary report, detection of fetal breathing motion with a combination of fetal thoracic motion and perinasal fluid currents was associated with normal lung development in four of five cases of diaphragmatic hernia. However, in one of the five cases, thoracic motion was not associated with perinasal fluid movement, and this fetus died at 1 day of age from pulmonary hypoplasia.[87]

Vascular Anomalies

Color Doppler sonography elucidates additional important information in fetal abnormalities associated with increased vascularity due to arteriovenous shunting. Color Doppler can reveal seemingly cystic spaces to be large vascular channels in the aneurysm of the vein of Galen and in the rare giant cavernous hemangioma of the liver[4,5,88] (Fig. 14–28). Furthermore, color Doppler identifies the dramatic increase in supplying and draining vessels of the aneurysm of the vein of Galen and of other masses, such as hemangioendothelioma of the liver and sacrococcygeal teratoma, obvious manifestations of the increased shunting of blood flow in these abnormalities[4,5,89,90] (Fig. 14–29). The potential for high-output heart failure has been monitored through serial measurements of cardiac output with overt hydrops occurring only above a certain threshold value.[90] Possibly, fetal surgery

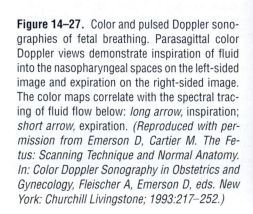

Figure 14–27. Color and pulsed Doppler sonographies of fetal breathing. Parasagittal color Doppler views demonstrate inspiration of fluid into the nasopharyngeal spaces on the left-sided image and expiration on the right-sided image. The color maps correlate with the spectral tracing of fluid flow below: *long arrow,* inspiration; *short arrow,* expiration. *(Reproduced with permission from Emerson D, Cartier M. The Fetus: Scanning Technique and Normal Anatomy. In: Color Doppler Sonography in Obstetrics and Gynecology, Fleischer A, Emerson D, eds. New York: Churchill Livingstone; 1993:217–252.)*

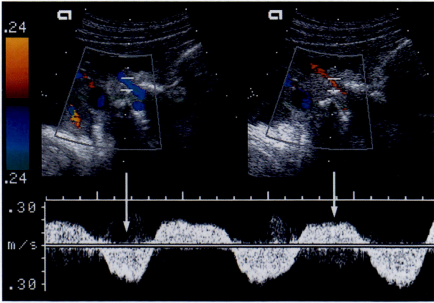

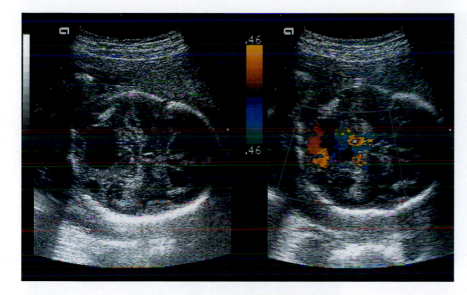

Figure 14–28. Vein of Galen aneurysm in a 22-week fetus. *(Left)* Ventriculomegaly and a posterior cystic mass. Although the vein of Galen aneurysm is a strong consideration, it is not the only abnormality in the differential diagnosis. *(Right)* The posterior cyst is shown to be filled with high-velocity blood flow and to be supplied by many small adjacent vessels on this color Doppler map. A specific diagnosis can now be made. *(Courtesy of Dr. Richard Felker, University of Tennessee, Memphis.)*

can be planned or delivery timed more rigorously in these conditions immediately prior to development of hydrops.[91]

Fetal Vessel Identification as Diagnostic Aid

Color Doppler delineation of certain fetal vessels can provide important secondary assistance in the diagnosis of some fetal abnormalities, even in cases where that vasculature is not directly related to the abnormality.

The perivesicle umbilical arteries are constant anatomic markers for the inferolateral walls of the urinary bladder. These vessels are generally not difficult to demonstrate and do not require the use of color Doppler for their clarification. The search for the fetal bladder, however, may be rendered rather difficult in a case of marked oligohydramnios or when a large mass distorts the fetal pelvic anatomy. The color Doppler map very efficiently targets the appropriate anatomic site to visualize urine in the bladder in these situations. Color

Doppler sonography of the perivesicle umbilical arteries is also a very efficient technique for confirming a single umbilical artery seen in the umbilical cord or for determining which is the absent umbilical artery (Fig. 14–30). An accessory technique is the demonstration of the renal artery as confirmatory evidence of an ectopic kidney, a sometimes difficult diagnosis because of similarities in sonographic appearances between kidneys and intestinal loops (Fig. 14–31). Furthermore, we and others have used color Doppler evidence of absent renal arteries to confirm the sonographic suspicion of renal agenesis[92]; however, the accuracy of this negative finding has not been rigorously proven.

Gray-scale imaging is excellent for the diagnosis and differentiating of abdominal wall defects. Color Doppler may prove useful, however, by delineating the insertion of the umbilical vessels into the omphalocele in a case of an eccentric insertion. In addition, the color map may clearly reveal the

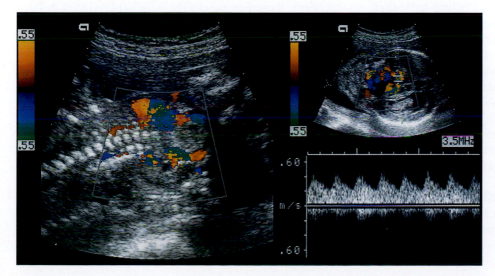

Figure 14–29. *(Left)* Tangle of supplying and draining vessels in the neck and posterior fossa demonstrated with color Doppler sonography. *(Right)* Pulsed Doppler interrogation reveals very low-impedance high-velocity arterial flow supplying the aneurysm. This reveals that the underlying nature of a vein of Galen aneurysm is an arteriovenous malformation. These Doppler appearances explain the common occurrence in this condition of fetal hydrops due to high-output heart failure. *(Courtesy of Dr. Richard Felker, University of Tennessee, Memphis.)*

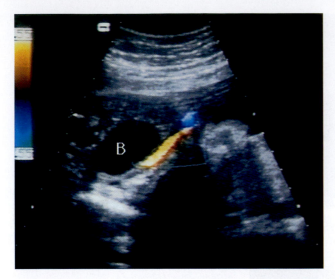

Figure 14–30. Color Doppler sonography demonstrates single umbilical artery *(yellow)* coursing along edge of urinary bladder (B) to the umbilicus. The umbilical vein is coded blue. This view is extremely useful for identifying which umbilical artery is absent in order to determine the dominant laterality of the fetus with abdominal heterotaxy. It is also a very effective view for localizing the urinary bladder in technically difficult cases. *(Reproduced with permission from Emerson D. Placenta and Umbilical Cord. In: Color Doppler Sonography in Obstetrics and Gynecology, Fleischer A, Emerson D, eds. New York: Churchill Livingstone; 1993:287–308.)*

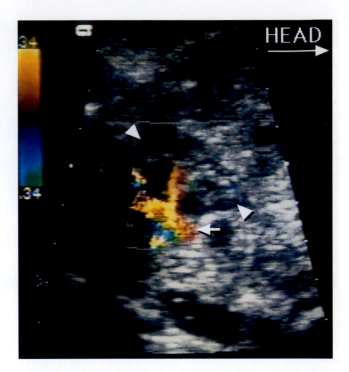

Figure 14–31. Color Doppler sonographic confirmation of suspected fetal ectopic kidney. Pelvic kidney is seen in this coronal view of the pelvis, although bowel loops can sometimes simulate this appearance. Color Doppler map reveals the renal artery branching off of the right common iliac artery and terminating in the renal pelvis. Pulsed Doppler demonstrated a typical renal artery waveform. *Arrow* points to the distal abdominal aorta just above the bifurcation. *(Reproduced with permission from Emerson D, Cartier M. Fetal Abnormalities and Malformations. In: Color Doppler Sonography in Obstetrics and Gynecology, Fleischer A, Emerson D, eds. New York; Churchill Livingstone; 1993;253–286.)*

normal umbilical insertion in a case of gastroschisis even when this area is obscured by the overlying herniated intestines on conventional sonography.

Color Doppler demonstration of intracranial fetal vascular anatomy may prove helpful in the diagnosis of agenesis of the corpus callosum and of cytomegalovirus infection.[93,94] In the case of agenesis of the corpus callosum, the color map reveals the loss of the normal sweep of the pericallosal artery and presence of radially extending branches of the anterior cerebral artery,[93] and, in a postnatal case describing intrauterine infection, Doppler revealed that abnormal branched echogenic linear foci within the brain were located in the distribution of the thalamostriate arteries.[94]

Amniotic band syndrome has numerous and varied presentations. Color Doppler may prove diagnostically helpful on occasion, as it did in one case seen in our laboratory. One fetal foot was swollen and a constricting ring was seen at the lower calf. The color flow map revealed arterial flow past the ring into the foot but no measurable venous flow from the foot past the ring. The diagnosis of amniotic band syndrome was made prior to the color Doppler interrogation, but our understanding of the pathophysiology was enhanced due to it.[95]

Blood Flow as an Indicator of Renal Functional Status

Color and pulsed Doppler measurements of renal blood flow would seem to provide an ideal quantitative handle on the increasing maturation of fetal kidneys throughout gestation and on their functional status when they are obstructed or structurally abnormal. Indeed, there is an inverse correlation between gestational age and pulsatility index.[71,96,97] Nevertheless, the increase in renal blood flow during the course of fetal life correlates directly with increasing cardiac output, with no increase occurring in the percentage of cardiac output.[71] Furthermore, there was no change in pulsatility index in fetal renal arteries during maternal indomethacin treatment, although the lack of Doppler findings may have been due to limiting the investigation to the first 24 hours of therapy.[98] In addition, although there is a recognized fall in urine output during states of high fetal activity, no changes in renal artery pulsatility index have been detectable.[99] In contrast, there is a significant transient fall in renal artery pulsatility index after intravascular transfusion, indicating that Doppler can detect in utero changes related to increased renal flow and urine production.[100] Renal artery resistance has been found to be elevated in growth retardation and oligohydramnios, but there is disagreement regarding the extent of change.[96,101–103] Although there is a trend toward elevated renal artery pulsatility index in fetal hydronephrosis and multicystic dysplastic kidneys, this does not appear to offer clinical benefit because most values fall within the normal reference range.[92]

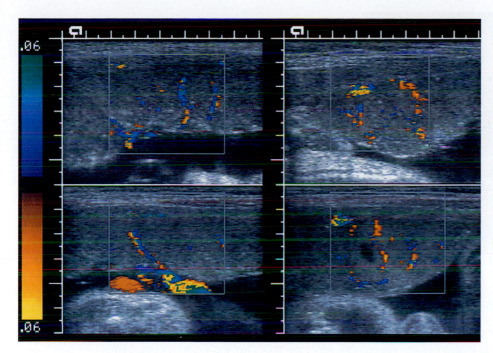

Figure 14–32. Placental vasculature is well demonstrated with color Doppler sonography. Umbilical artery and vein are seen at the cord insertion site into the placenta in the *left lower* image. Umbilical arteries course within the chorionic plate and into the substance of the placenta as arteries of the main stem villi in the *left upper* image. Maternal spiral arterioles are seen at the decidual surface of the placenta and coursing deep into the placenta in the *right upper* image. Additional maternal arterial vessels *(coded orange)* descend into the placenta in the *bottom right* image. Maternal flow can sometimes be seen entering the central anechoic spaces of the placenta. *(Reproduced with permission from Emerson D. Placenta and Umbilical Cord. In: Color Doppler Sonography in Obstetrics and Gynecology, Fleischer A, Emerson D, eds. New York: Churchill Livingstone; 1993:287–308.)*

CORD AND PLACENTA

Conventional real-time sonography provides excellent visualization of the placenta and umbilical cord. The three vessels of the cord, the body of the placenta, the chorionic plate vessels, and the subplacental complex of vessels are all clearly demonstrated. Nevertheless, there are situations in which color Doppler sonography may provide clinically important additional information. By detecting both fetal and maternal vessels as they penetrate the placenta (Fig. 14–32), there is hope of ultimately developing better techniques to grade placental function.[104]

Umbilical Cord

Color Doppler sonography assists in the diagnosis of a single umbilical artery when conventional sonographic imaging is compromised by oligohydramnios or early gestational age.[72,105] Color Doppler can assist in the measurement of amniotic fluid volume by demonstrating otherwise unseen or poorly seen loops of cord within amniotic fluid pockets. Umbilical cord in abnormal or in potentially high-risk locations (prolapsed cord, nuchal cord) is more easily recognized on the color flow map (Fig. 14–33). Cord masses, such as cysts and umbilical vein or artery aneurysms, may be more fully investigated with the addition of color Doppler sonography. Of particular importance are the relation of the mass and the umbilical vessels and the possibility of vascular compromise.[105,106] As described earlier, color Doppler depiction of the umbilical cord insertion may be clinically important in the case of abdominal wall defects. Color Doppler sonography of the umbilical cord may provide supplementary diagnostic information for certain fetal abnormalities,

such as a short stretched cord in the limb–body wall complex and reversed flow to an acardiac twin.[107,108]

Placenta

Color Doppler sonography provides clinically useful information in three conditions: chorioangioma, vasa previa, and

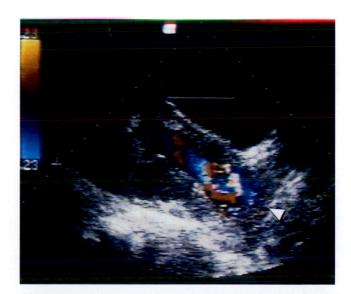

Figure 14–33. Sagittal view of cervix in a patient with premature labor, cervical dilatation *(arrowhead)*, and prolapsed cord. Color Doppler sonography made the cord considerably more visible, although this was detected with conventional real-time sonography. *(Reproduced with permission from Emerson D. Placenta and Umbilical Cord. In: Color Doppler Sonography in Obstetrics and Gynecology, Fleischer A, Emerson D, eds. New York: Churchill Livingstone; 1993:287–308.)*

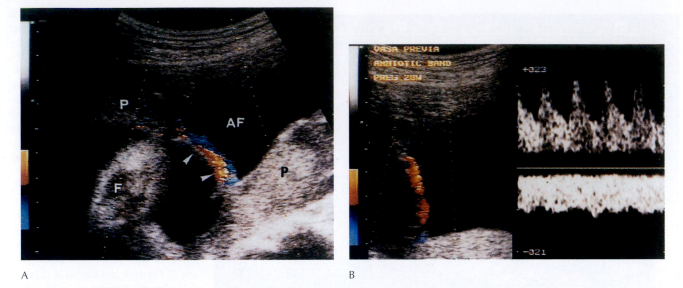

A   B

Figure 14–34. Vasa previa. **(A)** Conventional sonography demonstrated a band of tissue *(arrowheads)* traversing the lower uterine cavity between the posterior main body of the placenta and the anterior succenturiate lobe (P). Color Doppler reveals umbilical artery *(red)* and vein *(blue)* within the shelf. AF, amniotic fluid; F, fetus. **(B)** Pulsed Doppler interrogation within the shelf identifies typical umbilical artery and vein waveforms. *(Reproduced with permission from Hsieh FJ, Chen HF, Ko TM, et al. J Ultrasound Med. 1991;10:397–399.)*

placenta accreta. Chorioangiomas, which are complex or solid masses of the placenta, are relatively nonspecific on conventional ultrasound due to commonly occurring irregularities of the placenta and thrombosed venous lakes. Color Doppler sonography may assist in this diagnosis by demonstrating the suspected mass to be a vascular tumor with fetal arterial waveforms.[109,110]

In vasa previa, placental vessels pass through the amniotic cavity near the cervix outside of the placenta and cord. It may be associated with a velamentous insertion of the cord or a succinturiate lobe. There is great risk of fetal mortality during labor due to compression or tearing of these vessels. Conventional sonography can detect this abnormality but color and pulsed Doppler techniques are important in confirming the findings[111–114] (Fig. 14–34A and B).

Placenta accreta is a potentially life-threatening condition for the mother in which the placenta infiltrates into the substance of the myometrium to various degrees, forming an abnormal attachment to the uterus. In the accreta subtype, there is partial loss of the decidua basalis. In increta, there is complete loss of the decidua basalis and partial invasion of the myometrium; and in percreta, there is complete invasion of the myometrium. Prospective diagnosis is extremely important, but, unfortunately, despite some useful sonographic signs and relevant clinical and historical features, the condition is probably significantly underdiagnosed. Color Doppler sonography supplements the conventional sonographic signs, probably adding some diagnostic accuracy to the diagnosis, although its contribution to diagnostic sensitivity is not known. Color Doppler demonstrates loss of the vascularity typically seen in the hypoechoic subplacental zone and may

reveal multiple abnormal intraplacental lakes with pulsatile and laminar flow[115,116] (Fig. 14–35).

In addition to these indications, there is hope that with the advent of some new technologies, such as color Doppler

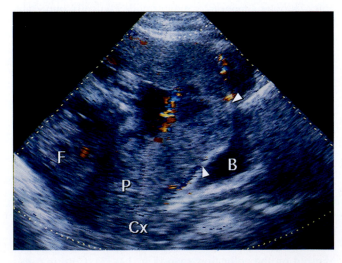

Figure 14–35. Sagittal color Doppler sonogram of placenta accreta. Anterior placenta (P) extends down over the cervix (Cx). The absence of subplacental vessels in the region between the *arrowheads* is abnormal and indicates presence of accreta. This corresponded to the area that was devoid of the normal hypoechoic myometrium and could not be identified on conventional real-time sonography. F, fetus; B, bladder. *(Courtesy of Delores Pretorius, MD, San Diego; reproduced with permission from Emerson D. Placenta and Umbilical Cord. In: Color Doppler Sonography in Obstetrics and Gynecology, Fleischer A, Emerson D, eds. New York: Churchill Livingstone; 1993:287–308.)*

energy and ultrasound contrast agents, there will be new methods to improve the diagnosis of placental infarction and abruption and the quantification of overall placental flow.

REFERENCES

1. Emerson DS, Cartier MS, Altieri LA, et al. Diagnostic efficacy of endovaginal color Doppler flow imaging in an ectopic pregnancy screening program. *Radiology*. 1992;183:413–420.

2. Trudinger BJ, Cook CM, Giles WB, et al. Fetal umbilical artery velocity waveforms and subsequent neonatal outcome. *Br J Obstet Gynaecol*. 1991;98:378–384.

3. Gembruch U, Knopfle G, Chatterjee M, et al. Prenatal diagnosis of atrioventricular canal malformations with up-to-date echocardiographic technology: Report of 14 cases. *Am Heart J*. 1991;121:1489–1497.

4. Ishimatsu J, Yoshimura O, Tetsuou M, et al. Evaluation of an aneurysm of the vein of Galen in utero by pulsed and color Doppler ultrasonography. *Am J Obstet Gynecol*. 1991;164:743–744.

5. Jeanty P, Kepple D, Roussis P, et al. In utero detection of cardiac failure from an aneurysm of the vein of Galen. *Am J Obstet Gynecol*. 1990;163:50–51.

6. Cartier MS, Emerson D, Plappert T, et al. Hypoplastic left heart with absence of the aortic valve: Prenatal diagnosis using two-dimensional and pulsed Doppler echocardiography. *J Clin Ultrasound*. 1987;15:463–468.

7. Chan FY, Woo SK, Ghosh A, et al. Prenatal diagnosis of congenital fetal arrhythmias by simultaneous pulsed Doppler velocimetry of the fetal abdominal aorta and inferior vena cava. *Obstet Gynecol*. 1990;76:200–205.

8. De Vore G, Horenstein J. Simultaneous Doppler recording of the pulmonary artery and vein: A new technique for the evaluation of a fetal arrhythmia. *J Ultrasound Med*. 1993;12:669–671.

9. Sauerbrei E. Lung sequestration. Duplex Doppler diagnosis at 19 weeks gestation. *J Ultrasound Med*. 1991;10:105–105.

10. Newman B. Real-time ultrasound and color Doppler imaging in pulmonary sequestration. *Pediatrics*. 1990;86:620–623.

11. Copel JA, Morotti R, Hobbins JC, et al. The antenatal diagnosis of congenital heart disease using fetal echocardiography: Is color flow mapping necessary? *Obstet Gynecol*. 1991;78:1–8.

12. Cartier M, Emerson D, Felker R, et al. Color flow Doppler for evaluation of abnormal fetal pulmonary blood flow. *J Ultrasound Med*. 1993;12:S54.

13. DiSessa T, Emerson D, Felker R, et al. Anomalous systemic and pulmonary venous pathways diagnosed in utero by ultrasound. *J Ultrasound Med*. 1990;9:311–317.

14. Emerson D, Becker J, Felker R, et al. Pulmonary venous connection, total anomalous. *Fetus*. 1993;3:7474-1–7474-6.

15. Burns PN, Principles of Doppler and color flow. *Radiol Med (Torino)*. 1993;85:3–16.

16. Maulik D. Hemodynamic interpretation of the arterial Doppler waveform. *Ultrasound Obstet Gynecol*. 1993;3:219–227.

17. Arduini D, Rizzo G, Boccolini MR, et al. Functional assessment of uteroplacental and fetal circulations by means of color Doppler ultrasonography. *J Ultrasound Med*. 1990;9:249–253.

18. Harrington K, Campbell S. Doppler ultrasound in prenatal prediction and diagnosis. *Curr Opin Obstet Gynecol*. 1992;4:264–272.

19. Bosward KL, Barnett SB, Wood AK, et al. Heating of guinea-pig fetal brain during exposure to pulsed ultrasound. *Ultrasound Med Biol*. 1993;19:415–424.

20. Barnett SB, Kossoff G, Edwards MJ. International perspectives on safety and standardization of diagnostic pulsed ultrasound in medicine. *Ultrasound Obstet Gynecol*. 1993;3:287–294.

21. Jauniaux E, Jurkovic D, Campbell S. In vivo investigations of the anatomy and the physiology of early human placental circulations. *Ultrasound Obstet Gynecol*. 1991;1:435–445.

22. Emerson D, Altieri L, Cartier M. Transabdominal and endovaginal ultrasound in ectopic pregnancy, In: Stovall T, ed. *Extrauterine Pregnancy: Clinical Diagnosis and Management*. New York: McGraw-Hill; 1993:137–178.

23. Stovall TG, Ling FW, Buster JE. Outpatient chemotherapy of unruptured ectopic pregnancy. *Fertil Steril*. 1989;51:435–438.

24. Pellerito JS, Taylor KJ, Quedens CC, et al. Ectopic pregnancy: Evaluation with endovaginal color flow imaging. *Radiology*. 1992;183:407–411.

25. Kadar N, De Vore G, Romero R. Discriminatory hCG zone: Its use in the sonographic evaluation for ectopic pregnancy. *Obstet Gynecol*. 1981;581:156–161.

26. Bree RL, Edwards M, Bohm VM, et al. Transvaginal sonography in the evaluation of normal early pregnancy: Correlation with hCG level. *AJR*. 1989;153:75–79.

27. Emerson D. Unpublished data, 1991.

28. Abramovici H, Auslender R, Lewin A, et al. Gestational-pseudogestational sac: A new ultrasonic criterion for differential diagnosis. *Am J Obstet Gynecol*. 1983;145:377–379.

29. Nyberg DA, Filly RA, Laing FC, et al. Ectopic pregnancy. Diagnosis by sonography correlated with quantitative hCG levels. *J Ultrasound Med*. 1987;6:145–150.

30. Cacciatore B, Ylostalo P, Stenman UH, et al. Suspected ectopic pregnancy: Ultrasound findings and hCG levels assessed by an immunofluorometric assay. *Br J Obstet Gynaecol*. 1988;95:497–502.

31. Jurkovic D, Bourne TH, Jauniaux E, et al. Transvaginal color Doppler study of blood flow in ectopic pregnancies. *Fertil Steril*. 1992;57:68–73.

32. Kurjak A, Zalud I, Schulman H. Ectopic pregnancy: Transvaginal color Doppler of trophoblastic flow in questionable adnexa. *J Ultrasound Med*. 1991;10:685–689.

33. Altieri L, Cartier M, Emerson D, et al. Endovaginal color flow Doppler in the early intrauterine pregnancy: Correlation with peritrophoblastic velocities, sac size, and hCG. *Radiology*. 1990;177(P):193.

34. Emerson D, Felker R. Early intrauterine pregnancy. In: Fleischer A, Emerson D, eds. *Color Doppler Sonography in Obstetrics and Gynecology*. New York: Churchill Livingstone; 1993:169–192.

35. Taylor KJ, Ramos IM, Feyock AL, et al. Ectopic pregnancy: Duplex Doppler evaluation. *Radiology*. 1989;173:93–97.

36. Tekay A. Jouppila P. Color Doppler flow as an indicator of trophoblastic activity in tubal pregnancies detected by transvaginal ultrasound. *Obstet Gynecol*. 1992;80:995–999.

37. Emerson D, Cartier M, Felker R, et al. Predicting treatment response to methotrexate using morphologic and Doppler sonographic characteristics of ectopic masses. *J Ultrasound Med*. 1993;12:S59–S60.

38. Stovall TG, Ling FW, Cope BJ, et al. Preventing ruptured

ectopic pregnancy with a single serum progesterone. *Am J Obstet Gynecol.* 1989;160:1425–1428.

39. Taylor K, Schwartz P, Kohorn E. Gestational trophoblastic neoplasia: Diagnosis with Doppler US. *Radiology.* 1987;165: 445–448.

40. Shimamoto K, Sakuma S, Ishigaki T, et al. Intratumoral blood flow: Evaluation with color Doppler echography. *Radiology.* 1987;165:683–685.

41. Kurjak A, Zalud I. Transvaginal color Doppler for evaluating gynecologic pathology of the pelvis. *Ultraschall Med.* 1990;11:164–168.

42. Jauniaux E, de Lannoy E, Moscoso G, et al. Prenatal diagnosis of molar pathologies coexisting with a fetus. Review of the recent literature and a case report. *J Gynecol Obstet Biol Reprod (Paris).* 1990;19:941–946.

43. Kurjak A, Zalud I, Salihagic A, et al. Transvaginal color Doppler in the assessment of abnormal early pregnancy. *J Perinat Med.* 1991;19:155–165.

44. Desai RK, Desberg AL. Diagnosis of gestational trophoblastic disease: Value of endovaginal color flow Doppler sonography. *AJR.* 1991;157:787–788.

45. Chau M, Chan F, Pun T, et al. Perforation of the uterus by an invasive mole using color Doppler ultrasound: Case report. *Ultrasound Obstet Gynecol.* 1993;3:51–53.

46. Kurjak A, Crvenkovic G, Salihagic A, et al. The assessment of normal early pregnancy by transvaginal color Doppler ultrasonography. *J Clin Ultrasound.* 1993;21:3–8.

47. Emerson D, Cartier M. The fetus: Scanning technique and normal anatomy. In: Fleischer A, Emerson D, eds. *Color Doppler Sonography in Obstetrics and Gynecology.* New York: Churchill Livingstone; 1993:217–252.

48. Chen HY, Chang FM, Huang HC, et al. Antenatal fetal blood flow in the descending aorta and in the umbilical vein and their ratio in normal pregnancy. *Ultrasound Med Biol.* 1988;14:263–268.

49. Rizzo G, Arduini D, Romanini C. Inferior vena cava flow velocity waveforms in appropriate- and small-for-gestational-age fetuses. *Am J Obstet Gynecol.* 1992;166:1271–1280.

50. Huisman TW, Stewart PA, Wladimiroff JW, et al. Flow velocity waveforms in the ductus venosus, umbilical vein and inferior vena cava in normal human fetuses at 12–15 weeks of gestation. *Ultrasound Med Biol.* 1993;19:441–445.

51. Gill R, Kossoff G, Warren P, et al. Umbilical venous flow in normal and complicated pregnancy. *Ultrasound Med Biol.* 1984;10:349–363.

52. Emerson D, Cartier M, Brown D, et al. Shunting of umbilical vein blood via the ductus venosus: Fetal Doppler study. *Radiology.* 1989;173(P):249.

53. Gudmundsson S, Huhta JC, Wood DC, et al. Venous Doppler ultrasonography in the fetus with nonimmune hydrops. *Am J Obstet Gynecol.* 1991;164:33–37.

54. Indik J, Chen V, Reed K. Association of umbilical venous with inferior vena cava blood flow velocities. *Obstet Gynecol.* 1991;77:551–557.

55. Kiserud T, Eik NS, Blaas HG, et al. Ultrasonographic velocimetry of the fetal ductus venosus. *Lancet.* 1991;338: 1412–1414.

56. De Vore G, Horenstein J. Ductus venosus index: A method for evaluating right ventricular preload in the second-trimester fetus. *Ultrasound Obstet Gynecol.* 1993;3:338–342.

57. Kanzaki T, Chiba Y. Evaluation of the preload condition of the fetus by inferior vena caval blood flow pattern. *Fetal Diagn Ther.* 1990;5:168–174.

58. Reed K, Sahn D, Scagnelli S, et al. Doppler echocardiographic studies of diastolic function in the human fetal heart: Changes during gestation. *J Am Coll Cardiol.* 1986;8:391–395.

59. Reed K, Meijboom E, Sahn D, et al. Cardiac Doppler flow velocities in human fetuses. *Circulation.* 1986;73:41–46.

60. Wladimiroff JW, Huisman TW, Stewart PA. Fetal cardiac flow velocities in the late first trimester of pregnancy: A transvaginal Doppler study. *J Am Coll Cardiol.* 1991;17:1357–1359.

61. Emerson D, Cartier M, De Vore G. et al. Distal pulmonary artery branches in the fetus: New observations with color flow and pulsed Doppler. *J Ultrasound Med.* 1991;10(S): S19.

62. Arbeille PH, Tranquart F, Berson M, et al. Visualization of the fetal circle of Willis and intracerebral arteries by colorcoded Doppler. *Eur J Obstet Gynecol Reprod Biol.* 1989;32:195–198.

63. Arbeille P, Body G, Fignon A, et al. Doppler assessment of the intracerebral circulation of the fetus. *Clin Phys Physiol Meas.* 1989;10:51–57.

64. Meerman RJ, van Bel F, van Zwieten PH, et al. Fetal and neonatal cerebral blood velocity in the normal fetus and neonate: A longitudinal Doppler ultrasound study. *Early Hum Dev.* 1990;24:209–217.

65. Hata T, Mari G, Reiter AA. Doppler velocity waveforms of blood flow in the fetal renal artery in a case of Meckel syndrome. *AJR.* 1991;156.

66. Mari G. Regional cerebral flow velocity waveforms in the human fetus. *J Ultrasound Med.* 1994;13:343–346.

67. Cartier M, Emerson D, Felker R, et al. Color and pulsed Doppler of the fetal superior mesenteric artery. *J Ultrasound Med.* 1992;11:S531.

68. Griffin D, Bilardo K, Masini L, et al. Doppler blood flow waveforms in the descending thoracic aorta of the human fetus. *Br J Obstet Gynaecol.* 1984;91:997–1006.

69. Tonge H, Wladimiroff J, Noordam M, et al. Blood flow velocity waveforms in the descending fetal aorta: Comparison between normal and growth retarded pregnancies. *Obstet Gynecol.* 1986;67:851–855.

70. Veille JC, Figueroa JP, Mueller Heubach E. Validation of noninvasive fetal renal artery flow measurement by pulsed Doppler in the lamb. *Am J Obstet Gynecol.* 1992;167:1663–1667.

71. Veille JC, Hanson RA, Tatum K, et al. Quantitative assessment of human fetal renal blood flow. *Am J Obstet Gynecol.* 1993;169:1399–1402.

72. Bonilla-Musoles F, Raga F, Ballester M, et al. Early detection of embryonic malformations by transvaginal and color Doppler sonography. *J Ultrasound Med.* 1994;13: 347–356.

73. De Vore GR, Horenstein J, Siassi B, et al. Fetal echocardiography. VII: Doppler color flow mapping: A new technique for the diagnosis of congenital heart disease. *Am J Obstet Gynecol.* 1987;156:1054–1064.

74. Gembruch U, Chatterjee MS, Bald R, et al. Color Doppler flow mapping of fetal heart. *J Perinat Med.* 1991;19:27–32.

75. Cartier M, Emerson D, Felker R, et al. Contribution of color Doppler in prenatal evaluation of congenital cardiac anomalies. *J Ultrasound Med.* 1992;11:S22.

76. Copel JA, Hobbins JC, Kleinman CS. Doppler echocardiography and color flow mapping. *Obstet Gynecol Clin North Am.* 1991;18:845–851.

77. Gembruch U, Knöpfle G, Bald R, et al. Early diagnosis of fetal congenital heart disease by transvaginal echocardiography. *Ultrasound Obstet Gynecol.* 1993;3:310–317.

78. Akita A, Harima N, Nawata S, et al. Two-dimensional and Doppler echocardiographic evaluation of intrauterine blood flow dynamics in the fetuses with a ventricular septal defect. *Acta Obstet Gynaecol Jpn.* 1991;43:1606–1612.

79. Gembruch U, Bald R, Hansmann M. Color-coded M-mode Doppler echocardiography in the diagnosis of fetal arrhythmia. *Geburtshilfe Frauenheilkd.* 1990;50:286–290.

80. Gembruch U, Chatterjee M, Bald R, et al. Prenatal diagnosis of aortic atresia by colour Doppler flow mapping. *Prenat Diagn.* 1990;10:211–217.

81. Gembruch U, Weinraub Z, Bald R, et al. Flow analysis in the pulmonary trunc in fetuses with tetralogy of Fallot by colour Doppler flow mapping; two case reports. *Eur J Obstet Gynecol Reprod Biol.* 1990;35:259–265.

82. Emerson D, Cartier M. The fetal pulmonary circulation. In: Copel J, Reed K, eds. *Doppler Ultrasound in Obstetrics and Gynecology.* New York: Raven Press; 1995:307–323.

83. Botash R, Spirt B. Color Doppler imaging aids in the prenatal diagnosis of congenital diaphragmatic hernia. *J Ultrasound Med.* 1993;12:359–361.

84. Isaacson G, Birnholz JC. Human fetal upper respiratory tract function as revealed by ultrasonography. *Ann Otol Rhinol Laryngol.* 1991;100:743–747.

85. Birnholz J, Isaacson G. Fetal nose breathing. *Radiology.* 1990;177(P):194.

86. Badalian SS, Chao CR, Fox HE, et al. Fetal breathing-related nasal fluid flow velocity in uncomplicated pregnancies. *Am J Obstet Gynecol.* 1993;169:563–567.

87. Fox H, Badalian S, Timor-Tritsch I, et al. Fetal upper respiratory tract function in cases of antenatally diagnosed congenital diaphragmatic hernia: Preliminary observations. *Ultrasound Obstet Gynecol.* 1993;3:164–167.

88. Lasser D, Preis O, Dor N, et al. Antenatal diagnosis of giant cystic cavernous hemangioma by Doppler velocimetry. *Obstet Gynecol.* 1988;42:476–477.

89. Gonen R, Fong K, Chiasson DA. Prenatal sonographic diagnosis of hepatic hemangioendothelioma with secondary non-immune hydrops fetalis. *Obstet Gynecol.* 1989;73:485–487.

90. Schmidt KG, Silverman NH, Harrison MR, et al. High-output cardiac failure in fetuses with large sacrococcygeal teratoma: Diagnosis by echocardiography and Doppler ultrasound. *J Pediatr.* 1989;114:1023–1028.

91. Langer JC, Harrison MR, Schmidt KG, et al. Fetal hydrops and death from sacrococcygeal teratoma: Rationale for fetal surgery. *Am J Obstet Gynecol.* 1989;160:1145–1150.

92. Wladimiroff JW, Heydanus R, Stewart PA, et al. Fetal renal artery flow velocity waveforms in the presence of congenital renal tract anomalies. *Prenat Diagn.* 1993;13:545–549.

93. Pilu G, Sandri G, Perola A, et al. Sonography of fetal agenesis of the corpus callosum: A survey of 35 cases. *Ultrasound Obstet Gynecol.* 1993;3:318–329.

94. Toma P, Magnano GM, Mezzano P, et al. Cerebral ultrasound images in prenatal cytomegalovirus infection. *Neuroradiology.* 1989;31:278–279.

95. Emerson D, Cartier M. Fetal abnormalities and malformations. In: Fleischer A, Emerson D, eds. *Color Doppler Sonography in Obstetrics and Gynecology.* New York: Churchill Livingstone; 1993:253–286.

96. Vyas S, Nicolaides KH, Campbell S. Renal artery flow-velocity waveforms in normal and hypoxemic fetuses. *Am J Obstet Gynecol.* 1989;161:168–172.

97. Cartier M, Emerson D, Felker R, et al. Pulsed Doppler waveforms of renal arteries in the fetus. *J Ultrasound Med.* 1990; 9:S32.

98. Mari G, Moise KJJ, Deter RL, et al. Doppler assessment of the renal blood flow velocity waveform during indomethacin therapy for preterm labor and polyhydramnios. *Obstet Gynecol.* 1990;75:199–201.

99. Oosterhof H, Lander M, Aarnoudse JG. Behavioral states and Doppler velocimetry of the renal artery in the near term human fetus. *Early Hum Dev.* 1993;33:183–189.

100. Mari G, Moise KJ, Deter R, et al. Doppler assessment of renal blood flow velocity waveforms in the anemic fetus before and after intravascular transfusion for severe red cell alloimmunization. *J Clin Ultrasound.* 1991;19:15–19.

101. Maeda K, Takeuchi Y. Fetal renal arterial blood velocity waveforms detected with color-flow mapping and pulsed Doppler flowmetry in intrauterine growth retardation. *J Clin Ultrasound.* 1990;18:527–531.

102. Akita A, Okada O, Saito T, et al. Evaluation of the renal artery in the fetuses with growth retardation and oligohydramnios by two dimensional Doppler ultrasonography. *Nippon Sanka Fujinka Gakkai Zasshi.* 1991;43:1554–1560.

103. Tanabe R. Doppler ultrasonographic assessment of fetal renal artery blood flow velocity waveforms in intrauterine growth retarded fetuses. *Kurume Med J.* 1992;39:203–208.

104. Jauniaux E, Jurkovic D, Campbell S, et al. Investigation of placental circulations by color Doppler ultrasonography. *Am J Obstet Gynecol.* 1991;164:486–488.

105. Jauniaux E, Campbell S, Vyas S. The use of color Doppler imaging for prenatal diagnosis of umbilical cord anomalies: Report of three cases. *Am J Obstet Gynecol.* 1989;161: 1195–1197.

106. Siddiqi TA, Bendon R, Schultz DM, et al. Umbilical artery aneurysm: Prenatal diagnosis and management. *Obstet Gynecol.* 1992;80:530–533.

107. Donnenfeld AE, van de Woestijne J, Craparo F, et al. The normal fetus of an acardiac twin pregnancy: Perinatal management based on echocardiographic and sonographic evaluation. *Prenat Diagn.* 1991;11:235–244.

108. Ishimatsu J, Nakanami H, Hamada T, et al. Color and pulsed Doppler ultrasonography of reversed umbilical blood flow in an acardiac twin. *Asia Oceania J Obstet Gynaecol.* 1993;19: 271–275.

109. Jauniaux E, Jurkovic D, Kurjak A, et al. Assessment of placental development and function. In: Kurjak A, ed. *Transvaginal Color Doppler.* Park Ridge, NJ: Parthenon Publishing Group; 1991:53–65.

110. Hirata GI, Masaki DI, O'Toole M, et al. Color flow mapping and Doppler velocimetry in the diagnosis and management of a placental chorioangioma associated with nonimmune fetal hydrops. *Obstet Gynecol.* 1993;81: 850–852.

111. Harding JA, Lewis DF, Major CA, et al. Color flow Doppler—

A useful instrument in the diagnosis of vasa previa. *Am J Obstet Gynecol*. 1990;163:1566–1568.

112. Nelson LH, Melone PJ, King M. Diagnosis of vasa previa with transvaginal and color flow Doppler ultrasound. *Obstet Gynecol*. 1990;76:506–509.

113. Hsieh FJ, Chen HF, Ko TM, et al. Antenatal diagnosis of vasa previa by color-flow mapping. *J Ultrasound Med*. 1991;10:397–399.

114. Arts H, van Eyck J. Antenatal diagnosis of vasa previa by transvaginal color Doppler sonography. *Ultrasound Obstet Gynecol*. 1993;3:276–278.

115. Guy G, Peisner D, Timor-Tritsch I. Ultrasonographic evaluation of uteroplacental blood flow patterns of abnormally lo-cated and adherent placentas. *Am J Obstet Gynecol*. 1990;163:723–727.

116. Hoffman-Tretin J, Koenigsberg M, Rabin A, et al. Placenta accreta: Additional sonographic observations. *J Ultrasound Med*. 1992;11:29–34.

117. Emerson D, Felker R. Ectopic pregnancy. In: Fleischer A, Emerson D, eds. *Color Doppler Sonography in Obstetrics and Gynecology*. New York: Churchill Livingstone; 1993:193–216.

118. Emerson D. Placenta and umbilical cord. In: Fleischer A, Emerson D, eds. *Color Doppler Sonography in Obstetrics and Gynecology*. New York: Churchill Livingstone; 1993:287–308.

15

Prenatal Detection of Anatomic Congenital Anomalies

Luís F. Gonçalves • Roberto Romero • Eli Maymon •
Percy Pacora • Katherine Bianco • Philippe Jeanty

The detection of anatomic congenital anomalies is one of the goals of prenatal care.[1] The information required for diagnosis and management of the obstetric patient with a fetal congenital anomaly demands knowledge in a variety of disciplines, including diagnostic imaging, obstetrics, genetics, pediatric surgery, anatomy, embryology, and teratology. Many health care professionals involved in diagnostic imaging have had limited exposure to the other fields. The purpose of this chapter is to introduce the reader to the section on congenital anomalies in this text. It provides an overview of the definition and magnitude of the problem and pathogenic mechanisms of gross congenital anomalies. The principles of prenatal diagnosis with ultrasound, the use of ultrasound as a screening tool for the detection of congenital anomalies, and the management options once a congenital anomaly has been detected are discussed.

DEFINITIONS

A congenital anomaly consists of a departure from the normal anatomic architecture of an organ or system. Anomalies may result from an intrinsically abnormal primordium or anlage of an organ or from a normal primordium that is affected during development by extrinsic forces.[2-4] Growing interest in prenatal development coupled with the need for a uniform nomenclature to refer to errors in morphogenesis led an international working group to propose a set of terms useful in the classification of anatomic congenital anomalies. Individual alterations of form or structure can be classified as malformations, deformations, and disruptions.

Malformation

A *malformation* is a morphologic defect of an organ, part of an organ, or a larger area of the body resulting from an intrinsically abnormal developmental process. The term *intrinsically abnormal developmental process* refers to an abnormality in the primordium (anlage) of the organ. This abnormality may not be identifiable in early stages of development. The typical example is a limb bud that appears normal in early embryonic life but later develops an extra digit. Malformations can be considered the result of a developmental arrest of the primordium (incomplete morphogenesis), redundant morphogenesis, or aberrant morphogenesis (Fig. 15–1). Examples of these types of malformations are listed in Table 15–1. Although malformations often occur during the embryonic period (until the ninth postmenstrual week),[5] some may also arise during later stages of development. A general

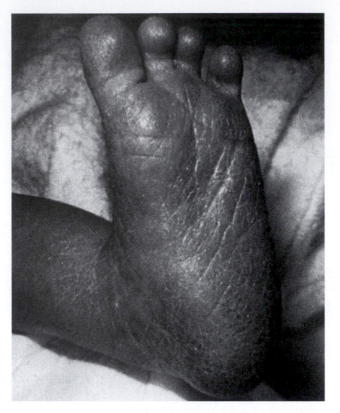

Figure 15–1. An example of malformation because of incomplete morphogenesis (four digits on this foot).

principle is that the earlier the malformation is initiated, the more complex the resulting anomaly (or anomalies).

Deformation

It should be stressed that it is not always possible to assign an anomaly to a specific class. In fact, malformations, de-

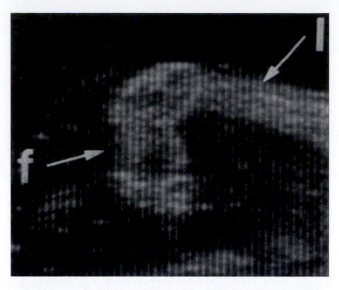

Figure 15–2. Clubfoot, an example of deformation. l, leg; f, foot. *(Reproduced with permission from Jeanty P, Romero R.* Obstetrical Ultrasound. *New York: McGraw-Hill; 1984.)*

formations, and disruptions may overlap (see definition of sequences later in this section).

Deformation refers to an abnormal form, shape, or position of part of the body caused by nondisruptive mechanical forces. The primordium of the organ is normal, but development is affected by mechanical forces that are extrinsic or intrinsic to the fetus. For example, a clubfoot deformity (Fig. 15–2) may be the result of intrauterine constraint due to oligohydramnios (extrinsic force) or lack of movement due to the neural defect associated with spina bifida (intrinsic force). Table 15–2 presents common forces leading to deformations. Four main factors influence the pathogenesis of deformations: pressure, fetal plasticity, fetal mobility, and the rate of fetal growth.[6–9] Deformations tend to occur late in gestation,

TABLE 15–1. ABNORMAL MORPHOGENESIS RESULTING IN MALFORMATIONS

Types of Abnormal Morphogenesis	Examples of Malformation	Relative Frequency as a Class
Incomplete morphogenesis		Common
Lack of development	Absent nostril, renal agenesis	
Hypoplasia	Microcephaly, micrognathia	
Incomplete closure	Cleft palate, iris coloboma	
Incomplete separation	Syndactyly	
Incomplete septation	Ventricular septal defect	
Incomplete migration	Exstrophy of the cloaca	
Incomplete rotation	Malrotated gut	
Incomplete resolution of early form	Choanal atresia, Meckel diverticulum	
Persistence of early location	Low-set ears, undescended testes	
Redundant morphogenesis	Supernumerary ear tag, polydactyly	Uncommon
Aberrant morphogenesis	Mediastinal thyroid gland, paratesticular spleen	Rare

Reproduced with permission from Cohen MM. The Child with Multiple Birth Defects. New York: Raven Press; 1982:2.

TABLE 15–2. CAUSES OF DEFORMATIONS

Extrinsic
   Maternal
      Small maternal size
      Small maternal pelvis
      Uterine malformation (e.g., bicornuate uterus)
      Uterine leiomyoma
   Fetal
      Early pelvic engagement of the fetal head
      Unusual fetal position
      Oligohydramnios
      Large fetus, rapid growth
      Multiple fetuses
Intrinsic
   Malformational
      Central nervous system malformations (e.g., spina bifida)
      Urinary tract malformations (e.g., bilateral renal agenesis
         or severe polycystic kidneys that may cause
         oligohydramnios and its sequence)
   Functional
      Congenital hypotonia secondary to neuromuscular disorders
      (e.g., arthrogryposis)

Derived from Cohen MM. The Child with Multiple Birth Defects. New York, Raven Press; 1982:10. Smith DW. In: Schaffer AJ, Markowitz M, eds. Major Problems in Clinical Pediatrics, vol 21. Philadelphia: WB Saunders, 1981:101.

because during this time, there is rapid fetal growth in a potentially constraining intrauterine environment.[6–11] Removal of the mechanical force responsible for the deformation results in normalization or improvement of the anomaly. Spontaneous resolution after birth occurs in approximately 90% of deformations.[12] Table 15–3 compares malformations and deformations. In general, the term *malformation* describes defects that are likely to have arisen during organogenesis, and the term *deformation* is reserved for defects arising after the embryonic period.

Disruption

A *disruption* is a morphologic defect of an organ, part of an organ, or a larger region of the body resulting from a breakdown or interference with an originally normal developmen-

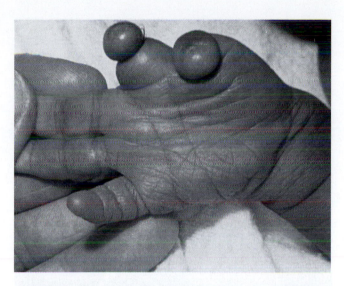

Figure 15–3. Amputation of fingers in an infant with amniotic band syndrome (disruption).

tal process. A typical example of this type of anomaly is digital amputation associated with amniotic band syndrome (Fig. 15–3).[13–15] Disruptions are sporadic events.

Dysplasia

Another concept frequently used by dysmorphologists is that of *dysplasia,* a term referring to abnormal organization of cells into tissue(s) and its morphologic result(s). The term *dysplasia* in pathology refers to a anaplastic process. Its use in dysmorphology is broader and refers to any type of tissue disorganization. Osteogenesis imperfecta is a dysplasia in which the primary disorder affects collagen; and thus, structures containing significant quantities of the particular type of defective collagen are affected.

The Fetus With Multiple Anomalies

A fetus may have multiple anomalies. This association may occur simply by chance or may be part of a pathogenetically related event. A set of terms has been coined to describe the relationship between coexistent anomalies: *polytopic field defect, sequence, syndrome,* and *association.*

Polytopic Field Defect. A *polytopic field defect* is a group of anomalies derived from the disturbance of a single developmental field. A developmental field is a region or part of an embryo that responds as a unit to embryonic interactions and results in complex or multiple anatomic structures. Opitz discussed in detail the meaning and implications of the concept of developmental field defects.[4,16–19] The embryo is omnipotent (the primary field) up to a certain time, during which further organization and differentiation occur in a number of different developmental autonomous areas (secondary fields). Disturbances in a developmental field may result in multiple, and usually contiguous, anomalies (monotopic field

TABLE 15–3. COMPARISON OF MALFORMATIONS AND DEFORMATIONS

	Malformation	Deformation
Time of occurrence	Embryonic period	Fetal period
Level of disturbance	Organ	Region
Incidence before 20th week	5% (estimated)	0.1%
Incidence after 28th week	3.7%	2.0%
Perinatal mortality	+ (41%)	– (6%)
Spontaneous correction	—	+
Correction	—	+

Derived from Cohen MM. The Child with Multiple Birth Defects. New York, Raven Press; 1982:10. Dunn PM. Proc R Soc Med. 1972;65:735.

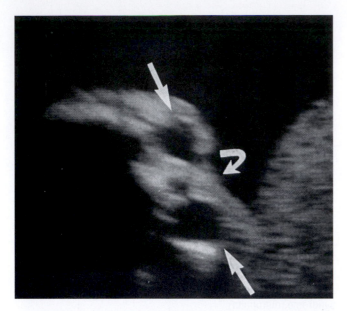

Figure 15–4. Axial scan at the level of the orbits in a holoprosencephalic fetus, showing hypotelorism (between *straight arrows*) and absence of the nasal bridge *(curved arrow)*. *(Reproduced with permission from Pilu G, et al.* Am J Perinatol. *1987;4:41.)*

defects) or multiple, distantly located anomalies (polytopic field defects). An example of a monotopic field defect is holoprosencephaly, where there are coexistent abnormalities of the face and central nervous system (Figs. 15–4 and 15–5). Abnormalities in the acrorenal field are frequently cited as illustrative examples of polytopic field defects. There are at least 24 different genetic conditions in which both kidneys

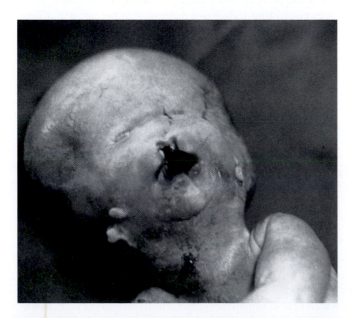

Figure 15–5. Postnatal appearance of the fetus shown in Figure 15–4, showing the classic stigmata of holoprosencephaly with medial cleft palate. *(Reproduced with permission from Pilu G, et al.* Am J Perinatol. *1987;4:41.)*

and limbs are involved, a fact that has been explained by invoking a relationship between the mesonephros and limb buds during embryogenesis. This concept is supported by the proximity between these two structures in early life and by experiments showing an inductive effect of mesonephros on proliferation and differentiation of limb bud cartilage. A complete map of the developmental fields of the human embryo is not available but could be constructed by classifying all human malformations and searching for causal heterogeneity among them. Opitz[17] proposed that, each time a certain malformation is seen in at least two causally different conditions, a developmental field has been identified, because identical structure means identical development, independent of differences in causal mechanisms. Mammalian primordia have only a limited number of responses to various dysmorphogenetic insults. The existence of developmental fields limits the possibility of independent responses from different structures of the organism.

Sequence. A *sequence* is a pattern of multiple anomalies derived from a single known or presumed prior anomaly or mechanical factor. Thus, there are malformations, deformations, and disruption sequences. The spectrum of anomalies of holoprosencephaly is an example of a *malformation sequence*. The precordal mesoderm is responsible for cleavage of the prosencephalon and normal development of the median facial structures. A primary defect of the precordal mesoderm leads to defects in both the brain and the face. In the brain, there is incomplete division of the cerebral hemispheres and underlying structures. Anomalies of the face include different degrees of hypoplasia of the median central structures (cyclopia, ethmocephaly, cebocephaly, and median cleft lip).

Severe oligohydramnios may lead to intrauterine constraint and a typical *deformation sequence* that includes abnormal positioning of limbs (club foot), breech presentation, Potter facies, growth deficiency, amnion nodosum, and pulmonary hypoplasia.[20–24]

Early amniotic rupture with the formation of amniotic bands may lead to a *disruption sequence* including amputations of fingers, bizarre facial clefts, and asymmetric encephaloceles (Fig. 15–6).[15,25–32]

Syndrome. A *syndrome* is a pattern of multiple anomalies thought to be pathogenetically related and not known to represent a single sequence or a polytopic field defect. The term *syndrome* is frequently employed to refer to a single cause such as Down's syndrome. The difference between a malformation sequence and a malformation syndrome is best understood with an example. Isolated holoprosencephaly is a malformation sequence. However, if holoprosencephaly occurs with other anomalies in an infant with trisomy 13 or Meckel syndrome, the condition is a malformation syndrome.

Association. An *association* refers to a nonrandom occurrence in two or more individuals of multiple anomalies not

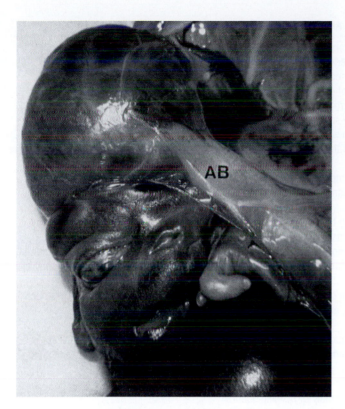

Figure 15–6. Amniotic band syndrome. An amniotic band is seen inserting on the fetal head. There is great division of the fetal face. The hand is forced against the fetal face and deformed. AB, amniotic band.

known to represent a polytopic field defect, a sequence, or a syndrome. The term *association* carries a purely statistical connotation and not a pathogenetic or causal implication. With increasing knowledge, associations may become syndromes or polytopic field defects.

Familiarity with these terms is important because correct classification of an anomaly has implications for clinical diagnosis, management, and genetic counseling.[2,10] Disruptions are sporadic events and, therefore, do not tend to recur in future pregnancies. The recurrence rate of deformations depends on the cause of the mechanical force leading to the anomaly. If the etiology of the abnormal mechanical force is a fetal malformation (e.g., spina bifida), the recurrence risk is different than if the abnormal force were related to a leiomyoma.[11] The diagnosis of a malformation suggests a chromosomal abnormality, a monogenic defect, or a multifactorial disorder.[4,10,33–35] Table 15–4[36] presents a brief glossary of terms used to describe congenital anomalies, including some of the terms discussed above.

CLASSIFICATION OF ANOMALIES

Although there are several systems to classify congenital anomalies, an easy and practical method is to divide them into major and minor. A *major anomaly* is one with a medical, surgical, or cosmetic importance and with impact on morbidity and mortality. A *minor anomaly* is one that does not have a serious surgical, medical, or cosmetic significance and does not affect normal life expectancy or lifestyle. Obviously, this classification is subjective and arbitrary. There is an overlap between minor anomalies and normal anatomic or phenotypic variants. A phenotypic variant occurs with a frequency of more than 4% in the general population, whereas minor anomalies occur at a rate of less than 4%. Clearly, this is also an arbitrary definition. Some ageneses are common enough to be considered "normal" anatomic variants (i.e., absence of the muscle palmaris longus or upper lateral incisor). The importance of minor anomalies is that they may serve as indicators of altered morphogenesis and more serious defects. Ninety percent of infants with three or more minor anomalies will have a major anomaly.[37] Thus, the identification of several minor anomalies requires a careful search for hidden anomalies, in particular cardiac, renal, and vertebral disorders. Tables 15–5 and 15–6 have been compiled from the pediatric and genetic literature and display the most common major and minor anomalies, respectively.[10,37–44]

A practical problem in clinical genetics is the classification of a "funny-looking kid" who has several dysmorphologic features that may correspond to multiple minor anomalies or multiple normal developmental variants. The two approaches that have been considered helpful are the analysis of family resemblance and analysis of associated anomalies. On close inspection, the child with multiple phenotypic variants will resemble some other family members. In contrast, the child with multiple minor anomalies due to aneuploidy should not look like other family members. The child with multiple phenotypic anomalies also should not have other major external or internal anomalies.

Ultrasonographic Markers

Anatomic defects observed by ultrasound may raise the suspicion of a more complex set of anomalies or chromosomal disorders. A lemon-shaped head, for example, is commonly associated with spina bifida, whereas an atrioventricular canal is a major cardiac defect associated with Down's syndrome.

Some minor anomalies may also carry a higher risk of chromosomal disorders. They are collectively called *markers*. A few have such a strong association with chromosomal anomalies that their identification per se is an indication for fetal karyotyping (e.g., increased nuchal translucency thickness).[45] Other markers are very common and usually not associated with any handicap. For example, mild hydronephrosis or choroid plexus cysts, when found in isolation, does not carry such a high risk for chromosomal anomalies to warrant the performance of invasive procedures. These markers, however, should prompt a thorough evaluation of the fetus for other anomalies before considering the need for fetal karyotyping. Table 15–7 presents a list of major anatomic defects and markers for chromosomal anomalies detectable by prenatal ultrasound.[46]

TABLE 15–4. GLOSSARY OF TERMS USED TO DESCRIBE CONGENITAL ANOMALIES

Anomaly	Deviation from the normal with regard to form, structure, or position
Aplasia	Complete absence of cellular proliferation
Hypoplasia	Results from insufficient or decreased cellular growth
Dysplasia	Abnormal growth or development of cells, causing disorganized cellular structure
Agenesis	Failure of a structure or organ to form
Dysgenesis	Defective development, resulting in some type of disorganization
Atrophy	Degeneration of cells that results in wasting or a decreased size
Hypotrophy	Undergrowth or the failure to reach the normal size
Hypertrophy	Overgrowth of a structure or organ
Genotype	Refers to an organism's genetic composition
Phenotype	Outward physical appearance or genetic makeup of an individual; the direct result of the genotype and, in some cases, the environment
Congenital	Refers to conditions present at birth that may or may not be genetic
Genetic	An inherited but not always congenital condition
Malformation	A birth defect due to an intrinsic abnormality or incomplete development; can be genetic, environmental, or multifactorial and typically occurs before 10 weeks of gestation; cleft lip and/or cleft palate may be classified as malformations
Disruption	An interference with formation of an otherwise normal structure and a result from external forces such as amniotic bands or teratogens; may be the result of environmental agents or mechanical concerns
Deformation	In contrast to a disruption, a deformation occurs after the normal formation of an organ or structure; it is the result of compression, constriction, or immobility, e.g., clubfeet due to oligohydramnios; in some cases, it may have a genetic cause
Etiology	Underlying cause of an anomaly
Pathogenesis	Specific mechanism by which an anomaly or disease occurs
Syndrome, genetic	A group of features seen together with common, specific etiology
Syndrome, complex	Composite of multiple features
Spectrum	Considered complex, with considerable variation
Association	Nonrandom occurrence of multiple features, with no known etiology, e.g., VACTERL and CHARGE
Sequence	Pattern of anomalies from a single anomaly or factor, e.g., Potter sequence versus syndrome
Teratogen	An environmental agent that causes a morphologic abnormality after fertilization but before delivery
Mendelian	Conditions, typically single gene, inherited in the manner conceived by Gregor Mendel
Multifactorial	Caused by both genetic and environmental factors
Sporadic	Occurring by chance, not hereditary

Adapted with permission from Evans M, Lampinen J. In: Levi S, Chervenak FA, eds. Ultrasound Screening for Fetal Anomalies: Is It Worth It? Volume 847. New York: Annals of the New York Academy of Science; 1998:1–2.

INCIDENCE OF CONGENITAL ANOMALIES

The precise incidence of congenital anomalies is difficult to determine. Accurate documentation depends on many factors including 1) age at examination (prenatal period, newborn period, infancy, or later in life),[38,39,43] 2) the experience of the observer (e.g., general pediatrician versus dysmorphologist),[17] 3) the definition of an anomaly (major, minor, normal phenotypic variation),[37,47,48] 4) the type of examination (body surface examination, extensive examination including evaluation of internal organs), and 5) ethnic, geographic, and social variations in the incidence of individual malformations.[46–51] Follow-up of infants is extremely important because only one-third of congenital anomalies are recognized in the newborn period.[48]

One of the first attempts to determine the incidence of congenital major and minor anomalies at birth was conducted by Marden et al.[37] These investigators, particularly interested in dysmorphology, examined 4412 newborns during the first 2 days of birth. A body surface examination that did not include auscultation of the heart and abdominal palpation as standard procedures was performed in all infants. A buccal smear for sex chromatin was also obtained. The incidence of major and minor anomalies was 2.04% and 14.7%, respectively. Among the 20 newborns having two or more minor defects, 90% had one or more major anomalies. Chromosomal aneuploidy was detected by buccal smear and phenotype examination in 4 of 1000 infants. Using data from the Collaborative Perinatal Project of the National Institute of Neurological and Communicative Disorders and Stroke, Chung and Myrianthopoulos reported the incidence of anomalies in a population of 52,332 liveborns.[52] Table 15–8 shows the incidence of major, minor, and multiple anomalies, sequences, and syndromes in their study. Table 15–9 presents the

TABLE 15–5. MAJOR ANOMALIES

Central nervous system
Hydrocephalus
Anencephaly
Microcephaly
Meningocele
Encephalocele
Macrocephaly
Cebocephaly

Craniofacial
Craniostenosis
Micrognathia
Choanal atresia
Hypertelorism, hypotelorism
Protruding forehead
Beaklike nose
Absent ramus of mandible
Cleft lip or cleft palate
Low nasal bridge
Broad nasal bridge
Prognathism
Macroglossia
Cranial asymmetry

Eye
Cataract or corneal opacity
Coloboma of iris
Microphthalmia
Myopia
Blue sclerae
Glaucoma
Microcornea
Retinal dysplasia
Anophthalmos
Cyclopia
Aniridia

Auricle (ear)
Low-set ear, severe
Low ear canal
Severely malformed

Skin
Webbed neck
Multiple hemangiomas

Kidney
Polycystic kidney
Hydronephrosis
Horseshoe kidney
Duplicated ureters
Bilateral renal agenesis
Multicystic kidney disease
Megaureter
Prune-belly syndrome
Ureteropelvic junction
  obstruction
Posterior urethral valves

Heart
Atrial septal defect
Ventricular septal defect
Tetralogy of Fallot
Atrioventricular defects
Univentricular heart
Hypoplastic left heart
  syndrome
Hypoplastic right ventricle
Complete transposition of
  the great vessels
Corrected transposition of
  the great vessels
Double outlet right
  ventricle
Pulmonic stenosis
Aortic stenosis
Cardiomyopathies
Total anomalous pulmonary
  venous return
Ectopia cordis
Tumors of the heart
Single ventricle
Supravalvular aortic
  stenosis
Asymmetrical septal
  hypertrophy
Endocardial fibroelastosis

(Heart continued)

Truncus arteriosus
Coarctation and tubular
  hypoplasia of the aortic
  arch
Ebstein's anomaly
Cardiosplenic syndromes

Gastrointestinal tract
Intestinal atresia
Imperforate anus
Omphalocele
Gastroschisis
Hepatomegaly
Splenomegaly
Pyloric stenosis
Malrotation of colon
Anal atresia with
  rectovestibular fistula
Biliary atresia
Megacystis–microcolon–
  intestinal–hypoperistalsis
  syndrome

Genital tract
Severe hypospadias
Common cloaca
Abdominal
  cryptorchidism
Inguinal cryptorchidism
Ambiguous genitalia
Bifid scrotum
Unicornuate uterus
Absence of uterus
Double vagina
Duplication or anomalous
  insertion of fallopian tubes
Hypoplastic ovaries
Uterine cysts
Vaginal atresia
Ovarian cysts

Skeleton
Absence of radius
Absence of fibula
Short femur
Malleable bones
Congenital dislocated
  hips
Sacral agenesis
Sirenomelia
Hypoplasia of clavicles
Small thoracic cage
Rib defects
Scoliosis, kyphosis
Short limbs
Elbow dysplasia
Narrow pelvis
Joint imitation and/or
  contractures
Absence of pubic rami
Vertebral malformation
Hemivertebrae
Phocomelia
Demineralization of bones

Hand
Polydactyly
Syndactyly
Clinodactyly
Complete cutaneous
  syndactyly
Absence of thumbs
Short hands
Absence of all metacarpals
Absence of distal phalanx
Broad fingers
Steeter's bands and deformity
Ectrodactyly
Oligodactyly

Foot
Polydactyly
Syndactyly
Equinovarus/clubfoot
Severe calcaneovalgus
Absence of nails

Other
Sacral teratoma
Absence of sternocleidomastoid
  muscle

TABLE 15–6. MINOR ANOMALIES

Craniofacial		Abdominal	
Borderline small mandible	Lower lip pits	Unusual diastasis recti	Meckel's diverticulum
Flat occiput, bony occipital spur	Microstomia	Umbilical hernia	Heterotopic pancreatic or splenic tissue
Prominent occiput	Macrostomia	**Genital**	
Small or short nose	Cleft or irregular tongue	Ectopic testicles in femoral locale	Hypogenitalism
Prominent nose	Anodontia, hypodentia	Micropenis	Hypoplasia of labia majora
Hypoplasia of nares	Irregular placement of teeth	**Skin**	
Abnormal filtrum	Neonatal teeth	Hemangioma	Lasse, redundant skin
Prominent full lips	Dental cysts	Pigmented nevi	Cutis marmorate
Eye		Mongoloid spots	Telangiectasis
Inner epicanthal folds	Prominent eyes	"Café au lait"	Hirsutism
Upward lateral slant of palpebral fissures	Ptosis of eyelid	High placed nipples	Deep sacral dimple, pilonidal cyst
Short palpebral fissures	Strabismus	Alopecia of scalp	Eczemalike skin disorder
Small inner canthal distance	Nystagmus		
Sparse eyebrows	Lens dislocation	**Hand**	
Shallow orbital ridges	Retinal pigmentation	Simian creases	Rudimentary polydactyly
Prominent supraorbital ridges	Iris: unusual patterning or coloration	Other crease patterns	Duplication of the thumb nail
Ear		Clinodactyly fifth finger	Clenched hand
Lack of usual fold or helix	Double lobules	**Foot**	
Severe slant away from eye	Incomplete helix	Partial syndactyly	Posterior prominence of heel
Preauricular or auricular skin tags	Absent tragus	Recessed fifth toes	Prominent calcaneous
Small ears, large ears, asymmetrical size	Separate lobule	**Other skeletal**	
Auricular sinus		Prominent sternum	Genu recurvatum
Heart		Depressed sternum	Cubitus valgus
Premature atrial and ventricular contractions	Atrioventricular block	Shieldlike chest	Joint hypermobility or lax ligaments
Supraventricular tachyarrythmias			

incidence of congenital anomalies in livebirths, fetal deaths, and neonatal deaths.[48] When all types of morphologic anomalies were considered, the incidence was 15% among live-born infants. Males were affected more frequently than females. The excess was attributed to a differential incidence of major anomalies because the prevalence of minor anomalies was not different between the genders.

MORBIDITY, MORTALITY, AND BURDEN OF CONGENITAL ANOMALIES TO SOCIETY

A substantial fall in maternal and infant mortality rates was achieved during the 20th century. Environmental interventions, improvements in nutrition, advances in clinical medicine, wider access to health care, increased surveillance and monitoring of disease, better education, and higher living standards contributed to this accomplishment. From 1915 through 1997, while the United States experienced a

93% drop in infant mortality (from approximately 100 per 1000 to 7.2 per 1000 live births),[53] the relative contribution of congenital anomalies to the perinatal death rate increased. In 1995, according to the Centers for Disease Control and Prevention, birth defects were the leading cause of infant mortality in the United States.[54,55] From 1968 to 1995, the proportion of infant deaths attributable to birth defects increased from 15 to 22%.[56,57] Similarly, in Scotland, the overall perinatal mortality declined by 75% between 1939 and 1941 and between 1974 and 1976, but over the same 37-year time span, the contribution of congenital anomalies to perinatal mortality increased from 10 to 25%.[58]

There is also an increased awareness about the role of congenital disease in determining morbidity. It has been estimated that at least 1% of all diseases requiring hospital admissions have a genetic basis or genetic contribution; as many as one of every four hospitalized children has a disease that is at least partly genetically determined, and approximately 1 of every 20 children is affected by a disorder that is completely genetic in origin.[59] The burden to the individual and

TABLE 15–7. ULTRASONOGRAPHIC MARKERS FOR CHROMOSOMAL DISORDERS

Ultrasonographic Marker	Chromosomal Anomaly
Skull/brain	
Absent corpus callosum	Trisomy 18
Brachycephaly	Trisomies 21, 18, 13 and monosomy 45,X0
Choroid plexus cysts	Trisomies 18 and 21
Enlarged cisterna magna	Trisomies 21, 18, and 13
Holoprosencephaly	Trisomy 13
Microcephaly	Trisomy 13, monosomy 45,X0
Posterior fossa cyst	Trisomies 21, 18, and 13
Strawberry-shaped head	Trisomy 18
Ventriculomegaly	Trisomies 21 and 18 and triploidy
Face/neck	
Cystic hygroma	Monosomy 45,X0
Facial cleft	Trisomies 18 and 13
Increased nuchal translucency	Trisomies 21, 18, 13 and monosomy 45,X0
Micrognathia	Trisomy 18 and triploidy
Nuchal edema	Trisomies 21, 18, and 13
Chest	
Cardiac abnormality	Trisomies 21, 18, 13, triploidy and monosomy 45,X0
Diaphragmatic hernia	Trisomies 18 and 13
Echogenic foci in the heart	Trisomy 21
Abdomen	
Collapsed stomach	Trisomies 21 and 18
Duodenal atresia	Trisomy 21
Hyperechogenic fetal bowel	Trisomy 21
Omphalocele	Trisomies 18 and 13
Urinary tract	
Mild hydronephrosis	Trisomies 21, 18, 13 and monosomy 45,X0
Other renal anomalies	Trisomies 21, 18, 13 and triploidy
Other	
Hydrops	Trisomy 21 and monosomy 45,X0
Small for gestational age	Trisomy 18, triploidy, and monosomy 45,X0
Relatively short femur	Trisomies 21, 18, triploidy, and monosomy 45,X0
Clinodactyly	Trisomy 21
Overlapping fingers	Trisomy 18
Polydactyly	Trisomy 13
Syndactyly	Triploidy
Talipes	Trisomies 18 and 13 and triploidy

TABLE 15–8. TYPES OF ANOMALIES IN LIVEBORN SINGLETONS

	n	%
No anomalies	44,214	84.49
Single major	3446	6.58
Single minor	3801	7.26
Multiple major	450	0.86
Multiple minor	119	0.23
Sequences	156	0.30
Syndromes	146	0.28
Total	52,332	100.00

Reproduced with permission from Chung CS, Myrianthopoulos NC. Am J Med Genet. *1987;27:508.*

the risk of death and in all parameters of evaluated postnatal morbidity. The authors estimated that if major congenital anomalies did not occur, a reduction of 16% in postnatal mortality to age 7 years could be achieved. Infants with congenital anomalies also impose an economic burden to society and contribute stress to the family nucleus. For example, the incidence of divorce and sibling social maladjustment is greater in families of children with spina bifida than in families of infants without congenital anomalies.[60,61]

CAUSES AND RECURRENCE RISK OF CONGENITAL ANOMALIES

Causative factors for congenital malformations may be identified in approximately 40% of the cases and are usually divided into four major groups: single gene disorders, chromosome abnormalities, multifactorial conditions (involving both environmental and genetic components), and environmental factors.[62]

Approximately 7.5% of all congenital malformations are caused by a single gene mutation.[63] Autosomal mutations occur when the gene is located in a non–sex chromosome and may be either dominant (e.g., adult polycystic kidney disease, achondroplasia, hypochondroplasia, Treacher–Collins syndrome, Holt–Oram syndrome) or recessive (e.g., Meckel–Gruber syndrome, achondrogenesis, short-rib polydactyly syndrome, camptomelic dysplasia). Autosomal dominant conditions have a recurrence risk of 50% for the subsequent offspring, whereas autosomal recessive conditions have a recurrence risk of 25%. The term *X-linked disorder* is reserved for single gene mutations in the X chromosome (e.g., fragile X syndrome, Pena–Shokeir syndrome, otopalatodigital syndrome). In this case, women are symptomless carriers, and the disease is usually manifested only in males.

Chromosomal anomalies are responsible for about 6% of all serious congenital malformations among liveborn infants. They may be numerical or structural in nature. Polyploidy is an example of a numerical chromosomal anomaly, with one or more extra sets of 23 chromosomes added to the

society imposed by congenital anomalies has been examined by Chung and Myrianthopoulos.[52] Table 15–10 illustrates the rates for postnatal mortality, neurologic abnormality at 7 years of follow-up, psychological deficit at age 7 years, and the requirement for major surgery for infants with different types of congenital anomalies. Infants with anomalies detected within the first year have a significant increase in

TABLE 15–9. INCIDENCE OF MALFORMATIONS IN LIVEBIRTHS, FETAL AND NEONATAL DEATHS, AND DEATHS UP TO 1 YEAR

	n Individuals	n Malformations	% Malformations
Live births	51,096	7856	15.27
Fetal deaths	1004	82	8.17
Neonatal deaths	877	255	29.08
Deaths from 28 days to 1 year	417	98	23.50
Total deaths	2298	435	18.93

Modified from Myrianthopoulos NC, Chung CS. Birth Defects: Original Article Series 1980;11:11.

normal diploid karyotype (e.g., triploidy: 69,XXX, 69,XXY, or 69,XYY). Approximately 20% of all abortuses have a polyploid karyotype.[64] Trisomies occur in approximately 55% of abortuses and 98% of newborns with chromosomal abnormalities and are characterized by the presence of an extra chromosome (e.g., trisomy 21, trisomy 18, and trisomy 13).[64] When one whole chromosome is missing, the abnormality is known as monosomy (e.g., Turner's syndrome: 45,X0). Deletions are examples of structural chromosomal derangements in which part of a chromosome arm is lost (e.g., 5p–, or cri-du-chat, syndrome). Exchange of chromosome segments may occur in the absence of gene loss and may be either translocations or inversions. Although carriers of balanced translocations are phenotypically normal, they are at increased risk of producing genetically unbalanced gametes and abnormal offspring.[65]

Multifactorial conditions are responsible for 20% of malformations in liveborn fetuses. Examples of malformations with a multifactorial inheritance include spina bifida and congenital dislocation of the hip. These anomalies are the result of interactions between a relatively large number of genes with similar effects and nongenetic, usually undefined, factors.[63,65,69]

A study conducted in Norway attempted to sort out environmental and genetic factors as causes of congenital anomalies.[66] A total of 371,933 mothers whose first and second births were recorded in a population-based registry were studied. The investigators attempted to estimate the recurrence risk of congenital anomalies in the second pregnancy of women whose first baby was affected by a congenital anomaly in order to dissect the contribution of environmental factors. They also examined the effects of changing partner or city of residence between the first and second completed pregnancies in the recurrence risk of congenital anomalies. The results of this study showed that the recurrence risk of any congenital anomaly in the second pregnancy was at least 2.4 times higher for those who had a previous anomalous baby. Six different defect categories accounted for more than two-thirds of all the defects (Table 15–11). Mothers of babies affected by cleft lip, cardiac defects, limb defects, clubfoot, and genital defects had a significantly higher risk having a second child with a similar defect. Changing partner between

TABLE 15–10. MORTALITY AND MORBIDITY RATES IN INFANTS WITH CONGENITAL ANOMALIES AGAINST NO-ANOMALIES GROUPS

	Postnatal Mortality to 7 Years	Neurologic Abnormality, 1–7 Years	Psychiatric Deficits at Age 7 Years	Major Surgery to 7 Years
Total population	0.030	0.054	0.183	—
No anomaly	0.026	0.035	0.049	0.162
Minor only	0.015*	0.046†	0.059‡	0.196*
Multiple major	0.058*	0.064*	0.069*	0.367*
Single major	0.116*	0.109*	0.152*	0.492*
Sequences	0.442*	0.211*	0.159*	0.583*
Syndromes	0.288*	0.733*	0.720*	0.378*
All anomalies	0.052*	0.069*	0.078*	0.292*
Major anomalies, sequences, syndromes	0.087*	0.092*	0.097*	0.386*

*$p \leq 0.001$.
†$p \leq 0.01$.
‡$p \leq 0.05$.
Reproduced with permission from Chung CS, Myrianthopoulos NC. Am J Med Genet. 1987;27:510.

TABLE 15–11. RISK OF SIMILAR AND DISSIMILAR BIRTH DEFECTS IN SECOND INFANTS OF MOTHERS WITH AN AFFECTED FIRST INFANT

| Defect in First Infant | *n* at Risk | Second Infant | | | | | |
| | | Similar Defects | | | Dissimilar Defects | | |
		Observed	Expected	Relative Risk*	Observed	Expected	Relative Risk*
Clubfoot	2784	100	14.7	7.3 (5.9–9.1)	59	42.0	1.4 (1.0–1.7)
Genital defect	1447	25	5.1	4.9 (3.2–7.3)	35	24.2	1.5 (1.0–2.0)
Limb defect	957	25	2.2	11.3 (7.2–17)	41	17.1	2.4 (1.7–3.3)
Cardiac defect	567	6	1.0	6.0 (2.2–13)	11	10.5	1.1 (0.5–1.9)
Total cleft lip	436	18	0.6	31.4 (19–52)	10	8.2	1.2 (0.6–2.2)
Isolated cleft lip	144	3	0.1	44.5 (9.0–134)	2	2.9	0.7 (0.1–2.5)
All combined†	9192	201	26.4	7.6 (6.5–8.0)	249	164.6	1.5 (1.3–1.7)

*95% confidence intervals are given in parentheses.
†Includes 23 categories of isolated and multiple birth defects. In addition to those listed in the table, the categories were anencephaly; spina bifida; hydrocephalus; other central nervous system defects; eye defects; ear, face, or neck defects; circulatory system defects; respiratory system defects; esophageal defects; abdominal wall defects; anal defects; renal defects; axial defects; skin, hair, and nail defects; other birth defects; Down's syndrome; and other chromosomal syndromes.
Reproduced with permission from Lie RT, et al. N Engl J Med. 1994;331:1–4.

the first and second pregnancies did not affect the recurrence risk. However, those who remained in the same municipality during the second pregnancy had an 11.6 times higher risk of having a baby with the same birth defect as the previous malformed one [27.3 per 1000 (115 of 4200) versus 2.3 per 1000 (454 of 192,999); relative risk = 11.6, 95% confidence interval = 9.3 to 14.0]. These observations indicate that currently unidentified environmental factors may be responsible for birth defects and that identification of potential teratogens may lead to the development of preventive measures. It is estimated that, on average, 60 to 70% of pregnant women use from 3 to 10 medications during pregnancy and that 20 to 30% of pregnant women abuse some chemical substance during pregnancy.[67] Currently, 2 to 3% of the spectrum of congenital malformations is attributed to teratogens,[68] with most malformations resulting from exposures during days 18 to 40 postconception, except for the palate, central nervous system, and genital structures, that can be affected at later stages of development.[69] Table 15–12 lists known human teratogens and the respective anomalies associated with prenatal exposure to them. The Food and Drug Administration lists five categories of labeling for drug use in pregnancy.

Category A. Controlled studies in women have failed to demonstrate a risk to the fetus in the first trimester, and the possibility of fetal harm appears remote.

Category B. Animal studies have not indicated a risk to the fetus, and there are no controlled human studies or animal studies to show an adverse effect on the fetus, but well-controlled studies in pregnant women have failed to demonstrate a risk to the fetus.

Category C. Studies have shown the drug to have animal teratogenic or embryocidal effects, but there are no controlled

studies in women or no studies are available in animals or women.

Category D. Positive evidence of human fetal risk exists, but benefits in certain situations (e.g., life-threatening situations or serious diseases for which safer drugs cannot be used or are ineffective) may make use of the drug acceptable despite its risks.

Category X. Studies in animals or humans have demonstrated fetal abnormalities, or there is evidence of fetal risk based on human experience, or both, and the risk clearly outweighs any possible benefit.

ULTRASOUND DIAGNOSIS OF CONGENITAL ANOMALIES

The first reports of prenatal recognition of congenital anomalies with ultrasound were published in 1961 by Donald and Brown[70] and in 1964 by Sunden.[71] Sunden documented identification of three cases of "acrania." Subsequently, the first prenatal diagnosis of a congenital anomaly with ultrasound that altered obstetric management was reported by Campbell et al. in 1972.[72]

The cardinal principle behind the diagnosis of congenital anomalies with ultrasound is recognition of a departure from normal fetal anatomy. Congenital anomalies are generally recognized with ultrasound by one of the following means: 1) absence of a normal anatomic structure; 2) a disruption of the contour, shape, location, sonographic texture, or size of a normal anatomic structure; 3) presence of an abnormal structure; 4) abnormal fetal biometry; or 5) abnormal fetal motion.

TABLE 15–12. KNOWN AND POTENTIAL HUMAN TERATOGENS*

Teratogen Category	Specific Agent	Reported Effects or Associations	Risk
Alcohol		Fetal alcohol syndrome: IUGR, maxillary hypoplasia, reduction in width of palpebral fissure, microcephaly, mental retardation	High for alcohol consumption of 6 oz or more per day; lower exposures also can induce detrimental effects
Amphetamines		Congenital heart disease, IUGR	
Analgesics and antypyretic drugs	Aspirin	Prolonged gestation; increased risk of maternal and fetal hemorrhage	
	Acetaminophen	Maternal and fetal renal toxicity with chronic ingestion of high doses	
	Nonsteroid antiinflammatory drugs	Constriction of the ductus arteriosus	
Analgesics (narcotics)	Codeine	Respiratory system malformations	Risk not clearly defined because of confounders such as lifestyle and use of multiple drugs; risk of medical use appears to carry little, if any, fetal risk
Androgens		Masculinization of the female embryo, clitoromegaly with or without fusion of labia minora	Effects are dose and stage dependent; stimulates growth and differentiation of sex steroid receptor–containing tissue
Angiotensin-converting enzyme inhibitors		IUGR, oligohydramnios, pulmonary hypoplasia, skull hypoplasia, neonatal anuria, and neonatal death	Risk when used during the second or third trimester over prolonged periods; no teratogenic effect or abortigenic effect when used in the first trimester
Antibiotics	Cloramphenicol	Neonatal cardiovascular collapse in women treated near term	
	Nitrofurantoin	Hemolysis, anemia, hyperbilirubinemia, especially in glucose-6-phosphate-dehydrogenase-deficient infants	
	Streptomycin; gentamicin, tobramycin, amikacin	Interference with hearing by affecting the eighth nerve	Relatively low-risk phenomenon, mainly associated with long-term maternal exposure
	Sulfonamides	Increased bilirubin levels in the newborn and increased risk for kernicterus in exposures near term	
	Tetracycline	Bone and tooth staining	Effects seen only if exposure is late in the first or during second or third trimester because tetracyclines have to interact with calcified tissue
Anticonvulsants	Carbamazepine	Upslanting palpebral fissures, epicanthal folds, short nose with long philtrum, fingernail hypoplasia, developmental delay	
	Diphenylhydantoin	Microcephaly, mental retardation, cleft lip/palate, hypoplastic nails, and distal phalanges	Associations documented only with chronic exposure; risk of malformation appears no greater than 10%; short-term therapy (i.e., prophylaxis of a head injury) is not associated with a substantially increased risk

(Continued)

TABLE 15–12. *(continued)*

Teratogen Category	Specific Agent	Reported Effects or Associations	Risk
	Oxazolidine-2,4-diones: trimethadione, methadione	V-shaped eyebrows, low-set ears with anteriorly folded helix, high-arched palate, irregular teeth, CNS anomalies, severe developmental delay	Characteristic facial features documented only with chronic exposure
	Valproic acid	Neural tube defects and facial dysmorphology	Small head size and developmental delay have been reported with high doses. Risk of spina bifida is approximately 1%. Risk of facial dysmorphology may be greater
Antihistamines	Diphenhydramine	Genitourinary malformation	Not a lot of data on these compounds
Azathioprine		Abortion	
Busulfan		Slunted growth, corneal opacities, cleft palate, hypoplasia of ovaries, thyroid and parathyroids	Dependability of evidence is doubtful
Caffeine		Excessive consumption (>300 mg/day) is associated with IUGR and embryonic loss in some studies	
Chorionic villus sampling		Limb reduction defects of the congenital amputation type; orofacial malformations	For chorionic villus sampling performed <9 weeks
Cocaine		Microcephaly, vascular disruptive phenomena (limb amputations and cerebral infarction), IUGR, neurobehavioral abnormalities, preterm delivery, fetal loss	Low for disruptive phenomena and high for deleterious effects on fetal outcome
Ciclophosphamide		Ectrodactyly, syndactyly, cardiovascular anomalies, other minor anomalies, IUGR	Dose related; at the lowest therapetic dose the risk is small
Chloroquine		Deafness	Dependability of evidence: suggestive
Diethylstilbestrol		Clear cell adenocarcinoma of the vagina	1:1000 to 1:10,000 of female fetuses exposed *in utero*
		Vaginal adenosis	75% of female fetuses exposed before 9 weeks
		Increased incidence of genitourinary lesions and infertility in males	
		Increased risk of prematurity	
Electromagnetic fields	Video display terminals		No increased risk of abortion or malformations
	Power lines		Small or nonexistent
	Appliances		Small or nonexistent
Folic acid antagonists	Aminopterin, Methotrexate	Microcephaly, hydrocephaly, cleft palate, meningomyelocele, IUGR, abnormal cranial ossification, reduction in derivatives of first branchial arch, mental retardation, postnatal growth retardation	
Infectious agents	Cytomegalovirus	IUGR, brain damage with mental retardation, characteristic parenchymal calcification	Fetal infection in approximately 20% of maternal infections; risk of brain damage is moderate after fetal infection in early pregnancy
	Herpes simplex	Generalized organ infections, microcephaly, hepatitis, eye defects, vesicular rash	Risk of abortion agreed to be increased after herpes simplex 2 infection

(Continued)

TABLE 15–12. *(continued)*

Teratogen Category	Specific Agent	Reported Effects or Associations	Risk
	HIV	Symptomatic maternal HIV infection, other sexually transmitted diseases and opportunistic infections may increase the risk of low birth weight, postnatal CNS deterioration, and perinatal morbidity	Overall risk of vertical transmission is 25–40%
	Parvovirus B19	Hydrops fetalis and fetal death	
	Rubella virus	Mental retardation, deafness, cardiovascular malformations, cataracts, glaucoma, microphthalmia	>80% for infection <12 weeks; 54% for infection at 13–14 weeks; 25% at the end of the second trimester; 100% at term
		Diabetes mellitus or rubella panencephalitis may develop later in life	
	Syphilis	Maculopapular rash, hepatosplenomegaly, deformed nails, osteochondritis at joints of extremities, congenital neurosyphilis, abnormal epiphyses, chorioretinitis	
	Toxoplasmosis	Hydrocephaly, microphthalmia, chorioretinitis	
	Varicella zoster	Skin and muscle defects, IUGR, limb-reduction defects	No measurable increase risk of early teratogenic effects Risk of severe neonatal infection is high if maternal infection occurs in last week of pregnancy
	Venezuelan equine encephalitis	Hydranencephaly, microphthalmia, CNS destructive lesions, luxation of hip	
Lead		Levels < 50 μg%: developing CNS in the fetus and child maybe susceptible to lead toxicity resulting in decreased IQ and behavioral effects Levels > 50 μg%: in children, result in anemia and encephalopathy; may have serious effects on CNS development	
Lithium carbonate		Increased incidence of Ebstein's anomaly and other heart and great vessel defects on	Clear teratogenic effect in animals; effects in humans still unclear Increased risk on early reports The strength of the association has diminished with publication of more studies
Mepivacaine		Bradycardia, death	Dependability of evidence: conclusive
Methyl mercury		Minamata disease: cerebral palsy, microcephaly, mental retardation, blindness, cerebellar hypoplasia	At low exposure, the teratogenic effect predominates
Methylene blue		Intestinal atresia Hemolytic anemia and jaundice in neonatal period	Risk still not clear for intestinal atresia after intraamniotic injection
Misoprostol		Limb reduction defects and Möbius syndrome	

(Continued)

TABLE 15–12. *(continued)*

Teratogen Category	Specific Agent	Reported Effects or Associations	Risk
D-penicillamine		Custis laxa, hyperflexibility of joints	Low risk; condition appears to be reversible
Polychlorinated biphenyls		Cola-colored babies: pigmentation of gums, nails and groin, hypoplastic deformed nails; IUGR, abnormal skull calcification	Body residues in exposed women can affect pigmentation in offspring for up to 4 years after exposure
Progestins		Masculinization of female embryo exposed to high doses of some testosterone-derived progestins	Dose of progestins present in modern oral contraceptives presents no masculinization or feminization risks; no risks for nongenital malformations
Radiation (external irradiation)		Microcephaly, mental retardation, eye anomalies, IUGR, visceral malformations	Risk is dependent on dose and time of exposure; exposures from diagnostic procedures present no increased risk of abortion, IUGR or malformations; no measurable risk from exposures $\leq$ 5 rad (50 mGy) of x-rays at any stage of pregnancy; exposure of the pregnant uterus to therapeutic doses of ionizing radiation used in radiation therapy significantly increases the risk of aborting the embryo; the fetus is more resistant after the 8th week of development
Radioactive isotopes		Fetal thyroid hypoplasia	I^{131} Radioisotopes used for diagnosis present no risk for inducing abortion
Retinoids, systemic	Isotretinoin, etretinate	CNS, cardioaortic, ear and clefting defects; microtia, anotia, thymic aplasia, other branchial and aortic arch abnormalities and certain congenital heart malformations	
Retinoids, topical	Tretinoin	Epidemiologic studies, animal studies and absorption studies in humans do not suggest a teratogenic risk	
Smoking and nicotine		Placental lesions, IUGR, increased postnatal morbidity and mortality	
Thalidomide		Limb-reduction defects (preaxial preferential effects, phocomelia); facial hemangioma; esophageal, duodenal or anal atresia; anomalies of the external ears, eyes, kidneys and heart; increased incidence of neonatal and infant mortalitiy	
Thyroid	Iodides, radioiodine, antithyroid drugs (propylthiouracil), iodine deficiency	Fetal hypothyroidism or goiter with variable neurologic and aural damage	
Toluene abuse		IUGR, craniofacial anomalies, microcephaly	Occupational exposures should present an increase in the teratogenic or abortigenic risk
Vitamin A		CNS, cardioaortic, ear and clefting defects; microtia, anotia, thymic aplasia, other branchial and aortic arch abnormalities and certain congenital heart malformations	Exposures < 10,000 IU present no risk to the fetus

(Continued)

TABLE 15–12. *(continued)*

Teratogen Category	Specific Agent	Reported Effects or Associations	Risk
Vitamin D		Supravalvular aortic stenosis, elfin facies and mental retardation	The quality of information upon which the association is suspected is poor; risk may be increased
Warfarin derivatives		Nasal hypoplasia, stippling of secondary epiphysis, IUGR, anomalies of eyes, hands and neck, variable CNS anatomic defects (absence of corpus callosum, hydrocephalus, asymmetric brain hypoplasia)	10–25% risk from exposure during 8–14 weeks' gestation

*Compiled from studies by Mattison and Macina,[67] Brent and Beckman,[69] and Kliegman.[222]
CNS, central nervous system; IUGR, intrauterine growth retardation.

Inability to identify a normal structure such as the fetal stomach or calvarium suggests esophageal atresia and ancencephaly or acrania, respectively. A localized defect in the calvarium indicates the presence of a cephalocele. A displaced stomach into the chest is diagnostic of a diaphragmatic hernia. This condition is suspected because of a displacement of the heart within the chest even before visualization of the stomach or intestine in an abnormal location. Duodenal atresia is diagnosed by identifying a "double-bubble" sign (abnormal morphology of the stomach). Fetal tumors are typically identified when an additional structure is visualized that alters fetal anatomy. Abnormal biometry is used for the recognition of disorders characterized by fetal disproportion such as skeletal dysplasias and microcephaly. Absence of motion also identifies infants at risk for arthrogryposis multiplex congenita or other neuromuscular congenital disorders.

The sonographic recognition of congenital anomalies depends on knowledge of embryology, fetal anatomy, ultrasound resolution, and natural history of the disorder (Figs. 15–7 and 15–8). Improvements in ultrasonographic resolution, transvaginal probes, color Doppler technology, and three-dimensional imaging have led to an ever-increasing recognition of congenital anomalies. Although differences in maternal body habitus, fetal position, and ultrasonographic expertise among centers performing obstetric ultrasound may preclude visualization of minor abnormalities in every case, prenatal diagnosis of small defects such as simian crease, skin tags, and epicanthal folds[73] have been reported. Prenatal detection of minor anomalies, usually recognized only by a body surface examination of the newborn, is expected to improve with technologic advancements such as three-dimensional ultrasound.[74–80] Further, prenatal diagnosis of congenital malformations during the first trimester should improve as a result of implementation of nuchal translucency screening programs for the detection of chromosomal anomalies.[45,81–87] The reader should bear in mind the potential limitations of prenatal diagnosis at this stage. Because

of the embryologic timetable, some defects may not be diagnosed during the first trimester. For example, physiologic midgut herniation might hamper prenatal diagnosis of small omphaloceles before 12 weeks (Figs. 15–9 and 15–10).[88–90] Another example of limitation for early prenatal diagnosis is the case of infantile polycystic kidney disease (IPKD). This defect is recognized by signs of *in utero* renal failure, such as oligohydramnios and a nonvisualized bladder, coupled with enlarged hyperechogenic kidneys. However, sonographic observations have demonstrated that kidney measurements and function may be normal in early fetal life when IPKD is present. Therefore, the diagnosis of IPKD is not always possible before the 24th week of gestation.[91,92]

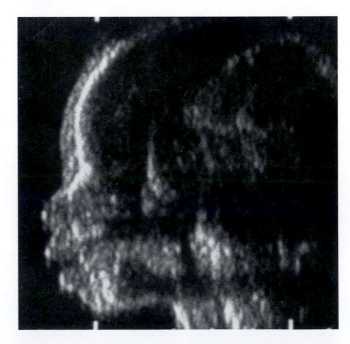

Figure 15–7. Normal fetal profile at 25 weeks. *(Reproduced with permission from Pilu G, et al. Am J Obstet Gynecol. 1986;155:45.)*

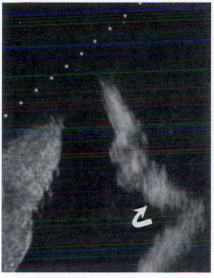

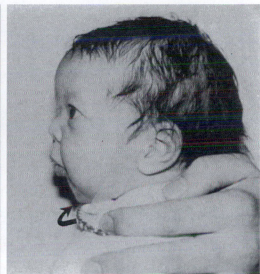

Figure 15–8. (A) Midsagittal scan of the face of a 34- to 33-week fetus with Robin's anomalad. Micrognathia is evident. **(B)** A side view of the infant is provided for comparison. *(Reproduced with permission from Pilu G, et al. Am J Obstet Gynecol. 1986;154:630.)*

A   B

ACCURACY OF PRENATAL ULTRASOUND IN THE DETECTION OF CONGENITAL ANOMALIES

Second-Trimester Ultrasound

The accuracy of ultrasound to detect congenital anomalies has been the subject of considerable debate in the literature. Although inaccuracy is intrinsic to the diagnostic process in medicine and cannot be completely eliminated, it is imperative to inform patients of what to expect from the avail-

able diagnostic tools. Because the ability to detect congenital anomalies is directly dependent on operator skills, patients who desire prenatal diagnosis of congenital anomalies should be referred to centers capable of performing to their expectations.

Table 15–13 shows detection rates for congenital anomalies from routine ultrasound screening programs.[93–106] Detection rates for populations at high risk are shown in Table 15–14.[107–114] Sensitivity (i.e., the ability to detect an anomaly when it is actually present at autopsy or at birth) ranged from 16 to 92% for pregnancies undergoing routine ultrasound screening. Lower detection rates (16% and 21%) have been reported from earlier multicenter trials including laboratories with different levels of ultrasonographic

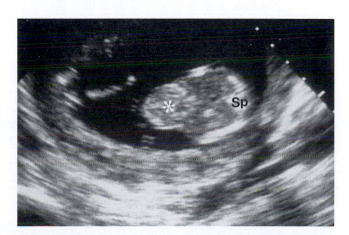

Figure 15–10. Prenatal diagnosis of an omphalocele at 15 weeks of gestation. Transverse scan of the abdomen at the level of the umbilicus demonstrates the lesion (∗). Sp, spine.

Figure 15–9. Longitudinal scan showing the insertion of the umbilical cord in the abdomen of a first trimester fetus.

TABLE 15–13. COMPARISON OF STUDIES EVALUATING THE ACCURACY IN DETECTING CONGENITAL ANOMALIES BY ROUTINE ULTRASOUND SCREENING BEFORE 24 WEEKS

Study	Subjects (Period)	Age in Weeks	Prevalence of Anomalies	Sensitivity*	Specificity*	PPV*	NPV*
Saari-Kemmppainen et al.[93]	4073 (1986–1987)	16–20	0.99%	40% (18/45)	99.8% (4636/4646)	64.3% (18/28)	99% (4636/4663)
Levi et al.[94]	16,072 (1984–1989)	12–20	1.61%	20.8% (54/259)	100% (15,972/15,972)	100% (54/54)	98.7% (15,972/16,177)
Rosendahl and Kivenen[95]	9012 (1980–1988)	<24	1.03%	39.8% (37/93)	†	†	†
Chitty et al.[98]	8432 (1988–1989)	<24	1.36%	74.4% (93/125)	99.9% (8305/8307)	97.9% (93/95)	99.6% (8305/8337)
Carrera[96]	? (1970–1991)		3.03%	78.3% (788/?)	99% (?/?)	?	?
Shirley et al.[97]	6183 (1989–1991)	19	1.36%	60.7% (51/84)	99.9% (6098/6099)	98.1% (51/52)	99.5% (6098/6131)
Luck[99]	8523 (1988–1991)	19	1.48%	84.3% (140/166)	99.9% (8355/8357)	98.6% (140/142)	99.7% (8355/8381)
RADIUS† (detected <24 weeks)[100]	7685 (1987–1991)	15–22	2.4%	16.6% (31/187)	99.9% (7382/7388)	83.8% (31/37)	97.9% (7382/7538)
Eurenius et al.[105]	8324 (1990–1992)	15–22	1.74%	22.1% (32/145)	99.8% (8159/8179)	61.5% (32/52)	98.0% (8159/8324)
Smith and Hau[104]	246,481 (1989–1994)	18–22	1.13%	92% (230/251)‡	‡	†	†
Skupski et al.[101]	860 (1990–1994)	18–20	0.5%§	75% (3/4)	100% (856/856)	100% (3/3)	99.9% (856/857)
VanDorsten et al.[102]	2031 (1993–1996)	15–22	3.0	75.0% (45/60)	99.9% (1969/1971)	95.7% (45/47)	99.2% (1969/1984)
Magriples and Copel[103]	911 (Not reported)	16–20	3.1	71.4% (20/28)	99.4% (878/883)	80.0% (20/25)	99.1% (878/886)
EUROFETUS[106]	Not reported (1990–1993)	Second and third trimester	Not reported	61.4% (2262/36,889)	†	†	†

*Ratios are presented in parentheses. NPV, negative predictive value; PPV, positive predictive value.
†The data presented reflects the fact that, although 7685 pregnancies were randomized to have routine examinations performed at 15–22 and 31–35 weeks, only 7575 actually had sonograms performed.
‡Reported detection rate for nine structural anomalies with scans performed at 18–21 weeks (anencephaly, spina bifida, encephalocele, hidrocephaly, hypoplastic ventricle, diaphragmatic hernia, exomphalos, gastroschisis, renal agenesis).
§Major anomalies detectable by prenatal ultrasonography.

TABLE 15–14. ACCURACY OF PRENATAL ULTRASOUND IN DETECTING CONGENITAL ANOMALIES, REGARDLESS OF THE INDICATION FOR SONOGRAM AND TIMING OF THE DIAGNOSIS

Study	Subjects (Period)	Age in Weeks	Prevalence*	Type of Study	Sensitivity*	Specificity*	PPV*	NPV*
Hill et al.[107]	5420 (1979–1983)	Second and third trimesters	1.2% (64/5420)	Prospective	28% (18/64)	100% (5356/5356)	100% (18/18)	99% (5356/5402)
Lys et al.[108]	8316 (1986)	Entire pregnancy	2.3% (190/8316)	Retrospective case control	14% (27/190)	98% (187/190)	—	—
Mida et al.[109]	1000 (1989)	Entire pregnancy	4.5% (45/1000)	Prospective	11% (5/45)	100% (952/955)	63% (5/8)	96% (952/992)
Sabbagha et al.[110]†	615 (1980–1983)		13.2% (81/615)	Prospective	95% (78/81)	99% (530/534)	95% (78/82)	99% (530/533)
Sollie et al.[111]†	494 (1980–1985)		20.6% (102/494)	Prospective	86% (88/102)	100% (392/392)	100% (88/88)	97% (392/476)
Manchester et al.[112]‡	257 (1988)	>16	82.5% (212/257)	Prospective	99% (211/212)	91% (41/45)	98% (211/215)	98% (41/42)
Gonçalves et al.[113]§	574 (1987–1991)		8.7% (574/6616)	Retrospective case control	53% (152/287)	99% (285/287)	—	—
Ott et al.[114]	1338 (1990–1991)	Entire pregnancy	9.3%	Retrospective	70% (87/125)	98% (1194/1213)	82% (87/106)	98% (1194/1232)

*Ratios are presented in parentheses. NPV, negative predictive value; PPV, positive predictive value.
†Patients referred because of high risk or suspected congenital anomalies in previous examinations. The study by Sabbagha et al. includes only major congenital anomalies; it does not include eye malformations, face, neck, cardiovascular, respiratory, genital, or aneuploidies.
‡Patients were referred because of an anomaly suspected during previous ultrasonographic examination in other institutions.
§Two hundred eighty-seven cases were excluded because they had conditions that, although considered anomalies in newborns, are normal in fetuses (patent ductus arteriosus; undescended testicles; others were excluded because the anomalies were considered undetectable by prenatal ultrasound (pigmentation defects of the skin and eye).

expertise. Studies enrolling only pregnancies at high risk (those with a previous ultrasound suggestive of congenital anomalies, positive family history, or teratogen exposure) have reported higher detection rates because of selection bias. Most studies published in the last 5 years from specialized centers have reported sensitivities in the range of 60 to 80% for major anomalies. It is our opinion that this should be the minimum acceptable standard for centers offering prenatal diagnosis.

Although a false-negative diagnosis may leave the family with the emotional, medical, social, and economic burdens imposed by a child born with a congenital anomaly, false-positive diagnoses may be equally ominous because they may lead to termination of a pregnancy with a normal fetus. Specificity is the statistical parameter that measures the ability to rule out a diagnosis when it is not present, being inversely related to the rate of false-positive diagnoses. Contrary to the nonuniform detection rates for congenital anomalies mentioned above, specificity was invariably high in all studies, no matter the type of population scanned or the ultrasonographic expertise of those performing the examinations (Tables 15–13 and 15–14).

Detection rates for specific anomalies have been determined in a group of 287 fetuses with 467 anomalies. Lethal anomalies were correctly diagnosed in 89% of the cases, followed by 77% of those requiring neonatal intensive care unit (NICU) admission and 30% of minor anomalies. Anencephaly, acrania, iniencephaly, hydrocephalus, cystic adenomatoid malformation of the lung, extralobar lung sequestration, abnormalities of situs, cardiac rhabdomyomas, atresia of the small intestine, diaphragmatic hernia, omphalocele, bilateral renal agenesis, congenital ureteral obstruction, hy-dronephrosis, congenital urethral obstruction, hydrops, and sacrococcygeal teratoma were correctly identified in every case. Defects of the cardiovascular system, cleft lip and/or palate, microcephalus, and hypospadias/epispadias were among the anomalies most frequently missed by ultrasonography. Similar results have been reported by other investigators.

The specific prenatal detection rate for congenital heart anomalies is another important issue. The livebirth incidence of congenital heart disease is estimated as 0.8 to 0.9%, and 20 to 30% of perinatal deaths may be attributed to congenital heart disease.[115] As it will be discussed later in this chapter, prenatal diagnosis followed by delivery in specialized centers may significantly improve perinatal outcome. Most of the studies with low detection rates performed unsatisfactorily in the detection of congenital heart defects. Table 15–15 summarizes reports on the accuracy of ultrasound for detecting congenital heart anomalies.[116–131] As expected, sensitivity was higher in single centers that implemented intensive training programs for the examination of the fetal heart, with systematic inclusion of the four-chamber view and outflow tracts as part of the routine examination as well as analysis of blood flow by color Doppler imaging. Most cases of ventricular hypoplasia, tetralogy of Fallot, transposition of the great arteries, and endocardial cushion defects should be accurately diagnosed. Anomalies that are still missed with relative frequency include atrial septal defects, ventricular septal defects, valvar stenoses, and abnormal pulmonary venous return. False-positive diagnoses in some series were high, but they corresponded to small ventricular septal defects that are likely to close spontaneously before or after birth.

TABLE 15–15. ACCURACY OF FETAL ECHOCARDIOGRAPHY IN DETECTING HEART DEFECTS

Study	Subjects (Population)	Age in Weeks	Prevalence	Sensitivity	Specificity	PPV	NPV
Sandor et al.[116]	124 (High risk)		10.5%	62%	100%	100%	96%
Benacerraf et al.[117]	49 (Affected fetuses)		—	57%	—	—	—
Copel et al.[118]	1022 (High risk)		7.34%	92%	99%	96%	99%
Crawford et al.[119]	989 (High risk)		9.2%	81%	—	99%	—
Callan et al.[120]	303 (High risk)		7.59%	91%	99%	84%	99%
Bromley et al.[121]	69 (Affected fetuses)	≥18	—	83%	—	—	—
Achiron et al.[122]	5347 (Low risk)		0.39%	82%	100%	95%	99%
Rustico et al.[123]	7024 (Low risk)	20–22	0.93%	35.4%	99.9%	74.2%	99.4%
Ott[124]	1136 (Low risk)	15–40	1.23%	14.3%	99.0%	14.3%	99.0%
Ott[124]	886 (High risk)	15–40	1.81%	62.5%	99.8%	83.3%	99.3%
Giancotti et al.[125]	736 (High risk)	18–22	3.6%	90%	99%	96%	99%
Stümpflen et al.[126]	3085 (Unselected)	18–28	1.69%	88.5%	100%	100%	99.8%
Buskens et al.[127]	5319 (Low risk; four-chamber only)	16–24	1.2%	4.4%	99.9%	28.6%	99.2%
Todros et al.[128]	8299 (Low risk; four-chamber only)	≥18	0.48%	15%	99.9%	50%	99.6%
Klein et al.[130]	97,245 (Low risk)	—	0.32%	34.8%	—	—	—
Stoll et al.[129]	92,021 (Low risk)	≥18	0.85%	13.7%	99.9%	99.0%	75.3%
Hafner et al.[131]	6541 (Low risk)	21–22	1.3%	43.8%	99.7%	70.9%	99.2%

NPV, negative predictive value; PPV, positive predictive value.

TABLE 15–16. ACCURACY OF FIRST TRIMESTER TRANSVAGINAL ULTRASOUND TO DETECT CONGENITAL ANOMALIES

| Study | Subjects | Age in Weeks | Prevalence | Sensitivity* | | | Total Detection Rate* |
				1st Trimester	2nd Trimester	3rd Trimester	
Yagel et al.[144]	536	13–16	8.6%	71.7% (33/46)	17.4% (8/46)		89.1% (41/46)
Hernádi and Töröcsik[145]	3991	12	0.9%	40.8% (20/49)	18.4% (9/49)	20.4% (10/49)	79.6% (39/49)
D'Ottavio et al.[146]	4080	13–15	2.1%	61.4% (54/88)	37.3% (24/88)		88.6%
Economides[147]	6000	11–14	Not stated	68%	13%		85%

*Ratios are given in parentheses.

First-Trimester Ultrasound

Improvements in transvaginal ultrasound technology and the discovery of a strong association between increased nuchal translucency thickness and chromosomal anomalies has fueled interest in first-trimester prenatal diagnosis. Early diagnosis is a desirable goal of prenatal care because it allows detection in nonviable pregnancies, accurate determination of chorionicity in twin pregnancies, and early pregnancy termination for selected anomalies. In the following sections, prenatal detection rates for diagnosis of congenital anomalies in the first trimester and the role of nuchal translucency thickness as a screening test for aneuploidies are reviewed.

Prenatal Detection of Congenital Anomalies During the First Trimester.

Since the introduction of transvaginal probes and the first reports of anomaly detection in the first trimester,[132–134] several centers have reported their experience with prenatal diagnosis at this gestational period.[135–147] It has been shown that 6%, 75%, 96%, 98%, and 98% of the fetal structures can be imaged by transvaginal ultrasound by 10, 11, 12, 13, and 14 weeks, respectively. Accordingly, 13 weeks has been proposed as the optimal time to perform nuchal translucency measurements and conduct the first-trimester anatomic evaluation.[148] Table 15–16 summarizes studies that have evaluated the diagnostic accuracy of first-trimester ultrasound for detection of congenital anomalies. Examinations performed in the first trimester can detect about 60% of the major congenital anomalies and another 20% can be picked up during the second-trimester scan, bringing the combined detection rate for congenital anomalies to approximately 80%.

Although there are potential advantages in detecting serious congenital anomalies in early pregnancy, these advantages should be balanced against the possible drawbacks. The desirable goals of early diagnosis are the avoidance of late termination of pregnancy in cases of severe malformations and the possibility of introducing more effective therapeutic strategies for treatable conditions. Pitfalls include the identification of malformed fetuses destined to miscarry spontaneously[149–151] and an increased rate of false-positive diagnoses because abnormalities such as isolated cystic hygroma, hydronephrosis, and ventricular septal defects may regress spontaneously over the remainder of the pregnancy.[144]

Ultrasound Screening With Nuchal Translucency Thickness.

Nuchal translucency is a collection of fluid observed at the back of the fetus during the first trimester (Fig. 15–11). Fetuses with increased nuchal translucency thickness are at

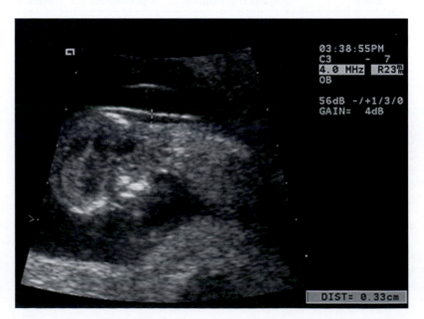

Figure 15–11. Sagittal section of a 13-week fetus showing a normal nuchal translucency.

greater risk for having a chromosomal abnormality, mainly trisomy 21, followed by trisomies 18 and 13. Those fetuses with an increased nuchal translucency and normal karyotype have a greater risk of cardiac defects, diaphragmatic hernia, omphalocele, body stalk anomaly, and fetal akinesia deformation sequence. Some rare skeletal dysplasias and genetic syndromes, usually found in fewer than 1 per 10,000 pregnancies, may also be more prevalent among fetuses with an increased nuchal translucency thickness.[152] Among the possible mechanisms to explain an increase in nuchal translucency thickness are 1) cardiac failure in association with abnormalities of the heart and great arteries; 2) venous congestion in the head and neck due to constriction of the fetal body in amnion rupture sequence or superior mediastinal compression found in diaphragmatic hernia or the narrow chest in skeletal dysplasia; 3) altered composition of the extracellular matrix; 4) abnormal or delayed development of the lymphatic system; 5) failure of lymphatic drainage due to impaired fetal movements in various neuromuscular disorders; 6) fetal anemia or hypoproteinemia; and 7) congenital infection, acting through anemia or cardiac dysfunction.[153]

Several studies have examined the value of increased nuchal translucency thickness as a screening test to identify fetuses with Down's syndrome. A full discussion of this subject is beyond the scope of this chapter, and the reader is referred to Chapter 5 in this book. The largest study to date was published by the Fetal Medicine Foundation First Trimester Screening group.[45] The investigators evaluated nuchal translucency thickness screening between 10 and 14 weeks in 96,127 women with singleton pregnancies. Among these pregnancies, 326 (3.4 per 1000) were affected by trisomy 21 and 325 (3.4 per 1000) by other chromosomal abnormalities. Nuchal translucency thickness was above the 95th centile of the normal range for crown–rump length in 4.4% (4209 of 95,476) of the normal pregnancies, in 71.8% (234 of 326) of those with trisomy 21, and in 70.5% (229 of 325) of those with other chromosomal defects. It was estimated that screening with nuchal translucency thickness alone would detect 77% [95% confidence interval (CI) = 72 to 82] of the fetuses with trisomy 21 for a screen-positive rate of 5%. The addition of first-trimester biochemical markers [pregnancy associated plasma protein-A (PAPP-A) and free β-human chorionic gonadotrophin (β-hCG)] is expected to increase the detection rate of trisomy 21 to 90%, maintaining a screen-positive rate of 5%.[154]

Legal Implications of Accuracy Studies
Malpractice suits related to fetal anomalies are the most common type of litigation involving ultrasound (75% of the cases) in the United States.[155] Other frequent claims are related to gynecologic ultrasound (15%) and abdominal ultrasound (10%). The most frequent claim is missing an anomaly on a sonogram performed for a standard indication, such as dating.

From this discussion, it should be clear that *a normal ultrasound scan does not guarantee that a fetus will be born normal*. Physicians performing obstetric ultrasound should inform their patients about this, preferably in writing, as a visible statement in the front page of the ultrasonographic report. Several technical difficulties may impair the adequate anatomic study of a fetus: maternal obesity, abnormalities in amniotic fluid volume, fetal position during the examination, and the time frame in which the examination is performed (to name a few). For instance, diaphragmatic hernia (a major structural abnormality, with life-threatening implications) is frequently missed in scans performed before 24 weeks. The same holds true for a number of other anomalies including duodenal atresia, esophageal atresia, coarctation of the aorta, hydronephrosis, clubfeet, and hydrocephaly. Structures that have not been satisfactorily imaged during the examination should also be clearly described in the report.

MANAGEMENT PRINCIPLES IN THE DETECTION OF CONGENITAL ANOMALIES
The following issues need to be considered in a program of prenatal diagnosis of anatomic congenital anomalies.

Offering Prenatal Diagnosis
When a patient seeks prenatal diagnosis for a specific congenital anomaly, it is imperative to learn whether this type of prenatal diagnosis has ever been reported. Gestational age and specific sonographic findings used for the diagnosis must be carefully reviewed. Caution is advised with claims reported in the literature. In many instances, the title of the case report claims that a specific prenatal diagnosis has been made, when only recognition of an abnormal finding without a precise antenatal diagnosis has occurred. Knowledge of the spectrum of the disease, including associated anomalies and natural history of the disorder, is also required. Unless there is a great deal of experience (e.g., spina bifida), patients must be informed that the diagnostic accuracy of ultrasound for that specific disorder is not known and that false-positive and false-negative diagnoses may occur. The implications of these potential diagnostic errors must also be discussed. For medicolegal considerations, it may be wise to document such discussions in the medical record.

Work-Up of an Abnormal Finding
One of every five newborns affected with a birth defect has more than one major anatomic abnormality, and this association is often of critical prognostic importance.[48,52] Therefore, the identification of any anomaly in a fetus must prompt a careful search for other associated abnormalities. Echocardiography and fetal karyotype determinations must be considered. The association between congenital heart disease and extracardiac anomalies has been demonstrated in a recent series showing that 23% of fetuses referred for

echocardiography because of an extracardiac anomaly had congenital heart disease. The relationship between different types of congenital heart disease and various extracardiac anomalies has been reviewed elsewhere.[156,157] Chromosome abnormalities had been previously documented in the pediatric literature in infants with congenital anomalies. Approximately one-third of fetuses with structural anomalies have a chromosome disorder.[90–93,158–161] The information derived from amniocentesis may allow more informed counseling and influence obstetric management. Amniocentesis has been the standard method for obtaining material for karyotype determination, but placental biopsy and percutaneous fetal blood sampling are used when a rapid answer is desired or additional studies from fetal blood are indicated.[162,163]

Pregnancy Termination

In a country where pregnancy termination is available for social as well as medical reasons, this option is offered to mothers carrying an anomalous fetus. The gestational age limit at which termination of pregnancy can be offered differs across countries and across states in the United States. Some clinicians and ethicists believe that elective termination of pregnancy in the third trimester can be offered to some mothers carrying a fetus with a uniformly lethal condition for which prenatal diagnosis is certain (i.e., anencephaly). Recently, these infants have become a potential source of organs for transplantation, an option that raises serious ethical and practical medical questions.[164,165]

Site, Mode, and Timing of Delivery

Delivery of fetuses with congenital anomalies should ideally occur in a center with a newborn special care unit. Pediatricians may face unexpected complications posed by undiagnosed associated anomalies. An interdisciplinary team composed of specialists in maternal–fetal medicine, diagnostic imaging, neonatology, and human genetics should be available for consultation. Depending on the specific nature of the anomaly, other specialists such as a pediatric surgeon, pediatric cardiologist, cardiovascular surgeon, and neurosurgeon may also be required. Paramedical personnel, such as a social worker, are also important in providing emotional support to the family.

Some anomalies may alter the method of delivery. Conjoined twins, giant omphaloceles, giant sacrococcygeal tumors, and severe hydrocephaly are examples of these conditions. The optimal method of delivery for other anomalies such as omphaloceles, gastroschisis, and myelomeningocele has not been determined.[166–170] Some disorders, that are not uniformly lethal but are frequently associated with neonatal death or serious neurologic handicap require careful discussion with the parents to define management in the event of fetal distress. For these conditions, some favor a nonaggressive management approach because analysis of the risk to benefit ratio is slanted toward maternal well-being; therefore, some

clinicians would advise against a cesarean section. However, the final decision rests with the parents.

Delivery of an infant with a congenital anomaly should ideally occur at term. Surgical corrective procedures would be delayed by respiratory distress syndrome or other problems of prematurity. Early delivery may be considered for some rare conditions that worsen *in utero*.

Surgical Fetal Therapy

Although lethal congenital anomalies are best managed by pregnancy termination, others such as ductal-dependent cardiac anomalies and abdominal wall defects may benefit from maternal transport and delivery in tertiary care centers, where pediatric cardiologists and surgeons are available for immediate assessment and intervention. Fetal surgery is a natural step toward the treatment of simple anatomic conditions with high neonatal mortality or long-term morbidity.[171–176] Although a detailed discussion of this subject is beyond the scope of this chapter, a list of congenital anomalies that may benefit from *in utero* surgical correction is presented in Table 15–17. Percutaneous ultrasonographically guided procedures are generally used in the treatment of lower urinary tract obstruction (vesicoamniotic shunts) and chylothorax (thoracoamniotic shunts). Percutaneous balloon valvuloplasty has been attempted in fetuses with aortic or pulmonic valve stenosis.[177,178] Open fetal surgery has been performed with some success in fetuses with diaphragmatic hernia, cystic adenomatoid malformation of the lung, lower urinary tract obstruction, and sacrococcygeal teratoma. Developments in fetoscopy have made it possible to perform endoscopic surgical procedures *in utero*. Ligation of the umbilical cord of the acardiac twin in the twin-reversed arterial perfusion syndrome,[110–113,179–182] laser photocoagulation of communicating chorionic vessels in twin-to-twin transfusion syndrome,[114–119,183–188] endoscopic ablation of posterior urethral valves,[189] tracheal occlusion in diaphragmatic hernia,[190,191] and lysis of amniotic bands[192] have been successfully performed endoscopically. Despite the promising

TABLE 15–17. DEFECTS THAT MAY REQUIRE IN UTERO TREATMENT

Obstructive uropathy
Acqueductal stenosis
Twin-to-twin transfusion
Congenital diaphragmatic hernia
Sacrococcygeal teratoma
Myelomeningocele
Congenital cystic adenomatoid malformation
Congenital hydrothorax
Tracheal atresia, stenosis, obstruction by tumor
Hydrops not associated with chromosomal and structural anomalies
Amniotic band syndrome
Congenital heart disease

results, all of these procedures are still experimental and should only be performed in centers that are committed to a program of continuing research. These centers should work in close collaboration with pediatric surgeons, perinatal obstetricians, sonographers, echocardiographers, neonatologists, intensive care specialists, geneticists, ethicists, and neonatal/obstetric nurses. They should also be committed to being reviewed by institutional review boards and to publish all their results (bad and good).[175]

SHOULD EVERY PREGNANT PATIENT HAVE AN ULTRASOUND EXAMINATION?

There has been continuous debate concerning the routine use of ultrasound in obstetrics. Whereas some, including a consensus conference sponsored by the National Institutes of Health, have favored selective use of ultrasound for a number of indications, others have opposed its routine use during pregnancy.[93,100,193–200]

The RADIUS study was the largest randomized clinical trial of routine ultrasound screening during pregnancy. The trial was conducted in the United States and recruited patients from 109 practices [81 private, 15 academic, and 13 health maintenance organizations (HMOs)]. Ultrasound examinations were conducted in 28 laboratories equipped with state-of-the-art equipment and using a rigid, uniform scanning protocol. The examinations were performed by 60 different technicians and subsequently reviewed by 94 sonologists (including 2 of the trial investigators, 13 maternal–fetal medicine specialists, and 75 radiologists). In-service training, review of the first 25 sonograms performed by each sonographer and sonologist, and additional training and review, if necessary, were provided by one of the senior investigators. The content of the examinations consisted of identification of the number of fetuses, presentation, placental location, amniotic fluid volume, biparietal diameter, head circumference, abdominal circumferences, femur length, and an anatomic survey including intracranial anatomy, four-chamber view of the heart, demonstration of the spine in transverse and coronal planes, stomach, kidneys, bladder, umbilical cord insertion, and all extremities. A total of 15,530 women were randomly allocated to have either two ultrasound examinations (at 15 to 22 weeks and at 31 to 35 weeks) or ultrasound only if indicated. The objective of the first scan was to detect gestational age errors, multiple pregnancies, and major malformations, and the second examination was conducted to detect fetal growth disorders (intrauterine growth retardation, macrosomia) and anomalies that appear late or were unrecognized in the early scan. The study was designed to test the hypothesis that routine ultrasound screening during pregnancy would decrease the perinatal death rate or the rate of moderate and severe neonatal complications.[194] The secondary objective of the study was to test whether routine ultrasound screening during pregnancy could improve maternal management

and outcome.[195] The results showed no difference in the rate of adverse perinatal outcome between patients allocated to routine ultrasound screening and those in the control group. Similarly, there was no difference in the rate of adverse maternal outcome and rates of induced abortion, amniocentesis, tests of fetal well-being, external version, induction of labor, cesarean section, and duration of hospitalization. Patients allocated to the ultrasound screening group had a lower rate of tocolysis and post-term pregnancies.

A meta-analysis of four previously conducted randomized clinical trials[93,196–198] published in the *British Medical Journal*[199] included data from 15,935 pregnancies (7992 allocated to routine sonography versus 7943 allocated to selective scanning). This meta-analysis showed that women allocated to routine ultrasound screening had a higher detection rate of small-for-gestational-age (SGA) infants, multiple pregnancy, and severe malformations when compared with women who had ultrasound only if indicated. More importantly, the perinatal mortality rate was significantly lower in patients allocated to routine scanning (Fig. 15–12). This effect was largely attributable to the contribution of the Helsinki trial,[93] which reported a 49.2% reduction in perinatal mortality (from 9.0 per 1000 to 4.6 per 1000) in women who underwent routine sonography. The investigators considered that the lower perinatal mortality "was due to improved early detection of malformations which led to induced abortions."

Why the Discrepancy Between the Results of the Two Studies?

Many of the conclusions of the RADIUS study are questionable, and we will provide the evidence to support our view in the following paragraphs.[201–203] In brief, we believe that the results of the RADIUS study failed to demonstrate a decrease in perinatal or maternal morbidity and mortality because of poor performance in the detection of congenital malformations, lack of statistical power and uniform management protocols to detect a reduction in cesarean section rates for post-term pregnancies, and lack of statistical power

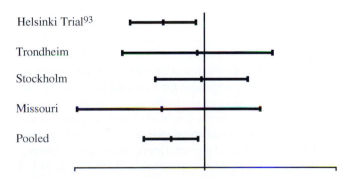

Figure 15–12. Impact of routine ultrasound screening during pregnancy according to a meta-analysis of four randomized clinical trials. The results (from top down) are from the Helsinki, Trondheim, Stockholm, and Missouri trials and the pooled estimate.

TABLE 15–18. ACCURACY OF THE RADIUS STUDY TO DETECT CONGENITAL MALFORMATIONS

	Routine Scan (%)	Control (%)	p	Relative Risk (95% CI)
Before 24 weeks	31/187 (16.6)	8/163 (4.9)	<0.001	3.4 (1.6–7.2)
All gestational ages	65/187 (34.8)	18/163 (11.0)	<0.01	3.2 (2.0–5.1)

CI, confidence interval.

to detect an improvement in maternal or perinatal outcome in multiple gestations.

Detection of Congenital Anomalies. Table 15–18 shows that routine scanning was better than *ultrasound when indicated* in the detection of congenital anomalies in the RADIUS study.[100] The difference was significant both before and after 24 weeks of gestation (the limit for pregnancy termination in most of the United States). However, the higher detection rate did not translate into improved perinatal outcome. Several factors may be responsible for this lack of improvement. First, the detection rate of congenital anomalies in the study group [16.6% (31 of 187)] was extremely low and does not represent the current diagnostic capabilities of ultrasound. Table 15–18 is a compilation of published studies in which ultrasound was used as a screening method for the detection of anomalies before 24 weeks of gestation.[93,100] Excluding the results of the RADIUS study from this table, 52,229 pregnancies were screened in six different European centers, with an overall sensitivity of 50.9% (393 of 772). The difference between the sensitivity of the RADIUS study and that of this combined series is highly significant (16.6% versus 50.9%, 95% CI = 3.40 to 8.04, $p < 0.00001$). This low sensitivity may be largely attributed to the extremely poor performance of nontertiary care centers, which conducted 63% of the examinations. Despite the careful study design, detection rates were significantly higher for tertiary care centers when compared with community hospitals and office-based facilities [35% (19 of 54) versus 13% (8 of 64); relative detection rate = 2.7, 95% CI = 1.3 to 5.8]. Nontertiary care centers were unable to detect any craniofacial, cardiac, gastrointestinal, and skeletal anomalies.[100]

The meta-analysis conducted by Bucher and Schmidt[199] indicated that routine sonography in the Helsinki trial[93] reduced perinatal mortality, mainly because a substantial proportion of women diagnosed to have fetuses with congenital anomalies chose to terminate their pregnancies. Indeed, the livebirth rate (number of livebirths per pregnancy) was not different between patients allocated to routine scanning and those allocated to ultrasound if indicated.[199] Therefore, routine ultrasound reduced perinatal mortality simply by placing the deaths that would have occurred in the perinatal period in a different category, namely pregnancy terminations.[203]

Correction of Dating Errors. The correct assessment of gestational age has two potential advantages: 1) reduction of

unnecessary administration of tocolysis because of incorrect diagnosis of preterm labor and 2) improvement of outcome and management of post-term pregnancy.

In the RADIUS study, women routinely scanned received tocolysis less frequently than women having ultrasound only if indicated (3.41% versus 4.22%, $p < 0.01$).[194] Because the rate of preterm delivery was similar in the two groups, it can be concluded that routine sonography decreased the rate of unnecessary tocolysis. Such a gain is desirable because tocolysis is expensive and risky. Indeed, cardiovascular side effects induced by beta-adrenergic agents have been implicated as a cause of iatrogenic maternal death of patients in premature labor.[204]

Similarly, women allocated to routine scanning had a lower rate of post-term gestation (10.1% versus 21.4% above 41 weeks, $p < 0.001$; 3.2% versus 4.6% above 42 weeks, $p < 0.001$).[195] These findings are consistent with the results of the Helsinki trial, in which ultrasound reduced the rate of post-term gestation (above 42 weeks) from 5.9 to 2.9% $p < 0.01$.[93] It has been demonstrated by a large randomized clinical trial that routine induction of labor in post-term gestations with prostaglandin E_2 reduces the cesarean section rate by 3.3 percentage points (from 24.5 to 21.1%) when compared with expectant management.[205] This benefit could not be demonstrated in the context of the RADIUS study, in part because routine induction of labor was not the standard of care for post-term gestations enrolled in the trial. Also, although the rate of adverse perinatal outcome was 40% lower in the patients allocated to routine sonography (1.6% versus 2.6%, respectively), this difference was not statistically significant. This is not surprising because the study would need at least 6848 post-term patients to detect this difference with 80% power. The RADIUS study had only 592 post-term gestations and thus a power of less than 12%. Similarly, 5202 patients would have been required to detect a significant reduction (24.5 to 21.2%) in the rate of cesarean section for post-term gestations with 80% power.[201,203]

Detection of Multiple Pregnancies. The RADIUS study found that routine ultrasound was significantly better than *ultrasound when indicated* in the detection of multiple gestations before 26 weeks of gestation [98.5% (67 of 68) versus 62.3% (38 of 61); odds ratio = 40.5, $p < 0.001$].[194] Moreover, 13.1% (8 of 61) of twins born to patients in the control group did not have the diagnosis made until delivery admission. However, the improved diagnosis did not result in improved perinatal or maternal outcome and management. Did the

RADIUS study have the power to detect a difference between the two groups?

The rate of adverse perinatal outcome in multiple gestations was 25% (17 of 68) in patients allocated to routine ultrasound versus 37.7% (23 of 61) in those in the control group. The difference was not statistically significant (relative risk = 0.8, 95% CI = 0.39 to 1.11, $p = 0.13$). However, the RADIUS study had less than 36% power to detect this difference. Four hundred forty-eight twin gestations would be required to test the hypothesis; the RADIUS study had only 129.[203]

Detection of Growth Disorders. The RADIUS study found no difference in the birth rate of SGA infants (defined as birth weight below the 10th percentile for age) between the screening and control groups (2.3% for each group).[194] This is not surprising because ultrasound is a diagnostic and not a therapeutic tool. There are no reasons to expect that performing a diagnostic ultrasound by itself can correct a fetal growth disorder. To assess the value of routine ultrasound, we need to know the detection rate of SGA and macrosomia in each study group. However, such information has not been provided in the three reports of the RADIUS study. Assessment of the value, or lack thereof, of routine ultrasound in the diagnosis of SGA requires information about the potential consequences of false-negative and false-positive diagnoses of SGA in each of the study groups. The statement that there was no difference in perinatal outcome between patients having routine ultrasound versus patients having *ultrasound when indicated* does not answer this question.

Cost of a Routine Screening Program. It has been estimated by the authors of the RADIUS study that a policy of universal ultrasound screening during pregnancy would increase health costs by more than $1 billion. They have reasoned that screening 4,000,000 pregnant women in the United States at a rate of 1.6 scans per patient at a cost of $200.00 per scan

would cost more than $1 billion. Even if the number of patients screened were restricted to 40% of the women who would not have a formal indication for routine scanning, it would still cost $500 million.[194]

The available data from the RADIUS study indicate that the majority of pregnant women will have had an ultrasound examination during pregnancy.[194] First, 60.5% (32,317 of 53,367) of women screened for the trial were considered ineligible to participate because they had indications to be scanned. The authors did not provide information about when these examinations were performed, although we suspect that a large number were conducted in the second and third trimesters and could have been used to screen for congenital anomalies. Second, an additional 6% of women (3,163 of 53,376) declined consent. Although the reasons for this have not been stated, a fraction might not have wanted to give up prenatal diagnosis with ultrasound to participate in a research project. An additional 4.4% (2357 of 53,367) were lost to follow-up before randomization. Among the women randomized to the control group, 45% had an ultrasound examination for established indications. Thus, it can be inferred that 6988 of the 15,530 women (45%) eligible for randomization would have had an ultrasound examination for established indications. Based on this figure, we have estimated that at least 74% of women would have an ultrasound examination during pregnancy and most of them at a gestational age when they could have been screened for congenital anomalies. Therefore, the argument of universal screening only applies to the remaining patients (approximately 26 to 30%).

Another approach to examine the issue of cost effectiveness is to compare the cost of detecting a congenital anomaly with ultrasound with other screening programs that are part of the standard prenatal care. DeVore[206] compared the cost of detecting an anomaly with ultrasound screening performed by individuals with different ultrasonographic skill to the cost of maternal serum α-fetoprotein (MSAFP) screening (Table 15–19). If ultrasound screening is performed by

TABLE 15–19. COST PER DETECTED MALFORMED FETUS USING PRENATAL SCREENING TESTS IN LOW-RISK POPULATIONS

	Total Diagnostic Procedures Performed	Total Cost of Diagnostic Procedures (1994 dollars)	Rate of Detection of Major Fetal Malformations *(n)*	Cost for Detection of a Malformed Fetus
California MSAFP screening program (1986–1990)	1,057,941	$56,070,873 ($53/test)*	1.31/1000 (1390)	$40,338
RADIUS study (1987–1991; second-trimester ultrasound screening)	7281	$1,456,200 ($200/test)	3.6/1000 (26)	$56,008
Tertiary centers	2658	$531,600 ($200/test)	6.8/1000 (18)	$29,533
Nontertiary centers	4623	$924,600 ($200/test)	1.7/1000 (8)	$115,575

*The cost includes MSAFP for all patients and the following for all patients with an elevated or low MSAFP: genetic counseling, ultrasound examination, amniocentesis, amniotic fluid α-fetoprotein, and karyotype.
MSAFP, maternal serum α-fetoprotein.
Derived from DeVore G. Obstet Gynecol 1994;84:622.

individuals who have a diagnostic rate similar to that reported for tertiary care centers participating in the RADIUS study, the cost of detecting a malformed fetus would be $10,805 less than the cost of detecting an anomaly with MSAFP screening. If screening is performed by individuals whose diagnostic rates are similar to those reported for nontertiary centers, the cost would be $75,237 higher than the cost of MSAFP screening. To offer a cost-effective program of routine ultrasound screening during pregnancy, DeVore proposed that physicians should be reimbursed by second-trimester ultrasound exams based on their reported diagnostic skills. Vintzileos et al.[207] evaluated the possible economic impact of offering targeted ultrasonography instead of routine amniocentesis for patients with elevated MSAFP in the United States. Their hypothesis was that the cost of universal amniocentesis in patients with an elevated concentration of MSAFP in the second trimester should be at least equal to the cost of universal targeted ultrasonography, with amniocentesis used only for those with abnormalities on a sonogram. The cost of universal targeted ultrasonography would include the cost of all normal ultrasound examinations, the cost of amniocentesis for those with abnormal ultrasonographic results, and the lifetime cost of caring for all live infants with spina bifida. They estimated the annual cost of genetic amniocentesis in patients with elevated MSAFP to range from US $90 million to US $214 million, if the therapeutic abortion rates were 100% and 50%, respectively. The annual cost of targeted ultrasonography for patients with elevated MSAFP, considering a detection rate of 90% (the worst possible scenario given the sensitivities reported in the literature), would be US $54 million and US $165 million, if the therapeutic abortion rates were 100% and 50%, respectively (this estimate includes both the cost of sonograms and the cost of amniocentesis performed because of abnormal ultrasonographic results). In addition to the cost benefit, they estimated that 268 fetal losses would be prevented each year because of avoidance of invasive prenatal diagnostic testing in a substantial number of fetuses. They concluded that ultrasound for detection of congenital anomalies is cost-effective, provided that it is performed in tertiary care centers.

IMPACT OF PRENATAL DIAGNOSIS ON THE BIRTH PREVALENCE AND OUTCOME OF FETUSES WITH CONGENITAL ANOMALIES

We have briefly outlined the capabilities of ultrasound as a tool to diagnose congenital anomalies. The examination is accurate, provided it is performed by skilled operators with appropriate equipment. Quality prenatal ultrasound diagnosis is a reality in many institutions, and, in our view, there is no reason it should not be standard practice.

We have also described the possible courses of action once an anomaly has been diagnosed: prenatal treatment, delivery in a tertiary care center, or pregnancy termination.

Fetal surgery is still an experimental procedure performed in a few specialized centers. The number of cases treated is too small to draw definitive conclusions; however, if fetal surgery proves beneficial in larger series and becomes widely available, early prenatal diagnosis of congenital diaphragmatic hernia, urinary tract obstruction, twin-to-twin transfusion syndrome, acardiac twins, amniotic bands, sacrococcygeal teratoma, and spina bifida could have a positive impact on the long-term morbidity and mortality of fetuses affected by these conditions.[208]

Maternal transport to centers equipped with neonatal intensive care and surgical capabilities may have a measurable impact on perinatal outcome for selected defects. Teratomas, anterior cystic hygromas, and thyroid masses may significantly obstruct the neonatal airway and require tracheal intubation on the mother's abdomen before umbilical cord clamping.[209] Likewise, prenatal diagnosis of severe cardiac anomalies and delivery in specialized centers may have a measurable impact on perinatal outcome. It has been suggested that as many as 200 infants die each year in the United Kingdom with unrecognized congenital heart disease, that approximately 100 die from isolated unsuspected cardiac abnormalities, and that among those fetuses, half have reparable lesions.[210] Chang et al.[211] evaluated prenatal diagnosis and referral of fetuses with critical left ventricular outflow tract obstruction for delivery and postnatal treatment in a tertiary care center. Among 22 fetuses with severe left outflow tract obstruction (hypoplastic left heart syndrome, $n = 16$; valvular aortic stenosis, $n = 2$; common atrioventricular canal with subaortic stenosis, $n = 3$; and single ventricle with subaortic stenosis, $n = 1$), fetal echocardiography predicted critical obstruction in all but one patient. Seventeen patients underwent cardiac surgery as neonates, and 77% (13 of 17) of them survived. One patient had a successful balloon aortic valvotomy for critical aortic stenosis but died later of sepsis. Copel et al.[212] also reported improved survival for prenatally diagnosed fetuses undergoing biventricular heart repair in a specialized center (96% versus 76%, $p < 0.05$). For other congenital anomalies, evidence that prenatal diagnosis with planned delivery in tertiary care centers improves outcome is lacking. Skari et al.[213] found no improvement in neonatal morbidity and mortality when comparing prenatally versus postnatally diagnosed fetuses with diaphragmatic hernia, abdominal wall defects, myelomeningocele, and bladder exstrophy. Neonatal survival rate was 77% (10 of 13) for the prenatally diagnosed versus 96% (22 of 23) for the postnatally diagnosed fetuses ($p = 0.12$). In addition, no differences were observed in the length of hospital stay or in time spent on ventilatory support or parenteral nutrition. Dillon and Renwick[214] reported similar observations in 56 fetuses with gastroschisis and in 43 with omphalocele. Fourteen fetuses with gastroschisis and 10 with omphalocele were not diagnosed prenatally. Delivery of these babies away from the regional pediatric surgery center did not adversely affect perinatal outcome.

At present, termination of pregnancy is still the most prevalent change in management resulting from prenatal diagnosis. Zimmer et al.[215] reported a rise in the number of pregnancy terminations [from 0.35% (17 of 4762) to 0.86% (42 of 4841), $p > 0.01$] as a result of improved detection rates of congenital anomalies (from 53.9 to 79.6%, $p < 0.001$) over a 5-year period. The improved detection rates followed by action at diagnosis resulted in a significant decrease in the incidence of newborns with congenital anomalies [from 1.95% (93 of 4762) to 1.34% (65 of 4841), $p < 0.01$]. Data from the Hawaii Birth Defects Program also showed a significant decrease in birth prevalence rates of anencephaly, spina bifida, encephalocele, and trisomies 21, 18, and 13 between 1987 and 1996 as a result of prenatal diagnosis followed by pregnancy termination.[216] The 1998 report from the International Clearing House for Birth Defects Monitoring Systems (ICBDMS)* showed a significant reduction in the birth prevalence of neural tube defects in the majority of participating centers (Atlanta,[217] Canada, Australia, New Zealand, England, France, Spain, Italy, Norway, Netherlands, Finland, Czech Republic, Hungary, Israel, and Japan). This reduction was attributed to pregnancy termination of anencephaly and spina bifida after prenatal diagnosis.[218] The exceptions were centers located in countries where pregnancy termination is presently illegal (Mexico and many South American countries). A decrease in the prevalence of hypoplastic left heart syndrome was observed in the United Kingdom as a result of routine screening of cardiac anomalies with the four-chamber view.[219] Similar findings were reported in France, where a decreased prevalence at birth of major congenital cardiac defects was observed as a result of prenatal diagnosis followed by termination of severe cases.[130] In Boston, Massachusetts, at the Brigham and Women's Hospital, an active birth defect surveillance system registered a significant drop in live births with cardiovascular malformations as a result of improvements in ultrasound detection rates.[220]

An unquantified potential benefit to parents of a fetus affected by congenital anomalies is a team approach to prenatal diagnosis and management. Prenatal diagnosis allows full discussion of the case with specialized services such as neonatal intensive care, pediatric surgery, and clinical genetics before delivery. There is more time for information to be understood, questions answered, and professional psychological assistance as well as family support obtained. Prenatal diagnosis followed by specilized team counseling should avoid unprepared, critical decisions regarding the infant to be made in the setting of labor or immediately after delivery.[221]

If detection of congenital anomalies is one of the goals of prenatal care, it seems that routine ultrasound examination is the best available tool to accomplish this objective. We

have described the potential advantages of accurate prenatal diagnosis.

Innovations in ultrasound technology and research are changing the practice of prenatal diagnosis. In the next few years, we will see an increasing number of centers performing quality ultrasonographic diagnosis in the first trimester. Ultrasound will likely have a predominant role in screening for chromosomal anomalies because of nuchal translucency, and refinements in syndromic diagnoses will likely happen as a result of three-dimensional technology. Sonographers should master the skills of examining the fetal heart and should be able to examine the fetus in detail the first trimester.

We and others[200] favor routine obstetric ultrasound for all pregnancies, provided it is performed properly.

ACKNOWLEDGMENTS

This work was supported by a grant from the Walter Scott Foundation for Medical Research.

REFERENCES

1. Romero R, Oyarzun E, Sirtori M, Hobbins JC. Detection and management of anatomic congenital anomalies. A new obstetric challenge. *Obstet Gynecol Clin North Am.* 1988;15:215.
2. Spranger J, Benirschke K, Hall J, et al. Errors of morphogenesis: Concepts and terms. *J Pediatr.* 1982;100:160.
3. Jones KL. *Smith's Recognizable Patterns of Human Deformation.* Philadelphia: WB Saunders; 1988.
4. Opitz JM, Herrman J, Petterson JC, et al. Terminological, diagnostic, nosological and anatomical-developmental aspects of developmental defects in man. I. Terminological and epistemological considerations. *Am J Med Genet.* 1979;3:71.
5. Moore KL. *The Developing Human: Clinically Oriented Embryology.* Philadelphia: WB Saunders; 1982.
6. Dunn PM. Congenital postural deformities: Perinatal associations. *Proc R Soc Med.* 1972;65:735.
7. Dunn PM. Congenital postural deformities: Further perinatal associations. *Proc R Soc Med.* 1974;67:32.
8. Dunn PM. Congenital sternomastoid torticollis: An intrauterine postural deformity. *Arch Dis Child.* 1974;49:824.
9. Hall JG. In utero movement and use of limbs are necessary for normal growth: A study of individuals with arthrogryposis. In: *Prog Clin Biol Res.* 1985;200:155.
10. Cohen MM. *The Child With Multiple Birth Defects.* New York: Raven Press; 1982.
11. Romero R, Chervenak FA, Devore G, et al. Fetal head deformation and congenital torticollis associated with a uterine tumor. *Am J Obstet Gynecol.* 1981;141:839.
12. Dunn PM. Congenital postural deformities. *Br Med Bull.* 1976;32:71.
13. Baker CJ, Rudolph AJ. Congenital ring constrictions and intrauterine amputations. *Am J Dis Child.* 1971;121:393.
14. Torpin R. *Fetal Malformations Caused By Amnion Rupture During Gestation.* Springfield, Ill: Charles C. Thomas; 1968.

---

*ICBDMS is a nongovernmental association, officially related to the World Health Organization, representing more than 30 birth defects monitoring systems in 34 countries.

15. Higginbottom MC, Jones KL, Hall BD, Smith DW. The amniotic band disruption complex: Timing of amniotic rupture and variable spectra of consequent defects. *J Pediatr.* 1979;95:544.

16. Opitz JM. The developmental analysis of human congenital anomalies. In: Papadatos CJ, Bartsocas CS, eds. *Skeletal Dysplasias.* New York: Alan R. Liss; 1982:15.

17. Opitz JM. What the general pediatrician should know about developmental anomalies. *Pediatr Rev.* 1982;3:267.

18. Opitz JM. The developmental field concept in clinical genetics. *J Pediatr.* 1982;101:805.

19. Opitz JM, Lewin SO. The developmental field concept in pediatric pathology—Especially with respect to fistular alhypoplasia and the DiGeorge anomaly. *Birth Defects.* 1987;23:277.

20. Smith DW. Recognizable patterns of human deformation: Identification and management of mechanical effects on morphogenesis. In: Schaffer AJ, Markowitz M, eds. *Major Problems in Clinical Pediatrics, vol 21.* Philadelphia: WB Saunders; 1981:85.

21. Smith DW, Jones KL. Recognizable patterns of human malformation: Genetic, embryologic and clinical aspects. In: Markowitz M, ed. *Major Problems in Clinical Pediatrics, vol 12.* Philadelphia: WB Saunders; 1982:484.

22. Sivit CJ, Hill MC, Larsen JW, et al. The sonographic evaluation of fetal anomalies in oligohydramnios between 16 and 30 weeks gestation. *AJR.* 1986;146:1277.

23. Perlman M, Levin M. Fetal pulmonary hypoplasia, anuria and oligohydramnios: Clinicopathologic observations and review of the literature. *Am J Obstet Gynecol.* 1974;118:119.

24. Thomas IT, Smith DW. Oligohydramnios, cause of the nonrenal features of Potter's syndrome, including pulmonary hypoplasia. *J Pediatr.* 1974;84:811.

25. Smith DW. Recognizable patterns of human deformation: Identification and management of mechanical effects on morphogenesis. In: Schaffer AJ, Markowitz M, eds. *Major Clinical Problem in Clinical Pediatrics, vol 21.* Philadelphia: WB Saunders; 1981:90.

26. Smith DW, Jones KL. Recognizable patterns of human malformation: Genetic, embryologic and clinical aspects. In: Markowitz M, ed. *Major Problems in Clinical Pediatrics, vol 12.* Philadelphia: WB Saunders; 1982:488.

27. Fiske CE, Filly RA, Golbus MS. Prenatal ultrasound diagnosis of amniotic band syndrome. *J Ultrasound Med.* 1982;1:45.

28. Hughes RM, Benzie RJ, Thomson CL. Amniotic band syndrome causing fetal deformity. *Prenat Diagn.* 1984;4:447.

29. Mahony BS, Filly RA, Callen PW, et al. The amniotic band syndrome: Antenatal sonographic diagnosis and potential pitfalls. *Am J Obstet Gynecol.* 1985;152:63.

30. Seeds JW, Cefalo RC, Herbert WN. Amniotic band syndrome. *Am J Obstet Gynecol.* 1982;144:243.

31. Torpin R. Amniochorionic mesoblastic fibrous strings and amniotic bands: Associated constricting fetal malformation of fetal death. *Am J Obstet Gynecol.* 1965;91:65.

32. Worthern NJ, Lawrence D, Bustillo M. Amniotic band syndrome: Antepartum ultrasonic diagnosis of discordant anencephaly. *J Clin Ultrasound.* 1980;8:453.

33. Jones KI, Jones MC. A clinical approach to the dysmorphic child. In: Emery AEH, Rimoin DL, eds. *Principles and Practice of Medical Genetics.* Edinburgh: Churchill Livingstone; 1983;152.

34. Optiz JM, Herrman J, Peternson JC, et al. Terminological, diagnostic, nosological, and anatomical developmental aspects of developmental defects in man. II: Patient evaluation, delineation, and nosology of developmental defects—An overview. *Am J Med Genet.* 1981;3:107.

35. Epstein CJ. *The Consequence of Chromosome Imbalance: Principles, Mechanisms, and Models, vol 1.* Cambridge: Cambridge University Press; 1986.

36. Evans M, Lampinen J. What is an anomaly. In: Levi S, Chervenak FA, eds. *Ultrasound Screening for Fetal Anomalies: Is It Worth It? vol 847.* New York: Annals of the New York Academy of Sciences, 1998:1.

37. Marden PM, Smith DW, McDonald MJ. Congenital anomalies in the newborn infant, including minor variations: A study of 4,412 babies by surface examination for anomalies and buccal smear for sex chromatin. *J Pediatr.* 1964;64:358.

38. Emery AEH, Rimoin D, eds. *Principles and Practice of Medical Genetics.* Edinburgh: Churchill Livingstone; 1983.

39. Kaback MM. *Genetic Issues in Pediatric and Obstetric Practice.* Chicago: Year Book Medical Publishers; 1981.

40. Smith DW, Jones KL. Recognizable patterns of human malformation: Genetic, embryologic and clinical aspects. In: Markowitz M, ed. *Major Problems in Clinical Pediatrics, vol 7.* Philadelphia: WB Saunders; 1982:1.

41. Harrison MR, Golbus MS, Filly RA. *The Unborn Patient: Prenatal Diagnosis and Treatment.* Oralando: Grune & Stratton; 1984.

42. Romero R, Pilu G, Jeanty P, et al. *Prenatal Diagnosis of Congenital Anomalies.* Norwalk, CT: Appleton & Lange; 1988.

43. Milunsky A, ed. *Genetic Disorders and the Fetus. Diagnosis, Prevention and Treatment,* 2nd ed. New York: Plenum; 1986.

44. Papadatos CJ, Bartsocas CS. Endocrine genetics and genetics of growth. In: Back N, Brewer GJ, Eijsvoogel VP, eds. *Progress in Clinical and Biological Research, vol 200.* New York: Alan R. Liss; 1985:1.

45. Snijders RJM, Noble P, Sebire N, et al. UK multicentre project on assessment of risk of trisomy 21 by maternal age and fetal nuchal-translucency thickness at 10–14 weeks of gestation. *Lancet.* 1998;351:343.

46. Pilu G, Nicolaides KH. Features of chromosomal defects. In: Pilu G, Nicolaides KH, eds. *Diagnosis of Fetal Abnormalities: The 18–23 Week Scan.* London: Parthenon Publishing Group; 1999:99.

47. Hook EB, Marden PM, Reiss NP, Smith DW. Some aspects of the epidemiology of human minor birth defects and morphological variants in a completely ascertained newborn population (Madison study). *Teratology.* 1976;13:47.

48. Myrianthopoulos NC, Chung CS. Congenital malformations in singletons: Epidemiologic survey. In: Bergman D, ed. *Birth Defects, vol 11.* New York: Stratton Inter-count Med Book Corp, 1974:1.

49. Christianson RE, van den Berg BJ, Milkovich L, Oechsli FW. Incidence of congenital anomalies among white and black live births with long-term follow-up. *Am J Public Health.* 1981;71:1333.

50. Greenberg F, James LM, Oakley GP. Estimates of birth relevance rates of spina bifida in the United States from computer-generated maps. *Am J Obstet Gynecol.* 1983;145:570.

51. Terry PB, Bissenden JG, Condie RG, Mathew PM. Ethnic differences in congenital malformations. *Arch Dis Child.* 1985;60:866.

52. Chung CS, Myrianthopoulos NC. Congenital anomalies: Mortality and morbidity, burden and classification. *Am J Med Genet.* 1987;27:505.

53. Centers for Disease Control. Achievements in public health, 1900–1999: Healthier mothers and babies. *MMWR.* 1999; 48(38):849.

54. Centers for Disease Control. Contribution of birth defects to infant mortality—United States, 1986. *MMWR.* 1989;38:633.

55. Anderson RN, Kochanek KD, Murphy SL. *Report of the Final Mortality Statistics, 1995.* Monthly Vital Statistics Report, vol 45, no. 11, suppl 2. Hyattsville, MD: US Department of Health and Human Services, Centers for Disease Control, National Center for Health Statistics, 1997.

56. National Center for Health Statistics. *Vital Statistics of the United States, 1968, vol II, Mortality, Part A.* Health Services and Mental Health Administration Publication No. (HSM) 72-1101. Rockville, MD: US Department of Health, Education and Wellfare, Public Health Service, Centers for Disease Control, 1972.

57. Ventura SJ, Martin JA, Curtin SC, Mathews TJ. *Report of Final Natality Statistics, 1995.* Monthly Vital Statistics Report, vol 45, no. 11, suppl 2. Hyattsville, MD: US Department of Health and Human Services, Centers for Disease Control, National Center for Health Statistics, 1997.

58. Leck I. Fetal malformations. In: Barron SL, Thomson AM, eds. *Obstetrical Epidemiology.* London: Academic Press; 1983;263.

59. Emery AEH, Rimoin D. Nature and incidence of genetic disease. In: Emery AEH, Rimoin D, eds. *Principles and Practice of Medical Genetics.* Edinburgh: Churchill Livingstone; 1983;1.

60. Lorber J. The effect of spina bifida on family life. In: Beard RW, ed. *Diagnosis and Management of Neural Tube Defects.* London: Royal College of Obstetricians and Gynaecologists; 1978;133.

61. Main DM, Mennuti MT. Neural tube defects: Issues in prenatal diagnosis and counseling. *Obstet Gynecol.* 1986;67:1.

62. Fraser FC. Relation of animal studies to the problem in man. In: Wilson JH, Fraser FC, eds. *Handbook of Teratology, vol 1.* New York: Plenum; 1977:75.

63. Kalter H, Warkany J. Congenital malformations: Etiologic factors and their role in prevention (first of two parts). *N Engl J Med.* 1983;308:424.

64. Jones KL. *Smith's Recognizable Patterns of Human Malformation.* Philadelphia: WB Saunders; 1988.

65. Daker M, Bobrow M. Screening for genetic disease and fetal anomaly during pregnancy. In: Chalmers I, Enkin M, Keirse MJNC, eds. *Effective Care in Pregnancy and Childbirth.* Oxford: Oxford University Press; 1989;366.

66. Lie RT, Wilcox AJ, Skjærven R. A population-based study of the risk of recurrence of birth defects. *N Engl J Med.* 1994;331:1.

67. Mattison DR, Macina OT. Characterizing risks for developmental toxicity: Effects of drugs and chemicals on the fetus. In: Reece EA, Hobbins JC, eds. *Medicine of the Fetus and Mother.* Philadelphia: Lippincot-Raven, 1999:327.

68. Finnel RH. Teratology: General considerations and principles. *J Allergy Clin Immunol.* 1999;103:S337.

69. Brent RL, Beckman DA. Prescribed drugs, therapeutic agents and fetal teratogenesis. In: Reece EA, Hobbins JC, eds. *Medicine of the Fetus and Mother.* Philadelphia: Lippincot-Raven; 1999:289.

70. Donald I, Brown TG. Localization using physical devices, radioisotopes and radiographic methods. I: Demonstration of tissue interfaces within the body by ultrasonic echo sounding. *Br J Radiol.* 1961;34:539.

71. Sunden B. The diagnostic value of ultrasound in obstetrics and gynecology. *Acta Obstet Gynecol Scand.* 1964;43:121.

72. Campbell S, Holt EM, Johnstone FD, May P. Anencephaly: Early ultrasonic diagnosis and active management. *Lancet.* 1972;2:1226.

73. Shapiro I, Degani S, Timor-Tritsch I. Prenatal sonographic diagnosis of inner epicanthal fold: A new marker of chromosomal abnormalities. Abstract 26, presented at the IV World Congress of Ultrasound in Obstetrics and Gynecology, Budapest, Hungary, 1994.

74. Merz E. Application of transvaginal and abdominal three-dimensional ultrasound for the detection or exclusion of malformations of the fetal face. *Ultrasound Obstet Gynecol.* 1997;4:237.

75. Chan L, Uerpairojkit B, Reece EA. Diagnosis of congenital malformations using two-dimensional and three-dimensional ultrasonography. *Obstet Gynecol Clin.* 1997;24:49.

76. Platt LD, Santulli T Jr, Carlson DE, et al. Three-dimensional ultrasonography in obstetrics and gynecology: Preliminary experience. *Am J Obstet Gynecol.* 1998;178:1199.

77. Shih JC, Shyu MK, Lee CN, et al. Antenatal depiction of the fetal ear with three-dimensional ultrasonography. *Obstet Gynecol.* 1998;91:500.

78. Merz E. Three-dimensional ultrasound—A requirement for prenatal diagnosis? *Ultrasound Obstet Gynecol.* 1998;12:225.

79. Merz E. Prenatal diagnosis of ambiguous gender using three-dimensional sonography. *Ultrasound Obstet Gynecol.* 1999;13:217.

80. Baba K, Okai T, Kozuma S, Taketani Y. Fetal abnormalities: Evaluation with real-time processible three-dimensional US—Preliminary report. *Radiology.* 1999;211:441.

81. Cullen MT, Green J, Whetham J, et al. Transvaginal ultrasonographic detection of congenital anomalies in the first trimester. *Am J Obstet Gynecol.* 1990;163:466.

82. Rottem S, Bronshtein M. Transvaginal sonographic diagnosis of congenital anomalies between 9 and 16 weeks, menstrual age. *J Clin Ultrasound.* 1990;18:307.

83. Bronshtein M, Zimmer EZ, Milo S, et al. Fetal cardiac abnormalities detected by transvaginal sonography at 12–16 weeks' gestation. *Obstet Gynecol.* 1991;78:374.

84. Gembruch U, Knöpfle G, Chatterjee M, et al. Prenatal diagnosis of atrioventricular canal malformations with up-to-date echocardiographic technology: Report of 14 cases. *Am Heart J.* 1991;121:1489.

85. Gembruch U, Knöpfle G, Chatterjee M, et al. First-trimester diagnosis of fetal congenital heart disease by transvaginal two-dimensional and Doppler echocardiography. *Obstet Gynecol.* 1990;75:496.

86. Henshaw RC, Smith APM, Smith NC, Murray GI. Multiple fetal anomalies in the first trimester; detection using transvaginal ultrasound and therapeutic abortion using mifepristone (RU486) in conjunction with gemeprost vaginal pessaries. *Br J Obstet Gynaecol.* 1992;99:258.

87. Bronshtein M, Zimmer EZ, Gerlis M, et al. Early ultrasound diagnosis of fetal congenital heart defects in high-risk and low-risk pregnancies. *Obstet Gynecol.* 1993;82:225.

88. Schmidt W, Yarkoni S, Crelin ES, Hobbins JC. Sonographic visualization of physiologic anterior abdominal wall hernia in the fist trimester. *Obstet Gynecol.* 1987;69:911.

89. Curtis JA, Watson L. Sonographic diagnosis of omphalocele in the first trimester of fetal gestation. *J Ultrasound Med.* 1988;7:97.

90. Blas HGK. The examination of the embryo and early fetus: How and by whom? *Ultrasound Obstet Gynecol.* 1999;14:153.

91. Romero R, Cullen M, Jeanty P, et al. The diagnosis of congenital renal anomalies with ultrasound. II: Infantile polycystic kidney disease. *Am J Obstet Gynecol.* 1984;150:259.

92. Simpson JL, Sabbagha RE, Elias S, et al. Failure to detect polycystic kidneys in utero by second trimester ultrasonography. *Hum Genet.* 1982;60:259.

93. Saari-Kemppainen A, Karjalainen O, Ylostalo P, Heinonen OP. Ultrasound screening and perinatal mortality: Controlled trial of systematic one-stage screening in pregnancy. The Helsinki Ultrasound Trial. *Lancet.* 1990;336:387.

94. Levi S, Hyjazi Y, Schaaps JP, et al. Sensitivity and specificity of routine antenatal screening for congenital anomalies by ultrasound: The Belgian multicentric study. *Ultrasound Obstet Gynecol.* 1991;1:102.

95. Rosendahl H, Kivenen S. Antenatal detection of congenital malformations by routine ultrasonography. *Obstet Gynecol.* 1989;73:947.

96. Carrera JM. Routine prenatal ultrasound screening for fetal abnormalities: 22 years' experience. *Ultrasound Obstet Gynecol.* 1995;5:174.

97. Shirley IM, Bottomley F, Robinson VP. Routine radiographer screening for fetal abnormalities by ultrasound in an unselected low risk population. *Br J Radiol.* 1992;65:564.

98. Chitty LS, Hunt GH, Moore J, Lobb MO. Effectiveness of routine ultrasonography in detecting fetal structural abnormalities in a low risk population. *Br Med J.* 1991;303:1165.

99. Luck CA. Value of routine ultrasound scanning at 19 weeks: A four year study of 8,849 deliveries. *Br Med J.* 1992;304:1474.

100. Crane JP, LeFevre ML, Winborn RC, et al. A randomized trial of prenatal ultrasonographic screening: Impact on the detection, management, and outcome of anomalous fetuses. *Am J Obstet Gynecol.* 1994;171:392.

101. Skupski DW, Newman S, Edersheim T, et al. The impact of routine obstetric ultrasonographic screening in a low-risk population. *Am J Obstet Gynecol.* 1996;175:1142.

102. VanDorsten JP, Hulsey TC, Newman RB, Menard MK. Fetal anomaly detection by second-trimester ultrasonography in a tertiary center. *Am J Obstet Gynecol.* 1998;178:742.

103. Magriples U, Copel JA. Accurate detection of anomalies by routine ultrasonography in an indigent clinic population. *Am J Obstet Gynecol.* 1998;179:978.

104. Smith NC, Hau C. A six year study of the antenatal detection of fetal abnormality in six Scottish health boards. *Br J Obstet Gynaecol.* 1999;106:206.

105. Eurenius K, Axelsson O, Cnattingius S, et al. Second trimester ultrasound screening performed by midwives; sensitivity for detection of fetal anomalies. *Acta Obstet Gynecol Scand.* 1999;78:98.

106. Grandjean H, Larroque D, Levi S, EUROFETUS team. Sensitivity of routine ultrasound screening of prengnancies in the Eurofetus database. *Ann N Y Acad Sci.* 1998;847:118.

107. Hill LM, Breckle R, Gehrking WC. Prenatal detection of congenital malformations by ultrasonography. *Am J Obstet Gynecol.* 1985;151:44.

108. Lys F, De Wals P, Borlee-Grimee I, et al. Evaluation of routine ultrasound examination for the prenatal diagnosis of malformation. *Eur J Obstet Gynecol Reprod Biol.* 1989;30:101.

109. Mida M, Gondry J, Verhoest P, et al. Évaluation de l'écographie. A propos d'une série en continu de 100 grossess. *Rev Gynecol Obstet.* 1989;84:627.

110. Sabbagha RE, Shikh Z, Tamura RK, et al. Predictive value, sensitivity and specificity of ultrasonic targeted imaging for fetal anomalies in gravid women at high risk for birth defects. *Am J Obstet Gynecol.* 1985;152:822.

111. Sollie JE, van Geijn HP, Arts NFT. Validity of a selective policy for ultrasound examination of fetal congenital anomalies. *Eur J Obstet Gynecol Reprod Biol.* 1988;27:125.

112. Manchester DK, Pretorius DH, Avery C, et al. Accuracy of ultrasound diagnoses in pregnancies complicated by suspected fetal anomalies. *Prenat Diagn.* 1988;8:109.

113. Gonçalves LF, Jeanty P, Piper JM. The accuracy of ultrasonography in detecting congenital malformations. *Am J Obstet Gynecol.* 1994;171:1606.

114. Ott WJ, Arias F, Sheldon G, et al. Comprehensive ultrasound examination in a private perinatal practice. *Am J Perinatol.* 1995;12:385.

115. Achiron R, Glaser J, Gelernetr I, et al. Extended fetal echocardiographic examination for detecting cardiac malformation in low-risk pregnancies. *Br Med J.* 1992;304:671.

116. Sandor GG, Farquarson D, Wittmann B, et al. Fetal echocardiography: Results in high-risk patients. *Obstet Gyencol.* 1986;67:358.

117. Benacerraf BR, Pober BR, Sanders SP. Accuracy of fetal echocardiography. *Radiology.* 1987;165:847.

118. Copel JA, Pilu G, Green J, et al. Fetal echocardiographic screening for congenital heart disease: The importance of the four-chamber view. *Am J Obstet Gynecol.* 1987;157:648.

119. Crawford D, Chita SK, Allan SD. Prenatal detection of congenital heart disease: Factors affecting obstetrical management and survival. *Am J Obstet Gynecol.* 1988;169:352.

120. Callan NA, Maggio M, Steger S, Kan JS. Fetal echocardiography: Indications for referral, prenatal diagnoses and outcomes. *Am J Perinatol.* 1991;8:390.

121. Bromley B, Estroff JA, Sanders SP, et al. Fetal echocardiography: Accuracy and limitations in a population at high and low risk for heart defects. *Am J Obstet Gynecol.* 1992;166:1473.

122. Achiron R, Glaser J, Gelernter I, et al. Extended fetal echocardiographic examination for detecting cardiac malformations in low risk pregnancies. *Br Med J.* 1992;304:671.

123. Rustico MA, Benettoni A, D'Ottavio GD, et al. Fetal heart screening in low-risk pregnancies. *Ultrasound Obstet Gynecol.* 1995;6:313.

124. Ott WJ. The accuracy of antenatal fetal echocardiography screening in high- and low-risk patients. *Am J Obstet Gynecol.* 1995;172:1741.

125. Giancotti A, Torcia F, Giampa G, et al. Prenatal evaluation of congenital heart disease in high-risk pregnancies. *Clin Exp Obstet Gynecol.* 1995;12:225.

126. Stümpflen I, Stümpflen A, Wimmer M, Bernaschek G. Effect

of detailed fetal echocardiography as part of routine prenatal ultrasonographic screening on detection of congenital heart disease. *Lancet.* 1996;348:854.

127. Buskens E, Grobbee DE, Frohn-Mulder IME, et al. Efficacy of routine fetal ultrasound screening for congenital heart disease in normal pregnancy. *Circulation.* 1996;94:67.

128. Todros T, Faggiano F, Chiappa E, et al. Accuracy of routine ultrasonography in screening heart disease prenatally. Gruppo Piomontese for Prenatal Screening of Congenital Heart Disease. *Prenat Diagn.* 1997;17:901.

129. Stoll C, Alembik Y, Dott B, et al. Evaluation of prenatal diagnosis of congenital heart disease. *Prenat Diagn.* 1998;18:801.

130. Klein SK, Cans C, Robert E, Jouk PS. Efficacy of routine fetal ultrasound screening for heart disease in Isere County, France. *Prenat Diagn.* 1999;19:318.

131. Hafner E, Scholler J, Schuchter K, et al. Detection of fetal congenital heart disease in a low-risk population. *Prenat Diagn.* 1999;18:808.

132. Benacerraf BR, Lister JE, DuPonte BL. First-trimester diagnosis of fetal abnormalities. A report of three cases. *J Reprod Med.* 1988;33:777.

133. Rottem S, Bronshtein M. Transvaginal sonographic diagnosis of congenital anomalies between 9 weeks and 16 weeks menstrual age. *J Clin Ultrasound.* 1990;18:307.

134. Cullen MT, Green J, Whetham J, et al. Transvaginal ultrasonographic detection of congenital anomalies in the first trimester. *Am J Obstet Gynecol.* 1990;163:466.

135. Rottem S, Bronshtein M, Thaler I, Brandes JM. First trimester transvaginal sonographic diagnosis of fetal anomalies. *Lancet.* 1989;1:444.

136. Achiron R, Tadmor O. Screening for fetal anomalies during the first trimester of pregnancy: Transvaginal versus transabdominal sonography. *Ultrasound Obstet Gynecol.* 1991;1:186.

137. Bronshtein M, Zimmer EZ, Milo S, et al. Fetal cardiac abnormalities detected by transvaginal sonography at 12–16 weeks' gestation. *Obstet Gynecol.* 1991;78:374.

138. Gembruch U, Knöpfle G, Chatterjee M, et al. Prenatal diagnosis of atrioventricular canal malformations with up-to-date echocardiographic technology: Report of 14 cases. *Am Heart J.* 1991;121:1489.

139. Gembruch U, Knöpfle G, Chatterjee M, et al. First-trimester diagnosis of fetal congenital heart disease by transvaginal two-dimensional and Doppler echocardiography. *Obstet Gynecol.* 1990;75:496.

140. Henshaw RC, Smith APM, Smith NC, Murray GI. Multiple fetal anomalies in the first trimester, detection using transvaginal ultrasound and therapeutic abortion using mifepristone (RU486) in conjunction with gemeprost vaginal pessaries. *Br J Obstet Gynecol.* 1992;99:258.

141. Bronshtein M, Zimmer EZ, Gerlis M, et al. Early ultrasound diagnosis of fetal congenital heart defects in high-risk and low-risk pregnancies. *Obstet Gynecol.* 1993;82:225.

142. Bonilla-Musoles FM, Raga F, Ballester MJ, Serra V. Early detection of embryonic malformations by transvaginal and color Doppler sonography. *J Ultrasound Med.* 1994;13:347.

143. D'Ottavio G, Meir YJ, Rustico MA, et al. Pilot screening for fetal malformations: Possibilities and limits of transvaginal sonography. *J Ultrasound Med.* 1995;14:575.

144. Yagel S, Achiron R, Ron M, et al. Transvaginal ultrasonogra-

phy cannot be used alone for targeted organ ultrasonographic examination in a high-risk population. *Am J Obstet Gynecol.* 1995;172:971.

145. Hernádi L, Töröcsik M. Screening for fetal anomalies in the 12th week of pregnancy by transvaginal sonography in an unselected population. *Prenat Diagn.* 1997;17:753.

146. D'Ottavio GG, Mandruzzato G, Meir YJ, et al. Comparison of first and second trimester screening for fetal anomalies. *Ann N Y Acad Sci.* 1998;847:200.

147. Whitlow BJ, Chatzipapas IK, Lazanakis ML, et al. The value of sonography in early pregnancy for the detection of fetal abnormalities in an unselected population. *Br J Obstet Gynaecol.* 1999;106:929.

148. Whitlow BJ, Economides DL. The optimal gestational age to examine fetal anatomy and measure nuchal translucency in the first trimester. *Ultrasound Obstet Gynecol.* 1998;11:258.

149. Macintosh MCM, Wald NJ, Chard T, et al. The selective miscarriage of Down's syndrome from 10 weeks of pregnancy. *Br J Obstet Gynaecol.* 1996;103:1171.

150. Snijders RJM, Sebire NJ, Nicolaides KH. Maternal age and gestational age specific risk from chromosomal defects. *Ultrasound Obstet Gynecol.* 1995;6:250.

151. Blanch G, Quenby S, Ballantyne ES, et al. Embryonic abnormalities at medical termination of pregnancy with mifepristone and misoprostol during first trimester: Observational study. *Br Med J.* 1998;316:1712.

152. Souka A, Heath V. Increased nuchal translucency with normal karyotype. In: Nicolaides KH, Sebire NJ, Snijders RJM, eds. *The 11–14 Week Scan: The Diagnosis of Fetal Abnormalities.* New York: Parthenon Publishing; 1999:67.

153. Von Kaisenberg C, Hyett J. Pathophysiology of increased nuchal translucency. In: Nicolaides KH, Sebire NJ, Snijders RJM, eds. *The 11–14 Week Scan: The Diagnosis of Fetal Abnormalities.* New York: Parthenon Publishing; 1999:109.

154. Brizot ML, Noble P. Nuchal translucency and maternal serum biochemistry. In: Nicolaides KH, Sebire NJ, Snijders RJM, eds. *The 11–14 Week Scan: The Diagnosis of Fetal Abnormalities.* New York: Parthenon Publishing; 1999:38.

155. Sanders RC. Legal problems related to obstetrical ultrasound. *Ann N Y Acad Sci.* 1998;847:220.

156. Copel JA, Pilu G, Kleinman CS. Congenital heart disease and extracardiac anomalies: Associations and indications for fetal echocardiography. *Am J Obstet Gynecol.* 1986;154:1121.

157. Copel JA, Pilu G, Green J, et al. Fetal echocardiographic screening for congenital heart disease: The importance of the four-chamber view. *Am J Obstet Gynecol.* 1987;157:648.

158. Platt LD, DeVore GR, Lopez E, et al. Role of amniocentesis in ultrasound-detected fetal malformations. *Obstet Gynecol.* 1986;68:153.

159. Williamson RA, Weiner CP, Patil S, et al. Abnormal pregnancy sonogram: Selective indication for fetal karyotype. *Obstet Gynecol.* 1987;69:15.

160. Palmer CG, Miles JH, Howard-Peebles PN, et al. Fetal karyotype following ascertainment of fetal anomalies by ultrasound. *Prenat Diagn.* 1987;7:551.

161. Epstein CJ. *The Consequences of Chromosome Imbalance: Principles, Mechanisms and Models.* Cambridge: Cambridge University Press; 1986:3.

162. Romero R, Hobbins JC, Mahoney MJ. Fetal blood sampling

and fetoscopy. In: Milunsky A, ed. *Genetic Disorders and the Fetus.* New York: Plenum; 1986:571.

163. Nicolaides KH, Rodeck C, Gosden CM. Rapid karyotyping in non-lethal fetal malformations. *Lancet.* 1986;1:283.

164. Holzgreve W, Beller FK, Buchhols B, et al. Kidney transplantation from anencephalic donors. *N Engl J Med.* 1987;316:1069.

165. McCullagh P. *The Foetus as Transplant Donor; Scientific, Social and Ethical Perspective.* Chichester, England: Wiley; 1987.

166. Hill LM. Sonographic detection of fetal gastrointestinal anomalies. *Ultrasound Q.* 1988;6:35.

167. Chervenak FA, Duncan C, Ment L, et al. Perinatal management of meningomyelocele. *Obstet Gynecol.* 1985;53:376.

168. Ralis ZA. Traumatizing effect of breech delivery on infants with spina bifida. *J Pediatr.* 19875;87:613.

169. Stark G, Drummond M. Spina bifida as an obstetric problem. *Dev Med Chil Neurol.* 1970;22(suppl):157.

170. Bensen JT, Dillard RG, Burton BK. Open spina bifida: Does cesarean section delivery improve prognosis? *Obstet Gynecol.* 1988;71:532.

171. Nicolaides KH. Fetal therapy. *Curr Opin Obstet Gynecol.* 1990;2:268.

172. Nicolini U. Prenatal diagnosis and fetal therapy. *Curr Opin Obstet Gynecol.* 1993;5:50.

173. Evans MI, Adzick NS, Johnson MP, et al. Fetal therapy—1994. *Curr Opin Obstet Gynecol.* 1994;6:58.

174. Merrill DC, Weiner C. Fetal medicine. *Curr Opin Obstet Gynecol.* 1992;4:273.

175. Adzick NS, Harrison MR. Fetal surgical therapy. *Lancet.* 1994;343:897.

176. Albanese CT, Harrison MR. Surgical treatment for fetal disease. *Ann N Y Acad Sci.* 1998;847:74.

177. Chaoui R, Bollmann R, Göldner B, Rogalsky V. Aortic balloon valvuloplasty in the human fetus under ultrasonographic guidance: A report of two cases. Abstract 266, presented at the IV World Congress of Ultrasound in Obstetrics and Gynecology, Budapest, Hungary, 1994.

178. Maxwell D, Allan L, Tynan MJ. Balloon dilatation of the aortic valve in the fetus: A report of two cases. *Br Heart J.* 1991;65:256.

179. McCurdy CM, Childers JM, Seeds JW. Ligation of the umbilical cord of an acardiac-acephalus twin with an endoscopic intrauterine technique. *Obstet Gynecol.* 1993;82:708.

180. Quintero RA, Reich H, Puder KS, et al. Umbilical cord ligation of an acardiac twin by fetoscopy at 19 weeks of gestation. *N Engl J Med.* 1994;330:469.

181. Quintero RA, Gonçalves LF, Berry S, et al. Endoscopic and ultrasound-guided umbilical cord ligation in abnormal monochorionic twin gestations. Abstract 122a, presented at the IV World Congress of Ultrasound in Obstetrics and Gynecology, Budapest, Hungary, 1994.

182. Ville Y, Hyett JA, Vandenbussche F, Nicolaides KH. Endoscopic laser coagulation of umbilical cord vessels in twin reversed arterial perfusion sequence. *Ultrasound Obstet Gynecol.* 1994;4:1.

183. De Lia JE, Cruikshank DP, Keye WR. Fetoscopic neodymium: YAG laser occlusion of placental vessels in severe twin–twin transfusion syndrome. *Obstet Gynecol.* 1990;75:1046.

184. De Lia JE, Kuhlmann, Hartad T, Cruikshank D. Twin–twin transfusion syndrome treated by fetoscopic neodymium: YAG laser occlusion in chorioangiopagus. *Am J Obstet Gynecol.* 1993;168:308.

185. Ville Y, Hecher K, Ogg D, et al. Successful outcome after Nd:YAG laser separation of chorioangiopagus-twins under sonoendoscopic control. *Ultrasound Obstet Gynecol.* 1992;2:429.

186. De Lia JE, Cruikshank DP. Feticide versus laser surgery for twin–twin transfusion syndrome. *Am J Obstet Gynecol.* 1994;170:1480.

187. Quintero RA, Gonçalves LF, Guevara F, et al. Color Doppler-guided coagulation of abnormal communicating vessels in twin–twin transfusion syndrome. Abstract 122b, presented at the IV World Congress of Ultrasound in Obstetrics and Gynecology, Budapest, Hungary, 1994.

188. Ville Y, Hyett J, Hecher K, Nicolaides KH. Management of severe twin–twin transfusion syndrome: Amniodrainage compared to endoscopic surgery. Abstract 196, presented at the IV World Congress of Ultrasound in Obstetrics and Gynecology, Budapest, Hungary, 1994.

189. Quintero RA, Reich H, Gonçalves LF, et al. Human endoscopic fetal surgery. Abstract 195, presented at the IV World Congress of Ultrasound in Obstetrics and Gynecology, Budapest, Hungary, 1994.

190. VanderWall KJ, Bruch SW, Meuli M, et al. Fetal endoscopic ('FETENDO') tracheal clip. *J Pediatr Surg.* 1996;31:1101.

191. Harrison MR, Mychaliska GB, Albanese CT, et al. Correction of congenital diaphragmatic hernia in utero. IX: Fetuses with poor prognosis (liver herniation and low lung-to-head ratio) can be served by fetoscopic temporary tracheal occlusion. *J Pediatr Surg.* 1998;33:1017.

192. Quintero RA, Morales WJ, Phillips J, et al. In utero lysis of amniotic bands. *Ultrasound Obstet Gynecol.* 1997;10:316.

193. *Diagnostic Ultrasound Imaging in Pregnancy.* Washington, DC: National Institutes of Health; 1984.

194. Ewigman BG, Crane JP, Frigoletto FD, et al. A randomized trial of prenatal ultrasound screening in a low risk population: Impact on perinatal outcome. *N Engl J Med.* 1993;329:7 812.

195. LeFevre ML, Bain RP, Ewigman BG, et al. A randomized trial of prenatal ultrasound screening: Impact on maternal management and outcome. *Am J Obstet Gynecol.* 1993;169:483.

196. Waldestrom U, Nilsson S, Fall O, et al. Effects of routine one-stage ultrasound screening in pregnancy: A randomized controlled trial. *Lancet.* 1988;2:585.

197. Bakketeing LS, Jacobsen G, Brodtkorb CJ, et al. Randomized controlled trial of ultrasonographic screening in pregnancy. *Lancet.* 1984;2:207.

198. Ewigman B, LeFebre M, Hesser J. A randomized trial of routine prenatal ultrasound. *Obstet Gynecol.* 1990;76:189.

199. Bucher HC, Schmidt JG. Does routine ultrasound scanning improve outcome in pregnancy? Meta-analysis of various outcome measures. *Br Med J.* 1993;307:13.

200. Levi S, Chervenak FA. Preface: Ultrasound screening for fetal anomalies, is it worth it? Screening revisited after the EUROFETUS data. *Ann N Y Acad Sci.* 1998;847:ix.

201. Romero R. Routine obstetrical ultrasound (editorial). *Ultrasound Obstet Gynecol.* 1993;3:303.

202. Romero R, Gonçalves LF, Gomez R. Equal time: Should ultrasound be routine. *Contemp Obstet Gynecol.* 1993;11:9.

203. Gonçalves LF, Romero R. A critical appraisal of the RADIUS study. *Fetus.* 1993;3:8000-7.

204. Hudgens DR, Conradi SE. Sudden death associated with terbutaline sulfate administration. *Am J Obstet Gynecol.* 1993;169:120.

205. Hannah ME, Hannah WJ, Hellmann J, et al. Induction of labor as compared with serial antenatal monitoring in post-term pregnancy: A randomized controlled trial. *N Engl J Med.* 1992;326:1587.

206. DeVore GR. Clinical commentary: The routine antenatal diagnostic imaging with ultrasound study: Another perspective. *Obstet Gynecol.* 1994;84:622.

207. Vintzileos AM, Ananth CV, Fisher AJ, et al. Cost–benefit analysis of targeted ultrasonography for prenatal detection of spina bifida in patients with an elevated concentration of second-trimester maternal serum alpha-fetoprotein. *Am J Obstet Gynecol.* 1999;10:1227.

208. Albanese CT, Harrison MR. Surgical treatment for fetal disease: The state of the art. *Ann N Y Acad Sci.* 1998;847:74.

209. Zerella JT, Finberg FJ. Obstruction of the neonatal airway from teratomas. *Surg Gynecol Obstet.* 1990;170:126.

210. Abu-Harb M, Hey E, Wren C. Death in infancy from unrecognized congenital heart disease. *Arch Dis Child.* 1994;71:3.

211. Chang AC, Huhta JC, Yoon GY, et al. Diagnosis, transport, and outcome in fetuses with left ventricular outflow tract obstruction. *J Thorac Cardiovasc Surg.* 1991;102:841.

212. Copel JA, Tan AS, Kleinman CS. Does a prenatal diagnosis of congenital heart disease alter short-term outcome? *Ultrasound Obstet Gynecol.* 1997;10:237.

213. Skari H, Bjornland K, Bjornstad-Ostensen A, et al. Consequences of prenatal ultrasound diagnosis: A preliminary report on neonates with congenital malformations. *Acta Obstet Gynecol Scand.* 1998;77:635.

214. Dillon E, Renwick M. The antenatal diagnosis and management of abdominal wall defects: The northern region experience. *Clin Radiol.* 1995;50:855.

215. Zimmer EZ, Avraham Z, Sujoy P, et al. The influence of prenatal ultrasound on the prevalence of congenital anomalies at birth. *Prenat Diagn.* 1997;17:623.

216. Forrester MB, Merr RD, Yoon PW. Impact of prenatal diagnosis and selective termination on the prevalence of selected birth defects in Hawaii. *Am J Epidemiol.* 1998;148:1206.

217. Roberts HE, Moore CA, Cragan JD, et al. Impact of prenatal diagnosis on the birth prevalence of neural tube defects, Atlanta, 1990–1991. *Pediatrics.* 1995;96:880.

218. International Clearing House for Birth Defects Monitoring Systems. *Annual Report 1998.* Rome: The International Centre for Birth Defects; 1998.

219. Allan LD, Cook A, Sullivan I, Sharland GK. Hypoplastic left heart syndrome: Effects of fetal echocardiography on birth prevalence. *Lancet.* 1991;337:959.

220. Lin AE, Herring AH, Amstutz KS, et al. Cardiovascular malformation: Changes in prevalence and birth status, 1972–1990. *Am J Med Genet.* 1999;84:102.

221. Wilkins-Haug L. Considerations for delivery of infants with congenital abnormalities. *Obstet Gynecol Clin.* 1999;25:399.

222. Kliegman RM. Maternal medication and the fetus. In: Behrman RE, Kliegman RM, Arvin AM, eds. *Nelson Textbook of Pediatrics,* 15th ed. Philadelphia: WB Saunders; 1996:448.

16

Prenatal Diagnosis of Cerebrospinal Anomalies

*Gianluigi Pilu • Roberto Romero • Sandro Gabrielli •
Antonella Perolo • Luciano Bovicelli*

The prevalence of congenital anomalies of the central nervous system (CNS) varies depending on ethnicity, type of ascertainment, and length of follow-up. Long-term follow-up studies in the United States and Europe have suggested an incidence of about 1 in 100 births.[1,2] The CNS was the first to be investigated *in utero* with diagnostic ultrasound. Anencephaly was the first congenital anomaly to be recognized by this technique before viability.[3] Since then, the investigation of the fetal neural axis has remained a central issue in antenatal sonography. Such an interest is explained by a number of reasons. Central nervous system anomalies are frequent and often have a severe prognosis. In many cases, these anomalies have a genetic background, and consequently, many couples at risk demand antenatal diagnosis. Modern, high-resolution ultrasound equipment has a unique potential in evaluating normal and abnormal anatomy of the fetal neural axis from the very early stages of development, but identification of selected anomalies remains a challenge in many cases. In this chapter, the sonographic investigation of the fetal brain and the identification of CNS anomalies are reviewed.

SONOGRAPHY OF THE DEVELOPING FETAL BRAIN

Transvaginal high-frequency high-resolution probes show in great detail details of the developing cerebrum (Figs. 16–1 and 16–2). The interested reader is referred to specific publications on this subject.[4–6]

In the midtrimester, an adequate survey of fetal brain morphology can be performed by using two axial planes that are easily and rapidly obtained in most pregnancies (Fig. 16–3).[7] From cephalad to caudad, these views demonstrate the lateral ventricles and choroid plexuses, the diencephalon and surrounding structures, and the posterior fossa. Coronal and sagittal views are more difficult to obtain and often require a transvaginal scan. However, these views may become necessary in targeted examinations for a proper evaluation of the midline structures and to assess the symmetry of the two hemispheres.[8]

VENTRICULOMEGALY

The incidence of congenital enlargement of the cerebral ventricles ranges from 0.3 to 1.5 in 1000 births.[2] This range

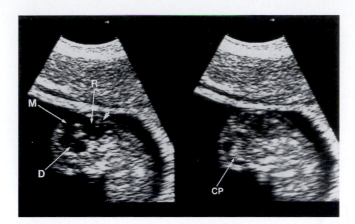

Figure 16–1. Transvaginal sonography of the cephalic pole at 10 weeks' gestation. The primary cerebral vesicles are seen. In the *left panel,* a midsagittal view demonstrates the rostrad diencephalic vesicle (D), the intermediate mesencephalic vesicle (M), and the caudad rhombencephalic vesicle (R) that appear as sonolucent spaces with a typically convoluted pattern. The developing choroid plexus fold of the fourth ventricle is seen dissecting the rhombencephalic vesicle *(arrowhead).* In the *right panel,* a more lateral view demonstrates the small glomus of the developing choroid plexus (CP) marking the telencephalic vesicle.

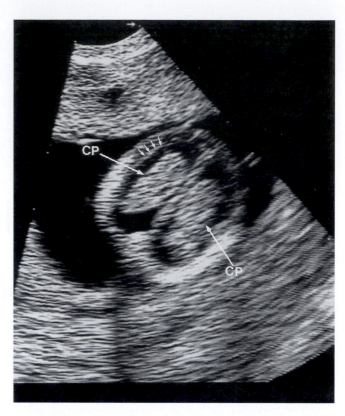

Figure 16–2. Transvaginal sonogram. At 12 weeks' gestation the brightly echogenic choroid plexuses (CP) dominate the intracranial cavity. The thin sonolucent cortex is also demonstrated *(arrows).*

may represent an underestimation because most available surveys are based on clinical ascertainment, and, in many cases, enlarged ventricles are presumably asymptomatic at birth.

The cerebral lateral ventricles have a complex tridimensional architecture that undergoes major developmental changes throughout gestation. It is not surprising that sonographic assessment of these structures have been the object of many studies and that many different approaches to the definition and diagnosis of fetal ventriculomegaly have been proposed. Reference charts have been established for the different portions of the lateral ventricles, measured in both standard axial planes and coronal and sagittal sections.[9–12] However, measurement of the transverse diameter of the ventricular atrium at the level of the glomus of the choroid plexus is favored at present (Fig. 16–4).[7,13] In general, this measurement is easily obtained and has been found to be highly reproducible.[14] Different studies have reported very similar results in the midtrimester, with a mean value of the atrial width of approximately 7 mm and a standard deviation of about 1 mm. There is less agreement on the normal values in the third trimester.[15] Some degree of asymmetry of the lateral ventricles exists in the human fetal brain and is detectable *in utero.*[16] Male fetuses have slightly but significantly larger measurements than female fetuses.[17,18]

The term *borderline ventriculomegaly* is commonly used to refer to cases with an atrial width of 10 to 15 mm. This finding is associated with an increased risk of heterogeneous nervous and non-CNS anomalies. When isolated, border-

line ventriculomegaly has no consequences, in most cases. However, in a minority of cases, this finding may be the earliest manifestation of brain damage from heterogeneous causes including primary cerebral maldevelopment (e.g., obstructive hydrocephalus, lissencephaly) and destructive lesions (e.g., periventricular leukomalacia) deriving from hypoxia or infections. A review of 234 cases showed an abnormal outcome in 23% of cases.[15] Perinatal death occurred in 4%, usually in association with severe growth retardation, premature delivery, or intrauterine infections. Chromosomal anomalies, primarily trisomy 21, were present in 4%; malformations were undetected at a second-trimester sonogram in 9%; and neurologic sequelae, mostly a delay in cognitive or motor development of mild to moderate severity, were present in 11%. The risk of an abnormal neurologic outcome was increased in females versus males, when the atrial width was 12 mm or more, and when the diagnosis was made in the second trimester rather than later in gestation. Borderline ventriculomegaly may be unilateral, and it has been suggested that in this case it is usually a benign finding. However, the data are limited, and chromosomal aberrations and neurologic sequelae have been documented even in these infants.[19]

The optimal management of isolated borderline ventriculomegaly remains uncertain. Although it is unclear

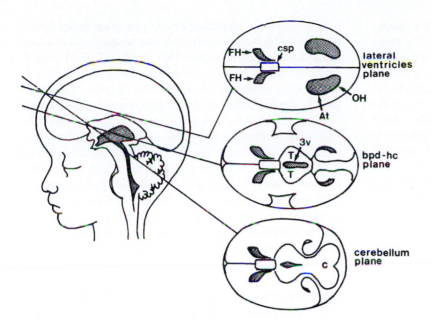

Figure 16–3. Schematic representation of three scanning planes that allow visualization of the relevant intracranial fetal anatomy. From rostrad to caudad, the first plane demonstrates the lateral ventricles; the second plane is used to measure biparietal diameter (bpd) and head circumference (hc); the third plane reveals the cerebellum within the posterior fossa. FH, Frontal Horns; csp, cavitas septi pellucidum; At, Atrium; OH, Occipital Horn; T, Thalami; 3v, third ventricle; c, cerebellum.

whether or not this finding is an independent risk factor for aneuploidy, it would seem prudent to offer a procedure for fetal karyotyping. A TORCH screen is also commonly recommended, although an association has not been demonstrated thus far. Isolated borderline ventriculomegaly may be the harbinger of severe cerebral lesions that cannot be predicted in early gestation. This occurs rarely, but it is obviously a reason for major concern. Fetal magnetic resonance imaging (MRI) has recently been employed to diagnose subtle cerebral maldevelopment in fetuses with borderline ventriculomegaly.[20] Unfortunately, the diagnostic capability of this technique before fetal viability is still relatively undetermined.

Overt enlargement of the cerebral lateral ventricles, or *hydrocephalus*, is usually defined on the basis of an atrial width of more than 15 mm in the second and third trimesters. Although fetal hydrocephalus may be an isolated finding, it is found more frequently with other cerebral anomalies, usually neural tube defects and midline anomalies. Fetuses with isolated overt ventriculomegaly diagnosed *in utero* at our

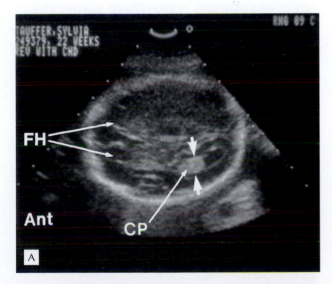

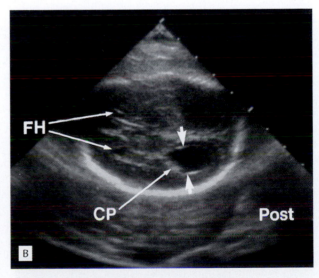

Figure 16–4. Axial scans at similar levels in a normal fetus and in a fetus with hydrocephalus. **(A)** Normalcy is indicated by brightly echogenic choroid plexus (CP) that entirely fills the lumen of the atrium, being closely apposed to both medial and lateral walls of the ventricle *(arrowheads).* **(B)** Hydrocephalus is attested by anterior displacement of the shrunken choroid plexus that appears clearly detached from the medial wall of the ventricle. FH, Frontal Horns of Lateral Ventricles; Ant, Anterior; Post, Posterior.

institution were usually found at birth to have either *acqueductal* stenosis or communicating hydrocephalus. The prognosis of this condition remains unclear. Extrapolation of data from available pediatric series has limitations. In a review of the prenatal literature, isolated ventriculomegaly was associated with a postnatal survival rate of 70%, and 59% of the survivors had a normal developmental quotient at follow-up.[21]

Congenital hydrocephalus has genetic implications. It should be stressed that the experience thus far indicates that antenatal ultrasound is unreliable for predicting the recurrence of isolated hydrocephalus, in particular the X-linked variety, because in many cases enlargement of the lateral ventricles only develops late in gestation or after birth.[22] DNA analysis for the X-linked variety is now available and should be considered, although the exact sensitivity remains to be determined.[23]

NEURAL TUBE DEFECTS

The diagnosis of anencephaly is easy during the midtrimester and relies on the demonstration of the absence of the cranial vault. Although the fetal head can be positively identified by vaginal sonography as early as the 7th week of gestation, the diagnosis may be difficult in the first trimester. Anencephaly is considered to be the final stage of acrania, as a consequence of disruption of abnormal brain tissue unprotected by the calvarium.[24,25] A cephalic pole, albeit overtly abnormal, therefore is usually present in early gestation. A recent prospective study has suggested, however, that anencephaly can be reliably predicted even at 10 to 14 weeks of gestation (Fig. 16–5).[26]

Sonographic identification of open *spina bifida* is usually possible during the early midtrimester but requires expertise and meticolous scanning (Figs. 16–6 and 16–7). Examination of the fetal head can assist the sonologist in the difficult task of diagnosing this lesion. Variable degrees of displacement of the cerebellar vermis, fourth ventricle, and medulla oblongata through the foramen magnum inside the upper cervical canal (a condition referred to as Arnold–Chiari or Chiari type II malformation) is present in virtually all cases and results in obliteration of the cisterna magna and in the small size and abnormal shape of the cerebellum that is impacted deep into the posterior fossa.[27] The term *banana sign* is commonly used to define this condition. Frontal bossing (lemon sign) is also frequently present (Fig. 16–8). A variable degree of ventricular enlargement is present in virtually all cases of open spina bifida at birth but in fewer than 70% of cases in midtrimester (Fig. 16–9). The sensitivity of this cranial sign in identifying spina bifida exceeds 99%.[28] The available evidence suggests that false-negative findings are probably limited only to cases with skin-covered lesions, which tend to offer a much better prognosis. False-positive findings are virtually nonexistent for the cerebellar signs. However, the lemon sign is found in 1 to 2% of normal fetuses.

The accuracy of ultrasound in the diagnosis of spina bifida depends on the experience of the operator, the quality of the equipment, and the time dedicated to the scan. The accuracy of referral centers is close to 100%. The accuracy of routine nontargeted examinations is uncertain. The largest prospective studies on low-risk patients have reported

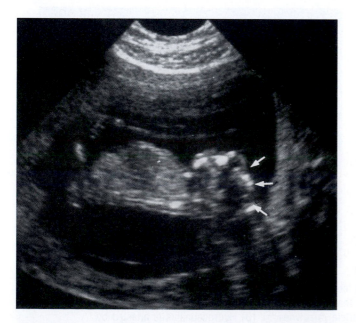

Figure 16–5. Transvaginal sonography demonstrates absence of the cephalic pole *(arrows)* in a 12-week fetus. This is anencephaly.

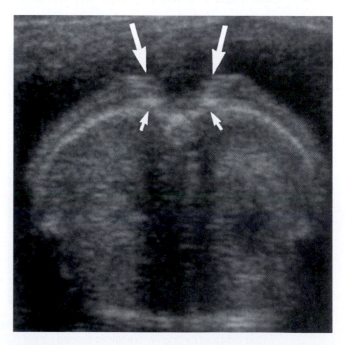

Figure 16–6. Transverse scan of the fetal trunk in a fetus with spina bifida. *Large arrows* indicate a soft tissue defect; *small arrows* indicate widely separated ossification centers of the posterior processes.

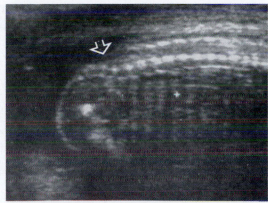

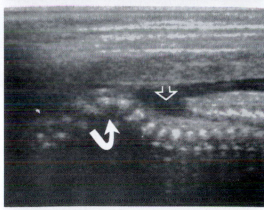

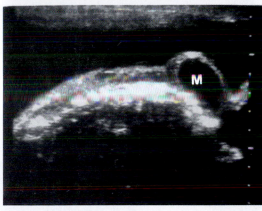

Figure 16–7. Sagittal views demonstrating spectrum of spina bifida. From *top* to *bottom*, sacral spina bifida *(open arrow)*, thoracolumbar spina bifida *(open arrow)* with severe associated kyphoscoliosis, and complete rachischisis with cervical meningocele (M). *(Reproduced with permission from Pilu G, Romero R, Reece EA, et al. Am J Obstet Gynecol. 1988;158:1052.)*

conflicting results. In the two largest studies performed in Belgium, presumably without maternal serum α-fetoprotein screening, the sensitivities were 30 and 40%.[29,30] In the RADIUS trial, in which routine ultrasound was performed in conjunction with maternal α-fetoprotein screening, the sensitivity was 80%.[31] In one retrospective study conducted in the United Kingdom, the estimated sensitivity was higher for serum α-fetoprotein screening (84 to 92%) than for

ultrasound screening (70 to 84%).[32] In all of these studies, it is unclear whether the cranial signs of fetal spina bifida were systematically examined. In a more recent retrospective multicenter study employing cranial signs, the sensitivity of ultrasound was 85%.[33] Nevertheless, the available evidence thus far indicates that maternal serum α-fetoprotein screening, which is the standard of care in many European countries and in the United States, has a marginally greater sensitivity than ultrasound.

Different strategies for α-fetoprotein screening in pregnancy exist, and the interested reader is referred to specific publications on this subject.[34,35] One important problem that has not been solved is the evaluation of patients with a positive screening test. Expert sonography, also known in the United States as a level II ultrasound examination, has virtually 100% diagnostic accuracy for malformations associated with increased maternal serum α-fetoprotein,[36] and amniocentesis does carry some risk to the fetus. Consequently, some centers have elected to limit examination of patients with positive screen tests to ultrasound.[34] Others prefer to perform amniocentesis to select patients for level II examinations because of various considerations; the most important ones being the decrease in the need for expert sonographic examinations and the availability of ancillary tests performed on amniotic fluid such as the presence of acetylcholinesterase.[35]

MIDLINE ANOMALIES

The *holoprosencephalies* are complex abnormalities of the forebrain that are postulated to derive from a failure in the diverticulation of the embryonic prosencephalon. These conditions are characterized mainly by abnormal midline separation of the cerebral hemispheres and diencephalic structures. The most widely accepted classification of these disorders recognized three major varieties: alobar, semilobar, and lobar. Alobar and semilobar holoprosencephalies are associated almost invariably with typical facial abnormalities including cyclopia, hypotelorism, and median cleft lip. The incidence of holoprosencephaly at birth is uncertain, but this anomaly has been found in 1 of 250 voluntary terminations of pregnancy,[37] suggesting a high intrauterine fatality rate. The etiology is heterogeneous. In most cases, the anomaly is isolated and sporadic. In other cases, chromosomal abnormalities are found (trisomy 13 and polyploidy)[38] as are other congenital anatomic deformities such as anencephaly, Dandy–Walker malformation, encephalocele, and DiGeorge and Meckel syndromes. Several familial cases suggest genetic inheritance with autosomal dominant transmission.

Prenatal diagnosis of alobar and semilobar holoprosencephalies depends on the demonstration of a single rudimentary cerebral ventricle (Fig. 16–10). Additional findings include the presence of a cyst on the top of the brain, also

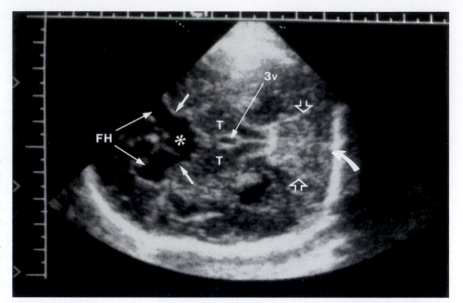

Figure 16–8. Axial view of the head in a fetus with spina bifida. Transverse diameter of the cerebellum *(open arrows)* is decreased and the cisterna magna is obliterated *(curved arrow)*. The ample communication (∗) between enlarged frontal horns (FH) secondary to disruption of the cavum septum pellucidi, and the square appearance of the ventricles, secondary to hypertrophy of caudate nucleus *(straight arrows)*, are typical signs of Arnold–Chiari malformation. T, Thalami; 3v, third ventricle.

referred to as the *dorsal sac,* and typical facial anomalies.[39,40] The diagnosis has been made as early as the first trimester.[41] Recognition of the lobar variety has also been reported. Diagnosis requires a midcoronal scan demonstrating the absence of the cavum septum pellucidum and central fusion of the frontal horns, which have a flat squared roof and communicate amply with the inferior third ventricle (Fig. 16–11).[42] The presence of the fused fornices, which appear as a linear structure running within the third ventricle from the anterior to the posterior commissure, is a frequent and very specific finding with this condition.[43] Mild to overt ventriculomegaly is usually present and the face is normal.

The invariably poor prognosis for infants affected by alobar and semilobar holoprosencephalies is well established. The outcome of infants with the lobar variety is uncertain. Severe obstructive hydrocephalus, usually deriving from a concomitant acqueductal stenosis, is frequently found. Thus far, cases diagnosed *in utero* have demonstrated extremely poor neurologic development.[42]

Agenesis of the corpus callosum is an anomaly of uncertain prevalence and clinical significance. The incidence differs among studies, depending on the population investigated and the method of ascertainment. Estimates of 0.3 to 0.7% in the general population and of 2 to 3% in the developmentally disabled are usually quoted. The etiology is

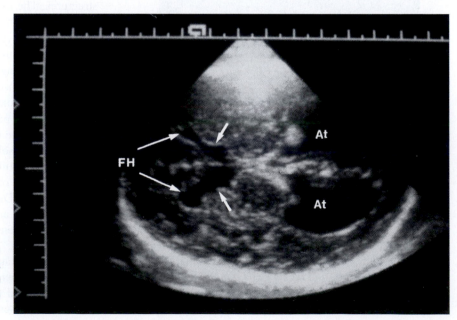

Figure 16–9. Hydrocephalus in a fetus with spina bifida. Hypertrophy of the caudate nucleus *(arrows)* results in a typical square appearance of the frontal horns (FH). At, Atria of lateral ventricles.

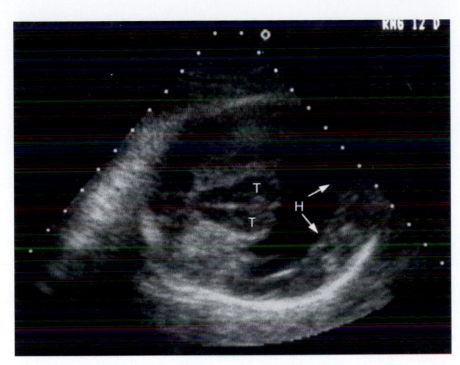

Figure 16–10. Axial view of the fetal head demonstrating a central rudimentary single ventricle (H), lined anteriorly by pancaked frontal cortex and posteriorly by bulblike thalami (T). The third ventricle cannot be demonstrated. This is alobar holoprosencephaly. *(Reproduced with permission from Pilu G, Romero R, Rizzo N, et al. Am J Perinatol. 1987;4:41.)*

heterogenous. Genetic factors are probably important. Autosomal dominant, autosomal recessive, and sex-linked transmission have all been documented. Agenesis of the corpus callosum is also a part of many Mendelian syndromes. The

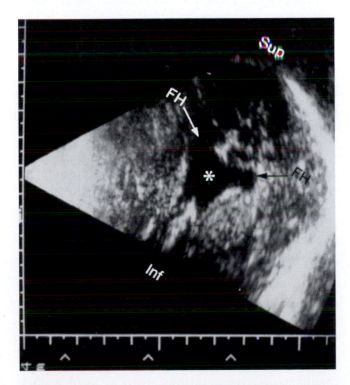

Figure 16–11. Coronal view of the head demonstrating frontal horns (FH) that have a flat roof and amply communicate (∗). This is lobar holoprosencephaly. Sup, superior; Inf, inferior.

high frequency of associated malformations suggests that agenesis of the corpus callosum is often a part of a widespread developmental disturbance. In one antenatal series, anatomic anomalies were present in 50% of cases, most frequently Dandy–Walker malformation and congenital heart disease. An abnormal karyotype (trisomy 18 and 8) was found in 20%.[44]

Agenesis of the corpus callosum is associated with subtle findings, and the diagnosis of this condition is a challenge even for expert sonologists, in particular before 20 weeks.[45] Development of the corpus callosum is a late event in cerebral ontogenesis that takes place between 12 and 18 weeks of gestation; before 18 weeks, the diagnosis is probably impossible in most cases. In routine examinations performed after this time, failure to visualize the cavum septum pellucidum or an increased atrial width should suggest the possibility of agenesis of the corpus callosum (Fig. 16–12).

Once a suspicion has been formulated, more specific findings can be searched for. Direct demonstration of the absence of the corpus callosum is possible by midcoronal and midsagittal scans (Fig. 16–13). These views are at times difficult to obtain, in particular, fetuses in vertex presentation. Nevertheless, vaginal sonography is of great advantage in such cases.[44]

Agenesis of the corpus callosum may be either complete or partial. In the latter case, also referred to as *dysgenesis of the corpus callosum,* the caudad portion (splenium and body) is missing to different degrees. Complete agenesis is commonly regarded as a malformation deriving from faulty embryogenesis, whereas partial agenesis may represent both a true malformation and a disruptive event occurring at any time during pregnancy. Furthermore, the sonographic

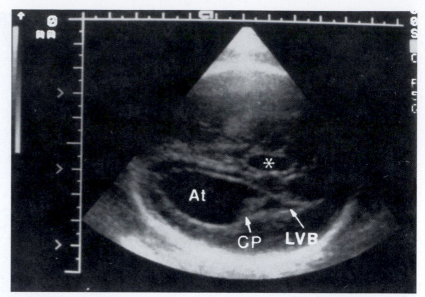

Figure 16–12. Axial view of the head demonstrating a striking enlargement of the atria (At) and wide separation of the bodies of lateral ventricles (LVB). Cystic structure on midline (∗) is the upwardly displaced third ventricle. This is agenesis of the corpus callosum. CP, Choroid Plexus.

findings associated with partial agenesis are probably more subtle than those with the complete form. Therefore, antenatal diagnosis will not be possible in all cases.

The prognosis of isolated agenesis of the corpus callosum remains unclear. Many authorities believe that agenesis of the corpus callosum has little consequence on neurologic development. However, no specific risk figures are available at present. A total of 30 infants with a prenatal diagnosis of isolated agenesis of the corpus callosum (no other malformations demonstrable at sonography and a normal karyotype) and a postnatal follow-up from a few months to 11 years has been reported thus far. A normal or borderline development was present in 26 cases, or 87%.[46,47]

The term *Dandy–Walker syndrome* was introduced to indicate the association of 1) ventriculomegaly of variable degree, 2) a large cisterna magna, and 3) a defect in the cerebellar vermis through which the cyst communicates with the fourth ventricle.

In more recent years, different definitions have been proposed to indicate a group of posterior fossa abnormalities similar to those of the classic Dandy–Walker syndrome. Most of these definitions refer with the following findings: 1) cystic dilatation of the fourth venticle, 2) dysgenesis of the cerebellar vermis, and 3) a high position of the tentorium. At present, the term *Dandy–Walker complex* is used to indicate a spectrum of anomalies of the posterior fossa that are classified by axial computed tomography as follows: classic Dandy–Walker malformation (enlarged posterior fossa, complete or partial agenesis of the cerebellar vermis, elevated tentorium), Dandy–Walker variant (variable hypoplasia of the cerebellar vermis with or without enlargement of the posterior fossa), and megacisterna magna (enlarged cisterna magna with integrity of both cerebellar vermis and fourth ventricle). This classification was challenged after the introduction of MRI. For a number of reasons, the axial scans traditionally employed in computed tomography do not have

the capability of clearly assessing the status of the cerebellar vermis and may underestimate or overestimate the size of the defect. The excellent resolution of sagittal planes made possible by MRI has demonstrated that the classification based on computed tomography axial planes is inadequate to describe the anatomic derangement encountered in the Dandy–Walker complex. Some degree of vermian dysgenesis can be found in all cases, even with megacisterna magna, whereas classic Dandy–Walker malformation and Dandy–Walker variant have so many similarities that a clear-cut distinction is often impossible.[48]

Although hydrocephalus has been classically considered an essential diagnostic element of this condition, more recent evidence suggests that, even with classic Dandy–Walker, ventriculomegaly is not overtly present at birth in most patients but develops usually in the first months of life.[49]

The Dandy–Walker malformation has an estimated prevalence of about 1 in 30,000 births and has been found in 4 to 12% of all cases of infantile hydrocephalus.[50] The incidence of Dandy–Walker variant and megacisterna magna is unknown.

The Dandy–Walker malformation is frequently associated with other neural defects, usually ventriculomegaly, and other midline anomalies such as agenesis of the corpus callosum, holoprosencephaly, and cephaloceles. Other deformities include polycystic kidneys, cardiovascular defects, and facial clefting. Postnatal studies indicate a frequency of associated malformation ranging between 50 and 70%.

The sonographic diagnosis of classic Dandy–Walker malformation is straightforward from midgestation (Fig. 16–14)[51] and has been reported as early as 14 weeks by using vaginal sonography.[52] In the transcerebellar view, an enlarged cisterna magna is connected to the area of the fourth ventricle through a defect in the cerebellar vermis. Borderline to overt ventriculomegaly and other neural and extraneural malformations are frequently present.

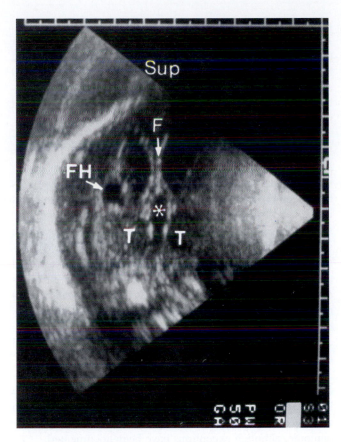

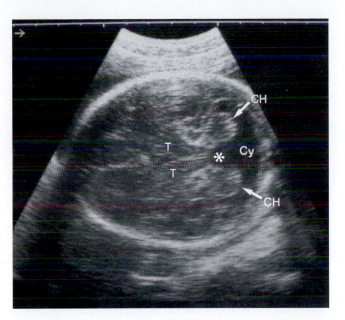

Figure 16–14. The fourth ventricle (∗) amply communicates with a cystic cisterna magna (Cy) through a wide defect of the cerebellar vermis. Cerebellar hemispheres (CH) are widely separated. This is Dandy–Walker malformation. T, Thalami.

Figure 16–13. Coronal scan of the head in the same case as Figure 16–12. Absence of corpus callosum is clearly demonstrated by visualization of the falx cerebri (F) that comes in close contact with the upwardly displaced third ventricle (∗). Note the wide distance between midline and frontal horn (FH), distal to the transducer. T, Thalami; Sup, superior.

However, in cases with partial agenesis of the vermis confined to the inferior portion, the traditional transcerebellar view can appear normal, and meticulous scanning may be required to identify the defect. Demonstration (in a lower section) that the inferior cerebellar vermis separates the fourth ventricle from the cisterna magna is required to rule out this condition.

Criteria for a definitive diagnosis of megacisterna magna and Dandy–Walker variant in the fetus have not been firmly established. The former condition should be suspected when the cisterna magna has a depth greater than 10 mm,[53] and the latter when a thin communication is found between the fourth ventricle and the cisterna magna.[54] Caution is warranted in making these diagnoses. In the early second trimester, the sonographic appearance of the normal cerebellar development can resemble pathology; the relatively large fourth ventricle and the incompletely formed inferior cerebellar vermis may give the false impression of a vermian defect.[55,56] Therefore, it is not prudent to diagnose a defect in the vermis at this gestational age. A follow-up scan at 18 weeks or later is recommended, even in the second and

third trimesters. A scanning angle too steep may create the impression of an excessively large cisterna magna and even of a vermian defect.[57,58] The origin of this artifact is unclear. It has been speculated that it may be caused by fluid within the vallecula cerebelli that tends to expand slightly in the anterior aspect, and it has a very thin membranous roof. The juxtaposition of the vallecula with the adjacent cerebellar tonsils creates the impression of a connection between the fourth ventricle and the cisterna magna, similar to that described by computed tomography studies of Dandy–Walker variant. Visualization of the posterior fossa in the median plane may be helpful in these cases because it allows the visualization of the vermis in the sagittal plane, but it is unlikely that even this approach will allow an accurate identification of subtle dysgenesis of the cerebellum such as those described in postnatal MRI studies. In our experience, the vast majority of fetuses with either an isolated enlargement of the cisterna magna or an image suggestive of a small vermian defect was found to be entirely normal at birth by both neuroimaging and clinical evaluation. On the other hand, despite meticulous multiplanar imaging, we have been unable to demonstrate any cerebellar defect in a fetus that had a borderline cisterna magna who was found at birth to have Dandy–Walker variant and overt ventriculomegaly requiring a shunt.

On the basis of both the available evidence and our own experience, we believe that antenatal sonography allows a certain diagnosis only of the most severe anatomic varieties of the Dandy–Walker complex, that is, those characterized by both an enlarged cisterna magna and a wide defect in the cerebellar vermis; commonly referred to as classic

Dandy–Walker malformation. Experience thus far is limited with less severe varieties. It is usually impossible to solve antenatally the doubt of either a large cisterna magna or a small inferior defect of the vermis.

Classic Dandy–Walker malformation is usually clinically manifest within the first year of life, with symptoms of hydrocephalus or other neurologic symptoms. Mortality rates as high as 24% have been reported in the first neurosurgical series, but, because of advances in pediatric anesthesia and surgical techniques, deaths have become less common. Prognosis regarding the intellectual development in survivors is controversial. Given the low frequency of this condition, only limited series are available. Nevertheless, subnormal intelligence has been reported in 40 to 70% of cases.[49,50,59]

The clinical significance of Dandy–Walker variant and megacisterna magna is uncertain. These conditions are frequently seen in association with neurologic compromise, but no clear-cut prognostic data exist. Prenatal series have documented a frequent association with other malformations or chromosomal aberrations.[53,54]

DESTRUCTIVE CEREBRAL LESIONS

Congenital *porencephaly* is defined as the presence of cystic cavities within the brain matter. The cavities may communicate with the ventricular system, the subarachnoid space, or both. Loss of cerebral tissue may derive from a morphogenetic disorder (true porencephaly or schizencephaly). More frequently, it is the consequence of an intrauterine disruption (pseudoporencephaly or encephaloclastic porencephaly). The developmental form may be bilateral and symmetrical and is frequently associated with microcephaly. In pseudoporencephaly a unilateral lesion is usually found (Fig. 16–15). In both cases, there is a wide variability in the size of the lesion. Cerebrospinal fluid turnover is often impaired, and hydrocephalus is present. *Hydranencephaly* can be regarded as an extreme form of pseudoporencephaly. Most of the cerebral hemispheres are replaced by fluid. The brainstem and rhomboencephalic structures are usually spared (Fig. 16–16). The head may be small, of normal size, or extremely enlarged. The etiology is heterogeneous. Congenital infections including toxoplasmosis and cytomegalovirus and intrauterine strangulation or occlusion of the internal carotid arteries have been reported. *Schizencephaly* is associated with clefts in the fetal brain connecting the lateral ventricles with the subarachnoid space and is often found with absence of the septum pellucidum. *Encephaloclastic porencephaly* is characterized by an intraparenchymal cyst often connected with the lateral ventricles, the subarachnoid space, or both and is almost constantly associated with ventriculomegaly. Accurate antenatal diagnosis of both *schizencephaly* and *porencephaly* has been reported.[60] It should be stressed that porencephaly is a disruption that usually occurs only in the third trimester.

The outcome of infants with congenital destructive process of the brain is dictated by the size and location of the lesion. Extensive porencephaly, particularly when associated with hydrocephalus or microcephaly, tends to have a poor outcome, although exceptions have been documented.

DISORDERS OF NERVE CELL PROLIFERATION

The association between decreased head size and reduction of both brain mass and total cell number in *microcephalic*

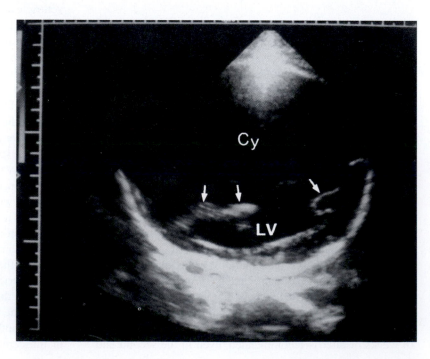

Figure 16–15. Porencephaly. There is gross distortion of intracranial anatomy and a conspicuous shift of midline echo *(arrows)*. A fluid-filled collection replaces the cerebral hemisphere close to the transducer and amply communicates with the contralateral lateral ventricle (LV). Cy, Cyst.

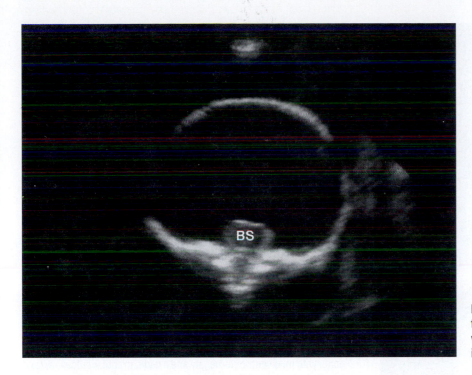

Figure 16–16. Coronal scan of the head of a third trimester fetus. Brain stem (BS) bulges within fluid that fills the intracranial cavity. This is hydranencephaly.

infants is well established. However, the threshold of abnormalcy is uncertain. Some authors have suggested employing a head circumference below −2 standard deviations from the mean as diagnostic criterion. Others prefer to consider head circumference below −3 standard deviations as abnormal. The incidence of microcephaly obviously differs in different surveys, depending on the definition used to identify the lesion.

Microcephaly should not be considered a single clinical entity but rather a symptom of many etiologic disturbances. The clinical subdivision proposed by Book et al.[61] distinguishes between those cases resulting from environmental insults (infections, anoxia, radiations, etc.) and genetic microcephaly, which includes all those cases in which microcephaly is inherited as a Mendelian trait, either alone or as a part of a recognized syndrome.

Microcephaly is characterized by a typical disproportion in size between the skull and the face. The forehead is sloping. The brain is small, with the cerebral hemispheres affected to a greater extent than the diencephalic and rhombencephalic structures. Abnormal convolutional patterns, including macrogyria, microgyria, and agyria, are frequently found. The ventricles may be enlarged. Microcephaly is frequently found in cases of porencephaly, lissencephaly, and holoprosencephaly.

Many difficulties arise in attempting to identify fetal microcephaly.[62] The usefulness of head measurements alone is limited by incorrect dating or intrauterine growth retardation. Furthermore, the natural history of fetal microcephaly is largely unknown. A progressive development of the lesion interfering with early recognition has been described.

A comparison of biometric parameters such as the ratio of the head circumference to the abdominal circumference and the ratio of the femur length to the biparietal diameter has been suggested.[63] Nevertheless, both false-positive and false-negative diagnoses occur frequently.[64] It is clear that the predictive value of ultrasound biometry has limitations. A qualitative evaluation of the intracranial structures is a useful adjunct to biometry because many cases of microcephaly are associated with morphologic derangements in particular with ventriculomegaly, schizencephaly, and disorders of ventral induction.[65] A nomogram of the normal dimensions of the frontal lobes has been developed and may prove useful.[66] Recently, in two midtrimester fetuses with microcephaly, transvaginal sonography showed aberrant findings including large subarachnoid spaces and a rudimentary shape of the lateral ventricles. Demonstration of a sloping forehead also increases the index of suspicion (Fig. 16–17).[67]

The outcome of microcephaly is uncertain. In a study of 28 infants with head circumference below −2 standard deviations from the mean, only 50% were mentally retarded.[68] In another study of infants with a head circumference between −2 and −3 standard deviations from the mean 18% of cases were mentally retarded and infants with a head circumference below −3 standard deviations from the mean were mentally retarded in 72% of cases.[69] It is clear that a small head size does not necessarily imply mental retardation.

Megalencephaly, an abnormally large brain, is usually found in individuals of normal and even superior intelligence, but it may be associated with mental retardation and neurologic impairment.[70] Obstetric and pediatric sonographers

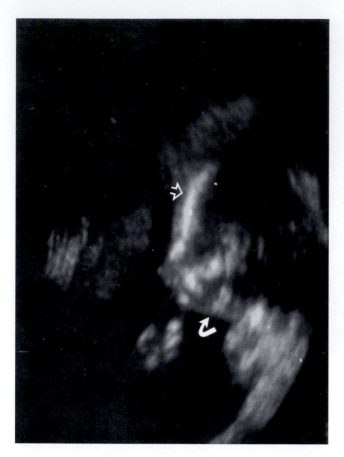

Figure 16–17. In this midtrimester fetus with microcephaly and multiple anomalies, a sagittal view of the face reveals a sloping forehead *(open arrow)* and striking micrognathia *(curved arrow)*. *(Reproduced with permission from Romero R, Pilu G, Jeanty P, et al. Prenatal Diagnosis of Congenital Anomalies. Norwalk, CT: Appleton & Lange; 1987.)*

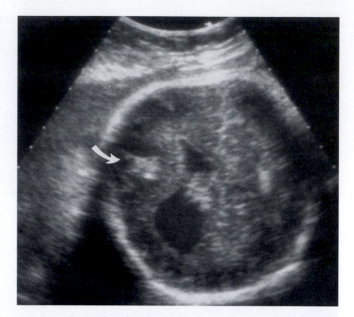

Figure 16–18. Unilateral megalencephaly. A coronal sonogram of the head of a third trimester fetus demonstrates a shift of the midline echo, with mild ventriculomegaly and a wide, irregular sulcus *(arrow)* within the surface of the predominant hemisphere.

are frequently challenged by the problem of megalencephaly, a condition that should be suspected in the presence of abnormally large head measurements without evidence of hydrocephalus or intracranial masses. In such cases, examination of the parents may be helpful because asymptomatic megalencephaly is frequently familial.

Unilateral megalencephaly is a rare anomaly of unknown etiology characterized by overgrowth of one lobe or an entire hemisphere and has been occasionally associated with hemigigantism of the body. Anatomic dissection in these cases shows aberrant convolutional patterns, ectopic nodules of gray matter, and a diffuse increase in neuronal size. Sonographic findings include enlargement of one cerebral hemisphere in the absence of a mass effect, a shift of the midline structures, and mild ipsilateral ventriculomegaly (Fig. 16–18). Although a rare condition, unilateral megalencephaly has been identified *in utero* with sonography,[71] and it should be considered in the differential diagnosis of conditions associated with a shift of the midline echo, which also include porencephaly and congenital brain tumors. Mental

retardation and uncontrolled seizures have been described in affected infants.

CONCLUSIONS

Modern ultrasound equipment has a unique role in the evaluation of the normal and abnormal fetal CNS from very early in pregnancy. A large number of congenital anomalies can be consistently recognized. Criteria for identification of nervous malformations are well established. Transvaginal sonography is extending antenatal diagnosis to very early gestation. It should be stressed that some cerebral anomalies are the consequence of disruptions or developmental disorders. Failure to diagnose severe cerebral lesions in early gestation has been documented in several publications.[45,60,62] Postnatal ascertainment of many cerebral anomalies is difficult and requires long-term follow-up studies. Two large prospective studies, the RADIUS trial and the EUROFETUS study, have reported a sensitivity in the range of 80% for the detection of CNS malformations.[45,72] However, postnatal ascertainment was based mostly on clinical examination of infants in the first days after birth. Thus, these results should be interpreted with caution. Eventually, when a fetal CNS anomaly is detected, counseling the parents and devising a sensible obstetric management is frequently difficult. Some CNS anomalies have outcomes that can be predicted with reasonable precision. This is certainly the case with catastrophic lesions such as anencephaly and severe holoprosencephaly and with anomalies that are invariably detected at birth such as spina bifida.

However, many conditions can be identified *in utero* but have an unclear natural history. Agenesis of the corpus callosum, minor forms of holoprosencephaly, and intracranial cysts are remarkable examples of this. Fetal sonography can also identify new entities that were previously undescribed, the most remarkable example being borderline cerebral ventriculomegaly. It is important to note that at present there is quite a dramatic discrepancy between the diagnostic capability of antenatal ultrasound, which is high and the understanding of the prognostic implications of anatomic alterations, which is limited from many points of view.

REFERENCES

1. McIntosh R, Merritt KK, Richards MR. The incidence of congenital anomalies. A study of 5,964 pregnancies. *Pediatrics.* 1954;14:505–510.

2. Myrianthopoulos NC. Epidemiology of central nervous system malformations. In: Vinken PJ, Bruyn GW, eds. *Handbook of Clinical Neurology.* Amsterdam: Elsevier; 1977:139–171.

3. Campbell S, Johnstone FD, Holt EM. Anencephaly: Early ultrasonic diagnosis and active management. *Lancet.* 1972;2:1226.

4. Timor-Tritsch IE, Monteagudo A, Warren WB. Transvaginal sonography of the central nervous system in the first and early second trimester. *Am J Obstet Gynecol.* 1991;164:1689–1693.

5. Blaas HG, Eik-Nes SH, Kiserud T, Hellerik LR. Early development of the forebrain and midbrain: A longitudinal ultrasonographic study from 7 to 12 weeks of gestation. *Ultrasound Obstet Gynecol.* 1994;4:183–192.

6. Blaas HG, Eik-Nes SH, Kiserud T, Hellerik LR. Early development of the hindbrain: A longitudinal ultrasonographic study from 7 to 12 weeks of gestation. *Ultrasound Obstet Gynecol.* 1995;5:151–160.

7. Filly RA, Cardoza JD, Goldstein RB, Barkovich AJ. Detection of fetal central nervous system anomalies. A practical level of effort for a routine sonogram. *Radiology.* 1989;172:403–410.

8. Timor Tritsch IE, Monteagudo A. Transvaginal neurosonography: Standardization of the planes and sections by anatomic landmarks. *Ultrasound Obstet Gynecol.* 1996;8:42–50.

9. Goldstein I, Reece EA, Pilu G, et al. Sonographic development of the normal developmental anatomy of fetal cerebral ventricles: I. The frontal horns. *Obstet Gynecol.* 1988;72:588–592.

10. Goldstein I, Reece EA, Pilu G, Hobbins JC. Sonographic evaluation of the normal developmental anatomy of the fetal cerebral ventricles. IV: The posterior horn. *Am J Perinatol.* 1990;7:79–83.

11. Pilu G, Reece EA, Goldstein I, et al. Sonographic evaluation of the normal developmental anatomy of the fetal cerebral ventricles: II. The atria. *Obstet Gynecol.* 1989;73:250–255.

12. Monteagudo A, Timor Tritsch IE, Moomjy M. Nomograms of the lateral ventricles using transvaginal sonography. *J Ultrasound Med.* 1993;12:265–269.

13. Cardoza JD, Goldstein RB, Filly RA. Exclusion of fetal ventriculomegaly with a single measurement: The width of the lateral ventricular atrium. *Radiology.* 1988;169:711–714.

14. Heiserman J, Filly RA, Goldstein RB. The effect of measurement errors on the sonographic evaluation of ventriculomegaly. *J Ultrasound Med.* 1991;10:121–124.

15. Pilu G, Falco P, Gabrielli S, et al. The clinical significance of fetal isolated cerebral borderline ventriculomegaly: Report of 31 cases and review of the literature. *Ultrasound Obstet Gynecol.* 1999;14:320–326.

16. Achiron R, Yagel S, Rotstein Z, et al. Cerebral lateral ventricular asymmetry: Is this a normal ultrasonographic finding in the fetal brain? *Obstet Gynecol.* 1997;89:233–237.

17. Patel MD, Goldstein RB, Tung S, Filly RA. Fetal cerebral ventricular atrium: Difference in size according to sex. *Radiology.* 1995;194:713–715.

18. Nadel AS, Benacerraf BR. Lateral ventricular atrium: Larger in male than female fetuses. *Int J Gynecol Obstet.* 1995;51:123–126.

19. Lipitz A, Malinger G, Meizner I, et al. Outcome of fetuses with isolated borderline unilateral ventriculomegaly diagnosed at mid-gestation. *Ultrasound Obstet Gynecol.* 1998;12:23–26.

20. Greco P, Resta M, Vimercati A, et al. Antenatal diagnosis of isolated lissencephaly by ultrasound and magnetic resonance imaging. *Ultrasound Obstet Gynecol.* 1998;12:276–279.

21. Gupta JK, Bryce F, Lilford RJ. Management of apparently isolated fetal ventriculomegaly. *Obstet Gynecol Surv.* 1994;49:716–722.

22. Rogers JC, Danks DM. Prenatal diagnosis of sex-linked hydrocephalus. *Prenat Diagn.* 1983;3:269–273.

23. Serville F, Benit P, Saugier P, et al. Prenatal exclusion of X-linked hydrocephalus-stenosis of the aceduct of Sylvius sequence using closely linked DNA markers. *Prenat Diagn.* 1993;13:435–439.

24. Bronshtein M, Ornoy A. Acrania: Anencephaly resulting from secondary degeneration of a closed neural tube. Two cases in the same family. *J Clin Ultrasound.* 1991;19:230–232.

25. Timor-Tritsch IE, Greenebaum E, Monteagudo A, Baxi L. Exencephaly–anencephaly sequence: Proof by ultrasound imaging and amniotic fluid cytology. *J Mater Fetal Med.* 1996;5:182–185.

26. Johnson SP, Sebire NJ, Snijders RJM, et al. Ultrasound screening for anencephaly at 10–14 weeks. *Ultrasound Obstet Gynecol.* 1997;9:14–18.

27. Nicolaides KH, Campbell S, Gabbe SG, Guidetti R. Ultrasound screening for spina bifida: Cranial and cerebellar signs. *Lancet.* 1986;2:72–74.

28. Watson WJ, Cheschier NC, Katz VL, Seeds JW. The role of ultrasound in the evaluation of patients with elevated maternal serum alpha-fetoprotein: A review. *Obstet Gynecol.* 1991;78:123–128.

29. Levi S, Hijazi Y, Schaaps JP, et al. Sensitivity and specificity of routine antenatal screening for congenital anomalies by ultrasound: The Belgian multicentric study. *Ultrasound Obstet Gynecol.* 1991;1:102–110.

30. Levi S, Schaaps JP, De Havay P, et al. End-result of routine ultrasound screening for congenital anomalies: The Belgian multicentric study. *Ultrasound Obstet Gynecol.* 1995;5:366–371.

31. Ewigman BG, Crane JP, Frigoletto FD, et al. Effect of prenatal ultrasound screening on perinatal outcome. *N Engl J Med.* 1993;329:821–826.

32. Williamson P, Alberman E, Rodeck C, et al. Antecedent circumstances surrounding neural tube defect births in 1990–91.

The Steering Committee of the National Confidential Enquiry into Counselling for Genetic Disorders. *Br J Obstet Gynaecol.* 1997;104:51–55.

33. Sebire NJ, Noble PL, Thorpe-Beeston JG, et al. Presence of the 'lemon' sign in fetuses with spina bifida at the 10–14-week scan. *Ultrasound Obstet Gynecol.* 1997;10:403–407.

34. Nadel AS, Norton ME, Wilkins-Haug L. Cost-effectiveness of strategies used in the evaluation of pregnancies complicated by elevated maternal serum alpha-fetoprotein levels. *Obstet Gynecol.* 1997;89:660–665.

35. Filly RA, Callen PW, Goldstein RB. Alpha-fetoprotein screening programs: What every obstetric sonologist should know. *Radiology.* 1993;188:1–9.

36. Nadel AS, Green JK, Holmes LB, et al. Absence of need for amniocentesis in patients with elevated levels of maternal serum alphafetoprotein and normal ultrasonographic examinations. *N Engl J Med.* 1990;323:557–561.

37. Matsunaga E, Shiota Y. Holoprosencephaly in human embryos: Epidemiological studies of 150 cases. *Teratology.* 1977;16: 261–265.

38. Rizzo N, Pittalis MC, Pilu G, et al. Prenatal karyotyping in malformed fetuses. *Prenat Diagn.* 1990;10:17–21.

39. Filly RA, Chinn DH, Callen PW. Alobar holoprosencephaly. Ultrasonographic prenatal diagnosis. *Radiology.* 1984;151: 455–459.

40. Pilu G, Reece EA, Romero R, et al. Prenatal diagnosis of craniofacial malformations by sonography. *Am J Obstet Gynecol.* 1986;155:45–49.

41. Turner CD, Silva S, Jeanty P. Prenatal diagnosis of alobar holoprosencephaly at 10 weeks' gestation. *Ultrasound Obstet Gynecol.* 1993;3:360–362.

42. Pilu G, Sandri F, Perolo A, et al. Prenatal diagnosis of lobar holoprosencephaly. *Ultrasound Obstet Gynecol.* 1992;2: 88–92.

43. Pilu G, Ambrosetto P, Sandri F, et al. Intraventricular fused fornices: A specific sign of fetal lobar holoprosencephaly. *Ultrasound Obstet Gynecol.* 1994;4:65–68.

44. Pilu G, Sandri F, Perolo A, et al. Sonography of fetal agenesis of the corpus callosum: A survey of 35 cases. *Ultrasound Obstet Gynecol.* 1993;3:318–325.

45. Bennett GL, Bromley B, Benacerraf BR. Agenesis of the corpus callosum: Prenatal detection is usually not possible before 22 weeks of gestation. *Radiology.* 1993;199:447–451.

46. Gupta JK, Lilford RJ. Assessment and management of fetal agenesis of the corpus callosum. *Prenat Diagn.* 1995;15: 301–308.

47. Vergani P, Ghidini A, Strobelt N, et al. Prognostic indicators in the prenatal diagnosis of agenesis of the corpus callosum. *Am J Obstet Gynecol.* 1994;170:753–758.

48. Barkovich AJ, Kjos BO, Normal D. Revised classification of the posterior fossa cysts and cystlike malformations based on the results of multiplanar MR imaging. *AJNR.* 1989;10: 977–988.

49. Hirsch JF, Pierre Kahn A, Reiner D, et al. The Dandy–Walker malformation. A review of 40 cases. *J Neurosurg.* 1984;61: 515–522.

50. Osenbach RK, Menezes AH. Diagnosis and management of the Dandy–Walker malformation: 30 years of experience. *Pediatr Neurosurg.* 1991;18:179–185.

51. Pilu G, Goldstein I, Reece EA, et al. Sonography of fetal

Dandy–Walker malformation: A reappraisal. *Ultrasound Obstet Gynecol.* 1992;2:151–156.

52. Achiron R, Achiron A. Transvaginal ultrasonic assessment of the early fetal brain. *Ultrasound Obstet Gynecol.* 1991;1: 336–342.

53. Nyberg DA, Mahony BS, Hegge FN, et al. Enlarged cisterna magna and the Dandy–Walker malformation: Factors associated with chromosome abnormalities. *Obstet Gynecol.* 1991; 77:436–442.

54. Estroff JA, Scott MR, Benacerraf BR. Dandy–Walker variant: Prenatal sonographic diagnosis and clinical outcome. *Radiology.* 1992;185:755–758.

55. Bromley B, Nadel AS, Pauker S, et al. Closure of the cerebellar vermis: Evaluation with second trimester US. *Radiology.* 1994;193:761–763.

56. Babcock CJ, Chong BW, Salamat MS, et al. Sonographic anatomy of the developing cerebellum: Normal embryology can resemble pathology. *AJR.* 1996;166:427–433.

57. Mahony BS, Callen PW, Filly RA, Hoddick WK. The fetal cisterna magna. *Radiology.* 1984;153:773–776.

58. Laing FC, Frates MC, Brown DL, et al. Sonography of the fetal posterior fossa: False appearance of mega-cisterna magna and Dandy–Walker variant. *Radiology.* 1994;192:247–251.

59. Sawaya R, McLaurin RL. Dandy–Walker syndrome: Clinical analysis of 23 cases. *J Neurosurg.* 1981;55:89–93.

60. Pilu G, Falco P, Perolo A, et al. Differential diagnosis and outcome of fetal intracranial hypoechoic lesions: Report of 21 cases. *Ultrasound Obstet Gynecol.* 1997;9:229–235.

61. Book JA, Schut JW, Reed SC. A clinical and genetical study of microcephaly. *Am J Ment Def.* 1953;57:637–675.

62. Bromley B, Benacerraf BR. Difficulties in the prenatal diagnosis of microcephaly. *J Ultrasound Med.* 1995;14:303–307.

63. Chervenak FA, Jeanty P, Cantraine F, et al. The diagnosis of fetal microcephaly. *Am J Obstet Gynecol.* 1984;149:512–517.

64. Chervenak FA, Rosenberg J, Brightman RC, et al. A prospective study of the accuracy of ultrasound in predicting fetal microcephaly. *Obstet Gynecol.* 1987;69:908–910.

65. Jaworski M, Hersh JH, Donat J, et al. Computed tomography of the head in the evaluation of microcephaly. *Pediatrics.* 1986;78:1064–1069.

66. Goldstein I, Reece EA, Pilu G, et al. Sonographic assessment of the fetal frontal lobe: A potential tool for the diagnosis of microcephaly. *Am J Obstet Gynecol.* 1988;158:1057–1061.

67. Pilu G, Falco P, Milano V, et al. Prenatal diagnosis of microcephaly assisted by vaginal sonography and power Doppler. *Ultrasound Obstet Gynecol.* 1998;11:357–359.

68. Avery GB, Menses L, Lodge A. The clinical significance of measurement microcephaly. *Am J Dis Child* 1972;123: 214–220.

69. Martin HP. Microcephaly and mental retardation. *Am J Dis Child.* 1970;119:128–132.

70. DeMyer W. Megalencephaly in children. Clinical syndromes, genetic patterns, and differential diagnosis from other causes of megalencephaly. *Neurology.* 1972;22:634–638.

71. Sandri F, Pilu G, Dallacasa P, et al. Sonography of unilateral megalencephaly in the fetus and newborn infant. *Am J Perinatol.* 1991;8:18–21.

72. Grandjean H, Larroque D, Levi S. The performance of routine ultrasonographic screening of pregnancies in the Eurofetus Study. *Am J Obstet Gynecol.* 1999;181:446–454.

17

Neck and Chest Fetal Anomalies

Philippe Jeanty • Luís F. Gonçalves

NECK

Cystic Hygroma

Cystic hygroma is a disease that results from nonfusion of the lymphatic vessels, usually at the back of the neck.[1-6] The obstruction leads to considerable enlargement and the formation of cysts. Most of these cysts are located in the back of the neck (Fig. 17–1), but some can be found in other areas, such as the thoracic inlet (see section under Chest) and even in the abdomen. Cystic hygroma can be either an isolated finding or part of a syndrome, such as Turner's syndrome, or some trisomy, such as trisomy 13, 18, or 21.

The extent of abnormality associated with a cystic hygroma is variable. In some more benign cases, a few cysts are visible in the back of the neck; in more dramatic cases, a dissection of the skin of the fetus is created by the cysts, and the fetus is "wrapped" by multiple cysts. The condition can be so severe that at the time the peripheral fluid collections may be mistaken for pockets for amniotic fluid (Fig. 17–2).

Amniotic fluid and severe cystic hygroma can be differentiated by the fact that in cystic hygroma there are septations that are not present in amniotic fluid. Further, the fetus does not move because it is encased in the edematous collection. The spontaneous evolution is usually for the enlargement of the cyst; however, in a few cases a communication can spontaneously occur that reconnects the cyst with the normal lymphatic system, and the cysts can drain normally and disappear. In such cases, the fetus will present at delivery with a web neck or extra skin folds, but with no evidence of cystic malformation. The multiple cysts are separated by septation and fibrous strands that correspond to tissue that has been compressed by the enlargement of the cyst. Those septations are characteristic and help distinguish this condition from cephaloceles. Because of the association between cystic hygroma and chromosomal abnormalities, an amniocentesis or percutaneous umbilical blood sampling should be performed in these fetuses. One of the most common abnormalities associated with cystic hydroma is Turner's syndrome. Therefore, whenever a cystic hygroma is discovered, some further examination of the aortic arch should be performed to search for coarctation of the aorta. Other associated abnormalities, such as horseshoe kidneys and bicuspid aortic valves, should also be searched for in the fetuses.

A differential diagnosis of a milder case of cystic hygroma is occipital encephaloceles. Cephaloceles are associated with a break in the calvarium, whereas this is not present in cystic hygromas. Further, cephaloceles can usually be differentiated by a lack of septation within the cystic mass and their lack of downward extension over the neck and shoulders of the fetus (Fig. 17–3).

Prognosis. In the severe form of cystic hygroma with hydrops and oligohydramnios, the prognosis is usually fatal, with fetal demise often occurring *in utero*. In the milder cases

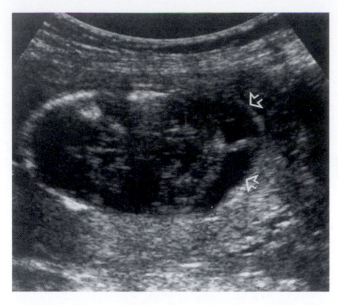

Figure 17–1. Fluid-containing masses *(arrows)* in the back of the neck of a fetus, with a septation in the middle. These are characteristic of the mild form of cystic hygroma.

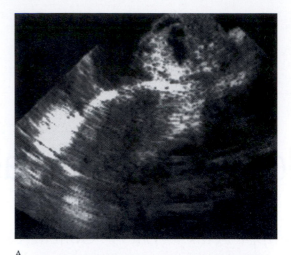

A

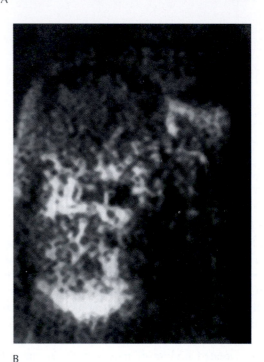

B

Figure 17–3. Longitudinal views of the mass **(A)** and its relation with the head and chest **(B)**. Note the heterogenicity of the mass. *(Reprinted with permission from De Catte L, De Backer A, Goosens A, et al. The Fetus. 1992;2:2381.)*

in which the fetus can be delivered alive, surgery can be attempted to palliate the defect; however, even in these favorable cases, the defects induced by the cysts, such as mandibular, occipital, and vertebral bone deformities, will remain a problem. Others, such as facial nerve palsy, are difficult to compensate for or correct.

In a few cases the hygroma may disappear. We had a few such fetuses with normal karyotype. Careful sonographic evaluation of the fetus at about 18 weeks' gestational age revealed no anomalies and no evidence of hydrops. The case that we have described indicates that these cystic hygromas can undergo spontaneous resolution, possibly because of delayed development of a communication between the jugular lymphatic sac and the venous system. This observation may have an impact on the counseling of affected patients. Several recent communications have highlighted that the presence of

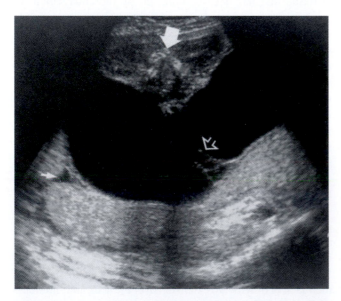

Figure 17–2. Extensive cystic hygroma. The fetal neck *(large arrows)* is compressed against the anterior portion of the maternal abdomen. The "amniotic fluid" is, in fact, fluid in the cyst. One can observe septation *(open arrow)*. The real amniotic fluid is compressed in a tiny corner (highlighted by *small left arrow*).

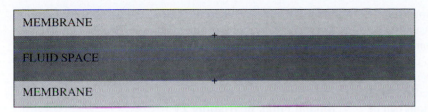

Figure 17–4. Diagram showing proper caliper placement for measurement of the nuchal translucency thickness.

small hygroma, nuchal blebs, or nuchal folds measuring no more than 3 mm in the first trimester was associated with a 1% to 3% risk of aneuploidy.

Nuchal Translucency

Nuchal translucency is the accumulation of fluid in the back of the neck of human fetuses, usually observed by ultrasound after 9 weeks of menstrual age.[7–9] Nuchal translucency thickness can be consistently measured between 10 and 14 weeks in fetuses with a crown–rump length (CRL) between 38 and 84 mm. Increased nuchal translucency thickness is associated with a higher risk of chromosomal anomalies (in particular trisomy 21) and other nonchromosomal anomalies and syndromes, discussed below.[7,10]

In trisomy 21, excessive accumulation of fluid may be explained by an overexpression of type VI collagen coded by a gene in chromosome 21, resulting in a connective tissue with a more elastic composition. Excessive fluid accumulation may also occur when fetal movements are impaired (e.g., in fetal akinesia sequence), in intrathoracic or extrathoracic compression syndromes, and in cardiac anomalies associated with early heart failure.[7,11] Nuchal translucency is more consistently observed between 10 and 14 weeks because, at this stage, the lymphatic system is still developing and the placental peripheral resistance is high. After 14 weeks, placental vascular resistance drops and the lymphatic system is developed enough to drain away the excessive fluid.

Measuring the nuchal translucency thickness should be straightforward. The following guidelines should be followed to accurately assess fetal risk:

- measurements may be taken either with the transvaginal or transabdominal probe, provided that a clear sagittal section of the fetus is obtained;
- the image must be magnified such that the fetus occupies at least 75% of the screen;
- calipers should be positioned to measure the maximum thickness of the subcutaneous translucency between the skin and the soft tissue overlying the cervical spine (Fig. 17–4);
- it is also important, when the fetus is lying on its back and close to the amniotic membrane, to wait until it moves, so that the space between the fetal back and the amniotic membrane is not mistakenly measured as nuchal translucency.

Figure 17–5 shows a nomogram of nuchal translucency measurements by CRL. From this graph, it can be concluded that nuchal translucency thickness increases with CRL and, hence, with gestational age. The median and 95th percentile of nuchal translucency thickness at a CRL of 38 mm are 1.3 and 2.2 mm, respectively, and at a CRL of 84 mm, 1.9 and 2.8 mm, respectively. Nuchal translucency thickness measurements below 2.5 mm are considered normal (or below 3 mm when using instruments that give measurements rounded to the nearest millimeter). However, because the likelihood of trisomy 21 differs according to the degree by which a given nuchal translucency thickness measurement deviates from the normal median (the thicker the nuchal translucency, the higher the risk of trisomy 21), a more precise estimate of the trisomy 21[8] risk for any given pregnancy may be achieved by taking into consideration all variables

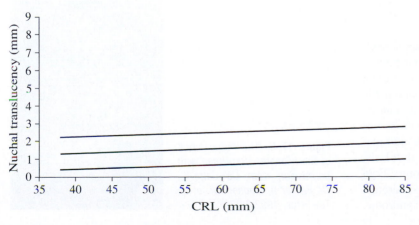

Figure 17–5. Nomogram of nuchal translucency thickness by crown-rump-length (CRL). *(Adapted from Pandya PP, Snyders RJM, Johnson SP, et al.* Br J Obstet Gynaecol. *1995;102:957.)*

involved, including maternal age,[12] CRL, previous family history, and nuchal translucency thickness measurements. This approach is known as *sequential risk assessment*.[8] The age-specific risk for trisomy 21 is multiplied by a likelihood ratio depending on how much the nuchal translucency thickness measurement deviates from the normal median for a given CRL (delta value). Two hypothetical situations can be used to illustrate this point. Suppose a 13-week pregnancy in a 34-year-old woman: the CRL is 65 mm, nuchal translucency thickness is 2.9 mm, median nuchal translucency for the given CRL is 1.7[8] mm, and the delta value is 1.2 mm (2.9 to 1.7 mm). The likelihood ratio, in this case, would be 4.51,[8] which would then be multiplied by the age-specific risk for trisomy 21 (1 in 475), thereby increasing the previous risk to 1 in 105. With the same example, use a nuchal translucency thickness of 2.5 mm; the delta value is now 0.8 mm, the likelihood ratio is 9.91, and the age-specific adjusted risk of trisomy 21 at birth, in this case, drops to 1 in 522. A slight change of 0.4 mm in the measurement changes risk assessment completely.

Once the concept of serial risk assessment is grasped, we shall examine the performance of nuchal translucency thickness as a screening test for trisomy 21 in the first trimester. Several studies evaluating the role of nuchal translucency thickness have been published in the English-language literature.[7,8,13–16] The largest study to date was conducted by the Fetal Medicine Foundation First Trimester Screening Group and published at *The Lancet* in 1998.[17] Among 96,127 women of median age 31 years (range of 14 to 49 years), the estimated trisomy 21 risk, from maternal age and fetal nuchal translucency thickness, was 1 in 300 or higher in 7907 (8.3%) of 95,476 normal pregnancies, 268 (82.2%) of 326 with trisomy 21, and 253 (77.9%) of 325 with other chromosomal defects. For a cutoff estimated trisomy 21 risk of 1 in 300, the sensitivity of the test was 82.2% (268 of 326), the false-positive rate was 8.3% (7907 of 95,476), the positive predictive value was 3.2% (268 of 8428), and the negative predictive value was 99.9% (87,569 of 87,699). For a false-positive rate of 5%, the sensitivity was 77% (95% confidence interval = 72 to 82). Therefore, nuchal translucency thickness screening has the potential to detect approximately 80% of trisomy 21–affected fetuses, with a 5% false-positive rate when offered to women with estimated risk equal or higher than 1 in 300.

Another important aspect of nuchal translucency screening is the documented association of an abnormal finding with an increased prevalence of some nonchromosomal anomalies and syndromes: cardiac defects, diaphragmatic hernia, omphalocele, body stalk anomaly, and fetal akinesia deformation sequence. Other documented associations under investigation are achondrogenesis type II, achondroplasia, Beckwith–Wiedeman syndrome, campomelic dysplasia, ectrodatyly–ectodermal dysplasis–clefting syndrome, Fryn syndrome, GM1 gangliosidosis, hydrolethalus syndrome, Jarcho–Levin syndrome, Jeune syndrome, Joubert syndrome, Meckel–Gruber syndrome, Nance–Sweeney syndrome, Noonan syndrome, Roberts syndrome, Smith–Lemli–Opitz syndrome, spinal muscular atrophy type 1, thanatophoric dysplasis, trigonocephaly "C" syndrome, VACTER association, and Zellweger syndrome.

Nuchal Folds in Trisomy 21

The presence of a nuchal thickening greater than 5 to 6 mm is considered a risk factor for trisomy 21.

Teratoma of the Neck[18]

Teratomas are benign cystic, semicystic, or solid tumors (Figs. 17–3 and 17–6). They are composed of multiple tissues foreign to the part from which they arise and are derived from all three germ cell layers. Lesions of this kind, arising in the anterior and posterior triangles of the neck, excluding those involving the base of the skull and cervical spine, are defined as *cervical teratomas*. Subclassification of these tumors into thyroid and cervical teratomas on the basis of either the presence or absence of a normal thyroid gland or their blood supply is of no clinical interest and has been abandoned. In nearly all cases of anteriorly originating cervical teratomas, a close relation with the thyroid gland can be observed.

Prevalence. Perinatal neoplasms represent only 2.6% of all tumors observed in children. Among these perinatal masses, 35% are teratomas, 80% of which are localized at the sacro-coccygeal site, causing anatomic and functional distortion of the urogenital and anorectal region. Cervical teratomas are much rarer. In a large series of 4257 childhood neoplasms, only 4 teratomas of the neck were recorded, representing an incidence of less than 0.1%.[19,20] This extreme rarity is reflected in the literature, where, at present, approximately 165 cases of perinatal cervical teratoma have been reported. Moreover, the number of prenatally diagnosed cases is small.

Etiology. The etiology is unknown, and only one report has described the occurrence of a cervical teratoma in siblings born 10 years apart.[21]

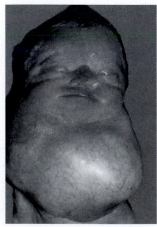

Figure 17–6. The appearance of the neonate. *(Reprinted with permission from De Catte L, De Backer A, Goosens A, et al. The Fetus. 1992;2:2381.)*

Pathogenesis. The constant relation of the cervical teratoma with the thyroid gland, by actual replacement of the thyroid tissue, involvement by direct continuity, or intimate attachment of the tumor to the gland's capsule, has led some investigators to state that all teratomas originating in the anterior portion of the neck arise from embryonic cells in the primitive anlage of the thyroid gland. Because of the extreme rarity of the intrathyroid origin of the cervical teratomas, however, other investigators regard the relation with the gland as merely fortuitous.

Pathology. Histologically, the vast majority of these tumors (68%) are composed of neural tissue. In approximately 36% of these tumors, thyroid tissue is found as a part of the tumor, whereas in nearly 15% the thyroid is present as a pseudocapsule. The cystic, fluid-filled parts of the tumor are held responsible for the rapid expansion. Malignancy by invasive growth and metastatic spread have been reported in five cases; however, malignant degeneration could be observed more frequently in teratomas of the neck occurring in teenagers and adults.

Laboratory Tests. Only scanty information on fetal hematologic and biochemical parameters is available. A high level of amniotic fluid -fetoprotein (AFP) occurred in one case of malignant cervical teratoma. Increased neonatal serum AFP levels were observed twice in a large benign teratoma of the neck and in one case of a sacrococcygeal teratoma. The rapidly growing embryonic tissue in the neoplasms may increase these serum AFP levels. Fetal erythroblast count was significantly raised without deterioration of the other hematologic parameters.

Diagnosis. The anterior or anterolateral appearance, the mixed solid–cystic composition, and the small echogenic reflections, which indicate the presence of cartilage, calcifications, or both, suggest a teratoma.

Differential Diagnosis. Differentiation with other cervical masses is often difficult, but it is very important. Color and pulsed Doppler investigations are both helpful in the differentiation of a hemangioma. Fetal tachycardia, in association with a bilobed, a solid anterior neck mass, suggests the presence of a fetal goiter, which is confirmed by a raised amniotic fluid thyroid-stimulating hormone level.

Prognosis and Complications. Despite the fact that most of these tumors are histologically benign, fetal and neonatal outcome is often compromised. The incidences of polyhydramnios, preterm delivery, and perinatal death have, respectively, been reported as 25%, 17%, and 43%.[20] In very large cervical teratomas (larger than 80 mm at the largest diameter), prematurity and dystocia or cesarean section rates increase to more than 50%. Fetal deglutition impairment is responsible for the associated polyhydramnios. Deviation of the

larynx and trachea results in compression of the esophagus and inhibits fetal swallowing. Smaller teratomas (50 mm), in which the contribution of the volume of the mass to the compression is questionable, are also frequently associated with hydramnios. Perhaps hypoglossal nerve compression by the expanding tumor mass adds to the deglutition problem.

Management. The anterior localization and the semisolid appearance of these tumors can provoke an upper airway obstruction, which is the most urgent neonatal emergency, requiring immediate intervention. When anticipated by ultrasound, the necessary equipment can be mobilized at the time of the cesarean section to deal with these respiratory difficulties. The use of a laryngoscope and a McGill forceps, a guidewire, or both by an experienced neonatologist may not always overcome the intubation problem. Extreme compression and deviation of the trachea may require bronchoscopic exploration to prevent perforation.

In small tumors, emergency tracheotomy may secure adequate ventilatory support. Repeated prenatal needling of the cystic components may also reduce the tumor mass and facilitate neonatal surgery. Moreover, just before delivery, this needling may reduce the compression of the larynx and trachea to favor intubation.

A recent report has proposed the use of an extracorporeal membrane oxygenation system by cannulation of the umbilical arteries and vein and the support of fetal circulation.[22] This procedure creates time to explore the fetal larynx and trachea without asphyxiating the newborn. In cases of major obstruction, temporary blood oxygenation allows immediate surgical neck exploration to establish adequate ventilation.

Others have used magnetic resonance imaging (MRI) and ultrasound to plan the operation on placental support (OOPS) and *ex utero* intrapartum treatment (EXIT) procedures and found them useful.[23–25]

Large teratomas of the neck, although rarely in fetal life, represent a perinatal mortality risk. After prenatal diagnosis, a multidisciplinary approach is necessary to cope with the immediate neonatal respiratory threat.

Goiter

Goiters have rarely been detected in fetuses. They usually occur in fetuses of mothers treated for a thyroid condition, whether the mother is eu-, hypo-, or hyperthyroid. Under proper postnatal management, they disappear and are of little significance. Prenatally, however, they may compress the esophagus and cause polyhydramnios. When this is found, one must suspect that the trachea of the fetus is also compressed, and the pediatric resuscitation team should be available at birth.

Intrapharyngeal and Intraoral Teratoma

These will also appear as heterogeneous anterior neck masses that grow rapidly. Like neck teratoma, they can cause head deflexion and polyhydramnios.[26]

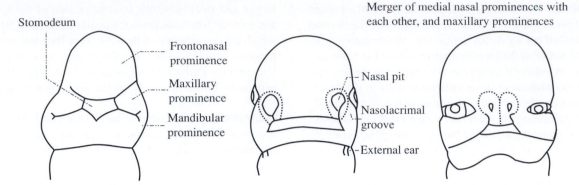

Figure 17–7. Schematic representation of facial development at days 24, 33, and 48 postconception. Mesenchymal cells of neural crest origin migrate into the mandibular prominence, forming the precursor of the lower jaw. The migration of the ears to their adult site is actually secondary to rapid proliferation of cells destined to form the mandible and differential growth of the cranium. *(Reprinted with permission from Joffe GM, Izquierdo LA, Del Valle GO, et al. The Fetus. 1991;1:7448.)*

Agnathia–Microstomia–Synotia (Otocephaly) and Agnathia–Holoprosencephaly[27]

Agnathia–microstomia–synotia is defined as absence or hypoplasia of the mandible, proximity of the temporal bones, and abnormal position of the ears. When complicated by holoprosencephaly, it is referred to as *agnathia–holoprosencephaly*. This is a rare malformation that may represent an autosomal recessive defect.

Embryology. Facial development occurs in the human embryo mainly between the fifth and eighth weeks postconception. Surrounding the primitive stomodeum are the frontonasal prominence superiorly, maxillary prominence of the first branchial arch laterally, and the mandibular prominence (also first branchial arch derivatives) interiorly (Fig. 17–7).

The mandible is the first part of the face to form. It is thought to arise from proliferation and migration of mesenchyme, possibly of neural crest origin. The medial ends of the mandibular prominence merge in the midline by the beginning of the fifth week of gestation postconception. The maxillae form during the sixth and seventh weeks of gestation by the merging of the maxillary prominences with each other and the frontonasal prominence along the nasolacrimal groove.

Ultrasound Appearance. The prenatal findings include an extreme micrognathia, the presence of ears on the front and lateral aspects of the neck, the inability to obtain the "cleft lip" view, and accessory findings, such as polyhydramnios (from failure to swallow) and holoprosencephaly.

The infant shown in Figure 17–8 demonstrates clefting of both the upper lip and palate in addition to the rare median cleft of the lower lip. The upper cleft can be explained on the basis of failure of migration of mesenchyme of the maxillary prominence, resulting in bilateral clefting. The cleft of the lower lip is secondary to total absence of development of the mandibular prominence, which also resulted in complete absence of the mandible.

Because the maxillary mesenchymal migration did not occur, the ears did not undergo "migration" to their usual position and remained in their original embryonic location.

Associated Anomalies. Aside from holoprosencephaly, cephalocele, midline proboscis, hypoplastic tongue, tracheoesophageal fistula, cardiac anomalies, and adrenal hypoplasia can also be found.

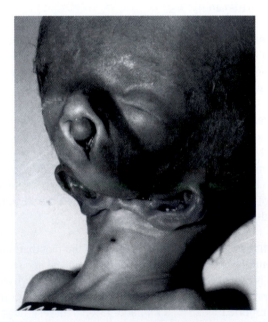

Figure 17–8. Gross findings at the time of autopsy showed ears fused in the midline, complete absence of the mandible, and clefting of both lips. *(Reprinted with permission from Joffe GM, Izquierdo LA, Del Valle GO, et al. The Fetus. 1991;1:7448.)*

Differential Diagnosis. The differential diagnosis of agnathia–holoprosencephaly includes agnathia–microstomia–synotia (no holoprosencephaly) and Robin's anomalad. This is another disorder of formation of the mandible that is characterized by mandibular hypoplasia, posterior cleft palate, and posterior displacement of the tongue. The key to distinguishing agnathia–microstomia–synotia from Robin's anomalad using ultrasonography is localization of the ears. The ears remain in the midline over the neck in agnathia–microstomia–synotia, whereas some degree of "migration" does occur in Robin's anomalad.

CHEST

Cystic Adenomatoid Malformation[28]

Congenital cystic adenomatoid malformation (CCAM) is a pulmonary developmental anomaly that may give rise to a full spectrum of clinical presentations. The following sections outline the reasons for the different presentations and discuss the embryology, pathogenesis, antenatal ultrasonographic findings, and differential diagnosis.

Embryology. The lower respiratory system begins its development approximately 26 days after conception. The laryngotracheal groove develops longitudinally in the floor of the primitive pharynx and is the forerunner of the larynx, trachea, bronchi, and terminal bronchioles. At 6 weeks postconception, the endodermally derived terminal bronchioles induce the surrounding splanchnic mesenchyme to begin development of the respiratory component of the bronchopulmonary segment. The pseudoglandular period (5 to 17 weeks postconception) is so named because histologically the developing lung has a glandlike appearance. This is the period of development of the bronchiolar divisions with differentiation into the air-conducting system. As will be seen later, the histologic appearance of type III CCAM is quite similar to the appearance of the developing lung in the pseudoglandular period. The canalicular period (16 to 25 weeks) resembles type II CCAM. During this period of time, the lumina of the bronchi and bronchioles become larger, and the lung tissue becomes well vascularized. Respiration is possible at the end of this period, with the presence of some terminal sacs (primitive alveoli). During the terminal sac period (24 weeks to birth), proliferation of terminal sacs occurs with marked thinning of the epithelium. Capillaries bulge into the sacs, beginning the facilitation of gas exchange. During the alveolar period (late fetal period to 8 years of life), the lining of the terminal sacs attenuates to an extremely thin layer of squamous epithelium. According to Moore, "characteristic mature alveoli do not form for some time after birth."[29]

Pathogenesis. The first report of CCAM in the English-language literature was presented by Ch'in and Tang in 1949.[30] They described a case report of the disease and reviewed the 10 other cases that had been described in the world literature up to that time. The findings in the majority of these 11 cases were similar to those of most case reports found today. The disease is almost exclusively limited to one lung, with bilateral involvement being extremely rare. In addition, usually only one lobe of the affected lung is involved. If the bronchus leading to the affected lobe is traced, it is noted to end blindly. The early descriptions of the histologic findings described small and large cysts lined by columnar and cuboidal epithelium. Larger cysts were noted to have elastic fibers and smooth muscle in their walls. Almost all of the cases described in the early literature noted a lack of cartilage surrounding the cystic structures. Some investigators noted the presence of tall columnar epithelium that resembled gastric mucosa. Associated findings reported in the early literature almost always included "the constancy of general anasarca," with most investigators noting compression of the venae cavae secondary to marked mediastinal shift. Polyhydramnios was a feature common to most of the early case descriptions. Ch'in and Tang's[30] early description of the pathologic findings forms the basis of our understanding of the disease today. They stated that "the essential feature is an excessive overgrowth of the bronchioles, especially the terminal bronchioles, which causes the marked enlargement of the lobe, while the development of the alveoli is completely suppressed except at the periphery."[30] They compared the entity to a hamartoma but noted that it lacked certain elements found in normal lung, such as cartilage and mucous glands.

The next major review of the pathogenesis of cystic adenomatoid malformation was reported by Stocker et al. in 1977.[31] They stated that by 1975, 70 cases had been reported in the literature, including those of Ch'in and Tang. Their review was of 38 cases found in the files of the Armed Forces Institute of Pathology between 1917 and 1975. In the review of these cases, they noted a male-to-female ratio of 1 to 7. Twenty of these infants were preterm, 15 were term, and 3 were unknown. Nine of the 38 infants were stillborn. In contrast to the series of Ch'in and Tang, 10 of these infants had other congenital anomalies. These anomalies included truncus arteriosus, hydrocephalus, deformity of the clavicle or cervical and thoracic spine, jejunal atresia, diaphragmatic hernia, bilateral renal agenesis, tetralogy of Fallot, sirenomeli (including agenesis of ureters, bladder, urethra, uterus, cervix, vagina, gallbladder, descending colon, sigmoid colon and rectum, and imperforate anus), ventricular septal defect, and tracheoesophageal fistula. Interestingly, anasarca was not noted in any of these cases. In 12 liveborn infants, partial or total pulmonary lobectomy was performed; 11 of these infants survived. Unilateral pulmonary involvement was again the rule, and in 19 cases a single lobe was involved, whereas in 10 cases two or more lobes were affected. The major contribution of this review was to define three distinct variants of CCAM based on gross and microscopic examination.

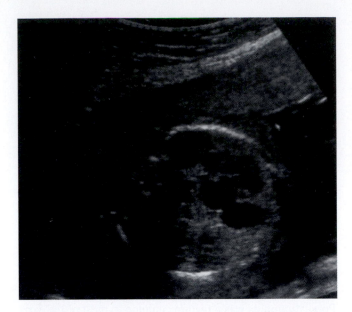

Figure 17–9. Numerous cysts in the chest that represent type I cystic adenomatoid malformation. Some of the cysts were drained under ultrasound guidance but reappeared within 48 h.

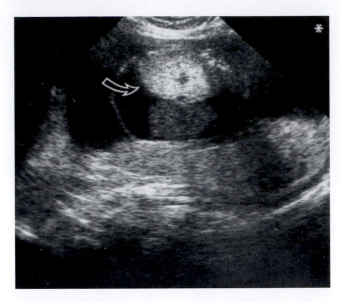

Figure 17–10. This echogenic mass *(arrow)* associated with pleural effusion represents type III cystic adenomatoid malformation of the lung.

Type I Cysts. Type I cysts (19 cases) are notable for their large size (up to 7 cm in diameter) (Fig. 17–9). These cysts are lined by pseudostratified columnar epithelium with numerous polypoid projections. They overlie a thick wall of smooth muscle and elastic tissue. Mucus-producing cells are occasionally noted. Stocker et al.[31] noted that, in 2 of 19 cases, an island of cartilage was noted near the area where the cysts communicated with the normal bronchial tree. Smaller cysts were also noted in these lesions and were lined by cuboidal to columnar epithelium. The smaller cysts were noted to contain less smooth muscle and elastic tissue than the larger cysts. Of note was the appearance of alveoluslike structures adjacent to or communicating with the larger cysts. These alveoluslike structures were lined with cells that were indistinguishable from these of alveolar lining cells, but the structures were 2 to 10 times larger than normal alveoli. Blood vessels were reportedly normal.

Type II Cysts. The type II lesion has smaller cysts, usually smaller than 1 cm in largest diameter. These cysts are lined by cuboidal to tall columnar epithelium that rarely demonstrate pseudostratification. The walls of these cysts are composed of a thin layer of connective tissue containing discontinuous bands of smooth muscle and elastic tissue rarely more than three to four cell layers thick. Mucus cells are not present in type II lesions. Of note was the finding of striated muscle between cysts in two of these cases. Cartilage was seen only as a normal component of bronchi located adjacent to the lesion.[31] Blood vessels are normal in the type II lesion.

Type III Cysts. The type III lesions (three cases in this series) were noted to be firm, bulky masses of lung tissue on gross inspection (Fig. 17–10).[31] Histologically, these lesions were described as having cysts that were 2 to 5 mm in largest diameter. These cysts resembled bronchioles in size and distribution and were lined by ciliated cuboidal epithelium. The cyst walls were composed of thin, even layers of smooth muscle. The bulk of the lesion, aside from the cysts, consisted of irregularly shaped alveolus-sized structures lined by nonciliated cuboidal epithelium. Reference was made to their resemblance to the glandlike structures seen during the pseudoglandular period of embryonic development (5 to 17 weeks). Mucogenic cells and cartilage were not present.

In the series of Stocker et al.[31] the clinical course of 16 liveborn infants with type I lesions was described. Seven became symptomatic on the first day of life, two between days 1 and 7, and the remainder between 1 and 4 weeks of life. Ten of the cases of type II lesion had associated anomalies (outlined previously). All of these infants were symptomatic on the first day of life.

Type I and type III lesions were noted to be bulky lesions and thus produced the greatest degree of mediastinal shift.

There were only two liveborn infants with type III lesions in this series,[31] and they were noted to be symptomatic on the first day of life.

Stocker et al. attempted to correlate the type of lesion with the time in embryogenesis at which the insult may have occurred. The type I lesion, with its more mature findings of pseudostratification of epithelium, thick wall of smooth muscle surrounding the larger cysts, mucous glands, and rare foci of cartilage, may occur as late as 49 days postconception.

Type II lesions were frequently associated with other severe congenital anomalies in this series, suggesting earlier timing of aberrant differentiation, probably before 31 days postconception. Type III lesions, with their pseudoglandular appearance, probably develop early in embryogenesis.

By 1978, Ostor and Fortune[32] stated that the number of cases reported in the English-language literature had risen to 142, including those of Stocker et al. Ostor and Fortune took a different view of the embryogenesis of the disease and stated that the insult probably occurred later in gestation (16 to 20 weeks). They stated that the presence of normal alveoli at the periphery of the lesion, with abnormal growth in the center of the lesion, implies failure of canalization of terminal bronchioles and subsequent inability to connect the conducting and respiratory elements. Stated another way, the endodermally derived conducting branches fail to connect with the mesodermally derived respiratory branches that cluster about their tips.

In 1979, Bale[33] suggested that, whereas researchers disagreed as to the exact nature of the disease (overgrowth, hyperplasia, or hamartoma) and the embryologic timing of pathogenesis (early embryonic period versus 16 to 20 weeks), all agreed that the defect occurred at the level of bronchiole. Therefore, she suggested that the disease be termed *congenital bronchiolar malformation.*

In 1980, Krous et al.[34] reported a case of a neonatal demise that was found on autopsy to have a type II CCAM and bilateral renal agenesis. They noted that theirs was the third case in the literature in which bilaterality of the disease process was noted. They also noted that the usual findings in bilateral renal agenesis (facial and limb positional defects; i.e., Potter's syndrome) were mild. They used scanning electron microscopy to demonstrate abundant type 2 pneumocytes within the lesions. Because the cysts were noted to communicate with the normal bronchial tree, they speculated that pulmonary fluid production by the cysts mitigated the usual findings with bilateral renal agenesis. They speculated that the polyhydramnios often found in CCAM is secondary to fluid production by the type 2 pneumocytes lining the cysts.

Others have speculated that the polyhydramnios usually seen in this disease may be due to decreased swallowing secondary to esophageal compression or decreased absorption of lung fluid by the hypoplastic, malformed lungs.

Some investigators prefer to classify the type of lesion as microcystic (cysts smaller than 5 mm in diameter) and macrocystic (cysts equal to or greater than 5 mm in diameter).[35] These investigators propose that poorer prognosis in microcystic disease is secondary to the development of hydrops and hypoplasia of normal lung tissue.

Antenatal Diagnosis. The first description of CCAM recorded in the ultrasound literature was in 1975 by Garrett et al.[36] By 1981, there were three published cases of antenatal ultrasonographic diagnosis of CCAM. In type III CCAM, a large echogenic lesion produces marked mediastinal shift.

The solid, echogenic appearance of the type III lesion is in contrast to the fluid-filled cysts characteristic of type I and type II lesions because of the innumerable interfaces that give a solid appearance quite anologous to that of infantile polycystic kidney.

The differential diagnosis of CCAM includes extralobar and intralobar pulmonary sequestration, bronchogenic cyst, and mediastinal lesions, such as enterogenous cyst, neurenteric cyst, or cystic teratoma.

Sauerbrei[37] recently described the use of duplex Doppler imaging to establish the diagnosis of pulmonary sequestration and to distinguish between extralobar sequestration (ELS) and intralobar sequestration (ILS). He described the antenatal diagnosis of a fetal pulmonary mass that is hyperechoic (differential diagnosis includes type III CCAM) but demonstrates a vessel coursing between the mass and the peritoneal cavity. Duplex Doppler examination of the vessel showed arterial flow from the peritoneal cavity into the mass and venous flow in the opposite direction, which is typical of ELS. Because ELS and ILS may mimic CCAM in ultrasound appearance, it is important to diligently search for an anomalous blood supply when attempting to make the diagnosis.

There have been cases reported in the literature in which diagnosis of CCAM has been made with ultrasound in which the mass apparently regressed on serial scans. Saltzman et al. stated that "it is difficult to tell whether this apparent improvement resulted from actual shrinking of the lung mass or whether the overall normal fetal growth without growth of the mass gave the illusion of a smaller lesion."[38]

Cystic adenomatoid malformation is most often confused with congenital diaphragmatic hernia when evaluating with ultrasound.

In Utero Therapy for Congenital Cystic Adenomatoid Malformation. *In utero* therapy may hold promise for fetuses with CCAM, even in the presence of hydrops. The first reported case of successful drainage of this type of pulmonary cyst occurred in 1987 by Nicolaides et al.[39] Treatment is usually by placement of a "double-pigtail" catheter for continuous drainage (instead of repeat taps). Although there may be some benefit in type I CCAM, the natural evolution of type I is usually favorable and the benefit of the treatment is not clearly established. *In utero* treatment should probably be reserved for cases with associated hydrops in view of the poor prognosis of fetuses born with hydrops.

In 1990, Harrison et al.[40] described the *in utero* resection of CCAM in two fetuses at 27 and 23 weeks' gestational age. The first case was technically successful; however, cesarean section was necessary at 28 weeks of gestation secondary to worsening preeclampsia. Establishment of placentomegaly before fetal pulmonary resection resulted in worsening maternal hyperdynamic status that failed to resolve after the fetal surgical therapy. Because there was not enough time to allow expansion of normal lung tissue after surgical resection of the CCAM, the neonate succumbed to respiratory insufficiency.

In the second case, the period of time between successful resection of the CCAM and delivery of the neonate was 6 weeks. Despite delivery at 30 weeks of gestation, this infant was well at 5 months of age.

Lung Cyst

Isolated bronchogenic cysts are rare and benign when small. They should be differentiated from other cystic structures, such as pericardial cysts, neurenteric cysts, and duplication of the esophagus.

Laryngeal Atresia[42]

Congenital laryngeal atresia is a rare upper airway obstruction. It leads to death unless a surgical airway is immediately established.

Embryology. The development of the larynx begins in the fourth week of embryonic life with the formation of a primitive glottis, the laryngeal aditus, in the floor of the foregut. Anterior to the aditus is the primordium of the epiglottis and posteriorly is the narrow pharyngotracheal duct, connecting the pharynx with the tracheal lumen. Smith and Graham described three types of laryngeal atresia[56] (Fig. 17–11).

Type I: Supra and Infraglottic. The arytenoid cartilages and the paired muscles are fused across the midline. The cricoid is conical and the vestibule is absent.

Type II: Infraglottic. This type is characterized by a dome-shaped cricoid cartilage including the lumen; the arytenoids, vestibule, and vocal cords are normal.

Type III: Glottic. The vestibule and cricoid cartilage are normal. The glottis is occluded by an anterior membrane of fibrous connective tissue and muscle and by a posterior bar of cartilage formed by fusion of the arytenoids at their vocal processes.

Pathogenesis. An arrest of the normal development of the larynx during embryonic life seems to be the cause of the lack of its canalization. The three different types of atresia previously described are not absolute, but rather are gradations of a continuous spectrum, and indicate that the arrest has happened in different stages of embryonic development. Walander[43] showed that the laryngotracheal development of 8-, 12-, and 20-mm rat embryos is similar to the three stages described by Smith and Graham.[56]

Diagnosis. One of the most common findings is pulmonary hyperplasia. The lungs are enlarged by volume and weight, but their general histology is normal. They have been shown to consist of an increased amount of tissue and not simply an accumulation of lung secretion caused by the laryngeal obstruction. The extension of the pulmonary hyperplasia correlates with the degree of laryngeal obstruction. Gatti et al. demonstrated that complete atresia leads to enlarged lungs with dilatation of the trachea and bronchi, whereas a partial laryngeal obstruction is associated with lungs of normal size at autopsy.[44] The heart and great vessels are compressed, and cardiac failure from obstructed venous return is almost always present with different degrees of ascites and hydrops.

Polyhydramnios is commonly associated with laryngeal atresia and is attributable to the decreased fetal swallowing of amniotic fluid, from compression of the esophagus by the lung, from compression of the stomach by ascites, or from both.

The ultrasonographic diagnosis *in utero* has only been made in cases of complete atresia. The diagnosis is based on indirect signs or consequences of the total airway obstruction, such as bulky lungs (Figs. 17–12 through 17–15), fetal hydrops and ascites, polyhydramnios, and so forth. The failure to recognize incomplete atresia is probably due to a lack of pulmonary distention. Recognition of the characteristic changes may be difficult in the early second trimester. Only a half-dozen cases of laryngeal atresia have been diagnosed *in utero* with ultrasound; most cases have only been recognized at birth. The diagnosis must be suspected if a newborn infant, normal at the time of birth, develops severe cyanosis and respiratory distress after ligation of the cord and an attempt at endotracheal intubation is unsuccessful. In such instances, only an immediate tracheotomy will save the newborn.

Differential Diagnosis. Cystic adenomatoid malformation of the lung, type III, creates a large solid mass affecting an entire lobe, with a bulky appearance of the whole lung. Similarly, the less common bronchial atresia presents with an enlarged echogenic lung. Rarely, these two conditions can be bilateral. When bilateral, they can be differentiated from laryngeal atresia by the presence of a fluid-filled trachea in laryngeal atresia. Other differential diagnoses include laryngeal stenosis and hypoplasia, laryngeal membrane, and tracheal atresia.

Associated Anomalies. Sometimes laryngeal atresia can also occur in the context of a rare congenital syndrome, such as Fraser syndrome (an autosomal recessive disorder whose most consistent feature is cryptophthalmos, but includes other anomalies of the ears, nose, genitalia, and skeleton, and mental retardation) or 47,XXX chromosome constitution.

Prognosis. The prognosis of larynx atresia is poor if an immediate diagnosis is not made or when other severe anomalies are associated. Only very few cases of surviving newborns have been reported in the literature; one of these is in good health at 10 months of age, with no obvious neurologic defects, despite an anoxia of 15 min at birth.

Management. When not diagnosed promptly at birth, complete larynx atresia is a fatal malformation. In about half of the cases, other severe anomalies are associated. In these

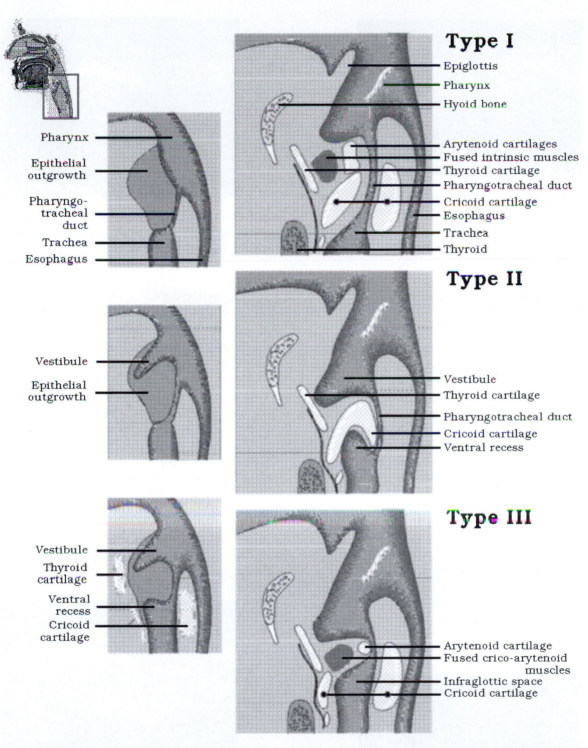

Figure 17–11. Embryology of the larynx in the rat embryo (8 to 20 mm) and corresponding stages of developmental arrest in the human. Type I is supraglottic and infraglottic. The arytenoid cartilages and the paired muscles are fused across the midline. The cricoid is conical, and the vestibule is absent. Type II is infraglottic. It is characterized by a dome-shaped cricoid cartilage occluding the lumen. The arytenoids, vestibule, and vocal cords are normal. Type III is a glottic obstruction. The vetibule and cricoid cartilage are normal. The glottis is occluded by an anterior membrane of fibrous connective tissue and muscle and by a posterior bar of cartilage formed by fusion of the arytenoids at their vocal processes. *(Reprinted with permission from Valcamonico A, Gonçalves LF, Jeanty P. The Fetus. 1992;2:7483.)*

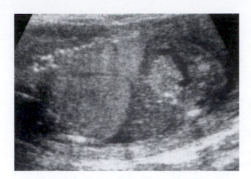

Figure 17–12. Bilaterally enlarged echogenic lungs that depress the diaphragm. *(Reprinted with permission from Valcamonico A, Gonçalves LF, Jeanty P. The Fetus. 1992;2:7483.)*

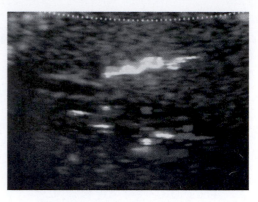

Figure 17–14. Color Doppler distinguishes the fluid-filled trachea from the aorta. *(Reprinted with permission from Valcamonico A, Gonçalves LF, Jeanty P. The Fetus. 1992;2:7483.)*

cases, the prognosis is very poor, and the option of pregnancy termination can be offered.

Chylothorax

Chylothorax is an accumulation of lymph inside the chest within dilated lymphatics.[45–51] Pleural effusions are covered under a separate heading under chronic abnormalities and fetal hydrops. Chylothorax can be either symmetric or asymmetric (Fig. 17–16). It may be associated with ascites. When this is the case, it is difficult to differentiate from anasarca.

Chylothorax can be associated with trisomy 21, congenital pulmonary lymphangiectasis, tracheoesophageal fistula, and extralobar sequestration. Fetal lymph is perfectly clear because it does not contain any fat droplets. (These will only be present when the child absorbs milk.) Therefore, the diagnosis between chylothorax and pleural effusion is often difficult. The diagnosis should be suggested when other causes of hydrops are excluded and when the fetal heart is observed to be normal. Some physicians have attempted to drain chylothoraces under ultrasound guidance, but the benefit of this procedure is not clearly established.

Lung Sequestration[52]

Pulmonary sequestrations may be an isolated finding or part of a constellation of anomalies. A large majority of patients are symptomatic and are diagnosed within the first 6 months of life; however, 10% are found incidentally in asymptomatic individuals. The sequestrations were isolated findings in all five of our cases. The four neonates who underwent surgery have had uncomplicated postoperative courses, and the fifth case has been followed up expectantly.

Diagnosis. The typical appearance of a subdiaphragmatic sequestration is a nonpulsatile, hemogeneous well-circumscribed, hyperechoic mass in the fetal abdomen or retroperitoneum (Fig. 17–17). Ninety percent of the extralobar sequestrations are localized to the left side of the fetal abdomen. Cystic areas are commonly found within the lesion. Duplex Doppler may be helpful to demonstrate the systemic arterial

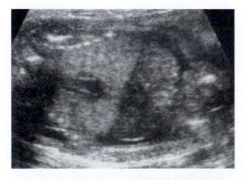

Figure 17–13. The heart is compressed between the lungs. *(Reprinted with permission from Valcamonico A, Gonçalves LF, Jeanty P. The Fetus. 1992;2:7483.)*

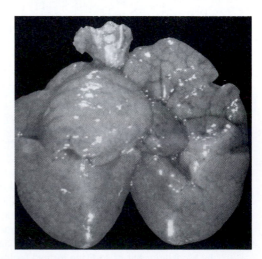

Figure 17–15. The lungs at autopsy. Note the compressed heart. *(Reprinted with permission from Valcamonico A, Gonçalves LF, Jeanty P. The Fetus. 1992;2:7483.)*

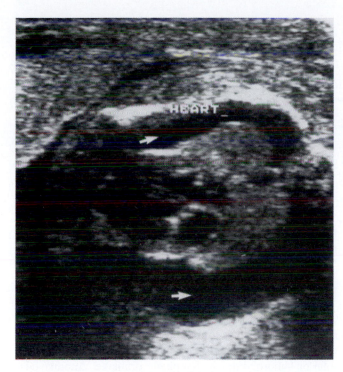

Figure 17–16. Chylothoraces *(arrows)* in a fetus with Down syndrome. Notice that, although the chylothorax is bilateral, it is predominant on the right side.

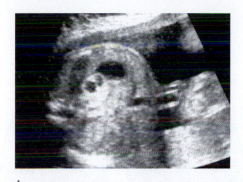

A

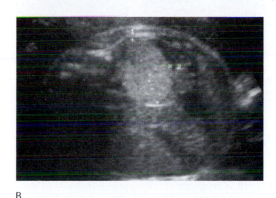

B

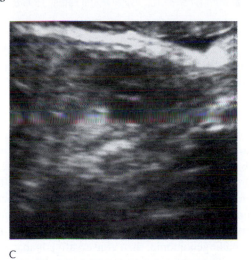

C

Figure 17–17. Several examples of infradiaphragmatic lung sequestrations. **(A–C)** Note that the masses are hyperechoic, are smooth, and partly surround the aorta. *(Reprinted with permission from Wheeler TC, Jeanty P. The Fetus. 1993;3:7485.)*

blood supply, and color flow Doppler can define the venous drainage pattern.

Embryology. The normal lung develops from the primitive laryngotracheal groove, which arises on the ventral aspect of the primitive foregut between 5 and 6 weeks of embryologic development. The lung bud undergoes multiple divisions to give rise to the tracheobronchial tree. An aberrant lung bud may develop in the embryonic foregut distal to the tracheobronchial bud. This pluripotential mass of tissue migrates distally, with its blood supply giving rise to the sequestration. Late origination from the elongated foregut results in an extralobar sequestration invested in its own pleura (Fig. 17–18). The original connection with the foregut typically involutes, but persistence will allow communication with the gastrointestinal tract.

Pathology. Microscopically, extralobar sequestrations resemble normal lungs except that there is diffuse dilatation of parenchymal structures. The bronchioles, alveolar ducts, and alveoli are dilated and tortuous. Congenital cystic adenomatoid malformation has been described in 15 to 25% of extralobar sequestrations. Gross examination typically reveals a single ovoid or pyramidal lesion ranging from 3 to 6 cm. The blood supply typically arises from the systemic arteries. Vascular supplies originating from the thoracic or abdominal aorta have been noted in 80% of cases. Venous drainage of extralobar sequestrations are usually through the azygous and hemiazygous systems.

Differential Diagnosis. Several entities must be considered in addition to pulmonary sequestration when an echogenic mass is visualized beneath or within the diaphragm. Neuroglastoma, teratoma, adrenal hemorrhage, or foregut duplication should be considered in the differential diagnosis. Multiple cysts within the mass may be noted with associated

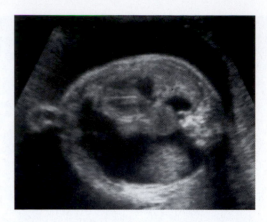

Figure 17–19. Left pleural effusion with cardiac displacement to the right. Note the retromediastinal herniation and the displacement of the descending aorta to the right. The heart is also compressed. *(Reprinted with permission from Boiskin I, Brunner JP, Jeanty P. The Fetus. 1991;1:7485.)*

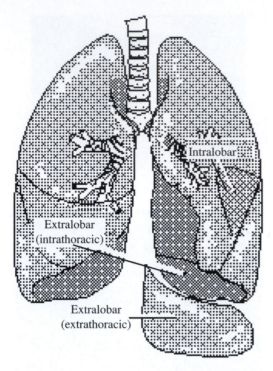

Figure 17–18. Classification of lung sequestrations. *(Reprinted with permission from Wheeler TC, Jeanty P. The Fetus. 1993;3:7485.)*

effusion is less clear. This may be related to either an increased arterial pressure gradient across the sequestered lung lobe or abnormalities in lymphatic drainage. Another possibility is torsion of the lung sequestration about its pedicle with preserved arterial flow and interrupted venous flow.[45–51]

CCAM. Duplex and color flow Doppler may provide additional information by demonstrating vascular flow from the abdominal aorta.

Diagnosis. Findings that should alert the examiner include a shift of the mediastinum and increased lung echogenicity. A pulmonary sequestration appears as a solid, well-defined echogenic nonpulsatile intrathoracic mass separate from the heart (Figs. 17–19 through 17–23). The lesion occurs most commonly on the left in the posterior or basal portions. Prominent vessels, in particular an anomalous systemic artery arising from the aorta, extending into the mass will confirm the diagnosis.

Therapy and Prognosis. Prenatal intervention was neither indicated nor required in the five cases presented. Intrauterine drainage of large pleural effusions associated with an extralobar sequestration has been shown to reverse fetal hydrops. In the postpartum period, surgical resection is usually performed in elective fashion. Some researchers advocate observation rather than immediate operation as an acceptable alternative. If the sequestration is nonaerated and angiography is pathogenomonic, then conservative management is acceptable. The prognosis for patients with subdiaphragmatic pulmonary sequestration is generally favorable. Associated congenital anomalies carry a worse prognosis, particularly if there is associated pulmonary hypoplasia.

Lung Sequestration with Torsion[35]
Pleural effusions in the fetus may occur as an isolated abnormality or in association with more serious conditions, such as immune or nonimmune hydrops.[35]

The association among extralobar pulmonary sequestration, fetal hydrops, and polyhydramnios is rare. Mass effect and mediastinal shift with resultant partial venous obstruction and low cardiac output have been postulated as a cause for the hydrops.[19,27] The cause for the unilateral pleural

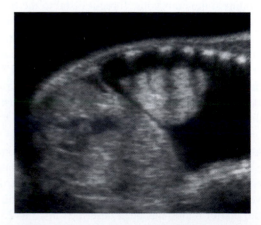

Figure 17–20. Sagittal view that demonstrates the sequestrum and the effusion. A small amount of ascites is seen below the diaphragm. *(Reprinted with permission from Boiskin I, Brunner JP, Jeanty P. The Fetus. 1991;1:7485.)*

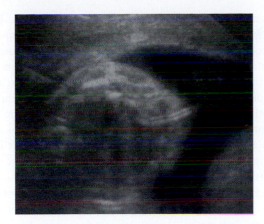

Figure 17–21. The shunt in place after aspiration of the pleural fluid. The shunt is inserted in the anterolateral chest. *(Reprinted with permission from Boiskin I, Brunner JP, Jeanty P. The Fetus. 1991;1:7485.)*

Embryology. The most accepted theory on the origin of pulmonary sequestrations was proposed by Eppinger and Schawerstein in 1902 and subsequently supported by others.[53] According to their view, an aberrant lung bud develops in the embryonic foregut distal to the normal tracheobronchial bud. This pluripotential mass of tissue acquires its own blood supply and migrates distally, giving rise to the sequestration. Whether the latter will be intralobar or extralobar is determined at the time at which the aberrant bud develops. An early origin of the abnormal bud in the short primitive foregut will be carried distally by the normal lung and incorporated as an intralobar sequestration. A late origin from the elongated foregut will remain outside the lung (extralobar). It is speculated that the communication between the aberrant bud and foregut outgrows its vascular supply and undergoes involution.

Pathology. The gross appearance of a pulmonary sequestration is similar to that of normal lung parenchyma. Histolog-

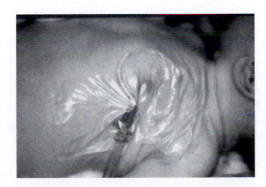

Figure 17–22. After delivery, the shunt is connected to a suction apparatus. *(Reprinted with permission from Boiskin I, Brunner JP, Jeanty P. The Fetus. 1991;1:7485.)*

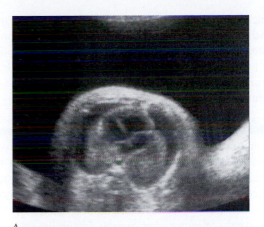

A

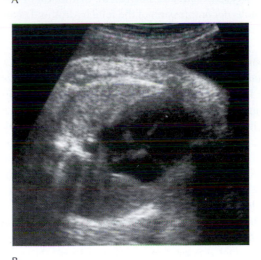

B

Figure 17–23. **(A)** Axial view at 34 weeks of gestation demonstrates bilateral pleural effusions **(B)** that are no longer visible at 37 weeks. *(Reprinted with permission from Sherer DM, Abramowicz JS, Woods JR. The Fetus. 1991;1:7488.)*

ically, numerous dilated bronchioles, alveolar ducts, alveoli, and lymphatics are seen. Occasionally, cysts are present and lined by ciliated columnar epithelium. Blood supply is from the systemic circulation by arteries from the aorta or intercostal arteries. The feeding arteries from the aorta pass through the pulmonary ligament. The venous drainage is to the systemic system via the azygous or hemiazygous veins. Ninety percent are on the left side, and 80% are located in the posterior costophrenic sulcus adjacent to the lower esophagus.

Differential Diagnosis. Several entities must be included in the differential diagnosis of a solid lung mass of increased echogenicity diagnosed on antenatal ultrasound. These include pulmonary sequestration, type III CCAM, and bronchial atresia. Pathologically, CCAM is described as macrocystic, medium-sized, cystic, and solid. Type III is the rarest and has microcysts showing a solid appearance on ultrasound examination. Congenital bronchial atresia is another echogenic pulmonary mass lesion. It is found most commonly in the upper lobes and rarely in the lower lobes. Occasionally, anechoic areas within the mass representing dilated mucus-filled bronchi are seen.

Prognosis. Until now, no neonatal survival of more than a few hours after birth has been reported. We had two patients with successful intrauterine treatment, both of which had drainage. In the first case, the drainage of the pleural effusion may have played no role because it was performed just hours before delivery; however, in the second case, it allowed 4 more weeks of intrauterine growth. Institution of early and continuous decompression of the fetal hydrothorax can result in a successful outcome.

Pleural Effusions

Prenatal pleural effusion may be part of a generalized hydropic fetal condition of immune or nonimmune origin, accompanying a structural anomaly or, more rarely, an isolated finding. Fetal pleural effusions diagnosed in the late second or third trimester with spontaneous resolution have rarely been reported. The following paragraph describes a case[54] in which marked bilateral pleural effusion, noted first at 34 weeks, subsequently underwent complete spontaneous resolution at 37 weeks with good neonatal outcome.

The etiology of fetal pleural effusions is wide and includes hydrops fetalis of immune and nonimmune origin and chromosomal abnormalities, such as trisomy 21 and monosomy X. Isolated pleural effusions usually are associated with an underlying structural anomaly: pulmonary lymphangiectasia, CCAM of the lung, bronchopulmonary sequestration, diaphragmatic hernia, chest wall hemartoma, or pulmonary vein atresia. Possible etiologies of transient pleural effusions may be undetected fetal infection, brief episodes of fetal cardiac failure associated with undocumented arrhythmias, or transient decreases in fetal colloid osmotic pressure.

Complications and Outcome. The major complication of large persistent pleural effusions is prevention of normal lung growth and development, often resulting in pulmonary hypoplasia. Prognostic parameters for the infant with fetal pleural effusions are 1) gestational age at diagnosis and delivery, 2) whether the pleural effusions are persistent or whether spontaneous resolution occurs, 3) whether or not the case is complicated by hydrops, and 4) whether involvement is uni- or bilateral. Better outcomes are associated with later gestational age at diagnosis and delivery. In addition, fetuses with isolated unilateral pleural effusions without hydrops or with spontaneous resolution before delivery have enhanced survival rates.

Management. An array of invasive prenatal decompression techniques exist and are considered feasible in cases thought to be at risk for developing pulmonary hypoplasis. These procedures include repeated fetal thoracentesis, fetal tube thoracostomy (pleuroamniotic drain), or fetal thoracomaternal cutaneous shunting. All of these procedures carry the complication risks associated with surgical procedures; infections, preterm labor, clogging of shunts, etc. The difficulty in predicting pulmonary hypoplasia is the key issue in the management of the fetus with massive pleural effusions. This difficulty is enhanced in cases in which one does not know the length of time the effusions have existed. Cases of spontaneous resolution of fetal pleural effusions emphasize the importance of exercising clinical judgment and sonographic follow-up prior to embarking on prenatal surgical decompression.

Cervicomediastinal and Axillary Cystic Hygromas[55]

These are also called lymphatic hamartomas, (cystic) lymphangioma, hygroma colli cysticum, and jugular lymphatic obstructive sequence. These are uni- or multilocular lymphatic hamartomas ranging in size from several millimeters to 80 mm and containing a clear or cloudy fluidlike lymph. They occur in 1.6 per 10,000 pregnancies to 0.8% of pregnancies at risk for having a structural anomaly.[56]

Pathogenesis. There are at least three theories to explain the origin of cystic hygroma. The first theory suggests that an early jugular–lymphatic obstructive sequence could cause hydrops fetalis, pterygium colli, and cystic hygroma. This obstruction impedes communication between the jugular–lymphatic sacs and the internal jugular vein. Other researchers[57,58] believe that cystic hygroma is caused by an abnormal embryonic sequestration of lymphatic tissue and its subsequent failure to join normal lymphatic channels. A third theory[59] suggests that abnormal budding of the lymphatics occurs between 6 and 9 weeks of gestation. These then canalize to form lymph-filled cysts. Of these three theories, the first seems the most likely; however, the other two theories could be applied to noncervical lymphangiomyomatosis.

Location. In most cases, cystic hygromas are localized in the neck (Figs. 17–24 through 17–26). The biggest masses can be so large as to reach the floor of the mouth and the tongue. They can also reach the cheek, parotid, axilla, and mediastinum. In their descent toward the mediastinum, they follow the phrenic nerve between the subclavian vessels.[60] Cystic hygromas confined to the mediastinum are rare; they usually represent mediastinal invasion by cervical hygroma and are found in about 2 to 3% of cases.

Types. Lymphangiomas are made up of lymphatic vessels and are, fundamentally, endothelial cells limiting spaces and supporting connective tissue. There are three groups:

- *simple lymphangioma,* formed by lymphatic capillaries.

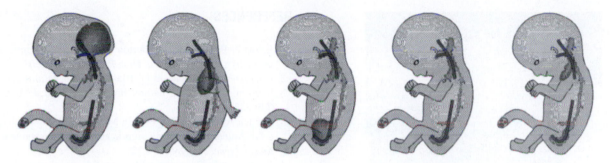

Figure 17–24. Distribution of cystic hygromas. The most common regions are *(from left to right)* the neck (75%); followed by the axillary region (20%); retroperitoneum and abdominal viscera (2%); limbs, bones, and mesentery (2%); and cervicomediastinum (1%). *(Reprinted with permission from Suma V, Marini A, Gamba P, et al. The Fetus. 1992;2:2281.)*

- *cavernous lymphangioma*, formed by bigger lymphatic vessels with a fibrous adventitia.
- *cystic lymphangioma*, commonly called *hygroma*, formed by multiple cysts ranging from a few millimeters to several centimeters in size.

These cysts are filled with lymphlike clear or muddy fluid. No communication exists between the lymphatic system and a cystic hygroma. Cystic hygromas have a predilection for local infiltration of the dermis, subcutaneous tissue, and soft tissue; occasionally, they are widespread. The neck, axilla, and chest may be particularly prone to this infiltrative behavior because of the local prevalence of major muscular and neurovascular bundles loosely embedded in fat.

About 50% of these are present at birth, and up to 90% became evident by 2 years of age. The incidence of cystic hygroma is approximately 1.6 per 10,000 pregnancies or 0.8% of pregnancies at risk for a structural anomaly.

Associated Anomalies. Although the cystic hygroma may be isolated, in many cases it is associated with hydrops fetalis.

Chromosomal defects, in particular monosomy X (Turner syndrome) and a wide variety of anatomic abnormalities, are found in more than 80% of the fetuses.

Ultrasound Diagnosis. The characteristic sonographic appearance shows asymmetric, multiseptate, thin-walled cystic masses localized in the axilla. Occasionally, the cystic mass may have a more complex echotexture, with cystic and solid components. This occurs when the obstructed lymphatic channels are among muscle and fibrous tissue or when portions of the abnormal lymphatic tissue remain clumped together.

Differential Diagnosis. The differential diagnosis should consider the possible masses involving the chest, such as cervical teratoma.

Prognosis. The prognosis depends on the presence or absence of associated hydrops, chromosomal aberrations, and anatomic defects.

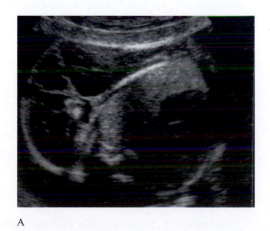
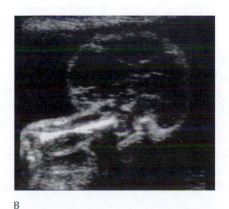

A   B

Figure 17–25. (A) View of the chest and right arm at 26 weeks. A multicystic mass surrounds the humerus and extends to the chest wall. **(B)** Humerus and the cystic mass at its proximal end. *(Reprinted with permission from Suma V, Marini A, Gamba P, et al. The Fetus. 1992;2:2286.)*

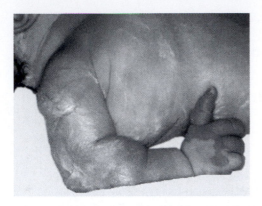

Figure 17–26. Cystic hygroma of the axillary region at birth. *(Reprinted with permission from Suma V, Marini A, Gamba P, et al. The Fetus. 1992;2:2281.)*

Spontaneous resolution of a cystic hygroma of the neck in a fetus affected by Turner syndrome and in a fetus with normal karyotype has been described. The presence of hydrops fetalis or lymphangiectasia indicates a serious prognosis, with a mortality rate of 100% within a few weeks from diagnosis. Two recent reports have suggested that isolated cystic hydroma in a typical location in the neck or axilla may have a better prognosis.[61,62] In the literature, 32 cases of cystic hygroma in children have been reported. In 12 cases, the hygroma was localized in the neck; in the remaining cases, it was in rare sites. Of these, 6 had hygromas in the axilla and chest wall, 5 in the mesentery, and 9 had lymphangiomas localized in various uncommon sites, such as cervicomediastinum, retroperiotoneum, scrotum, and multiple sites.

The complete excision of the cystic mass was possible in 23 cases. In another 7 cases, only partial removal was possible because of the size of the cystic mass. Two of the 23 patients who underwent complete excision died during the postoperative period. It appears that the prognosis for these babies depends largely on the anatomic location, the size of the tumors, and the ability of the pediatric surgeon to remove the masses.

Obstetric Management. When a prenatal diagnosis of cystic hygroma is made, the determination of the karyotype is recommended in all cases. Serial sonograms to assess the growth of the mass and monitoring for the development of hydrops should aid in the management of the pregnancy and are useful in the counseling of future pregnancies.

In the fetus with associated hydrops, the chance of survival is small; therefore, a nonagressive approach is advisable. The option of pregnancy termination should be offered before viability.

If there is a small, isolated cystic hygroma, no modification of standard obstetric management is required. When large lesions are present, a cesarean section may be advisable.

REFERENCES

1. Byrne J, Blanc WA, Warburton D, et al. The significance of cystic hygroma in fetuses. *Hum Pathol.* 1984;15:61.
2. Chervenak FA, Isaacson G, Blakemore KJ, et al. Fetal cystic hygroma. Cause and natural histgory. *N Engl J Med.* 1983; 309:822.
3. Garden AS, Benzie RJ, Miskin M, et al. Fetal cystic hygroma colli: Antenatal diagnosis, significance, and management. *Am J Obstet Gynecol.* 1986;154:221.
4. Newman DE, Cooperberg PL. Genetics of sonographically detected intrauterine fetal cystic hygromas. *J Can Assoc Radiol.* 1984;35:77.
5. Pearce JM, Griffin D, Campbell S. The differential prenatal diagnosis of cystic hygromata and encephalocele by ultrasound examination. *J Clin Ultrasound.* 1985;13:317.
6. Seashore JH, Gardiner LJ, Ariyan S. Management of giant cystic hygromas in infants. *Am J Surg.* 1985;149:459.
7. Nicolaides KH, Azar G, Byrne D, et al. Fetal nuchal translucency; ultrasound screening for chromosomal defects in the first trimester of pregnancy. *Br Med J.* 1992;304:867.
8. Nicolaides KH, Brizot ML, Snijders RJM. Fetal nuchal translucency thickness; ultrasound screening for fetal trisomy in the first trimester of pregnancy. *Br J Obstet Gynaecol.* 1994;101;782.
9. Pandya PP, Snijders RJM, Johnson SP, et al. Screening for fetal trisomies by maternal age and fetal nuchal translucency thickness at 10 to 14 weeks of gestation. *Br J Obstet Gynecol.* 1995;102:957.
10. Souka AP, Snijders RJM, Novakov A, et al. Defects and syndromes in chromosomally normal fetuses with increased nuchal translucency thickness at 10–14 aweeks of gestation. *Ultrasound Obstet Gynecol.* 1998;11:391.
11. *Br Med J.* 1999;318:81.
12. Snijders RJM, Holzgreve W, Cuckle H, Nicolaides KH. Maternal age-specific risks for trisomies at 9–14 weeks gestation. *Prenat Diagn.* 1994;14:543.
13. Ville Y, Lalondrelle C, Doumerc S. First-trimester diagnosis of nuchal anomalies: Significance and fetal outcome. *Ultrasound Obstet Gynecol.* 1992;2:314.
14. Szabeo J, Gellen J, Szemere G. First-trimester ultrasound screening for fetal aneuploidies in women over 35 and under 35 years of age. *Ultrasound Obstet Gynecol.* 1995;5:161.
15. Taipale P, Hillesman V, Salonen R, Ylostalo P. Increased nuchal translucency as a marker for fetal chromosomal defects. *N Engl J Med.* 1997;337:1654.
16. Snijders RJ, Johnson S, Sebire NJ, et al. First-trimester ultrasound screening for chromosomal defects. *Ultrasound Obstet Gynecol.* 1996;7:216.
17. Snijders RJ, Noble P, Sebire N, et al. UK multicentre project on assessment of risk of trisomy 21 by maternal age and fetal nuchal-translucency thickness at 10–14 weeks of gestation. *Lancet.* 1998;351:343.
18. De Catte L, De Backer A, Goosens A, et al. Teratoma, neck. *Fetus.* 1992;2:2381.
19. Mahony BS, Hegge FN. The face and neck. In: Nyberg DA, Mahony BS, Pretorious DH, eds. *Diagnostic Ultrasound of Fetal Anomalies.* Chicago: Year Book Medical Publishers; 1990: 203.

20. Jordan RB, Gauderer MW. Cervical teratomas: An analysis. Literature review and proposed classification. *J Pediatr Surg.* 1988;23:583.

21. Gonzalez-Crussi F. Teratomas of the neck. In: *Atlas of Tumor Pathology: Extragonadal Teratomas.* Washington, DC: Armed Forces Institute of Pathology; 1984;118.

22. Kelly MF, Berenholz L, Rizzo KA, et al. Approach for oxygenation of the newborn with airway obstruction due to a cervical mass. *Ann Otol Rhinol Laryngol.* 1990;99:179.

23. Skarsgard ED, Chitkara U, Krane EJ, et al. The OOPS procedure (operation on placental support): *In utero* airway management of the fetus with prenatally diagnosed tracheal obstruction. *J Pediatr Surg.* 1996;31:826.

24. Hubbard AM, Crombleholme TM, Adzick NS. Prenatal MRI evaluation of giant neck masses in preparation for the fetal exit procedure. *Am J Perinatol.* 1998;15:253.

25. Liechty KW, Crombleholme TM, Flake AW, et al. Intrapartum airway management for giant fetal neck masses: The EXIT (*ex utero* intrapartum treatment) procedure. *Am J Obstet Gynecol.* 1997;177:870.

26. Chescheir NC, Kuller JA, Wells SR, et al. Perinatal management of a lingual teratoma. *Obstet Gynecol.* 1996;87(5 Pt 2):848.

27. Joffe GM, Izquierdo LA, Del Valle GO, et al. Agnathia–holoprosencephaly. *Fetus.* 1991;1:7448.

28. Joffe GM, Izquierdo LA, Del Valle GO, et al. Congenital lobar adenomatosis, type I. *Fetus.* 1991;1:7484.

29. Moore KL. *The Developing Human: Clinically Oriented Embryology,* 4th ed. Philadelphia: WB Saunders; 1998.

30. Ch'in KY, Tang MY. Congenital adenomatoid malformation of one lobe of a lung with general anasarca. *Arch Pathol.* 1949;48:221:155.

31. Stocker JT, Madewell JE, Drake RM. Congenital cystic adenomatoid malformation of the lung. *Hum Pathol.* 1977;82:155.

32. Ostor AG, Fortune DW. Congenital cystic adenomatoid malformation of the lung. *Am J Clin Pathol.* 1978;70:595.

33. Bale PM. Congenital cystic malformation of the lung. *Am J Clin Pathol.* 1979;71:411.

34. Krous HF, Harper PE, Perlman M. Congenital cystic adenomatoid malformation in bilateral renal agenesis. *Arch Pathol Lab Med.* 1980;104:368.

35. Boiskin I, Brunner JP, Jeanty P. Lung extralobar intrathoracic sequestration, torsion. *Fetus.* 1991;1:7485.

36. Garrett WJ, Kossoff G, Lawrence R. Gray-scale echography in the diagnosis of hydrops due to fetal lung tumor. *J Clin Ultrasound.* 1975;3:45.

37. Sauerbrei E. Lung sequestration. *J Ultrasound Med.* 1991;10:101.

38. Salzman DH, Adzick SN, Benacerraf BR. Fetal cystic adenomatoid malformation of the lungs: Apparent improvement in utero. *Obstet Gynecol.* 1988;71:1000.

39. Nicolaides KH, Blott M, Greenough A. Chronic drainage of fetal pulmonary cyst. *Lancet.* 1987;i:618.

40. Harrison MR, Adzick NS, Jennings RW, et al. Antenatal intervention for congenital cystic adenomatoid malformation. *Lancet.* 1990;336:965.

41. Valcamonico A, Gonçalves LF, Jeanty P. Larynx, atresia. *Fetus.* 1992;2:7483.

42. Silver MM, Thurston W, Patrik JE. Perinatal pulmonary hyperplasia due to laryngeal atresia. *Hum Pathol.* 1988;19:110.

43. Walander A. Prenatal development of the epithelial primordium of the larynx in rat. *Acta Anat (Basel).* 1950;10(suppl):2.

44. Gatti WM, MacDonald E, Orfei E, et al. Congenital laryngeal atresia. *Laryngoscope.* 1987;97:966.

45. Benacerraf BR, Frigoletto FD. Mid-trimester fetal thoracentesis. *J Clin Ultrasound.* 1985;13:202.

46. Bliek AJ, Mulholland DJ. Extralobar lung sequestration associated with fatal neonatal respiratory distress. *Thorax.* 1971;26:125.

47. Defoort P, Thiery M. Antenatal diagnosis of congenital chylothorax by gray scale sonography. *J Clin Ultrasound.* 1978;6:4.

48. Hunter WS, Becraft DMQ. Congenital pulmonary lymphangiectasis associated with pleural effusions. *Arch Dis Child.* 1984;59:278.

49. Jaffa AJ, Barak S, Kaysar N, et al. Case report. Antenatal diagnosis of bilateral congenital chylothorax with pericardial effusion. *Acta Obstet Gynecol Scand.* 1985;64:455.

50. Koffler H, Papile LA, Burstein RL. Congenital chylothorax: Two cases associated with maternal polyhydramnios. *Am J Dis Child.* 1978;132:638.

51. Schmidt W, Harms E, Wolf D. Successful prenatal treatment of nonimmune hydrops fetalis due to congenital chylothorax. Case report. *Br J Obstet Gynaecol.* 1985;92:685.

52. Wheeler TC, Jeanty P. Lung sequestration, extralobar subdiaphragmatic. *Fetus* 1993;3:7485.

53. Stocker JT. Sequestrations of the lung. *Semin Diagn Pathol.* 1986;3:106.

54. Sherer DM, Abramowicz JS, Woods JR. Pleural effusion, bilateral transient. *Fetus.* 1991;1:7488.

55. Suma V, Marini A, Gamba P. et al. Cystic hygroma, axillary, cervicomediastinal. *Fetus.* 1992;2:2281.

56. Smith DW, Graham JM. Jugular lymphatic obstruction sequence. In: Jones, *Recognizable Pattern of Human Malformation: Genetic Embryologic and Clinical Aspects.* Philadelphia: WB Saunders; 1982;472.

57. Goetsch E. Hygroma colli cysticum and hygroma axillae: Pathologic and clinical study and report of twelve cases. *Arch Surg.* 1938;36:394.

58. Phillips H, McGaham J. Intrauterine fetal cystic hygroma; Sonographic detection. *AJR.* 1981;136:799.

59. Lee K, Klein T. Surgery of cysts and tumors of the neck. In: Paparella M, Snunriek D, eds. *Otolaryngology.* Philadelphia: WB Saunders; 1980;2987.

60. Csicsko JF, Grosfeld JL. Cervico mediastinal hygroma with pulmonary hypoplasia in the newborn. *Am J Dis Child.* 1974;128:577.

61. Hoffman-Tretin J, Koenigsberg M, Ziprkowski M. Antenatal demonstration of axillary cystic hygroma. *J Ultrasound Med.* 1988;7:233.

62. Benacerraf BR, Frigoletto FD. Prenatal sonographic diagnosis of isolated congenital cystic hygroma unassociated with lymphedema or other morphologic abnormalities. *J Ultrasound Med.* 1987;6:63.

Sonography of the Fetal Gastrointestinal System

Barbara S. Hertzberg • Mark A. Kliewer • James D. Bowie

Prenatal sonography can detect a wide variety of fetal gastrointestinal abnormalities. This chapter examines the sonographic findings of the gastrointestinal disorders that can be recognized *in utero,* with an emphasis on potential diagnostic pitfalls that arise from confusion with normal anatomy, anatomic variants, and pathologic processes elsewhere in the fetus.

GENERAL PRINCIPLES

The routine obstetric survey often provides clues to the presence of a fetal gastrointestinal disorder. Gastrointestinal pathology can declare itself either as an abnormal finding or as the absence of a normal finding. Therefore, the sonologist must be alert to the presence of polyhydramnios, fetal ascites, too many fluid-filled structures in the abdomen, intraabdominal calcifications, and the absence of a fluid-filled stomach.

Although polyhydramnios may be a sign of gastrointestinal tract obstruction, increased amniotic fluid volume occurs in a variety of disorders and is frequently a nonspecific finding with no identifiable etiology.[1,2] As a first approximation, mildly increased amniotic fluid volume in the singleton pregnancy has maternal causes(e.g., diabetes or isoimmunization disorders) in 20% of cases, has fetal causes in 20%, and is idiopathic in 60%.[3] The frequency of fetal anomalies, however, increases with the severity of the polyhydramnios.[4] With severe polyhydramnios, the likelihood of fetal anomalies is 75% or greater.[4,5] Gastrointestinal abnormalities are among the most common fetal causes of increased amniotic fluid and account for approximately one third of such cases in singleton pregnancies.[4] Polyhydramnios develops with fetal gastrointestinal tract obstruction if the amniotic fluid swallowed by the fetus cannot be effectively reabsorbed and, therefore, is left to accumulate in the amniotic cavity.[6] Thus, polyhydramnios is more common with high rather than with low gastrointestinal tract obstructions.

Like polyhydramnios, fetal ascites can be the result of a gastrointestinal abnormality but is a nonspecific finding. Ascites occurs in conjunction with immune and nonimmune hydrops, *in utero* infection, gastrointestinal or urinary tract obstruction with perforation, abdominal tumors, and, rarely, spontaneous perforation of the common bile duct or chyloperitoneum.[7,8] Large quantities of fetal ascites are relatively easy to diagnose with antenatal sonography, but when smaller amounts of ascites are suspected, the possibility of pseudoascites should also be considered.[9–11] *Pseudoascites* refers to an echogenic band around the perimeter

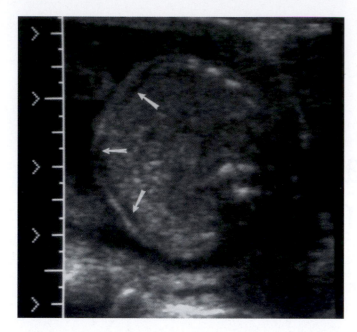

Figure 18–1. Axial view of a normal fetal abdomen showing a thin hypoechoic rim just inside the outer margin of the abdominal wall *(arrows).* This echogenic area is referred to as "pseudoascites" and is thought to represent abdominal wall musculature.

of the anterior and lateral aspects of the fetal abdomen, corresponding to the abdominal wall musculature (Fig. 18–1). Although this hypoechoic rim of abdominal muscles can mimic true ascites, it is confined to the anterior and lateral aspects of the abdomen and can frequently be followed to muscle insertions on the ribs. In contrast to pseudoascites, true ascites tends to surround organs, collect in peritoneal recesses, and outline the falciform ligament, greater omentum, and umbilical vessels as they enter the abdomen (Figs. 18–2 and 18–3).

Accurate recognition of dilated loops of bowel requires a familiarity with the appearance of the fluid-filled structures

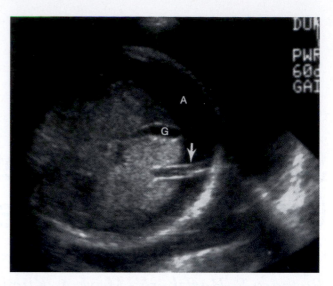

Figure 18–3. Transverse section of the fetal abdomen reveals ascites (A) surrounding the umbilical vein *(arrow).* G, gallbladder.

normally found in the fetal abdomen. These include the stomach, gallbladder, urinary bladder, and portal vein. Later in pregnancy, the fetal colon accounts for many of the hypoechoic areas seen in the abdomen. The sonologist should attempt to identify each echo-free area found in the fetal abdomen. If an unexplained cystic structure is seen, the organ of origin should be determined when possible. The fetal kidneys are the most common source of fluid collections or masses in the fetal abdomen and are particularly implicated when the abnormal area touches the spine. A wide variety of other processes unrelated to the bowel and kidney can, however, also cause abnormal fluid collections, and at times it is not possible to localize the proximate organ with certainty. Other possible sources include the ovaries (cyst or teratoma), uterus (hydrometrocolpos), urinary bladder

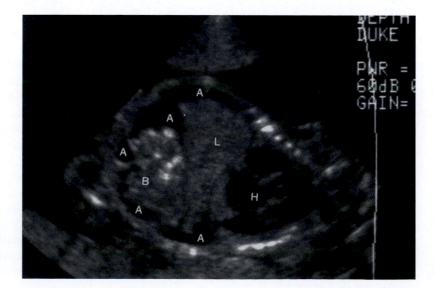

Figure 18–2. Coronal scan of a fetus with ascites and multiple congenital anomalies, demonstrating true ascites (A) surrounding organs and collecting in peritoneal recesses. L, liver; H, heart; B, bowel.

(obstructed), spine (anterior meningocele or sacrococcygeal teratoma), biliary tree (choledochal cyst), omentum or mesentery (omental or mesenteric cyst), and liver (hepatic cyst). Identification of peristalsis, demonstration of a connection to the stomach, or a characteristic tubular shape suggest a gastrointestinal etiology.

ESOPHAGUS AND STOMACH

The normal fetal esophagus is occasionally visualized by prenatal sonography as a tubular echogenic structure in the neck and posterior chest.[12] It often exhibits a multilayered pattern.

The most commonly identified esophageal anomaly is esophageal atresia. This malformation results in an abrupt termination of the esophagus as a blind pouch. In approximately 90% of cases, esophageal atresia is associated with a tracheoesophageal fistula, which most often connects the trachea to the distal esophagus. Additional abnormalities occur in a high percentage of fetuses with esophageal atresia, and these include cardiac, chromosomal, gastrointestinal, genitourinary, and central nervous system lesions.[13] The VACTERL complex of vertebral, anal, cardiovascular, tracheoesophageal, renal, radial, and limb malformations is perhaps the best-known grouping of anomalies associated with tracheoesophageal lesions.

The sonographic diagnosis of esophageal atresia is based on the demonstration of polyhydramnios in association with an inability to visualize a fluid-filled fetal stomach in its normal location in the left upper quadrant[14] (Fig. 18–4). Rarely, a fluid-filled pouch corresponding to the atretic segment of the esophagus is seen in the neck.[15] Unfortunately, esophageal atresia cannot be diagnosed or excluded simply by inspecting for a fetal stomach. Because the majority of fetuses with esophageal atresia also have a tracheoesophageal fistula, the stomach can be visualized if fluid crosses from the trachea into the stomach through the fistula.[16] In this subset, the stomach can be seen in almost 60% of fetuses. Conversely, the combination of polyhydramnios and gastric nonvisualization is only seen in approximately one-third of fetuses with a tracheoesophageal fistula, underscoring how difficult it can be to make an antenatal diagnosis of esophageal atresia if the fetus also has such a fistula. Further confounding the antenatal diagnosis, rarely, a fluid-filled stomach can be identified in the fetus with esophageal atresia without a tracheoesophageal fistula. This is probably the consequence of distention of the stomach by intrinsic gastric secretions.

The fluid-filled stomach is consistently imaged in the left upper quadrant by 14 to 15 menstrual weeks, although it is often seen earlier.[17] Failure to see fluid in the stomach is unusual in normal fetuses beyond this stage of gestation and should prompt a follow-up examination. Nonvisualization of the stomach can occasionally occur in normal pregnancies as a transient finding, although the frequency with which this occurs is not well established. In one recent series, transient nonvisualization was detected in 9 of 995 fetuses and was associated with a normal outcome in all but 1 infant. In contradistinction, another study reported abnormal outcomes in 4 of 12 (33%) fetuses with transient gastric nonvisualization.[18,19] More recently, no congenital anomalies were found in 14 fetuses with transient gastric nonvisualization, although two of these pregnancies ended in spontaneous abortion at 20 weeks.[20] The stomach normally changes in size as it fills and empties during the course of an ultrasound examination, so failure to visualize the stomach of a healthy

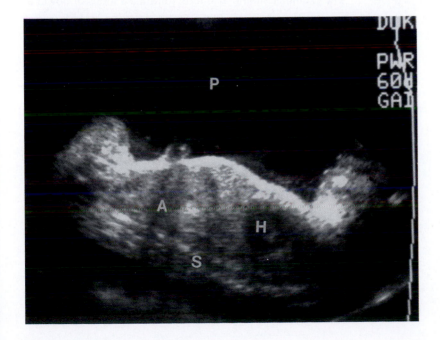

Figure 18–4. Parasagittal scan to the left of midline. Note marked polyhydramnios (P) and absence of a fluid-filled stomach in this fetus with esophageal atresia but no tracheoesophageal fistula. A, abdomen; H, heart; S, spine.

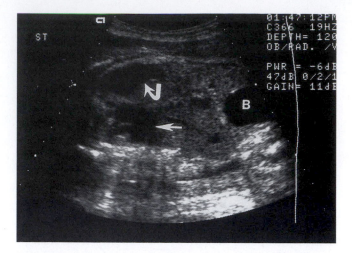

Figure 18–5. Oblique coronal image of the thorax, abdomen; and pelvis of a fetus with a diaphragmatic hernia. The stomach *(curved arrow)* is not seen in its expected location in the left upper quadrant but is instead seen in the thorax, adjacent to the heart *(straight arrow)*. B, bladder.

fetus is likely due to scanning during a period of physiologic emptying.[18,19,21]

A stomach that appears significantly smaller than expected can also signal an underlying abnormality. A small stomach that persists on follow-up should prompt a detailed morphologic survey. In a recent series, 27 of 52 (52%) fetuses with a small stomach had an abnormal outcome.[23] However, if a small stomach is observed as an isolated, transient finding with normalization of gastric size on a follow-up scan, the outcome is more likely to be normal: all 12 fetuses with an isolated, transiently small stomach in the aforementioned series had a normal outcome.[23] Identification of a small or absent stomach is more likely to be associated with a poor

outcome when observed at after 24 weeks than when seen earlier in gestation.[23]

Besides being a potential sign of esophageal atresia or a normal variant, nonvisualization of the stomach or visualization of a small stomach also occurs in a variety of other pathologic conditions.[18–20,22,23] One of the most common causes of gastric nonvisualization is oligohydramnios. In this setting, the fetal stomach is simply not distended with fluid because of the general paucity of amniotic fluid available for the fetus to swallow. Oligohydramnios likely accounts for published descriptions of gastric nonvisualization in a wide variety of conditions, including genitourinary tract abnormalities, chromosomal abnormalities, and intrauterine growth retardation. Gastric nonvisualization can also be related to impairment of the normal swallowing mechanism. This is the likely explanation for gastric nonvisualization in fetuses with central nervous system abnormalities, facial clefts, and neuromuscular disorders. Finally, the stomach may be distended with fluid but not recognized if it is displaced from its expected location in the left upper quadrant, as occurs in the fetus with a diaphragmatic hernia or a situs abnormality (Fig. 18–5).

Prenatal sonography occasionally detects echogenic masses in the fetal stomach (Fig. 18–6). These have been termed *gastric pseudomasses* because they are usually transient conglomerations of swallowed cells and cell fragments.[24] A pseudomass in the fetal stomach should not be misinterpreted as a pathologic mass, such as a gastric neoplasm. Moreover, gastric pseudomasses usually do not indicate the presence of an associated pathology. They can, however, be produced by swallowed intraamniotic blood after amniocentesis or placental abruption.[25] With this in mind, the uterus should be carefully scanned for evidence of placental abruption when a gastric pseudomass is detected. The examiner should also look for dilated loops of bowel in

Figure 18–6. Coronal image of a normal fetus shows two echogenic collections *(arrows)* in the stomach. These "gastric pseudomasses" are usually a transient finding without pathologic significance, although the likelihood of detecting gastric pseudomasses is increased in the fetus with bowel obstruction. Gastric pseudomasses can also be seen when the fetus swallows intraamniotic blood. C, colon.

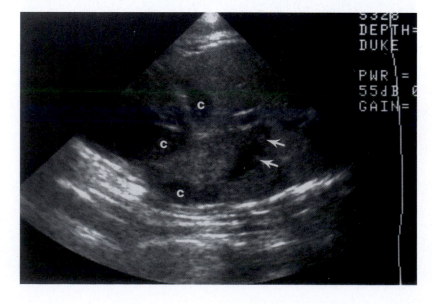

the fetal abdomen because the likelihood of detecting debris or pseudomasses in the stomach is increased in fetuses with delayed intestinal transport due to bowel obstruction. In the absence of clinical or sonographic evidence of placental abruption or fetal abnormalities, an isolated gastric pseudomass can generally be interpreted as a normal variant not requiring further workup.

Other stomach abnormalities that can be detected *in utero* include gastric outlet obstructions, such as pyloric web, atresia or stenosis, and congenital hiatal hernia.[26–32] Hypertrophic pyloric stenosis typically does not present until several weeks after birth, but rarely it can be associated with antenatal gastric dilation.[26–30] Recognizing abnormal dilation can be difficult because the normal fetal stomach has a wide range of sizes.[26] Ancillary findings include polyhydramnios, gastric wall thickening, a funnel-shaped narrowing of the gastric antrum, and a shapeless lesser curvature.[26,27] Congenital hiatal hernia is also a potentially difficult diagnosis to make *in utero* because it can resemble a congenital diaphragmatic hernia in which only a portion of the stomach has herniated into the chest. Therefore, both hiatal hernia and diaphragmatic hernia can result in a cystic structure in the thorax that is in continuity with the stomach. The specific diagnosis of hiatal hernia should be considered, however, when only a small part of the stomach resides in the thorax and ancillary findings characteristic of a diaphragmatic hernia are notably absent, such as mediastinal shift, decreased abdominal circumference, polyhydramnios, pleural or pericardial effusion, and other structural abnormalities.[28] It is important to distinguish these two entities because hiatal hernia has a better prognosis than diaphragmatic hernia, is not associated with chromosomal or structural anomalies, and is not considered a potential indication for *in utero* surgery.

DUODENUM

Duodenal atresia is the most common type of congenital small bowel obstruction. Most cases are thought to represent a developmental error resulting from failure to recanalize the duodenal lumen during the 11th week of gestation. Duodenal atresia is associated with a high incidence of associated anomalies, including congenital heart disease, esophageal atresia, imperforate anus, small bowel atresia, biliary atresia, and renal and vertebral anomalies.[33–35] In addition, at least 20 to 30% of fetuses with duodenal atresia have trisomy 21.[33]

Prenatal diagnosis of duodenal obstruction is based on sonographic demonstration of polyhydramnios in association with a fluid-filled "double bubble" in the upper part of the fetal abdomen (Fig. 18–7). The double bubble is produced by a distended stomach in the upper left quadrant connecting to a large duodenal bulb on the right. In contrast, a fluid-distended duodenum is only rarely recognized in a normal

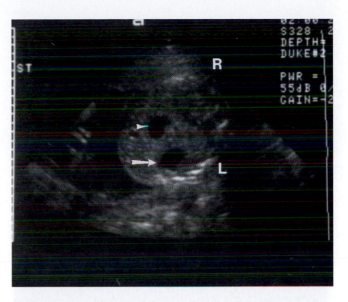

Figure 18–7. Axial image of a fetus with duodenal atresia shows a "double bubble" sign due to fluid in the stomach *(arrow)* in the left upper quadrant and a dilated duodenal bulb *(arrowhead)* on the right. L, toward fetal left; R, toward fetal right.

fetus, and when it is seen, it should be a transient finding which resolves in 10 to 15 mins either way.[36,37] The double-bubble sign observed *in utero* is analogous to the gas-filled double bubble seen on postpartum radiographs of infants with duodenal atresia. Antenatal ultrasound identification of the double-bubble sign has been established as early as 14 to 15 weeks,[37,38] although, in many cases, the diagnosis is not recognized until the third trimester.

Demonstration of two fluid-filled bubbles in the upper part of the fetal abdomen is not, however, found exclusively with duodenal atresia. The term *double bubble* implies duodenal obstruction and should not be used when other competing diagnoses are more likely. In the fetus with duodenal atresia, the second bubble will be in the expected location of the duodenal bulb, which is typically in the center of the abdomen, just to the right of midline. If the second bubble is not in an appropriate location for the duodenal bulb, the differential diagnosis depends on the appearance and location of the abnormal cystic structure. For example, a cyst in the left upper quadrant could be imaged in the same scan plane as the fetal stomach and, therefore, resemble the double bubble, but it would more likely be a renal cyst, splenic cyst (Fig. 18–8), or gastric duplication cyst.[39–41] Even if the second cyst is in the right midabdomen in an appropriate location for the duodenal bulb, it is important to try to determine whether there is continuity between the two fluid-filled structures, as would be expected with the stomach emptying into an enlarged duodenum (Fig. 18–9). If a connection cannot be shown, a number of other possibilities should be considered. The most common of these is a choledochal cyst, although other potential explanations for a right upper quadrant cyst include a renal, hepatic, omental, duplication, or ovarian

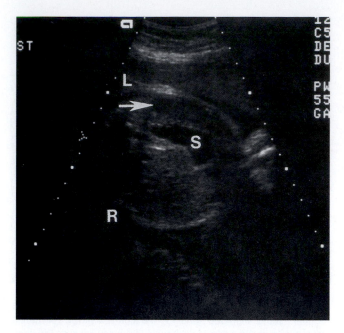

Figure 18–8. "Pseudo-double bubble" sign due to visualization of a splenic cyst *(arrow)* and the fetal stomach (S) on the same image. L, toward fetal left; R, toward fetal right.

cyst.[42–45] One other potential pitfall is to bisect an otherwise normal fetal stomach in an oblique scan plane, giving the spurious appearance of a double bubble[46] (Fig. 18–10A). This misrepresentation can be corrected by scanning the abdomen in a true transverse plane, so as to demonstrate the typical tapering configuration of the gastric antrum (Fig. 18–10B).

The double-bubble sign is not specific for duodenal atresia but simply indicates the presence of an obstructive process

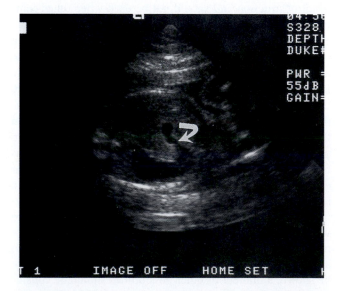

Figure 18–9. Oblique image of the abdomen of a fetus with duodenal atresia shows connection *(arrow)* between the stomach and an enlarged duodenal bulb.

in the duodenum. Other possible causes of duodenal obstruction include a duodenal web, annular pancreas,[47] preduodenal portal vein,[48] duodenal stenosis, Ladd's bands, volvulus, or obstruction from an intestinal duplication.

Rarely, duodenal atresia and esophageal atresia occur in combination without an associated tracheoesophageal fistula. This results in formation of a closed loop of bowel comprising the distal esophagus, stomach, and duodenum. Dilation of this closed loop tends to occur earlier and be far more severe than in isolated duodenal atresia because of massive accumulation of gastric and biliary secretions. Antenatal ultrasound may demonstrate an extremely distended C-shaped abdominal fluid collection, which is thought to be characteristic of this combination of anomalies when seen in the second trimester.[49,50] If the fluid collection extends into the thorax, the differential diagnosis should also include congenital diaphragmatic hernia.[49,51]

SMALL BOWEL AND ECHOGENIC BOWEL

Small bowel loops can occasionally be seen in the normal fetus, but they usually are not demonstrated without a special effort. Individual segments of small bowel should not exceed approximately 7 mm in diameter or 15 mm in length and are usually considerably smaller than these values.[52,53] The small bowel is often seen in active peristalsis and changes in configuration during real-time observation.

The sonographic diagnosis of small bowel obstruction relies on demonstration of multiple interconnecting, overdistended bowel loops. The number of dilated loops depends on the level of obstruction: The lower the level of obstruction, the more loops are seen (Fig. 18–11A and B). The peristalsis observed in obstructed small bowel loops may appear more vigorous when compared with peristalsis in unobstructed bowel.[53,54] Identification of such peristalsis can help substantiate that an abnormal structure is bowel. Polyhydramnios occurs in association with many cases of jejunal and ileal obstruction, and it is more common with higher levels of obstruction.

A variety of different processes can be mistaken for dilated small bowel. These include the cysts in an enlarged multicystic dysplastic kidney (Fig. 18–12), a dilated tortuous ureter, and normal-caliber large bowel. When small bowel obstruction is suspected, the kidneys should be examined carefully to ensure that the abnormal, fluid-containing structures are not renal in origin. Likewise, the possibility of a dilated ureter should be excluded by evaluating the location and course of the abnormal structures for subtle connections to the kidney or bladder. Normal-caliber large bowel can usually be distinguished from obstructed small bowel on the basis of its peripheral location and course, which corresponds to that of the postnatal colon and rectosigmoid. At times, however, distinction between normal colon and dilated small bowel can be difficult to make. Serial scans may be helpful when there

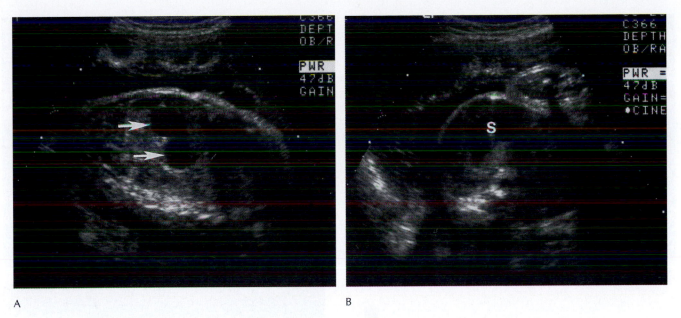

Figure 18–10. (A) Apparent double bubble sign *(arrows)* produced by imaging the normal fetal stomach in an oblique scan plane. **(B)** When the transducer is rotated into a true axial plane, a normal-appearing fetal stomach (S) is seen.

is reason to suspect a bowel obstruction but early sonograms are normal: Duodenal and small bowel obstructions are often not apparent by sonography until the late second trimester or early third trimester.[55]

Prenatal small bowel dilation occurs in a variety of disorders, including both obstructive and nonobstructive etiologies. The most common obstructive cause of small bowel dilation is intestinal atresia.[56] Small bowel atresia is usually related to an *in utero* vascular accident. There are several morphologically different types of atresias, the most common of which results in blind ends of bowel separated from each other by a gap. Other varieties include a membrane obstructing otherwise intact bowel, blind ends of bowel connected by a fibrous band, multiple atresias, and the "apple peel atresia," which refers to diffuse atresia affecting a long segment of bowel. Unlike duodenal atresia, small bowel atresia is associated with a low rate of extragastrointestinal and chromosomal abnormalities. Additional gastrointestinal tract abnormalities, such as volvulus, malrotation, and duplication are relatively common, however. These other intestinal abnormalities also can cause antenatal small bowel obstruction in the absence of atresia.[57,58] A "whirlpool" or "snail" sign in which a dilated loop of bowel is wrapped around itself has been observed in some cases of volvulus.[57]

Another well-known source of antenatal small bowel obstruction is meconium ileus. Meconium ileus is a specific type of distal small bowel obstruction unique to fetuses with cystic fibrosis. The bowel obstruction in fetuses with cystic fibrosis is thought to result from impaction of abnormally thickened, viscous meconium. In addition to dilated loops of small bowel, fetuses with cystic fibrosis can exhibit a variety of other telling findings by prenatal sonography, including polyhydramnios, meconium peritonitis, an inconspicuous gallbladder, abnormal areas of increased abdominal echogenicity, and decreased prominence of the colon due to microcolon.[59–66] These findings, however, are nonspecific. Hyperechoic areas in the fetal abdomen can be particularly difficult to characterize and interpret.

These hyperechoic areas in the fetal abdomen have been described in a variety of normal and abnormal processes other than cystic fibrosis. A single echogenic masslike area is seen transiently in the pelvis and lower abdomen of many normal fetuses in the mid-second trimester[67,68] (Fig. 18–13). Although it is clear that such an area is not an abdominal mass, there is disagreement as to whether or not such areas can be dismissed as normal variants in all cases. Other sources of increased abdominal echogenicity that should cause relatively little concern include hyperechoic colonic meconium in an otherwise normal fetus near term and hyperechoic bowel contents in the fetus who has swallowed intraamniotic blood.[69,70] Rarely, increased intestinal echogenicity may be due to ingestion of gas-forming bacteria from the amniotic fluid in the setting of chorioamnionitis.[71] Otherwise, the fetal bowel should never contain air.

Regions of increased abdominal echogenicity, particularly during the second trimester, have more recently been associated with an increased prevalence of a variety of unfavorable outcomes including cystic fibrosis; chromosomal abnormalities, such as triploidy and trisomies 13, 18, and 21; cytomegalovirus infection; intestinal obstruction; anorectal malformation; severe intrauterine growth retardation; and fetal demise.[61,64,72–82] The prevalence of these

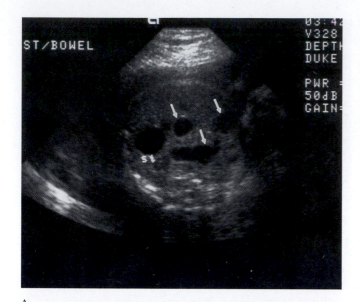

A

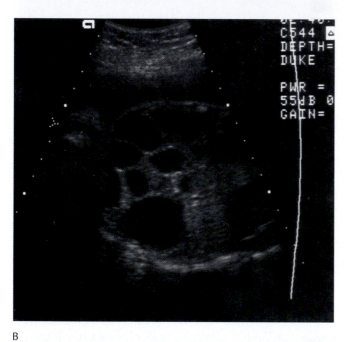

B

Figure 18–11. (A) A few dilated loops of small bowel *(arrows)* are seen in a fetus with proximal jejunal atresia. ST, stomach. **(B)** Multiple loops of dilated small bowel in a fetus with distal jejunal atresia. Note the increased number of dilated loops compared with **A**.

abnormal outcomes seems to be greatest in fetuses exhibiting the most extreme levels of abdominal hyperechogenicity; that is, when the area is at least as echogenic as bone. Despite these alarming reports, increased abdominal echogenicity should be interpreted with caution because many fetuses with this finding are normal.[22] Moreover, echogenicity is a subjective finding that differs with the observer, scan plane, transducer frequency, and other technical factors. Further studies will be necessary before consensus can

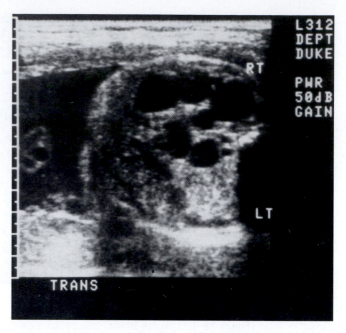

Figure 18–12. Axial image of the abdomen of a fetus with a right multicystic dysplastic kidney. Note the similarity in appearance of the renal cysts to the obstructed dilated loops of small bowel in Figure 18-11B. RT, toward fetal right; LT, toward fetal left.

be reached regarding the appropriate management of the second-trimester fetus with hyperechoic bowel. Among the unresolved questions to be addressed is whether or not additional antenatal diagnostic tests, such as follow-up sonography, fetal karyotype analysis, DNA testing for cystic fibrosis, and third-trimester monitoring for fetal growth and well-being, should be routinely offered to the parents of these fetuses.

Nonobstructive etiologies of small bowel obstruction are relatively unusual and include congenital chloridorrhea and megacystis–microcolon–intestinal hypoperistalsis syndrome.[83–87] Bowel dilation in congenital chloridorrhea is related to impaired transport of chloride from the distal ileum and colon. Dilation in megacystis–microcolon–intestinal hypoperistalsis syndrome is thought to be related to decreased peristalsis due to an intrinsic abnormality of smooth muscle. In this syndrome, dilation of the urinary bladder, rather than of the bowel, tends to be the most frequent and striking finding antenatally.[83–85] Even so, the diagnosis should be considered, particularly when the combination of dilated bowel and urinary bladder is seen.[83,84]

LARGE BOWEL

Large bowel obstruction is generally more difficult to diagnose than small bowel obstruction because there is considerable variability in the diameter of the normal fetal colon. As early as 22 menstrual weeks, the fetal colon can be seen

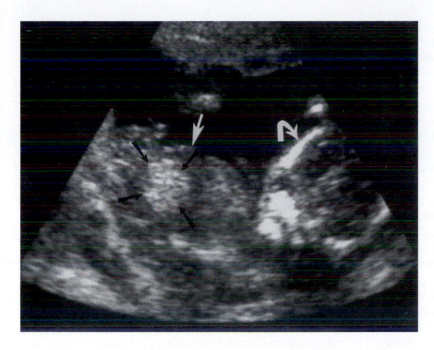

Figure 18–13. Coronal scan of a normal 16-week fetus demonstrates a focal area of increased echogenicity *(black arrows)* in the lower abdomen. Although this is frequently a normal variant, areas of increased abdominal echogenicity have been associated with unfavorable outcomes, such as cystic fibrosis, chromosomal abnormalities, cytomegalovirus infection, and severe intrauterine growth retardation. *Curved white arrow*, fetal head: *straight white arrow*, fetal abdomen.

as a tubular structure around the perimeter of the abdomen, which follows the expected course of the colon in the abdomen and the rectosigmoid in the pelvis.[52,53] In contrast, small bowel will be much smaller in caliber and more centrally located. Small bowel can often be seen to actively peristalse during real-time evaluation. During the latter part of the third trimester, the normal fetal colon can be particularly prominent and striking (Fig. 18–14) and could be mistaken as abnormal. The contents of the colon are usually less echogenic than adjacent abdominal structures but can be hyperechoic during the third trimester.[69,70] The mean diameter of the colon increases approximately linearly with menstrual age, but there is wide variation in size around the mean at any

given age. Therefore, the colon diameters of normal fetuses can overlap those of fetuses with abnormally distended large bowel. Near term, the normal fetal colon may measure up to 18 mm or more in diameter.[52]

Dilated colon has been detected antenatally in fetuses with meconium plug syndrome, Hirschsprung's disease, and anorectal malformation, but diagnosing a pathologically dilated colon can be problematic considering the wide variation in size and appearance of the normal fetal colon.[88,92] Bowel dilation in the meconium plug syndrome is due to transient colonic obstruction from meconium in the distal colon. Meconium plug syndrome occurs in both normal fetuses and those with cystic fibrosis. Hirschsprung's disease

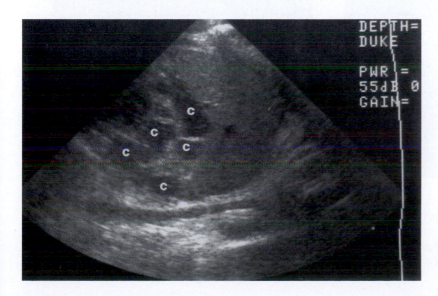

Figure 18–14. Coronal scan of a normal fetus near term demonstrating a meconium-filled colon (C). Note how prominent the colon can be late in the third trimester.

is due to congenital absence of the ganglion cells of the myenteric plexus. The involved segment of bowel extends proximally from the anus to involve different lengths of the colon. Because the aganglionic segment is unable to transmit peristaltic contractions normally, there is a functional obstruction that results in dilation of bowel proximal to the affected segment. Hirschsprung's disease usually is not apparent before birth, although antenatal detection has been rarely described.[89,90] Findings that can be seen antenatally include polyhydramnios and multiple loops of dilated fetal bowel.[89,90]

Anorectal malformation refers to a spectrum of abnormalities of hindgut termination including imperforate anus anal agenesis, anorectal agenesis, and rectal atresia. These lesions are associated with a high incidence of additional anomalies and are commonly found as a component of the VACTERL syndrome or the caudal regression syndrome (renal agenesis or dysplasia, sacral agenesis, lower extremity hypoplasia). Anorectal malformations also occur in complex abnormalities of cloacal development, such as persistent cloaca and cloacal exstrophy. The malformations are divided into two groups depending on the location of atresia. High lesions terminate above the levator sling, are commonly associated with a fistula to the genitourinary system, and require an abdominal surgical approach. Low malformations terminate below the levator sling in an orifice on the perineum or inside the posterior vaginal fourchette, and are usually treated with a perineal surgical approach.

Antenatal ultrasound shows dilated fetal colon or hyperechoic areas in the abdomen in some fetuses with anorectal malformation.[77,78,92–96] Even so, the sensitivity of ultrasound for detecting colonic and anorectal obstruction is poor.[92,97,98] The likelihood of sonographic visualization of dilated bowel in the fetus with an anorectal malformation increases as pregnancy progresses.[69] Identification of a dilated V- or U-shaped segment of bowel in the fetal pelvis or lower abdomen is though to be particularly suggestive of anorectal malformation[92,99] Intraluminal intestinal or bladder calcifications have also been described, usually in fetuses with a fistula between the gastrointestinal and urinary tracts. These calcifications are thought to form because of the mixing of urine and meconium.[92,100–102]

The normal meconium-filled rectum is occasionally mistaken for a presacral mass[103,104] (Fig. 18–15A). This error, which has been termed the *presacral pseudomass,* is readily disclosed by rotating the transducer into an oblique plane to demonstrate a connection between the presumed mass and the sigmoid colon (Fig. 18–15B).

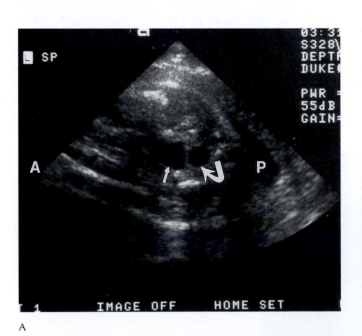

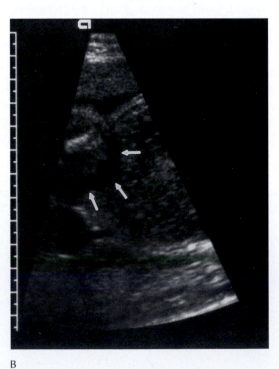

Figure 18–15. **(A)** Axial image through the pelvis of a fetus referred from an outside institution to evaluate a "presacral mass." Two hypoechoic structures are seen. The anterior one represents the fetal bladder *(straight arrow),* but the posterior one *(curved arrow)* had been thought to be abnormal. **(B)** Oblique scan through the questionable area in **A** shows that it is not a mass but the rectum. Note the typical configuration of the rectosigmoid *(arrows).*

PERITONEAL CAVITY AND ABDOMINAL CALCIFICATIONS

Meconium peritonitis is a chemical peritonitis resulting from intrauterine bowel perforation. Common underlying disorders include small bowel atresia, meconium ileus, volvulus, and intussusception, but many cases are idiopathic. Because fetal meconium is sterile, *in utero* leakage of bowel contents does not lead to bacterial contamination.[105] Prognosis is variable and depends to a large extent on the underlying etiology and presence of associated abnormalities. Some affected fetuses are asymptomatic postpartum and have a normal outcome, and their condition presumably would have remained undetected after birth had they not undergone antenatal sonography.[106]

The antenatal ultrasound findings in fetuses with meconium peritonitis are variable. Intraperitoneal calcifications are considered to be the most characteristic of the antenatal ultrasound findings. These calcifications develop because intraperitoneal meconium incites an inflammatory reaction that stimulates formation of fibrotic tissue, which then calcifies. The calcifications are highly echogenic and can be punctate, linear, or clumped foci. Because of the small size of these calcifications, posterior shadowing may or may not be seen (Fig. 18–16A and B). Rarely, calcifications can extend into the thorax through one of the permanent (caval, esophageal, and aortic hiatuses) or temporary (left and right pleuroperitoneal canals, foramen of Morgagni) openings in the diaphragm.[107,108]

Although abdominal calcifications are considered characteristic of meconium peritonitis, the identification of calcification in the fetal abdomen does not always indicate that the fetus has meconium peritonitis. Other potential etiologies of such calcifications include liver and spleen calcification (hepatic necrosis, *in utero* infection, such as cytomegalovirus or toxoplasmosis or idiopathic), a calcified neoplasm (teratoma or neuroblastoma), or intraluminal calcifications in the fetus with anal atresia.[91,92,109–112] Meconium peritonitis can be distinguished from these other etiologies if the calcifications are peritoneal in distribution. This said, because the liver occupies such a large portion of the fetal abdomen, it can be difficult to unequivocally locate the calcifications to the peritoneum or to the liver. There are, however, several telltale sonographic clues that strongly favor a peritoneal distribution: The punctate foci are found only around the expected margin of the liver and not in the substance of the liver itself; the calcifications line up or form sheets along the diaphragm (Fig. 18–17), and the calcifications are seen in the scrotum of a male fetus. Calcification in the scrotum is particularly telling because the processus vaginalis connects the scrotal sac to the peritoneal cavity late in pregnancy.[113]

A number of other sonographic findings can also be seen in fetuses with meconium peritonitis. These include polyhydramnios, dilated loops of bowel, fetal ascites, echogenic ascites with mass effect on organs, inguinal hernia, and

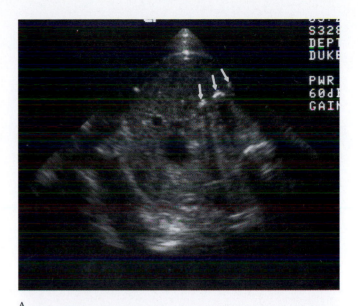

A

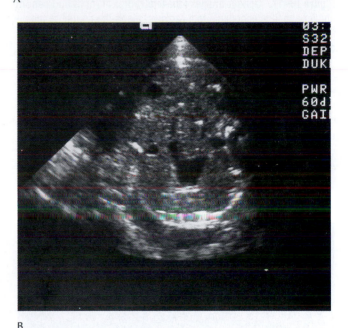

B

Figure 18–16. (A) Axial image of abdomen of a fetus with meconium peritonitis shows scattered highly echogenic foci *(arrows)* with posterior shadowing. **(B)** Although the majority of the echogenic foci in this fetus does not shadow, the foci are nevertheless typical in appearance for meconium peritonitis calcifications.

meconium pseudocyst.[107,114] Antenatally detected inguinal hernias have been described both in association with meconium peritonitis and as an isolated findings.[115–116] *Meconium pseudocyst* refers to a focal cystic cavity formed from extruded intestinal contents that have been walled off by matted bowel loops and fibrous tissue.[107,117–119] Sonographic imaging of a meconium pseudocyst shows an irregular, thickwalled cystic abdominal mass that may contain debris, septations, calcifications, or all of these (Fig. 18–18). The origin

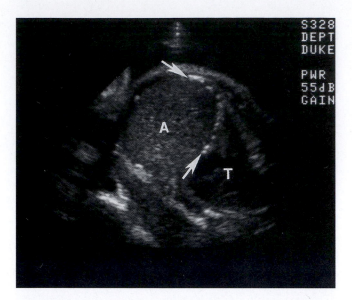

Figure 18–17. Oblique image of the fetal thorax (T) and abdomen (A) shows punctate echogenic foci *(arrows)* along the course of the diaphragm, a distribution that favors meconium peritonitis over hepatic calcifications.

of such a mass may be obscure, however, because the differential diagnosis of a cystic mass in the fetal abdomen is wide and includes obstructed urinary bladder, ovarian cyst, duplication cyst, teratoma, mesenteric cyst, renal cyst, choledochal cyst, and hydrometrocolpos. Nonetheless, if intraperitoneal

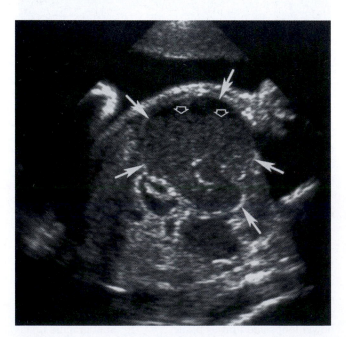

Figure 18–18. Oblique image through the abdomen of a fetus with meconium peritonitis demonstrating a large meconium pseudocyst *(solid arrows)* with a fluid debris level *(open arrows).*

calcifications are associated with the complicated cystic mass, a confident diagnosis of meconium peritonitis with meconium pseudocyst can be made.

Congenital duplication cysts can develop anywhere along the gastrointestinal tract. Duplications of the esophagus, stomach, and small bowel have been detected by antenatal sonography, as have intestinal duplication cysts located in the retroperitoneum apparently unassociated with bowel.[39–41,43–45,120–125] In some cases, only evidence of the bowel obstruction caused by the cyst, rather than the cyst itself, will be seen.[120] Even when the duplication cyst is seen, the ultrasound appearance is usually not specific, and the differential diagnosis depends on the location of the cyst. For example, the differential diagnosis of a gastric duplication cyst includes choledochal cyst[121] and duodenal atresia, but that of a small bowel duplication cyst would include mesenteric, omental, and ovarian cysts. Although most intestinal duplications are isolated abnormalities, there is a slightly increased overall incidence of associated congenital anomalies, particularly vertebral lesions.[39,125]

Mesenteric and omental cysts could also potentially be detected *in utero* and should be considered in the differential diagnosis of a cystic intraabdominal lesion in the fetus.[13] These are rare lesions, which can be unilocular or multilocular.

VENTRAL ABDOMINAL WALL

The most commonly identified ventral abdominal wall defects are omphalocele and gastroschisis. Both of these are associated with exteriorization of abdominal contents, but omphalocele is a midline defect in which abdominal contents herniate through the umbilicus, whereas gastroschisis is a paraumbilical defect that involves all layers of the abdominal wall. Distinction between these two conditions has important prognostic implications and can usually be accomplished sonographically. Gastroschisis is usually an isolated entity, rarely associated with anomalies other than intestinal malrotation and secondary gastrointestinal lesions. In contrast, fetuses with omphalocele are at high risk for additional anomalies including cardiac defects, genitourinary lesions, neural tube abnormalities, gastrointestinal anomalies, and chromosomal aneuploidies. Prenatal identification of an omphalocele should prompt a careful search for additional abnormalities and consideration of fetal karyotyping. Omphaloceles are found as a component of a variety of congenital syndromes, most notably, Beckwith–Wiedemann syndrome (omphalocele, macroglossia, organomegaly, and neonatal hypoglycemia), pentalogy of Cantrell (midline supraumbilical abdominal defect, sternal defect, deficiency of diaphragmatic pericardium, deficiency of anterior diaphragm, and intracardiac anomaly), and cloacal exstrophy (OEIS complex: omphalocele, exstrophy of the bladder, imperforate anus, and spina bifida).[95,126–133]

Abdominal wall defects are also important components of amniotic band syndrome and limb–body wall complex. If an abdominal wall defect satisfies the criteria for gastroschisis but is found in an unusual location or is associated with evisceration of organs other than bowel, then amniotic band syndrome and limb–body wall complex should be considered as potential explanations.[34–136] The amniotic band syndrome consists of a spectrum of congenital malformations that can range from relatively mild extremity deformities, such as lymphedema in digits or constriction rings in limbs, to groups of complex, often lethal anomalies, such as facial clefts in unusual orientations, abdominal wall defects, bizarre spine and head defects, and limb reduction anomalies. A leading theory for the pathogenesis of amniotic band syndrome ascribes the formation of the offending intrauterine bands to the rupture of the amnion. To be sure, intrauterine bands or membranes are frequently detected in association with the fetal lesions. Limb–body wall complex is a complex fetal malformation consisting of severe cranial-defects (encephalocele or exencephaly), facial clefts, large body wall defects involving the thorax, abdomen, or both, limb defects, scoliosis, internal malformations, and short umbilical cord.[136] It is not clear whether limb–body wall complex is categorically distinct from amniotic band syndrome or whether it represents a severe form of amniotic band syndrome.

A variety of ultrasound findings can be used to separate omphalocele and gastroschisis. A membrane consisting of amnion and peritoneum surrounds the herniated contents of an omphalocele (Fig. 18–19), but no covering membrane is found in gastroschisis because it is formed from a full thickness abdominal wall defect that allows herniated bowel loops to float freely in the amniotic fluid (Fig. 18–20). In cases of omphalocele, the umbilical cord inserts into the herniated mass or the surrounding membrane (Fig. 18–19), whereas in cases of gastroschisis the cord inserts normally into the fetal abdomen (Fig. 18–21). Unprotected by a membrane and at risk for ischemic events, the eviscerated bowel in gastroschisis is prone to secondary complications, such as thickening and fibrosis. Rarely, the membrane surrounding an omphalocele ruptures, which obfuscates the distinction between the two entities.[137] In most fetuses with gastroschisis, only the small bowel is eviscerated, whereas omphaloceles can include the liver and other organs in addition to intestinal loops (Fig. 18–19). In fact, sonographic demonstration that the liver has herniated through an abdominal wall defect is considered strong evidence for an omphalocele.[138] The site of the defect is also potentially helpful: The defect is in the midline with omphalocele, but off-midline, usually to the right, with gastroschisis. Confidently localizing the site of the defect can be difficult, particularly late in gestation, so the other distinguishing features tend to be more useful. Ascites will only be visualized in the fetus with an omphalocele (Fig. 18–19) because the absence of a covering membrane in gastroschisis allows ascitic fluid to escape into the surrounding amniotic

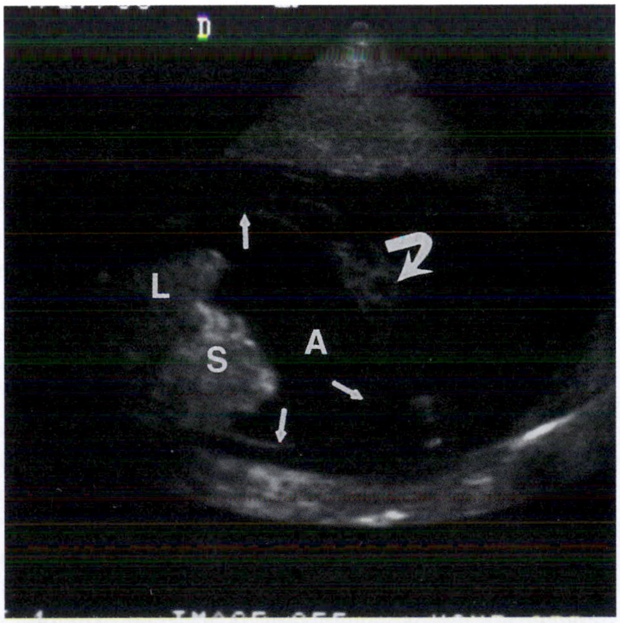

Figure 18–19. Scan through the eviscerated contents of an omphalocele shows both the liver (L) and the small bowel (S) surrounded by ascites (A) and a membrane *(straight arrows)*. Note the insertion of the umbilical cord *(curved arrow)* onto the membrane surrounding the omphalocele.

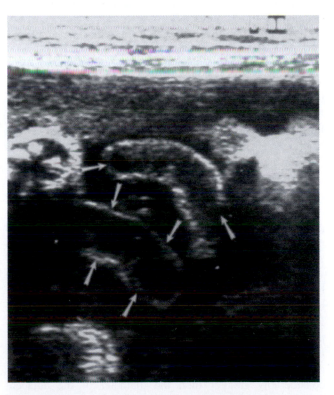

Figure 18–20. Fetus with gastroschisis. Sonogram shows dilated thick-walled bowel loops floating freely in the amniotic cavity without a covering membrane. *(Courtesy of Mary Warner, MD.)*

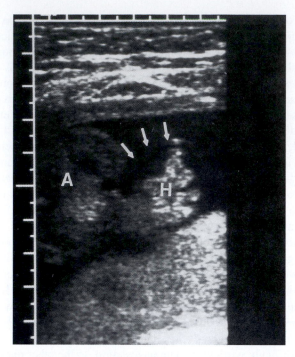

Figure 18–21. Fetus with gastroschisis. Note normal insertion of umbilical cord *(arrows)* into the fetal abdomen (A). H, herniated bowel.

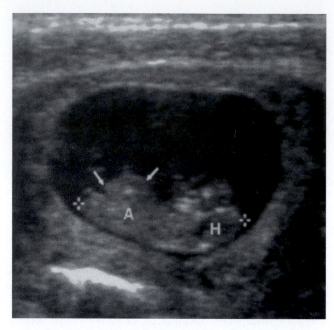

Figure 18–22. Sagittal scan of a normal 10-week embryo shows a masslike protrusion from the fetal abdomen (A) due to a bowel that has migrated into the base of the umbilical cord *(arrows)*. This migration occurs as a normal embryologic event during the first trimester and should not be mistaken for an omphalocele or gastroschisis. H, head.

fluid.[138] Occasionally, a lesion will have some features of omphalocele and some features of gastroschisis and cannot be unambiguously classified.[139]

Although intuitively it would seem that the smaller an omphalocele, the better the prognosis, this is often not the case.[140] The anomalies associated with omphalocele are often more life-threatening than the omphalocele itself and determine the prognosis.[140,141] In the absence of other anomalies, fetal outcome can be good even when an omphalocele is large.[141] Furthermore, omphaloceles that contain only bowel have a much higher likelihood of karyotype abnormalities than those that also contain liver.[140,142,143]

There are a number of potential pitfalls in the diagnosis of abdominal wall defects, the most commonplace of which relates to normal embryologic development. The bowel migrates into the umbilical cord during the period of rapid elongation of the midgut at approximately 8 menstrual weeks and returns to the abdominal cavity by 12 menstrual weeks.[144–147] This transient herniation is often detected with high-resolution sonographic equipment and could potentially be mistaken for an omphalocele or gastroschisis (Fig. 18–22). It can be particularly difficult to distinguish between omphalocele and normal midgut herniation.[148] The umbilical cord protrusion arising from normal developmental events typically measures less than 7 mm in diameter, is considerably smaller than the diameter of the adjacent fetal abdomen, and is not commonly seen after the fetus reaches a crown–rump length of approximately 44 mm (11.2 weeks).[149,150] If an abdominal wall mass is well within

these dimensions and is clearly localized to the base of the umbilical cord, it is likely to represent the normal process of midgut herniation. Any abdominal wall protrusion approaching or exceeding these limits, however, merits follow-up to exclude a true ventral abdominal wall defect. The likelihood of a pathologic abdominal wall defect increases with the diameter of the protrusion; however, even though omphalocele can be suspected with very large herniations,[151] a definitive diagnosis probably should not be offered during the first trimester until these criteria are validated in large prospective studies. In contrast, the normal process of midgut herniation need not be a serious consideration if the mass of herniated bowel is clearly separate from the umbilical cord insertion and is not covered by a membrane. These latter findings are diagnostic of gastroschisis even during the first trimester.[152,153]

Overdiagnosis of ventral abdominal wall defects also occurs when the umbilical cord, an umbilical cord mass, or a skin lesion on the fetal abdomen, such as a hemangioma, is mistaken for herniated bowel.[154,155] Doppler is helpful in distinguishing between umbilical cord and bowel. If the fetal abdomen is compressed between the uterine walls by oligohydramnios, a uterine contraction, or the fetal extremities, its shape can be distorted so as to spuriously resemble an abdominal wall defect. This apperance has been referred to as a *pseudo-omphalocele*[156] (Fig. 18–23). A true omphalocele should form an acute angle with the abdominal wall, whereas pseudo-omphalocele will form an obtuse angle with the

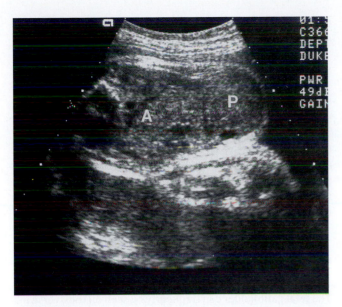

Figure 18–23. Oblique image of the fetal abdomen (A) demonstrating a "pseudo-omphalocele" (P). This normal variant occurs when the fetal abdomen is scanned obliquely or is compressed between the uterine walls.

abdominal wall. Rarely, an umbilical hernia may be observed *in utero*.[157]

False negatives are a common problem in the antenatal diagnosis of ventral abdominal wall defects.[158,159] Small defects can be missed when oligohydramnios or fetal position makes it difficult to define the boundaries of the abdominal wall and umbilical cord insertion, but even large defects are sometimes overlooked. The usual reason for missing a large defect is that the herniated bowel was assumed to represent a normal structure, such as the umbilical cord.[154] It is important to try to determine the identity of any structures floating freely in the amniotic fluid. Color Doppler imaging can be decisive when a particular structure could represent the umbilical cord.

LIVER, SPLEEN, AND PANCREAS

Nomograms of fetal liver length are available for evaluation of suspected abnormalities of liver size.[160–162] Fetal liver measurements are usually obtained in a longitudinal plane, from the dome of the right hemidiaphragm to the tip of the right lobe. The liver progressively increases in size throughout a normal gestation. It is particularly sensitive to fetal growth abnormalities and has been shown to be disproportionately small in fetuses with intrauterine growth retardation.[161] In contrast, hepatomegaly occurs with severe isoimmunization disorders, other forms of fetal anemia, *in utero* infection, fetal congestive heart failure, neoplasms, metabolic disorders, and macrosomia.[161,162,164,165] The severity of hepatomegaly has been shown to correlate with the severity of isoimmunization

disorders, and it has even been sugested that fetal liver measurements can be useful in assessing the need for transfusion in isoimmunized pregnancies. There are, however, relatively few studies on sonographic determination of liver size, so the impact of interobserver variability and other technical factors has not been well studied. The left lobe of the fetal liver is disproportionately large compared with the right lobe.[166] This may be a consequence of the normal fetal circulation: The left lobe receives more oxygenated blood than the right because of direct drainage of the umbilical vein into the left portal vein.[166,167]

Anternatal detection of fetal liver masses is a relatively uncommon occurrence, although a variety of different types of fetal liver masses have been described. These have included benign vascular tumors (hemangioendothelioma and hemangioma), mesenchymal hamartoma, adenoma, and metastatic neuroblastoma.[108,168–178] Sonographically detected fetal liver masses exhibit a variety of gray-scale ultrasound features and can be solid, cystic (unilocular or multilocular), or complex (containing both cystic and solid components). In general, these various gray-scale patterns are not specific for a particular type of liver mass. The association of hydrops with a fetal liver mass, however, suggests the possibility of high output failure from arteriovenous shunting in a vascular tumor, such as a hemangioendothelioma or hemangioma. This could potentially be confirmed by Doppler. Likewise, calcification within a fetal liver mass suggests the diagnosis of metastatic neuroblastoma or of a hemangioma.[108,178] Although we know of no antenatally detected cases of hepatoblastoma, it seems likely it will eventually be identified *in utero* because it is the most common primary hepatic malignancy in infancy. In children, these tumors are generally heterogeneous in echogenicity. The most common etiology for a cystic mass in the liver is a choledochal cyst (discussed later). Other rare but possible explanations for a liver cyst include a mesenchymal hamartoma or a solitary nonparasitic cyst.[179,180]

Hepatic calcifications are occasionally identified antenatally. The differential diagnosis for fetal liver calcification includes intrauterine infection such as toxoplasmosis or cytomegalovirus, tumors such as metastatic neuroblastoma, and ischemic hepatic necrosis.[109–112,181–183] When the hepatic calcification is seen as an isolated finding and *in utero* infection or neoplasia can be excluded, the outcome is often normal.[111,112] Care should be given to accurately locate the calcifications to the liver or the peritoneum because the latter indicates meconium peritonitis.

The fetal spleen can be visualized on transverse scans as a homogeneous solid structure posterolateral to the stomach (Fig. 18–24). Although most conspicuous late in gestation, it can be imaged in many second- and third-trimester fetuses with a concerted effort. The spleen tends to be less echogenic than the surrounding abdominal contents. As is the case with the liver, tables of normal values are available for analyzing fetal spleen measurements.[184–186] Splenomegaly has been detected *in utero* in conjunction with congenital

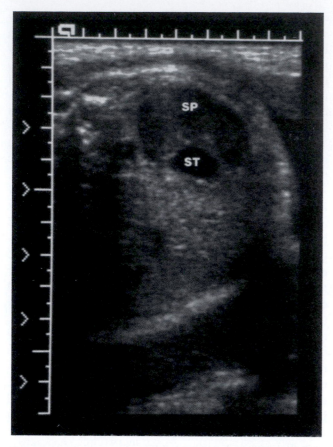

Figure 18–24. Transverse scan of a normal fetus at term demonstrating the spleen (SP) posterolateral to the fetal stomach (ST).

syphilis, cytomegalovirus infection, and severely affected isoimmunized fetuses.[181,186,187] Splenic measurements have been used in the management of isoimmunized pregnancies to predict the severity of fetal anemia.[184] Congenital splenic

cysts have been identified antenatally and likely represent endothelial inclusion cysts.[188]

The fetal pancreas is not usually seen during routine obstetric scanning, but it can be identified with effort in some second- and third-trimester fetuses.[158] Pancreatic visualization is enhanced if scans are performed in an oblique transverse plane and the fetal spine is oriented posteriorly in the maternal abdomen. Although pancreatic pathology could potentially be detected by antenatal sonography, there is little if any literature regarding antenatal detection of pancreatic abnormalities to date. The pancreas is known to hypertrophy in infants born to diabetic women and decrease in size in fetuses with intrauterine growth retardation.[189]

GALLBLADDER AND BILE DUCTS

The fetal gallbladder can frequently be seen on transverse images as an ovoid or teardrop, fluid-filled structure between the right and left lobes of the liver (Fig. 18–25). It extends anteriorly almost to the anterior abdominal wall. The gallbladder is thought to play a passive role in the fetus and does not exhibit significant volume changes after administration of a glucose load or fatty meal to the fasting mother.[190] Although nonvisualization of the fetal gallbladder has been associated with cystic fibrosis, biliary atresia, and gallbladder agenesis, most fetuses with a nonvisualized gallbladder are normal.[66,191,192] The gallbladder increases in size progressively with advancing gestational age until the gallbladder size plateaus in the mid third trimester.[192–194] Other gallbladder anomalies that have been described *in utero* include left-sided gallbladder and septated gallbladder,[160] but gallbladder anomalies as a group are only rarely detected prenatally.

Cholelithiasis can be detected *in utero*.[195–200] As in the adult, material in the fetal gallbladder exhibits a variety of

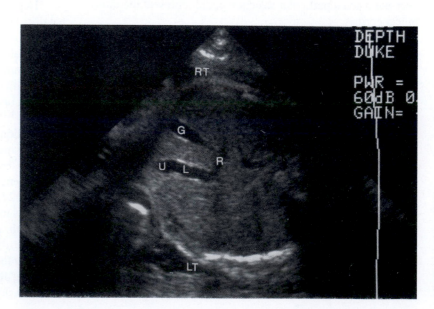

Figure 18–25. Axial scan through the abdomen of a normal fetus showing the typical configuration and location of the gallbladder (G) and portal veins. U, umbilical portion of portal vein; RT, right side of fetus; LT, left side of fetus; L, left portal vein; R, right portal vein.

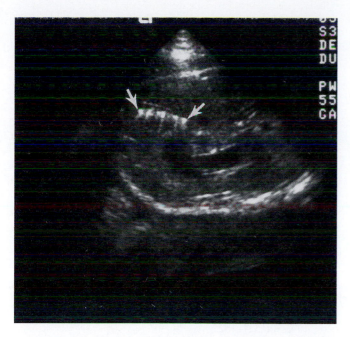

Figure 18–26. Oblique image of the fetal abdomen showing echogenic foci *(arrows)* in the gallbladder with distal comet-tail artifacts.

different appearances including echogenic foci with distal shadowing or comet-tail artifacts (Fig. 18–26), echogenic foci without distal artifacts, or layering low-level echoes similar to sludge.[196–198] Unlike in adults, however, many cases of fetal gallstones spontaneously resolve.[196–200] Even those that do persist do not usually become clinically significant. The etiology of fetal cholelithiasis is not clear, and in most reported cases, no predisposing factors were identified.

A choledochal cyst is a localized dilation of the biliary system. The most common form of choledochal cyst is dilation of the common bile duct. By antenatal sonography, the choledochal cyst is depicted as a fluid-filled mass in the right upper quadrant.[42,201–206] When the gallbladder is depicted on the same scan plane as the choledochal cyst, an image of two fluid-filled right upper quadrant masses will be produced. Choledochal cysts have been detected as early as 15 weeks' gestation.[204] The differential diagnosis of a cystic mass in the right upper quadrant is wide and includes choledochal cyst, duodenal atresia, a dilated bowel loop, omental and mesenteric cysts, and cysts of the liver, ovary, kidney, and pancreas. The specific diagnosis of choledochal cyst is suggested when a tubular structure(s) representing a dilated bile duct is identified communicating with the right upper quadrant cystic mass. This finding is more commonly seen postpartum than *in utero.*[42,202,204] Caroli's disease (communicating cavernous ectasia of the biliary tree) can occur in association with a choledochal cyst. It has been detected by antenatal sonography as multiple large cystic structures in continuity with each other. If right upper quadrant cystic structures are seen in association with bilaterally enlarged kidneys and oligohydramnios, the combination of Caroli's

disease and infantile polycystic kidney disease should be considered.[207]

REFERENCES

1. Golan A, Welman I, Saller Y, et al. Hydramnios in singleton pregnancy: Sonographic prevalence and etiology. *Gynecol Obstet Invest.* 1993;35:91–93.
2. Smith CV, Plambeck RD, Rayburn WF, et al. Relation of mild idiopathic polyhydramnios to perinatal outcome. *Obstet Gynecol.* 1992;79:387–389.
3. Alexander ES, Spitz HB, Clark RA. Sonography of polyhydramnios. *AJR.* 1982;138:343.
4. Damato N, Filly RA, Goldstein RB, et al. Frequency of fetal anomalies in sonographically detected polyhydramnios. *J Ultrasound Med.* 1993;12:11–15.
5. Barkin SZ, Pretorius DH, Beckett MK, et al. Severe polyhydramnios: Incidence of anomalies. *AJR.* 1987;148:155.
6. Phelan JP, Martin GI. Polyhydramnios: Fetal and neonatal implications. *Clin Perinatol.* 1989;16:987–994.
7. Sarno AP Jr, Bruner JP, Southgate WM. Congenital chyloperitoneum as a cause of isolated fetal ascites. *Obstet Gynecol.* 1990;76:955–957.
8. Chilukuri S, Bonet V, Cobb M. Antenatal spontaneous perforation of the extrahepatic biliary tree. *Am J Obstet Gynecol.* 1990;163:1201–1202.
9. Rosenthal SJ, Filly RA, Callen PW, et al. Fetal pseudoascites. *Radiology.* 1979;131:195.
10. Hashimoto BE, Filly RA, Callen PW, et al. Fetal pseudoascites. Further anatomic observations. *J Ultrasound Med.* 1986; 5:151.
11. Gross BH, Callen PW, Filly RA. Ultrasound appearance of fetal greater omentum. *J Ultrasound Med.* 1982;1:67.
12. Avni EF, Rypens F, Milaire J. Fetal esophagus: Normal sonographic appearance. *J Ultrasound Med.* 1994;13:175–180.
13. Romero R, Pilu G, Jeanty P, et al. The gastrointestinal tract and intrabdominal organs. In: *Prenatal Diagnosis of Congenital Anomalies.* Norwalk, CT: Appleton & Lange; 1988:233.
14. Eyheremendy E, Fister M. Antenatal real-time diagnosis of esophageal atresia. *J Clin Ultrasound.* 1983;11:395–397.
15. Kalache KD, Chaoui R, Hau H, Bollmann R. The upper neck pouch sign: A prenatal sonographic marker for esophageal atresia. *Ultrasound Obstet Gynecol.* 1998;11:138–140.
16. Pretorius DH, Drose JA, Dennis MA, et al. Tracheoesophageal fistula in utero: Twenty-two cases. *J Ultrasound Med.* 1987;6:509–513.
17. Nagata S, Koyanagi T, Horimoto N, et al. Chronological development of the fetal stomach assessed using real-time ultrasound. *Early Hum Dev.* 1990;22:15–22.
18. Millener PB, Anderson NG, Chisholm RJ. Prognostic significance of nonvisualization of the fetal stomach by sonography. *AJR.* 1993;160:827–830.
19. Pretorius DH, Gosink BB, Clautice-Engle T, et al. Sonographic evaluation of the fetal stomach: Significance of nonvisualization. *AJR.* 1988;151:987–989.
20. Brumfield CG, Davis RO, Owen J, et al. Pregnancy outcomes following sonographic nonvisualization of the fetal stomach. *Obstet Gynecol.* 1998;91:905–908.

21. Zimmer EZ, Chao CR, Abramovich G, et al. Fetal stomach measurements: Not reproducible by the same observer. *J Ultrasound Med.* 1992;11:663–665.

22. Perez CG, Goldstein RB. Sonographic borderlands in the fetal abdomen. *Semin Ultrasound CT MRI.* 1998;19:336–346.

23. McKenna KM, Goldstein RB, Stringer MD. Small or absent fetal stomach: Prognostic significance. *Radiology.* 1995;197:729–733.

24. Fakhry J, Shapiro LR, Schechter A, et al. Fetal gastric pseudomasses. *J Ultrasound Med.* 1987;6:177–180.

25. Walker JM, Ferguson DD. The sonographic appearance of blood in the fetal stomach and its association with placental abruption. *J Ultrasound Med.* 1988;7:155–161.

26. Hasegawa T, Kubota A, Imura K, et al. Prenatal diagnosis of congenital pyloric atresia. *J Clin Ultrasound.* 1993;21:278–281.

27. Hershkovitz E, Steiner Z, Shinwell ES, et al. Prenatal ultrasonic diagnosis of nonhypertrophic pyloric stenosis associated with intestinal malrotation. *J Clin Ultrasound.* 1994;22:52–54.

28. Bahado-Singh RO, Romero R, Vecchio M, et al. Prenatal diagnosis of congenital hiatal hernia. *J Ultrasound Med.* 1992;11:297–300.

29. Katz S, Basel D, Branski D. Prenatal gastric dilatation and infantile hypertrophic pyloric stenosis. *J Pediatr Surg.* 1988;23:1021–1022.

30. Peled Y, Hod M, Friedman S, et al. Prenatal diagnosis of familial congenital pyloric atresia. *Prenat Diagn.* 1992;12:151–154.

31. Bonin B, Gruslin A, Simpson NAB, et al. Second trimester prenatal diagnosis of congenital gastric outlet obstruction. *J Ultrasound Med.* 1998;17:403–406.

32. Sharony R, Sinow R, Asch M, et al. Prenatal ultrasound diagnosis of gastric outlet obstruction due to a pyloric web. *Prenat Diagn.* 1995;15:56–59.

33. Miro J, Bard H. Congenital atresia and stenosis of the duodenum: The impact of a prenatal diagnosis. *Am J Obstet Gynecol.* 1988:158:555–559.

34. Hancock BJ, Wiseman NE. Congenital duodenal obstruction: The impact of an antenatal diagnosis. *J Pediatr Surg* 1989:24:1027–1031.

35. Romero R, Ghidini A, Costigan K, et al. Prenatal diagnosis of duodenal atresia: Does it make any difference? *Obstet Gynecol.* 1988;71:739–741.

36. Levine D, Goldstein RB, Cadrin C. Distention of the fetal duodenum: Abnormal findings? *J Ultrasound Med.* 1998;17:213–215.

37. Zimmer EZ, Bronshtein M. Early diagnosis of duodenal atresia and possible monographic pitfalls. *Prenatal Diagn.* 1996;16:564–566.

38. Petrikovsky BM. First-trimester diagnosis of duodenal atresia. *Am J Obstet Gynecol.* 1994;171:569–570.

39. Herman TE, Oser AB, McAlister WH. Tubular communicating duplications of esophagus and stomach. *Pediatr Radiol* 1991;21:494–496.

40. Özmen MN, Önderoglu L, Ciftci AO, et al. Prenatal diagnosis of gastric duplication cyst. *J Ultrasound Med.* 1997;16:219–222.

41. Richards DS, Langham MR, Anderson CD. The prenatal sonographic appearance of enteric duplication cysts. *Ultrasound Obstet Gynecol.* 1996;7:17–20.

42. Dewbury KC, Aluwihare MC, Birch SJ, et al. Prenatal ultrasound demonstration of a choledochal cyst. *Br J Radiol.* 1980;53:906.

43. Malone FD, Crombelholme TM, Nores JA, et al. Pitfalls in the "double bubble" sign: A case of congenital duodenal duplication. *Fetal Diagn Ther.* 1997;12:298–300.

44. Yamataka A, Pringle KC. A case with duodenal duplication cyst: Prenatal diagnosis and surgical management. *Fetal Diagn Ther.* 1998; 13:39–41.

45. Degani S, Mogilner JG, Shapiro I. In utero sonographic appearance of intestinal duplication cysts. *Ultrasound Obstet Gynecol.* 1995;5:415–418.

46. Gross BH, Filly RA. Potential for a normal fetal stomach to simulate the sonographic "double bubble" sign. *J Can Assoc Radiol.* 1982;33:39–40.

47. Pachi A, Maggi E, Giancotti A, et al. Ultrasound diagnosis of fetal annular pancreas. *J Perinat Med.* 1989;361–364.

48. Choi S-O, Park W-H. Preduodenal portal vein: A cause of prenatally diagnosed duodenal obstruction. *J Pediatr Surg.* 1995;30:1521–1522.

49. Estroff JA, Parad RB, Share JC, et al. Second trimester prenatal findings in duodenal and esophageal atresia without tracheoesophageal fistula. *J Ultrasound Med.* 1994;13:375–379.

50. Tsukerman GL, Krapiva GA, Kirillova IA. First-trimester diagnosis of duodenal stenosis associated with oesophageal atresia. *Prenat Diagn.* 1993;13:371–376.

51. Chitty LS, Goodman J, Seller MJ, et al. Esophageal and duodenal atresia in a fetus with Down's syndrome: Prenatal sonographic features. *Ultrasound Obstet Gynecol.* 1996;7:450–452.

52. Nyberg DA, Mack LA, Patten RM, et al. Fetal bowel. Normal sonographic findings. *J Ultrasound Med.* 1987;6:3–6.

53. Parulekar SG. Sonography of normal fetal bowel. *J Ultrasound Med.* 1991;10:211–220.

54. Langer JC, Adzick S, Filly RA, et al. Gastrointestinal tract obstruction in the fetus. *Arch Surg.* 1989;124:1183–1187.

55. Nelson LH, Clark CE, Fishburne JI, et al. Value of serial sonography in the in utero detection of duodenal atresia. *Obstet Gynecol.* 1982;59:657–660.

56. Weissman A, Goldstein I. Prenatal sonographic diagnosis and clinical management of small bowel obstruction. *Am J Perinatol.* 1993;10:215–216.

57. Miyakoski K, Tanaka M, Miyazaki T, et al. Prenatal ultrasound diagnosis of small-bowel torsion. *Obstet Gynecol.* 1998;91:802–803.

58. Yoo S-J, Park KW, Cho SY, et al. Definitive diagnosis of intestinal volvulus in utero. *Ultrasound Obstet Gynecol.* 1999; 13:200–203.

59. Lince DM, Pretorius DH, Manco-Johnson ML, et al. The clinical significance of increased echogenicity in the fetal abdomen. *AJR.* 1985;145:683–686.

60. Estroff JA, Parad RB, Benacerraf BR. Prevalence of cystic fibrosis in fetuses with dilated bowel. *Radiology:* 1992;183:677–680.

61. Dicke JM, Crane JP. Sonographically detected hyperechoic fetal bowel: Significance and implications for pregnancy management. *Obstet Gynecol.* 1992;80:778–782.

62. Muller F, Aubry MC, Gasser B, et al. Prenatal diagnosis of cystic fibrosis. II. Meconium ileus in affected fetuses. *Prenat Diagn*. 1985;5:109.

63. Nyberg DA, Hastrup W, Watts H, et al. Dilated fetal bowel: A sonographic sign of cystic fibrosis. *J Ultrasound Med*. 1987;6:257–260.

64. Hogge WA, Hogge JS, Boehm CD, et al. Increased echogenicity in the fetal abdomen: Use of DNA analysis to establish a diagnosis of cystic fibrosis. *J Ultrasound Med*. 1993;12:451–454.

65. Caspi B, Elchalal U, Lancet M, et al. Prenatal diagnosis of cystic fibrosis: Ultrasonographic appearance of meconium ileus in the fetus. *Prenat Diagn*. 1988;8:379–382.

66. Duchatel F, Muller F, Oury JF, et al. Prenatal diagnosis of cystic fibrosis: Ultrasonography of the gallbladder at 17–19 weeks of gestation. *Fetal Diagn Ther*. 1993;8:28–36.

67. Fakhry J, Reiser M, Shapiro LR, et al. Increased echogenicity in the lower fetal abdomen: A common normal variant in the second trimester. *J Ultrasound Med*. 1986;5:489–492.

68. Manco LG, Nuran FA, Sohnen H, et al. Fetal small bowel simulating an abdominal mass at sonography. *J Clin Ultasound*. 1986;14:404–407.

69. Paulson EK, Hertzberg BS, Hyperechoic meconium in the third trimester fetus: An uncommon normal variant. *J Ultrasound Med*. 1991;10:677–680.

70. Fung ASL, Wilson S, Toi A, et al. Echogenic colonic meconium in the third trimester: A normal sonographic finding. *J Ultrasound Med*. 1992;11:676–678.

71. Caspi B, Elchalal U, Hagay Z, et al. Echogenicity of the fetal bowel due to gas accumulation. *J Ultrasound Med*. 1993; 4:231–233.

72. Nyberg DA, Dubinsky T, Resta RG, et al. Echogenic fetal bowel during the second trimester: Clinical importance. *Radiology*. 1993;188:527–531.

73. Scioscia AL, Pretorius DH, Budorick NE, et al. Second-trimester echogenic bowel and chromosomal abnormalities. *Am J Obstet Gynecol*. 1992;167:889–894.

74. Persutte WH. Second trimester hyperechogenicity in the lower abdomen of two fetuses with trisomy 21: Is there a correlation? *J Clin Ultrasound*. 1990;18:425–428.

75. Pletcher BA, Williams MK, Mulivor RA, et al. Intrauterine cytomegalovirus infection presenting as fetal meconium peritonitis. *Obstet Gynecol*. 1991;78:903–905.

76. Forouzan I. Fetal abdominal echogenic mass: An early sign of intrauterine cytomegalovirus infection. *Obstet Gynecol*. 1992;80:535–537.

77. Miller SF, Angtuaco TL, Quirk JG, et al. Anorectal atresia presenting as an abdominopelvic mass. *J Ultrasound Med*. 1990;9:669–672.

78. Hallak M, Reiter AA, Smith LG Jr, et al. Oligohydramnios and megacolon in a fetus with vesicorectal fistula and analurethral atresia: A case report. *Am J Obstet Gynecol*. 1992;167:79–81.

79. Stipoljev F, Sertic J, Kos M, et al. Incidence of chromosomopathies and cystic fibrosis mutations in second trimester fetuses with isolated hyperechoic bowel. *J Mater Fetal Med*. 1999;8:44–47.

80. Weiner Z. Congenital cytomegalovirus infection with oligohydramnios and echogenic bowel at 14 weeks' gestation. *J Ultrasound Med*. 1995;14:617–618.

81. Font GE, Solari M. Prenatal diagnosis of bowel obstruction initially manifested as isolated hyperechoic bowel. *J Ultrasound Med*. 1998;17:721–723.

82. Grignon A, Dubois J, Ouellet MC, et al. Echogenic dilated bowel loops before 21 weeks' gestation: A new entity. *AJR*. 1997;168:833–837.

83. Stamm E, King G, Thickman D. Megacystis–microcolon–intestinal hypoperistalsis syndrome: Prenatal identification in siblings and review of the literature. *J Ultrasound Med*. 1991;10:599–602.

84. Carlsson SÅ, Hökegård Mattsson LÅ: Megacystis–microcolon–intestinal hypoperistalsis syndrome—Antenatal appearance in two cases. *Acta Obstet Gynecol Scand*. 1992;71:645–648.

85. Young ID, McKeever PA, Brown LA, et al. Prenatal diagnosis of the megacystis–microcolon–intestinal hypoperistalsis syndrome. *J Med Genet*. 1989;26:403–406.

86. Langer JC, Winthrop AL, Burrows RF, et al. False diagnosis of intestinal obstruction in a fetus with congenital chloride diarrhea. *J Pediatr Surg*. 1991;26:1282–1284.

87. Lundkvist K, Ewald U, Lindgren PG. Congenital chloride diarrhoea: A prenatal differential diagnosis of small bowel atresia. *Acta Paediatr*. 1996;85:295–298.

88. Samuel N, Dicker D, Landman J, et al. Early diagnosis and intrauterine therapy of meconium plug syndrome in the fetus: Risks and benefits. *J Ultrasound Med*. 1986;5:425.

89. Vermesh M, Mayden KL, Confino E, et al. Prenatal sonographic diagnosis of Hirschsprung's disease. *J Ultrasound Med*. 1986;5:37.

90. Wrobleski D, Wesselhoeft C. Ultrasonic diagnosis of prenatal intestinal obstruction. *J Pediatr Surg*. 1979;14:598.

91. Shalev E, Weiner E, Zuckerman H: Prenatal ultrasound diagnosis of intestinal calcifications with imperforate anus. *Acta Obstet Gynecol Scand*. 1983;62:95–96.

92. Harris RD, Nyberg DA, Mack LA, et al. Anorectal atresia. Prenatal sonographic diagnosis. *AJR*. 1987;149:395.

93. Grant T, Newman M, Gould R, et al. Intraluminal colonic calcifications associated with anorectal atresia—Prenatal sonographic detection. *J Ultrasound Med*. 1990;9:411–413.

94. Lande IM, Hamilton EF. The antenatal sonographic visualization of cloacal dysgenesis. *J Ultrasound Med*. 1986;5:275.

95. Kutzner DK, Wilson WG, Hogge WA. OEIS complex (cloacal exstrophy): Prenatal diagnosis in the second trimester. *Prenat Diagn*. 1988;8:247–253.

96. Claiborne AK, Blocker SH, Martin CM, et al. Prenatal and postnatal sonographic delineation of gastrointestinal abnormalities in a case of the VATER syndrome. *J Ultrasound Med*. 1986;5:45.

97. Corteville JE, Gray DL, Langer JC. Bowel abnormalities in the fetus—Correlation of prenatal ultrasonographic findings with outcome. *Am J Obstet Gynecol*. 1996;175:724–729.

98. Stoll C, Alembik Y, Dott B, et al. Evaluation of prenatal diagnosis of congenital gastro-intestinal atresias. *Eur J Epidemiol*. 1996;12:611–616.

99. Hearn-Stebbins B, Sherer DM, Abramowicz JS, et al. Prenatal sonographic features associated with an imperforate anus and rectourethral fistula. *J Clin Ultrasound*. 1991;19:508–512.

100. Berdon WE, Baker DH, Wigger HJ, et al. Calcified intraluminal meconium in newborn males with imperforate anus. Enterolithiasis in the newborn. *AJR*. 1975;125:449.

101. Mandell J, Lillehei CW, Greene M, et al. The prenatal diagnosis of imperforate anus with rectourinary fistula: Dilated fetal colon with enterolithiasis. *J Pediatr Surg.* 1992;27:82–84.

102. Hill LM, Rivello D, Martin JG. Intraluminal bladder calcifications: An antenatal sign of an enterovesical fistula. *Obstet Gynecol.* 1990;76:500–502.

103. Karcnik T, Rubenstein JB, Swayne LC. The fetal presacral pseudomass: A normal sonographic variant. *J Ultrasound Med.* 1991;10:579–581.

104. Moreland SI III, Cohen MI, Leopold GR, et al. Third-trimester fetal sonography: Meconium simulating a presacral mass. *AJR.* 1988;150:379–380.

105. Brugman SM, Bjelland JJ, Thomasson JE, et al. Sonographic findings with radiologic correlation in meconium peritonitis. *J Clin Ultrasound.* 1979;7:305.

106. Estroff JA, Bromley B, Benacerraf BR. Fetal meconium peritonitis without sequelae. *Pediatr Radiol.* 1992;22:277–278.

107. Foster MA, Nyberg DA, Mahony BS, et al. Meconium peritonitis: Prenatal sonographic findings and their clinical significance. *Radiology.* 1987;165:661–665.

108. Kedar RP, Malde HM. Meconium thorax: Prenatal sonographic diagnosis. *J Ultrasound Med.* 1992;11:683–685.

109. Nguyen DL, Leonard JC. Ischemic hepatic necrosis: A cause of fetal liver calcification. *AJR.* 1986;147:596–597.

110. Jaffa AJ, Many A, Hartoov J, et al. Prenatal sonographic diagnosis of metastatic neuroblastoma: Report of a case and review of the literature. *Prenat Diagn.* 1993;13:73–77.

111. Koopman E, Wladimiroff JW. Fetal intrahepatic hyperechogenic foci: Prenatal ultrasound diagnosis and outcome. *Prenat Diagn.* 1998;18:339–342.

112. Achiron R, Seidman DS, Afek A, et al. Prenatal ultrasonographic diagnosis of fetal hepatic hyperechogenicities: Clinical significance and implications for management. *Ultrasound Obstet Gynecol.* 1996;7:251–255.

113. Kenney PJ, Spirt BA, Ellis DA, et al. Scrotal masses caused by meconium peritonitis: Prenatal sonographic diagnosis. *Radiology.* 1985;154:362.

114. Yankes JR, Bowie JD, Effmann EL, et al. Antenatal diagnosis of meconium peritonitis with inguinal hernias by ultrasonography—Therapeutic implications. *J Ultrasound Med.* 1988;7:221–223.

115. Ober KJ, Smith CV. Prenatal ultrasound diagnosis of a fetal inguinal hernia containing small bowel. *Obstet Gynecol.* 1991;78:905–906.

116. Meizner I, Levy A, Katz M, et al. Prenatal ultrasonographic diagnosis of fetal scrotal inguinal hernia. *Am J Obstet Gynecol.* 1992;166:907–909.

117. McGahan JP, Hanson F. Meconium peritonitis with accompanying pseudocyst: Prenatal sonographic diagnosis. *Radiology.* 1983;148:125–126.

118. Schwimer SR, Vanley GT, Reinke RT. Prenatal diagnosis of cystic meconium peritonitis. *J Clin Ultrasound.* 1984;12: 37–39.

119. Lauer JD, Cradock TV. Meconium pseudocyst: Prenatal sonographic and antenatal radiologic correlation. *J Ultrasound Med.* 1982;1:333–335.

120. Bidwell JK, Nelson A. Prenatal ultrasonic diagnosis of congenital duplication of the stomach. *J Ultrasound Med.* 1986;5: 589.

121. vanDam LJ, deGroot CJ, Hazebroek FWS, et al. Intrauterine demonstration of bowel duplication by ultrasound. *Eur J Obstet Gynecol Reprod Biol.* 1984;18:229.

122. Balén EM, Hernández-Lizoáin JL, Pardo F, et al. Giant jejunoileal duplication: Prenatal diagnosis and complete excision without intestinal resection. *J Pediatr Surg.* 1993;28: 1586–1588.

123. Goyert GL, Blitz D, Gibson P, et al. Prenatal diagnosis of duplication cyst of the pylorus. *Prenat Diagn.* 1991;11:483–486.

124. Jaquemark F, Palaric JC, Hervé DD, et al. Antenatal diagnosis of abdominothoracic alimentary tract duplication: A case report. *Surg Radiol Anat.* 1991;13:53–57.

125. Duncan BW, Adzick NS, Eraklis A. Retroperitoneal alimentary tract duplication detected in utero. *J Pediatr Surg.* 1992;27: 1231–1233.

126. Weinstein L, Anderson C. In utero diagnosis of Beckwith–Wiedemann syndrome by ultrasound. *Radiology.* 1980;134: 474.

127. Koontz WL, Shaw LA, Lavery JP. Antenatal sonographic appearance of Beckwith–Wiedemann syndrome. *J Clin Ultrasound.* 1986;14:67.

128. Baker ME, Rosenberg ER, Trofatter KF, et al. The in utero findings in twin pentalogy of Cantrell. *J Ultrasound Med.* 1984;3:525.

129. Fried AM, Woodring JH, Shier RW, et al. Omphalocele in limb/body wall deficiency syndrome: Atypical sonographic appearance. *J Clin Ultrasound.* 1982;10:400.

130. Viljoen DL, Jaquire Z, Woods DL. Prenatal diagnosis in autosomal dominant Beckwith–Wiedemann syndrome. *Prenat Diagn.* 1991;11:167–175.

131. Meizner I, Carmi R, Katz M, et al. In utero prenatal diagnosis of Beckwith–Wiedemann syndrome: A case report. *Eur J Obstet Gynecol Reprod Biol.* 1989;32:259–264.

132. Wieacker P, Wilhelm C, Greiner P, et al. Prenatal diagnosis of Wiedemann–Beckwith syndrome. *J Perinat Med.* 1989;17:351–355.

133. Ghidini A, Sirtori M, Romero R, et al. Prenatal diagnosis of pentalogy of Cantrell. *J Ultrasound Med.* 1988;7:567–572.

134. Mahony BS, Filly RA, Callen PW, et al. The amniotic band syndrome: Antenatal sonographic diagnosis and potential pitfalls. *Am J Obstet Gynecol.* 1985;152:63–68.

135. Seidman JD, Abbondanzo SL, Watkin WG, et al. Amniotic band syndrome. *Arch Pathol Lab Med.* 1989;113:891–897.

136. Patten RM, Van Allen M, Mack LA, et al. Limb–body wall complex: In utero sonographic diagnosis of a complicated fetal malformation. *AJR.* 1986;146:1019–1024.

137. Hansen LK, Pedersen SA, Kristoffersen K. Prenatal rupture of omphalocele. *J Clin Ultrasound.* 1987;15:191–193.

138. Bair JH, Russ PD, Pretorius DH, et al. Fetal omphalocele and gastroschisis: A review of 24 cases. *AJR.* 1986;147: 1047.

139. Perrella RR, Ragavendra N, Tessler FN, et al. Fetal abdominal wall mass detected on prenatal sonography: Gastroschisis vs omphalocele. *AJR.* 1991;157:1065–1066.

140. Hughes MD, Nyberg DA, Mack LA, et al. Fetal omphalocele: Prenatal US detection of concurrent anomalies and other predictors of outcome. *Radiology.* 1989;173:371–376.

141. Tucci M, Bard H. The associated anomalies that determine prognosis in congenital omphaloceles. *Am J Obstet Gynecol.* 1990;163:1646–1649.

142. Getachew MM, Goldstein RB, Edge VL, et al. Correlation

between omphalocele contents and karyotypic abnormalities: Sonographic study in 37 cases. *AJR.* 1991;158:133–136.

143. Nyberg DA, Fitzsimmons J, Mack LA, et al. Chromosomal abnormalities in fetuses with omphalocele—Significance of omphalocele contents. *J Ultrasound Med.* 1989;8:299–308.

144. Cyr DR, Mack LA, Schoenecker SA, et al. Bowel migration in the normal fetus: US detection. *Radiology.* 1986;161:119–121.

145. Schmidt W, Yarkoni S, Crelin E, et al. Sonographic visualization of physiologic anterior abdominal wall hernia in the first trimester. *Obstet Gynecol.* 1987;69:911–915.

146. Timor-Tritsch IE, Warren WB, Peisner DB, et al. First-trimester midgut herniation: A high-frequency transvaginal sonographic study. *Am J Obstet Gynecol.* 1989;161:831–833.

147. Bronshtein M, Yoffe N, Zimmer EZ. Transvaginal sonography at 5 to 14 weeks' gestation: Fetal stomach, abnormal cord insertion, and yolk sac. *Am J Perinatol.* 1992;9:344–347.

148. Gray DL, Martin CM, Crane JP. Differential diagnosis of first trimester ventral wall defect. *J Ultrasound Med.* 1989;8:255–258.

149. Bowerman RA. Sonography of fetal midgut herniation: Normal size criteria and correlation with crown–rump length. *J Ultrasound Med.* 1993;5:251–254.

150. Brown DL, Emerson DS, Shulman LP, et al. Sonographic diagnosis of omphalocele during 10th week of gestation. *AJR.* 1989;153:825–826.

151. Pagliano M, Mossetti M, Ragno P. Echographic diagnosis of omphalocele in the first trimester of pregnancy. *J Clin Ultrasound.* 1990;18:658–660.

152. Kushnir O, Izquierdo L, Vigil D, et al. Early transvaginal sonographic diagnosis of gastroschisis. *J Clin Ultrasound.* 1990;18:194–197.

153. Guzman ER. Early prenatal diagnosis of gastroschisis with transvaginal ultrasonography. *Am J Obstet Gynecol.* 1990;162:1253–1254.

154. Lindfors KK, McGahan JP, Walter JP. Fetal omphalocele and gastroschisis: Pitfalls in sonographic diagnosis. *AJR.* 1986;147:797–800.

155. Miller KA, Gauderer WL. Hemangioma of the umbilical cord mimicking an omphalocele. *J Pediatr Surg.* 1997;32:810–812.

156. Salzman L, Kuligowska E, Semine A. Pseudoomphalocele: Pitfall in fetal sonography. *AJR.* 1986:146:1283–1285.

157. Richards DS, Kays DW. Prenatal ultrasonographic diagnosis of a simple umbilical hernia. *J Ultrasound Med.* 1998;17:265–267.

158. Walkinshaw SA, Hebisch RG, Hey EN. How good is ultrasound in the detection and evaluation of anterior abdominal wall defects? *Br J Radiol.* 1992;65:298–301.

159. Roberts JP, Burge DM. Antenatal diagnosis of abdominal wall defects: A missed opportunity? *Arch Dis Child.* 1990;65:687–689.

160. Vintzileos AM, Neckles S, Campbell WA, et al. Fetal liver ultrasound measurement during normal pregnancy. *Obstet Gynecol.* 1985;66:477.

161. Roberts AB, Mitchell JM, Pattison NS. Fetal liver length in normal and isoimmunized pregnancies. *Am J Obstet Gynecol.* 1989;161:42–46.

162. Murao F, Senoh D, Takamiya O, et al. Ultrasonic evaluation of liver development in the fetus in utero. *Gynecol Obstet Invest.* 1989;28:198–201.

163. Murao F, Takamiya O, Yamamoto K, et al. Detection of intrauterine growth retardation based on measurements of size of the liver. *Gynecol Obstet Invest.* 1990;29:26–31.

164. Ghidini A, Sirtori M, Romero R, et al. Hepatosplenomegaly as the only prenatal finding in a fetus with pyruvate kinase deficiency anemia. *Am J Perinatol.* 1991;8:44–46.

165. Vintzileos AM, Campbell WA, Storlazzi E, et al. Fetal liver ultrasound measurements in isoimmunized pregnancies. *Obstet Gynecol.* 1986;68:162.

166. Champetier J, Yver R, Tomasella T. Functional anatomy of the liver of the human fetus: Applications to ultrasonography. *Surg Radiol Anat.* 1989;11:53–62.

167. Gross BH, Harter LP, Filly RA. Disproportionate left hepatic lobe size in the fetus: Ultrasonic demonstration. *J Ultrasound Med.* 1982;1:79.

168. Platt LD, DeVore GR, Benner P, et al. Antenatal diagnosis of a fetal liver mass. *J Ultrasound Med.* 1983;2:521.

169. Horgan JG, King DL, Taylor KJW. Sonographic detection of prenatal liver mass. *J Clin Gastroenterol.* 1984;6:277.

170. Nakamoto SK, Dreilinger A, Dattel B, et al. The sonographic appearance of hepatic hemangioma in utero. *J Ultrasound Med.* 1983;2:239.

171. Gonen R, Fong K, Chiasson DA. Prenatal sonographic diagnosis of hepatic hemangioendothelioma with secondary non-immune hydrops fetalis. *Obstet Gynecol.* 1989;73:485–487.

172. Sepúlveda WH, Donetch G, Giuliano A. Prenatal sonographic diagnosis of fetal hepatic hemangioma. *Eur J Obstet Gynecol Reprod Biol.* 1993;48:73–76.

173. Abuhamad AZ, Lewis D, Inati MN, et al. The use of color flow Doppler in the diagnosis of fetal hepatic hemangioma. *J Ultrasound Med.* 1993;4:223–226.

174. Hansen GC, Ragavendra N. Atypical mesenchymal hamartoma of the liver: Prenatal sonographic diagnosis (letter to the editor). *AJR.* 1992;158:921–922.

175. Hirata GI, Matsunaga ML, Medearis AL, et al. Ultrasonographic diagnosis of a fetal abdominal mass: A case of a mesenchymal liver hamartoma and a review of the literature. *Prenat Diagn.* 1990;10:507–512.

176. Marks F, Thomas P, Lustig I, et al. In utero sonographic description of a fetal liver adenoma. *J Ultrasound Med.* 1990;9:119–122.

177. Bejvan SM, Winter TC, Shields LE, et al. Prenatal evaluation of mesenchymal hamartoma of the liver: Gray scale and power Doppler sonographic imaging. *J Ultrasound Med.* 1997;16:227–229.

178. Dreyfus M, Baldauf J-J, Dadoun K, et al. Prenatal diagnosis of hepatic hemangioma. *Fetal Diagn Ther.* 1996;11:57–60.

179. Chung WM. Antenatal detection of hepatic cyst. *J Clin Ultrasound.* 1986;14:217.

180. Foucar E, Williamson RA, Yiu-Chiu V, et al. Mesenchymal hamartoma of the liver identified by fetal sonography. *AJR.* 1983;140:970.

181. Yamashita Y, Iwanaga R, Goto A. Congenital cytomegalovirus infection associated with fetal ascites and intrahepatic calcifications. *Acta Paediatr Scand.* 1989;78:965–967.

182. Liyanage IS, Katoch D. Ultrasonic prenatal diagnosis of liver metastases from adrenal neuroblastoma. *J Clin Ultrasound.* 1992;20:401–403.

183. Richards DS, Cruz AC, Dowdy KA. Prenatal diagnosis of fetal liver calcifications. *J Ultrasound Med.* 1988;7:691–694.

184. Oepkes D, Meerman RH, Vandenbussche FPHA, et al. Ultrasonographic fetal spleen measuremnts in red blood cell-alloimmunized pregnancies. *Am J Obstet Gynecol.* 1993;169: 121–128.

185. Aoki S, Hata T, Kitao M. Ultrasonographic assessment of fetal and neonatal spleen. *Am J Perinatol.* 1992;9:361–367.

186. Schmiddt W, Yarkoni S, Jeanty P, et al. Sonographic measurements of the fetal spleen: Clinical implications. *J Ultrasound Med.* 1985;4:667.

187. Eliezer S, Esler F, Ehud W, et al. Fetal splenomegaly, ultrasound diagnosis of cytomegalovirus infection: A case report. *J Clin Ultrasound.* 1984;12:520.

188. Lickman JP, Miller EI. Prenatal ultrasonic diagnosis of splenic cyst. *J Ultrasound Med.* 1988;7:637–638.

189. Hill LM, Peterson C, Rivello D, et al. Sonographic detection of the fetal pancreas. *J Clin Ultrasound.* 1989;17:475–479.

190. Jouppila P, Heikkinen J, Kirkinen P. Contractility of maternal and fetal gallbladder: An ultrasonic study. *J Clin Ultrasound.* 1985;13:461.

191. Bronshtein M, Abramovici WH, Filmar S, et al. Prenatal diagnosis of gall bladder anomalies—Report of 17 cases. *Prenat Diagn.* 1993;13:851–861.

192. Hertzberg BS, Kliewer MA, Maynor C, et al. Nonvisualization of the fetal gallbladder: Frequency and prognostic importance. *Radiology.* 1996;1999:679–682.

193. Chan L, Rao BK, Jiang Y, et al. Fetal gallbladder growth and development during gestation. *J Ultrasound Med.* 1995;14: 421–425.

194. Goldstein I, Tamir A, Weisman A, et al. Growth of the fetal gallbladder in normal pregnancies. *Ultrasound Obstet Gynecol.* 1994;4:289–293.

195. Beretsky I, Lankin DH. Diagnosis of fetal cholelithiasis using real-time high-resolution imaging employing digital detection. *J Ultrasound Med.* 1983;2:381.

196. Brown DL, Teele RL, Doubilet PM, et al. Echogenic material in the fetal gallbladder: Sonographic and clinical observations. *Radiology.* 1992;182:73–76.

197. Suchet IB, Labatte MF, Dyck CS, et al. Fetal cholelithiasis: A case report and review of the literature. *J Clin Ultrasound.* 1993;21:198–202.

198. Devonald KJ, Ellwood DA, Colditz PB. The variable appearances of fetal gallstones. *J Ultrasound Med.* 1992;11: 579–585.

199. Klingensmith WC III, Cioffi-Ragan DT. Fetal gallstones. *Radiology.* 1988;167:143–144.

200. Abbitt PL, McIlhenny J. Prenatal detection of gallstones. *J Clin Ultrasound.* 1990;18:202–204.

201. Frank JL, Hill MC, Chirathivat S, et al. Antenatal observation of a choledochal cyst by sonography. *AJR.* 1981;137: 166.

202. Elrad H, Mayden KL, Ahart S, et al. Prenatal ultrasound diagnosis of choledochal cyst. *J Ultrasound Med.* 1985;4: 553.

203. Howell CG, Templeton JM, Weiner S, et al. Antenatal diagnosis and early surgery for choledochal cyst. *J Pediatr Surg.* 1983;18:387.

204. Schroeder D, Smith L, Prain HC. Antenatal diagnosis of choledochal cyst at 15 weeks' gestation: Etiologic implications and management. *J Pediatr Surg.* 1989;24:936–938.

205. Brown DK, Kimura K, Sato Y, et al. Solitary intrahepatic biliary cyst: Diagnostic and therapeutic strategy. *J Pediatr Surg.* 1990;25:1248–1249.

206. Gallivan EK, Crombleholme M, D'Alton ME. Early prenatal diagnosis of choledochal cyst. *Prenat Diagn.* 1996;16: 934–937.

207. Hussman KL, Friedwald JP, Gollub MJ, et al. Caroli's disease associated with infantile polycystic kidney disease. *J Ultrasound Med.* 1991;10:235–237.

The Fetal Genitourinary System

Carol B. Benson • *Peter M. Doubilet*

The fetal kidneys begin developing within the pelvis at approximately 7 weeks of gestation from the metanephric mesoderm and the ureteric bud. The metanephric tissue develops into the nephrons of the kidney, and the ureteric bud differentiates into the collecting tubules, calyces, pelvis, and ureter. Between 7 and 11 weeks, as the fetal body grows in length, the kidneys ascend to their permanent position in the flank due to disproportionate growth of more caudal structures.[1–3]

Initially, the kidney is made up of several loosely connected lobes, each with a thin cortex. During the second trimester the lobes fuse, becoming less distinct, and the cortex thickens, leaving the kidney with a lobular contour that persists for several years after birth.[2–4] The kidneys begin to excrete urine at approximately 11 weeks of gestation, and from this age onward urine production increases progressively.

By the second trimester the kidneys become the major contributor to the amniotic fluid volume.[2,3] Adequate amniotic fluid volume is necessary for normal fetal pulmonary and skeletal development because it provides space for fetal growth and movement.[5] Therefore, a functioning urinary tract must be present for the lungs and skeleton to develop normally.[6]

Using transvaginal ultrasound, normal fetal kidneys can first be seen as early as 9 weeks of gestation and should always be visible by 13 weeks.[7,8] With transabdominal scanning, the kidneys may first be visible at 13 to 14 weeks of gestation and are seen in most patients by 16 to 18 weeks (Fig. 19–1). Delayed visibility may occur when factors such as maternal obesity or large uterine fibroids limit the fetal survey. The fetal bladder may be seen as early as 11 weeks with transvaginal scanning[7,8] and should be visible transabdominally by 16 weeks in virtually all patients.

The incidence of genitourinary anomalies at birth is 0.2 to 0.6%.[9,10] Genitourinary anomalies comprise approximately one-fourth of all congenital structural anomalies.[11] Anomalies of the genitourinary tract result from arrested development early in organogenesis, failure of normal ascent, obstruction of the collecting system or bladder outlet, and abnormal formation of renal tubules. These anomalies are most often isolated but may also occur in association with, or may cause, other fetal structural abnormalities. Associations between genitourinary and other organ system anomalies occur in a broad variety of inherited or sporadic syndromes, including chromosomal abnormalities.[2,3,12,13] In addition, urinary tract abnormalities that decrease urine production cause oligohydramnios, which may secondarily cause deformities involving other parts of the fetus. In particular, when severe oligohydramnios is present before 20 weeks of gestation, pulmonary hypoplasia, facial abnormalities, including flattened nose and low-set ears, and clubfeet or other limb positional abnormalities may result.[14,15]

Prenatal sonography can identify and characterize many anomalies of the genitourinary system. Ultrasound performed in the second and third trimesters detects at least 80 to 85% of genitourinary anomalies.[16,17] Prenatal diagnosis permits antenatal counseling and prompt postnatal evaluation and

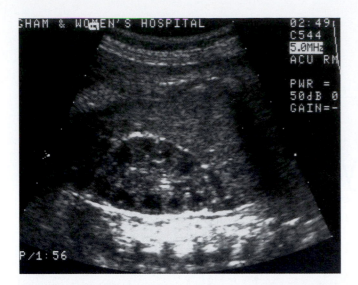

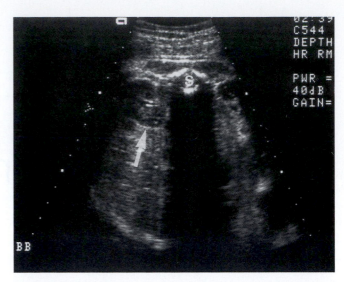

Figure 19–2. Unilateral renal agenesis. Transverse view at the level of the kidneys demonstrating one kidney *(arrow)* to the right of the spine (S) and no kidney on the left.

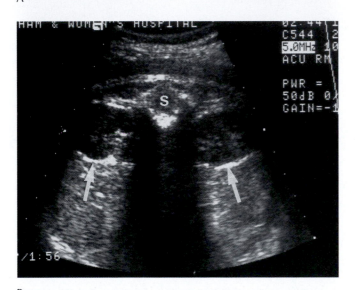

Figure 19–1. Normal kidneys. **(A)** Longitudinal scan of a normal kidney demonstrating its reniform shape with central sinus echoes and hypoechoic pyramids. **(B)** Transverse view of both kidneys *(arrows)*, one on either side of the spine (S), which casts a shadow between them.

treatment, thus avoiding the therapeutic delays that, before the availability of ultrasound, often led to impairment or loss of renal function.[18]

RENAL AGENESIS

Failure of development of the ureteric bud will lead to renal agenesis. Renal agenesis may be unilateral or bilateral. Unilateral agenesis occurs in approximately 0.3 per 1000 births and has an excellent prognosis. On prenatal ultrasound no kidney is seen in the renal fossa on the affected side and the contralateral kidney is large for gestational age (Fig. 19–2). It

is important not to mistake the ipsilateral adrenal, which may be flattened or "lying down," for a kidney. This error can be avoided by recognizing that the adrenal gland does not have central sinus echoes and does not have a reniform shape in the longitudinal plane. It is also important to scan the fetal pelvis to be sure the kidney is truly absent rather than in an ectopic location.[2,3,19–21]

Bilateral renal agenesis is a lethal anomaly in which there is failure of development of both kidneys. This condition occurs in approximately 1 to 4 per 10,000 births, with a male to female ratio of 2.5 to 1. When this anomaly is present, there is severe oligohydramnios from the early to mid–second trimester onward. Bilateral renal agenesis, together with the fetal deformities resulting from oligohydramnios—pulmonary hypoplasia, abnormal facies, and limb positional abnormalities—has been termed *Potter's syndrome*.[14] The neonate with bilateral agenesis typically dies shortly after birth from pulmonary hypoplasia. Recurrence in subsequent pregnancies is rare.

Sonographic diagnosis of bilateral agenesis is made on the basis of severe oligohydramnios and nonvisualization of the kidneys and urinary bladder (Fig. 19–3). Careful scanning is required before making the diagnosis because absence of surrounding amniotic fluid degrades the sonographic image. Other sonographic findings often seen with bilateral renal agenesis include dolichocephaly and a small thorax, both secondary to uterine compression from the absence of amniotic fluid.[2,3,15,19,22]

RENAL ECTOPIA

If one or both kidneys develop but fail to ascend normally into the renal fossa, one or both will ultimately reside in an

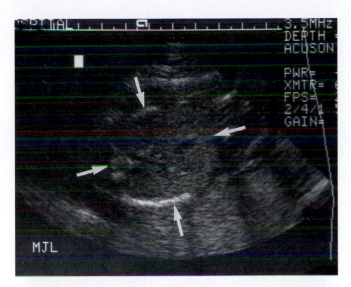

Figure 19–3. Bilateral renal agenesis. Transverse view of the fetal abdomen *(arrows)* demonstrating severe oligohydramnios and no kidneys.

ectopic location. This anomaly occurs in about 1 per 1200 births. The most common ectopic kidney is a pelvic kidney. Less commonly, a horseshoe kidney forms, in which the two kidneys are fused at their lower poles and ascend partially, such that their axes are altered and their lower poles extend

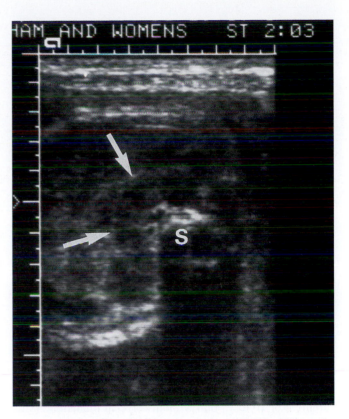

Figure 19–5. Horseshoe kidney. Transverse sonogram through the lower fetal abdomen showing renal parenchyma *(arrows)* joined together anterior to the spine (S).

across the midline of the lower abdomen. Occasionally, one kidney is crossfused to the lower pole of the contralateral kidney. Other ectopic kidneys, such as thoracic kidneys, are extremely rare.[2]

The sonographic findings with a pelvic kidney include a kidney in the pelvis adjacent to the urinary bladder and an empty renal fossa with a flattened adrenal gland (Fig. 19–4).[19,20,23] The pelvic kidney is at increased risk for urinary obstruction, and, therefore, hydronephrosis may be seen.[23] With crossfused ectopia, one renal fossa will be empty and the contralateral kidney will appear very long and may be unusual in shape. The lower moiety may be hydronephrotic or have cystic dysplasia secondary to obstruction.[24]

Sonographically, the location of the kidneys of a horseshoe kidney is lower in the abdomen, and the lower poles are displaced medially. Renal parenchyma may be seen extending across the midline in front of the fetal spine (Fig. 19–5).[2,25,26] These kidneys also have an increased incidence of obstruction and may have cystic dysplasia.[27]

HYDRONEPHROSIS

Dilatation of the fetal renal collecting system is the most common fetal abnormality detected by antenatal sonography. It

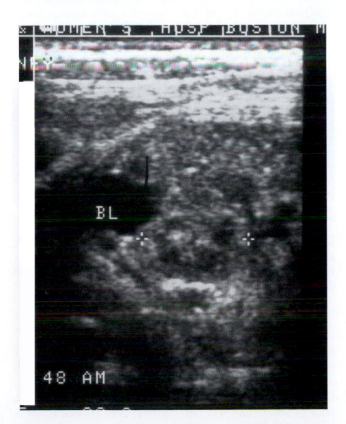

Figure 19–4. Pelvic kidney. Longitudinal view of the fetal pelvis showing a kidney (calipers) adjacent to the bladder (BL).

can result from obstruction of the urinary tract, vesicoureteral reflux, or deficient musculature in the walls of the urinary tract and abdomen *(prune belly syndrome)*. Urinary tract obstruction occurs most often at the level of the ureteropelvic junction but may also occur in the ureter, at the ureterovesical junction, or at the bladder outlet.

When fluid is seen in the renal pelvis by ultrasound, it is important to determine whether it represents hydronephrosis or is merely the small amount of fluid often seen in the normal renal pelvis in the second and third trimesters. Hydronephrosis should be diagnosed when there is caliectasis or the anteroposterior (AP) diameter of the renal pelvis, measured on a transverse view through the kidney, is at least 8 mm at 16 to 20 weeks or at least 10 mm after 20 weeks of gestation (Fig. 19–6). To avoid missing cases of evolving hydronephrosis, it is prudent to label a kidney with a renal pelvis of 4 to 7 mm at 16 to 20 weeks or of 5 to 9 mm after 20 weeks as possibly hydronephrotic and to follow the case either to resolution or to development of definite hydronephrosis. These criteria are based on studies that have shown that postnatal prognosis is related to prenatal AP diameter of the renal pelvis and the presence of caliectasis. When the AP measurement is less than 10 mm and no calyceal dilatation is seen, 94 to 97% of fetuses will be normal after birth. With an AP measurement of 10 to 15 mm without calyceal dilatation, 48 to 62% of fetuses will be normal and 39% will require medical or surgical intervention. With moderate to severe caliectasis, most fetuses will require surgery.[28–33]

When hydronephrosis is diagnosed, the ureters and bladder should be carefully evaluated, looking for ureteral dilatation, bladder distention, and urethral dilatation. It is also important to examine the contralateral kidney because renal anomalies are often bilateral.[3,13] In addition, amniotic fluid volume should be assessed, and a careful search made for other fetal anomalies.

When hydronephrosis is diagnosed in the second trimester, the possibility of a chromosomal abnormality, especially trisomy 21, must be entertained.[7,34–36] Up to one-fourth of fetuses with trisomy 21 have mild hydronephrosis in the second trimester as compared with 2 to 3% of normal fetuses. With isolated hydronephrosis in the absence of other abnormalities, the likelihood of trisomy 21 is approximately 1 in 340. The likelihood of a chromosomal abnormality is especially high when, in addition to hydronephrosis, the femur is small or there is a cardiac or gastrointestinal abnormality.[35,36]

An obstructed kidney is at risk for becoming dysplastic. The earlier and more complete the obstruction, the greater the likelihood and severity of dysplasia. Complete ureteral obstruction before 10 weeks results in a multicystic dysplastic kidney. When obstruction occurs after 10 weeks or is incomplete, the dysplastic kidney maintains a more reniform shape and is characterized sonographically by a thin echogenic renal parenchyma, often with small cysts. Sometimes hydronephrosis is present, in which case there is a di-

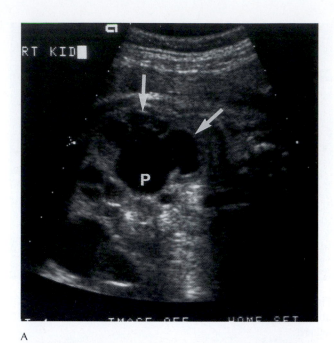

A

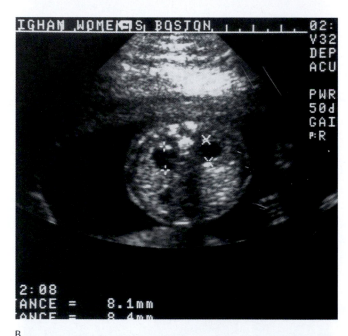

B

Figure 19–6. Hydronephrosis. **(A)** Coronal view of a hydronephrotic kidney showing a dilated renal pelvis (P) and dilated calyces *(arrows)*. **(B)** Transverse view of hydronephrotic kidneys with dilated renal pelvises measured anterior to posterior (calipers).

lated collecting system surrounded by abnormal-appearing renal tissue. In other cases, the dysplastic kidney is small and echogenic, with little or no fluid in the renal pelvis (Fig. 19–7). With any dysplastic kidney, renal function is poor or absent and will not improve, even if obstruction is corrected.[2,3,37]

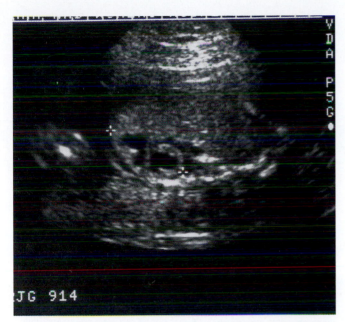

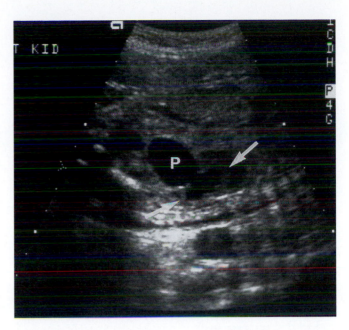

Figure 19–8. Ureteropelvic junction obstruction. Coronal view of kidney *(arrows)* obstructed at the ureteropelvic junction with a markedly dilated renal pelvis (P) and dilated intrarenal collecting system.

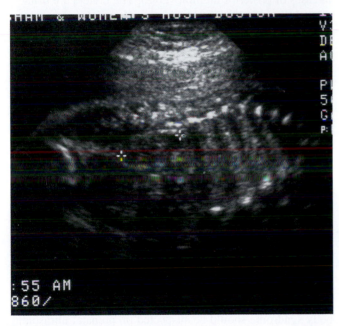

Figure 19–7. Dysplastic kidneys. **(A)** Calipers marking hydronephrotic dysplastic kidney with a thin echogenic renal cortex. **(B)** Calipers marking kidney is same patient 2 months later. The kidney is now small and dysplastic, with no hydronephrosis.

Ureteropelvic Junction Obstruction

Ureteropelvic junction (UPJ) obstruction is the most common cause of hydronephrosis in the neonate and affects males more than twice as often as females.[38,39] It is a functional obstruction and is bilateral in 30% of cases.[2,3,40–42] On ultrasound, a dilated renal pelvis is seen, with or without dilated

calyces (Fig. 19–8). The ureters are not dilated, and the amniotic fluid volume is usually normal.

Most kidneys with UPJ obstruction do not become dysplastic. Dysplasia does occur, however, in a minority of cases, typically those with severe or early-onset obstruction.[41] When dysplasia does occur, it is most often the hydronephrotic form, although it may evolve into the nonhydronephrotic variety. Development of dysplasia in a kidney with UPJ obstruction can be diagnosed when the parenchyma becomes abnormally echogenic or cystic.

Vesicoureteral Reflux

Vesicoureteral reflux, or reflux from the bladder into the ureter, results from an abnormal relation between the distal ureter and the bladder wall. Normally, the ureter traverses the bladder wall at a shallow angle, leading to a long intramural segment of ureter that acts as a valve preventing reflux. When the ureter has a steep, short course through the bladder wall, reflux results.[43] This abnormality is much more common among males than among females and is often bilateral.[44] It often resolves spontaneously within the first 1 to 2 years of life. Reflux that does not resolve spontaneously or is very severe at birth can be corrected surgically.

The sonographic findings of vesicoureteral reflux include hydronephrosis and hydroureter (Fig. 19–9).[45–47] In some cases, the hydronephrosis and hydroureter are present intermittently, with emptying and refilling every few minutes. In severe cases, the ureter may be markedly dilated and tortuous. Care must be taken not to mistake such a ureter for

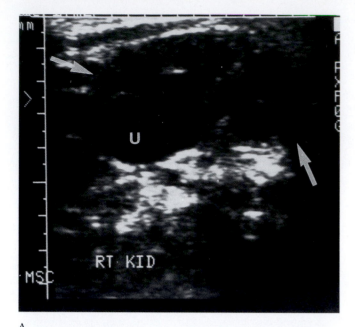

A

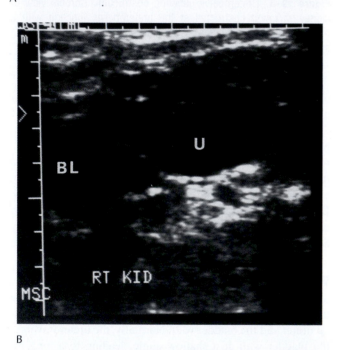

B

Figure 19–9. Hydronephrosis, hydroureter. **(A)** Coronal view of kidney *(arrows)* showing dilated calyces and a dilated proximal ureter (U). **(B)** Longitudinal view of the dilated ureter (U) to the bladder (BL).

a dilated bowel loop. This error can be avoided by following the dilated ureter proximally to the renal pelvis and distally to the bladder.

Primary Megaureter

Primary megaureter is a functional obstruction at the distal ureter, resulting from an aperistaltic distal ureteral seg-

ment. The prognosis is good. In mild cases no intervention is required, and in more severe cases corrective surgery can be performed.

The sonographic findings are hydronephrosis and hydroureter. The dilated ureter may be quite large, filling much of the lower abdomen, and may demonstrate peristalsis.[3,40,42] Because the combination of hydronephrosis and hydroureter is seen with both reflux and megaureter, the distinction between the two usually cannot be made *in utero* but must await postnatal evaluation with voiding cystourethrography and intravenous pyelography.

Bladder Outlet Obstruction

Bladder outlet obstruction occurs almost exclusively in males, most often as a result of posterior urethral valves. It may also occur with urethral atresia or caudal regression syndrome, both of which occur in males and females.[3,48,49] On ultrasound, regardless of cause, the urinary bladder is dilated and may have a thick wall. The posterior urethra may be dilated and appear as a projection from the bladder base, particularly in cases of posterior urethral valves. The ureters are usually dilated (Fig. 19–10). The kidneys have a variable appearance depending on the presence and extent of dysplasia. Possible appearances include hydronephrosis with normal-appearing renal parenchyma, hydronephrosis with echogenic or cystic renal parenchyma, or small shrunken kidneys with echogenic parenchyma. The kidneys may also appear normal or only mildly hydronephrotic when the urinary tract ruptures, thus decompressing itself. In these cases, fluid will be seen in the perinephric space or in the abdomen, in which case it is called *urine ascites* (Fig. 19–11).

Sonographic findings similar to those of bladder outlet obstruction may occur with prune belly syndrome. This entity occurs in males and is characterized by a deficiency of the abdominal musculature, the muscular walls of the urinary tract, and cryptorchidism. The two entities may, in fact, be related, in that some neonates diagnosed with prune belly syndrome may have had bladder outlet obstruction *in utero,* with distention of the urinary tract and abdominal wall, leading to muscle stretching and laxity. Prune belly syndrome should be suspected on prenatal ultrasound when, in addition to the findings seen with bladder outlet obstruction—distended bladder and bilateral hydronephrosis and hydroureter—the bladder wall is thin and the testicles are undescended.[43,50]

Megacystis megaureter may also appear sonographically similar to posterior urethral valves and prune belly syndrome. It is characterized by bilateral hydronephrosis and hydroureter and a dilated urinary bladder. Unlike the anomalies involving bladder outlet obstruction, the amniotic fluid volume with megacystis megaureter is usually normal or increased.[50–52]

The prognosis with bladder outlet obstruction is variable and is best predicted prenatally on the basis of amniotic fluid volume: the lower the fluid volume, the worse the prognosis.

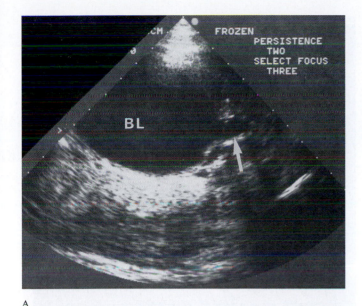

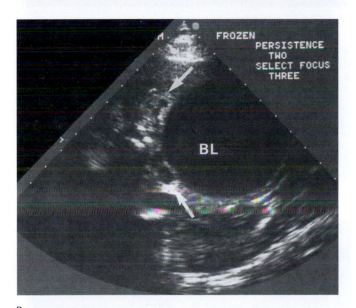

Figure 19–10. Posterior urethral valves. **(A)** Longitudinal view of pelvis showing enlarged bladder (BL) with dilated posterior urethra *(arrow).* **(B)** Transverse view of fetal abdomen showing markedly dilated bladder (BL) and small, echogenic, dysplastic kidneys *(arrows).*

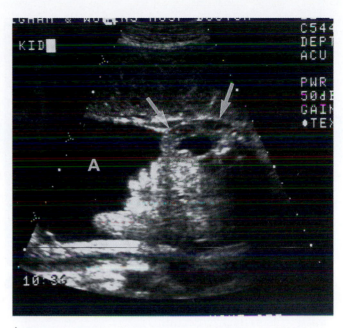

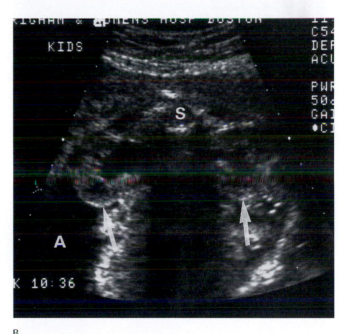

Figure 19–11. Posterior urethral valves with urine ascites. **(A)** Longitudinal view of the fetal abdomen showing severe oligohydramnios, a dysplastic kidney with hydronephrosis *(arrows),* and massive urine ascites (A). **(B)** Transverse view showing bilateral hydronephrotic kidneys *(arrows)* on either side of the spine (S) and ascites (A).

In particular, the prognosis is dismal when there is severe oligohydramnios.[50,51] In these cases, neonatal death may occur early from pulmonary insufficiency or later from renal insufficiency secondary to dysplasia.[3,48,49]

Prenatal treatment of bladder outlet obstruction has been successfully employed in a number of fetuses with this condition. Treatment involves creating a passageway for urine from the urinary tract to the amniotic cavity, by either percutaneously placing a shunt catheter from the fetal bladder

to the amniotic fluid space (Fig. 19–12) or open hysterotomy and fetal surgery to create bilateral ureterostomies.[52–54] Treatment can be considered in cases that meet the following selection criteria: 1) presence of oligohydramnios; 2) previable gestational age, normal-appearing renal parenchyma; 3) no other lethal anomalies, normal karyotype; and 4) normal

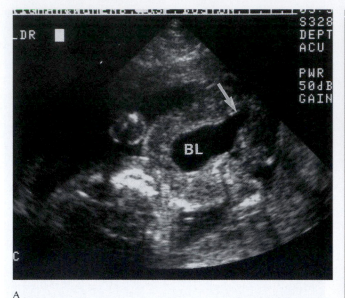

A

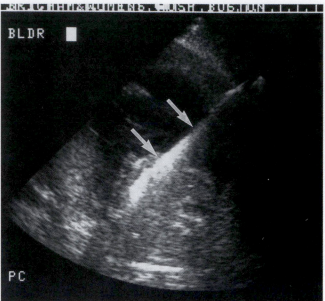

B

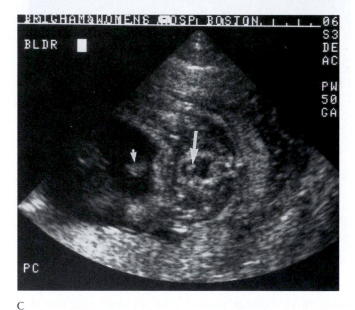

C

Figure 19–12. Shunt therapy for posterior urethral valves. **(A)** Sonogram of the fetal pelvis demonstrating dilated bladder (BL) with dilated posterior urethra *(arrow)*. There is moderate oligohydramnios. **(B)** Scan demonstrating a trocar *(arrows)* inserted transabdominally into the fetal bladder to facilitate placement of the shunt tubing. **(C)** Transverse view through the fetal pelvis after insertion of the shunt showing decompression of the bladder with tubing in place *(arrow)*. There is now minimal oligohydramnios. This sonogram also confirms that this is a male fetus *(arrowhead)*.

renal function, as determined by biochemical tests performed on urine percutaneously aspirated from the fetal bladder. Although only a small fraction of fetuses with bladder outlet obstruction will meet these stringent criteria, treatment in those that do meet them may lead to a viable infant with adequate pulmonary and renal function.

RENAL DUPLICATION

Duplication of the renal collecting system is a common abnormality that, unlike most urinary tract anomalies, affects females much more often than males.[55,56] In 83 to 90%, the duplication anomaly is unilateral.[56] When there is complete duplication of the ureter as well, the upper pole ureter typically implants ectopically, in a site caudal and medial to normal, and this ureter is often obstructed, and the lower pole ureter inserts orthotopically and may reflux. When the upper pole ureter implants ectopically in the bladder, there may be a ureterocele *(ectopic ureterocele)* bulging into the bladder lumen.

The diagnosis of duplication can be made by ultrasound when there is hydronephrosis that differentially affects the upper and lower poles of the kidney (Fig. 19–13). The hydronephrosis is most often limited to, or more severe in, the upper pole. The associated dilated ureter may also be seen,

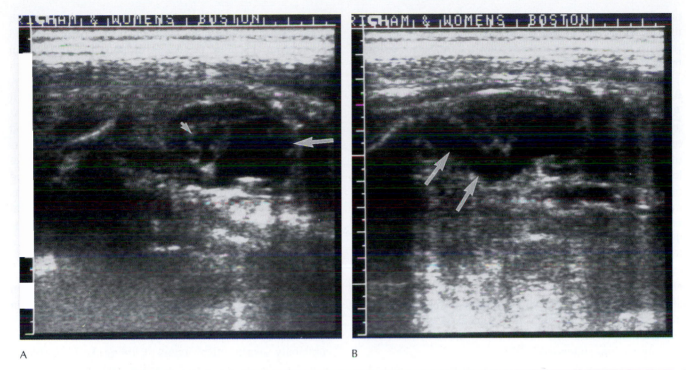

A   B

Figure 19–13. Renal duplication. **(A)** Coronal view of a kidney with a duplicated collecting system demonstrating disproportionate hydronephrosis of the upper pole calyces *(arrow)* as compared with the lower pole calyces *(arrowhead)*. **(B)** Longitudinal scan showing the dilated upper pole ureter *(arrows)* extending from obstructed upper pole of the kidney.

and occasionally an ectopic ureterocele will be seen in the urinary bladder.[55–57] The dilated upper pole collecting system may mimic a cyst or hydronephrosis of the entire kidney.[55]

MULTICYSTIC DYSPLASTIC KIDNEY

A multicystic dysplastic kidney is a form of renal dysplasia that results when there is complete obstruction or atresia at the level of the renal pelvis and infundibulum *(pelvoinfundibular atresia)* or of the proximal ureter before 10 weeks of gestation. The resulting dysplastic kidney is nonfunctional and is comprised of noncommunicating cysts of various sizes that replace the normal renal parenchyma. The multicystic dysplastic kidney is larger than a normal kidney. Contralateral renal abnormalities are seen in 40% of cases, the most common of which is ureteropelvic junction obstruction.[58] Rarely, multicystic dysplastic kidneys occur bilaterally. This is a fatal condition because it is functionally equivalent to bilateral renal agenesis.

On ultrasound, a multicystic dysplastic kidney appears as a mass in the renal fossa composed of multiple cysts of various sizes (Fig. 19–14).[2,3,37] Amniotic fluid volume is usually normal. The finding of low fluid volume should prompt a careful inspection of the contralateral kidney, with a search for obstruction, dysplasia, or agenesis.

HEREDITARY POLYCYSTIC KIDNEY DISEASE

Polycystic kidney disease may be inherited either as an autosomal recessive abnormality or as an autosomal dominant

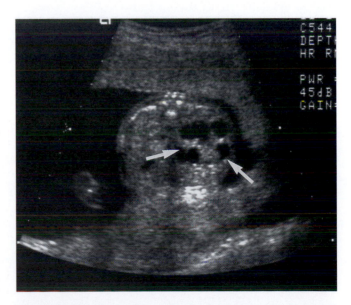

Figure 19–14. Multicystic dysplastic kidney. Transverse sonogram of fetal abdomen demonstrating dysplastic kidney as a cluster of cysts with a small amount of solid tissue *(arrows)* in the renal fossa.

one. The autosomal recessive form manifests itself early in life, in many cases *in utero.* The autosomal dominant form typically manifests itself in the second or third decade of life, but in rare cases may be evident *in utero.*[59–61]

Autosomal Recessive Polycystic Kidney Disease

Autosomal recessive polycystic kidney disease, previously termed *infantile polycystic kidney disease,* is an inherited disorder characterized by cystic dilatation of the renal tubules, often with associated hepatic fibrosis. The renal abnormality leads to impaired or absent renal function. This renal abnormality is usually evident *in utero,* but in some cases may not manifest itself until childhood. The age at presentation is related to the fraction of renal tubules that are affected. When 90% of renal tubules are involved, renal function is markedly impaired *in utero* and neonatal death is likely. Cases of autosomal recessive polycystic kidney disease that present in childhood may have only 10% of renal tubules affected. In all cases, the degree of hepatic fibrosis is inversely proportional to the degree of renal involvement. As a result, the hepatic component of the disease mostly affects those cases that survive into childhood.[59,60,62]

The changes in the kidneys caused by autosomal recessive polycystic kidney disease lead to enlargement of the kidneys with maintenance of their reniform shape. When the onset is prenatal, ultrasound will demonstrate enlarged kidneys with generalized increased echogenicity and enhanced through-transmission (Fig. 19–15). The bladder is often absent, and severe oligohydramnios may be present as early as 16 weeks of gestation. In these cases, the syndrome is lethal because of pulmonary hypoplasia secondary to the severe oligohydramnios. In cases in which renal impairment begins somewhat later, the kidneys may be enlarged with increased echogenicity, but the bladder may be present and oligohydramnios may be absent or may develop later in gestation.[59,60,62–64]

The finding of bilateral echogenic kidneys is not specific for autosomal recessive polycystic kidney disease. It may be seen with a number of other pathologic entities, including autosomal dominant polycystic kidney disease and various forms of renal dysplasia, and may also be a normal variant.[63] When echogenic kidneys are identified prenatally, it is important to look for the urinary bladder and assess the amniotic fluid volume. Follow-up prenatal scans and postnatal tests of renal function may provide additional information to distinguish a pathologic condition from a normal variant.

Autosomal Dominant Polycystic Kidney Disease

Autosomal dominant polycystic kidney disease most often presents in young adulthood but can occasionally be seen in the fetus or neonate. This syndrome is associated with multiple renal cysts, hypertension, and renal failure. Cysts are commonly seen in other organs including the liver, spleen, and pancreas. In the rare cases that present in the fetus, the sonographic appearance of the kidneys may be similar to that of autosomal recessive polycystic kidney disease, with enlarged echogenic kidneys. Cysts may occasionally be seen in the kidneys, and decreased amniotic fluid may be present.[59,61]

RENAL MASSES AND CYSTS

Solid masses and isolated cysts may be found in fetal kidneys, although both occur infrequently. The most common solid mass is a mesoblastic nephroma, which is a hamartoma of the kidney (Fig. 19–16). Rarely, a Wilm's tumor will be seen in the fetus.[43] Isolated cysts, seen sonographically as anechoic round lesions in the kidney (Fig. 19–17), must be distinguished from focal hydronephrosis, which most often affects the upper pole of a duplicated collecting system.

ABNORMALITIES OF THE URINARY BLADDER

Megacystis

Megacystis is an anomaly in which there is ineffective emptying of the urinary bladder, leading to marked dilatation of the bladder. With megacystis megaureter, hydronephrosis and hydroureter are also seen.[50–52] Megacystis occurs in females in association with deficient bowel peristalsis (*megacystis microcolon*) or in either sex due to a neurogenic bladder from a meningomyelocele.[42]

On ultrasound, the sonographic findings may mimic posterior urethral valves, with a large urinary bladder seen in the lower pelvis, diminished amniotic fluid, and hydronephrosis,

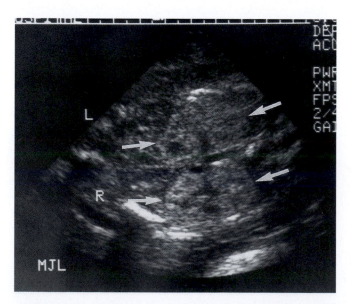

Figure 19–15. Autosomal recessive polycystic kidneys. Coronal sonogram showing both kidneys are enlarged and echogenic (*arrows*), and there is severe oligohydramnios.

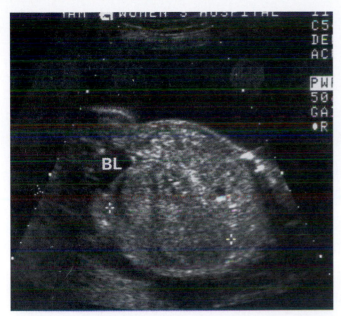

A

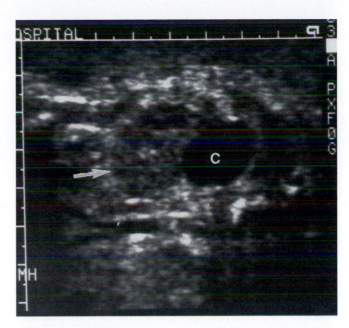

Figure 19–17. Renal cyst. Coronal view of kidney *(arrow)* containing an upper pole cyst (C).

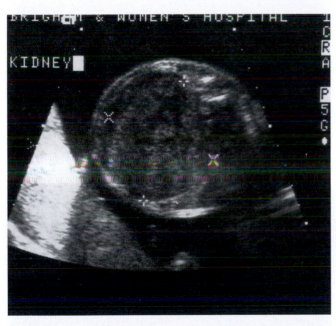

B

Figure 19–16. Mesoblastic nephroma. **(A)** Longitudinal sonogram showing large mass (calipers) arising from the renal fossa with compression on fetal bladder (BL). **(B)** Transverse view of the fetal abdomen demonstrating large renal mass (calipers) filling much of the fetal abdomen.

hydroureter. In less severe cases, the only finding is a dilated urinary bladder.[43]

Exstrophy

Failure of regression, or incomplete regression, of the cloacal membrane results in a spectrum of anomalies that ranges in severity from mild epispadius in males or labial separation in females, to cloacal exstrophy, a large defect in the lower anterior abdominal wall, bladder, and colon, with eversion of the bladder and distal colon. Cloacal exstrophy occurs sporadically and affects males twice as frequently as females.[65]

Intermediate in severity is exstrophy of the urinary bladder, in which there is a defect in the anterior abdominal and bladder walls, with eversion of the bladder. The symphysis pubis is splayed, and there are associated anomalies of the external genitalia, including labial separation and a bifid clitoris in females and epispadius in males.[65,66]

On ultrasound, bladder exstrophy may be suspected when there is absence of the urinary bladder, especially if there is also a soft tissue mass on the surface of the lower abdominal wall, representing exposed bladder mucosa. In some cases, however, fluid can be seen in the urinary bladder despite its opening to the amniotic cavity, and the diagnosis may be difficult to make.[43]

ABNORMALITIES OF THE REPRODUCTIVE SYSTEM AND EXTERNAL GENITALIA

Ovarian Cysts and Masses

Cysts occasionally develop in the ovary of a female fetus. Most are follicular cysts, but corpus luteal cysts, theca lutein cysts, teratomas, and cystadenomas may also occur. A cyst may grow throughout gestation in response to high estrogens in the maternal serum. Cysts also predispose the ovary to torsion. On ultrasound, an ovarian cyst is a simple cyst in the lower fetal abdomen (Fig. 19–18). It is indistinguishable from

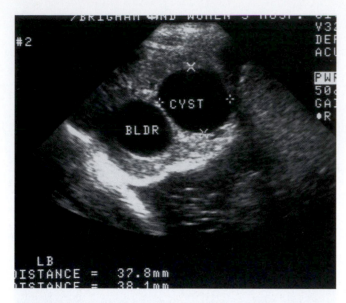

Figure 19–18. Ovarian cyst. Sonogram of fetal pelvis demonstrating a cyst (CYST) adjacent to the urinary bladder (BLDR).

a mesenteric cyst, omental cyst, gastrointestinal duplication cyst, or hydrometrocolpos. Ovarian torsion can be diagnosed if there is an acute change in a previously identified ovarian cyst with increase in size and development of echoes within the cyst (Fig. 19–19).[67,68]

Congenital solid ovarian masses are rare, most often being germ cell tumors. When present, they appear as solid masses in the lower abdomen.[43]

Hydrometrocolpos

Hydrometrocolpos is a condition in which the uterus and vagina are distended by cervical and vaginal secretions due to obstruction from imperforate hymen, transverse vaginal septum, or vaginal or cervical atresia. When the dilated uterus and vagina form a large pelvic mass, they may cause hydronephrosis and hydroureter. The sonographic appearance of hydrometrocolpos is a cystic pelvic mass, often with low level echoes, located posterior to the bladder and extending into the abdomen.[69] Because it is indistinguishable from other pelvic and lower abdominal cystic masses, precise diagnosis cannot be made until after birth.

Hydrocele

Collection of fluid between the layers of the tunica vaginalis in the scrotum is a hydrocele. It is easily diagnosed sonographically by identifying fluid within the scrotum, often outlining the testicles (Fig. 19–20). Hydroceles may be seen in association with ascites. When present as an isolated finding, they are of little or no clinical significance.

Cryptorchidism

Cryptorchidism, or undescended testicle, can be detected sonographically by failure to visualize the testicle within the scrotum. The testicles may not fully descend until late in pregnancy, so this finding may be present in at least 10% of fetuses in the early to mid–third trimester. Its incidence at term is 0.7%.[70] Although most often an isolated finding, it

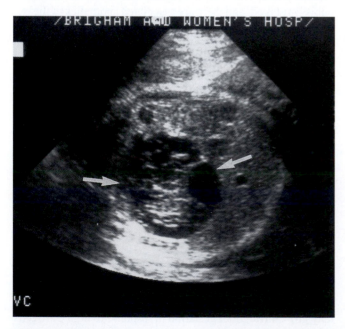

Figure 19–19. Ovarian torsion. Sonogram of fetal pelvis demonstrating a complex cystic mass *(arrows)* that represents a torsed ovary. Previous scans had shown a smaller, simple ovarian cyst.

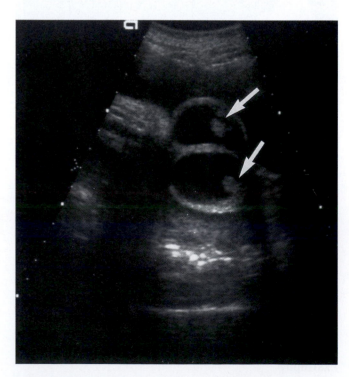

Figure 19–20. Hydroceles. Scan through the fetal scrotum demonstrating large hydroceles around the testicles *(arrows).*

can be seen in a variety of syndromes, including prune belly syndrome, Noonan's syndrome, and trisomies 13, 18, and 21.

Ambiguous Genitalia

Ambiguous genitalia refers to external genitalia that are not clearly of either sex. This can result from abnormal hormone levels, as in congenital adrenal hyperplasia, transplacental passage of hormones, and true hermaphroditism (presence of both ovarian and testicular tissue). Anomalies of the external genitalia that are not hormonally mediated can also occur (e.g., micropenis). These latter anomalies can be isolated; they may have associated urinary tract anomalies or chromosomal abnormalities; or they may occur as one component of a multiple malformation syndrome.[71]

Testicular Feminization

Testicular feminization is a condition characterized by female external genitalia in conjunction with a male karyotype (46,XY chromosomes). It results from a disorder in the androgen receptor, which renders the body unable to respond to testosterone. Affected fetuses produce testosterone at levels higher than normal, but the hormone has no effect and the fetus fails to develop male features. Prenatal diagnosis can be made in conjunction with genetic amniocentesis when the sonogram demonstrates female external genitalia and amniocentesis demonstrates a male karyotype.[72]

REFERENCES

1. Moore KL, Persaud TVN. *The Developing Human.* 5th ed. Philadelphia: WB Saunders; 1993.
2. Daneman A, Alton DJ. Radiographic manifestations of renal anomalies. *Radiol Clin North Am.* 1991;29:351–363.
3. Patten RM, Mack LA, Wang KY, Cyr DR. The fetal genitourinary tract. *Radiol Clin North Am.* 1990;28:115–130.
4. Patriquin H, Lefaivre JF, Lafortune M, et al. Fetal lobation: An anatomo-ultrasonographic correlation. *J Ultrasound Med.* 1990;9:191–197.
5. McNamara MF, McCurdy CM, Reed KL, et al. The relation between pulmonary hypoplasia and amniotic fluid volume: Lessons learned from discordant urinary tract anomalies in monoamniotic twins. *Obstet Gynecol.* 1995;85:867–869.
6. Brace RA, Wolf EJ. Normal amniotic fluid volume change throughout pregnancy. *Am J Obstet Gynecol.* 1989;161:382–388.
7. Bronshtein M, Yoffe N, Brandes JM, Blumenfeld Z. First and early second-trimester diagnosis of fetal urinary tract anomalies using transvaginal sonography. *Prenat Diagn.* 1990; 10:653–666.
8. Rosati P, Guariglia L. Transvaginal sonographic assessment of the fetal urinary tract in early pregnancy. *Ultrasound Obstet Gynecol.* 1996;7:95–100.
9. Stoll C, Alembik Y, Dott B, Roth MP. Prenatal detection of internal urinary system's anomalies. *Eur J Epidemiol.* 1995; 11:283–290.

10. Gloor JM, Ogburn PL, Breckle RJ, et al. Urinary tract anomalies detected by prenatal ultrasound examination at Mayo Clinic Rochester. *Mayo Clin Proc.* 1995;70:526–531.
11. Cusick EL, Didier F, Droulle P, Schmitt M. Mortality after an antenatal diagnosis of foetal uropathy. *J Pediatr Surg.* 1995;30:463–466.
12. Nicolaides KH, Cheng HH, Abbas A, et al. Fetal renal defects: Associated malformations and chromosomal defects. *Fetal Diagn Ther.* 1992;7:1–11.
13. Hammond DI. Prenatal diagnosis of urinary tract malformations. *Can Assoc Radiol J.* 1992;43:179–187.
14. Potter EL. Bilateral absence of ureters and kidneys, report of fifty cases. *Obstet Gynecol.* 1965;25:3–12.
15. Sanders RC, Blakemore K. Lethal fetal anomalies: Sonographic demonstration. *Radiology.* 1989;172:1–6.
16. Dillon E, Walton SM. The antenatal diagnosis of fetal abnormalities: A 10 year audit of influencing factors. *Br J Radiol.* 1997;70:341–346.
17. Stefos T, Plachouras N, Sotiriadis A, et al. Routine obstetrical ultrasound at 18–22 weeks: Our experience on 7,236 fetuses. *J Mater Fetal Med.* 1999;8:64–69.
18. Brown T, Mandell J, Lebowitz RL. Neonatal hydronephrosis in the era of sonography. *AJR.* 1987;148:959–963.
19. Hoffman CK, Filly RA, Callen PW. The "lying down" adrenal sign: A sonographic indicator of renal agenesis or ectopia in fetuses and neonates. *J Ultrasound Med.* 1992;11: 533–536.
20. Jeanty P, Romero R, Kepple D, et al. Prenatal diagnoses in unilateral empty renal fossa. *J Ultrasound Med.* 1990;9: 651–654.
21. Sherer DM, Thompson HO, Armstrong B, Woods JR. Prenatal sonographic diagnosis of unilateral fetal renal agenesis. *J Clin Ultrasound.* 1990;18:648–652.
22. Sherer DM, McAndrew JH, Liberto L, Woods JR. Recurring bilateral renal agenesis diagnosed by ultrasound with the aid of amnioinfusion at 18 weeks' gestation. *Am J Perinatol.* 1992;9:49–51.
23. Hill LM, Peterson CS. Antenatal diagnosis of fetal pelvic kidneys. *J Ultrasound Med.* 1987;6:393–396.
24. Siegel RL, Rosenfeld DL, Leiman S. Complete regression of a multicystic dysplastic kidney in the setting of renal crossed fused ectopia. *J Clin Ultrasound.* 1992;20:466–469.
25. Sherer DM, Cullen JBH, Thompson HO, et al. Prenatal sonographic findings associated with a fetal horseshoe kidney. *J Ultrasound Med.* 1990;9:477–479.
26. King KL, Kofinas AD, Simon NV, Clay D. Antenatal ultrasound diagnosis of fetal horseshoe kidney. *J Ultrasound Med.* 1991;19:643–644.
27. Van Every MJ. In utero detection of horseshoe kidney with unilateral multicystic dysplasia. *Urology.* 1992;40: 435–437.
28. Grignon A, Filion R, Filiatrault D, et al. Urinary tract dilatation in utero: Classification and clinical applications. *Radiology.* 1986;160:645–647.
29. Johnson CE, Elder JS, Judge NE, et al. The accuracy of antenatal ultrasonography in identifying renal abnormalities. *AJDC.* 1992;146:1181–1184.
30. Lepercq J, Beaudoin S, Bargy F. Outcome of 116 moderate renal pelvis dialations at prenatal ultrasonography. *Fetal Diagn Ther.* 1998;13:79–81.

31. Fasolato V, Poloniato A, Bianchi C, et al. Feto-neonatal ultrasonography to detect renal abnormalities: Evaluation of 1-year screening program. *Am J Perinatol.* 1998;15:161–164.
32. Podevin G, Mandelbrot L, Vuillard E, et al. Outcome of urological abnormalities prenatally diagnosed by ultrasound. *Fetal Diagn Ther.* 1996;11:181–190.
33. Nguyen HT, Kogan BA. Upper urinary tract obstruction: Experimental and clinical aspects. *Br J Urol.* 1998;81:13–21.
34. Blumfield CG, Davis RO, Joseph DB, Cosper P. Fetal obstructive uropathies. *J Reprod Med.* 1991;36:662–666.
35. Benacerraf BR, Mandell J, Estroff JA, et al. Fetal pyelectasis: A possible association with Down syndrome. *Obstet Gynecol.* 1990;76:58–60.
36. Corteville JE, Dicke JM, Crane JP. Fetal pyelectasis and Down syndrome: Is genetic amniocentesis warranted? *Obstet Gynecol.* 1992;79:770–772.
37. Blane CE, Barr M, DiPietro MA, et al. Renal obstructive dysplasia: Ultrasound diagnosis and therapeutic implications. *Pediatr Radiol.* 1991;21:274–277.
38. Bosman G, Reuss A, Nijman JM, Wladimiroff JW. Prenatal diagnosis, management and outcome of fetal uretero-pelvic junction obstruction. *Ultrasound Med Biol.* 1991;17:117–120.
39. Ebel KD. Uroradiology in the fetus and newborn: Diagnosis and follow-up of congenital obstruction of the urinary tract. *Pediatr Radiol.* 1998;28:630–635.
40. Cohen HL, Haller JO. Diagnostic sonography of the fetal genitourinary tract. *Urol Radiol.* 1987;9:88–98.
41. Kleiner B, Callen PW, Filly RA. Sonographic analysis of the fetus with ureteropelvic junction obstruction. *AJR.* 1987;148:359–363.
42. Louie A, Arger PH. Fetal genitourinary tract. *Semin Roentgen.* 1990;4:342–352.
43. Currarino G. The genitourinary tract. In: Silverman FN, ed. *Caffey's Pediatric X-ray Diagnosis*, 8th ed. Chicago: Year Book Medical Publishers; 1985:1690–1696.
44. Anderson PAM, Rickwood AMK. Features of primary vesicoureteric reflux detected by prenatal sonography. *Br J Urol.* 1991;67:267–271.
45. Zerin JM, Ritchey ML, Chang ACH. Incidental vesicoureteral reflux in neonates with antenatally detected hydronephrosis and other renal abnormalities. *Radiology.* 1993;187:157–160.
46. Paduano L, Giglio L, Bembi B, et al. Clinical outcome of fetal uropathy. I. Predictive value of prenatal echography positive for obstructive uropathy. *J Urol.* 1991;146:1094–1096.
47. Grignon A, Filiatrault D, Homsy Y, et al. Ureteropelvic junction stenosis: Antenatal ultrasonographic diagnosis, postnatal investigation and follow-up. *Radiology.* 1986;160:649–651.
48. Mahoney BS, Callen PW, Filly RA. Fetal urethral obstruction: US evaluation. *Radiology.* 1985;157:221–224.
49. Hayden SA, Russ PD, Pretorius DH, et al. Posterior urethral obstruction. *J Ultrasound Med.* 1988;7:371–375.
50. Montemarano H, Bulas DI, Rushton HG, Selby D. Bladder distention and pyelectasis in the male fetus: Causes, comparisons, and contrasts. *J Ultrasound Med.* 1998;17:743–749.
51. Abbott JF, Levine D, Wapner R. Posterior urethral valves: Inaccuracy of prenatal diagnosis. *Fetal Diagn Ther.* 1998;13:179–183.
52. Peters CA. Lower urinary tract obstruction: Clinical and experimental aspects. *Br J Urol.* 1998;81:22–32.
53. Manning FA, Harrison MR, Rodeck C. Special report. Catheter shunts for fetal hydronephrosis and hydrocephalus. *N Engl J Med.* 1986;315:336–340.
54. Golbus MS, Filly RA, Callen PW, et al. Fetal urinary tract obstruction: Management and selection for treatment. *Semin Perinatol.* 1985;9:91–97.
55. Winters WD, Lebowitz RL. Importance of prenatal detection of hydronephrosis of the upper pole. *AJR.* 1990;155:125–129.
56. Vergani P, Ceruti P, Locatelli A, et al. Accuracy of prenatal ultrasonographic diagnosis of duplex renal system. *J Ultrasound Med.* 1999;18:463–467.
57. Sherer DM, Menashe M, Lebensart P, et al. Sonographic diagnosis of unilateral fetal renal duplication with associated ectopic ureterocele. *J Clin Ultrasound.* 1989;17:371–373.
58. Kleiner B, Filly RA, Mack L, Callen PW. Multicystic dysplastic kidney: Observations of contralateral disease in the fetal population. *Radiology.* 1986;161:27–29.
59. Reuss A, Wladimiroff JW, Niermeyer MF. Sonographic clinical and genetic aspects of prenatal diagnosis of cystic kidney disease. *Ultrasound Med Biol.* 1991;17:687–694.
60. Reuss A, Wladimiroff JW, Stewart PA, Niermeijer MF. Prenatal diagnosis by ultrasound in pregnancies at risk for autosomal recessive polycystic kidney disease. *Ultrasound Med Biol.* 1990;16:355–359.
61. Pretorius DH, Lee E, Manco-Johnson ML, et al. Diagnosis of autosomal dominant polycystic kidney disease in utero and in the young infant. *J Ultrasound Med.* 1987;6:249–255.
62. Barth RA, Guillot AP, Capeless EL, Clemmons JW. Prenatal diagnosis of autosomal recessive polycystic kidney disease: Variable outcome within one family. *Am J Obstet Gynecol.* 1992;166:560–567.
63. Estroff JA, Mandell J, Benacerraf BR. Increased renal parenchymal echogenicity in the fetus: Importance and clinical outcome. *Radiology.* 1991;181:135–139.
64. Bronshtein M, Bar-Hava I, Blumenfeld A. Clues and pitfalls in the early prenatal diagnosis of 'late onset' infantile polycystic kidneys. *Prenat Diagn.* 1992;12:293–298.
65. Meglin AJ, Balotin RJ, Jelinek JS, et al. Cloacal exstrophy: Radiology findings in 13 patients. *AJR.* 1990;155:1267–1272.
66. Barth RA, Filly RA, Sondheimer FK. Prenatal sonographic findings in bladder exstrophy. *J Ultrasound Med.* 1990;9:359–361.
67. Meizner I, Levy A, Katz M, et al. Fetal ovarian cysts: Prenatal ultrasonographic detection and postnatal evaluation and treatment. *Am J Obstet Gynecol.* 1991;164:874–878.
68. Sherer DM, Shah YG, Eggers PC, Woods JR. Prenatal sonographic diagnosis and subsequent management of fetal adnexal torsion. *J Ultrasound.* 1990;9:161–163.
69. Russ PD, Zavitz WR, Pretorius DH, et al. Hydrometrocolpos, uterus didelphys, and septate vagina: An antenatal sonographic diagnosis. *J Ultrasound Med.* 1986;5:211–213.
70. Morse MJ, Whitmore WF. Neoplasms of the testis. In: Walsh PC, Gittes RF, Perlmutter AD, Stamey TA, eds. *Campbell's Urology.* Philadelphia: WB Saunders; 1986;1535–1582.
71. Cooper C, Mahony BS, Bowie JD, Pope II. Prenatal ultrasound diagnosis of ambiguous genitalia. *J Ultrasound Med.* 1985;4:433–436.
72. Stephens JD. Prenatal diagnosis of testicular feminization. *Lancet* 1984;2:1038.

20

Fetal Skeletal Anomalies

*Eli Maymon • Roberto Romero • Fabio Ghezzi • Percy Pacora •
Gianliugi Pilu • Philippe Jeanty*

Skeletal dysplasias are a heterogeneous group of disorders and result in abnormalities in the size and shape of various segments of the skeleton. In recent years, major advances have been made in identifying mutations associated with chondrodysplasias. This chapter reviews the recent progress made in this field, the birth prevalence and classification of skeletal dysplasias and provides an approach to the diagnosis of conditions identifiable at birth.

MOLECULAR GENETIC BASIS OF THE CHONDRODYSPLASIAS

The process of skeletal formation and growth includes the differentiation of mesenchymal cells to form cartilage for future bone endochondral ossification. The growth of the long bones occurs through differentiation of chondrocytes in the growth plates and intramembranous ossification.[1,2] Disruption in any of these processes results in skeletal abnormalities.[3] A wide range of phenotypes has been described in osteochondrodysplasias. However, recent advances in the understanding of the molecular basis of skeletal dysplasias indicate that a spectrum of phenotypes share a similar genetic basis.[4,5]

Although the familial tendency of chondrodysplasias has been known for many years, the molecular basis for a number of conditions has only recently been clarified.[6,7] (Table 20–1).

ABNORMAL MESENCHYMAL DIFFERENTIATION

Bone Morphogenetic Proteins

Bone morphogenetic proteins (BMPs) are products of a family of genes that play a role in regulating the early mesenchymal cell condensation into the chondrogenic and osteogenic cell lineages and in influencing the size and shape of skeletal elements.[8,9] BMPs have the ability to induce ectopic bone formation when implanted subcutaneously or in muscle.[10,11] BMPs have homology with the superfamily of transforming growth factors-beta.[12–14] Mutations in the cartilage-derived morphogenic protein-1 have been shown to cause acromesomelic chondrodysplasias, Hunter–Thompson type, and autosomal dominant brachydactyly type C.[15–18]

Mutation in Transcription Factor Genes

Transcription factors are a class of proteins that play an important role in regulatory gene expression. They bind to regulatory elements in DNA promotors or enhancers that result in stimulation or inhibition of gene transcription and mRNA formation.[19–21] They are arranged into distinct domains and are important for the development of the embryo. Mutations in the genes coding for this group of proteins may cause chondrodysplasias.

Homeotic (Hox) Genes. Homeotic change is the transformation of one body part into another. Homeotic, or Hox,

TABLE 20–1. MUTATIONS IN HUMAN SKELETAL DYSPLASIA

Gene	Syndrome
Disorders of mesenchymal condensation and differentiation	
SOX9	Campomelic dysplasia
HOX-13	Synpolydactyly
PAX-3	Waardenburg's syndrome
CDMP-1	Hunter–Thompson type acromesomelic dysplasia
	Brachydactyly type C
TBX-5	Holt–Oram syndrome
Disorders of maturation of cartilage	
FGFR1	Pfieffer's syndrome
	Apert's syndrome
	Jackson–Weiss syndrome
FGFR2	Crouzon's syndrome
	Thanatophoric dysplasia
	Achondroplasia
FGFR3	Hypochondroplasia
	Jansen's metaphyseal chondrodysplasia
PTHrPR	Blomstrand's osteochondrodysplasia
Disorders in collagenous and noncollagenous extracellular matrix	
COL1A1, A2	Osteogenesis imperfecta types I–IV
COL2A1	Achondrogenesis
	Hypochondrogenesis
	Kniest's dysplasia
	Stickler's dysplasia
COL9A2	Multiple epiphyseal dysplasia
COL10A1	Schmid's metaphyseal chondrodysplasia
COMP	Pseudoachondroplasia
DTDST	Achondrogenesis type IB
	Atelosteogenesis type II
	Diastrophic dysplasia

genes control the morphogenesis of body parts. These genes encode for a family of proteins (transcription factors) that have a DNA binding domain called the *homeodomain* or *homeobox*.[22–26] Transcription factors regulate gene expression by binding to DNA, and play a central role in skeletal pattern formation.[26–31] Inactivation or pathologic expression of these genes causes deletion or addition of skeletal elements.[29,30] Homeobox genes located in the 5′ section of the HoxA and HoxD complexes are required for proliferation of skeletal progenitor cells of the limb. Specific combinations of gene products determine the length of the upper arm (genes belonging to groups 9 and 10), the lower arm (groups 10, 11, and 12), and the digits (groups 11, 12, and 13).[32] Mutation in the HOXD-13 gene in humans causes synpolydactyly (webbing and insertion of an extra digit) in heterozygous individuals.[33] Pax (paired like homeobox-containing) genes are a gene family that share a sequence called *paired box* that codes for a protein domain with DNA binding properties.[34,35] This transcription factor is also involved in skeletal formation. Mutation in Pax-3 has been implicated

in Waardenburg's syndrome, an autosomal dominant skeletal dysplasia with craniofacial anomalies.[36–40] Mutation in another transcription factor gene, msx2, causes Boston type craniosynostosis.[41,42]

The SOX and TBX Genes. The gene responsible for campomelic dysplasia (CD) has been localized to chromosome 17.[43–45] A substantial fraction of XY patients with CD (75%) demonstrates sex reversal syndrome. The development of the testis in mammals requires the SRY (sex-determining region Y) gene,[46–49] and the protein encoded by this gene includes a high mobility group (HMG) domain, termed *HMG box*. This SRY HMG box binds to a specific DNA sequence that confers DNA transcription properties. Many other genes that encode proteins related to HMG boxes have been identified, and those that encode proteins with a similarity of more than 60% to the SRY HMG region have been termed *SOX* (SRY box).[50–52] The SRY gene exerts its effect by interacting with the adjacent SOX-9 gene.[53] SOX-9 is required for cartilage formation,[54,55] and mutations of the SOX-9 gene have been reported in several patients[56,57] indicating that both CD and sex reversal can be caused by this mutation.[56–67]

Holt–Oram syndrome is characterized by upper limb malformations and cardiac septation defects. Linkage studies have mapped the gene responsible for this condition to chromosome 12q2. Mutations in one of the human T-box transcription factor family (TBX5) underlie this skeletal disorder.[68–72]

ABNORMAL CHONDROCYTES MATURATION

Fibroblast Growth Factor Receptors

Fibroblast growth factors (FGFs) are a group of at least nine heparin binding polypeptide growth factors that have pleotropic effects on many different cell types at various stages of development.[73,74] The cellular responses to these proteins are mediated through cell surface receptors.[75] Different genes encode for different but highly homologous receptors. Fibroblast growth factor receptor (FGFR) mutations cause a spectrum of disorders linked to the degree of receptor activation.[76] Recurrent mutation of single amino acids in the transmembrane domain of FGFR3 causes a number of disorders. Achondroplasia, thanatophoric dysplasia, and hypochondroplasia are skeletal dysplasias resulting from mutations in FGFR3.[77–79] Graded activation of FGFR3 by mutations causes achondroplasia and thanatophoric dysplasia.[78] Achondroplasia, which is non-lethal, results from a glycine-to-arginine substitution at position 380 in the transmembrane domain of the tyrosine kinase receptor.[79] Distinct mutations in FGFR3 cause two different types of thanatophoric dysplasia.[80] Mutations in FGFR1 and FGFR2 have been described in Pfieffer's syndrome,[81] Apert's syndrome,[82–86] and Jackson–Weiss syndrome.[87] Crouzon's syndrome is associated with mutations in FGFR2.[88–93]

Parathyroid Hormone Related Protein Receptor

Jansen's metaphyseal chondrodysplasia is a short limb dwarfism caused by abnormal development of the growth plate. Hypercalcemia and hypophosphatemia with normal or low levels of parathyroid hormone (PTH) and PTH-related protein receptor (PTHrPR) characterize this disorder.[95] Schipani et al. identified a mutation of the gene encoding for this receptor in a patient with Jansen's metaphyseal chondrodysplasia.[96] The mutation results in a persistent activation of the receptor shared by these two hormones and leads to Jansen's metaphyseal chondrodysplasia.[97,98] The mutation results in a change of a histidine to an arginine residue (H223R), causing ligand independent activation of the receptor.[99,100] Recently, genomic DNA from an additional six patients with Jansen's disease was analyzed and revealed a second activation mutation in the PTH/PTHrPR.[101] This novel mutation causes a change of threonine to proline (T10P).[102,103] Blomstrand osteochondrodysplasia (BOCD) is a rare lethal skeletal dysplasia characterized by accelerated endochondral and intramembranous ossification.[104,105] Comparison of the characteristics of BOCD with type I PTH/PTHrPR)-ablated mice shows similarities that are most prominent in the growth plate. This overall similarity suggested that an inactivating mutation of the PTH/PTHrPR might be the underlying genetic defect causing BOCD. Inactivating mutations of the PTH/PTHrPR have recently been identified.[104–109]

DEFECTS OF EXTRACELLULAR MATRIX COMPONENTS

Collagen

Collagen is the most abundant extracellular matrix protein. It is synthesized from three promolecules known as α chains.[110,111] Type 1 collagen is a heterotrimer of one (α1) and two (α2) chains and is the most abundant protein in bone.[112] Type 2 collagen, a homotrimer, is the major structural component of cartilage. It also has a role in other structures: vitreous body, intervertebrate disc, and tectorial membrane of the inner ear.[113–115] Mutations in type 1 collagen gene locus α1 (COL1A1) and COL1A2 genes cause osteogenesis imperfecta.[116–124] The nature of the mutation and the consequent protein structure impacts the severity of the phenotype.[125] This impact decreases as the mutation shifts toward the amino terminal portion of the molecule. More than 30 mutations have been found at the type 2 collagen gene locus (COL2A1).[126–130] Mutations in other collagen types have been described with multiple epiphyseal dysplasia and Schmid's metaphyseal chondrodysplasia.[131–144] Table 20–1 presents the important mutations and the clinical phenotypes associated with them.

Cartilage Oligomeric Matrix Protein

Cartilage oligomeric matrix protein (COMP) is a noncollagenous component of cartilage matrix.[145] It is a pentamer of five identical subunits belonging to the thrombospondin family and is found in chondrocytes.[146–148] The gene for COMP was localized to chromosome 19. A mutation in the gene for COMP causes pseudohypochondrodysplasia, an autosomal dominant chondrodysplasia.[149–156]

DISORDERS OF PROTEOGLYCAN SULFATATION

Diastrophic dysplasia (DTD) is an autosomal recessive osteochondrodysplasia characterized by dwarfism,[157,158] spinal deformation,[159] and joint abnormalities.[160,161] Undersulfatation of proteoglycans in cartilage matrix,[162] abnormalities in chondrocytes and disorganization of collagen fibrils have been documented in this disorder.[161–164] The disease is highly prevalent in Finland.[165] The gene encoding for the sulfate transport protein is designated DTDST (diastrophic dysplasia sulfate transporter) and is the same gene for DTD (chromosome 5q). Mutations in this gene lead to defective sulfatation of proteoglycans.[166–168] Mutations in the DTDST have also been found in achondrogenesis IB and atelosteogenesis type II.[169–174]

BIRTH PREVALENCE AND CONTRIBUTION TO PERINATAL MORTALITY

The birth prevalence of skeletal dysplasias recognizable in the neonatal period, excluding limb amputations, has been estimated to be 2.4 per 10,000 births.[175] In a large series, 23% of affected infants were stillborn, and 32% died during the first week of life. The overall frequency of skeletal dysplasias among perinatal deaths was 9.1 per 1000. The birth prevalence of the different skeletal dysplasias and their relative frequency among perinatal deaths in this study are shown in Table 20–2. The four most common skeletal dysplasias found were thanatophoric dysplasia, achondroplasia, osteogenesis imperfecta, and achondrogenesis. Thanatophoric dysplasia and achondrogenesis accounted for 62% of all lethal skeletal dysplasias.[175] The most common nonlethal skeletal dysplasia was achondroplasia.

In another large series reporting the prevalence and classification of lethal neonatal skeletal dysplasias in western Scotland, the prevalence was 1.1 per 10,000 births, and the most frequently diagnosed conditions were thanatophoric dysplasia (1 per 42,000), osteogenesis imperfecta (1 per 56,000), chondrodysplasia punctata (1 per 84,000), campomelic syndrome (1 per 112,000), and achondrogenesis (1 per 112,000).[176] Rasmussen et al reported a prevalence of 2.14 cases per 10,000 deliveries in a longitudinal study that included elective pregnancy terminations, stillborn infants at more than 20 weeks of gestation, and liveborn infants diagnosed by the fifth day of life. The rate of lethal cases was 0.95 per 10,000 deliveries.[177] Table 20–3 shows the rate of the skeletal dysplasias per 10,000 births in 11 studies.

TABLE 20–2. BIRTH PREVALENCE (PER 10,000 TOTAL BIRTHS) OF SKELETAL DYSPLASIAS

	Birth Prevalence (per 10,000)	Frequency Among Perinatal Deaths
Thanatophoric dysplasia	0.69	1:246
Achondroplasia	0.37	—
Achondrogenesis	0.23	1:639
Osteogenesis imperfecta type II	0.18	1:799
Osteogenesis imperfecta (other types)	0.18	—
Asphyxiating thoracic dysplasia	0.14	1:3.196
Chondrodysplasia punctata	0.09	—
Campomelic dysplasia	0.05	1:3.196
Chondroectodermal dysplasia	0.05	1:3.196
Larsen's syndrome	0.05	—
Mesomelic dysplasia (Langer's type)	0.05	—
Others	0.46	1:800

Source: Camera and Mastroiacovo.[175]

CLASSIFICATION OF SKELETAL DYSPLASIAS

The fundamental problem with the classification of skeletal dysplasias is that the pathogenesis of these diseases is largely unknown.[178] To develop a uniform terminology, a group of experts met in Paris in 1977 and proposed an International Nomenclature for Skeletal Dysplasias based on descriptive findings of either clinical or radiologic nature.[179]

This nomenclature underwent a revision in 1992[180–182] and was reclassified using radiodiagnostic and morphologic criteria. The new classification grouped morphologically similar disorders into families of diseases based on presumed pathogenetic similarities. The International Working Group on Bone Dysplasias met in Los Angeles, California in 1997 to update the Paris nomenclature of Constitutional Disorders of Bone.[183–184] In the current revised nomenclature, families of disorders were rearranged based on recent etiopathogenetic information concerning the gene and/or protein defect. Disorders in which the defect is well documented were regrouped into distinct families based on the mutations. These include the "achondroplasia group" of disorders with mutation in FGFR3, the "diastrophic dysplasia group" of disorders with mutation in the DTDST gene, the "type II collagenopathies" with mutation in the type II collagen, and the "type XI collagenopathies" with mutation in COMP. Several new groups were added, including the "lethal skeletal dysplasias," the group with fragmented bones, and the "miscellaneous neonatal severe dysplasia" group. Other groups were renamed (Table 20–4).

Spranger and Maroteaux classified lethal osteochondrodysplasias in 11 groups based on radial and anatomic manifestations (Table 20–5). The purpose of this classification is to facilitate differential diagnosis, and the groups do not necessarily constitute pathogenetic "families."[185]

This chapter focuses primarily on the osteochondrodysplasias that are recognizable at birth. Although more than 200 skeletal dysplasias have been described and more will probably be identified as distinct entities, the number that can be recognized with the use of sonography in the antepartum period is considerably smaller. Most of these disorders result in short stature; the term *dwarfism* has been used to refer to this clinical condition. However, in this chapter, we use the term *dysplasia*.

TABLE 20–3. SUMMARY OF STUDIES OF OSTEOCHONDROPLASIAS

Reference	Rate per 10,000	Comment
Gustavon and Jorulf[684]	4.7	In newborns
Camera and Mastroiacovo[175]	2.4	In neonates
Connor et al.[176]	1.1	Lethal skeletal dysplasia in neonates
Weldner et al.[236]	7.5	
Orioli et al.[685]	2.3	First 3 days of life
Stoll et al.[686]	3.2	First 8 days of life
Anderson and Hauge[687]	1.5	Lethal chondrodysplasias only
Anderson[688]	7.6	Diagnosed in all ages
Kallen et al.[689]	1.6	No details about age
Rassmusen et al.[177]		
All cases	2.1	In first 5 days of life
Lethal chondrodysplasias	0.95	
Goredienko et al.[246]	3.1	

TABLE 20–4. INTERNATIONAL NOMENCLATURE OF CONSTITUTIONAL DISORDER OF BONE OSTEOCHONDRODYSPLASIAS

	Mode of Inheritance[1]	OMIM[2] Syndrome	Present at Birth	Chromosomal Locus	Gene	Protein	OMIM Gene/Protein
Achondroplasia group							
Thanatophoric dysplasia, type I	AD	187600	+	4p16.3	FGFR3	FGFR3	134934
Thanatophoric dysplasia, type II	AD	187610	+	4p16.3	FGFR3	FGFR3	134934
Achondroplasia	AD	100800	+	4p16.3	FGFR3	FGFR3	134934
Hypochondroplasia	AD	146000	−	4p16.3	FGFR3	FGFR3	134934
Other FGFR3 disorders							
Spondylodysplastic and other perinatally lethal groups							
Lethal platyspondylic skeletal dysplasias (San Diego type, Torrance type, Luton type)	SP	270230, 151210	+ +				
Achondrogenesis type 1A	AR	200600	+				
Metatropic dysplasia group							
Fibrochondrogenesis	AR	228520	+				
Schneckenbecken dysplasia	AR	269250	+				
Metatropic dysplasia (various forms)	AD	156530	+				
Short rib dysplasia (SRP) (with or without polydactyly) group							
SRP type I, Saldino–Noonan	AR	263530	+				
SRP type II, Majewski	AR	263520	+				
SRP type III, Verma–Naumoff	AR	263510	+				
SRP type IV, Beemer–Langer	AR	269860	+				
Asphyxiating thoracic dysplasia (Jeune)	AR	208500	+				
Chondroectodermal dyplasia (Ellis–van Creveld dysplasia)	AR	225500	+	4p16			
Atelosteogenesis-omodysplasia group							
Atelosteogenesis type I (includes "boomerang dysplasia")	SP	108720	+				
Omodysplasia I (Maroteaux)	AD	164745	+				
Omodysplasia II (Borochowitz)	AR	258315	+				
Otopalatodigital syndrome type II	XLR	304120	+				
Atelosteogenesis type III	SP	108721	+				
de la Chapelle dysplasia	AR	256050	+				
Diastrophic dysplasia group							
Diastrophic dysplasia	AR	222600	+	5q32-q33	DTDST	Sulfatate transporter	
Achondrogenesis 1B	AR	600972	+	5q32-q33	DTDST	Sulfatate transporter	
Atelosteogenesis type II	AR	256050	+	5q32-q33	DTDST	Sulfatate transporter	

(Continued)

TABLE 20–4. (continued)

	Mode of Inheritance[1]	OMIM[2] Syndrome	Present at Birth	Chromosomal Locus	Gene	Protein	OMIM Gene/Protein
Dyssegmental dysplasia group							
Dyssegmental dysplasia, Silverman–Handmaker type	AR	224410	+				
Dyssegmental dysplasia, Rolland–Desbuquois type	AR	224400	+				
Type II collagenopathies							
Achondrogenesis II (Langer–Saldino)	AD	200610	+	12q13.1-q13.3	COL2A1	Type II collagen	120140
Hypochondrogenesis	AD	200610	+	12q13.1-q13.3	COL2A1	Type II collagen	120140
Kniest's dysplasia	AD	156550	+	12q13.1-q13.3	COL2A1	Type II collagen	120140
Spondyloepiphyseal dysplasia (SED) congenita	AD	183900	+	12q13.1-q13.3	COL2A1	Type II collagen	120140
Spondyloepimetaphyseal dysplasia, Strudwick type	AD	184250	+	12q13.1-q13.3	COL2A1	Type II collagen	120140
SED with brachydactyly	AD		−	12q13.1-q13.3	COL2A1	Type II collagen	120140
Mild SED with premature onset arthrosis	AD		+	12q13.1-q13.3	COL2A1	Type II collagen	120140
Stickler's dysplasia (heterogeneous, some not linked to COL2A1)	AD	108300	+	12q13.1-q13.3	COL2A1	Type II collagen	120140
Type XI collagenopathies							
Stickler dysplasia (heterogeneous)	AD	184840	+	6p21	COL11A1	Type XI collagen	120280
Otospondylomegaepiphyseal dysplasia	AR	215150	+	6p21.3	COL11A2	Type XI collagen	120290
	AD		+	6p21.3	COL11A2	Type XI collagen	120290
Other spondyloepi-(meta)-physeal dysplasias [SE(M)D]							
X-linked SED tarda	XLD	313400	−	Xp22.2-p22.1			
Other late-onset SE(M)D (Irapa)	AR	271650	−				
Progressive pseudorheumatoid dysplasia	AR	208230	−				
Dyggve–Melchior–Clausen dysplasia	AR	223800	+				
Wolcott–Rallison dysplasia	AR	226980	−				
Immuno-osseous dysplasia, Schimke	AR	242900	+				
Opsismodysplasia	AR	258480	+				
Chondrodystrophic myotonia (Schwartz–Jampel), types 1 and 2	AR	258480	+	1q36-34			
SED with joint laxity	AR	255800	+				
Sponastrime dysplasia	AR	271640	+				
SEMD short limb, abnormal calcification	AR	271510	−				
	AR	271665	+				
Multiple epiphyseal dysplasias (MEDs) and pseudoachondroplasia							
Pseudoachondroplasia	AD	177170	−	19p12-13.1	COMP	COMP	600310

(Continued)

450

TABLE 20–4. (continued)

	Mode of Inheritance[1]	OMIM[2] Syndrome	Present at Birth	Chromosomal Locus	Gene	Protein	OMIM Gene/Protein
MED (Fairbanks and Ribbing types)	AD	132400	—		COMP	COMP	600310
Other MEDs	AD	600204	—	19p12-13.1	COL9A2	Type IX collagen	120260
	?	600969	—	1p32.2-33			
Chondrodysplasia punctata (stippled epiphyses group)							
Rhizomelic type	AR	215100	+	4p16-p14	PEX7	Peroxin-7	601757
Zellweger syndrome	AR	214100	+	7q11.23	PEX1		
	AR	214100	+	6p21.1	PEX6	Peroxin-6	601498
	AR	214100	+	7q11.23	PEX1	Peroxin-1	602136
	AR	214100	+	12	PEX5	Peroxin-5	
	AR	214100	+	8q21.1	PEX2	Peroxin-2	170993
Conradi–Hünermann type	XLD	302950	+	Xq28	CPXD		
X-linked recessive type	XLR	302940	+	Xp22.3	CPXR		
Brachytelephalangic type	XLR	302940	+	Xp22.32	ARSE	Arylsulfatase E	302950
Tibial–metacarpal type	AD	118651	+				
Vitamin K–dependent coagulation defect	AR	277450	+				
Other acquired and genetic disorders including warfarin embryopathy							
Metaphyseal dysplasias							
Jansen type	AD	156400	+	3p22-p21.1	PTHR	PTHR/PTHRP	168468
Schmid type	AD	156500	—	6q21-q22.3	COL10A1	COL10 α chain	120110
McKusick type (cartilage–hair hypoplasia)	AR	250250	+	9p13			
Metaphyseal anadysplasia	XLR?	309645	—				
Metaphyseal dysplasia with pancreatic insufficiency and cyclic neutropenia (Shwachman–Diamond)	AR	260400	—				
Adenosine deaminase deficiency	AD	102700	—	20q-13.11	ADA	Adenosine deaminase	102700
Metaphyseal chondrodysplasia, Spahr type	AR	250400	—				
Acroscyphodysplasia (various types)	AR	250215	—				
Spondylometaphyseal dysplasias (SMDs)							
Spondylometaphyseal dysplasia Kozlowski type	AD	184252	+				
SMD, Sutcliffe type	AD	184255	++				
SMD with severe genu valgum (includes Schmidt and Algerian types)	AD	184253	++				
SMD, Sedaghatian type	AR		+				

451

(Continued)

TABLE 20–4. *(continued)*

	Mode of Inheritance[1]	OMIM[2] Syndrome	Present at Birth	Chromosomal Locus	Gene	Protein	OMIM Gene/Protein
Mild SMD, different types that have not been well delineated			–				
Brachyolmia spondylodysplasias							
Hobaek (includes Toledo type)	AR	271530-630	–				
Maroteaux type	AR		–				
Autosomal dominant type	AD	113500	–				
Mesomelic dysplasias							
Dychondrosteosis (Leri–Weill)	AD	127300	–				
Langer type (homozygous dyschondrosteosis)	AR	249700	+				
Nievergelt type	AD	163400	+				
Kozlowski–Reardon type	AR		+				
Reinhardt–Pfeiffer type	AD	191400	+				
Werner type	AD		+				
Robinow type, dominant	AD	180700	–				
Robinow type, recessive	AR	268310	–				
Mesomelic dysplasia with synostoses	AD	600383	+				
Acromelic and acromesomelic dysplasias							
Acromicric dysplasia	AD	102370	+				
Geleophysic dysplasia	AR	231050	+				
Weill–Marchesani dysplasia	AR	277600	+				
Cranioectodermal dysplasia	AR	218330	+				
Trichorhinophalangeal dysplasia type I	AD	190350	+	8q24.12	TRPS1		
Trichorhinophalangeal dysplasia type II (Langer–Giedeon)	AD	150230	+	8q24.11-q24.13	TRPS1 + EXT1		
Trichorhinophalangeal dysplasia type III	AD	190351	+				
Grebe dysplasia	AR	200700	+	20q11.2	CDMP1	Cartilage-derived morphogenic protein 1	601146
Hunter–Thompson dysplasia	AR	201250	+	20q11.2	CDMP1	Cartilage-derived morphogenic protein 1	601146
Brachydactyly types A1–A4	AD	112500-800	+				
Brachydactyly type B	AD	113000	+				
Brachydactyly type C	AD	133100	+	21q11	CDMP1	Cartilage-derived morphogenic protein 1	601196

452

(Continued)

TABLE 20–4. (continued)

	Mode of Inheritance[1]	OMIM[2] Syndrome	Present at Birth	Chromosomal Locus	Gene	Protein	OMIM Gene/Protein
Brachydactyly type D	AD	113200	+	12q24			
Brachydactyly type E	AD	113000	−				
Pseudohypoparathyroidism (Albright hereditary osteodystrophy), various types; see OMIM				20q13	GNAS1	Guanine nucleotide binding protein of edenylate cyclase α subunit	139320
Acrodysostosis	SP (AD)	101800	−				
Saldino–Mainzer dysplasia	AR	266920	−				
Brachydactyly–hypertension dysplasia (Bilginturan)	AD	112410	+	12p			
Craniofacial conodysplasia	AD		+				
Angel-shaped phalango-epiphyseal dysplasia	AD	105835	+				
Acromesomelic dysplasia	AR	201250	+				
Other acromesomelic dysplasias							
Dysplasias with prominent membranous bone involvement							
Cleidocranial dysplasia	AD	119600	+	6p21	CBFA1	Core binding factor α1 subunit	600211
Osteodysplasty, Melnick–Needles	XLD	309350	−				
Precocious osteodysplasty (terHaar's dysplasia)	AR		+				
Yunis–Varon dysplasia	AR	216340	+				
Bent bone dysplasia group							
Campomeltic dysplasia	AD	114290	+	17q24.3-q25.1	SOX9	SRY-box 9	211970
Kyphomelic dysplasia	?AR	211350	+				
Stüve–Wiedemann dysplasia	AR	601559	+				
Multiple dislocations with dysplasias							
Larsen's syndrome	AD	150250	+	3p21.1-p14.1	LARI		
Larsen-like syndromes (including La Reunion Island)	AR	245600	+				
Desbuquois dysplasia	AR	251450	+				
Pseudodiastrophic dysplasia	AR	264180	+				
Dysostosis multiplex group							
Mucopolysaccharidosis IH	AR	252800	−	4p16.3	IDA	α-1-Iduronidase	
Mucopolysaccharidosis IS	AR	252800	−	4p16.3	IDA	α-1-Iduronidase	
Mucopolysaccharidosis II	XLR	309900	−	Xq27.3-q28	IDS	Iduronate-2-sulfatase	
Mucopolysaccharidosis IIIA	AR	252900	−	17q25.3	HSS	Heparan sulfate sulfatase	
Mucopolysaccharidosis IIIB	AR	252920	−	17q21		N-Ac-α-D-glucosaminidase	
Mucopolysaccharidosis IIIC	AR	252930	−			Ac-CoA: α-glucosaminidase-N-acetyltransferase	

(Continued)

TABLE 20–4. (continued)

Syndrome	Mode of Inheritance[1]	OMIM[2] Syndrome	Present at Birth	Chromosomal Locus	Gene	Protein	OMIM Gene/Protein
Mucopolysaccharidosis IIID	AR	252940	—	12q14	GNS	N-Ac-glucosamine-6-sulfatase	
Mucopolysaccharidosis IVA	AR	230500	—	16q24.3	GALNS	Galactose-6-sulfatase	
Mucopolysaccharidosis IVB	AR	230500	—	3p21.33	GLBI	β-Galactosidase	
Mucopolysaccharidosis VI	AR	253200	—	5q13.3	ARSB	Arylsulfatase B	
Mucopolysaccharidosis VII	AR	253200	—	7q21.11	GUSB	β-Glucuronidase	
Fucosidosis	AR	230000	—	1p34	FUCA	α-Fucosidase	
α-Mannosidosis	AR	248500	—	19p13.2-q12	MAN	α-Mannosidase	
β-Mannosidosis	AR	248510	—	4	MANB	β-Mannosidase	
Aspartylglucosaminuria	AR	208400	—	4q23-q27	AgA	Aspartylglucosaminidase	
GMI gangliosidosis, several forms	AR	230500	+	3p21-p14.2	GLB1	β-Galactosidase	
Sialidosis, several forms	AR	256550	+/−	6p21.3	NEU	α-Neuraminidase	
Sialic acid storage disease	AR	269920	+/−	6q14-q15	SIASD		
Galactosialidosis, several forms	AR	256540	+/−	20q13.1	PPGB	β-Galactosidase protective protein	
Multiple sulfatase deficiency	AR	272200	+/−			Multiple sulfatases	
Mucolipidosis II	AR	252500	+	4q21-23	GNPTA	N-Ac-Glucosamine-phosphotransferase	
Mucolipidosis III	AR	252600	—	4q21-23	GNPTA	N-Ac-Glucosamine-phosphotransferase	
Osteodysplastic slender bone group							
Type I osteodysplastic dysplasia	AR	210710	+				
Type II osteodysplastic dysplasia	AR	210720	+				
Microcephalic osteodysplastic dysplasia	AR						
Dysplasias with decreased bone density							
Osteogenesis imperfecta I (without opalescent teeth)	AD	166200	+/−	17q21	COL1A1	$\alpha(1)$I Procollagen	120150
Osteogenesis imperfecta I (with opalescent teeth)	AD	166240	+/−	17q21	COL1A1	$\alpha(1)$I Procollagen	120150
Osteogenesis imperfecta II	AD	166240	+/−	7q22.1	COL1A2	$\alpha(2)$I Procollagen	120160
	AD	166210	+	17q21	COL1A1	$\alpha(1)$I Procollagen	120150
	AD	166210	+	7q22.1	COL1A2	$\alpha(2)$I Procollagen	120160
	AR	259400	+	17q21	COL1A1	$\alpha(1)$I Procollagen	120150
Osteogenesis imperfecta III	AD	259420	+	17q21	COL1A1	$\alpha(1)$I Procollagen	120150
	AD	259420	+	7q22.1	COL1A2	$\alpha(2)$I Procollagen	120160
	AR	259420	+	7q22.1	COL1A2	$\alpha(2)$I Procollagen	120160
	AR	259420	+				
Osteogenesis imperfecta IV (without opalescent teeth)	AD	166220	+	7q22.1	COL1A2	$\alpha(2)$I Procollagen	120160
	AD	166220	+	17q21	COL1A1	$\alpha(1)$I Procollagen	120150
Osteogenesis imperfecta IV (with opalescent teeth)	AD	166220	+	7q22.1	COL1A2	$\alpha(2)$I Procollagen	120160

(Continued)

TABLE 20–4. *(continued)*

	Mode of Inheritance[1]	OMIM[2] Syndrome	Present at Birth	Chromosomal Locus	Gene	Protein	OMIM Gene/Protein
Cole–Carpenter dysplasia	AD	166220	+	17q21	COL1A1	$\alpha(1)$I Procollagen	120150
Bruck's dysplasia	SP	112240	+				
Singleton–Merton dysplasia	AR	259450	+				
Osteopenia with radiolucent lesions of the mandible	AD	166260		11q12-q13			
Osteoporosis-pseudoglioma dysplasia	AR	259770	−				
Geroderma osteodysplasticum	AR	231070	−				
Hyper-IGE syndrome with osteopenia	AR	147060	−				
Idiopathic juvenile osteoporosis	SP	259750	−				
Dysplasias with defective mineralization							
Hypophosphatasia, perinatal lethal and infantile forms	AR	241500	+	1p36.1-p34	ALPL	Alkaline phosphatase	171760
Hypophosphatasia, adult form	AD	146300	−	1p36.1-p34			
Hypophosphatemic rickets	XLD	307800	−	Xp22.2-p22.1	PHEX	X-linked hypophosphatemia protein	171760
Neonatal hyperparathyroidism	AR	239200	+	3q21-q24, 19p13.3	CASR	Calcium sensor	601199
Transient neonatal hyperparathyrodism with hypocalciuric hypercalcemia	AD	145980	+ +	3q21-q24 19p13.3	CASR	Calcium sensor	601199
Increased bone density without modification of bone shape							
Osteopetrosis							
Precocious type	AR	259700	+	11q12-13			
Delayed type	AD	166600	−	1p21			
Intermediate type	AR	259710	+				
With renal tubular acidosis	AR	259730	+	8q22	CA2	Carbonic anhydrase II	
Axial osteosclerosis							
Osteomesopyknosis	AD	166450	−				
With bamboo hair	AR	266500	−				
Pyknodysostosis	AR	265800	+	1q21	CTSK	Cathepsin K	601105
Osteosclerosis, Stanescu type	AD	122900	+				
Osteopathia striata							
Isolated	SP	166500	−				
With cranial sclerosis	AD	271510	+				
Sponastrime dysplasia	AR	155950	−				
Melorheostosis	SP		−				
Osteopoikilosis	AD	166700	−				

(Continued)

TABLE 20–4. *(continued)*

	Mode of Inheritance[1]	OMIM[2] Syndrome	Present at Birth	Chromosomal Locus	Gene	Protein	OMIM Gene/Protein
Mixed sclerosing bone dysplasia	SP		—				
van Buchem type	AR	239100	—				
Worth type	AD	144750	—				
Sclerosteosis	AR	269500	—				
With cerebellar hypoplasia	AR	213002	+				
Kenny–Caffey dysplasia	AD, AR	127000, 244460	—				
Osteoectasia with hyperphosphatasia (juvenile Paget's)	AR	239000	—				
Diaphyseal dysplasia with anemia	AR	231095	—				
Diaphyseal medullary stenosis with bone malignancy (Hardcastle)	AD	112250	—				
Increased bone density with metaphyseal involvement							
Pyle dysplasia	AR	265900	—				
Craniometaphyseal dysplasia							
Severe type	AR	218400	+	5p15.2-p14.2			
Mild type	AD	123000	—				
Other types							
Frontometaphyseal dysplasia	XLR	305620	—				
Dysosteosclerosis	AR	224300	—				
	XLR						
Oculodentoosseous dysplasia	AD	257850	+				
	AR	164200	+				
Trichodentoosseous dysplasia	AD	190320	—	17q21			
Neonatal severe osteosclerotic dysplasias							
Blomstrand's dysplasia	AR	215045	+				
Raine's dysplasia	?	259775	+				
Prenatal onset Caffey's disease	?AR	114000	+				
Lethal chondrodysplasias with fragmented bones							
Greenberg's dysplasia	AR	215140	+				
Dappled diaphyseal dysplasia	AR		+				
Astley-Kendall dysplasia	AR		+				
Disorganized development of cartilaginous and fibrous components of the skeleton							
Dysplasia epiphysealis hemimelica	SP	127800	—				
Multiple cartilaginous exostoses	AD	133700	—	8q23-q24.1	EXT1	Exostosin-1	
	AD	133701	—	11p12-p11	EXT2	Exostosin-2	
	AD	600209	—	19p	EXT3		
Enchondromatosis, Ollier	SP	166000	—				
Enchondromatosis with hemangiomata (Maffucci)	SP	166000	—				

(Continued)

TABLE 20-4. *(continued)*

	Mode of Inheritance[1]	OMIM[2] Syndrome	Present at Birth	Chromosomal Locus	Gene	Protein	OMIM Gene/Protein
Spondyloenchondromatosis	AR	271550	–				
Spondyloenchondromatosis with basal ganglia calcification	AR		–				
Dysspondyloenchondromatosis			–				
Metachondromatosis	AD	156250					
Osteoglophonic dysplasia	AD	166250	+				
Genochondromatosis	AD	166000	–				
Carpotarsal osteochondromatosis	AD	127820	–				
Fibrous dysplasia (McCune–Albright and others)	SP mosaic	174800	–	20q13	GNAS1	Guanine nucleotide protein, α subunit	139320
Jaffe–Campanucci	SP						
Fibrodysplasia ossificans progressiva	AD	135100	+	14q22-q23	BMP4	Bone morphogenic protein 4	112262
Cherubism	AD	118400	–				
Cherubism with gingival fibromatosis	AR	135300	–				
Osteolyses							
Multicentric predominantly carpal and tarsal in the hand							
Multicentric carpal–tarsal osteolysis with and without nephropathy	AD	166300	–				
Shinohara carpal–tarsal osteolysis			–				
Multicentric predominantly carpal, tarsal, and interphalangeal							
Francois's syndrome	AR	221800	–				
Winchester's syndrome	AR	277950	–				
Torg's syndrome	AR	259600	–				
Whyte–Hemingway carpal–tarsal phalangeal osteolyses	AD		–				
Predominantly distal phalanges							
Hadju–Cheney syndrome	AD	102500	–				
Giacci's familial neurogenic acroosteolysis	AR	201300	–				
Mandibulo acral syndrome	AR	248370	–				
Predominantly involving diaphyses and metaphyses							
Familial expansile osteolysis	AD	174810	–	18q21.1-q22			
Juvenile hyaline fibromatosis	AR	228600	+				
Patella dysplasias							
Nail patella dysplasia	AD	161200	–	9q34.1	NPS1		
Scyphopatellar dysplasia	AD		+				

[1] AD, autosomal dominant; AR, autosomal recessive; SP, spontaneous; XLD, X-linked dominant; XLR, X-linked recessive.
[2] OMIM, Online Mendelian Inheritance in Man.

457

TABLE 20–5. NOSOLOGY OF LETHAL OSTEOCHONDRODYSPLASIAS

1. Hypophosphatasia and morphologically similar disorders
   - 1.01 Hypophosphatasia
   - 1.02 Probable hypophosphatasia
   - 1.03 Lethal metaphyseal dysplasia
2. Chondrodysplasia punctata and similar disorders
   - 2.01 Rhizomelic chondrodysplasia punctata
   - 2.02 Lethal chondrodysplasia punctata, X-linked dominant
   - 2.03 Greenberg's dysplasia
   - 2.04 Dappled diaphysis dysplasia
3. Achondrogenesis and similar disorders
   - 3.01 Achondrogenesis IA (Houston Harris)
   - 3.02 Achondrogenesis IB (Fraccaro)
   - 3.03 New lethal osteochondrodysplasia
   - 3.04 Achondrogenesis II (Langer–Saldino)
   - 3.05 Hypochondrogenesis
4. Thanatophoric dysplasia and similar disorders
   - 4.01 Thanatophoric dysplasia, type 1
   - 4.02 Thanatophoric dysplasia, type 2
   - 4.03 Homozygous achondroplasia
   - 4.04 Lethal achondrodysplasia
   - 4.05 Glasgow variant
5. Platyspondylic lethal chondrodysplasias
   - 5.01 Platyspondylic chondrodysplasia, Torrance type
   - 5.02 Platyspondylic chondrodysplasia, San Diego type
   - 5.03 Platyspondylic chondrodysplasia, Luton type
   - 5.04 Platyspondylic chondrodysplasia, Shiraz type
   - 5.05 Opsismodysplasia
   - 5.06 Sixth form of platyspondylic chondrodysplasia
   - 5.07 Seventh form of platyspondylic chondrodysplasia
6. Short rib polydactyly syndromes
   - 6.01 Short rib–polydactyly syndrome, type I (Saldino–Noonan)
   - 6.02 Short rib–polydactyly syndrome, type II (Verma–Naumoff)
   - 6.03 Short rib–polydactyly syndrome, type III (Le Marec)
   - 6.04 Short rib–polydactyly syndrome, type IV (Yang)
   - 6.05 Short rib–polydactyly syndromes, type V
   - 6.06 Short rib–polydactyly syndrome, type VI (Majewski)
   - 6.07 Short rib–polydactyly syndrome, type VII (Beemer)
7. Lethal metatropic dysplasia and similar disorders
   - 7.01 Lethal metatropic dysplasia (hyperchondrogenesis)
   - 7.02 Isolated case
   - 7.03 Isolated case
   - 7.04 Fibrochondrogenesis
   - 7.05 Schneckenbecker's dysplasia
   - 7.06 Isolated case
   - 7.07 Isolated case
   - 7.08 Isolated case
8. Kniest-like disorders
   - 8.01 Dyssegmental dysplasia, Silverman type
   - 8.02 Dyssegmental dysplasia, Rolland–Desbuquois
   - 8.03 Lethal Kniest's disease
   - 8.04 Chondrodysplasia resembling Kniest's dysplasia
   - 8.05 Isolated case
   - 8.06 Blomstrand's chondrodysplasia
9. Lethal osteochondrodysplasias with pronounced diaphyseal abnormalities
   - 9.01 Campomelic's syndrome
   - 9.02 Stuve–Wiedemann syndrome
   - 9.03 Boomerang dysplasia
   - 9.04 Atelosteogenesis
   - 9.05 Disorder resembling atelosteogenesis
   - 9.06 de la Chappele's dysplasia
   - 9.07 McAlister's dysplasia
   - 9.08 Pseudodystrophic dysplasia
10. Osteogenesis imperfecta and similar disorders
    - 10.01 Osteogenesis imperfecta IIA
    - 10.02 Osteogenesis imperfecta IIB
    - 10.03 Osteogenesis imperfecta IIC
    - 10.04 Isolated case
    - 10.05 Astley–Kendall dysplasia
11. Lethal disorders with gracile bones
    - 11.01 Fetal hypokinesia phenotype
    - 11.02 Lethal osteochondrodysplasia with gracile bones
    - 11.03 Lethal osteochondrodysplasia with intrauterine overtibulation

Source: Spranger and Maroteaux.[185]

TERMINOLOGY FREQUENTLY USED IN THE DESCRIPTION OF BONE DYSPLASIAS

Shortening of the extremities can involve the entire limb (micromelia), the proximal segment (rhizomelia), the intermediate segment (mesomelia), or the distal segment (acromelia). The diagnosis of rhizomelia or mesomelia requires the comparison of the dimensions of the bones of the legs and forearm with those of the thigh and arm. Figures 20–1 and 20–2 show the relationship between the humerus and ulna and between the femur and tibia and can be used in the assessment of rhizomelia and mesomelia. Table 20–6 presents skeletal dysplasias characterized by rhizomelia, mesomelia, acromelia, and micromelia.

Several skeletal dysplasias feature alterations of the hands and feet. The term *polydactyly* refers to the presence of more than five digits. It is classified as postaxial if the extra digits are on the ulnar or fibular side and as preaxial if they are located on the radial or tibial side. *Syndactyly* refers to soft tissue or bony fusion of adjacent digits. *Clinodactyly* consists of permanent deviation of a finger (or fingers). The most common spinal abnormality seen in skeletal dysplasias is *platyspondylia*, which consists of flattening of the vertebrae (Fig. 20–3). Kyphosis and scoliosis can also be identified *in utero* (Fig. 20–4). Prenatal diagnoses of hemivertebra (Fig. 20–5) and coronal clefting of vertebral bodies have also been reported.[186]

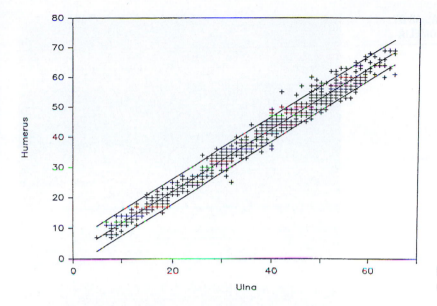

Figure 20–1. Relationship between the lengths of the ulna and the humerus.

BIOMETRY OF THE FETAL SKELETON IN THE DIAGNOSIS OF BONE DYSPLASIAS

Long bone biometry has been used extensively in the prediction of gestational age. Nomograms for this purpose use the long bone as the independent variable and the estimated fetal age as the dependent variable. However, the type of nomogram required to assess the normality of bone dimensions uses gestational age as the independent variable and the long bone as the dependent variable. For the proper use of these nomograms, the clinician must accurately know the gestational age of the fetus. Therefore, patients at risk for skeletal dysplasias should be advised to seek prenatal care at an early gestational age to assess all clinical estimators of

gestational age. Tables 20–7 and 20–8 present nomograms for the assessment of limb biometry for the upper and lower extremities, respectively. For patients presenting with uncertain gestational age, comparisons between limb dimensions and the head perimeter can be used (Figs. 20–6 and 20–7). While some investigators have employed the biparietal diameter for this purpose, the head perimeter has the advantage of being shape independent. A limitation of this approach is that it assumes that the cranium is not involved in the dysplastic process, and this may not be the case in some skeletal dysplasias.

The nomograms and figures in this chapter provide the mean and the 5th, and 95th percentiles of limb biometric parameters. The reader should be aware that 5% of the general

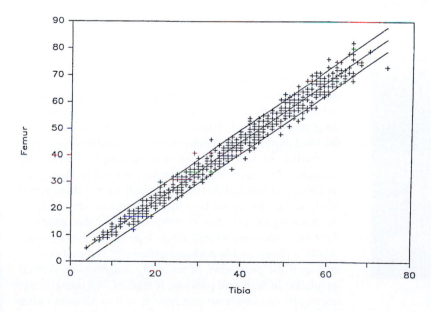

Figure 20–2. Relationship between the lengths of the tibia and the femur.

TABLE 20–6. CLASSIFICATION OF SKELETAL DYSPLASIAS BY RHIZOMELIA, MESOMELIA, ACROMELIA, AND MICROMELIA

Rhizomelia
Thanatophoric dysplasia
Atelosteogenesis
Chondrodysplasia punctata (thizomelic type)
Congenital short femur
Achondroplasia
Mesomelia
Mesomelic dysplasia (Langer, Reinhardt, and Robinow types)
Acromelia
Ellis–van Creveld syndrome (cohondroectodermal dysplasia)
Micromelia
Achondrogenesis
Atelosteogenesis
Short rib–polydactyly syndrome
Diastrophic dysplasia
Fibrochondrogenesis
Osteogenesis imperfecta (type II)
Kniest's dysplasia
Dyssegmental dysplasia
Robert's syndrome

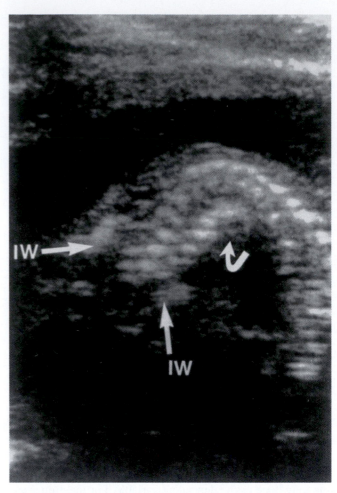

Figure 20–4. Coronal scan demonstrating severe scoliosis *(curved arrow).* IW, iliac wings.

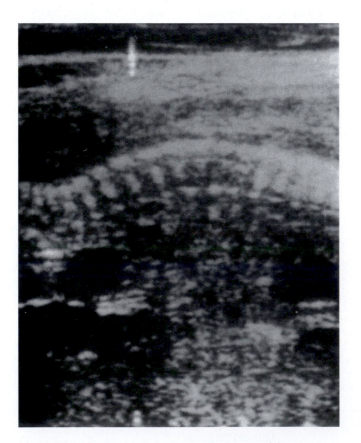

Figure 20–3. Sagittal scan of a fetus with platyspondyly.

population falls outside these boundaries. Ideally, a more stringent criterion, such as the 1st percentile of limb growth for gestational age, should be used for diagnosis. Unfortunately, none of the currently available nomograms have been based on the number of patients required to provide an accurate discrimination between the 5th and the 1st percentiles. However, most skeletal dysplasias diagnosed *in utero* or at birth are associated with dramatic long bone shortening, and under these circumstances, the precise boundary used (1st or 5th percentile) is not critical. An exception to this is achondroplasia, in which limb biometry is only mildly affected until the third trimester. Then abnormal growth can be detected by examining the slope of growth of femur length.[187] In a study including 127 cases of 17 skeletal dysplasias, Goncalves and Jeanty conducted discriminant analysis and showed that the femur length is the best biometric parameter to distinguish among the five most common disorders: thanatophoric dysplasia, osteogenesis imperfecta type II, achondrogenesis, achondroplasia, and hypochondroplasia.[188] Gabrieli et al.[189] evaluated the possibility of an early diagnosis of skeletal dysplasias in high-risk patients. A total of 149 consecutive, uncomplicated singleton pregnancies at 9 to 13 weeks after

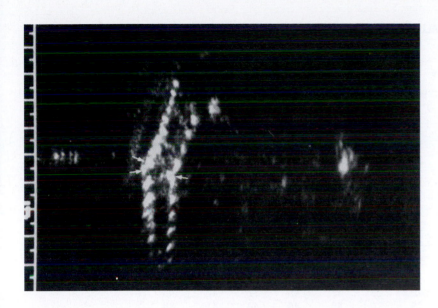

Figure 20–5. Hemivertebra. Longitudinal view of the lower thoracic spine showing the two abnormal ossification centers of the posterior elements, opposite a single ossification center. *(Reproduced with permission from Benacerraf BR, Greene MF, Barss VA. J Ultrasound Med. 1986;5:257.)*

TABLE 20–7. NORMAL VALUES FOR THE ARM (IN MILLIMETERS)

	Humerus			Ulna			Radius		
	Percentile			Percentile			Percentile		
Week	5th	50th	95th	5th	50th	95th	5th	50th	95th
12	—	9	—	—	7	—	—	7	—
13	6	11	16	5	10	15	6	10	14
14	9	14	19	8	13	18	8	13	17
15	12	17	22	11	16	21	11	15	20
16	15	20	25	13	18	23	13	18	22
17	18	22	27	16	21	26	14	20	26
18	20	25	30	19	24	29	15	22	29
19	23	28	33	21	26	31	20	24	29
20	25	30	35	24	29	34	22	27	32
21	28	33	38	26	31	36	24	29	33
22	30	35	40	28	33	38	27	31	34
23	33	38	42	31	36	41	26	32	39
24	35	40	45	33	38	43	26	34	42
25	37	42	47	35	40	45	31	36	41
26	39	44	49	37	42	47	32	37	43
27	41	46	51	39	44	49	33	39	45
28	43	48	53	41	46	51	33	40	48
29	45	50	55	43	48	53	36	42	47
30	47	51	56	44	49	54	36	43	49
31	48	53	58	46	51	56	38	44	50
32	50	55	60	48	53	58	37	45	53
33	51	56	61	49	54	59	41	46	51
34	53	58	63	51	56	61	40	47	53
35	54	59	64	52	57	62	41	48	54
36	56	61	65	53	58	63	39	48	57
37	57	62	67	55	60	65	45	49	53
38	59	63	68	56	61	66	45	49	54
39	60	65	70	57	62	67	45	50	54
40	61	66	71	58	63	68	46	50	55

TABLE 20–8. NORMAL VALUES FOR THE LEG (IN MILLIMETERS)

Week	Tibia Percentile			Fibula Percentile			Femur Percentile		
	5th	50th	95th	5th	50th	95th	5th	50th	95th
12	—	7	—	—	6	—	4	8	13
13	—	10	—	—	9	—	6	11	16
14	7	12	17	6	12	19	9	14	18
15	9	15	20	9	15	21	12	17	21
16	12	17	22	13	18	23	15	20	24
17	15	20	25	13	21	28	18	23	27
18	17	22	27	15	23	31	21	25	30
19	20	25	30	19	26	33	24	28	33
20	22	27	33	21	28	36	26	31	36
21	25	30	35	24	31	37	29	34	38
22	27	32	38	27	33	39	32	36	41
23	30	35	40	28	35	42	35	39	44
24	32	37	42	29	37	45	37	42	46
25	34	40	45	34	40	45	40	44	49
26	37	42	47	36	42	47	42	47	51
27	39	44	49	37	44	50	45	49	54
28	41	46	51	38	45	53	47	52	56
29	43	48	53	41	47	54	50	54	59
30	45	50	55	43	49	56	52	56	61
31	47	52	57	42	51	59	54	59	63
32	48	54	59	42	52	63	56	61	65
33	50	55	60	46	54	62	58	63	67
34	52	57	62	46	55	65	60	65	69
35	53	58	64	51	57	62	62	67	71
36	55	60	65	54	58	63	64	68	73
37	56	61	67	54	59	65	65	70	74
38	58	63	68	56	61	65	67	71	76
39	59	64	69	56	62	67	68	73	77
40	61	66	71	59	63	67	70	74	79

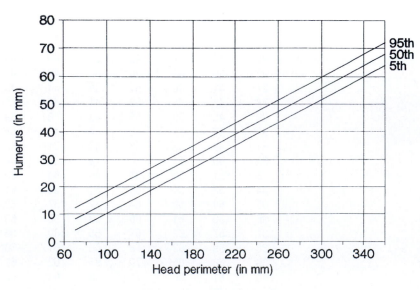

Figure 20–6. Relationship between the head perimeter and the length of the humerus.

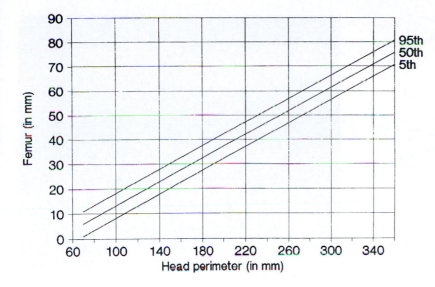

Figure 20–7. Relationship between the head perimeter and the length of the femur.

amenorrhea was included in the study. Transvaginal ultrasound was used to establish the relationship between femur length and menstrual age and between biparietal diameter and crown–rump length by using a polynomial regression. Eight patients with previous skeletal dysplasias were evaluated with serial examinations every 2 weeks between 10 and 11 weeks. A significant correlation between femur length and crown–rump length and biparietal diameter was found. Of the five cases with skeletal dysplasias, only two (one with recurrent osteogenesis imperfecta and one with recurrent achondrogenesis) were diagnosed in the first trimester. This study suggests that an early evaluation of the fetus and the correlation of femur length with crown–rump length and of femur length with biparietal diameter may be useful for early diagnosis of severe skeletal dysplasias. In less severe cases, biometric evaluation appears to be of limited value.

CLINICAL PRESENTATION

The challenge of the antenatal diagnosis of skeletal dysplasias generally presents itself in one of two ways: 1) a patient who has delivered an infant with a skeletal dysplasia and desires antenatal assessment of a subsequent pregnancy; or 2) the incidental finding of a shortened, bowed, or anomalous extremity during a routine sonographic examination. In patients at risk, the examination is easier when the particular phenotype is known. The inability to obtain reliable information concerning skeletal mineralization and the involvement of other systems (e.g., skin) with sonography is a limiting factor in the establishment of an accurate diagnosis after the identification of an incidental finding. Another limitation is the paucity of information about the *in utero* natural history of these disorders.

Despite these difficulties and limitations, there are good medical reasons for attempting an accurate prenatal diagno-

sis of skeletal dysplasias. A number of these disorders are uniformly lethal, and a confident antenatal diagnosis would present the patient with option of termination of the pregnancy. Table 20–9 lists these disorders. Other skeletal dysplasias are associated with mental retardation,[190] and this information is important in prenatal counseling. There is another group of disorders associated with thrombocytopenia and vaginal delivery may expose these infants to the risk of intracranial hemorrhage.

APPROACH TO THE DIAGNOSIS OF SKELETAL DYSPLASIAS

We propose the following systematic approach to the prenatal diagnosis of skeletal dysplasias:

Evaluation of Long Bones

All long bones should be measured in each extremity. Comparisons with other segments should be performed to establish whether the limb shortening is predominantly rhizomelic, mesomelic, or acromelic or whether it involves all segments (Fig. 20–8). A detailed examination of each bone is necessary to exclude the absence or hypoplasia of individual bones (fibula, tibia, scapula, and radius), which are frequently absent in certain conditions.[191–195]

TABLE 20–9. LETHAL SKELETAL DYSPLASIAS

Achondrogenesis
Thanatophoric dysplasia
Short rib–polydactyly syndromes (types I, II, and III)
Fibrochondrogenesis
Atelosteogenesis
Homozygous achondroplasia
Osteogenesis imperfecta, perinatal type
Hypophosphatasia

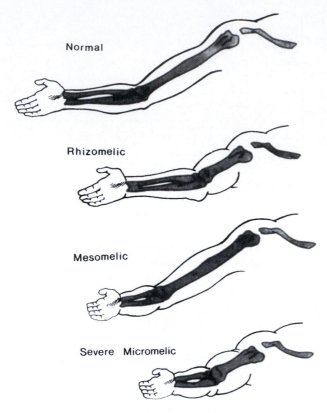

Normal

Rhizomelic

Mesomelic

Severe Micromelic

Figure 20–8. Varieties of short limb dysplasia according to the segment involved.

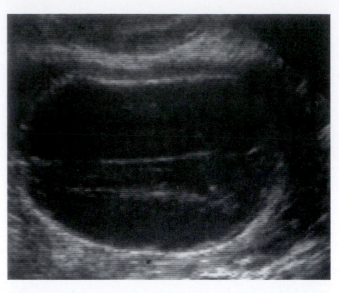

Figure 20–10. Sagittal scan of a fetus with severe demineralization of the calvarium.

An attempt should be made to characterize the degree of mineralization. This can be assessed by examining the acoustic shadow behind the bone and the echogenicity of the bone itself. Signs of demineralization are the visualization of an unusually prominent falx and the absent or decreased echogenicity of the spine. It should be stressed that there are limitations in the sonographic evaluation of mineralization using long bones and that other bones, such as the skull, may be better suited for this assessment (Figs. 20–9 and 20–10). The degree of long-bone curvature should be

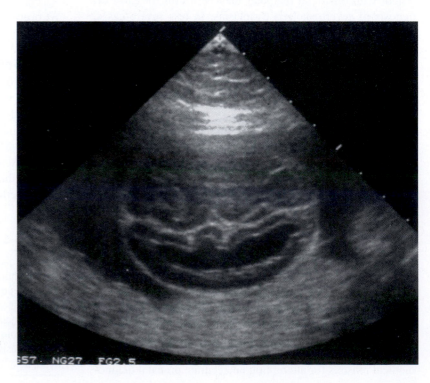

Figure 20–9. Demineralization of the skull in a case of congenital hypophosphatasia.

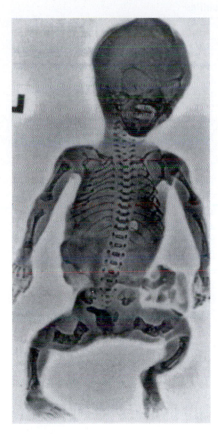

Figure 20–11. Osteogenesis imperfecta type II. Multiple fractures in long bones and ribs are present. Note the severe bowing and shortening of both femurs.

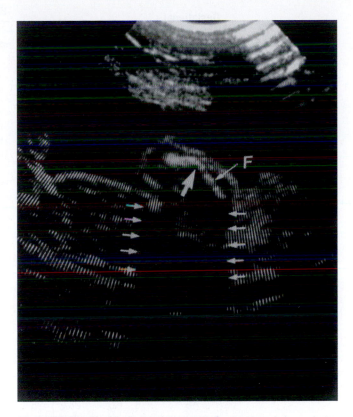

Figure 20–12. *In utero* fracture in a case of osteogenesis imperfecta. The *large arrow* corresponds to the fracture site. The *small arrows* outline the decreased shadowing cast by the bone. F, femur.

examined. At present, there is no objective means of assessing this sign, and experience is the only tool to assist the operator to discern the boundary between normality and abnormality. Campomelia (excessive bowing) is a characteristic of certain disorders (e.g., campomelic dysplasia). The possibility of fractures should also be considered, as they can be detected in some conditions (e.g., osteogenesis imperfecta) (Fig. 20–11). Fractures may be extremely subtle or may lead to angulation and separation of the segments of the affected bone (Fig. 20–12). The femur length-to-abdominal circumference ratio is helpful to predict fetal outcome when a possible skeletal dysplasia is suspected. A ratio below 0.16 has resulted in a lethal outcome. A ratio above 0.16 has predicted a nonlethal outcome.[196]

Evaluation of Thoracic Dimensions

Several skeletal dysplasias are associated with a hypoplastic thorax. Such a finding is extremely significant because chest restriction leads to pulmonary hypoplasia, a frequent cause of death in these conditions. The appropriateness of thoracic dimensions can be assessed by measuring the thoracic circumference at the level of the four-chamber view of the heart. The thoracic circumference can be measured or calculated by using the following formula:

thoracic circumference = (anteroposterior diameter
+ transverse diameter) × 1.57.

The thoracic length is measured from the boundary between the neck and the chest to the diaphragm. Tables 20–10 and 20–11 show nomograms used to evaluate the thoracic dimensions in fetuses with known gestational age. When gestational age is uncertain, age-independent ratios can be used. The thoracic-to-abdominal circumference ratio (normal value: 0.77 to 1.01) and the thoracic-to-head circumference ratio (normal value: 0.56 to 1.04) permit evaluation of the transverse thoracic dimensions.[197]

The rib cage perimeter (RCP) and thoracic circumference (TC) were measured in a prospective cross-sectional study of 88 patients with normal pregnancy and 8 cases known to have skeletal dysplasias.[198] The RCP-to-TC ratio is independent of gestational age (mean = 0.67 ± 0.04). In five cases of skeletal dysplasia, this ratio was decreased, and in one case it was increased.

Evaluation of thoracic dimensions is a critical part of the work-up because the cause of death in most lethal skeletal

TABLE 20–10. FETAL THORACIC CIRCUMFERENCE MEASUREMENTS (IN CENTIMETERS)

Gestational Age (wk)	n	Predictive Percentiles								
		2.5	5	10	25	50	75	90	95	97.5
16	6	5.9	6.4	7.0	8.0	9.1	10.3	11.3	11.9	12.4
17	22	6.8	7.3	7.9	8.9	10.0	11.2	12.2	12.8	13.3
18	31	7.7	8.2	8.8	9.8	11.0	12.1	13.1	13.7	14.2
19	21	8.6	9.1	9.7	10.7	11.9	13.0	14.0	14.6	15.1
20	20	9.5	10.0	10.6	11.7	12.8	13.9	15.0	15.5	16.0
21	30	10.4	11.0	11.6	12.6	13.7	14.8	15.8	16.4	16.9
22	18	11.3	11.9	12.5	13.5	14.6	15.7	16.7	17.3	17.8
23	21	12.2	12.8	13.4	14.4	15.5	16.6	17.6	18.2	18.8
24	27	13.2	13.7	14.3	15.3	16.4	17.5	18.5	19.1	19.7
25	20	14.1	14.6	15.2	16.2	17.3	18.4	19.4	20.0	20.6
26	25	15.0	15.5	16.1	17.1	18.2	19.3	20.3	21.0	21.5
27	24	15.9	16.4	17.0	18.0	19.1	20.2	21.3	21.9	22.4
28	24	16.8	17.3	17.9	18.9	20.0	21.2	22.2	22.8	23.3
29	24	17.7	18.2	18.8	19.8	21.0	22.1	23.1	23.7	24.2
30	27	18.6	19.1	19.7	20.7	21.9	23.0	24.0	24.6	25.1
31	24	19.5	20.0	20.6	21.6	22.8	23.9	24.9	25.5	26.0
32	28	20.4	20.9	21.5	22.6	23.7	24.8	25.8	26.4	26.9
33	27	21.3	21.8	22.5	23.5	24.6	25.7	26.7	27.3	27.8
34	25	22.2	22.8	23.4	24.4	25.5	26.6	27.6	28.2	28.7
35	20	23.1	23.7	24.3	25.3	26.4	27.5	28.5	29.1	29.6
36	23	24.0	24.6	25.2	26.2	27.3	28.4	29.4	30.0	30.6
37	22	24.9	25.5	26.1	27.1	28.2	29.3	30.3	30.9	31.5
38	21	25.9	26.4	27.0	28.0	29.1	30.2	31.2	31.9	32.4
39	7	26.8	27.3	27.9	28.9	30.0	31.1	32.2	32.8	33.3
40	6	27.7	28.2	28.8	29.8	20.9	32.1	33.1	33.7	34.2

TABLE 20–11. FETAL THORACIC LENGTH MEASUREMENTS (IN CENTIMETERS)

Gestational Age (wk)	n	Predictive Percentiles								
		2.5	5	10	25	50	75	90	95	97.5
16	6	0.9	1.1	1.3	1.6	2.0	2.4	2.8	3.1	3.2
17	22	1.1	1.3	1.5	1.8	2.2	2.6	3.0	3.2	3.4
18	31	1.3	1.4	1.7	2.0	2.4	2.8	3.2	3.4	3.6
19	21	1.4	1.6	1.8	2.2	2.7	3.0	3.4	3.6	3.8
20	20	1.6	1.8	2.0	2.4	2.8	3.2	3.6	3.8	4.0
21	30	1.8	2.0	2.2	2.6	3.0	3.4	3.7	4.0	4.1
22	18	2.0	2.2	2.4	2.8	3.2	3.6	3.9	4.1	4.3
23	21	2.2	2.4	2.6	3.0	3.4	3.8	4.1	4.3	4.5
24	27	2.4	2.6	2.8	3.1	3.5	3.9	4.3	4.5	4.7
25	20	2.6	2.8	3.0	3.3	3.7	4.1	4.5	4.7	4.9
26	25	2.8	2.9	3.2	3.5	3.9	4.3	4.7	4.9	5.1
27	24	2.9	3.1	3.3	3.7	4.1	4.5	4.9	5.1	5.3
28	24	3.1	3.3	3.5	3.9	4.3	4.7	5.0	5.4	5.4
29	24	3.3	3.5	3.7	4.1	4.5	4.9	5.2	5.5	5.6
30	27	3.5	3.7	3.9	4.3	4.7	5.1	5.4	5.6	5.8
31	24	3.7	3.9	4.1	4.5	4.9	5.3	5.6	5.8	6.0
32	28	3.9	4.1	4.3	4.6	5.0	5.4	5.8	6.0	6.2
33	27	4.1	4.3	4.5	4.8	5.2	5.6	6.0	6.2	6.4
34	25	4.2	4.4	4.7	5.0	5.4	5.8	6.2	6.4	6.6
35	20	4.4	4.6	4.8	5.2	5.6	6.0	6.4	6.6	6.8
36	23	4.6	4.8	5.0	5.4	5.8	6.2	6.5	6.8	7.0
37	22	4.8	5.0	5.2	5.6	6.0	6.4	6.7	7.0	7.1
38	21	5.0	5.2	5.4	5.8	6.2	6.5	6.9	7.1	7.3
39	7	5.2	5.4	5.6	6.0	6.4	6.7	7.1	7.3	7.5
40	6	5.4	5.6	5.8	6.1	6.5	6.9	7.3	7.5	7.7

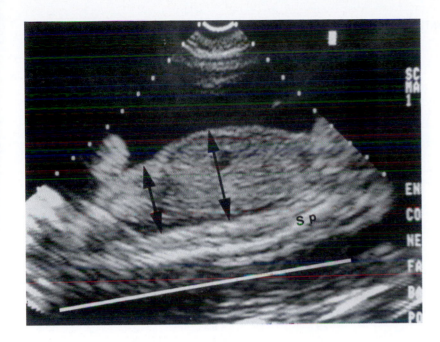

Figure 20–13. Longitudinal section of a fetus with thanatophoric dysplasia. Note the significant disproportion between the chest and abdomen. Sp, spine. *(Reproduced with permission from Jeanty P, Romero R. Obstetrical Ultrasound. New York: McGraw-Hill; 1983.)*

dysplasias is pulmonary hypoplasia secondary to an underdeveloped rib cage (Figs. 20–13 to 20–15). Table 20–12 lists skeletal dysplasias associated with altered thoracic dimensions.

Evaluation of Hands and Feet

Hands and feet should be examined to exclude polydactyly, brachydactyly (Fig. 20–16), and extreme postural deformities

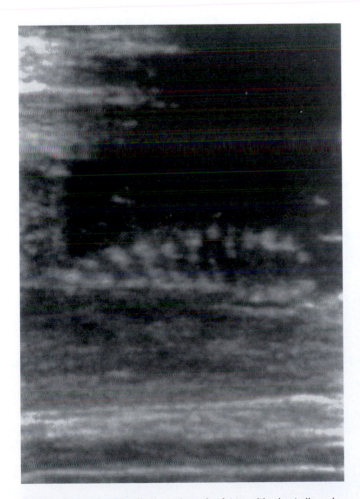

Figure 20–14. Longitudinal section of a fetus with short rib–polydactyly syndrome showing the very short ribs.

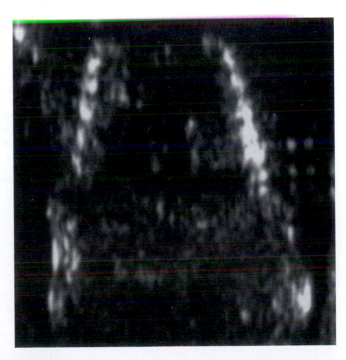

Figure 20–15. Coronal section of a fetus with short rib–polydactyly syndrome. Note the disproportion between the thoracic and abdominal cavities.

TABLE 20–12. SKELETAL DYSPLASIAS ASSOCIATED WITH ALTERED THORACIC DIMENSIONS

Long, narrow thorax
  Asphyxiating thoracic dysplasia (Jeune)
  Chondroectodermal dysplasia (Ellis–van Creveld)
  Metatropic dysplasia
  Fibrochondrogenesis
  Atelosteogenesis
  Camptomelic dysplasia
  Jarcho–Levin syndrome
  Achondrogenesis
  Osteogenesis imperfecta congenita
  Hypophosphatasia
  Dyssegmental dysplasia
  Cleidocranial dysplasia
Short thorax
  Osteogenesis imperfecta (type II)
  Kniest's dysplasia (metatropic dysplasia type II)
  Pena–Shokeir syndrome
Hypoplastic thorax
  Short rib–polydactyly syndrome (type I, type II)
  Thanatophoric dysplasia
  Cerebrocostomandibular syndrome
  Cleidocranial dysostosis syndrome
  Homozygous achondroplasia
  Melnick–Needles syndrome (osteodysplasty)
  Fibrochondrogenesis
  Otopalatodigital syndrome type II

TABLE 20–13. NOMOGRAM OF FETAL FOOT SIZE THROUGHOUT GESTATION (IN CENTIMETERS)

Gestational Age (wk)	Percentile		
	10th	50th	90th
14	1.6	1.8	2.1
15	1.6	1.9	2.2
16	1.8	2.2	2.8
17	1.9	2.2	2.2
18	1.9	2.7	3.0
19	2.5	3.0	3.9
20	3.3	3.3	3.3
21	2.4	2.4	2.4
22	2.5	3.6	4.0
23	4.1	4.1	4.0
24	4.6	4.6	4.6
25	4.0	4.7	5.3
26	4.0	4.7	5.4
27	4.5	5.0	5.6
28	5.1	5.3	5.5
29	4.9	5.4	5.8
30	6.1	6.1	6.1
31	5.1	5.6	5.2
32	5.4	5.7	6.2
33	5.9	5.9	5.9
34	6.0	6.5	7.1
35	7.1	7.1	7.1

such as those seen in diastrophic dysplasia. Table 20–13 shows a nomogram of the fetal foot size throughout gestation. Table 20–14 lists disorders associated with hand and foot deformities. Disproportion between hands and feet and the other parts of the extremity may also be a sign of a skeletal dysplasia. Figure 20–17 shows the relationship between femur length and foot length. The ratio of femur length to foot length is nearly constant from the 14th to the 40th weeks. The mean is 0.99 (SD = 0.06). A ratio below 0.87 should be considered abnormal.[199] Although fetuses with skeletal dysplasias have been reported to have abnormally low ratios,

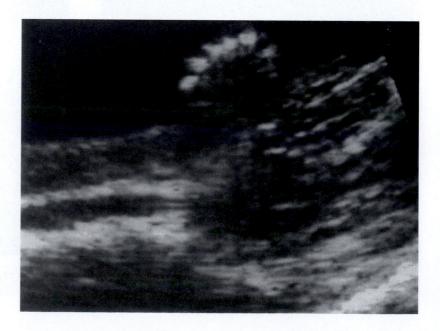

Figure 20–16. Transverse scan of a fetus with chondroectodermal dysplasia showing postaxial polydactyly. Six digits are easily identified.

TABLE 20–14. SKELETAL DYSPLASIAS ASSOCIATED WITH POLYDACTYLY AND SYNDACTYLY

Postaxial polydactyly
  Chondroectodermal dysplasia
  Short rib–polydactyly syndrome (type I, type II)
  Asphyxiating thoracic dysplasia
  Otopalatodigital syndrome
  Mesomelic dysplasia, Werner type (associated with absence
    of thumbs)
Preaxial polydactyly
  Chrondroectodermal dysplasia
  Short rib–polydactyly syndrome type II
  Carpenter's syndrome
Syndactyly
  Poland's syndrome
  Acrocephalosyndactylies (Carpenter's syndrome, Apert's
    syndrome)
  Otopalatodigital syndrome type II
  Mesomelic dysplasia, Werner type
  TAR syndrome
  Jarcho–Levin syndrome
  Robert's syndrome
Brachydactyly
  Mesomelic dysplasia, Robinow type
  Otopalatodigital syndrome
Hitchhiker thumbs
  Diastrophic dysplasia
Clubfoot deformity
  Diastrophic dysplasia
  Osteogenesis imperfecta
  Kniest dysplasia
  Spondyloepiphyseal congenita

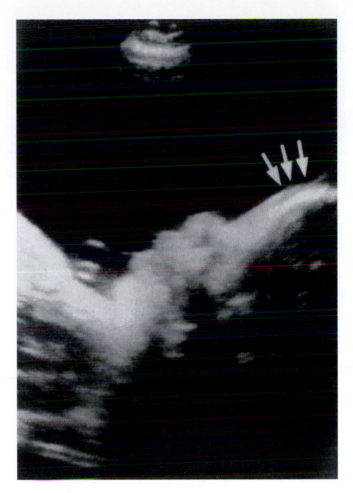

Figure 20–18. Frontal bossing in a sagittal scan. The *arrows* point to the prominent frontal bone.

more evidence is required to test the diagnostic value of this method.[200] It is expected that a small proportion of unaffected fetuses may have an abnormal ratio. As in the case of other limb biometric parameters, large deviations from the lower limit of normal are likely to be significant.

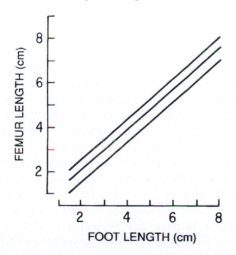

Figure 20–17. Relationship between femur length and foot length.

Evaluation of the Fetal Cranium

Several skeletal dysplasias are associated with defects of membranous ossification which affects skull bones. Orbits should be measured to exclude hypertelorism.[201,202] Other findings that should be noted or ruled out are micrognathia,[203] short upper lip, abnormally shaped ear,[204] frontal bossing (Fig. 20–18), and cloverleaf skull deformity (Figs. 20–19 to 20–20). Table 20–15 presents abnormalities of the skull and face associated with different skeletal dysplasias.

Evaluation of the Fetal Face

Sonographic examination of fetal facial features is of major importance in the assessment and diagnosis of skeletal dysplasias because many of these disorders are associated with typical facial abnormalities.[205] Sonographic evaluation of the fetal face is easily performed in a high percentage of patients from 16 to 20 weeks of gestation onward. The single, most reliable view in detecting facial abnormalities is the sagittal view. This view permits determination of midface hypoplasia, which occurs in several skeletal dysplasias, such

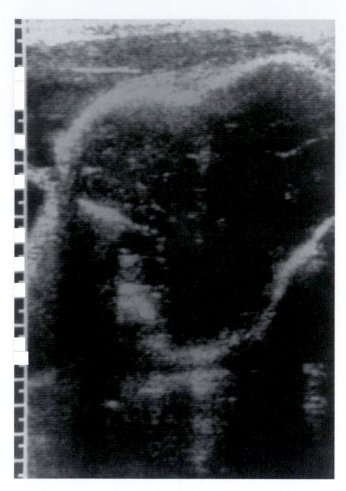

Figure 20–19. Coronal scan of the head of a fetus with thanatophoric dysplasia with cloverleaf skull.

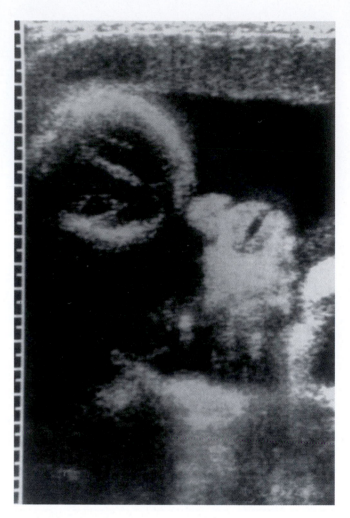

Figure 20–20. Frontal bossing in a fetus with cloverleaf skull. Note the prominent forehead. Under normal circumstances, the forehead is not visible on a scan that allows imaging of the mouth and nose.

as thanatophoric dysplasia, achondroplasia, campomelic dysplasia, osteogenesis imperfecta type I, and spondyloepiphyseal dysplasia congenita.[206,207]

In median clefting, the central portion of the upper lip is absent, and on the midline sagittal view, no upper lip will be seen. In bilateral cleft lip, the midline view will show a variable appearance, depending on the amount of residual premaxillary tissue present in the midline. In unilateral cleft lip, the midline sagittal scan may be relatively normal; the parasagittal view will demonstrate the cleft. This should be subsequently confirmed by scanning the coronal plane.

Cleft palate occurs in 66% of patients with cleft lip. Cleft palate is more difficult to diagnose with ultrasound because of shadowing of facial bones. Color flow Doppler sonography can be helpful in the diagnosis of cleft palate.[208] Micrognathia is also frequent in cases of skeletal dysyplasia[209–212] (Table 20–16). Nomograms of mandibular length throughout gestation are available.[213] (Table 20–17).

Intraorbital and interorbital diameters should be measured because hypertelorism may occur in cases of skeletal dysplasia (Table 20–18).

Evaluation of the Fetal Spine

Sonographic assessment of the fetal spine is a component in the examination of a fetus with suspected skeletal dysplasia. The following parameters should be assessed.

Vertebral Bodies. Fetal vertebral bodies are composed of three ossification centers representing the vertebral body and two laminae.[214–216] Abnormalities of the ossification center of the fetal vertebral body may result in bony defects, such as hemivertebrae (Fig. 20–5), butterfly vertebrae, or block vertebrae causing congenital scoliosis (Fig. 20–4). A study of the associated anomalies of 27 cases in which prenatal ultrasound detected hemivertebrae noted that, while 11 fetuses had no other abnormal findings, 16 fetuses had associated anomalies.[215] These anomalies included cardiac, gastrointestinal, renal, facial, extremity, and cranial. Seven fetuses had bilateral renal agenesis (Potter's syndrome). Only five of the fetuses with additional anomalies survived.

TABLE 20–15. SKELETAL DYSPLASIAS ASSOCIATED WITH SKULL AND FACE DEFORMITIES

Large head
  Achondroplasia
  Achondrogenesis
  Thanatophoric dysplasia
  Osteogenesis imperfecta
  Cleidocranial dysplasia
  Hypophosphatasia
  Campomelic dysplasia
  Short rib–polydactyly syndrome, type III
  Robinow's mesomelic dysplasia
  Otopalatodigital syndrome
Cloverleaf skull
  Thanatophoric dysplasia
  Campomelic dysplasia
Other craniostenosis
  Apert's syndrome
  Carpenter's syndrome
Congenital cataracts
  Condrodysplasia punctata
Cleft palate
  Asphyxiating thoracic dysplasia
  Kniest's dysplasia
  Distrophic dysplasia
  Spondyloepiphyseal dysplasia
  Campomelic dysplasia
  Jarcho–Levin syndrome
  Ellis–van Creveld syndrome
  Short rib–polydactyly syndrome, type II
  Metatropic dysplasia
  Otopalatodigital syndrome, type II
  Dyssegmental dysplasia
  Robert's syndrome
Short upper lip
  Chondroectodermal dysplasia
Micrognathia
  Campomelic dysplasia
  Distrophic dysplasia
  Weissenbacher–Zweymuller syndrome
  Otopalatodigital syndrome
  Pena–Shokier syndrome
  Thrombocytopenia with absent radii syndrome
  Langer's syndrome

TABLE 20–16. SKELETAL DYSPLASIAS ASSOCIATED WITH MICROGNATHIA

Camptomelic dysplasia
Diastrophic dysplasia
Otopalatodigital syndrome
Achondrogenesis
Mesomelic dysplasia
Pena–Shokeir syndrome
Treacher–Collins syndrome
Nager acrofacial dysostosis
Oromandibular limb hypogenesis
Goldenhar's syndrome
Atelosteogenesis
Hydrolethalus syndrome

in the vertebral bodies are believed to represent a localized splitting of the notochord due to adhesions between the ectoderm and endoderm during the embryonic period. These clefts range from a single cleft to multiple clefts. The presence of vertebral clefting in skeletal dysplasia was assessed by searching the database at the International Skeletal Dysplasia Registry.[220] Coronal and sagittal clefts were present in 40 different conditions. Coronal clefts were more common than

TABLE 20–17. NOMOGRAM OF MANDIBLE LENGTH THROUGHOUT GESTATION

GA (wk)	Lower PL	Mean	Upper PL
14	0.8	1.2	1.6
15	1.0	1.4	1.8
16	1.2	1.6	2.0
17	1.5	1.9	2.3
18	1.7	2.1	2.5
19	1.9	2.3	2.7
20	2.1	2.5	2.9
21	2.2	2.6	3.1
22	2.4	2.8	3.2
23	2.6	3.0	3.4
24	2.8	3.2	3.6
25	2.9	3.3	3.8
26	3.1	3.5	3.9
27	3.2	3.7	4.1
28	3.4	3.8	4.2
29	3.5	4.0	4.4
30	3.7	4.1	4.5
31	3.8	4.2	4.6
32	3.9	4.4	4.8
33	4.1	4.5	4.9
34	4.2	4.6	5.0
35	4.3	4.7	5.1
36	4.4	4.8	5.2
37	4.5	4.9	5.3
38	4.6	5.0	5.4
39	4.7	5.1	5.5

GA, gestational age; PL, prediction limit.

Platyspondyly may be diagnosed with current high resolution sonography[217] (Fig. 20–3). Rib defects are often associated with thoracic vertebral body anomalies.

Clefting of the vertebrae may be complete or incomplete, coronal or sagittal.[218] Coronal vertebral clefts are a result of lack of fusion between the anterior and posterior primary ossification centers after 16 weeks of gestation and can be observed by sonography *in utero*.[219,220] Sagittal clefts

TABLE 20–18. SKELETAL DYSPLASIAS ASSOCIATED WITH HYPERTELORISM

Otopalatodigital syndrome
Arthrogryposis multiplex congenita
Larsen's syndrome
Robert's syndrome
Cleidocranial dysostosis
Achondroplasia
Camptomelic dysplasia
Coffin syndrome
Klippel–Feil syndrome
Apert's syndrome
Sprengel's deformity
Mesomelic dysplasia
Holt–Oram syndrome

sagittal clefts and were located mainly in the thoracolumbar region. Clefts were most frequently observed in atelosteogenesis (88%), followed by chondroplasia punctata (79%), dyssegmental dysplasia (73%), Kniest dysplasia (63%), and short rib–polydactyly syndrome (53%).[220]

Spinal Curvature. The most common osseous anomaly causing scoliosis is the unilateral unsegmented bar with contralateral hemivertebrae.[215,221–225] Spinal dysraphism may occur with congenital scoliosis, and this possibility should be examined carefully. An apparent etiologic relationship exists between neural tube defects and other vertebral anomalies. Siblings of infants with congenital scoliosis have a 4% risk of neural tube defects.[225] This increased risk is present in siblings of children with a single hemivertebrae in addition to multiple vertebral anomalies (with or without neural arch defects). The differential diagnosis of fetal scoliosis includes neural tube defects, large abdominal wall defects, amniotic band syndrome, caudal regression, and hemivertebrae. Nonossification of the lumbar vertebral bodies has been detected in achondrogenesis.[226–228]

Evaluation of the Internal Organs

A detailed examination of the cardiovascular, genitourinary, gastrointestinal, and central nervous system organs should be performed in all fetuses with skeletal anomalies. Some syndromes present with specific abnormalities of the internal organs, thus helping in the differential diagnoses of these entities. For example, congenital heart disease is a prominent feature of Ellis–van Creveld syndrome and Holt–Oram syndrome.

Despite all efforts to establish an accurate prenatal diagnosis, a careful examination of the newborn is always required.[229] The evaluation should include a detailed physical examination performed by a geneticist or an individual with experience in the field of skeletal dysplasias and radiograms of the skeleton. The latter should include anterior, posterior, lateral, and Towne views of the skull and antero-

posterior views of the spine and extremities and scapula,[230] with separate films of hands and feet. Examination of the skeletal radiographs will permit a precise diagnosis in the majority of cases because the classification of skeletal dysplasias is largely based on radiographic findings. In lethal skeletal dysplasias, histologic examination of the chondroosseous tissue should be performed because this information may lead to a specific diagnosis. Chromosomal studies should be included because there is a specific group of constitutional bone disorders associated with cytogenetic abnormalities. Biochemical studies are helpful in rare instances (e.g., hypophosphatasia). DNA restrictions and enzymatic activity assays should be considered in those cases in which the phenotype suggests a metabolic disorder such as a mucopolysaccharidosis. The recent significant advance in identifying mutations responsible for dysplasias is useful for prenatal diagnosis by amniocentesis or chorionic villi sampling in patients at risk.[231] DNA should be saved in all cases.

Increased Nuchal Translucency and Skeletal Dysplasia. In chromosomally normal pregnancies, nuchal translucency (NT) thickness is associated with increased risk of major anomalies.[232–235] Recently, skeletal dysplasias have been associated with NT. In a multicenter screening project for trisomy 21 using the combination of maternal age and NT, 100,000 pregnancies were included.[232] An association between NT and a wide range of skeletal dysplasia was found among these patients. Several case reports and small series have also suggested that in chromosomally normal fetuses there may be an association between increased NT thickness and skeletal anomalies. Table 20–19 summarizes these data.

Role of Ultrasonography in the Detection of Skeletal Dysplasia. Several studies explored the role of ultrasound in the detection of skeletal dysplasias.[187,191,207,229,237–245] A prospective analysis of a high-risk population (15 women, 16 cases) carrying a genetic risk for skeletal dysplasias was conducted by Kurtz et al.[187] Based on ultrasonographic findings in the second trimester they were able to diagnose five abnormal fetuses of 16. Weldner et al. screened 12,453 patients in the second and third trimesters and estimated the prevalence of skeletal dysplasia as 7.5 per 10,000.[236] Sharony et al.[237] studied the accuracy of antenatal diagnosis of skeletal dysplasias. Fetuses and stillbirths were referred from other centers for suspected skeletal dysplasia. Most of the cases were sporadic, and the most common final diagnoses were osteogenesis imperfecta (16%) and thanatophoric dysplasia (14%). Gaffney et al. reported a series of 35 cases suspected for skeletal dysplasia. Using a systematic approach to ultrasound scanning in the second and third trimesters, they were able to predict the prognosis in 91% of cases, although an accurate diagnosis was made in only 31% of cases.[238]

In a large, high-risk pregnancy population (12,200) studied over 10 years with a wide range of gestational ages

TABLE 20–19. SKELETAL DYSPLASIAS ASSOCIATED WITH INCREASED THICKNESS OF NUCHAL TRANSLUCENCY

Skeletal Dysplasia	Reference
Campomelic dysplasia	Hafner et al.[690]
Achondrogenesis	Hewitt,[691] Soothill and Kyle,[692] Fisk et al.[693]
Sirinomelia	Hewitt[691]
Achondroplasia	Fukada et al.,[694] Hernadi and Torocsik[695]
Asphyxiating thoracic dysplasia	Ben Ami et al.,[696] Hsieh et al.[697]
Blomstrand's osteochondrodysplasia	den Hollander et al.[108]
Ectrodactyly ectodermal dysplasia	Leung et al.[698]
Fetal akinesia deformation sequence	Souka et al.,[234] Hyett et al.[699]
Jarcho–Levin syndrome	Eliyahu et al.,[700] Souka et al.[234]
Short rib–polydactyly syndrome	Hill and Leary[701]
Smith–Lemli–Opitz syndrome	Souka et al.,[234] Hyett et al.,[702] Maymon et al.,[703] Sharp et al.,[704] Hobbins et al.[705]
VATER association	Souka et al.[234]
Thanatophoric dysplasia	Souka et al.[234]

(between 9 and 40 weeks), there were 39 cases of skeletal dysplasia. Of the 39 cases, 30 (76.9%) were detected in the first and second trimesters.[246] Tretter et al.[247] identified 26 of 27 cases of lethal skeletal anomalies, and Hersh et al.[248] predicted lethality in 23 of 27 cases.

Recently, the sonographic features of skeletal dysplasias obtained by two-dimensional (2D) and three-dimensional (3D) ultrasound were compared in a series of seven cases. Three-dimensional was better than 2D sonography in depicting abnormal spatial relationships such as short ribs, splayed digits, and absent bones. In three of seven patients, 3D sonography provided additional information in the evaluation of skeletal dysplasias.[249]

OSTEOCHONDRODYSPLASIAS

A growing number of skeletal dysplasias have been recognized *in utero*. A complete account of each disorder is beyond the scope of this chapter. The following discussion presents only a few of the most common disorders relevant to prenatal diagnosis.

ACHONDROPLASIA, THANATOPHORIC DYSPLASIA, AND HYPOCHONDROPLASIA

These three chondrodysplasias are discussed in the same section because they are caused by mutation in FGFR3.[76,80,250–255]

The most common non-lethal skeletal dysplasia is achondroplasia, an autosomal dominant condition with a prevalence of 1 per 66,000. It is characterized by rhizomelic shortening, limb bowing, lordotic spine, and an enlarged head.[256] This disease is the result of anomalous growth of cartilage, followed by abnormal endochondral ossification,

which is responsible for the shortness of long bones. The bones of the hands and feet are short (brachydactyly). The head is large; a flattened nasal bridge, frontal bossing, and broad mandible are frequent features. The problems in the prenatal diagnosis of this condition have been discussed in detail by Kurtz et al.[257] Moreover, Modaff et al.[258] provided data about the frequency of the prenatal misdiagnosis of achondroplasia and illustrated the difficulty of making this specific prenatal diagnosis. They retrospectively collected data from 37 consecutive referrals of infants with achondroplasia in whom ultrasound was performed prenatally. Nine of 37 (24%) had a positive family history of achondroplasia; all nine were correctly diagnosed prenatally. Of the 28 with no family history of achondroplasia, 16 (57%) were recognized to have abnormalities on ultrasound but none were diagnosed with certainty. Five received an appropriate diagnosis of "most likely" achondroplasia and four others were given a nonspecific (but appropriate) diagnosis of some skeletal dysplasias, not otherwise specified. In seven instances (25%), an incorrect diagnosis of a lethal or very severe disorder was assigned.

The major difficulty in the antenatal diagnosis is that the long bone growth in this disease is not recognized in most cases until the third trimester of pregnancy. Therefore, it is usually not possible to detect this disorder in time for pregnancy termination.[259] However, prenatal diagnosis of achondroplasia is possible and has been reported.[260–262] The trident hand is a specific finding for achondroplasia.[263,264] A distinct difference in the femoral length growth curves of homozygous, heterozygous, and unaffected children of achondroplastic parents was described by Patel et al.[265] Prenatal diagnosis of achondroplasia using amniotic fluid has been reported recently using molecular techniques.[266] Heterozygous achondroplasia is compatible with normal intellectual development. However, cervicomedullary junction abnormalities that may lead to compression and place the infant with achondroplasia at risk for disability and death.[267] The disease is considered lethal in the homozygous state, however, a 37-month-old survivor has been reported.[268] The radiologic characteristics of homozygous achondroplasia lie between those of thanatophoric dysplasia and heterozygous achondroplasia. Administration of a growth hormone has been recently proposed for the treatment of achondroplasia.[269]

Tavormina et al.[270] recently identified a novel FGFR3 missense mutation in four unrelated individuals with skeletal dysplasias that approaches the severity observed in thanatophoric dysplasia type I. Three of the four individuals developed extensive areas of acanthosis nigricans beginning in early childhood, suffered from severe neurologic impairments, and have survived past infancy without prolonged life support measures. The FGFR3 mutation (A1949T: Lys650Met) occurs at the nucleotide adjacent to the Thanatophoric Dysplasia (TD) type II mutation (A1948G: Lys650Glu) and results in a different amino acid substitution. They referred to the phenotype caused by the Lys650Met mutation as "severe achondroplasia with developmental delay and acanthosis nigricans" (SADDAN) because it differs significantly from the phenotypes of other known FGFR3 mutations. It results in severe disturbances in endochondral bone growth that approach and overlap those observed in thanatophoric dysplasia type I. It is also associated with unusual bone deformities, such as femoral bowing with reverse (i.e., posterior apex), tibial and fibular bowing, and "ram's horn" bowing of the clavicle. In addition to the skeletal anomalies, progressive acanthosis nigricans, central nervous system structural anomalies, seizures, and severe developmental delays are observed in surviving SADDAN patients. This condition has not been associated with cloverleaf skull or craniosynostosis.[271]

Thanatophoric dysplasia is the most common lethal skeletal dysplasia in fetuses and neonates. It is characterized by extreme rhizomelia, a normal trunk length with a narrow thorax, and a large head with a prominent forehead. It occurs in 0.24 to 0.69 of 10,000 births.[80,176–178] Two subtypes have been identified: type 1, with typical bowed "telephone receiver" femurs[272] (Fig. 20–21) and without cloverleaf skull; and type 2, with severe cloverleaf skull (Fig. 20–19) and short, straight long bones.[180,273] However, mild cloverleaf skull has been described in type 1.[272,274–275] Distinct mutation in FGFR3 causes each one of these two types.[276–279] The differential diagnosis between the two depends on the radiographic findings and histology.[80] There is no agreement concerning the pattern of inheritance of this condition. Most cases of thanatophoric dysplasia (all cases of type 1 and most cases of type 2) are sporadic. Some familial cases of type 2 have been reported.[278–282] The prenatal sonographic findings depend on the specific variety.[220] The association of cloverleaf skull and micromelia is specific for thanatophoric dysplasia. Another skeletal dysplasia associated with cloverleaf skull is campomelic syndrome. However, micromelia is not a

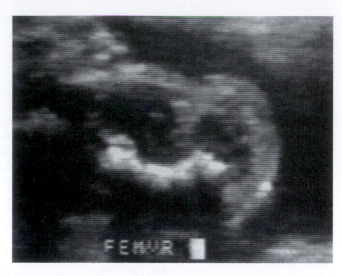

Figure 20–21. Bowed and short femur with the typical "telephone receiver" appearance.

feature of this condition. Cloverleaf skull may result from premature closure of the coronal and lambdoid sutures, defective development of the cranial base with secondary synostosis, or a primary developmental disorder of the brain with secondary deformation of the skull. Ventriculomegaly, macrocranium, and polyhydramnios are frequently seen. There is a relatively large calvarium with a prominent forehead (Fig. 20–18), a saddle nose, and hypertelorism. Additional findings are short ribs, platyspondyly (Fig. 20–3), and short and broad tubular bones in the hands and feet. The differential diagnoses include short rib–polydactyly syndrome, homozygous achondroplasia, and asphyxiating thoracic dysplasia (slight shortening of long bones and normal vertebrae). On review of the radiologic findings of several cases of thanatophoric dysplasia, Horton et al. were able to discern a group of distinct entities characterized by severe platyspondylia.[283] These disorders include the Torrance, San Diego, Lutton, and Shiraz types of platyspondylic lethal osteochondrodysplasias. Differential diagnosis among these entities is based on histologic and radiologic characteristics. Thanatophoric dysplasia is considered a lethal disorder, although survival of several months has been reported in some isolated cases.[282–287] Prenatal sonographic diagnosis has been documented on several occasions[288–296] and in one case in a triplet pregnancy.[297]

Prenatal diagnosis of thanatophoric dysplasia has recently been reported by using genomic DNA isolated from the amniotic fluid and polymerase chain reaction amplification. The common mutation, C → T mutation at nucleotide 742 in the FGFR3 gene, was identified by using restriction enzyme analysis.[298–300]

Hypochondroplasia is a disorder that results from a mutation in FGFR3[301–302] and resembles achondroplasia.[303] The incidence and prevalence have not been determined. Most cases occur sporadically as a result of a new mutation.[164] The differential diagnosis between these two conditions is based on the sparing of the head and the lack of tibial bowing in hypochondroplasia.[303–308] Although this condition is generally first detected during childhood, prenatal diagnosis in a patient at risk has been reported at 22 weeks.[260,308]

FIBROCHONDROGENESIS, ATELOSTEOGENESIS

Fibrochondrogenesis and atelosteogenesis have a clinical presentation similar to that of thanatophoric dysplasia. The differential diagnosis among these disorders *in utero* is extremely difficult. Fibrochondrogenesis is a very rare, lethal chondrodysplasia inherited with an autosomal recessive pattern and characterized by micromelia with significant metaphyseal flaring, normal head size, undermineralized skull, platyspondyly, clefting of the vertebral bodies, and narrow and bell-shaped thorax.[309,310] Metaphyseal flaring is not a feature of thanatophoric dysplasia.[311–314] This condition has been described in a consanguineous family.[315] Prenatal diagnosis by ultrasound has been accomplished.[316,317] Other conditions to be considered in the differential diagnosis include metatropic dysplasia and Kniest's dysplasia.

Atelosteogenesis is also a lethal chondrodysplasia characterized by severe micromelia (with hypoplasia of the distal segments of the humerus and femur), bowing of long bones, narrow chest with short ribs, coronal and sagittal vertebral clefts,[139] and dislocation at the level of the elbow and knee. Clubfoot deformities may also be present.[318] Three subtypes of atelosteogenesis have been described based on radiologic and pathologic findings.[319–322] Atelosteogenesis types I and III are sporadic; type II is inherited with an autosomal recessive pattern and is caused by mutation in DTDST.[169–171,323–325] It overlaps phenotypically and genetically with diastrophic dysplasia and achondrogenesis type 1B.[172–174] Differential diagnosis includes diastrophic dysplasia and de la Chapelle dysplasia.[326,327] Three cases of a lethal dysplasia termed "boomerang syndrome" ("boomerang like tibia") may actually represent the same disorder as atelosteogenesis type I.[328] Fibrochondrogenesis and atelosteogenesis are extremely rare, and only a few cases of each have been reported. Prenatal diagnosis of Atelosteogenesis has also been reported.[246,329–332]

ACHONDROGENESIS

Achondrogenesis, or anosteogenesis, is a lethal chondrodystrophy characterized by extreme micromelia, short trunk, and macrocrania. The birth prevalence is 0.09 to 0.23 per 10,000 births.[176,177,237,238,247] Traditionally, this disorder has been classified into two types: the more severe form, which is type I achondrogenesis (Parenti–Fraccaro), and type II achondrogenesis (Langer–Saldino). Recently, type I has been subdivided into two subtypes: type IA (Houston–Harris) and type IB (Fraccaro).[333–334] Hypochondrogenesis had been considered a separate disorder from achondrogenesis. However, evidence now suggests that hypochondrogenesis and achondrogenesis type II are phenotypic variants of the same disorder.[335–337] Indeed, clinically and radiologically, achondrogenesis type II, hypochondrogenesis, and neonatal spondyloepiphyseal dysplasia congenita are part of a spectrum of disease.[338] The fundamental biochemical disorder seems to be allelic mutations of the gene coding for type II procollagen.[339] A different classification dividing achondrogenesis into four types has been proposed by Whitley and Gorlin,[339] but this proposal has not yet gained wide acceptance.

Type IA achondrogenesis (Houston–Harris) is characterized by micromelia, lack of ossification of vertebral bodies, but ossification of the pedicles in the cervical and upper thoracic region, and short ribs with multiple fractures. The calvarium is demineralized. Type IB (Fraccaro), which is inherited as an autosomal recessive trait and is caused by mutation in DTDS gene,[170,340,341] but the calvarium is ossified, and fractured ribs are not seen. Although the vertebral bodies are minimally or not at all ossified, the pedicles show some ossification. Type II achondrogenesis is characterized by micromelia, lack of mineralization of all or many vertebral bodies, sacrum and ischion, enlarged calvarium with normal ossification, variable shortening of the ribs, and absence of fractures (Fig. 20–22).[342] Table 20–20 presents the characteristics of the different types of achondrogenesis. An association between cytic hygromas and achondrogenesis has been reported.[343–344]

Prenatal diagnosis should be suspected on the basis of micromelia, lack of vertebral ossification, and a large head

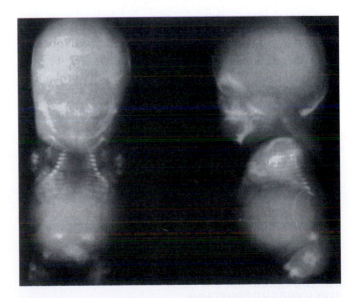

Figure 20–22. Frontal and lateral views in a case of achondrogenesis type II. There is no mineralization of the spine and ischial bones. The thorax is bell-shaped, with short and straight ribs and no fractures. Long bones are short, with metaphyseal flaring and cupping.

TABLE 20–20. RADIOLOGIC DIFFERENCES BETWEEN ACHONDROGENESIS TYPE I (A–B), TYPE II, AND HYPOCHONDROGENESIS

	Type IA (Houston–Harris)	Type IB (Fraccaro)	Type II (Langer–Saldino)	Hypochondrogenesis
Skull	Membranous calvarium	All parts of ossified skull well seen	Normal ossification	Normal ossification
Long bones	Extremely shortened with metaphyseal cupping and spurs "Rectangular bones"	Arms and legs shorter than with type IA, with minimal ossification; abundant metaphyseal spiking or spurring in lower leg bones "Square or stellate bones"	Short and bowed with metaphyseal flaring and cupping "Mushroom stem bones"	Less bowed and shortened with irregular or smooth metaphyses
Spine	Vertebral bodies unossified, with partly ossified pedicles	Vertebral bodies minimally or not ossified, pedicles ossified	Variable pattern of ossified or unossified vertebral bodies and pedicles	Thoracic and upper lumbar vertebral bodies ossified but still platyspondylic Cervical and lower lumbar bodies unossified
Pelvis	Poorly formed and ossified, with crenated iliac bones Ischial bones poorly ossified, pubic bones unossified	Iliac bones, same aspect as in type IA Ischial and pubic bones unossified	Halberd-like iliac bones with unossified ischial and pubic bones	Near-normally developed iliac bones with partial ossification of ischial bones and unossified pubic bones
Thorax	Short and barrel-shaped Short ribs with cupped metaphyses and multiple fractures	Same as in type IA, with unfractured ribs	Short and barrel- or bell-shaped with short unfractured ribs	Near normal but shallow cage with short unfractured ribs

Source: Spranger.[336]

with various degrees of ossification of calvarium.[345–349] Polyhydramnios and hydrops have been associated with achondrogenesis. However, sonographic examinations of most affected fetuses do not demonstrate fluid accumulation in body cavities. The hydropic appearance of these fetuses and neonates is probably attributable to redundancy of soft-tissue mass over a limited skeletal frame. Achondrogenesis type IA and type IB are inherited with an autosomal recessive pattern, whereas most cases of achondrogenesis type II and hypochondrogenesis have been sporadic (new autosomal dominant mutations). Some severe cases of type II achondrogenesis have an autosomal recessive pattern.[350]

Since the basic defect in achondrogenesis type IB was found, the diagnosis with molecular techniques is possible. The distinction between achondrogenesis type IB (which has a 25% risk for recurrence) and the more frequent autosomal dominant achondrogenesis type II which has lower recurrent risk (new mutation) is important for counseling. Couples at risk of having a child with achondrogenesis Type IB may take the advantage of molecular prenatal diagnosis by chorionic villus sampling.[170–172]

OSTEOGENESIS IMPERFECTA AND HYPOPHOSPHATASIA

Osteogenesis imperfecta and hypophosphatasia are discussed together because they are characterized by significant skeletal demineralization.

The term *osteogenesis imperfecta* (OI) was introduced more than a century ago to describe a newborn with extremely brittle bones (Fig. 20–23). Currently, the term refers to a heterogeneous group of disorders caused, in most cases, by mutations in one or two structural genes for type I procollagen.[119–124] Advanced paternal age is a risk factor for OI.[351] The prevalence of OI is 0.18 per 10,000 births.[176,177] The clinical heterogeneity in OI is due to the different mutations in the genes: COL1A1 and COL1A2.[119–123]

The most popular classification of OI is that proposed by Sillence et al.[352] In type I (autosomal dominant), patients have bone fragility, blue sclera (all ages), and hearing loss. There is osteoporosis and a normal calvarium; fractures range from none to multiple. Type II (new dominant mutations; fewer than 5% are autosomal recessive) is also known as the perinatal variety and is uniformly lethal. There is almost no ossification of the skull; beaded ribs; shortened, crumpled long bones; and multiple fractures are visible *in utero* (Fig. 20–11). The thorax is short but not narrow. Type II is subclassified into three subtypes (IIA, IIB, and IIC) according to radiologic criteria. Type III (autosomal recessive, rare) is a nonlethal variety characterized by blue sclera and multiple fractures present at birth. The sclera becomes white with time. The membranous skull is severely deossified and the long bones are mildly shortened but with marked angulations. Type IIB and type III OI are difficult to distinguish and may represent different degrees of severity of the same disorder.[353] Type IV (autosomal dominant) is the mildest form. Long bones and sclera are normal. There is mild to moderate osseous

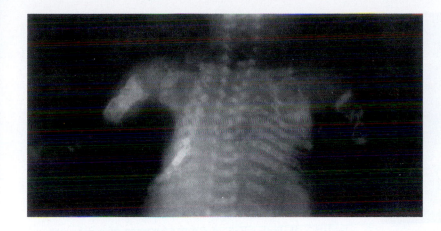

Figure 20–23. Osteogenesis imperfecta type IIA. Multiple skeletal fractures are present. Note the contiguous beading of the ribs and other long bones. The spine shows platyspondyly.

fragility, and 25% of these newborns have fractures. There is significant heterogeneity in the expression of the disease even within the same family.[354]

The natural history of OI *in utero* is quite variable. In some cases fractures and limb shortening can be observed in the early second trimester; in other cases abnormalities are not detectable until the third trimester.[355–357] Type IIA OI has been diagnosed as early as 15 weeks.[358,359] It seems that prenatal diagnosis of OI types IIB, IIC, and III may require a longer observation period because of the later onset of the disease.[360]

The prognosis for types I and IV is much better than that for types II and III. Antenatal diagnosis of OI type II has been reported several times.[361–364] Type I OI and type III OI diagnoses have also been reported.[365]

Collagen biosynthesis in cell culture from chorionic villi may serve as a way for prenatal diagnosis.[366,367] In a large study, Pepin et al.[368] reported the largest experience to date in the prenatal diagnosis of OI using biochemical techniques (107 cases). There were neither false negative nor false positive results. The time needed for diagnosis was 20 to 30 days when results relied on the use of biochemical techniques and 10 to 14 days when molecular strategies were used.

Hypophosphatasia is a rare autosomal recessive inherited disorder characterized by demineralization of bones and low alkaline phosphatase in serum and other tissues.[369] Alkaline phosphatase acts on pyrophosphate and other phosphate esters, leading to the accumulation of inorganic phosphates that are critical for the formation of bone crystals. Bone fragility is thought to be the result of deficient generation of bone crystals.[370]

Hypophosphatasia has been subdivided into three clinical types according to the age of onset: congenital–infantile, childhood, and adult.[371,372] The congenital–infantile and childhood varieties have an autosomal recessive pattern of inheritance, whereas the adult form is autosomal dominant. The congenital (neonatal) form is associated with early neonatal death or stillbirth.[373]

Fetuses with congenital hypophosphatasia have generalized demineralization of the skeleton, with shortening and bowing of tubular bones. Multiple fractures are present. The marked demineralization of the cranial vault results in deformation of the skull after external compression (Fig. 20–10). This sonographic sign is also present in some cases of OI type II and achondrogenesis type IA. Prenatal diagnosis of this condition has been reported using ultrasound[374,375] and by assaying alkaline phosphatase in tissue obtained by chorionic villous sampling[376] and alkaline phosphatase in amniotic fluid cell culture. Alkaline phosphatase measurement in amniotic fluid is not a reliable means of making a diagnosis of hypophosphatasia because most of the alkaline phosphatase in amniotic fluid is of intestinal origin.[377–378] The involved enzymes in hypophosphatasia are bone and liver alkaline phosphatases. These isoenzymes contribute to only 16% of the total amniotic fluid enzymatic activity.[179]

Prenatal molecular diagnosis of infantile hypophosphatasia using chorionic villus sampling has recently been reported.[380] A missense mutation has been identified in a case of neonatal hypophosphatasia.[381]

DIASTROPHIC DYSPLASIA

Diastrophic dysplasia is an autosomal recessive condition characterized by micromelia, clubfoot, hand deformities, multiple joint flexion contractures, and scoliosis.[382] Because of phenotypic variability, the diagnosis may be difficult at birth, and milder cases are diagnosed later.[383] The clinical features include rhizomelic-type limb shortening, contractures, hand deformities with abducted position of the thumbs ("hitchhiker thumb") (Figs. 20–24 and 20–25), and severe talipes equinovarus. The head is normal, but micrognathia and cleft palate may be present. This dysplasia is a generalized disorder of cartilage, with destruction of the cartilage matrix with formation of fibrous scar tissue and subsequent ossification. The latter process is responsible for the contractures. Mutation in the DTDST gene is associated with impaired sulfatation of proteoglycans and causes this disorder.[168]

The prenatal diagnosis of DTD has been made in patients at risk,[384–387] based on severe shortening and bowing

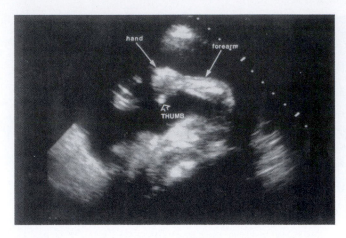

Figure 20–24. Longitudinal section of a right hand *in utero* demonstrating "hitchhiker thumb."

of all long bones.[388] This disorder has a wide spectrum of severity, and some cases may not be diagnosed *in utero*. This disease is not lethal. Intelligence and sexual development are unaffected. However, death in the neonatal period due to respiratory and spinal abnormalities and mental retardation

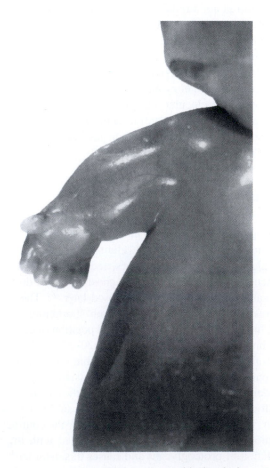

Figure 20–25. Hitchhiker thumb in diastrophic dysplasia.

have been reported in some patients. Differential diagnoses include arthrogryposis multiple congenita, atelosteogenesis type II, and pseudodiastrophic dysplasia. Pseudodiastrophic dysplasia has a presentation similar to that of DTD[389] and is inherited with an autosomal recessive pattern.[177] Histologic examination is required for a differential diagnosis. The distinctive morphologic abnormalities of the growth plate noted in DTD have not been observed in pseudodiastrophic dysplasia.

KNIEST'S SYNDROME

In 1952, Wilhelm Kniest reported a case of a 3.5-year-old girl with "skeletal changes showing a certain relationship to classical chondrodystrophy but differing in many of its manifestations."[390] His report separated this disorder from other chondrodystrophies which is known today as one of the type II collagenopathies.[391–394] This disorder is characterized by involvement of the spine (platyspondyly and coronal clefts) and tubular bones (shortened and metaphyseal flaring), with a broad and short thorax. There is a wide spectrum of disease.[395] The patient described by Kniest is still alive, although severely handicapped with short stature and blindness.[395] Molecular analysis of the patient's DNA showed a single base (G) deletion of the COL2A1 gene. Frequently, the disorder is compatible with life, however, death in the neonatal period has been reported.[396] Abnormalities of type II collagen are involved in the pathogenesis of the disease.[397] The term *Kniest-like disorders* is used to refer to a group of conditions that share histologic and radiologic characteristics with Kniest's syndrome but differ in terms of clinical presentation and inheritance.[398]

Dyssegmental dysplasia is another entity related to Kniest's dysplasia. Two distinct types of dyssegmental dysplasia have been recognized: the mild Rolland–Desbuquois form and the lethal Silverman—Handmaker form.[399–402] The latter is characterized by anarchic ossification of the vertebral bodies, metaphyseal flaring, and severe bowing of the long bones. The Rolland–Desbuquois type has essentially the same features, but the defects are much milder. Prenatal identification has been made in patients at risk.[403,404] A cephalocele is present in 50% of cases of the Silverman–Handmaker type of dysegmental dysplasia and has been attributed to defective segmentation at the level of the occiput. The disease is autosomal recessive. Other conditions associated with vertebral disorganization are Jarcho–Levin syndrome and mesomelic dysplasia.

CAMPOMELIC DYSPLASIA

Campomelic dysplasia (CMD) is a rare lethal disorder described first by Maroteaux in 1971.[405] The incidence ranges between 0.05 and 1.6 per 10,000 births. A unique aspect of CD is that 75% affected infants with male karyiotype present sex reversal syndrome and have female or ambiguous genitalia.[60,407] The histology of the gonads varies, from gonads with testicular differentiation to dysgenetic gonads with primary follicles. Recently, a single mutation in the SOX-9 gene has been reported in several patients with this disorder.[56,57,60,406,407] Campomelic dysplasia syndrome is characterized by bowing of the long bones of the lower extremities, an enlarged and elongated skull with a peculiar small facies, hypoplastic scapulae,[230,408–410] and several associated anomalies such as micrognathia, cleft palate, talipesequinovarus, congenital dislocation of hip, macrocephaly, micrognathia, hydrocephalus, hydronephrosis, and congenital heart defects.[411] The most significant features are bowing of the femur and tibia; other tubular bones are normal in length. The thorax is narrow and can be "bell-shaped." Cervical vertebrae are hypoplastic and poorly ossified.[411] In the largest clinical and genetic study including 36 patients with CMD, Mansour et al. concluded that CMD is considered an autosomal condition because females and males are both affected, and most cases are sporadic autosomal dominant mutations.[412] There are two "short bone varieties" of CMD, representing distinct syndromes: the normocephalic form is known as kyphomelic dysplasia, and the craniostenotic type which appears to be identical to Antley–Bixler syndrome. Differential diagnoses include OI, thanatophoric dysplasia, and hypophosphatasia. Antenatal diagnosis of CD has been reported in patients at risk.[413–416] The difficulties in the diagnosis have been discussed by Norghard et al.[416] and by Saunders et al.[417] The condition is frequently lethal in infancy, but some survivors have been reported.[413,418,419] The cause of death is respiratory distress referred to *tracheomalacia*, however, cleft palate, micrognatia, hypotonia and a small chest are also associated with this condition.[413]

SKELETAL DYSPLASIAS CHARACTERIZED BY A HYPOPLASTIC THORAX

The dysplastic process involves the ribs and other bones of the rib cages in many skeletal dysplasias. A reduction in thoracic dimensions leads to restriction of lung growth and, consequently, pulmonary hypoplasia. There is a specific group of dysplasias in which thoracic hypoplasia is a cardinal feature. These include asphyxiating thoracic dysplasia, Ellis–van Creveld syndrome, short-rib–polydactyly syndrome, and campomelic syndrome. Other disorders presenting with altered thoracic dimensions are thanatophoric dysplasia, atelosteogenesis, fibrochondrogenesis, achondrogenesis, and Jarcho–Levin syndrome (Fig. 20–26).[420]

Asphyxiating Thoracic Dysplasia
Asphyxiating thoracic dysplasia, originally described by Jeune et al.[421] and known as Jeune's syndrome, is a rare

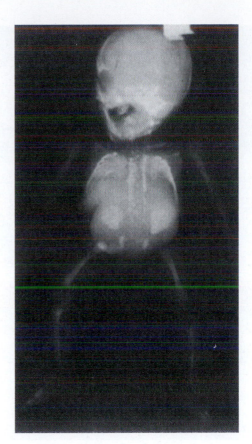

Figure 20–26. Jarcho–Levin syndrome. There is dramatic spinal shortening with disorganization of the vertebral bodies, a characteristic chest deformity ("crablike appearance" with posterior fusion and anterior flaring of the ribs), and unaffected long bones.

autosomal recessive skeletal disorder. Its prevalence is 0.14 per 10,000 births.[422–424] It is characterized by a narrow and bell-shaped thorax, with short, horizontal ribs. Long bones are normal or mildly shortened. Polydactyly and cleft lip and/or palate can occur in association and the presence of a proximal femoral ossification center at birth is also a characteristic finding.[425] Asphyxiating thoracic dysplasia has a wide spectrum of clinical manifestations, from lethal to mild forms; long-term survivors have been reported.[423,426–427] The clinical course for individuals surviving the neonatal period is complicated by respiratory distress of varying severity, nephropathy, hepatic and pancreatic problems.[428–430] Prenatal diagnosis with ultrasound has been reported.[431–438]

Short-Rib–Polydactyly Syndromes
Short-rib–polydactyly syndromes are a group of disorders characterized by micromelia, constricted thorax, and postaxial polydactyly[439–442] (Fig. 20–27). Traditionally, three different types have been recognized (Saldino–Noonan, Majewski, and Naumoff). These conditions have been

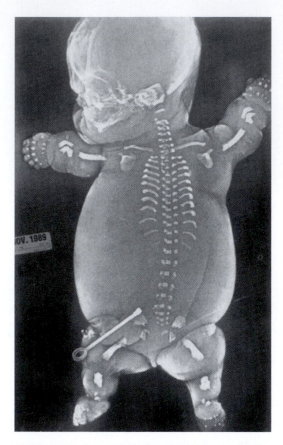

Figure 20–27. Short rib–polydactyly syndrome. There is severe shortening of all long bones, very short and horizontal ribs, and postaxial polydactyly in all four extremities. Note the angulation of the bones in the forearm.

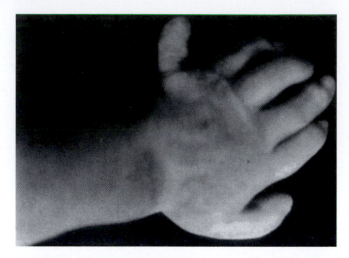

Figure 20–28. Postaxial polydactyly in a fetus with Ellis–van Creveld syndrome.

identified prenatally.[443–449] Table 20–21 shows the differential diagnoses and features of these conditions. Some authorities have expanded the definition of short-rib–polydactyly syndrome to encompass at least seven disorders, including the three previously mentioned entities, the Yang, Le Marec, and Beemer varieties, as well as asphyxiating thoracic dysplasia.[450–453] Spranger and Maroteaux indicated that the absence of polydactyly does not exclude the diagnosis of this entity.[185,454–456]

Chondroectodermal Dysplasia

Chondroectodermal dysplasia, also known as Ellis–van Creveld syndrome, is inherited with an autosomal recessive pattern.[457–462] It is characterized by acromesomelia with normal spine and skull, postaxial polydactyly (Fig. 20–28), long and narrow thorax with short ribs, and congenital heart disease (60% of cases).[463–469] Polydactyly is a consistent finding. The supernumerary digit usually has well-formed metacarpal and phalangeal bones. Survivors who reach adulthood present with short stature and normal intelligence. Prenatal diagnosis with ultrasound has been reported.[470–476] One third of affected individuals die in the postnatal period because of cardiopulmonary disease.[464–478]

LIMB DEFICIENCY OR CONGENITAL AMPUTATIONS

On occasion, the only identifiable anomaly is the absence of an extremity (limb deficiency) or a segment of an extremity (congenital amputation) (Table 20–22). These constitute a group of disorders different from osteochondrodysplasias. The overall incidence of congenital limb reduction deformities is approximately 0.49 per 10,000 births (Table 20–23).[479] It has been estimated that 51% of these limb reduction defects are simple transverse reduction deficiencies of one forearm or hand without associated anomalies. The remainder consists of multiple reduction deficiencies, associated with additional anomalies of the internal organs or craniofacial structures.[480]

Limb deficiencies can present alone or as part of a specific syndrome. An isolated limb deficiency of the upper extremity (e.g., distal segment of an arm) is generally an isolated anomaly. In contrast, congenital amputation of the leg generally occurs within the context of a syndrome, as do bilateral amputations or reduction of all limbs.[481] Isolated amputation of an extremity can be due to amniotic band syndrome, exposure to a teratogen, or a vascular accident. In most cases, the anomaly is sporadic, and the risk of recurrence is negligible. The sonographic findings have been reviewed recently.[482]

The following section reviews syndromes in which a limb amputation or deficiency is associated with other anomalies. We follow the classification proposed by Goldberg.[480]

SYNDROMES WITH ABSENT LIMBS AND FACIAL ANOMALIES

The aglossia–adactylia syndrome consists of transverse amputations of the limbs and malformations of the mouth, including micrognathia, vestigial tongue (hypoglossia), dental abnormalities, and ankylosis of the tongue to the hard palate,

TABLE 20–21. DISORDERS WITH THORACIC DYSPLASIA AND POLYDACTYLY

	Asphyxiating Thoracic Dysplasia (Jeune)	Chondroectodermal Dysplasia (Ellis–van Creveld)	Short Rib–Polydactyly Syndrome Type I (Saldino–Noonan)	Short Rib–Polydactyly Syndrome Type II (Majewski)	Short Rib Syndrome Type III (Naumoff)	Short Rib Syndrome Type IV (Beemer–Langer)
Relative prevalence	Common	Uncommon	Common	Extremely rare	Rare	Rare
Clinical features						
Thoracic constriction	++	+	+++	+++	+++	+++
Polydactyly	+	++	++	++	++	++
Limb shortening	+	++	+++	+	++	++
Congenital heart disease	−	++	++	++	−	
Other abnormalities	Renal disease	Ectodermal dysplasia	Genitourinary and gastrointestinal anomalies	Cleft lip and palate	Renal abnormality	Cleft lip and palate and genitourinary and gastrointestinal anomalies
Radiographic features						
Tubular bone shortening	+	+	+++	++	+++	++
Distinctive features in femora	−	−	Pointed ends	−	Marginal spurs	
Short, horizontal ribs	++	++	+++	+++	+++	+++
Vertical shortening of ilia and flat acetabula	++	++	++	−	++	
Defective ossification of vertebral bodies	−	−	++	−	+	++
Shortening of skull base	−	−	−	−	+	−

+, Not common; +++, most common; −, absent.
Reproduced with permission from Cremin BJ. Bone Dysplasias of Infancy: A Radiological Atlas. Berlin: Springer-Verlag; 1978.

TABLE 20–22. CONGENITAL AMPUTATIONS

Absent limb(s) only
  Single absent limb
  Multiple absent limbs
Absent limbs with rings
  Congenital ring constriction syndrome
Absent limbs and face anomaly
  Aglossia–adaclylia syndromes
  Möbius' syndrome
Absent limbs with other anomalies
  Ichthyosiform skin (CHILD syndrome)
  Fibula agenesis-complex brachydactyly (du Pan's syndrome)
  Splenogonadal fusion
  Skull and scalp defects (Adams–Oliver syndrome)
Phocomelia
  Thalidomide syndrome
  Thrombocytopenia with absent radii syndrome
  Robert's pseudothalidomide–SC syndrome
  Grebe's syndrome
Proximal femoral focal deficiency
  Femoral hypoplasia–unusual facies syndrome
  Femur–fibula–ulna complex
  Femur–tibia–radius complex
Split hand/split foot (SH/SF) syndromes
  Only SH/SF
  SH/SF and absent long bones
  Ectrodactyly, ectodermal dysplasia, cleft lip and palate syndrome
Others
  Split foot and triphalangeal thumb, autosomal dominant
  Split foot, or split hand and central polydactyly (see central polydactyly)
  SH/SF and congenital nystagmus (Karsch–Neugebauer syndrome)
  SH/SF and renel malformations (acrorenal syndrome)
  Split foot and mandibulofacial dysostosis (Fontaine's syndrome), autosomal dominant

Reproduced with permission from Goldberg MD. The Dysmorphic Child: An Orthopedic Perspective. New York: Raven Press; 1987.

TABLE 20–23. INCIDENCE OF DIFFERENT TYPES OF LIMB REDUCTION MALFORMATIONS IN HUNGARY, 1975–1977

Type	Total No.	Population Incidence (per 1000 Births)
Terminal transverse	79	0.14
Radial	13	0.09
Ulnar and fibular	41	0.11
Split hand and/or foot	20	0.04
Ring constriction	62	0.11
Total	274	0.49

Adapted from Bod M, Creizel A, Lenz W. Hum Genet. 1983;65:27.

the floor of the mouth, or the lips (glossopalatine ankylosis).[483] The spectrum of anomalies of the extremities is variable, ranging from absent digits to severe deficiencies of all four extremities. Intelligence is generally normal. The condition is sporadic and has been attributed to a vascular accident.[484,485] It includes Moebius's syndrome,[486] aglossia–adactylia syndrome, Hanhart's syndrome,[487–491] glossopalatine ankylosis syndrome, limb deficiency–splenogonadal fusion syndrome, and Charlie M's syndrome. There is confusion in the classification of these patients because of the associated anomalies and the frequency of overlapping features. Although some authors have considered Hanhart's syndrome and glossopalatine ankylosis syndrome as distinct entities, differential diagnosis is extremely difficult.[492]

The Mobius sequence consists of a number of facial anomalies attributed to paralysis of the sixth and seventh cranial nerves.[493] Limited jaw mobility and micrognathia are present.[494,495] Ptosis is also a common feature. The Mobius sequence is generally sporadic, but autosomal dominant and recessive forms have been described.[496,497] The associated limb reduction anomalies (25% of cases) are generally present in the upper extremities and range from transverse deficiencies to absent digits. Mental retardation occurs in 10% of cases.[496] The Mobius, Poland, and Klippel–Feil syndromes have been considered subclavian artery supply disruption sequences, based on the hypothesis that interruption of the early embryonic blood supply to the subclavian artery, vertebral artery, and/or their branches may lead to these conditions.[497–503]

Limb Reduction Defects Associated With Other Anomalies

Congenital hemidysplasia with ichthyosiform erythroderma and limb defects (CHILD syndrome) is a defect characterized by strict demarcation of skin lesions to one side of the midline.[504–506] The presence of unilateral defects of long bones is an important feature of the syndrome.[507] Limb deficiencies may differ, from hypoplasia of phalanges or metacarpals to complete absence of an extremity. The calvarium, scapulae, or ribs also may be involved. Zellweger's syndrome, chondrodysplasia punctata, and warfarin embryopathy may present with similar findings. Visceral anomalies include congenital heart disease,[507,508] absence of the thyroid, unilateral hydronephrosis, hydroureter, and unilateral absence of the kidney, fallopian tube, ovaries, and adrenal gland. The CHILD syndrome predominantly affects females (by a ratio of 19 to 1).[509,510]

Fibula aplasia complex brachydactyly (Du Pan's syndrome) is an extremely rare condition characterized by bilateral agenesis of the fibula with abnormalities of the metacarpals and proximal phalanges. Limb reduction defects can involve the lower extremities.[511] An autosomal recessive pattern of inheritance has been suggested.

The splenogonadal fusion syndrome is characterized by limb reduction defects and splenogonadal fusion.[512,513] Most reported cases have occurred in males.[514] Typically, there is a mass in the scrotum, and an ectopic spleen is identified during surgery.[515] There is a continuous type in which the normally located spleen is connected to the gonad by bands or cords of splenic tissue.[516] A review of 14 reported cases indicates that there is some overlap between this syndrome and aglossia–adactylia syndrome or Hanhart's syndrome.[517]

The Adams–Oliver syndrome is a group of disorders characterized by the association of limb reduction defects and scalp anomalies (aplasia cutis and deficiency of bony calvarium).[518] Sporadic and familial cases have been reported.

PHOCOMELIA

In phocomelia the extremities resemble those of a seal. Typically, the hands and feet are present, but the intervening arms and legs are absent. Hands and feet may be normal or abnormal. Three syndromes must be considered in the differential diagnosis of phocomelia: Robert's syndrome, some varieties of the thrombocytopenia with absent radius (TAR) syndrome, and Grebe's syndrome. Phocomelia also can be caused by exposure to thalidomide, but this is only of historical interest.[519] Recently, the diagnosis of phocomelia was reported with 3D ultrasound.[520]

Robert's syndrome is an autosomal recessive disorder characterized by the association of tetraphocomelia and facial dysmorphisms (hypertelorism, facial clefting defects, hypoplastic nasal alae).[521–523] The upper extremities are generally more severely affected than the lower extremities. The spine is not involved. Polyhydramnios has been noted, and other anomalies associated with the syndrome include horseshoe kidney, hydrocephaly, cephalocele, and spina bifida.[524] Prenatal diagnosis has been reported.[524]

Grebe's syndrome is a condition described among inbred Indian tribes from Brazil. It is an autosomal recessive disorder characterized by marked hypomelia of upper and lower limbs increasing in severity from proximal to distal segments.[525,526] In contrast to Robert's syndrome, the lower limbs are more affected than the upper extremities. Many affected fetuses die *in utero* or during the first year of life. Survivors have normal intelligence and develop normal secondary sexual characteristics. Antenatal diagnosis of Grebe's syndrome in twin pregnancy has been reported.[527]

Thrombocytopenia with absent radius syndrome is discussed in detail in the section on radial clubhand deformities.

Focal Proximal Femoral Deficiency, or Congenital Short Femur

Proximal femoral focal deficiency, or congenital short femur, refers to a group of disorders encompassing a wide range of congenital developmental anomalies of the femur. The disorder has been classified into five groups: type I, simple hypoplasia of the femur; type II, short femur with angulated shaft; type III, short femur with coxa vara (the most common); type IV, absent or defective proximal femur, and type V, absent or rudimentary femur.[528,529] One or both femurs can be affected, although the right femur is more frequently involved. Anomalies of the upper limbs can also be present and do not exclude the diagnosis.[176] The focal proximal femoral deficiency syndrome may be associated with umbilical or inguinal hernias. If both femurs are affected, it is important to examine the face carefully. The disorder may be femoral hypoplasia and unusual face syndrome,[530,531] which consists of bilateral femoral hypoplasia and facial defects, including short nose with broad tip, long philtrum, micrognathia, and cleft palate. Long bone abnormalities can extend to other segments of the lower extremities (absent fibula) and to the upper extremities. The syndrome is sporadic and has been associated with maternal diabetes mellitus. A familiar form has been described. This diagnosis has been made *in utero*.[532]

If the defect is unilateral, it may correspond to the femur–fibula–ulna or femur–tibia–radius complex. These two syndromes have different implications for genetic counseling: the former is nonfamilial, whereas the second has a strong genetic component.[533]

Split Hand and Foot Deformities

The term *split–hand–and foot syndrome* refers to a group of disorders characterized by splitting of the hand and foot into two parts. Other terms include *lobster claw deformity, ectrodactyly,* and *aborted fingers.*[534,535] The conditions are classified into typical and atypical varieties.[536] The typical form consists of the absence of both the finger and the metacarpal bone, resulting in a deep V-shaped central defect that clearly divides the hand into an ulnar and a radial part. It occurs in 1 per 90,000 live births and has a familial tendency (usually inherited with an autosomal dominant pattern).[537] The atypical variety is characterized by a much wider cleft formed by a defect of the metacarpals and the middle fingers. As a consequence, the cleft is U-shaped and wide, with only thumb and small finger remaining. It occurs in 1 per 150,000 live births.[538]

A complex system for the classification of these disorders, based on the distribution of remaining fingers, has been proposed.[539] However, this system is of limited value in differential diagnosis and syndrome classification. Split–hand–and foot deformities can occur as isolated anomalies or as part of a more complex syndrome. The syndromic types are the ones more frequently encountered.

The split–hand–and foot and absent long bones syndromes include two conditions in which there is split hand and aplasia of the tibia or split foot with aplasia of the ulna. However, skeletal anomalies are not limited to these bones; the clavicle, femur, and fibula can also be affected. The pattern of inheritance of these disorders has not been clearly determined. Autosomal dominant, recessive, and X-linked recessive patterns have been proposed.[540]

The ectrodactyly ectodermal dysplasia–cleft lip/palate syndrome is an autosomal dominant condition which generally involves the four extremities, with more severe deformities of the hands.[541,542] The spectrum of ectodermal defects is wide, and includes hypopigmentation, dry skin, sparse hair, and dental defects.[543–546] Tear duct anomalies and decreased lacrimal secretions may lead to chronic keratoconjunctivitis and severe loss of visual acuity.[547,548] The cleft lip is generally bilateral. Obstructive uropathy often occurs in this condition.[549] Intelligence is generally normal.[550]

A different group of syndromes involve associations of the split–hand–and foot deformities with other anomalies. These entities include split foot and triphalangeal thumb, split foot and hand and central polydactyly, Karsch–Neugebauer syndrome (split hand and foot with congenital nystagmus), acrorenal syndrome, and mandibulofacial dysostosis (Fontaine's syndrome).[551]

CLUBHANDS

Clubhand deformities are classified into two main categories: radial and ulnar. Radial clubhand includes a spectrum of disorders that encompass absent thumb, thumb hypoplasia, thin first metacarpal, and absent radius (Table 20–24). Ulnar clubhand is much less frequent than radial clubhand and the severity ranges from mild deviations of the hand of the ulnar side of the forearm to complete absence of the ulna. Although radial clubhand is frequently syndromic, ulnar clubhand is usually an isolated anomaly. Table 20–25 presents conditions that present with ulnar ray defects.

Whenever a clubhand is identified, it is important to conduct a thorough examination of the fetus and newborn to delineate associated anomalies that may suggest a syndrome. Fetal blood-sampling and fetal echocardiography are recommended. A complete blood cell count, including platelets, is important to establish the diagnosis of Fanconi's pancytopenia, TAR syndrome, and Aase's syndrome. A fetal karyotype is indicated because several chromosomal abnormalities (e.g., trisomy 18, trisomy 21, and other structural aberrations) have been reported in association with clubhand deformities. Congenital heart disease is an important feature of Holt–Oram syndrome, Lewis upper limb–cardiovascular syndrome, and some cases of TAR syndrome.

Radial Clubhand

The term *isolated radial clubhand* indicates that the clubhand is not part of a recognized syndrome.[552,553] However, this does not exclude that other anomalies may be present (e.g., scoliosis, congenital heart disease). Isolated nonsyndromic radial clubhand is generally a sporadic disorder.[553–556]

Radial clubhand may be part of the three syndromes characterized by hematologic abnormalities: Fanconi's pancytopenia, TAR syndrome, and Aase's syndrome.

Fanconi's anemia (pancytopenia) is an autosomal recessive disease characterized by the association of bone marrow failure (anemia, leukopenia, and thrombocytopenia)[557] and skeletal anomalies, including a radial clubhand with absent thumbs, radial hypoplasia, and a high frequency of chromosomal instability (demonstrated in amniotic fluid cells or fetal lymphocytes as a high frequency of chromosomal breakage after incubation with diepoxy-butane).[558–561] Approximately 25% of affected individuals do not have limb reduction anomalies. Associated findings include microcephaly, congenital dislocation of the hip, scoliosis, and cardiac, pulmonary, and gastrointestinal anomalies.[562–564] Intrauterine growth retardation is common. Up to 25% of the patients will show some degree of mental deficiency. It is assumed that the basic defect is related to the ability to repair DNA damage, in particular that of so-called DNA cross links. Currently, there are eight complementation groups in Fanconi's anemia (FA-A-FA-H), which indicate that at least eight independent genes can lead to Fanconi's anemia. Three of these genes have been identified: FANCA, FANCC, and FANCG.[565–566] Prenatal diagnosis has been reported many times.[567]

Thrombocytopenia with absent radius (TAR) syndrome is an autosomal recessive disorder characterized by thrombocytopenia (platelet count of less than 100,000/mm³)[568–572] and bilateral absence of the radius.[573,574] The thumb and metacarpals are always present. The ulna and humerus may be absent, and clubfoot deformities may be present. Congenital heart disease is present in 33% of cases (e.g., tetralogy of Fallot and septal defects). Delivery by cesarean section is recommended, because these fetuses are at risk for intracranial hemorrhage.[575,576] TAR has been successfully diagnosed *in utero* many times.[577–580]

Aase's syndrome is an autosomal recessive condition characterized by congenital hypoplastic anemia and a radial clubhand with bilateral triphalangeal thumb and a hypoplastic distal radius.[581–584] Cardiac defects (ventricular septal defects, coarctation of the aorta) may be present.[585] Triphalangeal thumbs are a feature of several bone dysostoses and malformation syndromes.[586] They may also occur in random association with other defects and as isolated, often familial, anomalies.[587] Other disorders with this condition are Holt–Oram syndrome, Diamond–Blackfan syndrome,[588,589] chromosomal abnormalities, and fetal hydantoin syndrome.

Holt–Oram syndrome is an autosomal dominant disorder characterized by congenital heart disease (mainly atrial septal defects, secundum type, and ventricular septal defects),[589–593] aplasia or hypoplasia of the radius, and triphalangeal or absent thumbs.[71,594] Limb defects are often asymmetric, with the left side being more affected than the right side. There is no correlation between the severity of the limb

TABLE 20–24. RADIAL RAY DEFECTS: A DIFFERENTIAL DIAGNOSIS OF CONGENITAL DEFICIENCY OF THE RADIUS AND RADIAL RAY

I. Isolated: nonsyndromatic

II. Syndromes with blood dyscrasias
   A. Fanconi's anemia
   B. Thrombocytopenia with absent radii syndrome
   C. Aase's syndrome: congenital anemia, nonopposable triphalangeal thumb, scaphoid and distal radius hypoplasia, radioulnar synostosis, short stature with narrow shoulders, autosomal recessive (see Diamond–Blackfan syndrome for a similar, perhaps identical, syndrome)

III. Syndromes with congenital heart disease
   A. Holt–Oram syndrome
   B. Lewis upper limb–cardiovascular syndrome: more extensive arm malformations and more complex heart anomalies than with Holt–Oram, but probably not a separate syndrome, autosomal dominant

IV. Syndromes with craniofacial abnormalities
   A. Nager acrofacial dysostosis
   B. Radial clubhand and cleft lip and/or cleft palate: sporadic
   C. Juberg–Hayward syndrome: cleft lip and palate, hypoplastic thumbs, short radius, radial head subluxation, autosomal recessive
   D. Baller–Gerold syndrome: craniosynostosis, bilateral radial clubhand, absent/hypoplastic thumb; autosomal recessive
   E. Rothmund–Thomson syndrome: prematurely aged skin changes, juvenile cataract, sparse gray hair, absent thumbs, radial clubhands, occasional knee dysplasia (see progeria syndromes)
   F. Duane–radial dysplasia syndrome: abnormal ocular movements: inability to abduct and eyeball retraction with adduction, radius and radial ray hypoplasia, vertebral anomalies, renal malformation, autosomal dominant (see Klippel–Feil variants)
   G. The IVIC syndrome (Instituto Venezolano de Investigaciones Cientificas): radial ray deficiency, hypoplastic or absent thumbs and radial clubhands, impaired hearing, abnormal movements of extraocular muscles with strabismus, autosomal dominant
   H. LARD syndrome (lacrimo-auriculo-radial-dental; Levy–Hollister): absent lacrimal structures, protuberant ears, thumb and radial ray hypoplasia, abnormal teeth, autosomal dominant
   I. Radial defects with ear anomalies and cranial nerve 7 dysfunction
   J. Radial hypoplasia, triphalangeal thumb, hypospadias, diastema of maxillary central incisors, autosomal dominant

V. Syndromes with congenital scoliosis
   A. The VATER association
   B. Goldenhar syndrome (oculoauriculovertebral dysplasia)
   C. Klippel–Feil syndrome

VI. Radial aplasia and chromosome aberrations

VII. Syndromes with mental retardation
   A. Seckel's syndrome (bird-headed dwarfism): microcephaly, beaklike protrusion of nose, mental retardation, absent/hypoplastic thumbs, bilateral dislocated hips

VIII. Thalidomide embryopathy (of historical interest, but some 60% had radial clubhand)

Reproduced with permission from Goldberg MD. The Dysmorphic Child: An Orthopedic Perspective. New York: Raven Press; 1987.

defects and the cardiac anomaly.[595,596] Indeed, some individuals have only a skeletal anomaly.[596] Other findings include hypertelorism, chest wall, and vertebral anomalies.[597–600] This condition has been diagnosed prenatally.[601,602] The mutation that causes Holt–Oram syndrome has recently been identified.[68,603] The upper limb–cardiovascular syndrome described by Lewis et al. is probably not a separate entity from the Holt–Oram syndrome.[604]

Radial clubhand is also associated with congenital scoliosis. The three syndromes that should be considered part of the differential diagnosis include VATER association, some cases of Goldenhar's syndrome, and Klippel–Feil syndrome.[605]

The VATER association is the result of defective mesodermal development during embryogenesis before the 35th day of gestation.[606–610] Typical findings are vertebral segmentation (70%), anal atresia (80%), tracheo-esophageal fistula (70%), esophageal atresia, and radial and renal defects (65% and 53%, respectively).[611,612] Other anomalies include a single umbilical artery (35%) and congenital heart disease, occurring in nearly 50% of patients.[613–618] The VATER association occurs sporadically, although recurrence within a sibship has been reported.[617] Prenatal diagnosis by sonography has been reported.[618]

Goldenhar's syndrome is characterized by hemifacial microsomia, vertebral anomalies, and radial defects.[619–623] Alterations in the morphogenesis of the first and second brachial arches result in hypoplasia of the malar, maxillary, or mandibular region, microtia, and ocular and oropharyngeal anomalies.[624–629] Prenatal diagnosis has been reported.[629]

Radial clubhand has been reported in association with several chromosomal anomalies, including trisomies 18 and 21, deletion of the long arm of 13, and ring formation of chromosome 4.[558,630,631]

TABLE 20–25. ULNAR RAY DEFECTS: A DIFFERENTIAL DIAGNOSIS OF CONGENITAL DEFICIENCY OF THE ULNA AND ULNAR RAY

I. Isolated: nonsyndromatic absent ulna

II. Ulna hypoplasia and skeletal deficiency elsewhere
   A. Ulna aplasia with lobster claw deformity of hand and/or foot, autosomal dominant
   B. Femur–fibula–ulna complex

III. Syndromes with ulna deficiency
   A. Cornelia de Lange's syndrome
   B. Miller syndrome (postaxial acrofacial dysostosis): absent ulna and ulnar rays and absent fourth and fifth toes; Treacher–Collins mandibulofacial hypoplasia, autosomal recessive; distinguish from Nagar preaxial acrofacial dysostosis
   C. Pallister ulnar–mammary syndrome: hypoplasia of ulna and ulnar rays; hypoplasia of the breast and absence of apocrine sweat glands, autosomal dominant
   D. Pillay syndrome (ophthalmomandibulomelic dysplasia): absent distal third of ulna, absent olecranon, hypoplastic trochlea and proximal radius, fusion of interphalangeal joints in ulnar fingers, knee dysplasia; corneal opacities, fusion of temporomandibular joint, autosomal dominant
   E. Weyers' oligodactyly syndrome: deficiency of ulna and ulnar rays, antecubital webbing, short sternum, malformed kidney and spleen, cleft lip and palate, sporadic
   F. Schnizel's syndrome: absent/hypoplastic fourth, fifth metacarpals and phalanges, hypogenitalism, anal atresia, autosomal dominant
   G. Mesometic dwarfism, Reinhardt–Pfeiffer type (ulno–fibula dysplasia): a generalized bone dysplasia but with a disproportionate hypoplasia of the ulna and fibula, autosomal dominant
   H. Mesomelic dwarfism, Langer's type: a generalized bone dysplasia, but with aplasia of the distal ulna and proximal fibula and hypoplasia of the mandible

Reproduced with permission from Goldberg MD. The Dysmorphic Child: An Orthopedic Perspective. New York: Raven Press; 1987.

Some disorders present with craniofacial abnormalities and radial clubhand deformities. These syndromes are sporadic and have many common features that make a specific prenatal diagnosis difficult. The most common craniofacial anomalies are cleft lip and palate. Uuspaa's study of 3225 cases with orofacial cleft showed a 2.8% association with upper extremity deformities.[632]

Ulnar clubhand occurs as an isolated, nonsyndromic anomaly in most cases. It can also be associated with a variety of syndromes (e.g., Poland's complex).[633]

POLYDACTYLY

Polydactyly is the presence of an additional digit.[634,635] The extra digit may range from a fleshy nubbin to a complete digit with controlled flexion and extension (Figs. 20–28 and 20–29). Polydactyly can be classified as postaxial (the most common form), preaxial, and central. Postaxial polydactyly occurs on the ulnar side of the hand and fibular side of the foot.[636–638] Preaxial polydactyly is present on the radial side of the hand and the tibial side of the foot[639] (Fig. 20–30).

Most cases reported isolated conditions with an autosomal dominant mode of inheritance. Some are part of a syndrome, usually an autosomal recessive one.[640–642] Preaxial polydactyly, especially a triphalangeal thumb, is most likely to be part of a syndrome. Central polydactyly consists of an extra digit that is usually hidden between the long and ring fingers. It is often bilateral and is inherited as an autosomal trait. It can be associated with other hand and foot malformations.[643–646]

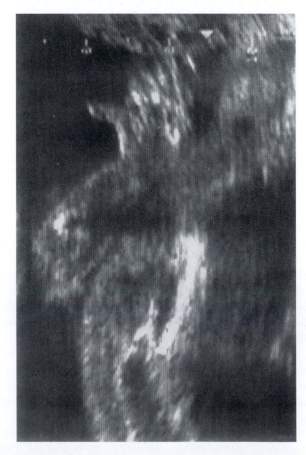

Figure 20–29. Sonographic image of the hand shown in Fig. 20–28. Note the abnormal angulation of the extra digit on the ulnar side of the forearm.

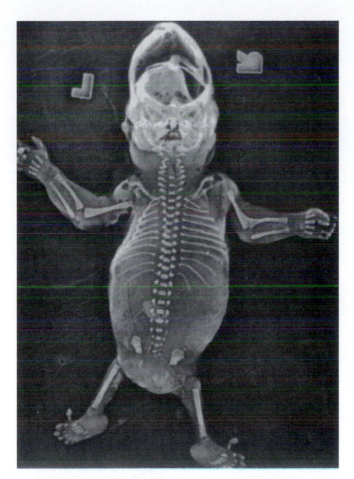

Figure 20–30. Unusual facies–femoral hypoplasia syndrome. Note the absence of the left femur and only a tiny portion of ossified bone on the right side. There is partial fusion of the tibia and fibula. Of interest is the presence of preaxial polydactyly in both feet.

ARTHROGRYPOSIS

The term *arthrogryposis multiplex congenita* (AMC) refers to multiple joint contractures present at birth in an intact skeleton.[647–649] Normal fetal movement between 7 and 8 weeks of gestation onward is important for the development of the joints; limitation of the fetal joint motion leads to the development of contractures and AMC.[650,651] This has been confirmed in animal models,[652] chick and rats embryos by using tubocurarin and butulism toxins,[653,654] inducing viral myopathy by coxakie A viruses,[655] and cross-section of the spinal cord.[656] Therefore, AMC is a syndrome, not a specific disorder. The incidence of the different underlying causes of AMC is variable in the literature. Neurologic, muscular, connective tissue, or skeletal abnormalities can lead to impaired fetal motion and AMC.[650,651] Table 20–26 shows motor systems that can lead to AMC. In a series of 74 children, Banker found that the most common cause of AMC was a neurogenic disorder followed by myopathic disorders.[657] Swinyard reported that central nervous system disorders are cause in 75% and muscle disorders in 10 to 15%

TABLE 20–26. DISORDERS OF THE DEVELOPING MOTOR SYSTEM ON ALL LEVELS, LEADING TO IMMOBILIZATION

Disorders of the developing neuromuscular system
Loss of anterior horn cells
Radicular disease with collagen proliferation
Peripheral neuropathy with neurofibromatosis
Congenital myasthenia
Neonatal myasthenia (maternal myasthenia gravis)
Amyoplasia congenita
Congenital muscular dystrophy
Central core disease
Congenital myotonic dystrophy
Glycogen accumulation myopathy
Disorders of developing connective tissue or connective tissue disease
Muscular and articular connective tissue dystrophy
Articular defects by mesenchymal dysplasia
Increased collagen synthesis
Disorders of developing medulla or medullar disease
Congenital spinal epidural hemorrhage
Congenital duplication of the spinal canal
Disorders of brain development (e.g., porencephaly or brain disease)
Congenital encephalopathy

based on autopsies of 75 cases of fetuses and newborns.[658] Quinn et al. reported that only 5 of 21 cases of lethal AMC were of neurogenic cause, 11 were myogenic and 5 were of uncertain etiology.[659] The condition is present in 0.03% live births,[660,661] The etiology of AMC may derive from hereditary conditions,[662–669] infectious agents, drugs, toxins, and fetal alcohol syndrome.[650,651,670] Maternal hyperthermia also has been associated with AMC.[671] Maternal antibodies specific for a fetal acetylcholine receptor have been recently reported to cause fetal AMC without evidence of maternal myasthenia gravis.[672,673] In addition, plasma from human mothers of fetuses with AMC when injected into pregnant mice causes deformities in offspring.[674] The pattern of inheritance depends on the specific cause of AMC.[675] In a series of 350 cases, Hall found that 46% of cases corresponded to a syndrome with no recurrence risk, 23% corresponded to disorders inherited with a mendelian pattern (autosomal dominant, recessive, or X-linked), 20% were unknown conditions, 6% were associated with environmental disorders, 3% were chromosomal, and 2% were multifactorial in origin.[676]

The recurrence risk differs depending on the underlying cause. Hall and Reed found that in 20% of 350 patients no diagnosis was made. They concluded that in this situation, the risk for recurrence is 4.7% if only the limbs are affected, 7% if the central nervous system is involved, and 1.4% if the limbs and another system are involved.[670]

The deformities are usually symmetric. In most cases of AMC, all four limbs are involved (Fig. 20–31), followed by deformities of the lower extremities only or bimelic involvement. The severity of the deformities increases distally

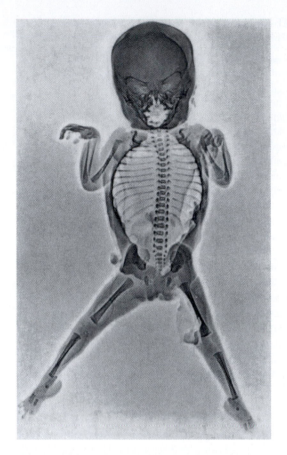

Figure 20–31. Arthrogryposis multiplex congenita. There is flexion of the upper limbs with hyperextension of the lower limbs.

in the involved limb, with the hands and feet typically being the most deformed.

Many congenital anomalies are associated with AMC. The most frequent are cleft palate, Klippel–Feil syndrome, meningomyelocele, and congenital heart disease. Ten percent of patients with AMC have associated anomalies of the central nervous system.[647]

The prenatal diagnosis of AMC with ultrasound has been reported in some cases.[677–682] The cardinal findings are absent fetal movement on real-time examination and severe flexion deformities.[678]

The prognosis of AMC depends on the specific cause. Although some cases are uniformly lethal, others are associated with mild to moderate handicap. Fahy and Hall, in a retrospective study of 828 cases, found that polyhydramnios is a poor prognostic sign.[683]

REFERENCES

1. Mundlos S, Olsen BR. Heritable diseases of the skeleton. Part I: Molecular insights into skeletal development—Transcription factors and signaling pathways. *FASEB J.* 1997;11:125–132.
2. Mundlos S, Olsen BR. Heritable diseases of the skeleton. Part II: Molecular insights into skeletal development—Matrix components and their homeostasis. *FASEB J.* 1997;11:227–233.
3. Frassica FJ, Inoue N, Vivolainen P, et al. Skeletal system: Biomechanical concepts and relationships to normal and abnormal conditions. *Semin Nucl Med.* 1997;27:321–327.
4. Gilbert-Barness E, Opitz JM. Abnormal bone development: Histopathology of skeletal dysplasias. *Birth Defects Orig Art Ser.* 1996;30:103–156.
5. Erlebacher A, Filvaroff EH, Gitelman SE, et al. Toward a molecular understanding of skeletal development [comment]. *Cell.* 1995;80:371–378.
6. Horton WA. Progress in human chondrodysplasias: Molecular genetics. *Ann N Y Acad Sci.* 1996;785:150–159.
7. Reardon W. Skeletal dysplasias detectable by DNA analysis. *Prenat Diagn.* 1996;16:1221–1236.
8. Wozney JM, Rosen V, Celeste AJ, et al. Novel regulators of bone formation: Molecular clones and activities. *Science.* 1988;242(4885):1528–1534.
9. Wozney JM. The bone morphogenetic protein family and osteogenesis. *Mol Reprod Dev.* 1992;32:160–167.
10. Rosen V, Thies RS, Lyons K. Signaling pathways in skeletal formation: A role for BMP receptors. *Ann N Y Acad Sci.* 1996;785:59–69.
11. Chang SC, Hoang B, Thomas JT, et al. Cartilage-derived morphogenetic proteins. New members of the transforming growth factor-beta superfamily predominantly expressed in long bones during human embryonic development. *J Biol Chem.* 1994;269:28227–28234.
12. Venkataraman G, Sasisekharan V, Cooney CL, et al. Complex flexibility of the transforming growth factor beta superfamily. *Proc Natl Acad Sci U S A.* 1995;92:5406–5410.
13. Kingsley DM, Bland AE, Grubber JM, et al. The mouse short ear skeletal morphogenesis locus is associated with defects in a bone morphogenetic member of the TGF beta superfamily. *Cell.* 1992;71:399–410.
14. Kingsley DM. The TGF-beta superfamily: New members, new receptors, and new genetic tests of function in different organisms. *Genes Dev.* 1994;8:133–146.
15. Langer LO Jr, Cervenka J, Camargo M. A severe autosomal recessive acromesomelic dysplasia, the Hunter–Thompson type, and comparison with the Grebe type. *Hum Genet.* 1989; 81:323–328.
16. Thomas JT, Lin K, Nandedkar M, et al. A human chondrodysplasia due to a mutation in a TGF-beta superfamily member. *Nat Genet.* 1996;12:315–317.
17. Robin NH, Gunay-Aygun M, Polinkovsky A, et al. Clinical and locus heterogeneity in brachydactyly type C. *Am J Med Genet.* 1997;68:369–377.
18. Polinkovsky A, Robin NH, Thomas JT, et al. Mutations in CDMP1 cause autosomal dominant brachydactyly type C. *Nat Genet.* 1997;17:18–19.
19. Latchman D. S. Transcription-factor mutations and disease. *N Engl J Med.* 1996;334:28–33.
20. Latchman DS. *Gene Regulation: A Eukaryotic Perspective,* 2nd ed. London: Chapman & Hall, 1998.
21. Papavassiliou AG. Molecular medicine. Transcription. *N Engl J Med.* 1995;332:45–47.
22. Manak JR, Mathies LD, Scott MP. Regulation of a decapentaplegic midgut enhancer by homeotic proteins. *Development.* 1994;120:3605–3619.

23. Manak JR, Scott MP. A class act: Conservation of homeo-domain protein functions. *Development.* 1994;(suppl):61–77.

24. Morgan BA, Tabin CJ. The role of Hox genes in limb development. *Curr Opin Genetic Dev.* 1993;4:668.

25. Morgan BA, Tabin C. Hox genes and growth: Early and late roles in limb bud morphogenesis. *Development.* 1994;(suppl): 181–186.

26. Morgan BA. Hox genes and embryonic development. *Poult Sci.* 1997;76:96–104.

27. Gehring WJ, Muller M, Affolter M, et al. The structure of the homeodomain and its functional implications. *Trends Genet.* 1990;6:323–329.

28. Gehring WJ. Exploring the homeobox. *Gene.* 1993;135:215–221.

29. Gehring WJ, Qian YQ, Billeter M, et al. Homeodomain–DNA recognition. *Cell.* 1994;78:211–223.

30. Gehring WJ, Affolter M, Burglin T. Homeodomain proteins. *Annu Rev Biochem.* 1994;63:487–526.

31. Dorn A, Affolter M, Gehring WJ, et al. Homeodomain proteins in development and therapy. *Pharmacol Ther.* 1994;61:155–184.

32. Zakany J, Duboule D. Hox genes in digit development and evolution. *Cell Tissue Res.* 1999;296:19–25.

33. Muragaki Y, Mundlos S, Upton J, et al. Altered growth and branching patterns in synpolydactyly caused by mutations in HOXD13 [see comments]. *Science.* 1996;272(5261):548–551.

34. Gruss P, Walther C. Pax in development. *Cell.* 1992;69: 719–722.

35. Chalepakis G, Tremblay P, Gruss P. Pax genes, mutants and molecular function. *J Cell Sci.* 1992;16(suppl):61–67.

36. Chalepakis G, Tremblay P, Gruss P. Pax-3 contains domains for transcription activation and transcription inhibition. *Proc Natl Acad Sci U S A.* 1994;91:12745–12749.

37. Tassabehji M, Read AP, Newton VE, et al. Waardenburg's syndrome patients have mutations in the human homo-logue of the Pax-3 paired box gene [see comments]. *Nature.* 1992;355(6361):635–636.

38. Tassabehji M, Read AP, Newton VE, et al. Mutations in the PAX3 gene causing Waardenburg syndrome type 1 and type 2. *Nat Genet.* 1993;3:26–30.

39. Tekin M, Tutar E, Arsan S, et al. Ophthalmo-acromelic syndrome: Report and review. *Am J Med Genet.* 2000;90:150–154.

40. Singer S, Bower C, Southall P, et al. Craniosynostosis in Western Australia. 1980–1994: A population-based study. *Am J Med Genet.* 1999;83:382–387.

41. Maas R, Chen YP, Bei M, et al. The role of Msx genes in mammalian development. *Ann N Y Acad Sci.* 1996;785:171–181.

42. Jabs EW, Muller U, Li X, et al. A mutation in the homeodomain of the human MSX2 gene in a family affected with autosomal dominant craniosynostosis. *Cell.* 1993;75:443–450.

43. Maraia R, Saal HM, Wangsa D. A chromosome 17q de novo paracentric inversion in a patient with campomelic dysplasia; case report and etiologic hypothesis. *Clin Genet.* 1991; 39:401–408.

44. Tommerup N, Schempp W, Meinecke P, et al. Assignment of an autosomal sex reversal locus (SRA1) and campomelic dysplasia (CMPD1) to 17q24.3-q25.1. *Nat Genet.* 1993;4: 170–174.

45. Wirth J, Wagner T, Meyer J, et al. Translocation breakpoints in three patients with campomelic dysplasia and autosomal sex reversal map more than 130 kb from SOX9. *Hum Genet.* 1996;97:186–193.

46. Ramkissoon Y, Goodfellow P. Early steps in mammalian sex determination. *Curr Opin Genet Dev.* 1996;6:316–321.

47. Denny P, Swift S, Connor F, et al. An SRY-related gene expressed during spermatogenesis in the mouse encodes a sequence-specific DNA-binding protein. *EMBO J.* 1992;11: 3705–3712.

48. Denny P, Swift S, Brand N, et al. A conserved family of genes related to the testis determining gene, SRY. *Nucleic Acids Res.* 1992;20:2887.

49. MacLean HE, Warne GL, Zajac JD. Intersex disorders: Shedding light on male sexual differentiation beyond SRY. *Clin Endocrinol.* 1997;46:101–108.

50. Ng LJ, Wheatley S, Muscat GE, et al. SOX9 binds DNA, activates transcription, and coexpresses with type II collagen during chondrogenesis in the mouse. *Dev Biol.* 1997;183:108–121.

51. Wright EM, Snopek B, Koopman P. Seven new members of the Sox gene family expressed during mouse development. *Nucleic Acids Res.* 1993;21:744.

52. Prior HM, Walter MA. SOX genes: Architects of development. *Mol Med.* 1996;2:405–412.

53. Stevanovic M, Lovell-Badge R, Collignon J, et al. SOX3 is an X-linked gene related to SRY. *Hum Mol Genet.* 1993;2:2013–2018.

54. Bi W, Deng JM, Zhang Z, et al. Sox9 is required for cartilage formation. *Nat Genet.* 1999;22:85–89.

55. Lefebvre V, de Crombrugghe B. Toward understanding SOX9 function in chondrocyte differentiation. *Matrix Biol.* 1998;16:529–540.

56. McDowall S, Argentaro A, Ranganathan S, et al. Functional and structural studies of wild type SOX9 and mutations causing campomelic dysplasia. *J Biol Chem.* 1999;274:24023–24030.

57. Hageman RM, Cameron FJ, Sinclair AH. Mutation analysis of the SOX9 gene in a patient with campomelic dysplasia. *Hum Mutat.* 1998;1(suppl):S112–S113.

58. Schafer AJ, Foster JW, Kwok C, et al. Campomelic dysplasia with XY sex reversal: Diverse phenotypes resulting from mutations in a single gene. *Ann N Y Acad Sci.* 1996;785: 137–149.

59. Schafer AJ, Dominguez-Steglich MA, Guioli S, et al. The role of SOX9 in autosomal sex reversal and campomelic dysplasia. *Phil Trans R Soc Lond B Biol Sci.* 1995;350(1333):271–278.

60. Foster JW, Dominguez-Steglich MA, Guioli S, et al. Campomelic dysplasia and autosomal sex reversal caused by mutations in an SRY-related gene. *Nature.* 1994;372(6506): 525–530.

61. Wagner T, Wirth J, Meyer J, et al. Autosomal sex reversal and campomelic dysplasia are caused by mutations in and around the SRY-related gene SOX9. *Cell.* 1994;79:1111–1120.

62. Cameron FJ, Hageman RM, Cooke-Yarborough C, et al. A novel germ line mutation in SOX9 causes familial campomelic dysplasia and sex reversal. *Hum Mol Genet.* 1996;5: 1625–1630.

63. Foster JW. Mutations in SOX9 cause both autosomal sex reversal and campomelic dysplasia. *Acta Paediatr Jpn.* 1996;38:405–411.

64. Kwok C, Weller PA, Guioli S, et al. Mutations in SOX9, the gene responsible for campomelic dysplasia and autosomal

sex reversal [see comments]. *Am J Hum Genet.* 1995; 57:1028–1036.

65. Ninomiya S, Isomura M, Narahara K, et al. Isolation of a testis-specific cDNA on chromosome 17q from a region adjacent to the breakpoint of t(12;17) observed in a patient with acampomelic campomelic dysplasia and sex reversal. *Hum Mol Genet.* 1996;5:69–72.

66. Meyer J, Sudbeck P, Held M, et al. Mutational analysis of the SOX9 gene in campomelic dysplasia and autosomal sex reversal: Lack of genotype/phenotype correlations. *Hum Mol Genet.* 1997;6:91–98.

67. Huang B, Wang S, Ning Y, et al. Autosomal XX sex reversal caused by duplication of SOX9. *Am J Med Genet.* 1999;87:349–353.

68. Basson CT, Bachinsky DR, Lin RC, et al. Mutations in human TBX5 cause limb and cardiac malformation in Holt–Oram syndrome. *Nat Genet.* 1997;15:30–35.

69. Basson CT, Cowley GS, Solomon SD, et al. The clinical and genetic spectrum of the Holt–Oram syndrome (heart–hand syndrome). *N Engl J Med.* 1994;330:885–891.

70. Basson CT, Huang T, Lin RC, et al. Different TBX5 interactions in heart and limb defined by Holt–Oram syndrome mutations. *Proc Natl Acad Sci U S A.* 1999;96:2919–2924.

71. Brockhoff CJ, Kober H, Tsilimingas N, et al. Holt–Oram syndrome. *Circulation.* 1999;99:1395–1396.

72. Shono S, Higa K, Kumano K, et al. Holt–Oram syndrome. *Br J Anaesth.* 1998;80:856–857.

73. Johnson DE, Williams LT. Structural and functional diversity in the FGF receptor multigene family. *Adv Cancer Res.* 1993;60:1–41.

74. Givol D, Yayon A. Complexity of FGF receptors: Genetic basis for structural diversity and functional specificity. *FASEB J.* 1992;6:3362–3369.

75. Deng C, Wynshaw-Boris A, Zhou F, et al. Fibroblast growth factor receptor 3 is a negative regulator of bone growth. *Cell.* 1996;84:911–921.

76. Bellus GA, McIntosh I, Smith EA, et al. A recurrent mutation in the tyrosine kinase domain of fibroblast growth factor receptor 3 causes hypochondroplasia. *Nat Genet.* 1995;10:357–359.

77. Bonaventure J, Rousseau F, Legeai-Mallet L, et al. Common mutations in the gene encoding fibroblast growth factor receptor 3 account for achondroplasia, hypochondroplasia and thanatophoric dysplasia. *Acta Paediatr.* 1996; 417(suppl):33–38.

78. Bonaventure J, Rousseau F, Legeai-Mallet L, et al. Common mutations in the fibroblast growth factor receptor 3 (FGFR 3) gene account for achondroplasia, hypochondroplasia, and thanatophoric dwarfism. *Am J Med Genet.* 1996;63: 148–154.

79. Bonaventure J, Rousseau F, Legeai-Mallet L, et al. Fibroblast growth factor receptors and hereditary abnormalities of bone growth. *Arch Pediatr.* 1997;4:112S–117S.

80. Wilcox WR, Tavormina PL, Krakow D, et al. Molecular, radiologic, and histopathologic correlations in thanatophoric dysplasia. *Am J Med Genet.* 1998;78:274–281.

81. Plomp AS, Hamel BC, Cobben JM, et al. Pfeiffer syndrome type 2: Further delineation and review of the literature. *Am J Med Genet.* 1998;75:245–251.

82. Passos-Bueno MR, Richieri-Costa A, Sertie AL, et al. Presence of the Apert canonical S252W FGFR2 mutation in a patient without severe syndactyly. *J Med Genet.* 1998;35: 677–679.

83. Everett ET, Britto DA, Ward RE, et al. A novel FGFR2 gene mutation in Crouzon syndrome associated with apparent nonpenetrance [in process citation]. *Cleft Palate Craniofac J.* 1999;36:533–541.

84. Tsai FJ, Tsai CH, Peng CT, et al. Molecular diagnosis of Apert syndrome in Chinese patients. *Chung Hua Min Kuo Hsiao Erh Ko I Hsueh Hui Tsa Chih.* 1999;40:31–33.

85. Oldridge M, Zackai EH, McDonald-McGinn DM, et al. De novo alu-element insertions in FGFR2 identify a distinct pathological basis for Apert syndrome. *Am J Hum Genet.* 1999;64:446–461.

86. Chang CC, Tsai FJ, Tsai HD, et al. Prenatal diagnosis of Apert syndrome. *Prenat Diagn.* 1998;18:621–625.

87. Jabs EW, Li X, Scott AF, et al. Jackson–Weiss and Crouzon syndromes are allelic with mutations in fibroblast growth factor receptor 2. *Nat Genet.* 1994;8:275–279.

88. Preston RA, Post JC, Keats BJB, et al. A gene for Crouzon craniofacial dysostosis maps to the long arm of chromosome 10. *Nat Genet.* 1994;7:149–153.

89. Reardon W, Winter RM, Rutland P, et al. Mutations in the fibroblast growth factor receptor 2 gene cause Crouzon syndrome. *Nat Genet.* 1994;8:98–103.

90. Rutland P, Pulleyn LJ, Reardon W, et al. Identical mutations in the FGFR2 gene caused both Pfeiffer and Crouzon syndrome phenotypes. *Nat Genet.* 1995;9:173–176.

91. Li X, Park WJ, Pyeritz R, et al. Effect on splicing of a silent FGFR2 mutation in Crouzon Syndrome. *Nat Genet.* 1995;9:232–233.

92. Malcolm S, Reardon W. Fibroblast growth factor receptor-2 mutations in craniosynostosis. *Ann N Y Acad Sci.* 1996;785: 164–169.

93. Muenke M, Gripp KW, McDonald-McGinn DM, et al. A unique point mutation in the fibroblast growth factor receptor 3 gene (FGFR3) defines a new craniosynostosis syndrome. *Am J Hum Genet.* 1997;60:555–564.

94. Orloff JJ, Kats Y, Urena P, et al. Further evidence for a novel receptor for amino-terminal parathyroid hormone-related protein on keratinocytes and squamous carcinoma cell lines. *Endocrinology.* 1995;136:3016–3023.

95. Schipani E, Kruse K, Juppner H. A constitutively active mutant PTH-PTHrP receptor in Jansen-type metaphyseal chondrodysplasia. *Science.* 1995;268(5207):98–100.

96. Schipani E, Weinstein LS, Bergwitz C, et al. Pseudohypoparathyroidism type Ib is not caused by mutations in the coding exons of the human parathyroid hormone (PTH)/PTH-related peptide receptor gene. *J Clin Endocrinol Metab.* 1995; 80:1611–1621.

97. Schipani E, Langman C, Hunzelman J, et al. A novel parathyroid hormone (PTH)/PTH-related peptide receptor mutation in Jansen's metaphyseal chondrodysplasia. *J Clin Endocrinol Metab.* 1999;84:3052–3057.

98. Juppner H, Schipani E. Receptors for parathyroid hormone and parathyroid hormone-related peptide: From molecular cloning to definition of diseases. *Curr Opin Nephrol Hypertens.* 1996;5:300–306.

99. Gardella TJ, Luck MD, Jensen GS, et al. Juppner inverse agonism of amino-terminally truncated parathyroid hormone (PTH) and PTH-related peptide (PTHrP) analogs revealed

with constitutively active mutant PTH/PTHrP receptors. *Endocrinology.* 1996;137:3936–3941.

100. Schipani E, Langman CB, Parfitt AM, et al. Constitutively activated receptors for parathyroid hormone and parathyroid hormone-related peptide in Jansen's metaphyseal chondrodysplasia. *N Engl J Med.* 1996;335:708–714.

101. Schipani E, Lanske B, Hunzelman J, et al. Targeted expression of constitutively active receptors for parathyroid hormone and parathyroid hormone-related peptide delays endochondral bone formation and rescues mice that lack parathyroid hormone-related peptide. *Proc Natl Acad Sci U S A.* 1997;94:13689–13694.

102. Schipani E, Jensen GS, Pincus J, et al. Constitutive activation of the cyclic adenosine 3′,5′-monophosphate signaling pathway by parathyroid hormone (PTH)/PTH-related peptide receptors mutated at the two loci for Jansen's metaphyseal chondrodysplasia. *Mol Endocrinol.* 1997;11:851–858.

103. Leroy JG, Keersmaeckers G, Coppens M, et al. Blomstrand lethal osteochondrodysplasia. *Am J Med Genet.* 1996;63:84–89.

104. Galera MF, de Silva Patricio FR, Lederman HM, et al. Blomstrand chondrodysplasia: A lethal sclerosing skeletal dysplasia. Case report and review. *Pediatr Radiol.* 1999;29:842–845.

105. Karperien M, et al. A frame-shift mutation in the type I parathyroid hormone (PTH)/PTH-related peptide receptor causing Blomstrand lethal osteochondrodysplasia. *J Clin Endocrinol Metab.* 1999;84:3713–3720.

106. Jobert AS, Zhang P, Convineau A, et al. Absence of functional receptors for parathyroid hormone and parathyroid hormone-related peptide in Blomstrand chondrodysplasia. *J Clin Invest.* 1998;102:34–40.

107. Karaplis AC, He B, Nguyen MT, et al. Inactivating mutation in the human parathyroid hormone receptor type 1 gene in Blomstrand chondrodysplasia [see comments]. *Endocrinology.* 1998;139:5255–5258.

108. den Hollander NS, van der Harten HJ, Vermeij-Keers C, et al. First-trimester diagnosis of Blomstrand lethal osteochondrodysplasia. *Am J Med Genet.* 1997;73:345–350.

109. Loshkajian A, Roume J, Stanesu V, et al. Familial Blomstrand chondrodysplasia with advanced skeletal maturation: Further delineation. *Am J Med Genet.* 1997;71:283–288.

110. Boskey AL, Wright TM, Blank RD. Collagen and bone strength. *J Bone Min Res.* 1999;14:330–335.

111. Collagen in health and disease [editorial]. *Lancet.* 1978;1(8073):1077–1079.

112. Kietly CM, Hopkinson I, Grant M. The collagen family: Structure, assembley and organization in the extracellular matrix. In: Royce PM, Steinmann B, eds. *Connective Tissue and Its Heritable Disorders.* New York: Wiley-Liss; 1993:85–102.

113. van der Rest M, Garrone R. Collagen family of proteins. *FASEB J.* 1991;5:2814.

114. Tillet E, Franc JM, Franc S, et al. The evolution of fibrillar collagens: A sea-pen collagen shares common features with vertebrate type V collagen. *Comp Biochem Physiol B Biochem Mol Biol.* 1996;113:239–246.

115. Ruggiero F, Comte J, Cabanas C, et al. Structural requirements for alpha 1 beta 1 and alpha 2 beta 1 integrin mediated cell adhesion to collagen V. *J Cell Sci.* 1996;109:1865–1874.

116. Mundlos S, Chan D, Weng YM, et al. Multiexon deletions in the type I collagen COL1A2 gene in osteogenesis imper-

fecta type IB. Molecules containing the shortened alpha2(I) chains show differential incorporation into the bone and skin extracellular matrix. *J Biol Chem.* 1996;271:21068–21074.

117. Bateman JF, Moeller I, Hannagan M, et al. Characterization of three osteogenesis imperfecta collagen alpha 1(1) glycine to serine mutations demonstrating a position-dependent gradient of phenotypic severity. *J Biochem.* 1992;288:131–135.

118. Cole WG, Dallgleish R. Perinatal lethal osteogenesis imperfecta. *J Med Genet.* 1995;32:284.

119. Wang Q, Orrison BM, Marini JC, et al. Two additional cases of osteogenesis imperfecta with substitutions for glycine in the alpha 2(I) collagen chain. *J Biol Chem.* 1993;268:25162–25167.

120. Willing MC, Pruchno CJ, Atkinson M, et al. Osteogenesis imperfecta type I is commonly due to a COL1A1 null allele of type I collagen. *Am J Hum Genet.* 1992;51:508–515.

121. Willing MC, Deschenes SP, Slayton RL, et al. Premature chain termination is a unifying mechanism for COL1A1 null alleles in osteogenesis imperfecta type 1 cell strains. *Am J Hum Genet.* 1996;59:799–809.

122. Dyne KM, Valli M, Forlina A, et al. Deficient expression of the small proteoglycan decorin in a case of severe/lethal osteogenesis imperfecta. *Am J Med Genet.* 1996;63:161–166.

123. Byers PH, Steiner RD. Osteogenesis imperfecta. *Annu Rev Med.* 1992;43:269–282.

124. Kuivaniemi H, Tromp G, Prockop DJ. Mutations in collagen genes: Causes of rare and some common diseases in humans. *FASEB J.* 1991;5:2052–2060.

125. Azouz EM, et al. Bone dysplasias: An introduction. *Can Assoc Radiol J.* 1998;49:105–109.

126. Spranger J, Winterpacht A, Zabel B, et al. The type II collagenopathies: A spectrum of chondrodysplasias. *Eur J Pediatr.* 1994;153:56–65.

127. Mortier GR, Weis M, Nuytinck L, et al. Report of five novel and one recurrent COL2A1 mutations with analysis of genotype–phenotype correlation in patients with a lethal type II collagen disorder. *J Med Genet.* 2000;37:263–271.

128. Chen L, Yang W, Cole WG. Recurrent transition at a CG dinucleotide in exon 12 of COL2A1 produces Kniest dysplasia with abnormal RNA splicing by chondrocytes and lymphoblasts and interruption of the triple helix of type II collagen. *Ann N Y Acad Sci.* 1996;785:234–237.

129. Cole WG. Abnormal skeletal growth in Kniest dysplasia caused by type II collagen mutations. *Clin Orthop.* 1997;341:162.

130. Ahmad NN, McDonald-McGinn DM, Dixon P, et al. PCR assay confirms diagnosis in syndrome with variably expressed phenotype: Mutation detection in Stickler syndrome. *J Med Genet.* 1996;33:678–681.

131. Deere M, Hollaroan Blanton S, Scott CI, et al. Genetic heterogencity in multiple epiphyseal dysplasia. *Am J Hum Genet.* 1995;56:698–704.

132. Briggs MD, Choi HC, Warman ML, et al. Genetic mapping of a locus for multiple epiphyseal dysplasia (EDM2) to a region of chromosome I containing a type IX collagen gene. *Am J Hum Genet.* 1994;55:678–684.

133. Chan D, Weng YM, Graham HK, et al. A nonsense mutation in the carboxyl-terminal domain of type X collagen causes haploinsufficiency in Schmid metaphyseal chondrodysplasia. *J Clin Invest.* 1998;101:1490–1499.

134. Pokharel RK, Alimsardjono H, Uno K, et al. A novel mutation substituting tryptophan with arginine in the carboxyl-terminal, non-collagenous domain of collagen X in a case of Schmid metaphyseal chondrodysplasia. *Biochem Biophys Res Commun.* 1995;217:1157–1162.

135. Ikegawa S, Nakamura K, Nagano A, et al. Mutations in the N-terminal lobular domain of the type X collagen gene (COL10A1) in patients with Schmid metaphyseal chondrodysplasia. *Hum Mutat.* 1997;9:131–135.

136. Wallis GA, Rash B, Sykes B, et al. Mutations within the gene encoding the alpha 1 (X) chain of type X collagen (COL10A1) cause metaphyseal chondrodysplasia Schmid type but not several other forms of metaphyseal chondrodysplasia. *J Med Genet.* 1996;33:450–457.

137. Vikkulal M, Mariman ECM, Lui VCH, et al. Autosomal dominant and recessive osteochondrodysplasias associated with the COL11A2 locus. *Cell.* 1995;80:431–437.

138. Li D, Lacerda A, Warman ML, et al. A fibrillar collagen gene, Col11a1, is essential for skeletal morphogenesis. *Cell.* 1995;10:80.

139. Chan D, Freddi S, Weng YM, et al. Interaction of collagen alpha 1(X) containing engineered NC1 mutations with normal alpha1(X) in vitro. Implications for the molecular basis of Schmid metaphyseal chondrodysplasia. *J Biol Chem.* 1999;274:13091–13097.

140. Marks DS, Gregory CA, Wallis GA, et al. Metaphyseal chondrodysplasia type Schmid mutations are predicted to occur in two distinct three-dimensional clusters within type X collagen NC1 domains that retain the ability to trimerize. *J Biol Chem.* 1999;274:3632–3641.

141. McLaughlin SH, Conn SN, Bulleid NJ. Folding and assembly of type X collagen mutants that cause metaphyseal chondrodysplasia-type Schmid. Evidence for co-assembly of the mutant and wild-type chains and binding to molecular chaperones. *J Biol Chem.* 1999;274:7570–7575.

142. Sawai H, Ida A, Nakata Y, et al. Novel missense mutation resulting in the substitution of tyrosine by cysteine at codon 597 of the type X collagen gene associated with Schmid metaphyseal chondrodysplasia. *J Hum Genet.* 1998;43:259–261.

143. Ikegawa S, Nishimura G, Nagai T, et al. Mutation of the type X collagen gene (COL10A1) causes spondylometaphyseal dysplasia. *Am J Hum Genet.* 1998;63:1659–1662.

144. Ikegawa S, Nakamura K, Nagano A, et al. Mutations in the N-terminal globular domain of the type X collagen gene (COL10A1) in patients with Schmid metaphyseal chondrodysplasia. *Hum Mutat.* 1997;9:131–135.

145. Smith RK, Zunino L, Webbon PM, et al. The distribution of cartilage oligomeric matrix protein (COMP) in tendon and its variation with tendon site, age and load. *Matrix Biol.* 1997;16:255–271.

146. Newton G, Weremowicz S, Morton CC, et al. Characterization of human and mouse cartilage oligomeric matrix protein. *Genomics.* 1994;24:435–439.

147. Lawler J, Hynes RO. The structure of human thrombospondin, and adhesive glycoprotein with multiple calcium-binding sites and homologies with several different proteins. *J Cell Biol.* 1986;103:1635–1648.

148. Olsen BR, Sillence DO, Tam PP, et al. Abnormal compartmentalization of cartilage matrix components in mice lacking collagen X: Implications for function. *J Cell Biol.* 1997;136:459–471.

149. Briggs MD, Hoffman SM, King LM, et al. Pseudoachondroplasia and multiple epiphyseal dysplasia due to mutations in the cartilage oligomeric matrix protein gene. *Nat Genet.* 1995;10:330–336.

150. Cohn DH, Briggs MD, King LM, et al. Ahmanson mutations in the cartilage oligomeric matrix protein (COMP) gene in pseudoachondroplasia and multiple epiphyseal dysplasia. *Ann N Y Acad Sci.* 1996;785:188–194.

151. Hecht JT, Nelson LD, Crowder E, et al. Mutations in exon 17B of cartilage oligomeric matrix protein (COMP) cause pseudoachondroplasia. *Nat Genet.* 1995;10:325–329.

152. Maddox BK, Keene DR, Sakai LY, et al. The fate of cartilage oligomeric matrix protein is determined by the cell type in the case of a novel mutation in pseudoachondroplasia. *J Biol Chem.* 1997;272:30993–30997.

153. Susic S, McGrory J, Ahier J, et al. Multiple epiphyseal dysplasia and psuedoachondroplasia due to novel mutations in the calmodulin-like repeats of cartilage oligomeric matrix protein. *Clin Genet.* 1997;51:219–224.

154. Deere M, Sanford T, Francomano CA, et al. Identification of nine novel mutations in cartilage oligomeric matrix protein in patients with pseudoachondroplasia and multiple epiphyseal dysplasia. *Am J Med Genet.* 1999;85:486–490.

155. Ikegawa S, Ohashi H, Nishimura G, et al. Novel and recurrent COMP (cartilage oligomeric matrix protein) mutations in pseudoachondroplasia and multiple epiphyseal dysplasia. *Hum Genet.* 1998;103:633–638.

156. Hecht JT, Deere M, Putnam E, et al. Characterization of cartilage oligomeric matrix protein (COMP) in human normal and pseudoachondroplasia musculoskeletal tissues. *Matrix Biol.* 1998;17:269–278.

157. Makitie O, Kaitila I. Growth in diastrophic dysplasia. *J Pediatr.* 1997;130:641–646.

158. Matsuyama Y, Winter RB, Lonstein JE. The spine in diastrophic dysplasia. The surgical arthrodesis of thoracic and lumbar deformities in 21 patients. *Spine.* 1999;24:2325–2331.

159. Remes V, Marttinen E, Poussa M, et al. Cervical kyphosis in diastrophic dysplasia. *Spine.* 1999;24:1990–1995.

160. Peltonen J, Vaara P, Marttinen E, et al. The knee joint in diastrophic dysplasia. A clinical and radiological study. *J Bone Joint Surg (Br).* 1999;81:625–631.

161. Vaara P, Peltonen J, Poussa M, et al. Development of the hip in diastrophic dysplasia. *J Bone Joint Surg (Br).* 1998;80:315–320.

162. Wallis GA. Cartilage disorders. The importance of being sulphated. *Curr Biol.* 1995;5:225–227.

163. Qureshi F, Jacques SM, Johnson SF, et al. Histopathology of fetal diastrophic dysplasia. *Am J Med Genet.* 1995;56:300–303.

164. Bailey AJ, Sims TJ, Stanesu V, et al. Abnormal collagen cross-linking in the cartilage of a diastrophic dysplasia patient. *Br J Rheumatol.* 1995;34:512–515.

165. Hastbacka J, Kerrebrock A, Mokkala K, et al. Identification of the Finnish founder mutation for diastrophic dysplasia (DTD). *Eur J Hum Genet.* 1999;7:664–670.

166. Hastbacka J, de la Chapelle A, Mahtani MM, et al. The diastrophic dysplasia gene encodes a novel sulfate transporter: Positional cloning by fine-structure linkage disequilibrium mapping. *Cell.* 1994;78:1073–1087.

167. Hastbacka J, Superti-Furga A, Wilcox WR. Sulfate transport in chondrodysplasia. *Ann N Y Acad Sci.* 1996;785: 131–136.

168. Superti-Furga A, Hastbacka J, Rossi A, et al. A family of chondrodysplasias caused by mutations in the diastrophic dysplasia sulfate transporter gene and associated with impaired sulfation of proteoglycans. *Ann N Y Acad. Sci.* 1996;785:195–201.

169. Superti-Furga A, Hastbacka J, Wilcox WR, et al. Achondrogenesis type IB is caused by mutations in the diastrophic dysplasia sulphate transporter gene. *Nat Genet.* 1996;12:100–102.

170. Superti-Furga A. Achondrogenesis type 1B. *J Med Genet.* 1996;33:957–961.

171. Hastbacka J, Superti-Furga A, Wilcox WR, et al. Atelosteogenesis type II is caused by mutations in the diastrophic dysplasia sulfate-transporter gene (DTDST): Evidence for a phenotypic series involving three chondrodysplasias. *Am J Hum Genet.* 1996;58:255–262.

172. Rossi A, van der Harten HJ, Beemer FA, et al. Phenotypic and genotypic overlap between atelosteogenesis type 2 and diastrophic dysplasia. *Hum Genet.* 1996;98:657–661.

173. Sillence D, Worthington S, Dixon J, et al. Atelosteogenesis syndromes: A review, with comments on their pathogenesis. *Pediatr Radiol.* 1997;27:388–396.

174. Newbury-Ecob R. Atelosteogenesis type 2. *J Med Genet.* 1998; 35:49–53.

175. Camera G, Mastroiacovo P. Birth prevalence of skeletal dysplasias in the Italian multicentric monitoring system for birth defects. In: Papadatos CJ, Bartsocas CS, eds. *Skeletal Dysplasias.* New York: Alan R. Liss; 1982:441.

176. Connor JM, Connor RAC, Sweet EM, et al. Lethal neonatal chondrodysplasias in the West of Scotland 1970–1983 with a description of a thanatophoric, dysplasialike, autosomal recessive disorder, Glasgow variant. *Am J Med Genet.* 1985; 22:243.

177. Rasmussen SA, Bieber FR, Benacerraf BR, et al. Epidemiology of osteochondrodysplasias: Changing trends due to advances in prenatal diagnosis. *Am J Med Genet.* 1996;61:49–58.

178. Spranger J. International nomenclature of constitutional bone diseases (the Paris nomenclature). *Fortschr Geb Rontgenstr Nuklearmed.* 1971;115:283–287.

179. International nomenclature of constitutional diseases of bone. Revision—May, 1977. *J Pediatr.* 1978;93:614–616.

180. International nomenclature of constitutional diseases of bone —Revision, May, 1983. *Australas Radiol.* 1986;30:163–167.

181. Spranger J. International classification of osteochondrodysplasias. *Eur J Pediatr.* 1992;151:407–415.

182. Lachman RS, Tiller GE, Graham JM Jr, et al. Collagen, genes and the skeletal dysplasias on the edge of a new era: A review and update. *Eur J Radiol.* 1992;14:1–10.

183. Lachman RS. Introduction and overview. *Pediatr Radiol.* 1998;28:735–736.

184. Lachman RS. International nomenclature and classification of the osteochondrodysplasias (1997). *Pediatr Radiol.* 1998; 28:737–744.

185. Spranger J, Maroteaux P. The lethal osteochondrodysplasias. *Adv Hum Genet.* 1989;19:1.

186. Benaceraff BR, Greene MF, Barss VA. Prenatal sonographic diagnosis of congenital hemivertebra. *J Ultrasound Med.* 1986; 5:257.

187. Kurtz AB, Wapner RJ. Ultrasonographic diagnosis of second

188. Goncalves L, Jeanty P. Fetal biometry of skeletal dysplasias: A multicentric study. *J Ultrasound Med.* 1994;13:977–985.

189. Gabrielli S, et al. Can transvaginal fetal biometry be considered a useful tool for early detection of skeletal dysplasias in high-risk patients? *Ultrasound Obstet Gynecol.* 1999;13:107–111.

190. Coffin GS, Siris E, Wegienka LC. Mental retardation with osteocartilaginous anomalies. *Am J Dis Child.* 1966;112:205.

191. Bowerman R, et al. Anomalies of the fetal skeleton: Sonographic findings. *AJR.* 1995;164:973–979.

192. Graham M. Congenital short femur: Prenatal sonographic diagnosis. *J Ultrasound Med.* 1985;4:361.

193. Pashayan H, Fraser FC, McIntyre JM, et al. Bilateral aplasia of the tibia, polydactyly and absent thumbs in father and daughter. *J Bone Joint Surg.* 1971;53B:495.

194. Filkins K, Russo J, Bilinki I, et al. Prenatal diagnosis of thrombocytopenia absent radius syndrome using ultrasound and fetoscopy. *Prenat Diagn.* 1984;4:139.

195. Luthy DA, Hall JG, Graham CB, et al. Prenatal diagnosis of thrombocytopenia with absent radii. *Clin Genet.* 1979;15: 495.

196. Rahemtullah A, McGillivray B, Wilson RD. Suspected skeletal dysplasias: Femur length to abdominal circumference ratio can be used in ultrasonographic prediction of fetal outcome. *Am J Obstet Gynecol.* 1997;177:864–869.

197. Chitkara U, Rosenberg J, Chervenak FA, et al. Prenatal sonographic assessment of the fetal thorax: Normal values. *Am J Obstet Gynecol.* 1987;156:1069.

198. Dugoff L, Coffin CT, Hobbins JC. Sonographic measurement of the fetal rib cage perimeter to thoracic circumference ratio: Application to prenatal diagnosis of skeletal dysplasias. *Ultrasound Obstet Gynecol.* 1997;10:269–271.

199. Campbell J, Henderson A, Campbell S. The fetal femur/foot length ratio: A new parameter to assess dysplastic limb reduction. *Obstet Gynecol.* 1989;72:181.

200. Hershey DW. The fetal femur/foot length ratio: A new parameter to assess dysplastic limb reduction. *Obstet Gynecol.* 1989;73:682.

201. Galli G. *Craniosynostosis.* Boca Raton: CRC Press; 1984.

202. Kozlowski K, Robertson F, Middleton R. Radiographic findings in Larsen's syndrome. *Aust Radiol.* 1974;18:336.

203. Pilu G, Romero R, Reece EA, et al. The prenatal diagnosis of Robin anomalad. *Am J Obstet Gynecol.* 1986;154:630.

204. Pilu G, Reece EA, Romero R, et al. Prenatal diagnosis of craniofacial malformations with ultrasonography. *Am J Obstet Gynecol.* 1986;155:45.

205. Turner GM, Twining P. The facial profile in the diagnosis of fetal abnormalities. *Clin Radiol.* 1993;47:389–395.

206. Escobar LF, Bixler D, Padilla LM, et al. Fetal craniofacial morphometrics: In utero evaluation at 16 weeks' gestation. *Obstet Gynecol.* 1988;72:674–679.

207. Escobar LF, Bixler D, Weaver DD, et al. Bone dysplasias: The prenatal diagnostic challenge. *Am J Med Genet.* 1990;36:488–494.

208. Aubry MC, Aubry JP. Prenatal diagnosis of cervico-facial malformations and tumors. *Rev Prat.* 1991;41:16–20.

209. Prows CA, Bender PL. Beyond Pierre Robin sequence. *Neonat Netw.* 1999;18:13–19.

210. Pilu G, Reece EA, Romero R, et al. Prenatal diagnosis of

trimester skeletal dysplasias: A prospective analysis in a high-risk population. *J Ultrasound Med.* 1983;2:99.

craniofacial malformations with ultrasonography. *Am J Obstet Gynecol.* 1986;155:45–50.

211. Bromley B, Benacerraf BR. Fetal micrognathia: Associated anomalies and outcome. *J Ultrasound Med.* 1994;13:529–533.

212. Chitty LS, Campbell S, Altman DG. Measurement of the fetal mandible—Feasibility and construction of a centile chart. *Prenat Diagn.* 1993;13:749–756.

213. Watson WJ, Katz VL. Sonographic measurement of the fetal mandible: Standards for normal pregnancy. *Am J Perinatol.* 1993;10:226–228.

214. Zelop CM, Pretorius DH, Benacerraf BR. Fetal hemivertebrae: Associated anomalies, significance, and outcome. *Obstet Gynecol.* 1993;81:412–416.

215. Abrams SL, Filly RA. Congenital vertebral malformations: Prenatal diagnosis using ultrasonography. *Radiology.* 1985;155:762.

216. Kozlowski K, Bieganski T, Gardner J, et al. Osteochondrodystrophies with marked platyspondyly and distinctive peripheral anomalies. *Pediatr Radiol.* 1999;29:1–5.

217. Wells TR, Landing BH, Bostwick FH. Studies of vertebral coronal cleft in rhizomelic chondrodysplasia punctata. *Pediatr Pathol.* 1992;12:593–600. Erratum: *Pediatr Pathol.* 1993; 13:123.

218. Nores JA, Rotmensch S, Romero R, et al. Atelosteogenesis type II: Sonographic and radiological correlation. *Prenat Diagn.* 1992;12:741–753.

219. Lachman RS. Fetal imaging in the skeletal dysplasias: Overview and experience. *Pediatr Radiol.* 1994;24:413–417.

220. Westvik J, Lachman RS. Coronal and sagittal clefts in skeletal dysplasias. *Pediatr Radiol.* 1998;28:764–770.

221. McMaster MJ. Occult intraspinal anomalies and congenital scoliosis. *J Bone Joint Surg (Am).* 1984;66:588–601.

222. McMaster MJ, David CV. Hemivertebra as a cause of scoliosis. A study of 104 patients. *J Bone Joint Surg (Br).* 1986;68:588–595.

223. McMaster MJ. Congenital scoliosis caused by a unilateral failure of vertebral segmentation with contralateral hemivertebrae. *Spine.* 1998;23:998–1005.

224. McMaster MJ, Singh H. Natural history of congenital kyphosis and kyphoscoliosis. A study of one hundred and twelve patients. *J Bone Joint Surg (Am).* 1999;81:1367–1383.

225. Connor JM, Conner AN, Connor RA, et al. Genetic aspects of early childhood scoliosis. *Am J Med Genet.* 1987;27:419–424.

226. Johnson VP, Petersen LP, Holzwarth DR, et al. Midtrimester prenatal diagnosis of achondrogenesis. *J Ultrasound Med.* 1984;3:223–226.

227. Mahony BS, Filly RA, Callen PW, et al. Thanatophoric dwarfism with the cloverleaf skull: A specific antenatal sonographic diagnosis. *J Ultrasound Med.* 1985;4:151–154.

228. Sorge G, Ruggieri M, Lachman RS. Spondyloperipheral dysplasia. *Am J Med Genet.* 1995;59:139–142.

229. Carvalho L, Soares M, Feijoo MJ, et al. A collaborative approach to the diagnosis of a lethal short limb skeletal dysplasia. *Genet Couns.* 1997;8:139–143.

230. Mortier GR, Rimoin DL, Lachman RS. The scapula as a window to the diagnosis of skeletal dysplasias. *Pediatr Radiol.* 1997;27:447–451.

231. Francomano CA. The genetic basis of dwarfism. *N Engl J Med.* 1995;332:58–59.

232. Nicolaides KH, Azar G, Byrne D, et al. Fetal nuchal translucency: Ultrasound screening for chromosomal defects in first trimester of pregnancy. *Br Med J.* 1992;304:867–869.

233. Brady AF, Pandya PP, Yuksel B, et al. Outcome of chromosomally normal livebirths with increased fetal nuchal translucency at 10–14 weeks' gestation. *J Med Genet.* 1998;35:222–224.

234. Souka AP, Snijders RJ, Novakov A, et al. Defects and syndromes in chromosomally normal fetuses with increased nuchal translucency thickness at 10–14 weeks of gestation. *Ultrasound Obstet Gynecol.* 1998;11:391–400.

235. Pandya PP, Kondylios A, Hilbert L, et al. Chromosomal defects and outcome in 1015 fetuses with increased nuchal translucency. *Ultrasound Obstet Gynecol.* 1995;5:15–19.

236. Weldner BM, Persson PH, Ivarsson SA. Prenatal diagnosis of dwarfism by ultrasound screening. *Arch Dis Child.* 1985;60:1070–1072.

237. Sharony R, Browne C, Lachman RS, et al. Prenatal diagnosis of the skeletal dysplasias. *Am J Obstet Gynecol.* 1993;169:668–675.

238. Gaffney G, Manning N, Boyd PA, et al. Prenatal sonographic diagnosis of skeletal dysplasias—A report of the diagnostic and prognostic accuracy in 35 cases. *Prenat Diagn.* 1998;18:357–362.

239. Spirt BA, Oliphant M, Gottlieb RH, et al. Prenatal sonographic evaluation of short-limbed dwarfism: An algorithmic approach. *Radio Graphics.* 1990;10:217–236.

240. Donnenfeld AE, Mennuti MT. Second trimester diagnosis of fetal skeletal dysplasias. *Obstet Gynecol Surv.* 1987;42: 199–217.

241. McGuire J, Manning F, Lange I, et al. Antenatal diagnosis of skeletal dysplasia using ultrasound. *Birth Defects Orig Art Ser.* 1987;23:367–384.

242. Pretorius DH, Rumack CM, Manco-Johnson ML, et al. Specific skeletal dysplasias in utero: Sonographic diagnosis. *Radiology.* 1986;159:237–242.

243. Rouse GA, Filly RA, Toomey F, Grube GL. Short-limb skeletal dysplasias: Evaluation of the fetal spine with sonography and radiography. *Radiology.* 1990;174:177–180.

244. Kurtz AB, Needleman L, Wapner RJ, et al. Usefulness of a short femur in the in utero detection of skeletal dysplasias. *Radiology.* 1990;177:197–200.

245. MacDonald MR, Welsh MP. Perinatal approach to skeletal dysplasia. *Nebr Med J.* 1995;80:334–335.

246. Gordienko IY, Grechanina EY, Sopko NI, et al. Prenatal diagnosis of osteochondrodysplasias in high risk pregnancy. *Am J Med Genet.* 1996;63:90–97.

247. Tretter AE, Saunders RC, Meyers CM, et al. Antenatal diagnosis of lethal skeletal dysplasias. *Am J Med Genet.* 1998;75:518–522.

248. Hersh JH, Angle B, Pietrantoni M, et al. Predictive value of fetal ultrasonography in the diagnosis of a lethal skeletal dysplasia. *South Med J.* 1998;91:1137–1142.

249. Garjian KV, Pretorius DH, Budorick NE, et al. Fetal skeletal dysplasia: Three-dimensional US—Initial experience. *Radiology.* 2000;214:717–723.

250. Lemyre E, Azouz EM, Teebi AS, et al. Bone dysplasia series. Achondroplasia, hypochondroplasia and thanatophoric dysplasia: Review and update. *Can Assoc Radiol J.* 1999;50:185–197.

251. Cohen MM Jr. Achondroplasia, hypochondroplasia and

thanatophoric dysplasia: Clinically related skeletal dysplasias that are also related at the molecular level. *Int J Oral Maxillofac Surg.* 1998;27:451–455.

252. Ozono K. Recent advances in molecular analysis of skeletal dysplasia. *Acta Paediatr Jpn.* 1997;39:491–498.

253. Wilkin DJ, Szabo JK, Cameron R, et al. Mutations in fibroblast growth-factor receptor 3 in sporadic cases of achondroplasia occur exclusively on the paternally derived chromosome. *Am J Hum Genet.* 1998;63:711–716.

254. Zhao P, Ma H, Wang Y, et al. Mutations of the fibroblast growth factor receptor 3 gene in achondroplasia. *Chung Hua I Hsueh I Chuan Hsueh Tsa Chih.* 1999;16:16–18.

255. Climent C, Lorda-Sanchez I, Urioste M, et al. Achondroplasia: Molecular study of 28 patients. *Med Clin (Barc).* 1998;110:492–494.

256. Ramaswami U, Rumsby G, Hindmarsh PC, et al. Genotype and phenotype in hypochondroplasia. *J Pediatr.* 1998;133:99–102.

257. Kurtz AB, Filly RA, Wapner RJ, et al. In utero analysis of heterozygous achondroplasia: Variable time of onset as detected by femur length measurements. *J Ultrasound Med.* 1986; 5:137.

258. Modaff P, Horton VK, Pauli RM. Errors in the prenatal diagnosis of children with achondroplasia. *Prenat Diagn.* 1996; 16:525–530.

259. Elejalde BR, de Elejalde MM, Hamilton PR, et al. Prenatal diagnosis in two pregnancies of an achondroplastic woman. *Am J Med Genet.* 1983;15:437.

260. Huggins MJ, Mernagh JR, Steele L, et al. Prenatal sonographic diagnosis of hypochondroplasia in a high-risk fetus. *Am J Med Genet.* 1999;87:226–229.

261. Chitayat D, Fernandez B, Gardner A, et al. Compound heterozygosity for the achondroplasia–hypochondroplasia FGFR3 mutations: Prenatal diagnosis and postnatal outcome. *Am J Med Genet.* 1999;84:401–405.

262. Mesoraca A, Pilu G, Porolo A, et al. Ultrasound and molecular mid-trimester prenatal diagnosis of de novo achondroplasia. *Prenat Diagn.* 1996;16:764–768.

263. Guzman ER, Day-Salvatore D, Westover T, et al. Prenatal ultrasonographic demonstration of the trident hand in heterozygous achondroplasia. *J Ultrasound Med.* 1994;13:63–66.

264. Cordone M, Lituania M, Bocchino G, et al. Ultrasonographic features in a case of heterozygous achondroplasia at 25 weeks' gestation. *Prenat Diagn.* 1993;13:395–401.

265. Patel MD, Filly RA. Homozygous achondroplasia: US distinction between homozygous, heterozygous, and unaffected fetuses in the second trimester. *Radiology.* 1995;196:541–545.

266. Sawai H, Komori S, Tanaka H, et al. Prenatal diagnosis of achondroplasia using the nested polymerase chain reaction with modified primer sets. *Fetal Diagn Ther.* 1996;11:407–413.

267. Lachman RS. Neurologic abnormalities in the skeletal dysplasias: A clinical and radiological perspective. *Am J Med Genet.* 1997;69:33–43.

268. Pauli RM, Conroy MM, Langer LO, et al. Homozygous achondroplasia with survival beyond infancy. *Am J Med Genet.* 1983;16:459.

269. Seino Y, Moriwake T, Tanaka H, et al. Molecular defects in achondroplasia and the effects of growth hormone treatment. *Acta Paediatr.* 1999;88(suppl):118–120.

270. Tavormina PL, Bellus GA, Webster MK, et al. A novel skeletal dysplasia with developmental delay and acanthosis nigricans is caused by a Lys650Met mutation in the fibroblast growth factor receptor 3 gene. *Am J Hum Genet.* 1999;64:722–731.

271. Bellus GA, Bamshad MJ, Przylepa KA, et al. Severe achondroplasia with developmental delay and acanthosis nigricans (SADDAN): Phenotypic analysis of a new skeletal dysplasia caused by a Lys650Met mutation in fibroblast growth factor receptor 3. *Am J Med Genet.* 1999;85:53–65.

272. Brodie SG, Kitoh H, Lipson M, et al. Thanatophoric dysplasia type I with syndactyly. *Am J Med Genet.* 1998;80:260–262.

273. Weber M, Johannisson R, Carstens C, et al. Thanatophoric dysplasia type II: New entity? *J Pediatr Orthop B.* 1998;7: 10–22.

274. Iannaccone G, Gerlini G. The so-called "cloverleaf skull syndrome": A report of three cases with a discussion of its relationships with thanatophoric dwarfism and craniostenosis. *Pediatr Radiol.* 1974;2:175.

275. Jasnosz KM, MacPherson TA. Perinatal pathology casebook. Thanatophoric dysplasia with cloverleaf skull. *J Perinatol.* 1993;13:162–164.

276. Vajo Z, Francomano CA, Wilkin DJ. The molecular and genetic basis of fibroblast growth factor receptor 3 disorders: The achondroplasia family of skeletal dysplasias, Muenke craniosynostosis, and Crouzon syndrome with acanthosis nigricans. *Endocr Rev.* 2000;21:23–39.

277. d'Avis PY, Robertson SC, Meyer AN, et al. Constitutive activation of fibroblast growth factor receptor 3 by mutations responsible for the lethal skeletal dysplasia thanatophoric dysplasia type I. *Cell Growth Differ.* 1998;9:71–78.

278. Tavormina PL, Shiang R, Thompson LM, et al. Thanatophoric dysplasia (types I and II) caused by distinct mutations in fibroblast growth factor receptor 3. *Nat Genet.* 1995;9:321–328.

279. Yang SS, Heidelberger KP, Brough AJ, et al. Lethal short-limbed chondrodysplasia in early infancy. In: Rosenberg HS, Boland RP, eds. *Perspectives in Pediatric Pathology.* Chicago: Year Book Medical Publishers; 1976:1.

280. McKusick VA, Francomano CA, Antonarakis SE. *Mendelian Inheritance in Man: Catalogs of Autosomal Dominant, Autosomal Recessive, and X-Linked Phenotypes,* 9th ed. Baltimore: Johns Hopkins University Press; 1990.

281. Partington MW, Gonzales-Crussi F, Khakee SG, et al. Cloverleaf skull and thanatophoric dwarfism, a report of four cases, two in the same sibship. *Arch Dis Child.* 1971;46:656.

282. Schild RL, Hunt GH, Moore J, et al. Antenatal sonographic diagnosis of thanatophoric dysplasia: A report of three cases and a review of the literature with special emphasis on the differential diagnosis. *Ultrasound Obstet Gynecol.* 1996;8:60–67.

283. Horton WA, Rimoin DL, Hollister DW, et al. Further heterogeneity within lethal neonatal short-limbed dwarfism: The platyspondylic types. *J Pediatr.* 1979;94:736.

284. Moir DH, Kozlowski K. Long survival in thanatophoric dwarfism. *Pediatr Radiol.* 1976;5:123.

285. Stensvold K, Ek J, Hovland AR. An infant with thanatophoric dwarfism surviving 169 days. *Clin Genet.* 1986;29:157.

286. Baker KM, Olson DS, Harding CO, Pauli RM. Long-term survival in typical thanatophoric dysplasia type 1. *Am J Med Genet.* 1997;70:427–436.

287. Dominguez R, Talmachoff P. Diagnostic imaging update in skeletaldysplasias. *Clin Imaging.* 1993;17:222–234.

288. Fink IJ, Filly RA, Callen PW, Fiske CC. Sonographic

diagnosis of thanatophoric dwarfism in utero. *J Ultrasound Med.* 1982;1:337.

289. Sun CC, Grumbach K, DeCosta DT, et al. Correlation of prenatal ultrasound diagnosis and pathologic findings in fetal anomalies. *Pediatr Dev Pathol.* 1999;2:131–142.

290. Beetham FGT, Reeves JS. Early ultrasound diagnosis of thanatophoric dwarfism. *J Clin Ultrasound.* 1984;12:43.

291. Burrows PE, Stannard MW, Pearrow J, et al. Early antenatal sonographic recognition of thanatophoric dysplasia with cloverleaf skull deformity. *AJR.* 1984;143:841.

292. Mahony BS, Filly RA, Callen PW, Golbus MS. Thanatophoric dwarfism with the cloverleaf skull: A specific antenatal sonographic diagnosis. *J Ultrasound Med.* 1985;4:151.

293. Elejald BR, de Elejalde MM. Thanatophoric dyplasia: Fetal manifestations and prenatal diagnosis. *Am J Med Genet.* 1985;22:669.

294. Weiner CP, Williamson RA, Bonsib SM. Sonographic diagnosis of cloverleaf skull and thanatophoric dysplasia in the second trimester. *J Clin Ultrasound.* 1986;14:463.

295. van der Harten JJ, Brons JTJ, Dijkstra PF, et al. Some variants of lethal neonatal short-limbed platyspondylic dysplasia: A radiologic, ultrasonographic, neuro-pathologic and histopathologic study of 22 cases. In: Brons JTJ, van der Harten JJ, eds. *Skeletal Dysplasias, Pre- and Postnatal Identification: An Ultrasonographic, Radiologic and Pathologic Study.* Amsterdam: Free University Hospital; 1988:111.

296. Chervenak FA, Blakemore KJ, Isaacson G, et al. Antenatal sonographic findings of thanatophoric dysplasia with cloverleaf skull. *Am J Obstet Gynecol.* 1983;146:984.

297. Oga M, Takai N, Yoshimatsu J, et al. Infant with thanatophoric dwarfism in triplet pregnancy. *Gynecol Obstet Invest.* 1995;39:274–276.

298. Sawai H, Komori S, Ida A, et al. Prenatal diagnosis of thanatophoric dysplasia by mutational analysis of the fibroblast growth factor receptor 3 gene and a proposed correction of previously published PCR results. *Prenat Diagn.* 1999;19:21–24.

299. Yuce MA, Yardim T, Kurtul M, et al. Prenatal diagnosis of thanatophoric dwarfism in second trimester. A case report. *Clin Exp Obstet Gynecol.* 1998;25:149–150.

300. Bellus GA, McIntosh I, Szabo J, et al. Hypochondroplasia: Molecular analysis of the fibroblast growth factor receptor 3 gene. *Ann N Y Acad Sci.* 1996;785:182–187.

301. Cohn DH. Mutations affecting multiple functional domains of FGFR3 cause different skeletal dysplasias: A personal retrospective in honor of John Wasmuth. *Ann N Y Acad Sci.* 1996;785:160–163.

302. Matsui Y, Yasui N, Kimura T, et al. Genotype phenotype correlation in achondroplasia and hypochondroplasia. *J Bone Joint Surg (Br).* 1998;80:1052–1056.

303. Hall BD, Spranger J. Hypochondroplasia: Clinical and radiological aspects in 39 cases. *Radiology.* 1979;133:95.

304. Scott CL. Achondroplastic and hypochondroplastic dwarfism. *Clin Orthop.* 1976;114:18.

305. Stoilov I, Kilpatrick MW, Tsipouras P, Costa T. Possible genetic heterogeneity in hypochondroplasia. *J Med Genet.* 1995;32:492–493.

306. Prinster C, Carrera P, Del Maschio M, et al. Comparison of clinical–radiological and molecular findings in hypochondroplasia. *Am J Med Genet.* 1998;75:109–112.

307. Angle B, Hersh JH, Christensen KM. Molecularly proven hypochondroplasia with cloverleaf skull deformity: A novel association. *Clin Genet.* 1998;54:417–420.

308. Stoll C, Manini, P, Bloch J, et al. Prenatal diagnosis of hypochondroplasia. *Prenat Diagn.* 1985;5:423.

309. Eteson DJ, Adomian GE, Ornoy A, et al. Fibrochondrogenesis: Radiologic and histologic studies. *Am J Med Genet.* 1984; 19:277.

310. Al-Gazali LI, Bakalinova D, Bakir M, Dawodu A. Fibrochondrogenesis: Clinical and radiological features. *Clin Dysmorphol.* 1997;6:157–163.

311. Hunt NC, Vujanic GM. Fibrochondrogenesis in a 17-week fetus: A case expanding the phenotype. *Am J Med Genet.* 1998 23;75:326–329.

312. Lazzaroni-Fossati F, Stanescu V, Stanescu R, et al. Fibrochondrogenesis. *Arch Fr Pediatr.* 1978;35:1096–1104.

313. Martinez-Frias ML, Garcia A, Cuevas J, et al. A new case of fibrochondrogenesis from Spain. *J Med Genet.* 1996;33: 429–431.

314. Whitley CB, Langer LO, Ophoven J, et al. Fibrochondrogenesis: Lethal, autosomal recessive chondrodysplasia with distinctive cartilage histopathology. *Am J Med Genet.* 1984;19: 265.

315. Al-Gazali LI, Bakir M, Dawodu A, et al. Recurrence of fibrochondrogenesis in a consanguineous family [letter]. *Clin Dysmorphol.* 1999;8:59–61.

316. Megarbane A, Haddad S, Berjaoui L. Prenatal ultrasonography: Clinical and radiological findings in a boy with fibrochondrogenesis. *Am J Perinatol.* 1998;15:403–407.

317. Bankier A, Fortune D, Duke J, et al. Fibrochondrogenesis in male twins at 24 weeks gestation. *Am J Med Genet.* 1991; 38:95–98.

318. Maroteaux P, Spranger J, Stanescu V, et al. Atelosteogenesis. *Am J Med Genet.* 1982;13:15.

319. Sillence D, Worthington S, Dixon J, et al. Atelosteogenesis syndromes: A review, with comments on their pathogenesis. *Pediatr Radiol.* 1997;27:388–396.

320. Sillence DO, Lachman RS, Jenkins T, et al. Spondylo-humero-femoral hypoplasia (giant cell chondroplasia). *Am J Med Genet.* 1982;13:7.

321. Yang SS, Roskamp JA, Liu CT. Two lethal chondrodysplasias with giant chondrocytes. *Am J Med Genet.* 1983;15:615.

322. McAlister WH, Crane JP, Bucy RP, et al. A new neonatal short-limbed dwarfism. *Skeletal Radiol.* 1985;13:271.

323. Sillence DO, Kozlowski K, Rogers JG, et al. Atelosteogenesis: Evidence for heterogeneity. *Pediatr Radiol.* 1987;17:112.

324. Stern HJ, Graham JM Jr, Lachman RS, et al. Atelosteogenesis type 3: A distinct skeletal dysplasia with features overlapping atelosteogenesis and oto-palato-digital syndrome type 2. *Am J Med Genet.* 1990;36:183–195.

325. Superti-Furga A, Neumann L, Riebel T, et al. Recessively inherited multiple epiphyseal dysplasia with normal stature, club foot, and double layered patella caused by a DTDST mutation. *J Med Genet.* 1999;36:621–624.

326. De la Chapelle A, Maroteaux P, Havu N, Granroth G. Une rare dysplasie osseuse letale de transmission recessive autosomique. *Arch Fr Pediatr.* 1972;29:759.

327. Whitley CB, Burke BA, Granroth G, Gorlin RJ. De la Chapelle dysplasia. *Am J Med Genet.* 1986;25:29.

328. Kozlowski K, Sillence D, Cortis-Jones R, Osborn R. Boomerang dysplasia. *Br J Radiol.* 1985;58:369.

329. Bejjani BA, Oberg KC, Wilkins I, et al. Prenatal ultrasonographic description and postnatal pathological findings in atelosteogenesis type 1. *Am J Med Genet.* 1998;79:392–395.

330. Chevernak FA, Isaacson G, Rosenberg JC, Kardon KB. Antenatal diagnosis of frontal cephalocele in a fetus with atelosteogenesis. *J Ultrasound Med.* 1986;5:111.

331. Herzberg AJ, Effmann EL, Bradford WD. Variant of atelosteogenesis? Report of a 20-week fetus. *Am J Med Genet.* 1988;29:883.

332. Schultz C, Langer LO, Laxova R, et al. Atelosteogenesis type III: Long term survival, prenatal diagnosis, and evidence for dominant transmission. *Am J Med Genet.* 1999;83:28–42.

333. Borochowitz J, Lachman R, Adomian E, et al. Achondrogenesis type I: Delineation of further heterogeneity and identification of two distinct subgroups. *J Pediatr.* 1988;112:23.

334. Borochowitz Z, Ornoy A, Lachman R, Rimoin DL. Achondrogenesis II—Hypochondrogenesis: Variability versus heterogeneity. *Am J Med Genet.* 1986;24:273.

335. Van der Harten HJ, Brons JTJ, Dijkstra PF, et al. Achondrogenesis, hypochondrogenesis, the spectrum of chondrogenesis imperfecta: A radiologic, ultrasonographic and histopathologic study of 23 cases. *Pediatr Pathol.* 1988;8:571.

336. Spranger J. Pattern recognition in bone dysplasias. In: Papadatos CJ, Bartsocas CS, eds. *Endocrine Genetics and Genetics of Growth.* New York: Alan R. Liss; 1985:315.

337. Godfrey M, Keene DR, Blank E, et al. Type II achondrogenesis–hypochondrogenesis: Morphologic and immunohistopathologic studies. *Am J Hum Genet.* 1988;43:894.

338. Murray LW, Rimoin DL. Abnormal type II collagen in the spondylepiphyseal dysplasias. *Pathol Immunopathol Res.* 1988;17:99.

339. Whitley CB, Gorlin RJ. Achondrogenesis: New nosology with evidence of genetic heterogeneity. *Radiology.* 1983;148:693.

340. Cai G, Nakayama M, Hiraki Y, et al. Mutational analysis of the DTDST gene in a fetus with achondrogenesis type 1B. *Am J Med Genet.* 1998;78:58–60.

341. Wenstrom KD, Williamson RA, Hoover WW, Grant SS. Achondrogenesis type II (Langer–Saldino) is associated with jugular lymphatic obstruction sequence. *Prenat Diagn.* 1989;9:527.

342. Won HS, Yoo HK, Lee PR, et al. A case of achondrogenesis type II associated with huge cystic hygroma: Prenatal diagnosis by ultrasonography [letter]. *Ultrasound Obstet Gynecol.* 1999;14:288–290.

343. Ozeren S, Yuksel A, Tukel T. Prenatal sonographic diagnosis of type I achondrogenesis with a large cystic hygroma [letter]. *Ultrasound Obstet Gynecol.* 1999;13:75–76.

344. Golbus MS, Hall BD, Filly RA, Poskanzer LB. Prenatal diagnosis of achondrogenesis. *J Pediatr.* 1977;91:464.

345. Johnson VP, Yiu-Chiu VS, Wierda DR, Holzwarth DR. Midtrimester prenatal diagnosis of achondrogenesis. *J Ultrasound Med.* 1984;3:223.

346. Mahony BS, Filly RA, Cooperberg PL. Antenatal sonographic diagnosis of achondrogenesis. *J Ultrasound Med.* 1984;3:333.

347. Glenn LW, Teng SSK. In utero sonographic diagnosis of achondrogenesis. *J Clin Ultrasound.* 1985;13:195.

348. Benacerraf B, Osathanondh R, Bieber FR. Achondrogenesis type I: Ultrasound diagnosis in utero. *J Clin Ultrasound.* 1984;12:357.

349. Smith WL, Breitweiser TD, Dinno N. In utero diagnosis of achondrogenesis, type I. *Clin Genet.* 1981;19:51.

350. Chen H, Liu CT, Yang SS. Achondrogenesis: A review with special consideration of achondrogenesis type II (Langer–Saldino). *Am J Med Genet.* 1981;10:379.

351. Orioli IM, Castilla EE, Scarano G, Mastroiacovo P. Effect of paternal age in achondroplasia, thanatophoric dysplasia, and osteogenesis imperfecta. *Am J Med Genet.* 1995;59:209–217.

352. Sillence DO, Senn A, Danks DM. Genetic heterogeneity in osteogenesis imperfecta. *J Med Genet.* 1979;16:101.

353. Sillence DO, Barlow KK, Cole WG, et al. Osteogenesis imperfecta type III. Delineation of the phenotype with reference to genetic heterogeneity. *Am J Med Genet.* 1986;23:821.

354. Andersen PE Jr, Hauge M. Osteogenesis imperfecta: A genetic, radiological, and epidemiological study. *Clin Genet.* 1989;36:250–255.

355. Bischoff H, Freitag P, Jundt G, et al. Type I osteogenesis imperfecta: Diagnostic difficulties. *Clin Rheumatol.* 1999;18:48–51.

356. Bishop NJ. Osteogenesis imperfecta calls for caution [letter; comment]. *Nat Med.* 1999;5:466–467.

357. Bulas DI, Stern HJ, Rosenbaum KN, et al. Variable prenatal appearance of osteaogenesis imperfecta. *J Ultrasound Med.* 1994;13:419–427.

358. Wax JR, Smith FJ, Floyd RC. Lethal osteogenesis imperfecta: Second trimester sonographic diagnosis in a twin gestation. *J Ultrasound Med.* 1994;13:711–713.

359. Robinson LP, Worthen NJ, Lachman RS, et al. Prenatal diagnosis of osteogenesis imperfecta type III. *Prenat Diagn.* 1987;7:7.

360. Mertz E, Goldhofer W. Sonographic diagnosis of lethal osteogenesis imperfecta in the second trimester: Case report and review. *J Clin Ultrasound.* 1986;14:380.

361. Brons JTJ, van der Harten JJ, Wladimiroff JW, et al. Prenatal ultrasonographic diagnosis of osteogenesis imperfecta. *Am J Obstet Gynecol.* 1988;159:176.

362. Elejalde BR, de Elejalde MM. Prenatal diagnosis of perinatally lethal osteogenesis imperfecta. *Am J Med Genet.* 1983;14:353.

363. Nuytinck L, Sayli BS, Karen W, et al. Prenatal diagnosis of osteogenesis imperfecta type I by COL1A1 null-allele testing. *Prenat Diagn.* 1999;19:873–875.

364. Chervenak FA, Romero R, Berkowitz RL, et al. Antenatal sonographic findings of osteogenesis imperfecta. *Am J Obstet Gynecol.* 1982;143:228.

365. Thompson EM. Non-invasive prenatal diagnosis of osteogenesis imperfecta. *Am J Med Genet.* 1993;45:201–206.

366. Munoz C, Filly RA, Golbus MS. Osteogenesis imperfecta type II: Prenatal sonographic diagnosis. *Radiology.* 1990;174:181–185.

367. Chamson A, Bertheas MF, Frey J. Collagen biosynthesis in cell culture from chorionic villi. *Prenat Diagn.* 1995;15:165–170.

368. Pepin M, Atkinson M, Starman BJ, Byers PH. Strategies and outcomes of prenatal diagnosis for osteogenesis imperfecta: A review of biochemical and molecular studies completed in 129 pregnancies. *Prenat Diagn.* 1997;17:559–570.

369. Mornet E, Muller F, Ngo S, et al. Correlation of alkaline phosphatase (ALP) determination and analysis of the tissue nonspecific ALP gene in prenatal diagnosis of severe hypophosphatasia. *Prenat Diagn.* 1999;19:755–757.

370. Vandevijver N, De Die-Smulders CE, Offermans JP, et al.

Lethal hypophosphatasia, spur type: Case report and fe-topathological study. *Genet Couns.* 1998;9:205–209.

371. Ramage IJ, Howatson AJ, Beattie TJ. Hypophosphatasia. *J Clin Pathol.* 1996;49:682.

372. Pauli RM, Modaff P, Sipes SL, et al. Mild hypophosphatasia mimicking severe osteogenesis imperfecta in utero: Bent but not broken. *Am J Med Genet.* 1999;86:434–438.

373. Terada S, Suzuki N, Ueno H, et al. A congenital lethal form of hypophosphatasia: Histologic and ultrastructural study. *Acta Obstet Gynecol Scand.* 1996;75:502–505.

374. Wladimiroff JW, Niermeijen MF, van der Harten JJ, et al. Early prenatal diagnosis of congenital hypophosphatasia: Case report. *Prenat Diagn.* 1985;5:47.

375. Warren RC, McKenzie CF, Rodeck CH, et al. First trimester diagnosis of hypophosphatasia with a monoclonal antibody to the liver/bone/kidney isoenzyme of alkaline phosphatase. *Lancet.* 1985;2:856.

376. Sato S, Matsuo N. Genetic analysis of hypophosphatasia. *Acta Paediatr Jpn.* 1997;39:528–532.

377. Rudd NL, Miskin M, Hoar DI, et al. Prenatal diagnosis of hypophosphatasia. *N Engl J Med.* 1976;1:146.

378. Rattenbury JM, Blau K, Sandler M, et al. Prenatal diagnosis of hypophosphatasia. *Lancet.* 1976;1:306.

379. Orimo H, Nakajima E, Hayashi Z, et al. First-trimester prenatal molecular diagnosis of infantile hypophosphatasia in a Japanese family. *Prenat Diagn.* 1996;16:559–563.

380. Henthorn PS, Whyte MP. Infantile hypophosphatasia: Successful prenatal assessment by testing for tissue-non-specific alkaline phosphatase isoenzyme gene mutations. *Prenat Diagn.* 1995;15:1001–1006.

381. Ozono K, Yamagata M, Michigami T, et al. Identification of novel missense mutations (Phe310Leu and Gly439Arg) in a neonatal case of hypophosphatasia. *J Clin Endocrinol Metab.* 1996;81:4458–4461.

382. Horton WA, Rimoin DL, Lachman RS, et al. The phenotypic variability of diastrophic dysplasia. *J Pediatr.* 1978;93:609.

383. Kaitila I, Ammala P, Karjalainen O, et al. Early prenatal detection of diastrophic dysplasia. *Prenat Diagn.* 1983;3:237.

384. Mantagos S, Weiss RR, Mahoney M, Hobbins JC. Prenatal diagnosis of diastrophic dwarfism. *Am J Obstet Gynecol.* 1981;139:1111.

385. Gembruch U, Niesen M, Kehrberg H, Hansmann M. Diastrophic dysplasia: A specific prenatal diagnosis by ultrasound. *Prenat Diagn.* 1988;8:539.

386. Gollop TR, Eigier A. Brief clinical report: Prenatal ultrasound diagnosis of diastrophic dysplasia at 16 weeks. *Am J Med Genet.* 1987;27:321.

387. Jung C, Sohn C, Sergi C. Case report: Prenatal diagnosis of diastrophic dysplasia by ultrasound at 21 weeks of gestation in a mother with massive obesity. *Prenat Diagn.* 1998;18:378–383.

388. Gustavson K-H, Holmgren G, Jagell S, Jorulf G. Lethal and non-lethal diastrophic dysplasia: A study of 14 Swedish cases. *Clin Genet.* 1985;28:321.

389. Eteson DJ, Beluffi G, Burgio GR, et al. Pseudodiastrophic dysplasia: A distinct newborn skeletal dysplasia. *J Pediatr.* 1986;109:635.

390. Kniest W. Zur Abgrenzung der Dysostosis enchondralis von der Chondrodystrophie. *Z Kinderheilk.* 1952;70:633–640.

391. Winterpacht A, Hilbert M, Schwarze U, et al. Kniest and Stickler dysplasia phenotypes caused by collagen type II gene (COL2A1) defect. *Nat Genet.* 1993;3:323–326.

392. Fernandes RJ, Wilkin DJ, Weis MA, et al. Incorporation of structurally defective type II collagen into cartilage matrix in Kniest chondrodysplasia. *Arch Biochem Biophys.* 1998;355:282–290.

393. Weis MA, Wilkin DJ, Kim HJ, et al. Structurally abnormal type II collagen in a severe form of Kniest dysplasia caused by an exon 24 skipping mutation. *J Biol Chem.* 1998;273:4761–4768.

394. Siggers D, Rimoin D, Dorst J, et al. The Kniest syndrome. *Birth Defects.* 1974;10:193.

395. Spranger J, Winterpacht A, Zabel B. Kniest dysplasia: Dr. W. Kniest, his patient, the molecular defect. *Am J Med Genet.* 1997;69:79–84.

396. Chen H, Yang SS, Gonzales E. Kniest dysplasia: Neonatal death with necropsy. *Am J Med Genet.* 1980;6:171.

397. Weis MA, Wilkin DJ, Kim HJ, et al. Structurally abnormal type II collagen in a severe form of Kniest dysplasia caused by an exon 24 skipping mutation. *J Biol Chem.* 1998;273:4761–4768.

398. Hooshang T, Ralph SL. *Radiology of Syndromes, Metabolic Disorders, and Skeletal Dysplasias*, 3rd ed. Chicago: Year Book Medical Publishers; 1983.

399. Handmaker SD, Campbell IA, Robinson LD, et al. Dyssegmental dwarfism: A new syndrome of lethal dwarfism. *Birth Defects.* 1977;13:79.

400. Stoll C, Langer B, Gasser B, et al. Sporadic case of dyssegmental dysplasia with antenatal presentation. *Genet Couns.* 1998;9:125–130.

401. Prabhu VG, Kozma C, Leftridge CA, et al. Dyssegmental dysplasia Silverman–Handmaker type in a consanguineous Druze Lebanese family: Long term survival and documentation of the natural history. *Am J Med Genet.* 1998;75:164–170.

402. Andersen PE Jr, Hauge M, Bang J. Dyssegmental dysplasia in siblings: Prenatal ultrasonic diagnosis. *Skeletal Radiol.* 1988;17:29.

403. Kim HJ, Costales F, Bouzouki M, Wallach RC. Prenatal diagnosis of dyssegmental dwarfism. *Prenat Diagn.* 1986;6:143.

404. Hsieh YY, Chang CC, Tsai HD, et al. Prenatal diagnosis of dyssegmental dysplasia. A case report. *J Reprod Med.* 1999;44:303–305.

405. Maroteaux P, Spranger J, Opitz JM, et al. The campomelic syndrome. *Presse Med.* 1971;79:1157–1162.

406. Goji K, Nishijima E, Tsugawa C, et al. Novel missense mutation in the HMG box of SOX9 gene in a Japanese XY male resulted in campomelic dysplasia and severe defect in masculinization. *Hum Mutat.* 1998;1(suppl):S114–S116.

407. Wunderle VM, Critcher R, Hastie N, et al. Deletion of long-range regulatory elements upstream of SOX9 causes campomelic dysplasia. *Proc Natl Acad Sci U S A.* 1998;95:10649–10654.

408. Aslan Y, Erduran E, Mocan H, et al. Campomelic dysplasia associated with mandibular clefting. *Genet Couns.* 1996;7:17–20.

409. Glass RB, Rosenbaum KN. Acampomelic campomelic dysplasia: Further radiographic variations. *Am J Med Genet.* 1997;69:29–32.

410. Soell J. Camptomelic dysplasia: A case study [in process citation]. *Neonat Netw.* 1999;18:41–48.

411. Houston CS, Opitz JM, Spranger JW, et al. The campomelic syndrome: Review, report of 17 cases, and follow-up on the currently 17-year-old boy first reported by Maroteaux et al, in 1971. *Am J Med Genet.* 1983;15:3–28.

412. Mansour S, Hall CM, Pembrey ME, Young ID. A clinical and genetic study of campomelic dysplasia. *J Med Genet.* 1995; 32:415–420.

413. Fryns JP, van der Berghe K, van Assche A, vanden Berghe H. Prenatal diagnosis of campomelic dwarfism. *Clin Genet.* 1981;19:199.

414. Winter R, Rosenkranz W, Hofmann H, et al. Prenatal diagnosis of campomelic dysplasia by ultrasonography. *Prenat Diagn.* 1985;5:1.

415. Balcar I, Bieber FR. Sonographic and radiologic findings in campomelic dysplasia. *AJR.* 1983;141:481.

416. Norgard M, Yankowitz J, Rhead W, et al. Prenatal ultrasound findings in hydrolethalus: Continuing difficulties in diagnosis. *Prenat Diagn.* 1996;16:173–179.

417. Saunders RC, Greyson-Fleg RT, Hogge WA, et al. Osteogenesis imperfecta and campomelic dysplasia: Difficulties in prenatal diagnosis. *J Ultrasound Med.* 1994;13: 691–700.

418. Beluffi G, Fraccaro M. Genetical and clinical aspects of campomelic dysplasia. *Prog Clin Biol Res.* 1982;104:53.

419. Cooke CT, Mulcahy MT, Cullity GJ, et al. Campomelic dysplasia with sex reversal: Morphological and cytogenetic studies of a case. *Pathology.* 1985;17:526–529.

420. Romero R, Ghidini A, Eswara MS, et al. Prenatal findings in a case of spondylocostal dysplasia type I (Jarcho–Levin syndrome). *Obstet Gynecol.* 1988;71:988.

421. Jeune M, Carron R. Dystrophic thoracique asphyxiante caractere familial. *Arch Fr Pediatr.* 1955;12:276–279.

422. Maarup LP, Host A. The Jeune syndrome, asphyxiating thoracic dysplasia. A review and description of 2 siblings. *Ugeskr Laeger.* 1985;147:1676–1678.

423. Capilupi B, Olappi G, Cornaglia AM, Novati GP. Asphyxiating thoracic dysplasia or Jeune's syndrome. Description of 2 mild familial cases. *Pediatr Med Chir.* 1996;18:529–532.

424. Kozlowski K, Masel J. Asphyxiating thoracic dystrophy without respiratory distress. Report of 2 cases of the latent form. *Pediatr Radiol.* 1976;5:30.

425. Friedman JM, Kaplan HG, Hall JG. The Jeune syndrome (asphyxiating thoracic dystrophy) in an adult. *Am J Med.* 1975;59:857.

426. Silengo M, Gianino P, Longo P, et al. Dandy-Walker complex in a child with Jeune's asphyxiating thoracic dystrophy. *Pediatr Radiol.* 2000;30(6):430.

427. Novakovic I, Kostic M, Popovic-Rolovic M, et al. Jeune's syndrome (3 case reports). *Srp Arh Celok Lek.* 1996;124(suppl 1): 244–246.

428. Katthofer B. Asphyxiating thoracic dysplasia (Jeune-syndrome)—A medical and nursing report. *Kinderkrankenschwester.* 1993;12:342–344.

429. Trabelsi M, Hammou-Jeddi A, Kammoun A, et al. Asphyxiating thoracic dysplasia associated with hepatic ductal hypoplasia, agenesis of the corpus callosum and Dandy–Walker syndrome. *Pediatrie.* 1990;45:35–38.

430. Hsieh YY, Hsu TY, Lee CC, et al. Prenatal diagnosis of thoracopelvic dysplasia. A case report. *J Reprod Med.* 1999;44: 737–740.

431. Elejalde BR, de Elejalde MM, Pansch D. Prenatal diagnosis of Jeune syndrome. *Am J Med Genet.* 1985;21:433.

432. Lipson M, Waskey J, Rice J, et al. Prenatal diagnosis of asphyxiating thoracic dysplasia. *Am J Med Genet.* 1984;18:273.

433. Schinzel A, Savoldelli G, Briner J, Schubiger G. Prenatal sonographic diagnosis of Jeune syndrome. *Radiology.* 1985;154: 777.

434. Ardura Fernandez J, Alvarez Gonzalez C, Rodriguez Fernandez M, et al. Asphyxiating thoracic dysplasia associated with proximal myopathy and arachnoid cyst. *An Esp Pediatr.* 1990;33:592–596.

435. Kapoor R, Saha MM, Gupta NC. Antenatal diagnosis of asphyxiating thoracic dysplasia. *Indian Pediatr.* 1989;26: 495–497.

436. Skiptunas SM, Weiner S. Early prenatal diagnosis of asphyxiating thoracic dysplasia (Jeune's syndrome). Value of fetal thoracic measurement. *J Ultrasound Med.* 1987;6:41–43.

437. Panero Lopez AL, Puyol Buil PJ, Belaustegui Cueto A, et al. Asphyxiating thoracic dysplasia in two dizygotic twins. *An Esp Pediatr.* 1987;26:453–456.

438. Schinzel A, Savoldelli G, Briner J, et al. Prenatal sonographic diagnosis of Jeune syndrome. *Radiology.* 1985;154: 777–778.

439. Lavanya R, Pratap K. Short rib polydactyly syndrome—A rare skeletal dysplasia. *Int J Gynaecol Obstet.* 1995;50:291–292.

440. Sarafoglou K, Funai EF, Fefferman N, et al. Short rib–polydactyly syndrome: More evidence of a continuous spectrum. *Clin Genet.* 1999;56:145–148.

441. Wladimiroff JW, Niermeijer MF, Laar J, et al. Prenatal diagnosis of skeletal dysplasia by real-time ultrasound. *Obstet Gynecol.* 1984;63:360.

442. Muller LM, Cremin BJ. Ultrasonic demonstration of fetal skeletal dysplasia. *SAMJ.* 1985;67:222.

443. Meizner I, Barnhard Y. Short-rib polydactyly syndrome (SRPS) type III diagnosed during routine prenatal ultrasonographic screening. A case report. *Prenat Diagn.* 1995;15: 665–668.

444. Montemarano H, Bulas DI, Chandra R, Tifft C. Prenatal diagnosis of glomerulocystic kidney disease in short-rib polydactyly syndrome type II, Majewski type. *Pediatr Radiol.* 1995;25:469–471.

445. Scarano G, Della Monica M, Capece G, et al. A case of short-rib syndrome without polydactyly in a stillborn: A new type? *Birth Defects Orig Art Ser.* 1996;30:95–101.

446. Fujisawa K. Saldino–Noonan syndrome (short rib polydactyly syndrome type I). *Ryoikibetsu Shokogun Shirizu.* 1996;15:297–299.

447. Majewski E, Ozturk B, Gillessen-Kaesbach G. Jeune syndrome with tongue lobulation and preaxial polydactyly, and Jeune syndrome with situs inversus and asplenia: Compound heterozygosity Jeune–Mohr and Jeune–Ivemark? *Am J Med Genet.* 1996;63:74–79.

448. Prudlo J, Stoltenburg-Didinger G, Jimenez E, et al. Central nervous system alterations in a case of short-rib polydactyly syndrome, Majewski type. *Dev Med Child Neurol.* 1993;35:158–162.

449. Cideciyan D, Rodriguez MM, Haun RL, et al. New findings in short rib syndrome. *Am J Med Genet.* 1993;46:255–259.

450. Tsai FJ, Tsai CH, Wang TR. Beemer–Langer type short rib–polydactyly syndrome: Report of two cases. *Chung Hua*

Min Kuo Hsiao Erh Ko I Hsueh Hui Tsa Chih. 1994;35: 331–334.

451. Myong NH, Park JW, Chi JG. Short-rib polydactyly syndrome, Beemer–Langer type, with bilateral huge polycystic renal dysplasia: An autopsy case. *J Kor Med Sci.* 1998;13:201–206.

452. Hentze S, Sergi C, Troeger J, et al. Short-rib-polydactyly syndrome type Verma–Naumoff–Le Marec in a fetus with histological hallmarks of type Saldino–Noonan but lacking internal organ abnormalities. *Am J Med Genet.* 1998;80:281–285.

453. Elcioglu N, Karatekin G, Sezgin B, et al. Short rib-polydactyly syndrome in twins: Beemer–Langer type with polydactyly. *Clin Genet.* 1996;50:159–163.

454. Scarano G, Della Monica M, Capece G, et al. A case of short-rib syndrome without polydactyly in a stillborn: A new type? *Birth Defects Orig Art Ser.* 1996;30:95–101.

455. Shindel B, Wise S. Recurrent short rib–polydactyly syndrome with unusual associations. *J Clin Ultrasound.* 1999;27: 143–146.

456. Wu MH, Kuo PL, Lin SJ. Prenatal diagnosis of recurrence of short rib–polydactyly syndrome. *Am J Med Genet.* 1995;55:279–284.

457. Ohdo S. Ellis–van Creveld syndrome. *Ryoikibetsu Shokogun Shirizu.* 1996;15:261–263.

458. Alcalde MM, Castillo JA, Garcia Urruticoechea P, et al. Ellis–van Creveld syndrome: An easy early diagnosis?. *Rev Esp Cardiol.* 1998;51:407–409.

459. Ortega Rodriguez J, Ferrer Ferran J, Fernandez Lopez A, et al. The Ellis–van Creveld syndrome (chondroectodermal dysplasia). Apropos a clinical case. *An Esp Pediatr.* 1999;50: 74–76.

460. McKusick VA, Egeland JA, Eldridge R, et al. Dwarfism in the Amish. The Ellis–van Creveld syndrome. *Bull Johns Hopkins Hosp.* 1964;115:306.

461. Polymeropoulos MH, Ide SE, Wright M, et al. The gene for the Ellis–van Creveld syndrome is located on chromosome 4p16. *Genomics.* 1996;35:1–5.

462. Wasant P, Waeteekul S, Rimoin DL, et al. Genetic skeletal dysplasia in Thailand: The Siriraj experience. *Southeast Asian J Trop Med Publ Health.* 1995;26(suppl 1):59–67.

463. Levin SE, Dansky R, Milner S, et al. Atrioventricular septal defect and type A postaxial polydactyly without other major associated anomalies: A specific association [see comments]. *Pediatr Cardiol.* 1995;16:242–246.

464. Digilio MC, Marino B, Giannotti A, et al. Single atrium, atrioventricular canal/postaxial hexodactyly indicating Ellis–van Creveld syndrome [letter; comment]. *Hum Genet.* 1995;96:251–253.

465. Chang YC, Wu JM, Lin SJ, et al. Common atrium with Ebstein's anomaly in a neonate with Ellis–van Creveld syndrome. *Chung Hua Min Kuo Hsiao Erh Ko I Hsueh Hui Tsa Chih.* 1995;36:50–52.

466. Yapar EG, Ekici E, Aydogdu T, et al. Diagnostic problems in a case with mucometrocolpos, polydactyly, congenital heart disease, and skeletal dysplasia. *Am J Med Genet.* 1996;66:343–346.

467. Digilio MC, Marino B, Giannotti A, et al. Atrioventricular canal defect and postaxial polydactyly indicating phenotypic overlap of Ellis–van Creveld and Kaufman–McKusick syndromes [letter; comment]. *Pediatr Cardiol.* 1997;18:74–75.

468. Horigome H, Hamada H, Sohda S, et al. Prenatal ultrasonic diagnosis of a case of Ellis–van Creveld syndrome with a single atrium. *Pediatr Radiol.* 1997;27:942–944.

469. Gelb BD. Molecular genetics of congenital heart disease. *Curr Opin Cardiol.* 1997;12:321–328.

470. Bui TH, Marsk L, Ekloef O, Theorell K. Prenatal diagnosis of chondroectodermal dysplasia with fetoscopy. *Prenat Diagn.* 1984;4:155.

471. Mahoney MJ, Hobbins JC. Prenatal diagnosis of chondroectodermal dysplasia (Ellis–van Creveld syndrome) with fetoscopy and ultrasound. *N Engl J Med.* 1977;297:258.

472. Zimmer EZ, Weinraub Z, Raijman A, et al. Antenatal diagnosis of a fetus with an extremely narrow thorax and short limb dwarfism. *J Clin Ultrasound.* 1984;12:112.

473. Tongsong T, Chanprapaph P. Prenatal sonographic diagnosis of Ellis–van Creveld syndrome. *J Clin Ultrasound.* 2000;28:38–41.

474. Guschmann M, Horn D, Gasiorek-Wiens A, et al. Ellis–van Creveld syndrome: Examination at 15 weeks' gestation. *Prenat Diagn.* 1999;19:879–883.

475. Torrente I, Mangino M, De Luca A, et al. First-trimester prenatal diagnosis of Ellis–van Creveld syndrome using linked microsatellite markers. *Prenat Diagn.* 1998;18:504.

476. Horigome H, Hamada H, Sohda S, et al. Prenatal ultrasonic diagnosis of a case of Ellis–van Creveld syndrome with a single atrium. *Pediatr Radiol.* 1997;27:942–944.

477. Bouguerra L, Turki R, Hichri A. Value of echocardiography in Ellis–Van Creveld syndrome. *Arch Pediatr.* 1995;2:1022.

478. Chang YC, Wu JM, Lin SJ, et al. Common atrium with Ebstein's anomaly in a neonate with Ellis–van Creveld syndrome. *Chung Hua Min Kuo Hsiao Erh Ko I Hsueh Hui Tsa Chih.* 1995;Jan–Feb;36(1):50–52.

479. Bod M, Creizel A, Lenz W. Incidence at birth of different types of limb reduction abnormalities in Hungary 1975–1977. *Hum Genet.* 1983;65:27.

480. Goldberg MJ. *The Dysmorphic Child: An Orthopedic Perspective.* New York: Raven Press; 1987.

481. Zhu J, Miao L, Xu C, et al. Analysis of 822 infants with limb reduction defect in China. *J West China Univ Med Sci.* 1996;27:400–403.

482. Bromley B, Benacerraf B. Abnormalities of the hands and feet in the fetus: Sonographic findings. *AJR.* 1995;165:1239–1243.

483. Emmanouil-Nikoloussi EN, Kerameos-Foroglou C. Developmental malformations of human tongue and associated syndromes [review]. *Bull Group Int Rech Sci Stomatol Odontol.* 1992;35:5–12.

484. Tunobileck E, Yalcin C, Atasu M. Aglossia–adactylia syndrome (special emphasis on the inheritance pattern). *Clin Genet.* 1977;11:421.

485. Lecannellier J, Vischer D. The aglossia–adactylia syndrome. *Helv Paediatr Acta.* 1976;31:77–84.

486. Marti-Herrero M, Cabrera-Lopez JC, Toledo L, et al. Moebius syndrome. Three different forms of presentation. *Rev Neurol.* 1998;27:975–978.

487. Canete Estrada R, Gil Rivas R, Alvarez Marcos R, et al. Hanhart syndrome (aglossia–adactylia syndrome). Report of two cases. *An Esp Pediatr.* 1990; 33:465–468.

488. Deffez JP, Rostand B, Allain P, et al. An unusual aglossia-adactylia syndrome. *Rev Stomatol Chir Maxillofac.* 1981;82: 241–246.

489. Cuvelier B, Cousin J, Pauli A, et al. Aglossia–adactylia

syndrome: Two new cases. *Ann Pediatr (Paris)*. 1981;28: 433–435.

490. Robinow M, Marsh JL, Edgerton MT, et al. Discordance in monozygotic twins for aglossia–adactylia, and possible clues to the pathogenesis of the syndrome. *Birth Defects Orig Art Ser*. 1978;14:223–230.

491. Grippaudo FR, Kennedy DC. Oromandibular–limb hypogenesis syndromes: A case of aglossia with an intraoral band. *Br J Plast Surg*. 1998;51:480–483.

492. Lammens M, Moerman Ph, Fryns JP, et al. Neuropathological findings in Moebius syndrome. *Clin Genet*. 1998;54:136–141.

493. d'Orey C, Melo MJ, Costa A, et al. Moebius syndrome in newborn infants (letter). *Arch Pediatr*. 1997;4:897–898.

494. Bonanni P, Guerrini R. Segmental facial myoclonus in Moebius syndrome [in process citation]. *Mov Disord*. 1999;14: 1021–1024.

495. Baraitser M. Genetics of Moebius syndrome. *J Med Genet*. 1977;14:415.

496. Abramson DL, Cohen MM Jr, Mulliken JB. Mobius syndrome: Classification and grading system. *Plast Reconstr Surg*. 1998;102:961–967.

497. Matsui A, Nakagawa M, Okuno M. Association of atrial septal defect with Poland–Moebius syndrome: Vascular disruption can be a common etiologic factor. A case report. *Angiology*. 1997;48:269–271.

498. Lipson AH, Gillerot Y, Tannenberg AE, Giurgea S. Two cases of maternal antenatal splenic rupture and hypotension associated with Moebius syndrome and cerebral palsy in offspring. Further evidence for a utero placental vascular aetiology for the Moebius syndrome and some cases of cerebral palsy. *Eur J Pediatr*. 1996;155:800–804.

499. Farina D, Gatto G, Leonessa L, et al. Poland syndrome: A case with a combination of syndromes. *Panminerva Med*. 1999; 41:259–260.

500. Larrandaburu M, Schuler L, Ehlers JA, et al. The occurrence of Poland and Poland–Moebius syndromes in the same family: Further evidence of their genetic component. *Clin Dysmorphol*. 1999;8:93–99.

501. Bavinck JN, Weaver DD. Subclavian artery supply disruption sequence: Hypothesis of a vascular etiology for Poland, Klippel–Feil, and Mobius anomalies. *Am J Med Genet*. 1986;23:903–918.

502. Brill CB, Peyster RG, Keller MS, et al. Isolation of the right subclavian artery with subclavian steal in a child with Klippel–Feil anomaly: An example of the subclavian artery supply disruption sequence. *Am J Med Genet*. 1987;26:933–940.

503. St. Charles S, DiMario FJ Jr, Grunnet ML. Mobius sequence: Further in vivo support for the subclavian artery supply disruption sequence. *Am J Med Genet*. 1993;47:289–293.

504. Hebert AA, Esterly NB, Holbrook KA, et al. The CHILD syndrome. Histologic and ultrastructural studies. *Arch Dermatol*. 1987;123:503–509.

505. Hashimoto K, Topper S, Sharata H, et al. CHILD syndrome: Analysis of abnormal keratinization and ultrastructure. *Pediatr Dermatol*. 1995;12:116–129.

506. Happle R, Koch H, Lenz W. The CHILD syndrome. Congenital hemidysplasia with ichthyosiform erythroderma and limb defects. *Eur J Pediatr*. 1980;134:27–33.

507. Hoeger PH, Adwani SS, Whitehead BF, et al. Ichthyosiform erythroderma and cardiomyopathy: Report of two cases and review of the literature. *Br J Dermatol*. 1998;139: 1055–1059.

508. Happle R, Effendy I, Megahed M, et al. CHILD syndrome in a boy. *Am J Med Genet*. 1996;62:192–194.

509. Happle R, Mittag H, Kuster W. The CHILD nevus: A distinct skin disorder [review]. *Dermatology*. 1995;191:210–216.

510. Holmes LB, Redline RW, Brown DL, et al. Absence/hypoplasia of tibia, polydactyly, retrocerebellar arachnoid cyst, and other anomalies: An autosomal recessive disorder. *J Med Genet*. 1995;32:896–900.

511. Lipson AH. Amelia of the arms and femur/fibula deficiency with splenogonadal fusion in a child born to a consanguineous couple. *Am J Med Genet*. 1995;55:265–268.

512. Vosshenrich R, Bartkowski R, Fischer U, et al. Splenogonadal fusion. *Rofo Fortschr Geb Rontgenstr Neuen Bildgeb Verfahr*. 1991;155:191–193.

513. Bonneau D, Roume J, Gonzalez M, et al. Splenogonadal fusion limb defect syndrome: Report of five new cases and review. *Am J Med Genet*. 1999;86:347–358.

514. Pauli RM, Greenlaw A. Limb deficiency and splenogonadal fusion. *Am J Med Genet*. 1982;13:81.

515. Bearss RW. Splenic–gonadal fusion. *Urology*. 1980;16:277.

516. Moore PJ, Hawkins EP, Galliani CA, et al. Splenogonadal fusion with limb deficiency and micrognathia [review]. *South Med J*. 1997;90:1152–1155.

517. Bonafede RP, Beighton P. Autosomal dominant inheritance of scalp defects with extrodactyly. *Am J Med Genet*. 1979; 3:35.

518. Fryns JP, Legius E, Demaerel P, et al. Congenital scalp defect, distal limb reduction anomalies, right spastic hemiplegia and hypoplasia of the left arteria cerebri media. Further evidence that interruption of early embryonic blood supply may result in Adams–Oliver (plus) syndrome. *Clin Genet*. 1996;50:505–509.

519. Claus GH, Newman CGH. The thalidomide syndrome: Risks of exposure and spectrum of malformations. *Teratology*. 1986; 13:555.

520. Lee A, Kratochwil A, Deutinger J, et al. Three-dimensional ultrasound in diagnosing phocomelia. *Ultrasound Obstet Gynecol*. 1995;5:238–240.

521. de Ravel TJ, Seftel MD, Wright CA. Tetra-amelia and splenogonadal fusion in Roberts syndrome. *Am J Med Genet*. 1997;68:185–189.

522. Sinha AK, Verma RS, Mani VJ. Clinical heterogeneity of skeletal dysplasia in Roberts syndrome: A review [see comments]. *Hum Hered*. 1994;44:121–126.

523. Waldenmaier C, Aldenhoff P, Klemm T. The Roberts' syndrome. *Hum Genet*. 1978;40:345.

524. Benzacken B, Savary JB, Manouvrier S, et al. Prenatal diagnosis of Roberts syndrome: Two new cases [see comments]. *Prenat Diagn*. 1996;16:125–130.

525. Rittler M, Higa S. Grebe syndrome: A second case with extremely severe manifestations. *J Med Genet*. 1997;34:1038.

526. Kulkarni ML, Kumar B, Nasser A, et al. Grebe syndrome: A very severely affected case [letter]. *J Med Genet*. 1995;32: 326–327.

527. Kulkarni ML, Kulkarni BM, Nasser PU. Antenatal diagnosis of Grebe syndrome in a twin pregnancy by ultrasound. *Indian Pediatr*. 1995;32:1007–1011.

528. Hamanishi C. Congenital short femur. *J Bone Joint Surg.* 1980;62:307.

529. Daentl DL, Smith DW, Scott C. Femoral hypoplasia—Unusual facie syndrome. *J Pediatr.* 1975;86:107.

530. Burn J, Winter RJ, Baraitser M, et al. The femoral hypoplasia—Unusual facies syndrome. *J Med Genet.* 1984;21:331.

531. Sanpera I Jr, Fixsen JA, Sparks LT, et al. Knee in congenital short femur. *J Pediatr Orthop B.* 1995;4:159–163.

532. Makino Y, Inoue T, Shirota K, et al. A case of congenital familial short femur diagnosed prenatally. *Fetal Diagn Ther.* 1998;13:206–208.

533. Gupta DKS, Gupta SK. Familial bilateral femoral focal deficiency. *J Bone Joint Surg.* 1984;66:1470.

534. Frey M, Williams J. What is your diagnosis? Radiographic diagnosis—Ectrodactyly. *J Am Vet Med Assoc.* 1995; 206:619–620.

535. Holmes LB, Redline RW, Brown DL, et al. Absence/hypoplasia of tibia, polydactyly, retrocerebellar arachnoid cyst, and other anomalies: An autosomal recessive disorder. *J Med Genet.* 1995;32:896–900.

536. Miura T, Suzuki M. Clinical differences between typical and atypical cleft hand. *J Hand Surg.* 1984;9:311.

537. Glicenstein J, Guero S, Haddad R. Median clefts of the hand. Classification and therapeutic indications apropos of 29 cases. *Ann Chir Main Memb Super.* 1995;14:253.

538. Tada K, Yonenobu K, Swanson AB. Congenital central ray deficiency in the hand—A survey of 59 cases and subclassification. *J Hand Surg.* 1981;6:434.

539. Van den Berghe H, Dequeker J, Fryns JP, et al. Familial occurrence of severe ulnar aplasia and lobster claw feet: A new syndrome. *Hum Genet.* 1978;42:109.

540. Verma IC, Joseph R, Bhargava S, et al. Split-hand and split-foot deformity inherited as an autosomal recessive trait. *Clin Genet.* 1976;9:8.

541. Roelfsema NM, Cobben JM. The EEC syndrome: A literature study. *Clin Dysmorphol.* 1996;5:115–17.

542. Rudiger RA, Haase W, Passarge E. Association of ectrodactyly, ectodermal dysplasia, and cleft lip–palate. *Am J Dis Child.* 1970;120:160.

543. Miller CI, Hashimoto K, Shwayder T, et al. What syndrome is this? Ectrodactyly, ectodermal dysplasia, and cleft palate (EEC) syndrome. *Pediatr Dermatol.* 1997;14:239–240.

544. Kasmann B, Ruprecht KW. Ocular manifestations in a father and son with EEC syndrome. *Graefes Arch Clin Exp Ophthalmol.* 1997;235:512–516.

545. Buss PW, Hughes HE, Clarke A. Twenty-four cases of the EEC syndrome: Clinical presentation and management. *J Med Genet.* 1995;32:716–723.

546. Krunic AL, Vesic SA, Goldner B, et al. Ectrodactyly, soft-tissue syndactyly, and nodulocystic acne: Coincidence or association? *Pediatr Dermatol.* 1997;14:31–35.

547. Gershoni-Baruch R, Goldscher D, Hochberg Z. Ectrodactyly–ectodermal dysplasia–clefting syndrome and hypothalamopituitary insufficiency. *Am J Med Genet.* 1997;68:168–172.

548. Maas SM, de Jong TP, Buss P, et al. EEC syndrome and genitourinary anomalies: An update. *Am J Med Genet.* 1996;63:472–478.

549. Leiter E, Lipson J. Genitourinary tract anomalies in lobster claw syndrome. *J Urol.* 1976;115:339.

550. Penchaszadeh VB, De Negrotti TC. Ectrodactyly–ectodermal dysplasia–clefting (EEC) syndrome: Dominant inheritance and variable expression. *J Med Genet.* 1976;13:281.

551. Halal F, Homsy M, Perreault G. Acro–renal–ocular syndrome: Autosomal dominant thumb hypoplasia, renal ectopia, and eye defect. *Am J Med Genet.* 1984;17:753.

552. Chan KM, Lamb DW. Triphalangeal thumb and five-fingered hand. *Hand.* 1983;15:329.

553. Wood VE. Congenital thumb deformities. *Clin Orthop.* 1985;195:7

554. Bujdoso G, Lenz W. Monodactylous splithand–splitfoot. *Eur J Pediatr.* 1980;133:207.

555. Blauth W, Sonnichsen S. Congenital clubhand. *Orthopade.* 1986;15:160–171.

556. Goldberg MJ, Meyn M. The radial clubhand. *Orthop Clin North Am.* 1976;7:341–349.

557. Carroll RE, Louis DS. Anomalies associated with radial dysplasia. *J Pediatr.* 1974;84:409.

558. Rotman MB, Manske PR. Radial clubhand and contralateral duplicated thumb. *J Hand Surg (Am).* 1994;19:361–363.

559. Grill F, Freilinger W, Strobl W. Treatment of a radial club hand. *Z Orthop Ihre Grenzgeb.* 1996;134:324–331.

560. Alter BP. Bone marrow failure syndromes. *Clin Lab Med.* 1999;19:113–133.

561. Glanz A, Fraser FC. Spectrum of anomalies in Fanconi anaemia. *J Med Genet.* 1982;19:412.

562. Nilsson LR. Chronic pancytopenia with multiple congenital abnormalities (Fanconi's anaemia). *Acta Paediatr.* 1960;49:518.

563. Bueno Lozano O, Bueno Martinez I, Jimenez Vidal A, et al. A girl with pancytopenia, short stature and minor skeletal abnormalities. *An Esp Pediatr.* 1997;46:409–410.

564. Prindull G, Stubbe P, Kratzer W. Fanconi's anemia. I. Case histories, clinical and laboratory findings in six affected siblings. *Z Kinderheilkd.* 1975;120:37–49.

565. Digweed M. Molecular basis of Fanconi's anemia. *Klin Padiatr.* 1999;211:192–197.

566. Lo Ten Foe JR, Rooimans MA, Bosnoyan-Collins L, et al. Expression cloning of a cDNA for the major Fanconi anaemia gene, FAA. *Nat Genet.* 1996;14:320–323.

567. Auerbach AD, Sagi M, Adler B. Fanconi anemia: Prenatal diagnosis in 30 fetuses at risk. *Pediatrics.* 1985;76:794.

568. Sekine I, Hagiwara T, Miyazaki H, et al. Thrombocytopenia with absent radii syndrome: Studies on serum thrombopoietin levels and megakaryopoiesis in vitro. *J Pediatr Hematol Oncol.* 1998;20:74–78.

569. Ballmaier M, Schulze H, Strauss G, et al. Thrombopoietin in patients with congenital thrombocytopenia and absent radii: Elevated serum levels, normal receptor expression, but defective reactivity to thrombopoietin. *Blood.* 1997;90:612–619.

570. Miceli Sopo S, Pesaresi MA, Celestini E, et al. Pathogenesis of thrombocytopenia in the TAR syndrome. *Am J Pediatr Hematol Oncol.* 1992;14:186–187.

571. de Alarcon PA, Graeve JA, Levine RF, et al. Thrombocytopenia and absent radii syndrome: Defective megakaryocytopoiesis–thrombocytopoiesis. *Am J Pediatr Hematol Oncol.* 1991;13:77–83.

572. Fromm B, Niethard FU, Marquardt E. Thrombocytopenia and absent radius (TAR) syndrome. *Int Orthop.* 1991;15:95–99.

573. Urban M, Opitz C, Bommer C, et al. Bilaterally cleft lip, limb defects, and haematological manifestations: Roberts syndrome versus TAR syndrome. *Am J Med Genet.* 1998;79: 155–160.

574. Hedberg VA, Lipton JM. Thrombocytopenia with absent radii: A review of 100 cases. *Am J Pediatr Hematol Oncol.* 1988;10:51.

575. de Vries LS, Connell J, Bydder GM, et al. Recurrent intracranial haemorrhages in utero in an infant with alloimmune thrombocytopenia. Case report. *Br J Obstet Gynaecol.* 1988;95:299.

576. Shelton SD, Paulyson K, Kay HH. Prenatal diagnosis of thrombocytopenia absent radius (TAR) syndrome and vaginal delivery. *Prenat Diagn.* 1999;19:54–57.

577. Ergur AR, Yergok YZ, Ertekin A, et al. Prenatal diagnosis of an uncommon syndrome: Thrombocytopenia absent radius (TAR). *Zentralbl Gynakol.* 1998;120:75–78.

578. Boute O, Depret-Mosser S, Vinatier D, et al. Prenatal diagnosis of thrombocytopenia–absent radius syndrome. *Fetal Diagn Ther.* 1996;11:224–230.

579. Weinblatt M, Petrikovsky B, Bialer M, et al. Prenatal evaluation and in utero platelet transfusion for thrombocytopenia absent radii syndrome. *Prenat Diagn.* 1994;14:892–896.

580. Donnenfeld AE, Wiseman B, Lavi E, et al. Prenatal diagnosis of thrombocytopenia absent radius syndrome by ultrasound and cordocentesis. *Prenat Diagn.* 1990;10:29–35.

581. Muis N, Beemer FA, van Dijken P, et al. The Aase syndrome. Case report and review of the literature. *Eur J Pediatr.* 1986;145:153–157.

582. Hing AV, Dowton SB. Aase syndrome: Novel radiographic features. *Am J Med Genet.* 1993;45:413–415.

583. Yetgin S, Balci S, Irken G, et al. Aase–Smith syndrome: Report of a new case with unusual features. *Turk J Pediatr.* 1994;36:239–242.

584. D'Avanzo M, Pistoia V, Santinelli R, et al. Heterogeneity of the erythropoietic defect in two cases of Aase–Smith syndrome. *Pediatr Hematol Oncol.* 1994;11:189–195.

585. Pfeiffer RA, Ambs E. The Aase syndrome: Hereditary autosomal recessive congenital erythropoiesis insufficiency and triphalangeal thumbs. *Monatsschr Kinderheilkd.* 1983; 131:235–237.

586. Higginbottom MC, Jones KL, Kung FH. The Aase syndrome in a female infant. *J Med Genet.* 1978;15:484.

587. Dror Y, Durie P, Marcon P, et al. Duplication of distal thumb phalanx in Shwachman–Diamond syndrome. *Am J Med Genet.* 1998;78:67–69.

588. McLennan AC, Chitty LS, Rissik J, et al. Prenatal diagnosis of Blackfan–Diamond syndrome: Case report and review of the literature. *Prenat Diagn.* 1996;16:349–353.

589. Schneider MD, Schwartz RJ. Heart or hand? Unmasking the basis for specific Holt–Oram phenotypes. *Proc Natl Acad Sci U S A.* 1999;96:2577–2578.

590. Wilson GN. Correlated heart/limb anomalies in mendelian syndromes provide evidence for a cardiomelic developmental field. *Am J Med Genet.* 1998;76:297–305.

591. Bennhagen RG, Menahem S. Holt–Oram syndrome and multiple ventricular septal defects: An association suggesting a possible genetic marker? *Cardiol Young.* 1998;8:128–130.

592. Bohm M. Holt–Oram syndrome. *Circulation.* 1998;98: 2636–2637.

593. James MA, McCarroll HR Jr, Manske PR. Characteristics of patients with hypoplastic thumbs. *J Hand Surg (Am).* 1996; 21:104–113.

594. Cachat F, Rapatsalahy A, Sekarski N, et al. Three different types of atrial septal defects in the same family. *Arch Mal Coeur Vaiss.* 1999;92:667–669.

595. Sletten LJ, Pierpont ME. Variation in severity of cardiac disease in Holt–Oram syndrome. *Am J Med Genet.* 1996;65:128–132.

596. Elbaum R, Royer M, Godart S. Radial club hand and Holt–Oram syndrome. *Acta Chir Belg.* 1995;95:229–236.

597. Zhang KZ, Sun QB, Tsung OC. Holt–Oram syndrome in China: A collective review of 18 cases. *Am Heart J.* 1986; 111:573.

598. Matsuoka R. Holt–Oram syndrome. *Ryoikibetsu Shokogun Shirizu.* 1996;15:267–270.

599. Newbury-Ecob RA, Leanage R, Raeburn JA, et al. Holt–Oram syndrome: A clinical genetic study. *J Med Genet.* 1996;33:300–307.

600. Brons JTJ, van Geijn HP, Wladimiroff JW. Prenatal ultrasonographic diagnosis of the Holt–Oram syndrome. *Prenat Diagn.* 1988;8:175.

601. Penne D, Delanote G, Breysem L, et al. The Holt–Oram syndrome: Radiological approach. *J Belge Radiol.* 1997;80: 118–119.

602. Muller LM, De Jong G, Van Heerden KM. The antenatal ultrasonographic detection of the Holt–Oram syndrome. *S Afr Med J.* 1985;68:313–315.

603. Li QY, Newbury-Ecob RA, Terrett JA, et al. Holt–Oram syndrome is caused by mutations in TBX5, a member of the Brachyury (T) gene family. *Nat Genet.* 1997;15:21–29.

604. Lewis KB, Bruce RA, Baum D, et al. The upper limb–cardiovascular syndrome. *JAMA.* 1965;193:1080.

605. Chemke J, Nisani R, Fischel RE. Absent ulna in the Klippel–Feil syndrome: An unusual associated malformation. *Clin Genet.* 1980;17:167.

606. Tentamy SA, Miller JD. Extending the scope of the VATER association: Definition of a VATER syndrome. *J Pediatr.* 1974;85:345.

607. Masuno M. VATER association (VACTERL association). *Ryoikibetsu Shokogun Shirizu.* 1996;15:309–310.

608. Huang LW, Chen MR, Lin SP, et al. The VATER association: Analysis of forty six cases without karyotyping. *Chung Hua Min Kuo Hsiao Erh Ko I Hsueh Hui Tsa Chih.* 1995;36:30–34.

609. Medina-Escobedo G, Ridaura-Sanz C. The VATER association. *Bol Med Hosp Infant Mex.* 1992;49:231–240.

610. Quillin SP, Gilula LA. Imaging rounds #111. VATER association. *Orthop Rev.* 1992;21:85, 88–89.

611. Corsello G, Maresi E, Corrao AM, et al. VATER/VACTERL association: Clinical variability and expanding phenotype including laryngeal stenosis. *Am J Med Genet.* 1992;44:813–815. Erratum: *Am J Med Genet.* 1993;47:118.

612. Quan L, Smith DW. The VATER association: Vertebral defects, anal atresia, tracheoesophageal fistula with esophageal atresia, radial dysplasia. *Birth Defects.* 1972;8:75.

613. Werner W, Beintker M, Schubert J, et al. The VATER syndrome from the urologic viewpoint. *Urologe A.* 1998;37:203–205.

614. Unuvar E, Oguz F, Sahin K, et al. Coexistence of VATER association and recurrent urolithiasis: A case report. *Pediatr Nephrol.* 1998;12:141–143.

615. Botto LD, Khoury MJ, Mastroiacovo P, et al. The spectrum of congenital anomalies of the VATER association: An international study. *Am J Med Genet.* 1997;71:8–15.

616. Özbey H, Özbey N. Association of ambiguous genitalia with VATER anomalies. *Pediatr Surg Int.* 1997;12:230.

617. Auchterlonie IA, White MP. Recurrence of the VATER association within a sibship. *Clin Genet.* 1982;21:122.

618. Tongsong T, Wanapirak C, Piyamongkol W, et al. Prenatal sonographic diagnosis of VATER association. *J Clin Ultrasound.* 1999;27:378–384.

619. Rollnick BR, Kaye C, Nagatoshi K, et al. Oculoauriculovertebral dysplasia and variants: Phenotypic characteristics of 294 patients. *Am J Med Genet.* 1987;26:361.

620. Lal P, Agrawal P, Krishna A. Goldenhar syndrome. *Indian Pediatr.* 1997;34:837–838.

621. Manfre L, Genuardi P, Tortorici M, et al. Absence of the common crus in Goldenhar syndrome. *Am J Neuroradiol.* 1997;18:773–775.

622. Altamar-Rios J. Goldenhar's syndrome: A case report. *An Otorrinolaringol Ibero Am.* 1998;25:491–497.

623. Ferraris S, Silengo M, Ponzone A, et al. Goldenhar anomaly in one of triplets derived from in vitro fertilization. *Am J Med Genet.* 1999;84:167–168.

624. Araneta MR, Moore CA, Olney RS, et al. Goldenhar syndrome among infants born in military hospitals to Gulf War veterans. *Teratology.* 1997;56:244–251.

625. Tekkok IH. Syringomyelia as a complication of Goldenhar syndrome [letter; comment]. *Childs Nerv Syst.* 1996;12:291.

626. Matsuo K. Oculoauriculovertebral syndrome (Goldenhar syndrome). *Ryoikibetsu Shokogun Shirizu.* 1996;15:287–288.

627. Ferraris S, Silengo M, Ponzone A, et al. Goldenhar anomaly in one of triplets derived from in vitro fertilization [letter]. *Am J Med Genet.* 1999;84:167–168.

628. Luchtenberg M, Blotiu A, Lindemann G, et al. Anomalies of the efferent lacrimal ducts in Goldenhar syndrome (news). *Klin Monatsbl Augenheilkd.* 1998;213:aA8–9.

629. Tamas DE, Mahony BS, Bowie JD, et al. Prenatal sonographic diagnosis of hemifacial microsomia (Goldenhar–Gorlin syndrome). *J Ultrasound Med.* 1986;5:461.

630. Swanson AB, Tada K, Yonenubo K. Ulnar ray deficiency: Its various manifestations. *J Hand Surg.* 1984;9A:658.

631. Gausewitz SH, Meals RA, Setocuchi Y. Severe limb deficiency in Poland's syndrome. *Clin Orthop.* 1984;185:9.

632. Uuspaa V. Upper extremity deformities associated with the orofacial clefts. *Scand J Plast Reconstr Surg.* 1978;12:157.

633. David TJ. Preaxial polydactyly and the Poland complex. *Am J Med Genet.* 1982;13:1333.

634. Graham TJ, Ress AM. Finger polydactyly. *Hand Clin.* 1998;14:49–64.

635. de la Torre J, Simpson RL. Complete digital duplication: A case report and review of ulnar polydactyly. *Ann Plast Surg.* 1998;40:76–79.

636. De Smet L. Ulnar dimelia. *Acta Orthop Belg.* 1999;65:382–384.

637. Kaplan BS, Bellah RD. Postaxial polydactyly, ulnar ray dysgenesis, and renal cystic dysplasia in sibs. *Am J Med Genet.* 1999;87:426–429.

638. Bader B, Grill F, Lamprecht E. Polydactyly of the foot. *Orthopade.* 1999;28:125–132.

639. Kleanthous JK, Kleanthous EM, Hahn PJ Jr. Polydactyly of the foot. Overview with case presentations. *J Am Podiatr Med Assoc.* 1998;88:493–499.

640. Castilla EE, Lugarinho R, da Graca Dutra M, et al. Associated anomalies in individuals with polydactyly. *Am J Med Genet.* 1998;80:459–465.

641. Zguricas J, Heutink P, Heredero L, et al. Genetic aspects of polydactyly. *Handchir Mikrochir Plast Chir.* 1996;28:171–175.

642. Zguricas J, Bakker WF, Heus H, et al. Genetics of limb development and congenital hand malformations. *Plast Reconstr Surg.* 1998;101:1126–1135.

643. Lowry RB. Variability in the Smith–Lemli–Opitz syndrome: Overlap with the Meckel syndrome. *Am J Med Genet.* 1983;14:429.

644. Goodman RM, Sternberg M, Shem-Tob Y, et al. Acrocephalopolysyndactyly type IV: A new genetic syndrome in 3 sibs. *Clin Genet.* 1979;15:209.

645. Khaldi F, Bennaceur B, Hammou A, et al. An autosomal recessive disorder with retardation of growth, mental deficiency, ptosis, pectus excavatum and camptodactyly. *Pediatr Radiol.* 1988;18:432.

646. Christophorou MN, Nicolaidou P. Median cleft lip, polydactyly, syndactyly and toe anomalies in a non-Indian infant. *Br J Plast Surg.* 1983;36:447.

647. Gordon N. Arthrogryposis multiplex congenita. *Brain Dev.* 1998;20:507–511.

648. Silberstein EP, Kakulas BA. Arthrogryposis multiplex congenita in Western Australia. *J Paediatr Child Health.* 1998;34:518–523.

649. Porter HJ. Lethal arthrogryposis multiplex congenita (fetal akinesia deformation sequence, FADS). *Pediatr Pathol Lab Med.* 1995;15:617–637.

650. Hall JG. Arthrogryposis multiplex congenita: Etiology, genetics, classification, diagnostic approach, and general aspects. *J Pediatr Orthop B.* 1997;6:159–166.

651. Swinyard CA, Bleck EE. The etiology of arthrogryposis (multiple congenital contracture). *Clin Orthop.* 1985;194:15.

652. Jacobson L, Polizzi A, Vincent A. An animal model of maternal antibody-mediated arthrogryposis multiplex congenita (AMC). *Ann N Y Acad Sci.* 1998;841:565–567.

653. Moessinger A. Fetal akynesia deformation sequence: An animal model. *Pediatrics.* 1983;72:857–863.

654. Drachman D, Coulombre A. Experimental clubfoot and arthrogryposis multiplex congenita. *Lancet.* 1962;ii:523–526.

655. Drachman D, Weiner L, Price D, et al. Experimental arthrogryposis caused by viral myopathy. *Arch Neurol.* 1976;33:362–367.

656. Drachman D, Sokoloff L. The role of movement in embryonic joint development. *Development.* 1966;14:401–420.

657. Banker BQ. Neuropathologic aspects of arthrogryposis multiplex congenita. *Clin Orthop.* 1985;194:30.

658. Swinyard C. Concepts of multiple congenital contractures (arthrogryposis) in man and animals. *Teratology.* 1982;25:247–258.

659. Quinn C, Wigglesworth J, Heckmatt J. Lethal arthrogryposis multiple congenita: A pathological study of 21 cases. *Histopathology.* 1991;19:155–162.

660. Thompson GH, Bilenker RM. Comprehensive management of arthrogryposis multiplex congenita. *Clin Orthop.* 1985;194:6.

661. Bürglen L, Amiel J, Viollet L, et al. Survival motor neuron gene deletion in the arthrogryposis multiplex congenita—Spinal muscular atrophy association. *J Clin Invest.* 1996;98:1130–1132.

662. Krakowiak PA, Quinn JR, Bohnsack JF, et al. A variant of Freeman–Sheldon syndrome maps to 11p 15.5-pter. *Am J Hum Genet.* 1997;60:426–432.

663. Shohat M, Lotan R, Magal N, et al. A gene for arthrogryposis multiplex congenita neuropathic type is linked to D5S394 on chromosome 5qter. *Am J Hum Genet.* 1997;61:1139–1143.

664. Herva R, Leisti J, Kirkinen P, et al. A lethal autosomal recessive syndrome of multiple congenital contractures. *Am J Med Genet.* 1985;20:431–439.

665. Lerman-Sagie T, Levi Y, Kidron D, et al. Brief clinical report: Syndrome of osteopetrosis and muscular degeneration associated with cerebro-oculo-facio-skeletal changes. *Am J Med Genet.* 1987;28:137–142.

666. Hennekam R, Barth P, van Lookeren Campagne W, et al. A family with severe X-linked arthrogryposis. *Eur J Pediatr.* 1991;150:656–660.

667. Illum N, Reske-Nielson E, Skovby F, et al. Lethal autosomal recessive arthrogryposis multiplex congenita with whistling face and calcifications of the nervous system. *Neuropediatrics.* 1988;19:186–192.

668. Zori RT, Gardner JL, Zhang J, et al. Newly described from of X-linked arthrogryposis maps to the long arm of the human X chromosome. *Am J Med Genet.* 1998;78:450–454.

669. Hall JG. Genetic aspects of arthrogryposis. *Clin Orthop.* 1985;194:44.

670. Hall J, Reed S. Teratogens associated with congenital contractures in humans and in animals. *Teratology.* 1982;25:173–191.

671. Smith D, Claren S, Harvey M. Hyperthermia as a possible teratogenic agent. *Pediatrics.* 1978;92:878–883.

672. Riemersma S, Vincent A, Beeson D, et al. Association of arthrogryposis multiplex congenita with maternal antibodies inhibiting fetal acetylcholine receptor function. *J Clin Invest.* 1996;98:2358–2363.

673. Vincent A, Newland C, Brueton L, et al. Arthrogryposis multiplex congenita with maternal autoantibodies specific for a fetal antigen. *Lancet.* 1995;346:24–25.

674. Jacobson L, Polizzi A, Morriss-Kay G, et al. Plasma from human mothers of fetuses with severe arthrogryposis multiplex congenita causes deformities in mice. *J Clin Invest.* 1999;103:1031–1038.

675. Rivera MR, Avila CA, Kofman-Alfaro S. Distal arthrogryposis type IIB: Probable autosomal recessive inheritance. *Clin Genet.* 1999;56:95–97.

676. Hall JG. An approach to research on congenital contractures. *Birth Defects Orig Art Ser.* 1984;20:8–30.

677. Gorczyca DP, McGahan JP, Kindfors KK, et al. Arthrogryposis multiplex congenita: Prenatal ultrasonographic diagnosis. *J Clin Ultrasound.* 1989;17:40.

678. Kirkinen P, Herva R, Leisti J. Early prenatal diagnosis of a lethal syndrome of multiple congenital contractures. *Prenat Diagn.* 1987;7:189.

679. Goldberg JD, Chervenak FA, Lipman RA, et al. Antenatal sonographic diagnosis of arthrogryposis multiplex congenita. *Prenat Diagn.* 1986;6:45.

680. Miskin M, Rothberg R, Rudd N, et al. Arthrogryposis multiplex congenita—Prenatal assessment with diagnostic ultrasound and fetoscopy. *J Pediatr.* 1979;95:463.

681. Socol ML, Sabbagha RE, Elias S, et al. Prenatal diagnosis of congenital muscular dystrophy producing arthrogryposis. *N Engl J Med.* 1985;313:1230.

682. Dudkiewicz I, Achiron R, Ganel A. Prenatal diagnosis of distal arthrogryposis type 1. *Skeletal Radiol.* 1999;28:233–235.

683. Fahy M, Hall J. A retrospective study of pregnancy complications among 828 cases of arthrogryposis. *Genet Couns.* 1990;1:3–11.

684. Gustavson KH, Jorulf H. Different types of osteochondrodysplasia in a consecutive series of newborns. *Helv Paediatr Acta.* 1975;30:307–314.

685. Orioli IM, Castilla EE, Barbosa-Neto JG. The birth prevalence rates for the skeletal dysplasias. *J Med Genet.* 1986;23:328–332.

686. Stoll C, Dott B, Roth MP, et al. Birth prevalence rates of skeletal dysplasias. *Clin Genet.* 1989;35:88–92.

687. Andersen PE Jr, Hauge M. Congenital generalised bone dysplasias: Clinical, radiological, and epidemiological study. *J Med Genet.* 1989;27:37–44.

688. Andersen PE Jr. Prevalence of lethal osteochondrodysplasias in Denmark. *Am J Med Genet.* 1989;32:484–489.

689. Kallen B, Knudsen LB, Mutchinick O, et al. Monitoring dominant germ cell mutations using skeletal dysplasias registered in malformation registries: An international feasibility study. *Int J Epidemiol.* 1993;22:107–115.

690. Hafner E, Schuchter K, Liebhart E, et al. Results of routine fetal nuchal translucency measurement at weeks 10–13 in 4233 unselected pregnant women. *Prenat Diagn.* 1998;18:29–34.

691. Hewitt B. Nuchal translucency in the first trimester. *Aust NZ J Obstet Gynaecol.* 1993;33:389–391.

692. Soothill P, Kyle P. Fetal nuchal translucency test for Down's syndrome [letter; comment]. *Lancet.* 1997;350(9091):1629.

693. Fisk NM, Vaughan J, Smidt M, et al. Transvaginal ultrasound recognition of nuchal edema in the first-trimester diagnosis of achondrogenesis. *J Clin Ultrasound.* 1991;19:586–590.

694. Fukada Y, Yasumizu T, Takizawa M, et al. The prognosis of fetuses with transient nuchal translucency in the first and early second trimester. *Acta Obstet Gynecol Scand.* 1997;76:913–916.

695. Hernadi L, Torocsik M. Screening for fetal anomalies in the 12th week of pregnancy by transvaginal sonography in an unselected population. *Prenat Diagn.* 1997;17:753–759.

696. Ben Ami M, Perlitz Y, Haddad S, et al. Increased nuchal translucency is associated with asphyxiating thoracic dysplasia. *Ultrasound Obstet Gynecol.* 1997;10:297–298.

697. Hsieh YY, Hsu TY, Lee CC, et al. Prenatal diagnosis of thoracopelvic dysplasia. A case report. *J Reprod Med.* 1999;44:737–740.

698. Leung KY, MacLachlan NA, Sepulveda W. Prenatal diagnosis of ectrodactyly: The 'lobster claw' anomaly. *Ultrasound Obstet Gynecol.* 1995;6:443–446.

699. Hyett J, Noble P, Sebire NJ, et al. Lethal congenital arthrogryposis presents with increased nuchal translucency at 10–14 weeks of gestation. *Ultrasound Obstet Gynecol.* 1997;9:310–313.

700. Eliyahu S, Weiner E, Lahav D, et al. Early sonographic

diagnosis of Jarcho–Levin syndrome: A prospective screening program in one family. *Ultrasound Obstet Gynecol.* 1997;9:314–318.

701. Hill LM, Leary J. Transvaginal sonographic diagnosis of short-rib polydactyly dysplasia at 13 weeks' gestation. *Prenat Diagn.* 1998;18:1198–1201.

702. Hyett JA, Clayton PT, Moscoso G, et al. Increased first trimester nuchal translucency as a prenatal manifestation of Smith–Lemli–Opitz syndrome. *Am J Med Genet.* 1995;58: 374–376.

703. Maymon R, Ogle RF, Chitty LS. Smith–Lemli–Opitz syndrome presenting with persisting nuchal oedema and non-immune hydrops. *Prenat Diagn.* 1999;19:105–107.

704. Sharp P, Haan E, Fletcher JM, et al. First-trimester diagnosis of Smith–Lemli–Opitz syndrome. *Prenat Diagn.* 1997;17:355–361.

705. Hobbins JC, Jones OW, Gottesfeld S, et al. Transvaginal ultrasonography and transabdominal embryoscopy in the first-trimester diagnosis of Smith–Lemli–Opitz syndrome, type II. *Am J Obstet Gynecol.* 1994;171:546–549.

21

Fetal Syndromes*

Sandra Rejane Silva • Philippe Jeanty

Congenital anomalies are typically organized by organ system. This is an excellent organization in that similar disorders are grouped together. However, the multisystem syndromes do not fit neatly in the organ category organization. Usually the most striking finding or the most unusual finding is the one that leads to the inclusion in one or another group, but with the more precise information that one can now acquire, it is time to organize syndromes as a separate subject.

In the following pages we review several syndromes that should be familiar to sonographers and sonologists either because they are fairly characteristic or common or because their recognition will impact the management of the pregnancy. The selection of the syndromes included is somewhat artificial, but all can be detected prenatally or will affect the pregnancy. Clearly, this review cannot be an exhaustive. The *Birth Defect Encyclopedia*[†] contained about 2000 syndromes and the OMIM[‡] recently passed the 10,000-syndrome landmark. Even for physicians dedicated to the subject, this is an unmanageable amount of information to grasp. Rather than attempt to read (let alone memorize) such a large body of knowledge, it is more important to learn how to investigate unusual cases. What are the critical findings? Once the observations are made, are there other anamnestic information of importance? Before rushing to do an amniocentesis, some review of a large database is usually indicated to suggest differential diagnoses and further tests (call the lab to see what test tube they want). The London Dysmorphology Database used to be the standard, but OMIM is clearly the easier one to use now. Even Medline,[§] with the use of Boolean operators (advanced search), is an excellent tool to identify rare conditions. These tools should be readily available on anyone's desk.

Another aspect of the prenatal diagnosis of syndromes that must be kept in mind is the fabulous progress of molecular genetics. Since the recognition of the disorders by the fibroblast growth factor receptor (FGFR), the classification of the skeletal dysplasia (see Achondroplasia) has been completely reorganized.[‖] These sources should be consulted because it is likely that a genetic or a biochemical test (see Smith-Lemli-Opitz Syndrome) can be made for these disorders that will establish the diagnosis with certainty.

An important aspect of prenatal diagnosis is the assistance to the parents in making management decisions. This is best done by providing them with contacts with support groups, and the Internet has revolutionized the

---

*This chapter was originally published at *www.TheFetus.net.* A copy of this chapter is included in Peter Callen's *Ultrasonography in Obstetrics and Gynecology,* 4th ed. Philadelphia: Saunders. All text copyrighted by Drs. Silva and Jeanty, and all illustrations copyrighted Philippe Jeanty, 1992–2000.

[†] Buyse ML, ed. *Birth Defects Encyclopedia.* Cambridge, MA: Blackwell Scientific; 1990.

[‡] http://www.ncbi.nlm.nih.gov/Omim/searchomim.html

[§] http://www.ncbi.nlm.nih.gov/PubMed/

[‖] http://www.csmc.edu/genetics/skeldys/nomenclature.html

communication between parents formerly isolated in small pockets all around the world. A good resource is National Organization for Rare Disorders (NORD),¶ but often a good search with a metacrawler will identify many more sites of interest. At the time of this writing, Copernic 2000** is an excellent metacrawler with a strong medical flavor.

Over the last 5 years the function of the sonologist has changed significantly from simply identifying some findings to being much more proactive in the making of the differential diagnosis and the establishment of management plans. Often the sonologist will be the first one to identify the disorder and will be the one to establish contacts with the genetics department, dysmorphology specialists, and the various cardiologists and surgeons. The ability to provide clear direction to the parents is important, and, in this time of turmoil for the family, being the reference point to which they can come back is important. We routinely provide searches and references to our patients and attempt to identify support groups so they can obtain information from other parents, which is often more realistic that the information provided within the health care system.

ACHONDROGENESIS

Definition. This group of lethal neonatal chondrodysplasia with short limb dysplasia contains several entities (see following section).

Synonyms. Type IA is the Houston–Harris type; *type IB* is the Parenti–Fraccaro type; *type II* is the Langer–Saldino type and is also called *chondrogenesis imperfecta, achondrogenesis hypochondrogenesis type II,* and was *type IB achondrogenesis.* There are two less common types III and IV. Types II and IV were isolated by Whitley and Gorlin on femoral measurement.[1] The validity of these two last types has been questioned, with type III probably representing type II and type IV probably representing hypochondrogenesis.[1] These essentially radiologic categories have been modified several times and are being replaced by genetic classification (see below) and thus are mainly of historical interest.

Incidence. Rare, with probably fewer than 100 cases reported.

Etiology. Autosomal recessive (type IB) and dominant (type II).

Diagnosis. Type I achondrogenesis (Fig. 21–1) is a severe chondrodystrophy characterized radiographically by poor ossification of the spine (Fig. 21–2) and pelvis bones, which results in stillbirth or early death.[2–5] The ultrasound

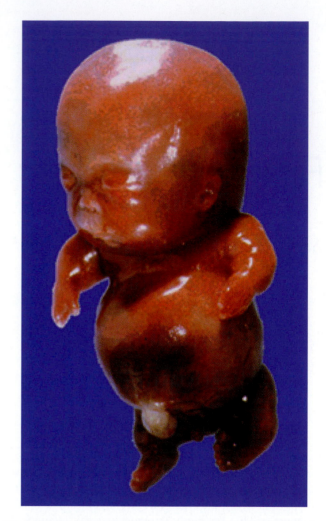

Figure 21–1. Almost absent mineralization of the spine (but not the spinal cord).

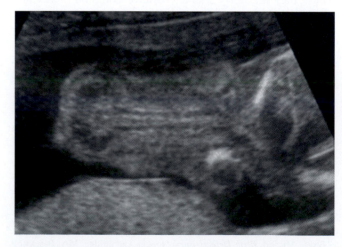

Figure 21–2. The appearance of transparent bones in which both corticals can be seen.

¶http://www.rarediseases.org/ or National Organization for Rare Disorders, Inc. P.O. Box 8923, New Fairfield, CT 06812-8923.
**http://www.copernic.com/

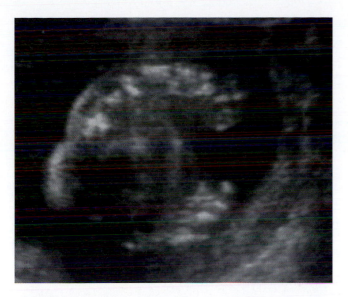

Figure 21–3. Micromelia with the arms not joining in front of the chest.

manifestation includes very short limbs (Fig. 21–3) and short thin ribs that may have fractures. The short ribs are responsible for the lethal pulmonary hypoplasia and the polyhydramnios from esophageal compression. The abnormal mineralization may or may not be manifested sonographically as bones that are very echogenic or in which both cortical sides can be imaged (Fig. 21–4). Normally, only the proximal cortical side is imaged, and the distal side is shadowed by the proximal side. *Type II* also presents with the same findings, but the mineralization deficit is less severe and the long bones less short.

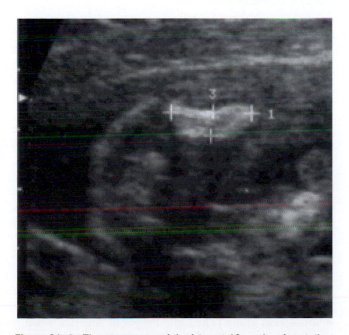

Figure 21–4. The appearance of the fetus at 19 weeks of gestation.

Genetic Anomalies. Type IA: Unknown. *Type IB:* Mutation in the gene for diastrophic dysplasia sulfate transporter (DTDST) gene on the long arm (loci 32–33) of chromosome.[5–8] The DTDST gene is recessively transmitted and is an allele of the diastrophic dysplasia gene. This is important because type II (see below) is an autosomal dominant mutation (and thus involves a new mutation for each case because the disease is lethal) and therefore has a much lower likelihood of recurrence than the 25% risk with type IB. The diagnosis can be made by chorionic villi sampling (CVS) in at-risk couples. Type II achondrogenesis is the Langer–Saldino type and is caused by new dominant mutation in the type II collagen (COL2A1) gene on chromosome 12.[9] Therefore, it is more related to hypochondroplasia, spondyloepiphyseal dysplasia, and Kniest–Stickler syndrome.[10] These may be allelic variants with hypochondrogenesis[11] related to achondrogenesis as hypochondroplasia is related to achondroplasia.

Differential Diagnosis. Osteogenesis imperfecta (OI; type II and occasionally type IIIc) and hypophosphatasia also present with demineralization, but the limb shortening is not usually as severe.

Prognosis. Lethal.

Management. Termination of pregnancy can be offered before viability. Standard prenatal care is not altered when continuation of the pregnancy is decided. Confirmation of diagnosis after birth is important for genetic counseling.

REFERENCES

1. Whitley CB, Gorlin RJ. Achondrogenesis: Nosology with evidence of genetic heterogeneity. *Radiology.* 1983;148:693–698.
2. Parenti GC. La anosteogenesi (una varieta della osteogenesi imperfetta). *Pathologica.* 1936;28:447–462.
3. Fraccaro M. Contributo allo studio delle malattie del mesenchima osteopoietico: l'acondrogenesi. *Folia Hered Pathol.* 1952;1:190–208.
4. Maroteaux P, Lamy M. Le diagnostic des nanismes chondrodystrophiques chez les nouveau-nes. *Arch Fr Pediatr.* 1968;25:241–262.
5. Langer LO Jr, Spranger JW, Greinacher I, Herdman RC. Thanatophoric dwarfism: A condition confused with achondroplasia in the neonate, with brief comments on achondrogenesis and homozygous achondroplasia. *Radiology.* 1969;92:285–294.
6. Superti-Furga A. A defect in the metabolic activation of sulfate in a patient with achondrogenesis type IB. *Am J Hum Genet.* 1994;55:1137–1145.
7. Superti-Furga A, Hastbacka J, Cohn DH, et al. Defective sulfation of proteoglycans in achondrogenesis type IB is caused by mutations in the DTDST gene: The disorder is allelic to diastrophic dysplasia (abstract). *Am J Hum Genet.* 1995;57:A48.

8. Superti-Furga A, Hastbacka J, Wilcox WR, et al. Achondrogenesis type IB is caused by mutations in the diastrophic dysplasia sulphate transporter gene. *Nat Genet.* 1996;12:100–102.

9. Rittler M, Orioli IM. Achondrogenesis type II with polydactyly. *Am J Med Genet.* 1995;59:157–160.

10. Spranger J. Pattern recognition in bone dysplasias. In: Papadatos CJ, Bartsocas CS, Spranger J, eds. *Endocrine Genetics and Genetics of Growth.* New York: Alan R. Liss; 1985:315–342.

11. Stanescu V, Stanescu R, Maroteaux P. Etude morphologique et biochimique du cartilage de croissance dans les osteochondrodysplasies. *Arch Fr Pediatr.* 1977;34:1–80.

ACHONDROPLASIA

Definition. Rhizomelic micromelia associated with frontal bossing and low nasal bridge.

Synonyms. None.

Incidence. Common in 0.5 to 1.5 per 10,000 births.

Etiology. Defective cartilaginous molding of the bone precursor.

Diagnosis. The micromelia is the most obvious finding, with limbs shorter than the 5th percentile after 20 weeks (Fig. 21–5). The frontal bossing and depressed nasal bridge can also be recognized (Fig. 21–6). Occasionally, more subtle anomalies such as the trident hand (an increased interspace between the 3rd and 4th digits) or the lack of widening of the lumbar canal can also be identified (Fig. 21–7).

Genetic Anomalies. Achondroplasia is an autosomal dominant skeletal dysplasia caused by mutation in the fibroblast

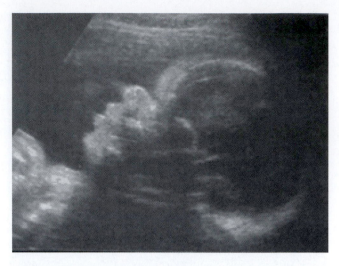

Figure 21–6. Frontal bossing.

growth factor receptor-3 gene, which is located on the short arm of chromosome 4 at the 16.3 locus.[1,2] Bellus et al. demonstrated that the anomaly was due to a glycine-to-arginine substitution at codon 380.[3] These papers are landmarks in our knowledge about skeletal dysplasias. Before these papers were published, skeletal dysplasias were almost strictly classified by radiologic criteria. These papers marked the beginning of an intense and successful search for gene mapping of skeletal dysplasia, many of which were subsequently recognized to result from alterations of fibroblast growth factors (FGF) I through III.

Differential Diagnosis. The differential diagnosis includes multiple conditions:

- thanatophoric dysplasia (narrower chest, platyspondyly, more severe micromelia, no trident hand, more severe polyhydramnios)
- achondrogenesis (very poor mineralization, with lack of echogenicity of the bones, more severe micromelia, more severe polyhydramnios)
- osteogenesis imperfecta type II (poor mineralization: often the proximal aspect of the brain is well seen through the "transparent" skull; variable micromelia, sometimes visible bone angulations from fractures, bell-shaped chest)
- diastrophic dysplasias (in which the micromelia is associated with joint contractures and in particular abnormal finger and toe positions)

Prognosis. Children with achondroplasia have normal intellectual achievements. The major problems are orthopedic (narrow spinal canal and foramen magnum). There is a vibrant support group (The Little People of America[4]) that is very active in resolving the problems of affected individuals.

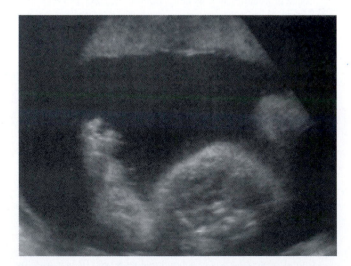

Figure 21–5. Short limb (in this image, the arm). Note the polyhydramnios (esophageal compression from short ribs).

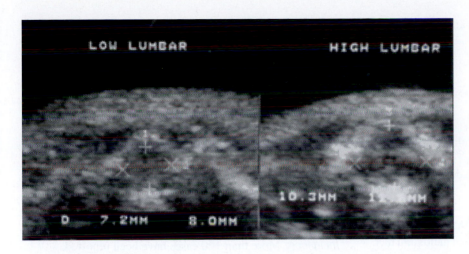

Figure 21–7. Lack of widening of the spinal canal.

Management. Although termination of pregnancy can be offered before viability, a majority of these children adapt well in society and lead productive lives.

REFERENCES

1. Velinov M, Slaugenhaupt SA, Stoilov I, et al. The gene for achondroplasia maps to the telomeric region of chromosome 4p. *Nat Genet.* 1994;6:318–321.
2. Le Merrer M, Rousseau F, Legeai-Mallet L, et al. A gene for achondroplasia—Hypochondroplasia maps to chromosome 4p. *Nat Genet.* 1994;6:314–317.
3. Bellus GA, Hefferon TW, Ortiz de Luna RI. Achondroplasia is defined by recurrent G380R mutations of FGFR3. *Am J Hum Genet.* 1995;56:368–373.
4. *http://www.lpaonline.org/welcome.html*

ACROFACIAL DYSOSTOSIS SYNDROMES

Definition. Nager's syndrome consists of limb anomalies including absence of the radius, synostosis of the radius and ulna, hypoplasia or absence of the thumbs, and severe micrognathia and malar hypoplasia.[1,2]

Synonyms. Mandibulofacial dysostosis, Treacher–Collins type, with limb anomalies; Nager acrofacial dysostosis. Rodriguez's lethal acrofacial dysostosis syndrome is a variant, with preaxial limb deficiencies, postaxial limb anomalies, severe hypoplasia of the shoulder and pelvic girdles, and cardiac and central nervous system (CNS) malformations.[3]

Incidence. Uncommon.

Etiology. Nager's syndrome may represent new mutations of an autosomal dominant trait.

Diagnosis. Severe micrognathia and the typical micromesomelia with the abnormal hand mainly suggest the diagnosis. Accessory anomalies have frequently been reported.

Genetic Anomalies. Nager's syndrome is on chromosome 9 (q32).[4]

Differential Diagnosis. Other disorders with micrognathia and distal ectromelia such as trisomy 18.

Prognosis. Lethal from lung hypoplasia due to severe mandibular hypoplasia.

Management. Termination of pregnancy can be offered before viability. Standard prenatal care is not altered when continuation of the pregnancy is decided. Confirmation of diagnosis after birth is important for genetic counseling.

REFERENCES

1. Slingenberg B. Misbildungen von Extremitaeten. *Virchows Arch Pathol Anat.* 1908;193:1–92.
2. Nager FR, de Reynier JP. Das Gehoerorgan bei den angeborenen Kopfmissbildungen. *Pract Otorhinolaryng.* 1948;10(suppl. 2):1–128.
3. Rodriguez JI, Palacios J, Urioste M. New acrofacial dysostosis syndrome in 3 sibs. *Am J Med Genet.* 1990;35:484–489.
4. Zori RT, Gray BA, Bent-Williams A, et al. Preaxial acrofacial dysostosis (Nager syndrome) associated with an inherited and apparently balanced X;9 translocation: prenatal and postnatal late replication studies. *Am J Med Genet.* 1993;46:379–383.

ACROMESOMELIC DYSPLASIA

Definition. Nonlethal short stature and short limb dysplasia that, as implied by the name, affects the forearms, hands, and feet. The radius is bowed. The wrist bones and phalanges are particularly short and square.[1-4]

Synonyms. None.

Incidence. Rare.

Etiology. Autosomal recessive for the regular[5] and acromesomelic dysplasia (Hunter–Thompson type; AMDH[6] for the severe form, due to a different cartilage-derived morphogenetic protein (CDMP).[7,8]

Diagnosis. The diagnosis is suggested by the finding for abnormal forearms and lower legs and abnormal hands and feet. The rest of the skeleton is not affected.

Genetic Anomalies. Acromesomelic dysplasia is caused by a mutation in CDMP-1 on chromosome 20.

Differential Diagnosis. Mesomelic dwarfism, Grebe's chondrodysplasia (only in a specific group of patients from a certain region of Brazil), and Nager's syndrome (but these have micrognathia).

Prognosis. Intellectual development has been reported as normal, and the orthopedic handicap is the major concern in these children.[3,9]

Management. Termination of pregnancy can be offered before viability. Standard prenatal care is not altered when continuation of the pregnancy is decided. Confirmation of diagnosis after birth is important for genetic counseling.

REFERENCES

1. Ferraz FG, Maroteaux P, Sousa JP, et al. Acromesomelic dwarfism: A new variation. *J Pediatr Orthop B*. 1997;6:27–32.
2. Campailla E, Maroteaux P. Acromesomelic dwarfism: Maroteaux–Martinelli–Campailla type. *Basic Life Sci*. 1988;48:177–178.
3. Stichelbout P, Pratz R, Lemaitre G, et al. Acromesomelic dysplasia. Apropos of a new case. *Arch Fr Pediatr*. 1984;41:487–489.
4. Hall CM, Stoker DJ, Robinson DC, Wilkinson DJ. Acromesomelic dwarfism. *Br J Radiol*. 1980;53:999–1003.
5. Langer LO Jr, Beals RK, Solomon IL, et al. Acromesomelic dwarfism: Manifestations in childhood. *Am J Med Genet*. 1977;1:87–100.
6. Hunter AG, Thompson MW. Acromesomelic dwarfism: Description of a patient and comparison with previously reported cases. *Hum Genet*. 1976;34:107–113.
7. Danda S, Phadke SR, Agarwal SS. Acromesomelic dwarfism: Report of a family with two affected siblings. *Ind Pediatr*. 1997;34:1127–1130.
8. Borrelli P, Fasanelli S, Marini R. Acromesomelic dwarfism

in a child with an interesting family history. *Pediatr Radiol*. 1983;13:165–168.
9. Pallister PD. A 59-year-old multiparous woman with acromesomelic dwarfism. *Am J Med Genet*. 1978;1:343–346.

AICARDI'S SYNDROMES

Definition. Aicardi's syndrome occurs in females and is associated with profound mental retardation, agenesis of the corpus callosum, chorioretinal lacunae, and infantile spasms.[1-3]

Synonyms. None.

Incidence. More than 100 cases have been reported.

Etiology. Unknown.

Diagnosis. Microophtalmia, choroid plexus cysts, choroid plexus papilloma, Dandy–Walker malformation, and dysgenesis of the corpus callosum can be recognized prenatally.[4,5]

Genetic Anomalies. Autosomal recessive inheritance or possibly an X-linked dominant disorder; lethal in the hemizygous male.[6,7]

Differential Diagnosis. Dysgenesis of the corpus callosum.

Prognosis. Poor, with most infants dying during the first few years. Those that survive are profoundly mentally retarded.

Management. Termination of pregnancy can be offered before viability. Standard prenatal care is not altered when continuation of the pregnancy is decided. Confirmation of diagnosis after birth is important for genetic counseling.

REFERENCES

1. Goutieres F, Aicardi J, Barth PG, Lebon P. Aicardi–Goutieres syndrome: An update and results of interferon-alpha studies. *Ann Neurol*. 1998;44:900–907.
2. Kato M, Ishii R, Honma A, et al. Brainstem lesion in Aicardi–Goutieres syndrome. *Pediatr Neurol*. 1998;19:145–147.
3. McEntagart M, Kamel H, Lebon P, King MD. Aicardi–Goutieres syndrome: An expanding phenotype. *Neuropediatrics*. 1998;29:163–167.
4. Uchiyama CM, Carey CM, Cherny WB, et al. Choroid plexus papilloma and cysts in the Aicardi syndrome: Case reports. *Pediatr Neurosurg*. 1997;27:100–104.
5. Aguiar MD, Cavalcanti M, Barbosa H, et al. Aicardi syndrome and choroid plexus papilloma: A rare association. Case report. *Arq Neuropsiquiatr*. 1996;54:313–317.
6. Hoag HM, Taylor SA, Duncan AM, Khalifa MM. Evidence that skewed X inactivation is not needed for the phenotypic expression of Aicardi syndrome. *Hum Genet*. 1997;100:459–464.

7. Costa T, Greer W, Rysiecki G, et al. Monozygotic twins discordant for Aicardi syndrome. *J Med Genet*. 1997;34:688–691.

ACQUIRED IMMUNODEFICIENCY SYNDROME (AIDS) EMBRYOPATHY

Definition. AIDS embryopathy is characterized by a group of dysmorphic features that manifests either before or after birth in offspring of women infected by the HIV virus. Transplacental infection occurs generally in early gestation.[1]

Synonym. Congenital AIDS, fetal AIDS, and fetal HIV infection.

Incidence. The transmission of HIV infection from mothers to newborns differs throughout the world, from 14.1% in Europe, to 28% in New York, 20% in San Francisco, and 45% in Africa.[2] Of all children infected with HIV virus, approximately 99% were infected from their mothers. Vertical transmission includes intrauterine, intrapartum, and postpartum (breastfeeding) infections. Intrauterine or transplacental infection accounts for 30 to 50% of the total. The incidence of AIDS embryopathy is uncertain and depends mainly on the severity of the maternal disease and early intrauterine transmission (the earlier the transmission, the higher risk of fetal compromise).

Etiology. The causative agent is the HIV virus.

Recurrence Risk. The risk of vertical transmission in another pregnancy will be the same if the fetus is exposed to the same risk factors (severity of maternal disease, high maternal viral load, low maternal CD4, maternal fever and anemia, prolonged ruptured of the membranes, membrane inflammation).

Diagnosis. Intrauterine diagnosis with invasive techniques is precluded to avoid fetal exposure to maternal blood and false-positive results due to maternal crossreaction. Ultrasonographic signs of fetal infection may be present, including fetal demise, growth retardation, microcephaly, and craniofacial abnormalities (present in 50 to 75% of affected cases; the characteristic facial appearance occurs after birth) including prominent, square, or boxlike forehead, lateral bossing, hypertelorism, flat nasal bridge, and short nose. Other findings that may be present at birth include long palpebral fissures, blue scleras, prominent upper vermilion border, short stature, large wide eyes, and well-formed philtrum.[3]

Associated Anomalies. Maternal opportunistic diseases, in particular infections that may also affect the fetus such as toxoplasmosis, cytomegalovirus, and parvovirus.

Differential Diagnosis. Other maternal viral infections, which can be excluded by maternal serology.

Prognosis. Until now, AIDS has been a uniformly lethal condition, with variable length of survival, which depends on multiple factors (maternal, infant, and viral). Mean survival ranges from 6.2 to 7.5 years, and only 70% reach 6 years of age.[4] Intrauterine death may occur in cases of severe maternal or fetal disease, in particular in those cases infected early in pregnancy.[5] The severity of congenital abnormalities seems to be associated with early fetal viremia (the earlier the infection, the more severe the compromise). Introduction of early antiviral therapy may reduce vertical transmission from 25 to 8%[6] and prolong the length of survival for those who are infected.

Management. Termination of pregnancy can be offered before viability for every patient infected with HIV virus. Monthly ultrasound evaluation throughout the pregnancy is recommended to search for growth restriction and structural anomalies. Maternal treatment consists of 100 mg zidovudine five times a day throughout the pregnancy; postnatal treatment of the newborn with the same regimen is mandatory.

REFERENCES

1. Nyhan WL. Structural abnormalities—A systematic approach to diagnosis in clinical symposia. *Ciba-Geigy Symp*. 1990;42:31–32.
2. Wara DW, Dorenbaum A. Pediatric AIDS: Perinatal transmission and early diagnosis. In: Sande MA, Volberding PA, eds. *The Medical Management of AIDS*. Philadelphia: WB Saunders; 1997;469–473.
3. Iosub S, Bamji M, Stone RK, et al. More on human immunodeficiency virus embryopathy. *Pediatrics*. 1987;80:512–516.
4. Ruiz Contreras J. Natural history of HIV infection in the child. *Allerg Immunopathol*. 1998;26:135–139.
5. Landers DV, Shannon MT. Management of pregnant women with HIV infection. In: Sande MA, Volberding PA, eds. *The Medical Management of AIDS*. Philadelphia: WB Saunders; 1997:459–468.
6. Connor E, Sperling R, Gelber R, et al. Reduction of maternal–infant transmission of human immunodeficiency virus type 1 with zidovudine treatment. *N Engl J Med*. 1994;331:1173–1180.

AMNIOTIC BAND SYNDROME

Definition. Amniotic band syndrome is a set of congenital malformations ranging from minor constriction rings and lymphedema of the digits to complex, bizarre multiple congenital anomalies that are attributed to amniotic bands that stick, entangle, and disrupt fetal parts.[1]

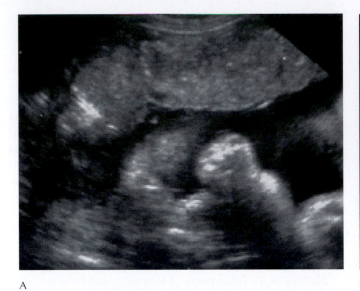

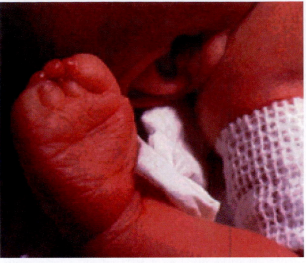

A   B

Figure 21–8. (A and **B)** Amputations of the fingers in a minor form of amniotic band. *(Reproduced with permission from Gonçalves LF, Jeanty P. The Fetus. 1992;2:1–6.)*

Synonyms. ADAM complex (amniotic deformities, adhesion, and mutilation), amniotic band sequence, amniotic disruption complex, annular grooves, congenital amputation, congenital constricting bands, Streeter bands, transverse terminal defects of limb,[2] aberrant tissue bands, amniochorionic mesoblastic fibrous strings, and amniotic bands.[3]

Prevalence. The prevalence is 7.7 per 10,000 live births,[2] but it can be as high as 178 per 10,000[4] for spontaneous abortions (male-to-female ratio, 1 to 1).

Etiology. Not precisely known. Some theories have been suggested, such as teratogenic, multifactorial, and genetic factors causing a rupture of the amnion.[5] Teratogenic effect of drugs such as methadone or lysergic acid diethylamide (LSD) may play an important role in many cases.[6–8]

Pathogenesis. Rupture of the amnion in early pregnancy leads to entrapment of fetal structures by "sticky" mesodermic bands that originate from the chorionic side of the amnion, followed by disruption.[4,9,10]

Diagnosis. The syndrome results in structural anomalies that differ from minor to lethal forms (Figs. 21–8 through 21–11). The most common findings are constriction rings around the digits, arms and legs; swelling of the extremities distal to the point of constriction; amputation of digits, arms, and legs; asymmetric face; facial clefts; cephalocele; anencephaly; multiple joint contractures; pterygium; clubfeet, clubhands, and pseudosyndactyly, microphthalmia, uveal coloboma, corneal metaplasia, and unilateral chorioretinal lacunae.[4,10–13]

Differential Diagnosis. Amniotic fold,[14] which can be differentiated because it does not "stick" to the body, and body stalk anomaly.

Prognosis. The more severe forms are lethal. Mild manifestations sometimes are just found at birth and do not have impact on survival.[4]

Recurrence Risk. No recurrence expected, except in rare sporadic familial cases, which have been reported in

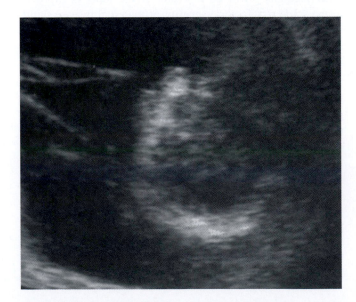

Figure 21–9. Strands of amnion *(arrows)* are attached and move with the forehead. *(Reproduced with permission from Gonçalves LF, Jeanty P. The Fetus. 1992;2:1–6.)*

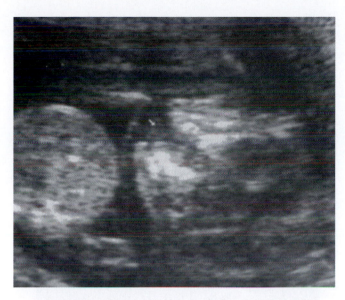

Figure 21–10. A large facial cleft *(white arrow)* extends to the lens of the left eye. *(Reproduced with permission from Gonçalves LF, Jeanty P. The Fetus. 1992;2:1–6.)*

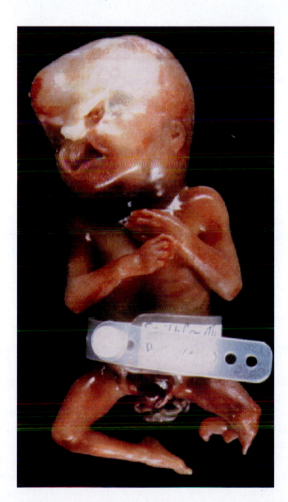

Figure 21–11. Multiple defects including facial clefts, cephalocele, amputations, and abdominal wall disruptions. *(Reproduced with permission from Gonçalves LF, Jeanty P. The Fetus. 1992;2:1–6.)*

association with epidermolysis bullosum and Ehler–Danlos syndrome.[2,15,16]

Management. Depends on the extent of the anomalies. Termination of pregnancy can be offered for the severe forms. Endoscopic release has recently been reported and may prove beneficial.[17]

REFERENCES

1. Goncalves LF, Jeanty P. Amniotic band syndrome. *The Fetus.* 1992;2:1–6.
2. Buyse ML. *Birth Defects Encyclopedia.* Cambridge, MA: Blackwell Scientific; 1990.
3. Seeds JW, Cefalo RC, Herbert WNP. Amniotic band syndrome. *Am J Obstet Gynecol.* 1982;144:243.
4. Nyberg DA, Mahony BS, Pretorius DH. *Diagnostic Ultrasound of Fetal Anomalies.* Littleton, MA: Year Book Medical; 1990.
5. Tadmor OP, Kreisberg GA, Achiron R, et al. Limb amputation in amniotic band syndrome: Serial ultrasonographic and Doppler observations. *Ultrasound Obstet Gynecol.* 1997;10:312–315.
6. Lockwood C, Ghidini A, Romero R, et al. Amniotic band syndrome in monozygotic twins: Prenatal diagnosis and pathogenesis. *Obstet Gynecol.* 1988;71:1012–1015.
7. Lockwood C, Ghidini A, Romero R, et al. Amniotic band syndrome: Reevaluation of its pathogenesis. *Am J Obstet Gynecol.* 1989;160:1030–1033.
8. Daly CA, Freeman J, Weston W, et al. Prenatal diagnosis of amniotic band syndrome in a methadone user: Review of the literature and a case report. *Ultrasound Obstet Gynecol.* 1996; 8;123–125.
9. Dimmick JE, Kalousek DK. *Developmental Pathology of the Embryo and Fetus.* Philadelphia: JB Lippincott; 1992.
10. Torpin R. *Fetal Malformations Caused by Amnion Rupture During Gestation.* Springfield, IL: Charles C. Thomas; 1968:1–76.
11. BenEzra D, Frucht Y. Uveal coloboma associated with amniotic band syndrome. *Can J Ophthalmol.* 1983;18:136–138.
12. BenEzra D, Frucht Y, Paez JH, et al. Amniotic band syndrome and strabismus. *J Pediatr Ophthalmol.* 1982;19:33–36.
13. Hashemi K, Traboulsi E, Chavis R, et al. Chorioretinal lacuna in the amniotic band syndrome. *J Pediatr Ophthalmol Strabismus.* 1991;28:238–239.
14. Randel SB, Filly RA, Callen PW, et al. Amniotic sheets. *Radiology.* 1988;166:633–636.
15. Marras A, Dessi C, Macciotta A. Epidermolysis bullosa and amniotic bands. *Am J Med Genet.* 1984;19:815.
16. Young ID, Lindenbaum RH, Thompson EM, et al. Amniotic band syndrome in connective tissue disorders. *Arch Dis Child.* 1985;60:1061–1063.
17. Quintero RA, Morales WJ, Phillips J, et al. In utero lysis of amniotic bands. *Ultrasound Obstet Gynecol.* 1997;10:316–320.

APERT'S SYNDROME

Definition. Apert's syndrome, or acrocephalosyndactyly, is a rare developmental deformity, characterized by craniofacial and limb malformations accompanied by variable degrees of mental retardation in 50% of cases.[1] Wheaton first described the syndrome in 1894, and Apert summarized the disorder, with a presentation of nine cases, in 1906.[2,3]

Incidence. The occurrence of Apert's syndrome is estimated to be 0.0625 to 0.1 per 10,000 live births.[4,5] Because of the high neonatal mortality rate, the prevalence in the general population is estimated at 5×10^{-6} to 1×10^{-5} per 10,000 live births. The male-to-female ratio is 1.

Etiology. Apert's syndrome is an autosomal disorder with dominant inheritance. Most of the cases are sporadic, resulting from fresh mutations (see below). Association with advanced paternal age has been described.[7]

Recurrence Risk. When resulting from a fresh mutation, the recurrence risk is improbable. If one parent carries the disorder, the recurrence risk is 50%.

Diagnosis. The most typical findings in Apert's syndrome are craniosynostosis (Fig. 21–12) (by synostosis of the coronal sutures), bilateral symmetric syndactyly of the limbs (mittenlike hands and feet), and midfacial hypoplasia. Additional features, which appear in variable frequency, include

- skeletal anomalies: short and broad head, high cranial vault (acrocephaly), prominent forehead (frontal bossing) (Fig. 21–13), hypertelorism and proptosis, depressed nasal bridge with parrot-beaked nose, hypoplastic maxillar, and prognathism.
- cardiac anomalies: pulmonic stenosis, overriding aorta, and ventricular septal defects.

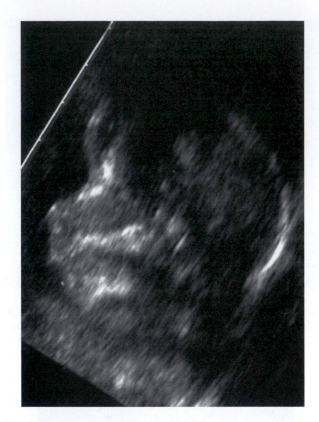

Figure 21–13. Exaggerated frontal bossing.

- central nervous system anomalies: hydrocephaly, malformation of the corpus callosum and limbic structures, gyral abnormalities, hypoplasia of the white matter, and heterotopic gray matter.

Polyhydramnios (caused by the decreased fetal swallowing) and variable degrees of mental retardation have also been found, and their occurrence and intensity seem to be correlated to the severity of central nervous system anomalies.[1,2,8]

The prenatal diagnosis by ultrasound and fetoscopy has been reported in all trimesters of pregnancy.[9,10] Increased nuchal fold at the first trimester may be a sonographic marker for the disorder.[11]

Genetic Anomalies. The most common mutations associated with Apert's syndrome are substitution S252W and P253R, which occur in the fibroblast growth factor receptor 2 genes.[12] Genetic molecular studies are recommended for the fetus (by chorionic villi sampling or amniocentesis) and parents when Apert's syndrome is suspected, in particular in those families affected for the first time.

A recent study correlates less severe craniofacial anomalies as well as more important limb anomalies to the mutation P253R.[13] Genetic evidence of abnormal expression of keratinocyte growth-factor receptor (KGFR) linked to the occurrence of limb deformities in Apert syndrome has also been suggested.[14]

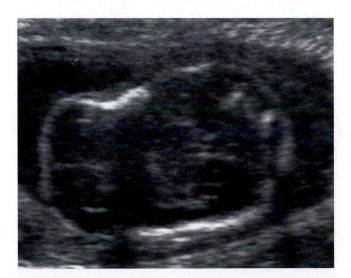

Figure 21–12. Craniosynostosis with narrowing of the skull at the level of the coronal suture.

Differential Diagnosis. Genetic syndromes also characterized by the presence of craniosynostosis such as Crouzon, Pfeiffer, Carpenter, and Saethre–Chotzen may be included in the differential diagnosis. Molecular genetic studies can exclude these disorders.[2]

Management. If diagnosed before viability, termination of pregnancy can be offered. After viability, standard obstetric management is not altered. Delivery in a tertiary center is recommended.

REFERENCES

1. Parent P, Le Guern H, Munck MR, Thoma M. Apert syndrome, an antenatal ultrasound detected case. *Genet Counsel.* 1994;5:297–301.
2. Kaufmann K, Baldinger S, Pratt L. Ultrasound detection of Apert syndrome: A case report and literature review. *Am J Perinat.* 1997;14:427–430.
3. Jones KL. Apert syndrome. In: Jones KL, ed. *Smith's Recognizable Patterns of Human Malformation.* Philadelphia: WB Saunders Company–Harcourt Brace and Company; 1997: 418–419.
4. Blank CE. Apert's syndrome (a type of acrocephalosyndactyly). Observations on a British series of thirty-nine cases. *Ann Hum Genet.* 1960;24:151–164.
5. Tunte W, Lenz W. Zur haufigkeit und mutations-rate des Apert-syndroms. *Hum Genet (Berlin),* 1967;4:101–111.
6. Cohen MM Jr, Kreiborg S, Lammer EJ, et al. Birth prevalence study of Apert syndrome. *Am J Med Genet.* 1992;42:655–659.
7. Erikson JD, Cohen MM Jr. A study of parental age effects on the occurrence of fresh mutations for the Apert syndrome. *Ann Hum Genet.* 1974;38:89–96.
8. Cohen MM, Kreibord S. The central nervous system in the Apert syndrome. *Am J Med Genet.* 1990;35:36–45.
9. Narayan H, Scott IV. Prenatal diagnosis of Apert's syndrome. *Prenat Diag.* 1991;10:187–192.
10. Leonard CO, Daikoku NH, Winn K. Prenatal fetoscopic diagnosis of the Apert syndrome. *Am J Med Genet.* 1982;11: 5–9.
11. Chenoweth-Mitchell C, Cohen GR. Prenatal sonographic findings of Apert syndrome. *J Clin Ultrasound.* 1994;22: 510–514.
12. Park WJ, Theda C, Maestri NE, et al. Analysis of phenotypic features and FGFR2 mutations in Apert syndrome. *Am J Hum Genet.* 1995;57:321–328.
13. von Gernet S, Golla A, Ehrenfels Y, Schuffenhauer S, Fairley JD. Genotype-phenotype analysis in Apert syndrome suggests opposite effects of the two recurrent mutations on syndactyly and outcome of craniofacial surgery. *Clin Genet.* 2000; 57:137–139.
14. Oldridge M, Zackai EH, McDonald-McGinn DM, et al. De novo Alu-element insertions in FGFR2 identify a distinct pathological basis for Apert syndrome. *Am J Hum Genet.* 1999;64: 446–461.

ARNOLD–CHIARI MALFORMATION

Definition. There are three types of Arnold–Chiari malformation. In type 1, just a lip of cerebellum is displaced downward with the tonsils, but the fourth ventricle remains in the posterior fossa. This is mainly an incidental computed tomographic (CT) discovery. Type 2 is usually involved in prenatal cases and is a congenital deformity characterized by displacement of cerebellar tonsils and parts of the cerebellum, fourth ventricle, pons, and medulla oblongata through the foramen magnum into the spinal canal. This is usually associated with hydrocephalus and meningomyelocele (Fig. 21–14). Type 3 is a more severe form, with large herniation of the posterior fossa content and myelomeningocle and hydrocephalus.[1]

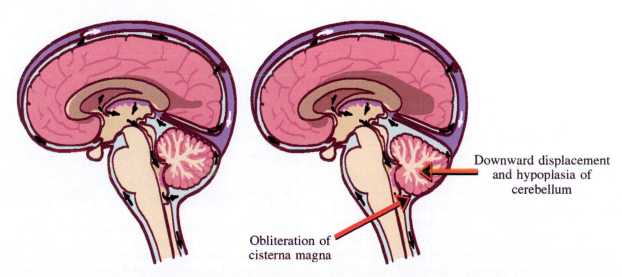

Downward displacement and hypoplasia of cerebellum

Obliteration of cisterna magna

Figure 21–14. Schematic drawing of the changes in Arnold–Chiari malformation type 2.

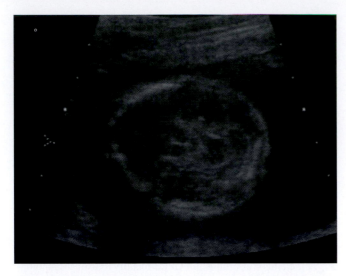

Figure 21–15. The banana sign. The lobes of the cerebellum have lost their lumpy appearance, and the vermian incisure is not as marked as normal.

Synonyms. The nickname "banana sign" (Fig. 21–15) has been applied to describe the deformity of the cerebellum.[3]

Incidence. Commonly associated with spina bifida but is otherwise rare.[2]

Etiology. Autosomal recessive for some forms.

Diagnosis. The displacement of the cerebellum deforms the lateral lobes (that lose their "round shape") and the vermian notch to appear more continuous (thus, the "banana" sign[3,4]). The diagnosis has been made as early as the first trimester.[5]

Genetic Anomalies. Unknown.

Differential Diagnosis. Nonobstructive hydrocephalus.

Associated Anomalies. Hydrocephaly from obstruction of the foramina of Magendie, synringomyelia, and distematomelia.

Prognosis. Poor due to the CNS anomalies.

Management. Termination of pregnancy can be offered before viability. For those affected by spina bifida, an experimental intrauterine repair done between 21 and 30 weeks of gestation has been proposed in a few centers in the United States (in the USA, call 800-RX-FETUS as well as at Vanderbilt University). Standard prenatal care is not altered when continuation of the pregnancy is decided. Confirmation of diagnosis after birth is important for genetic counseling.

REFERENCES

1. Lindenberg R, Walker BA. Arnold–Chiari malformation in sibs. *Birth Defects Original Artical Series.* 1971;VII:234–236.
2. Babcook CJ, Goldstein RB, Barth RA, et al. Prevalence of ventriculomegaly in association with myelomeningocele: Correlation with gestational age and severity of posterior fossa deformity. *Radiology.* 1994;190:703–707.
3. Nicolaides KH, Campbell S, Gabbe SG, Guidetti R. Ultrasound screening for spina bifida: Cranial and cerebellar signs. *Lancet.* 1986;2(8498):72–74.
4. Van den Hof MC, Nicolaides KH, Campbell J, Campbell S. Evaluation of the lemon and banana signs in one hundred thirty fetuses with open spina bifida. *Am J Obstet Gynecol.* 1990;162: 322–327.
5. Bernard JP, Suarez B, Rambaud C, et al. Prenatal diagnosis of neural tube defect before 12 weeks' gestation: Direct and indirect ultrasonographic semeiology. *Ultrasound Obstet Gynecol.* 1997; 10:406–409.

ARTHROGRYPOSIS MULTIPLEX CONGENITA

Definition. This heterogeneous set of conditions shares limitation of movements and joint ankylosis as main findings (Fig. 21–16).

Synonyms. Congenital contractures, fetal akinesia sequence, and Pena–Shokeir syndrome.

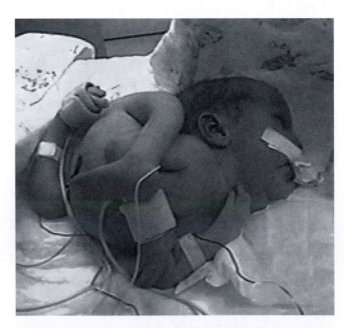

Figure 21–16. Newborn with congenital multiple arthrogryposis. Note the pronounced anomalies of the limbs, which are very rigid. Also note the linear fingers with a lack of visible flexion joints. The newborn died of respiratory failure a few hours after these images were obtained.

Incidence. Approximately 1 to 3 per 10,000 births.

Etiology. Possibly autosomal dominant.

Pathogenesis. Arthrogryposis results from decreased *in utero* motion, of neural,[1] muscular, connective tissue, or infectious origin.

Diagnosis. Although the anomalies are obvious when recognized and in particular when the baby is born, the prenatal diagnosis may be challenging when fluid is decreased, and the abnormal limb position appears attributable to the oligohydramnios. Some forms are associated with polyhydramnios and then the abnormal limb position (knocked knee, Fig. 21–17; genu recurvatum, clubfeet and hand) make the diagnosis easy. Polyhydramnios is often a manifestation of decreased swallowing, which may be part of the same pathogenesis as the arthrogryposis itself (muscular or neuronal deficit). An increase in nuchal lucency[2] and the characteristic decreased movement[3] can also be seen in the first trimester.

Genetic Anomalies. Several anomalies have been linked to the following sites: 5q35, 9p21–q21, and 11p15.5.

Differential Diagnosis. Trisomy 18, renal agenesis, and myotonic dystrophy may present, with some similar findings.

Associated Anomalies. Because of the heterogeneity of the conditions, numerous associated anomalies have been described including scoliosis, CNS anomalies, even seizures.[4]

Prognosis. The prognosis will depend on associated anomalies (respiratory limitations, scoliosis, etc.).

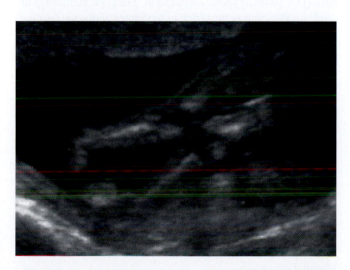

Figure 21–17. A different fetus with an abnormal and rigid position of the knee. The distance between the knee is less than that between the hips. Also note that both feet are inverted.

Management. Termination of pregnancy can be offered before viability. Standard prenatal care is not altered when continuation of the pregnancy is decided. Confirmation of diagnosis after birth is important for genetic counseling.

REFERENCES

1. Lammens M, Moerman P, Fryns JP, et al. Fetal akinesia sequence caused by nemaline myopathy. *Neuropediatrics.* 1997;28: 116–119.
2. Hyett J, Noble P, Sebire NJ, et al. Lethal congenital arthrogryposis presents with increased nuchal translucency at 10–14 weeks of gestation. *Ultrasound Obstet Gynecol.* 1997;9:310–313.
3. Ajayi RA, Keen CE, Knott PD. Ultrasound diagnosis of the Pena Shokeir phenotype at 14 weeks of pregnancy. *Prenat Diagn.* 1995;15:762–764.
4. Skupski DW, Sepulveda W, Udom-Rice I, et al. Fetal seizures: Further observations. *Obstet Gynecol.* 1996;88(4, pt 2):663–665.

ASPHYXIATING THORACIC DYSPLASIA

Definition. Autosomal recessive chondrodysplasia characterized by a small thorax, different degrees of rhizomelic brachymelia, polydactyly, pelvic abnormalities, and renal anomalies.

Synonyms. Jeune's syndrome.

Incidence. Unknown, usually affecting Caucasian babies.

Pathogenesis and Etiology. Autosomal recessive disorder.

Diagnosis. The most striking ultrasound finding is a very narrow chest with short limbs (Fig. 21–18). The limbs however, are not as short as those in other lethal conditions such as thanatophoric dysplasia, achondrogenesis, OI type 2, and the short rib polydactyly syndromes. The increase iliac wing angle, reported in the radiographic literature, has not been reported with ultrasound. Pancreatic cysts have been recognized in one case.[6]

Genetic Anomalies. Defect probably located on the short arm of chromosome 12.

Differential Diagnosis. Ellis van Crevelt's syndrome (short arm of chromosome 4) that presents mainly with cardiac rather than renal anomalies.

Prognosis. Despite the dreadful name, not all newborns are asphyxiated; with corrective surgery of the chest, some patient have had a fairly normal outcome.

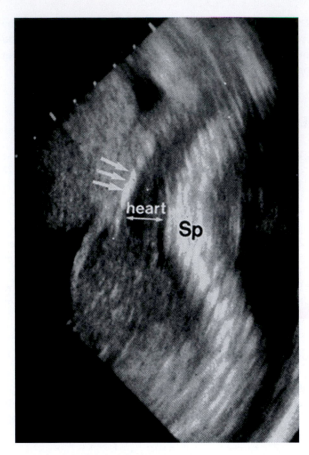

Figure 21–18. Longitudinal view of the chest and abdomen of a fetus with asphyxiating thoracic dysplasia. Note the constriction of the chest.

Management. Termination of pregnancy can be offered before viability. Standard prenatal care is not altered when continuation of the pregnancy is decided. Confirmation of diagnosis after birth is important for genetic counseling.

REFERENCES

1. Ben Ami M, Perlitz Y, Haddad S, Matilsky M. Increased nuchal translucency is associated with asphyxiating thoracic dysplasia. *Ultrasound Obstet Gynecol.* 1997;10:297–298.
2. Chen CP, Lin SP, Liu FF, et al. Prenatal diagnosis of asphyxiating thoracic dysplasia (Jeune syndrome). *Am J Perinatol.* 1996; 13:495–498.
3. Skiptunas SM, Weiner S. Early prenatal diagnosis of asphyxiating thoracic dysplasia (Jeune's syndrome). Value of fetal thoracic measurement. *J Ultrasound Med.* 1987;6:41–43.
4. Meinel K, Himmel D. Status of ultrasound and roentgen diagnosis in prenatal detection of osteochondrodysplasias. *Zentralbl Gynakol.* 1987;109:1303–1313.
5. Schinzel A, Savoldelli G, Briner J, Schubiger G. Prenatal sonographic diagnosis of Jeune syndrome. *Radiology.* 1985;154: 777–778.
6. Hopper MS, Boultbee JE, Watson AR. Polyhydramnios associated with congenital pancreatic cysts and asphyxiating thoracic dysplasia. A case report. *S Afr Med J.* 1979;56:32–33.

ASPLENIA–POLYSPLENIA SYNDROMES

Definition. This set of syndromes is caused by errors of lateralization of the primary field. It results (with simplifications) in a fetus with either a predominant right-sidedness and a isomeric left side (asplenia: a fetus whose left side is a mirror image of its right side) or left-sidedness and a isomeric right side (polysplenia: a fetus whose right side is a mirror image of its left side).[1,2] These fetuses are usually recognized because of the associated cardiac anomalies (see below).

Synonyms. Ivemark's syndrome.[3]

Incidence. Unknown, but not very rare.

Etiology. Autosomal recessive inheritance with male preponderance.

Diagnosis. The diagnosis is usually made by the recognition of the cardiac anomalies[4] (Fig. 21–19), in particular the presence of mesocardia (the axis of the interventricular septum being almost anteroposterior) with an endocardial cushion defect, an intrahepatic segment of the umbilical vein that is also oriented anteroposteriorly, and an odd-looking stomach (Fig. 21–20). The abnormal lobation of the lungs is difficult to recognize, and the only instance when it can be done is when a sliver of pleural fluid is infiltrated between the lobes. Another typical finding is the interruption of the inferior vena cava (IVC) with azygos continuation. The typical findings include an IVC that is posterior in the upper abdomen (instead of curving anteriorly to enter the right atrium) and the abrupt decrease in size of the IVC near the diaphragm. An enlarged azygos arch joining the superior vena cava (SVC) can also be recognized (Fig. 21–21). The presence of a persistent left SVC is rarely recognized, not because it is a challenging finding but because it is not sought.

Genetic Anomalies. Although it was that the syndrome resulted from possible mutations in the gene encoding connexin 43 (CX43),[5] this was not supported by subsequent studies.[6,7]

Differential Diagnosis. The cardiac anomalies (in particular endocardial cushion defect) without the syndrome and trisomy 18 may be included and should be included in the differential diagnosis.

Associated Anomalies. See Table 21–1.

Cardiac:
interruption of the IVC with azygous continuation
ASD-VSD
bilateral SVCs
endocardial cushion defects
anomalous pulmonary veinous return
left/right outflow obstruction
bilateral left atria

Lungs:
bilobated lobes
hyparteral bronchi
bronchi with a left-side morphology

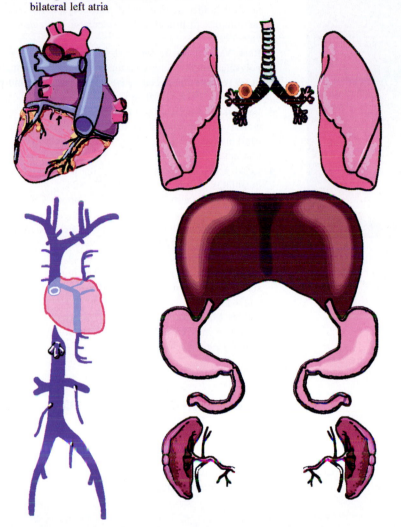

Gastrointestinal tract
midline symmetrical liver
absence of the gallbladder
abdominal heterotaxia
right / left-sided stomach
malrotation
polysplenia

Figure 21–19. Schematic drawing of the findings in polysplenia. *(Reproduced with permission from Fedrizzi R, Bruner J, Jeanty P. The Fetus. 1992;2:1–5.)*

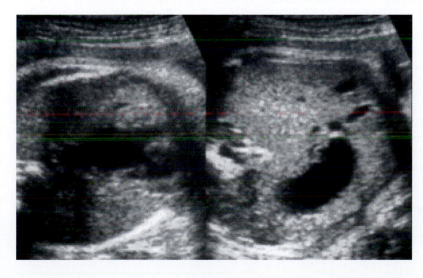

Figure 21–20. Polysplenia: dextrocardia with malrotation of the stomach on the right side. The apex of the heart is on the same side as the stomach. A complete form of endocardial cushion defect is noted, with a single atrium. *(Reproduced with permission from Fedrizzi R, Bruner J, Jeanty P. The Fetus. 1992;2:1–5.)*

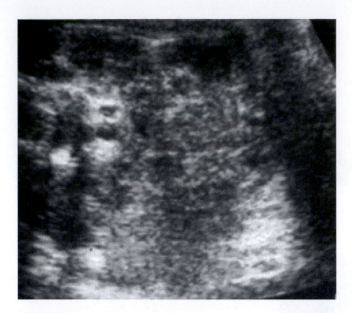

Figure 21–21. Horseshoe kidney in front of the great vessels. *(Reproduced with permission from Fedrizzi R, Bruner J, Jeanty P. The Fetus. 1992;2:1–5.)*

Prognosis. Asplenia tends to be a more severe disease because of the cyanotic heart lesions and the superimposed infections.

Management. Termination of pregnancy can be offered before viability. Standard prenatal care is not altered when continuation of the pregnancy is decided. Confirmation of diagnosis after birth is important for genetic counseling.

REFERENCES

1. Moller JH, Nakib A, Anderson RC, Edwards JE. Congenital cardiac disease associated with polysplenia, a developmental complex of bilateral 'left-sidedness.' *Circulation*. 1967;36: 789–799.
2. Rose V, Izukawa T, Moes CAF. Syndromes of asplenia and polysplenia: A review of cardiac and non-cardiac malformation in 60 cases with special reference to diagnosis and prognosis. *Br Heart J*. 1975;37:840–852.
3. Ivemark BI. Implications of agenesis of the spleen on the pathogenesis of cono-truncus anomalies in childhood: Analysis of the heart malformations in splenic agenesis syndrome, with fourteen new cases. *Acta Paediatr*. 1955;44 (suppl 104):1–110.
4. Cesko I, Hajdu J, Toth T, et al. Ivemark syndrome with asplenia in siblings. *J Pediatr*. 1997;130:822–824.
5. Britz-Cunningham SH, Shah MM, Zuppan CW, Fletcher WH. Mutations of the connexin 43 gap-junction gene in patients with heart malformations and defects of laterality. *N Engl J Med*. 1995;332:1323–1329.
6. Debrus S, Tuffery S, Matsuoka R, et al. Lack of evidence for connexin 43 gene mutations in human autosomal recessive lateralization defects. *J Molec Cell Cardiol*. 1997;29: 1423–1431.
7. Gebbia M, Towbin JA, Casey B. Failure to detect connexin 43 mutations in 38 cases of sporadic and familial heterotaxy. *Circulation*. 1996;94:1909–1912.

BECKWITH–WIEDEMANN SYNDROME

Definition. Beckwith–Wiedemann syndrome is a disorder first described by Beckwith in 1963[1] and by Wiedemann in 1964.[2] It is characterized by the classic triad of macrosomia, omphalocele, and macroglossia.

TABLE 21–1. ANOMALIES ASSOCIATED WITH ASPLENIA AND POLYSPLENIA SYNDROMES

	Asplenia	Polysplenia
Cardiovascular	Bilateral superior vena cava, anomalous pulmonary venous connections, absence of the coronary sinus, endocardial cushion defect, right ventricular outflow tract obstructions, transpositions of the great arteries, isomerism of the atria (both resemble a right atrium), atrial septal defects, the apex of the heart can be in either direction	Anomalous pulmonary venous return, interrupted inferior vena cava with (hemi)azygos continuation, atrial and ventricular septal defects, pulmonic stenosis, endocardial cushion defects (less severe than in asplenia)
Spleen	Splenic agenesis or more commonly hypotrophy	Multiple splenules
Lungs	Trilobated lungs with eparterial bronchus	Bilobated lungs with hyparterial bronchus
Liver	Decrease in the normal difference of size between the right and left lobe, independent hepatic vein on the opposite side of the inferior vena cava	
Stomach	Right sided or midline	
Bowel	Malrotation (the colon is posterior to the small bowel)	
Complications	Infections	

Synonym. Exomphalos–macroglossia–gigantism syndrome.

Incidence. The incidence has been estimated to be 0.72 per 10,000 births,[3] and more than 500 cases have been reported in the literature.[4]

Etiology. Sporadic in most cases, Beckwith–Wiedemann syndrome has an autosomal dominant inheritance, with incomplete penetrance and variable expressivity. Rearrangements involving the chromosome 11p15 region seems to be the mutation responsible for this disorder.[5]

Diagnosis. The detection of macrosomia, omphalocele (Fig. 21–22), and macroglossia associated with a normal karyotype makes the diagnosis of Beckwith–Wiedemann syndrome. Other features occurring in variable incidence include nephromegaly, hepatomegaly, polyhydramnios, ear lobe creases, diaphragmatic hernia, and cardiac defects.[6,7] Pancreatic cell hyperplasia may affect 30 to 50% of patients, causing hyperinsulinism and neonatal hypoglycemia on the second or third day of life.[8] A fairly typical finding also is a small ear lobe groove (Fig. 21–23).

Genetic Anomalies. Structural anomalies of the chromosome including paternal isodisomy of the 11p15.5 region, isodisomy of 11q, and uniparental disomy may be detected by cytogenetic studies.

Differential Diagnosis. Down's syndrome must be excluded by chromosomal analysis because of the occurrence of macro-

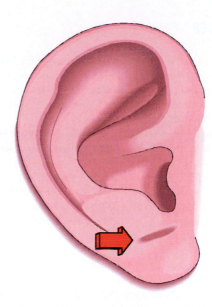

Figure 21–23. The ear lobe groove can be recognized when sought.

glosia in both conditions. Diabetic fetopathy is another cause of macrosomia and thus a differential diagnosis. Normal levels of maternal glucose exclude this possibility. Zellweger's syndrome can also combine liver and kidney enlargement and may be diagnosed prenatally by measuring fatty acid concentration and activity of marker enzymes.[9]

Complications. Untreated neonatal hypoglycemia is an important complication and may result in further cerebral dysfunction, such as seizures, mild to moderate mental retardation, or neonatal death in more severe cases.[10,11] Macroglosia can cause variable complications ranging from feeding difficulties to airway obstruction and death. Long-term complications includes high risk for abdominal tumors, in particular Wilm's tumor, hepatoblastoma, neuroblastoma, and adrenal cortical carcinoma.[3,11]

Prognosis. Neonatal mortality rate is approximately 21%, caused mainly by congestive heart failure.[3] Among those who survive, the prognosis is in general favorable, depending on the severity of the associated anomalies and long-term complications.

Management. When diagnosed before viability, termination can be offered. After viability, sonographic evaluation of fetal growth is suggested. When macrosomia is suspected, cesarean section may be offered because of the risk of shoulder dystocia. Delivery in a tertiary center is recommended for early abdominal wall defect repair and treatment of hypoglycemia. Sonographic screening for abdominal tumors each trimester is recommended during the first 6 years of life.[9]

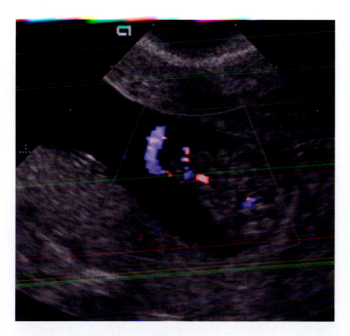

Figure 21–22. A typical omphalocele.

REFERENCES

1. Beckwith JB. Extreme cytomegaly of the adrenal fetal cortex, omphacele, hyperplasia of kidneys and pancreas, and Leydig-cell hyperplasia. Another syndrome? Presented at the annual meeting of the Western Society for Pediatric Research, Los Angeles, California, November 11, 1963.
2. Wiedemann HR. Complex malformatif. Familial avec hernie ombilicale et macroglossie-un "syndrome nouveau"? *J Hum Genet*. 1964;13:223–232.
3. Whisson CC, Whyte A, Ziesing P. Beckwith–Wiedemann syndrome: Antenatal diagnosis. *Aust Radiol*. 1994;38:130–131.
4. Viljoen DL, Jaquire Z, Wood DL. Prenatal diagnosis in autosomal dominant Beckwith–Wiedemann syndrome. *Prenat Diagn*. 1991;11:167–175.
5. Koufos A, Grundy P, Morgan K, et al. Familial Wiedemann–Beckwith syndrome and a second Wilms tumor locus both map to 11p15.5. *Am J Hum Genet*. 1989;44:711.
6. Fremond B, Poulain P, Odent S, et al. Prenatal detection of a congenital pancreatic cyst and Beckwith–Wiedemann syndrome. *Prenat Diagn*. 1997;17:276–280.
7. Ranzini AC, Day S, Turner T, et al. Intrauterine growth and ultrasound findings with Beckwith–Wiedemann syndrome. *Obstet Gynecol*. 1997;89:538–542.
8. Nyhan WL, Sakati NO. *Genetic and Malformation Syndromes in Clinical Medicine*. Chicago: Year Book Medical Publishers; 1976.
9. Nowotny T, Bollmann R, Pfeifer L, Windt E. Beckwith–Wiediemann syndrome: Difficulties with prenatal diagnosis. *Fetal Diagn Ther*. 1994;9:256–260.
10. Winter SC, Curry CJR, Smith C, et al. Prenatal diagnosis of the Beckwith–Wiedemann syndrome. *Am J Med Genet*. 1986;24:137–141.
11. Hewitt B, Bankier A. Prenatal ultrasound diagnosis of Beckwith–Wiedemann syndrome. *Aust NZ J Obstet Gynaecol*. 1994;34:488–490.

BILATERAL RENAL AGENESIS

Definition. Bilateral absence of the kidneys, usually associated with the oligohydramnios sequence.

Synonyms. Potter's syndrome (no longer used).

Incidence. One to two per 10,000 births.

Etiology. Occurence is usually sporadic, but 20 to 36% of bilateral renal agenesis (BRA) present a familial recurrence (possibly autosomal dominant, with incomplete penetrance and variable expression).

Pathogenesis. Results from a lack of induction of the metanephric blastema by the ureteral bud. The absence of kidney results in the absence of amniotic fluid after 12 to 13 weeks (before that, fluid is an exsudate or an extension of the intercellular fluid of the fetus). The oligohydramnios causes the pulmonary hypoplasia. In rare cases of monozygotic twin discordant for the renal agenesis, the pulmonary hypoplasia does not occur.[1-3]

Diagnosis. The diagnosis is first suggested by the absence of amniotic fluid and then by the absence of the bladder (Fig. 21–24) and the lack of kidneys.[4] Color Doppler has been found useful in identifying the lack of renal arteries[5] (Fig. 21–25). Before a final diagnosis is made, one should consider and, if possible, exclude the possibility of pelvic or ectopic kidneys, which could compress the bladder, and exclude the possibility of an ectopic ureter, which could explain the absence of a bladder.

Genetic Anomalies. Unknown.

Differential Diagnosis. Bilateral renal medullary cystic dysplasia and bilateral renal hypoplasia may appear as BRA.[6] Further, normal but nonfunctioning kidneys and abnormal placental implantation (e.g., on a uterine septum) can lead to the same presentation of severe oligohydramnios. This information is important to convey during patients' counseling: The concern is that not only the renal agenesis (which may be absent) but also the oligohydramnios will lead to pulmonary hypoplasia.

Associated Anomalies. Because this is a common anomaly, many different associations have been described (e.g., VACTERL, Meckel, chromosome 22 malformations). In

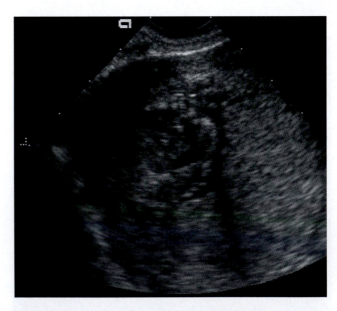

Figure 21–24. Anhydramnios at 15 weeks of gestation. This is actually not a bilateral renal agenesis, as is demonstrated in Fig. 21–25. This fetus had kidneys. Even with good equipment, the gray-scale diagnosis of the kidney is not always easy at this age, due in part to the oligohydramnios.

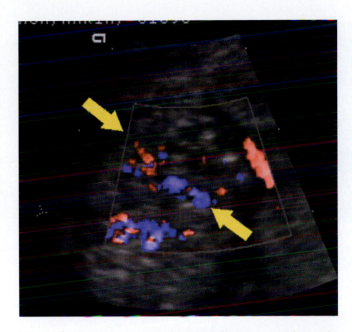

Figure 21–25. Bilateral renal arteries. Notice how much better the renal arteries are seen in color Doppler than are the actual kidneys. This teenage patient elected to continue the pregnancy but spontaneously miscarried a month later. The placenta was inserted on a uterine septum, severely limiting the rate of exchanges.

practice, most of these are difficult to identify by ultrasound because of the oligohydramnios.

Prognosis. Lethal.

Management. Many investigators have suggested the use of amnioinfusion or even intraabdominal infusion of saline to better visualize the anatomy.[7] Although there may be indications for such an aggressive approach in nonviable fetuses, these are quite uncommon, and the approach is not justified in the majority of cases. Termination of pregnancy can be offered before viability. Standard prenatal care is not altered when continuation of the pregnancy is decided. Confirmation of diagnosis after birth is important for genetic counseling.

REFERENCES

1. Lebel RR, Jones G, Israel J, Senica W. Renal agenesis without lung hypoplasia, Vacterl syndrome. *Fetus.* 1994;4:5–6.
2. Klinger G, Merlob P, Aloni D, et al. Normal pulmonary function in a monoamniotic twin discordant for bilateral renal agenesis: Report and review. *Am J Med Genet.* 1997;73:76–79.
3. Cilento BG Jr, Benacerraf BR, Mandell J. Prenatal and postnatal findings in monochorionic, monoamniotic twins discordant for bilateral renal agenesis-dysgenesis (perinatal lethal renal disease). *J Urol.* 1994;151:1034–1035.
4. Bronshtein M, Amit A, Achiron R, et al. The early prenatal sonographic diagnosis of renal agenesis: Techniques and possible pitfalls. *Prenat Diagn.* 1994;14:291–297.
5. Sepulveda W, Stagiannis KD, Flack NJ, Fisk NM. Accuracy of prenatal diagnosis of renal agenesis with color flow imaging in severe second-trimester oligohydramnios. *Am J Obstet Gynecol.* 1995;173;1788–1792.
6. Latini JM, Curtis MR, Cendron M, et al. Prenatal failure to visualize kidneys: A spectrum of disease. *Urology.* 1998;52:306–311.
7. Haeusler MC, Ryan G, Robson SC, et al. The use of saline solution as a contrast medium in suspected diaphragmatic hernia and renal agenesis. *Am J Obstet Gynecol.* 1993;168:1486–1492.

CAMPOMELIC DYSPLASIA

Definition. Campomelic dysplasia is a congenital disorder characterized by development of abnormal curvature of the long bones, particularly from lower extremities, such as the femur and tibiae.[1] Some investigators have classified the disease into two varieties: long limbed and short limbed, depending on the type of limbs involved in the pathologic process.[2]

Synonyms. Camptomelic dysplasia, campomelic syndrome, campomelic dwarfism, and congenital bowing of the limbs.[3]

Prevalence. The disorder affects 0.02 per 10,000 live births.[4] Sex reversal occurs in some genotypic males, with lack of the H-Y antigen. The phenotypic male-to-female ratio is approximately 1 to 2.3, and the karyotypic male-to-female ratio is approximately 2 to 1.[3]

Etiology. The transmission of campomelic dysplasia is unknown. Autosomal recessive inheritance is thought to be the most common pattern, although it may occur because of sporadic autosomal dominant mutation.[5]

Recurrence Risk. The risk depends on the etiology. If transmitted by an autosomal recessive pattern, the recurrence risk is 25%. If transmitted by an autosomal dominant pattern, the recurrence risk is 50% but most are new mutations.

Diagnosis. The most characteristic sign of campomelic dysplasia is the marked anterior bowing of the long bones, in particular the femur (Fig. 21–26A and B) and tibia. Severe angulation may mimic fractures. Other sonographic features that are commonly present include growth restriction, bell-shaped narrow chest, 11 pairs of ribs, hypoplasia of the midthoracic vertebral bodies, fibula, and scapula, scoliosis, shortness of the limbs, talipes equinovarus, tracheobronchomalacia, flat and small face, high forehead with prominent occiput, low nasal bridge, micrognathia, cleft of the soft palate, hypertelorism, low-set and malformed ears, hydrocephalus, and ambiguous genitalia.[6]

Genetic Anomaly. A mutation in SOX9, a sex-determining region of the Y (SRY) related gene, located at 17q24, seems

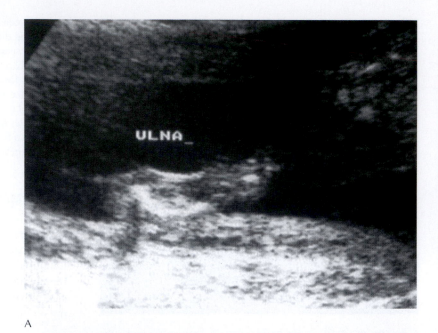

A

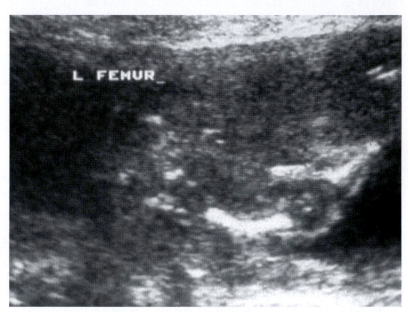

Figure 21–26. **(A** and **B)** Bowing of the tibia and femur. Note the gentle curve that sometimes differentiates these from the more acute angles of fetuses with osteogenesis imperfecta.

B

to be associated with the occurrence of both campomelic dysplasia and sex reversal.[7,8]

Pathogenesis. Although many theories have been proposed to explain the development of the anomalies present in this syndrome (in particular the bowing of the bones), the precise mechanism is not known. Some of the theories are: 1) mechanical stress due to faulty fetal position within the uterus[9]; 2) primary muscle imbalance and shortening, particularly of the calf muscles, causing secondary bending of the tibia[10]; 3) intrauterine fracture with subsequent healing[11]; 4) abnor-

mal vascular and cellular elements of perichondrium[12]; and 5) developmental disturbance in the cartilagineous phase of bone formation.[13]

Associated Anomalies. Polyhydramnios and anomalies from the central nervous, cardiac, and renal systems have been described prenataly.[6] After birth, hearing loss may occur.

Differential Diagnosis. Osteogenesis imperfecta types I and II, hypophosphatasia, unclassifiable varieties of congenital bowing of the long bones,[14] thanatophoric dysplasia, mesomelic dysplasia (Reinhart variety),[15] Roberts' syndrome and diastrophic dysplasia.[5]

Prognosis. Usually results in neonatal or infant death due to respiratory complications. Some survivors, including a male alive at 17 years, have been reported.[16]

Management. Before viability, the option of pregnancy termination should be offered. After viability, standard obstetric management is not altered, and respiratory function in the newborn must be supported.

REFERENCES

1. Valcamonico A, Jeanty P. Campomelic dysplasia. *Fetus.* 1992;2: 7544.
2. Khajavi A, Lachman R, Rimoin N, et al. Heterogeneity in the campomelic syndromes. Long and short bone varieties. *Radiology.* 1976;120:641–647.
3. Buyse ML. *Birth Defects Encyclopedia.* Cambridge, MA: Blackwell Scientific; 1990:252–253.
4. Urioste M, Arroyo A, Martinez-Frias ML. Campomelia, polycystic dysplasia and cervical lymphocele in two sibs. *Am J Med Genet.* 1991;41:475–477.
5. Benacerraf BR. Camptomelic dysplasia. In: Benacerraf BR, ed. *Ultrasound of Fetal Syndromes.* New York: Churchill Livinstone; 1998:168–169.
6. Huston CS, Opiz JM, Spranger JW, et al. The campomelic syndrome: Review, report of 17 cases, and follow-up on the currently 17-year-old boy first reported by Maroteaux et al. in 1971. *Am J Med Genet.* 1983;15:3–28.
7. Foster JW, Dominguez-Steglich MA, Guioni S, et al. Campomelic dysplasia and autosomal sex reversal caused by mutations in an SRY-related gene. *Nature.* 1994;372:525.
8. McDowall S, Argentaro A, Ranganathan S, et al. Functional and structural studies of wild type SOX9 and mutations causing campomelic dysplasia. *J Biol Chem.* 1999;274: 24023–24030.
9. Caffey J. Prenatal bowing and thickening of tubular bones with multiple cutaneous dimples in arms and legs: A congenital syndrome of mechanical origin. *Am J Dis Child.* 1947;74: 543–562.
10. Middleton DS. Studies of prenatal lesions of striated muscle as a cause of congenital deformities. *Edinb Med J.* 1934;41: 401–442.
11. Snure H. Intrauterine fracture. *Radiology.* 1929;13:362–365.
12. Bain AD, Barrett HS. Congenital bowing of the long bones: Report of a case. *Arch Dis Child.* 1959;34:516–524.
13. Lee FA, Isaacs H, Strauss J. The "campomelic" syndrome. *Am J Dis Child.* 1972;124:485–496.
14. Cordone M, Lituania M, Zampatti C, et al. In utero ultrasonographic features of campomelic dysplasia. *Prenat Diagn.* 1989;9:745–750.
15. Romero R, Pilu G, Jeanty P, et al. *Prenatal Diagnosis of Congenital Anomalies.* Norwalk, CT: Appleton & Lange; 1988.
16. Maroteaux P, Spranger J, Opiz JM, et al. Le syndrome campomelique. *Presse Med.* 1971;79:1157–1162.

CAUDAL REGRESSION SYNDROME

Definition. Caudal regression syndrome is a rare congenital defect, characterized by the absence of the sacrum and defects of different portions of lumbar spine, associated with anomalies from different systems.

Synonyms. Caudal dysplasia sequence and sacral agenesis.

Prevalence. From 0.1 to 0.25 per 10,000 in normal pregnancies and 200 to 250 times higher in diabetic pregnancies.[1]

Etiology. Unknown, but associated with maternal diabetes in 16% of affected cases.[2]

Recurrent Risk. This anomaly is not thought to be hereditary, and the recurrent risk is very small, although higher in diabetics.

Diagnosis. The sonographic findings are variable and depend on the extent and severity of the defect. It ranges from complete absence of the sacrum associated with abnormalities of the lumbar spine (Figs. 21–27 and 21–28) and lower extremities (such as clubbed feet and contractions of the knees, as shown in Fig. 21–29, and hips) to abnormalities of the sacrum, without associated defects.[3] The most typical findings are the absence of a few vertebrae, the shieldlike appearance of the fused or approximated iliac wings (Fig. 21–30), and the decrease interspace between the femoral heads. Some sections will intersect the fetus at such an angle so that no spine is

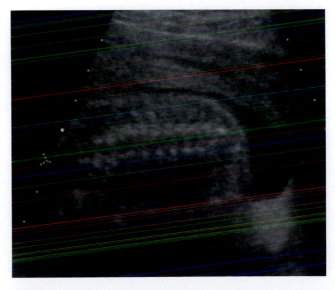

Figure 21–27. Although on superficial examination this image might pass for normal, on the caudal side of the image (on the right, because the ribs can be seen on the left side of the image) the spine terminates without the usual landmark of the iliac winds and sacrum.

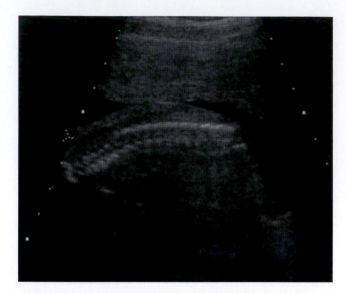

Figure 21–28. This same finding as that shown in Fig. 21–27 is even more striking on the sagittal view of the spine, where the distal end appears to have been "erased." This is the finding that caught the eye of an astute sonographer, who was puzzled by the spine "looking too short."

visible, a very striking and probably pathognomonic finding (Fig. 21–31). Decreased movement of the legs is frequently observed. First-trimester diagnosis may be hard to accomplish because of the incomplete ossification of the sacrum at that time. A short crown–rump length and abnormal appearance of the yolk sac have been proposed as early sonographic signs of caudal regression syndromes.[3]

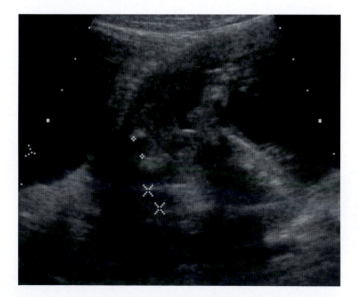

Figure 21–29. Webbing of the popliteal joint is very typical, but it is difficult to capture on a frozen image. By scanning meticulously over the popliteal region, the arciform shape of the soft tissue can be recognized.

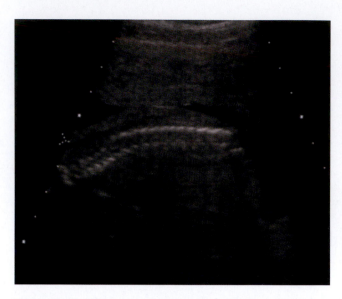

Figure 21–30. The lack of sacrum allows the iliac wings to be approximated, giving them a shieldlike appearance.

Genetic Anomaly. Unknown.

Pathogenesis. Disruption of the maturation of the caudal portion of the spinal cord complex before 4 weeks of gestation, leading to motricity deficits and neurologic impairment, differing from incontinence of urine and feces to complete neurologic loss.

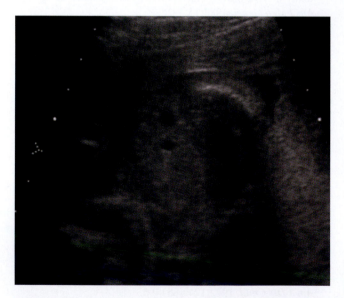

Figure 21–31. The spinal cord of this fetus is at about 2:00 (compare with the position of the iliac wings in Fig. 21–30). I do not know of any other condition that can provide this image of a cross-section through the fetal abdomen with no visible spine. None of the other differential diagnoses, such as achondrogenesis and the severest forms of osteogenesis imperfecta would present with the localized anomaly seen here.

Associated Anomalies. Anomalies of the central nervous, musculoskeletal, genitourinary, cardiac, respiratory, and gastrointestinal systems may be found in association with caudal regression syndrome.

Differential Diagnosis. Sirenomelia, which was thought to be the most severe form of caudal regression syndrome (today it is considered a different entity),[3] is the main differential diagnosis. Fusion of the lower extremities is a typical finding of sirenomelia.

Prognosis. Depends on the severity of the spinal defect and associated anomalies, but the vast majority of those who survive require urologic and orthopedic interventions. Severe forms are commonly associated with cardiac, renal, and respiratory problems, which are responsible for early neonatal death.

Management. If detected early, pregnancy termination can be offered. Standard prenatal care is not altered if continuation of the pregnancy is decided. If born alive, extensive surgery in a tertiary center is usually needed to repair the defects.

REFERENCES

1. Jaffe R, Zeituni M, Fejgin M. Caudal regression syndrome. *Fetus.* 1991;7561:1–3.
2. Jones KL. Caudal dysplasia sequence. In: Jones KL, ed. *Smith's Recognizable Patterns of Human Malformation.* Philadelphia: WB Saunders; 1998:635.
3. Benacerraf BR. Caudal regression syndrome and sirenomelia. In: Benacerraf BR, ed. *Ultrasound of Fetal Syndromes.* New York: Churchill Livingstone; 1998:250–254.

CEREBROHEPATORENAL SYNDROME

Definition. One of the four syndromes of the "peroxisome biogenesis disorders" resulting from anomalous enzymatic function of the metabolism of fatty acids due to deficient peroxisomes.

Synonyms. Zellweger's syndrome.

Incidence. From 0.2 to 0.25 per 10,000, male-to-female ratio is 1 to 1.

Etiology. Autosomal recessive with variable expression.

Diagnosis. The fetuses demonstrate growth restriction and hypotonicity. Abnormal head shape (bulging forehead, wide metopic suture), micrognathia, buphophtalmos (Fig. 21–32),

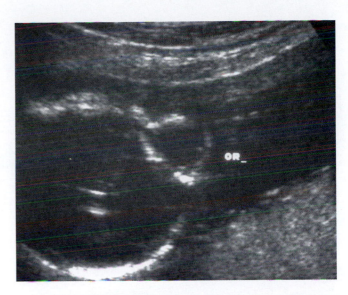

Figure 21–32. Buphophthalmos. Note the enlarged size of the eye.

CNS anomalies (hydrocephalus,[1] periventricular cysts[2]), hepatomegaly with dysgenesis,[3] cardiac anomalies, clinodactyly, and simian creases can also be detected prenatally. Biochemical studies using blood cells and fibroblasts can confirm the diagnosis by detection of reduced peroxisomes and abnormal lipid metabolism.

Genetic Anomalies. The probable locus is on the long arm of chromosome 7 in the 21 to 22 region. A genetic diagnosis can be performed by amniocentesis.[4]

Differential Diagnosis. Many aneuploidies may present with similar findings. Down's syndrome is commonly misdiagnosed, due to the overlapping of several structural findings.[3]

Prognosis. Most infants die within the first year.

Management. Termination of pregnancy can be offered before viability. Standard prenatal care is not altered when continuation of the pregnancy is decided. Confirmation of diagnosis after birth is important for genetic counseling.

REFERENCES

1. Nakai A, Shigematsu Y, Nishida K, et al. MRI findings of Zellweger syndrome. *Pediatr Neurol.* 1995;13:346–348.
2. Russel IM, van Sonderen L, van Straaten HL, Barth PG. Subependymal germinolytic cysts in Zellweger syndrome. *Pediatr Radiol.* 1995;25:254–255.
3. Jones KL. Zellweger syndrome. In: Jones KL, ed. *Smith's Recognizable Patterns of Human Malformation.* Philadelphia: WB Saunders; 1998:212–213.
4. Lazarow PB, Small GM, Santos M, et al. Zellweger syndrome

amniocytes: Morphological appearance and a simple sedimentation method for prenatal diagnosis. *Pediatr Res.* 1988;24: 63–67.

CLOVERLEAF SKULL OR KLEEBLATTSCHADEL

Definition. Cloverleaf skull or kleeblattschadel is a rare malformation caused by synostosis of multiple cranial sutures. It can be associated with hydrocephalus, proptosis, and hypoplasia of the midface and cranial base.

Synonyms. Craniosynostosis.

Incidence. Rare outside the associated syndromes (see below).

Etiology. Depend on the associated syndrome; most are de novo mutation of the $FGFR_{1-3}$.

Diagnosis. The findings are usually quite obvious, with the usual oval shape of the head at the level of the biparietal diameter (BPD) replaced by the trilobate skull: one frontal protrusion and two posterolateral protrusions.

Genetic Anomalies. Most are de novo mutations of the $FGFR_{1-3}$.

Differential Diagnosis. Hydrocephalus from other causes, although the head shape is usually normal.

Associated Anomalies. Many syndromes present with cloverleaf skull including most of the acrocephalopoly(syn)dactylies (Crouzon, Pfeiffer, Carpenter, Apert, etc.). It is also typical of the type II form of thanatophoric dysplasia (another FGFR mutation).

Prognosis. When associated with hydrocephalus, the outcome is usually poor, with frequent death in infancy.

Management. The surgical management of patients with cloverleaf skull deformity is aimed at relieving the intracranial hypertension and correcting the aesthetic appearance. By a process of repositioning and modifying segments of the skull, satisfactory results with regard to relief from intracranial hypertension and preservation of visual acuity and from the aesthetic viewpoint can now be achieved.[1,2]

REFERENCES

1. Zuccaro G, Dogliotti P, Bennum R, Monges J. Treatment of cloverleaf skull syndrome. *Childs Nerv Syst.* 1996;12:695–698.
2. Resnick DK, Pollack IF, Albright AL. Surgical management

of the cloverleaf skull deformity. *Pediatr Neurosurg.* 1995;22: 29–37.

FETAL ALCOHOL SYNDROME AND FETAL ALCOHOL EFFECTS

Definition. Children exposed to alcohol (more than 2.2 glasses of wine per day or the equivalent) *in utero* suffer from growth and mental retardation, physical abnormalities, and immune dysfunction.[1-3]

Synonyms. None.

Incidence. The incidence of fetal alcohol syndrome (FAS) ranges from 2 to 30 per 10,000 live births. This represents the most common form of mental retardation in the United States.

Etiology. Direct toxicity of alcohol and its metabolites cross the placenta and are not detoxified by the fetal liver.[4]

Diagnosis. The findings include microcephaly, long philtrum, small micrognathia, cleft palate, microphthalmia, malformed ears, atrial septal defect–ventricular septal defect (ASD–VSD), and growth retardation.

Genetic Anomalies. None.

Differential Diagnosis. Other conditions that involve growth retardation and microcephaly, such as TORCH infections and chromosomal anomalies.

Associated Anomalies. See Diagnosis.

Prognosis. Mental retardation and delay in growth that persist postnatally.[5,6]

Management. The management of these pregnancies should be aimed at reducing the alcohol consumption, although few programs have had much efficacy.

REFERENCES

1. Bradley KA, Badrinath S, Bush K, et al. Medical risks for women who drink alcohol. *J Gen Intern Med.* 1998;13:627–639.
2. Bagheri MM, Burd L, Martsolf JT, Klug MG. Fetal alcohol syndrome: Maternal and neonatal characteristics. *J Perinat Med.* 1998;26:263–269.
3. Allebeck P, Olsen J. Alcohol and fetal damage. *Alcohol Clin Exp Res.* 1998;22(7 suppl):329S–332S.
4. Zachman RD, Grummer MA. The interaction of ethanol and vitamin A as a potential mechanism for the pathogenesis of fetal alcohol syndrome. *Alcohol Clin Exp Res.* 1998;22:1544–1556.

5. Olson HC, Feldman JJ, Streissguth AP, et al. Neuropsychological deficits in adolescents with fetal alcohol syndrome: Clinical findings. *Alcohol Clin Exp Res.* 1998;22:1998–2012.

6. D'Apolito K. Substance abuse: Infant and childhood outcomes. *J Pediatr Nurs.* 1998;13:307–316.

FETAL CYTOMEGALOVIRUS INFECTION

Definition. Fetal cytomegalovirus (CMV) infection is a congenital disorder, characterized by hydrops, ascites, ventriculomegaly, and other findings caused by transplacental transmission of CMV to the fetus. The double-stranded DNA herpes group virus causes a mild infection or a mononucleosis-type illness in young healthy adults, chronic disease in older adults, and mild to severe congenital infection.[1]

Synonyms. Congenital CMV infection and congenital CMV infection.

Etiology. Cytomegalovirus (a double-stranded DNA herpes group virus).

Recurrence Risk. Considering that viral infection confers immunity in the vast majority, there is just a small theoretical risk of re-infection in another pregnancy.[2]

Incidence. Congenital CMV infection occurs in 0.2 to 2.2% of deliveries.[2] Approximately 5 to 10% of congenitally infected infants will demonstrate classical signs of illness at birth.[3,4] Few cases may have isolated findings such as ascites.

Diagnosis. Cytomegalovirus infection and other congenital infections should be suspected whenever nonimmune hydrops is found. Other suggestive findings that may be present are splenomegaly (Fig. 21–33), chorioretinitis (an echogenic lining to the vitreous body), occlusion of the foramen ovale (marked by decreased motion of the foramen ovale flap and thickening of the flap), signs of right heart overload from the premature closure), mild cerebral ventriculomegaly, intracranial calcifications, microcephaly, ascites, hyperechoic bowel, intrauterine growth retardation (IUGR), brain atrophy, and oligohydramnios. Most features are found by ultrasound examinations, around 20 weeks of gestation. Whenever maternal infection is confirmed, amniocentesis or cordocentesis is required for serologic studies (search for fetal specific IgM antibody), although it does not have 100% reliability. The diagnosis can also be made by histologic study of typical inclusion bodies in biopsy or autopsy specimens.[5]

Pathogenesis. The exact mode of transplacental passage is uncertain. The virus replicates in fetal tissues, producing inflammation, tissue necrosis, and organ dysfunction.[5] Cytomegalovirus hepatitis in the neonate can present with an intense inflammatory response involving the portal triads. In these cases, lobular disarray, degeneration of hepatocytes, and cholestasis are also seen.[6] The cause of ascites in congenital CMV infection is not certain. Contributing factors may include low serum protein levels due to hepatic dysfunction and portal obstruction resulting from periportal inflammation.[6]

Associated Anomalies. Isolated ascites is an uncommon but possible finding in fetuses with CMV infection. Cardiovascular, gastrointestinal, musculoskeletal, and ocular lesions may

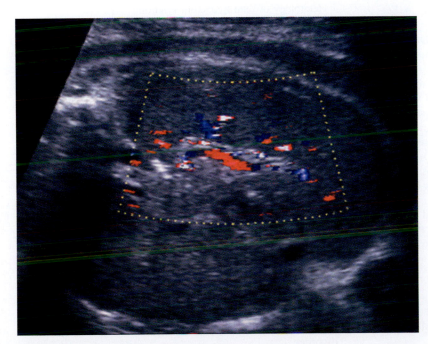

Figure 21–33. Splenomegaly. No measurements necessary. This spleen extends almost to the anterior abdominal wall.

be found in association with the classic features. Petechiae, neurosensory hearing loss, and poor intellectual development may also occur after birth.[1]

Differential Diagnosis. Because ascites is often the first manifestation of hydrops, the differential diagnosis for fetal ascites is essentially the same as with generalized hydrops, which includes mainly congenital infection. Conditions that present intracranial clacifications (such as tuberous sclerosis), hyperechoic bowel (cystic fibrosis and Down's syndrome), and hepatomegaly (primary liver disease or extramedullary hematopoiesis) should be considered.[1,7]

Prognosis. In general, neonates with symptomatic CMV infection do poorly, with a neonatal mortality rate as high as 30% and a high rate of neurologic handicap in survivors.[2,7] Cytomegalovirus hepatitis is reversible in survivors,[3] but mental retardation, motor handicaps, and hearing loss are expected long-term sequelae.

Management. Termination of pregnancy can be offered before viability. If continuing the pregnancy is decided, monthly follow-up with ultrasound is recommended to monitor growth restriction, hydrops, and other fetal manifestations. Decompression with paracentesis to remove fetal ascites may prevent pulmonary hypoplasia and improve the circulatory system in those cases severely affected.[8]

REFERENCES

1. Chriss-Price D, Lawrence SK, Jeanty P. Cytomegalovirus, splenomegaly. *Fetus.* 1994;4:5–8.
2. Stagno S, Whitley RJ. Herpesvirus infections of pregnancy. Part I: Cytomegalovirus and Epstein–Barr virus infections. *N Engl J Med.* 1985;313:1270–1274.
3. Stagno S. Cytomegalovirus. In: Remington JS, Klein JO, eds. *Infectious Diseases of the Fetus and Newborn Infant,* 3rd. ed. Philadelphia: WB Saunders; 1990:259–271.
4. Bale JF Jr. Human cytomegalovirus infection and disorders of the nervous system. *Arch Neurol.* 1984;41:310–320.
5. Richards DS, Preziosi M, Sexton C. Fetal CMV syndrome with ascites, hepatitis and negative serology. *Fetus.* 1992;2:7711.
6. Dehner LP. *Pediatric Surgical Pathology.* Baltimore: Williams and Wilkins; 1987:455–456.
7. Benacerraf BR. Cytomegalovirus (maternal infections). In: Benacerraf BR, ed. *Ultrasound of Fetal Syndromes.* New York: Churchill Livingstone; 1998:293–295.
8. Yamashita Y, Iwanaga R, Goto A, et al. Congenital cytomegalovirus infection associated with fetal ascites and intrahepatic calcifications. *Acta Paediatr Scand.* 1989;78:965–967.

FETAL HYDANTOIN SYNDROME

Definition. Effects due to maternal exposure to hydantoin anticonvulsant.

Synonyms. Dilantin, phenytoin, and a few other similar anticonvulsants are also included.

Incidence. From 7 to 10% of exposed infants.

Etiology. Alteration of enzymatic pathways.[1,2] Sibs exposed to similar amounts have been affected to different degrees.

Recurrence Risk. None.

Diagnosis. Growth retardation, microcephaly, hypoplasia of the distal phalanx of the fingers and toes, nail hypoplasia, typical facial appearance with a low nasal bridge, hirsutism, and cleft lip and palate, rib anomalies, and occasionally cardiac and genitourinary anomalies.[3–5]

Genetic Anomaly. None.

Associated Anomalies. None.

Differential Diagnosis. There are other causes of growth restriction and cardiac anomalies; thus, a TORCH titer and karyotype should be obtained.

Prognosis. Depends on the severity of the case.

Management. Switch the mother to a different medication if possible. Some prenatal testing may be possible.[6]

REFERENCES

1. Buehler BA, Rao V, Finnell RH. Biochemical and molecular teratology of fetal hydantoin syndrome. *Neurol Clin.* 1994;12: 741–748.
2. Finnell RH, Buehler BA, Kerr BM, et al. Clinical and experimental studies linking oxidative metabolism to phenytoin-induced teratogenesis. *Neurology.* 1992;42(suppl 5):25–31.
3. Sabry MA, Farag TI. Hand anomalies in fetal-hydantoin syndrome: From nail/phalangeal hypoplasia to unilateral acheiria. *Am J Med Genet.* 1996;62:410–412.
4. Ozkinay F, Yenigun A, Kantar M, et al. Two siblings with fetal hydantoin syndrome. *Turk J Pediatr.* 1998;40:273–278.
5. Adams J, Vorhees CV, Middaugh LD. Developmental neurotoxicity of anticonvulsants: Human and animal evidence on phenytoin. *Neurotoxicol Teratol.* 1990;12:203–214.
6. Buehler BA, Delimont D, van Waes M, Finnell RH. Prenatal prediction of risk of the fetal hydantoin syndrome. *N Engl J Med.* 1990;322:1567–1572.

FETAL LITHIUM EFFECTS

Definition. Cardiac anomaly (see below) and possible goiter due to maternal ingestion of lithium for manic depressive disorder.

Synonyms. None.

Incidence. Very rare.

Etiology. Maternal exposure to lithium. Reports in the 1970s associated the maternal use of lithium with Ebstein anomaly (with a 400% risk factor).[1-3] More recent data have not supported this finding.[4-6] The final answer is that there probably is a very small increase, but that it is infrequent enough that it should not be the cause for discontinuing treatment.

Recurrence Risk. None.

Diagnosis. Aside from the exceptional Ebstein anomaly, goiter, polyhydramnios,[7] and even stillbirth[8] have been reported.

Pathogenesis. Unknown.

Genetic Anomaly. None.

Associated Anomalies. None.

Differential Diagnosis. None.

Prognosis. Depends on the severity of the anomaly, if it exists.

Management. No alteration of management is indicated.

REFERENCES

1. Weinstein MR, Goldfield M. Cardiovascular malformations with lithium use during pregnancy. *Am J Psychiatry.* 1975;132: 529–531.
2. Park JM, Sridaromont S, Ledbetter EO, Terry WM. Ebstein's anomaly of the tricuspid valve associated with prenatal exposure to lithium carbonate. *Am J Dis Child.* 1980;134: 703–704.
3. Nora JJ, Nora AH, Toews WH. Lithium, Ebstein's anomaly, and other congenital heart defects. *Lancet.* 1974;2(7880): 594–595.
4. Cohen LS, Friedman JM, Jefferson JW, et al. A reevaluation of risk of in utero exposure to lithium. *JAMA.* 1994;271: 146–150.
5. Jacobson SJ, Jones K, Johnson K, et al. Prospective multicentre study of pregnancy outcome after lithium exposure during first trimester. *Lancet.* 1992;339(8792):530–533.
6. Zalzstein E, Koren G, Einarson T, Freedom RM. A case-control study on the association between first trimester exposure to lithium and Ebstein's anomaly. *Am J Cardiol.* 1990;65: 817–818.
7. Ang MS, Thorp JA, Parisi VM. Maternal lithium therapy and polyhydramnios. *Obstet Gynecol.* 1990;76(3, Pt 2):517–519.
8. Khandelwal SK, Sagar RS, Saxena S. Lithium in pregnancy and still birth: A case report. *Br J Psychiatry.* 1989;154:114–116.

FETAL RUBELLA SYNDROME

Definition. Fetal rubella syndrome is a congenital disorder resulting from primary maternal infection with the rubella virus (the fetus is infected by transplacental transmission) and is characterized mainly by deafness, mental retardation, congenital cataract, heart defects, and other structural anomalies that may be found with variable severity and frequency.

Synonym. Fetal rubella effects.[1]

Etiology. Rubella virus.

Recurrence Risk. None.

Incidence. Not precisely known. Administration of rubella vaccine has significantly reduced the incidence of maternal infection, although re-infection after vaccination is possible. The development of fetal infection reaches 50% among those exposed during the first trimester and 20% during the second trimester.[1,2]

Diagnosis. The most frequent sonographic findings in fetal rubella syndrome are cardiac malformations (in particular septal defects), eye defects (cataracts, microphtalmia), microcephaly, hepatomegaly, splenomegaly, and growth restriction. Deafness and mental retardation are expected after birth. The confirmation of fetal infection can be made by isolation of specific IgM in fetal blood.[3] Early diagnosis by isolation of rubella viral RNA from chorionic villus and amniotic fluid samples applying polymerase chain reaction has been proposed.[4] Because fetal ability to produce IgM antibodies is not completely developed until mid-second trimester, a negative test even in the 22nd to 23rd weeks does not completely exclude fetal infection.[4,5]

Associated Anomalies. Occasionally, the following anomalies can be associated with the classic findings of fetal rubella syndrome: renal disorders, hypospadias, cryptorchidism, meningocele, glaucoma, patent ductus arteriosus, and peripheral pulmonic stenosis.

Differential Diagnosis. All the conditions that can be associated with congenital hepatomegaly or cataract should be excluded. These conditions are congenital infections (such as CMV, toxoplasmosis, varicella, and syphilis), fetal anemia, fetal liver tumor, chondrodysplasia punctata, Neu-Laxova syndrome, Smith–Lemli–Optiz syndrome, and Walker–Walburg syndrome.[2]

Prognosis. Intrauterine death may occur. Postnatal impact of the intrauterine infection differs, from absence of any defect to all the anomalies mentioned above with variable severity. The agent may remain for years in the tissues, causing chronic infection and its complications (such as diabetes mellitus due to chronic viropathy of the pancreas).[1]

Management. Termination of pregnancy should be considered every time fetal infection is detected during the first trimester because of the severity of the condition in this group. After viability, monthly sonographic monitoring for growth and follow-up of the anomalies is recommended. PCR on amniotic fluid or fetal blood is indicated if a seroversion occurs before 18 weeks gestation. Therapeutic termination of pregnancy should be proposed if fetal infection is confirmed during the first and early second trimesters due to the severity of the condition in this group. After 18 weeks gestation, there is nearly no risk for the fetus: invasive procedures for antenatal diagnostic are not required and ultrasound surveillance is sufficient.[6]

REFERENCES

1. Jones KL. Fetal rubella effects. In: Jones KL, ed. *Smith's Recognizable Patterns of Human Malformation.* Philadelphia: WB Saunders; 1998:574–575.
2. Benacerraf BR. Rubella—Maternal infections. In: Benacerraf BR, ed. *Ultrasound of Fetal Syndromes.* New York: Churchill Livingstone. 1998:298–299.
3. Daffos F, Forestier F, Grangeot-Keros L, et al. Prenatal diagnosis of congenital rubella. *Lancet.* 1984;2:1–3.
4. Tanemura M, Suzumori K, Yagami Y, Katow S. Diagnosis of fetal rubella infection with reverse transcription and nested polymerase chain reaction: A study of 34 cases diagnosed in fetus. *Am J Obstet Gynecol.* 1995;174:579–582.
5. Enders G, Jonatha W. Prenatal diagnosis of intrauterine rubella. *Infection.* 1987;15:162–164.
6. Marret H, Golfier F, Di Maio M, Champion F, Attia-Sobol J, Raudrant D. Rubella in pregnancy. Management and prevention. *Presse Med.* 1999;28:2117–2122.

FETAL TOXOPLASMOSIS SYNDROME

Definition. *Toxoplasma gondii* is a ubiquitous parasite in mammals. Infection in the mother is usually asymptomatic, and a vast majority of patients are immune. However, 15 to 17% of primary maternal infections between the 7th and 14th weeks of gestation result in transmission to the fetus and may cause fetal anomalies.[1]

Synonyms. None.

Incidence. From 1 to 6 per 10,000 births (severe to subclinical infection). Half of the fetuses escape infection, one-third are have a subclinical infection, and only 10% have a severe infection.

Etiology. Infection.

Recurrence Risk. None.

Diagnosis. The findings include chorioretinitis, CNS abnormalities[2] (such as microcephaly, hydrocephalus,[3] encephalomyelitis, intracranial calcifications, seizures, and mental retardation), ascites,[4] and hepatosplenomegaly.[5,6] Although the diagnosis used to be made by serologic techniques and cultures,[7,8] it can now be done with polymerase chain reaction (PCR) detection of *Toxoplasma gondii* in fetal tissues.[9,10]

Pathogenesis. The fetus is infected hematogenously through the placenta during parasitemia in the mother.

Genetic Anomaly. None.

Associated Anomalies. See Diagnosis.

Differential Diagnosis. Other TORCH infections, although the absence of splenomegaly reduces the likelihood of CMV.

Prognosis. Approximately 75% of congenitally infected newborns are asymptomatic.

Management. The administration of specific antibiotherapy during pregnancy (spiramycine, sulfadiazine, pyrimethamine, and sulfonamides) significantly reduces the risk of fetal infection.[11]

REFERENCES

1. Pratlong F, Boulot P, Issert E, et al. Fetal diagnosis of toxoplasmosis in 190 women infected during pregnancy. *Prenat Diagn.* 1994;14:191–198.
2. Schwalbe J. Sonographic demonstration of intracranial changes in congenital toxoplasmosis. *Padiatr Grenzgeb.* 1988;27:239–244.
3. Cotty F, Carpentier MA, Descamps P, et al. Congenital toxoplasmosis with hydrocephalus diagnosed in utero: Outcome of treatment. *Arch Pediatr.* 1997;4:247–250.
4. Blaakaer J. Ultrasonic diagnosis of fetal ascites and toxoplasmosis. *Acta Obstet Gynecol Scand.* 1986;65:653–654.
5. Hrnjakovic-Cvjetkovic I, Jerant-Patic V, Cvjetkovic D, et al. Congenital toxoplasmosis. *Med Pregl.* 1998;51:140–145.
6. Abboud P, Harika G, Saniez D, et al. Ultrasonic signs of fetal toxoplasmosis. Review of the literature. *J Gynecol Obstet Biol Reprod (Paris).* 1995;24:733–738.
7. Pratlong F, Boulot P, Villena I, et al. Antenatal diagnosis of congenital toxoplasmosis: Evaluation of the biological parameters in a cohort of 286 patients. *Br J Obstet Gynaecol.* 1996;103:552–557.
8. Fricker-Hidalgo H, Pelloux H, Muet F, et al. Prenatal diagnosis of congenital toxoplasmosis: Comparative value of fetal blood and amniotic fluid using serological techniques and cultures. *Prenat Diagn.* 1997;17:831–835.
9. Pelloux H, Weiss J, Simon J, et al. A new set of primers for

the detection of *Toxoplasma gondii* in amniotic fluid using polymerase chain reaction. *FEMS Microbiol Lett.* 1996;138:11–15.

10. Toth T, Sziller I, Papp Z. PCR detection of *Toxoplasma gondii* in human fetal tissues. *Methods Mol Biol.* 1998;92:195–202.
11. Berrebi A, Kobuch WE, Bessieres MH, et al. Termination of pregnancy for maternal toxoplasmosis. *Lancet.* 1994;344(8914):36–39.

FETAL VALPROIC ACID EXPOSURE SYNDROME

Definition. The syndrome results from *in utero* exposure to valproic acid (an anticonvulsant), the major findings are spina bifida and cardiac anomalies.

Synonyms. Depakene™ exposure.

Incidence. Unknown but rare. Any epileptic pregnant mother has two to three times increased risk for congenital anomalies compared with the general population.[1] If exposure to valproic acid takes place between the 17th and 30th days after fertilization, the incidence of neural tube defects reaches 1 to 2%.[2]

Etiology. Exposure to valproic acid.[3]

Recurrence Risk. If the mother is exposed to valproic acid in a second pregnancy, the teratogenic effect will be the same.

Diagnosis. The findings include oral clefts, heart diseases, spina bifida, hypospadias and limb reductions[4,5]; IUGR, micrognathia, microcephaly, urogenital defects may be also present. Epilepsy and mental retardation may occur after birth.[6]

Pathogenesis. Unknown.

Genetic Anomaly. None.

Associated Anomalies. Anomalies from different systems have been reported in association with this syndrome, such as omphalocele, inguinal hernia, duodenal atresia, and scoliosis. Hyperbilirubinemia, hepatotoxicity, transient hyperglycinemia, afibrinogenemia, and fetal or neonatal distress may be found.[6]

Differential Diagnosis. Other neural tube defects. However, the clinical history in the presence of an association of spina bifida and cardiac anomaly should suggest the diagnosis.

Prognosis. Fetuses that presents major anomalies have a poor prognosis. Metabolic disturbances may also complicate the neonatal period.

Management. When detected in the second trimester, termination of the pregnancy can be offered. If the pregnancy is allowed to continue, no alteration of management is needed. Many new antiepileptic drugs have been introduced over the past few years, and switching the mother to one of those is recommended.

REFERENCES

1. Hanson JW, Buehler BA. Fetal hydantoin syndrome: Current status. *J Pediatr.* 1982;101:816–818.
2. Lemire RJ. Neural tube defects. *JAMA.* 1988;259:558–562.
3. Johannessen SI. Pharmacokinetics of valproate in pregnancy: Mother–foetus–newborn. *Pharm Weekbl Sci.* 1992;14:114–117.
4. Bradai R, Robert E. Prenatal ultrasonographic diagnosis in the epileptic mother on valproic acid. Retrospective study of 161 cases in the central eastern France register of congenital malformations. *J Gynecol Obstet Biol Reprod (Paris).* 1998;27:413–419.
5. Langer B, Haddad J, Gasser B, et al. Isolated fetal bilateral radial ray reduction associated with valproic acid usage. *Fetal Diagn Ther.* 1994;9:155–158.
6. Briggs GG, Freeman RK, Yaffe SJ. *Valproic Acid in Drugs in Pregnancy and Lactation.* Philadelphia: Williams & Wilkins; 1998:1092–1099.

FETAL VARICELLA ZOSTER

Definition. Fetal varicella zoster is a combination of abnormalities of multiple organs, caused by fetal contamination with maternal chickenpox infection.

Synonyms. Congenital varicella syndrome, varicella embryopathy, chicken pox, and herpes zoster.[1]

Incidence. The incidence of maternal infection with herpes virus *Varicella* is 7 per 10,000 pregnancies.[2] The risk of fetal involvement among all pregnant women infected with varicella during their gestation differs from 1 to 20%.[3,4]

Etiology. Herpes virus.

Recurrence Risk. Less than 1%.[1]

Diagnosis. Maternal infection, at anytime during pregnancy, exposes the fetus to a high risk of transplacental contamination and is indicative of fetal follow-up. The risk of fetal anomalies, however, is higher during the first and second trimesters. Sonographic signs of fetal disease include fetal demise, growth restriction, musculoskeletal abnormalities such as clubbed feet and abnormal position of the hands (caused by both necrosis and denervation of the affected tissue), limitation of limb extension due to cicatrices formation, cutaneous scars, limb hypoplasia, chorioretinitis, congenital

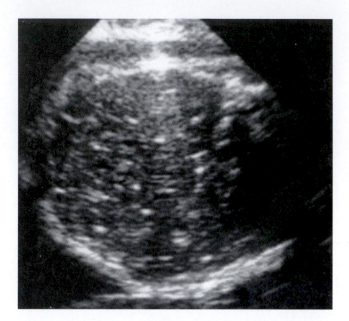

Figure 21–34. Transverse image of the fetal abdomen at 20 weeks of gestation showing multiple hyperechoic echoes in the liver. *(Reproduced with permission from Hayward I, Pretorius DH. The Fetus. 1992;2:5–6.)*

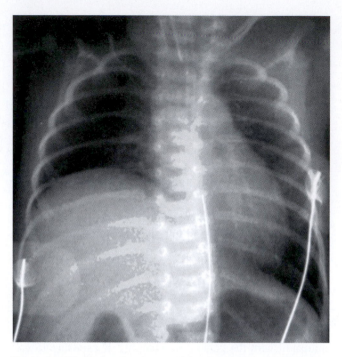

Figure 21–35. Transverse image of the abdomen immediately after birth showing scattered bright echoes throughout the liver. *(Reproduced with permission from Hayward I, Pretorius DH. The Fetus. 1992;2:5–6.)*

cataracts, microphthalmia, hydrops, polyhydramnios, hyperechogenic hepatic foci (Figs. 21–34 to 21–36), cerebral anomalies, such as ventriculomegaly or atrophy, and microcephaly (Figs. 21–37 and 21–38).[1,3] Isolation of the virus or specific IgM antibody in amniotic fluid or fetal blood is recommended for documentation of fetal infection.[3]

Pathogenesis. Direct damage to fetal tissues by neurotropic virus.

Associated Anomalies. Congenital anomalies from multiple organs with variable severity can be associated with varicella embryopathy (see above). Among survivors, development of mental retardation, seizures, and limitation of movements may occur after birth.[2]

Differential Diagnosis. Other viral infections, vascular accidents, and amniotic band syndrome.[1,2]

Prognosis. The severity of fetal involvement differs, from dermatologic lesions to lethal disseminated disease. Limited scarring tends to have an excellent prognosis. Fetal brain disruptions or severe maternal varicella with development of lethal maternal pneumonia or encephalitis have an extreme high risk for fetal demise. Mortality rates differ from 39 to 61%.[5] Early maternal infection (first and early second trimesters) has a higher association with fetal anomalies, and third-trimester infections have a higher risk for varicella zoster development at the neonatal period.[1]

Management. Termination of pregnancy can be offered before viability. If continuing the pregnancy is decided, periodic sonographic evaluation is recommended to search for fetal anomalies, limb contractures, and other signs of fetal compromise. Acyclovir is active against the varicella-zoster

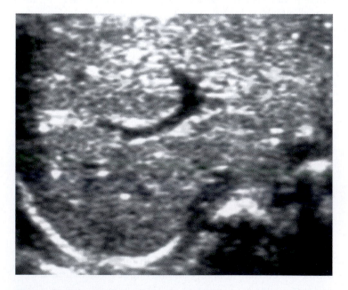

Figure 21–36. Chest radiograph of newborn showing elevation of the right hemidiaphragm and hypoplasia of the right clavicle. *(Reproduced with permission from Hayward I, Pretorius DH. The Fetus. 1992;2:5–6.)*

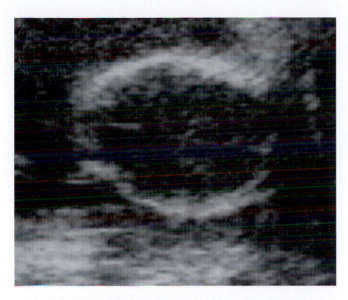

Figure 21–37. The brain of a fetus at 18 weeks of gestation and 2 weeks after maternal varicella. Note the normal appearance of the falx cerebri, choroid plexus, and cerebral hemispheres. *(Reproduced with permission from Lebel RR, Fernandez BB, Gibson L. The Fetus. 1992;2:1–4.)*

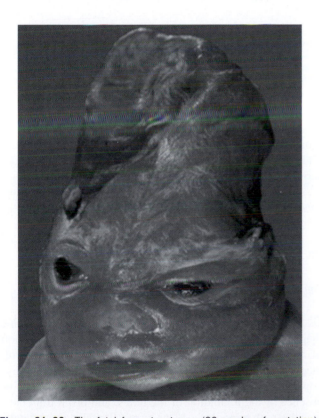

Figure 21–38. The fetal face at autopsy (26 weeks of gestation). Note the collapsed cranium, intact skin (very little maceration), disproportionate necrosis of the ocular globes, and flattened midface. *(Reproduced with permission from Lebel RR, Fernandez BB, Gibson L. The Fetus. 1992;2:1–4.)*

virus, and treatment is indicated in seriously ill adults and neonates.[6]

REFERENCES

1. Lebel RR, Fernandez BB, Gibson L. Varicella zoster; brain disruption. *Fetus*. 1992;2:1–4.
2. Benacerraf BR. Varicella (Maternal infections). In: Benacerraf BR, ed. *Ultrasound of Fetal Syndromes*. New York: Churchill Livingstone; 1998:302–304.
3. Hayward I, Pretorius DH. Varicella zoster. *Fetus*. 1992;2:5–6.
4. Trlifajova J, Benda R, Benes C. Effect of maternal infection on the outcome of pregnancy and the analysis of transplacental virus transmission. *Acta Virol*. 1986;30:249–255.
5. Hanshaw JB. Varicella-zoster infections. In: Hanshaw JB, ed. *Viral Diseases of the Fetus and Newborn*. Philadelphia: WB Saunders; 1985:161–174.
6. Chapman SJ. Varicella in pregnancy. *Semin Perinatol*. 1998;22:339–346.

FRASER'S SYNDROME

Definition. This syndrome combines acrofacial and urogenital malformations with or without cryptophthalmos. The four major characteristics are cryptophthalmos, syndactyly, genital anomalies, and affected siblings and eight minor characteristics (alterations of the nose, ears, larynx, oral clefts, umbilical hernia, renal agenesis either bilateral or unilateral, skeletal anomalies, and mental retardation) are part of the diagnosis of Fraser's syndrome.[1]

Synonyms. Cryptophthalmos syndactyly.

Incidence. Every 0.043 per 10,000 liveborn infants and 1.1 per 10,000 stillbirths.[1]

Etiology. Probably autosomal recessive because an unusual proportion of infants is born to consanguineous parents.[2]

Recurrence Risk. Twenty-five percent.

Diagnosis. The diagnosis has been suggested prenatally by the combination of obstructive uropathy, microphtalmia, syndactyly, pulmonary obstruction from laryngeal atresia (Fig. 21–39),[3] ascites,[4] fetal hydrops with nuchal edema,[5] and oligohydramnios.[6–8]

Pathogenesis. A defect of apoptosis has been suggested because several of the anomalies result from failure of programmed cell death (fusion of the eyelids, digits, larynx, and the vagina).[9]

Genetic Anomaly. Unknown.

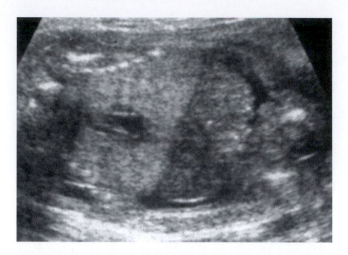

Figure 21–39. Laryngeal atresia (not in a fetus with Fraser's syndrome). Note the bulky echogenic lungs that invert the diaphragm and compress the heart. *(Reproduced with permission from Valcamonico A, Jeanty A. The Fetus. 1992;2:7483–7485.)*

Associated Anomalies. Cryptophthalmos; absent or malformed lacrimal ducts; middle and outer ear malformations; high palate; cleavage along the midplane of nares and tongue; hypertelorism; laryngeal stenosis; syndactyly; wide separation of symphysis pubis; displacement of umbilicus and nipples; primitive mesentery of small bowel; maldeveloped kidneys; fusion of labia and enlargement of clitoris; and bicornuate uterus and malformed fallopian tubes.[10]

Differential Diagnosis. Of the echogenic lungs; includes congenital diaphragmatic hernia, cystic adenomatoid malformation (type III), sequestrated lung, and tracheal or bronchial atresia. The differential diagnosis of the cryptophthalmos includes alobar holoprosencephaly, which should be easy to recognize from the simple hydrocephalus of the Fraser fetuses.

Prognosis. Fatal if laryngeal atresia or renal agenesis is present. If cryptophthalmos is the main sign, even surgical repair will yield very poor vision (20/200 and 20/360) in the rare correctable cases.[11]

Management. Depends on the predominant associated anomalies. Termination of the pregnancy can be recommended when renal agenesis or laryngeal atresia is present.

REFERENCES

1. Martinez-Frias ML, Bermejo Sanchez E, Felix V, et al. Fraser syndrome: Frequency in our environment and clinical–epidemiological aspects of a consecutive series of cases. *An Esp Pediatr.* 1998;48:634–638.

2. Ozgunen T, Evruke C, Kadayifci O, et al. Fraser syndrome. *Int J Gynaecol Obstet.* 1995;49:187–189.

3. Stevens CA, McClanahan C, Steck A, et al. Pulmonary hyperplasia in the Fraser cryptophthalmos syndrome. *Am J Med Genet.* 1994;52:427–431.

4. Lesniewicz R, Midro AT. Ultrasound diagnosis of four fetuses with Fraser syndrome during pregnancy. *Ginekol Pol.* 1998;69:152–157.

5. Fryns JP, van Schoubroeck D, Vandenberghe K, et al. Diagnostic echographic findings in cryptophthalmos syndrome (Fraser syndrome). *Prenat Diagn.* 1997;17:582–584.

6. Boyd PA, Keeling JW, Lindenbaum RH. Fraser syndrome (cryptophthalmos-syndactyly syndrome): A review of eleven cases with postmortem findings. *Am J Med Genet.* 1988;31:159–168.

7. Serville F, Carles D, Broussin B. Fraser syndrome: Prenatal ultrasonic detection. *Am J Med Genet.* 1989;32:561–563.

8. Schauer GM, Dunn LK, Godmilow L, et al. Prenatal diagnosis of Fraser syndrome at 18.5 weeks gestation, with autopsy findings at 19 weeks. *Am J Med Genet.* 1990;37:583–591.

9. Thomas IT, Frias JL, Felix V, et al. Isolated and syndromic cryptophthalmos. *Am J Med Genet.* 1986;25:85–98.

10. Fraser GR. Our genetical 'load': A review of some aspects of genetical variation. *Ann Hum Genet.* 1962;25:387–415.

11. Dibben K, Rabinowitz YS, Shorr N, Graham JM Jr. Surgical correction of incomplete cryptophthalmos in Fraser syndrome. *Am J Ophthalmol.* 1997;124:107–109.

FRYNS' SYNDROME

Definition. Fryns' syndrome is a rare congenital disorder characterized by dysmorphic facial features (coarse face with microphthalmia, hypertelorism, facial hair growth, cloudy corneas, broad and flat nasal bridge, cleft lip or palate, microretrognathia, and low-set ears), diaphragmatic hernia, distal limb hypoplasia, and pulmonary hypoplasia. The first description was published by Fryns et al. in 1979.[1]

Incidence. Unknown. Ayme et al. reported a prevalence of 0.7 per 10,000 births in France.[2]

Etiology. Autosomal recessive inheritance.[3]

Recurrence Risk. The recurrence risk is 25%.

Diagnosis. The phenotypic variability makes the sonographic diagnosis of Fryns' syndrome a challenge. The detection of typical facial dysmorphism (see above) associated with diaphragmatic hernia (a leading sonographic criteria), hypoplastic thorax with widely spaced nipples, hypoplasia or absence of the lobulation of the lungs, and distal limb deficiencies with hypoplasia of the terminal phalanges and nails should suggest Fryns syndrome. Development of polyhydramios late in the second trimester and normal or overgrowth of the fetus are also expected. The use of three-dimensional ultrasound may be helpful to precisely define the facial anomalies.[4] Although the frequency of cystic hygroma is not as high as the features mentioned above, this defect has been proposed as a sonographic first-trimester marker for recurrent cases.[5] Maternal and amniotic fluid α-fetoprotein levels may be elevated, in particular in fetuses that carry open defects.[6]

Genetic Anomaly. Until now, no specific DNA defect has been identified.[6]

Differential Diagnosis. The differential diagnosis includes trisomy 18 (which can be excluded by karyotype), Killian/Teschler–Nicole syndrome (mosaic tetrasomy 12p), Zellweger's syndrome (deficiency of peroxisomal enzyme), and Brachman–DeLange syndrome (usually associated with severe growth restriction).[4,6]

Associated Anomalies. Anomalies from skeletal, cardiac, central nervous, gastrointestinal, and genitourinary systems may be associated with Fryns' syndrome.[6]

Prognosis. Most affected infants are stillborn or die in the early neonatal period. The few reported surviving infants have severe mental and developmental retardation.[7]

Management. When detected before viability, termination of pregnancy can be offered. After viability, standard prenatal care is not altered.

REFERENCES

1. Fryns JP, Moerman F, Goddeeris P, et al. A new lethal syndrome with cloudy cornea, diaphragmatic defects, and distal limb deformities. *Hum Genet.* 1979;50:65–70.
2. Ayme S, Julian C, Gambarelli D, et al. Fryns syndrome, report on 8 new cases. *Clin Genet.* 1994;35:191–201.
3. Meinecke P, Fryns JP. The Fryns syndrome: Diaphragmatic defects, cranialfacial dysmorphism, and distal digital hypoplasia. Further evidence for autosomal recessive inheritance. *Clin Genet.* 1985;28:516–520.
4. Van Wymersch D, Favre R, Gasser B. Use of three-dimensional ultrasound to establish the prenatal diagnosis of Fryns syndrome. *Fetal Diagn Ther.* 1996;11:355–340.
5. Hösli IM, Tercanli S, Rehder H, Holzgreve W. Cystic hygroma as an early first trimester ultrasound marker for recurrent Fryns syndrome. *Ultrasound Obstet Gynecol.* 1997;10:422–424.
6. Sheffield JS, Twickler DM, Timmons C, et al. Fryns syndrome: Prenatal diagnosis and pathologic correlation. *J Ultrasound Med.* 1998;17:585–589.
7. Jones KL. Fryns syndrome. In: Jones KL, ed. *Smith's Recognizable Patterns of Human Malformation.* Philadelphia: WB Saunders; 1998:210–211.

GOLDENHAR'S SYNDROME

Definition. This syndrome is associated with hemifacial microsomia, epibulbar dermoids, preauricular appendages, transverse facial clefts, asymmetry of skull, and vertebral anomalies (vertebral segmentation errors).

Synonyms. Oculo-auricolo-vertebral dysplasia, Goldenhar–Gorlin syndrome, facio-auriculo-vertebral dysplasia.

Incidence. Every 0.2 per 10,000 births.[1]

Etiology. Probably sporadic, with rare cases suggesting an autosomal recessive (AR) or dominant (AD) inheritance.

Recurrence Risk. Probably none unless in an AD or AR kindred.

Diagnosis. The diagnosis is usually made by observing the facial asymmetry (Figs. 21–40A and B) (likely to become more common with three-dimensional ultrasound) or a maxillar cleft (Fig. 21–41) in association with unilateral microphthalmia (Figs. 21–42A and B).[2,3] Other findings include cardiac or urinary anomalies (see below) or lipoma of the corpus callosum.

Pathogenesis. Possible fetal hemorrhage in the region of the first and second branchial arches at the time when the blood supply of these arches switches from the stapedial artery to the external carotid artery.[4]

Genetic Anomaly. Unknown.

Associated Anomalies. Tracheoesophageal fistula,[5] epibulbar dermoids, syringohydromelia, neurodevelopmental delay,[6] tetralogy of Fallot,[7] ventricular septal defect, asplenia syndrome, ventricular inversion associated with double outlet right ventricle, pulmonary atresia with ventricular septal defects, double outlet right ventricle, and infradiaphragmatic total anomalous pulmonary venous connection,[8] ectopic or fused kidneys, renal agenesis, vesicoureteral reflux, ureteropelvic junction obstruction, ureteral duplication, and multicystic kidney.[9]

Differential Diagnosis. Kaufman's syndrome (oculo-cerebrofacial syndrome), acrofacial dysostosis, and the Charge association.

Prognosis. Aside from the mental handicap, these patient may have many complications due to upper airways problems and vertebral complications.

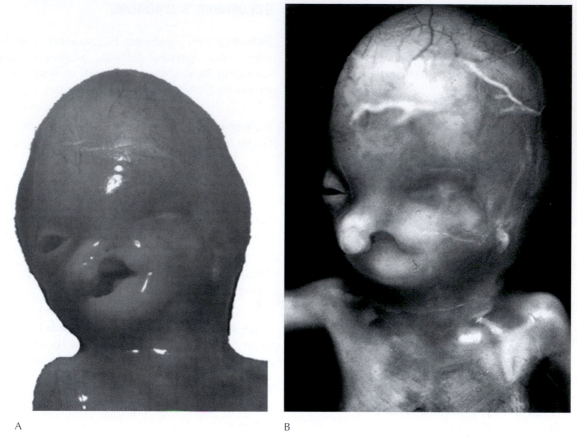

A   B

Figure 21–40. (A and **B)** Asymmetry of the face with hypoplasia of the left side and cleft. *(Courtesy of Dr. Luc de Catte, Belgium.)*

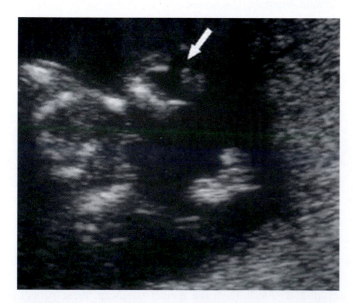

Figure 21–41. The maxillary cleft. *(Courtesy of Dr. Luc de Catte, Belgium.)*

Management. When the diagnosis is recognized in the early stages of gestation, termination of pregnancy may be offered. In the perinatal period, the management will attempt cosmetic improvements.

REFERENCES

1. Morrison PJ, Mulholland HC, Craig BG, Nevin NC. Cardio-vascular abnormalities in the oculo-auriculo-vertebral spectrum (Goldenhar syndrome). *Am J Med Genet.* 1992;44:425–428.
2. De Catte L, Laubach M, Legein J, Goossens A. Early prenatal diagnosis of oculoauriculovertebral dysplasia or the Goldenhar syndrome. *Ultrasound Obstet Gynecol.* 1996;8:422–424.
3. Stoll C, Viville B, Treisser A, Gasser B. A family with dominant oculoauriculovertebral spectrum. *Am J Med Genet.* 1998; 78:345–349.
4. Ryan CA, Finer NN, Ives E. Discordance of signs in monozygotic twins concordant for the Goldenhar anomaly. *Am J Med Genet.* 1988;29:755–761.
5. Sutphen R, Galan-Gomez E, Cortada X, et al. Tracheoesophageal

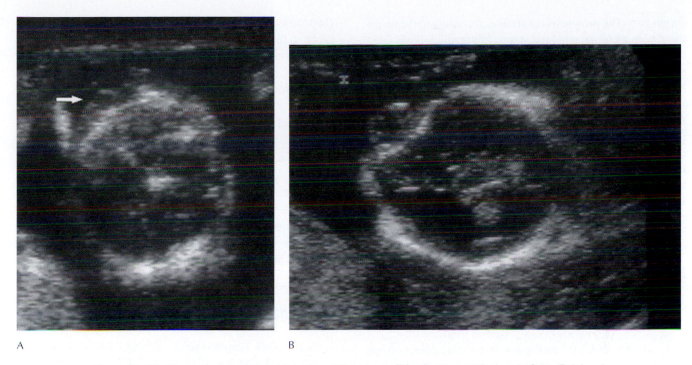

Figure 21–42. The normal eye **(A)** and the microphthalmic eye **(B)**. *(Courtesy of Dr. Luc de Catte, Belgium.)*

anomalies in oculoauriculovertebral (Goldenhar) spectrum. *Clin Genet.* 1995;48:66–71.

6. Cohen MS, Samango-Sprouse CA, Stern HJ, et al. Neurodevelopmental profile of infants and toddlers with oculo-auriculovertebral spectrum and the correlation of prognosis with physical findings. *Am J Med Genet.* 1995;60:535–540.

7. Sharma SN, Shrivastava S, Rao IM. Goldenhar syndrome with tetralogy of Fallot. *Indian Heart J.* 1993;45:223.

8. Kumar A, Friedman JM, Taylor GP, Patterson MW. Pattern of cardiac malformation in oculoauriculovertebral spectrum. *Am J Med Genet.* 1993;46:423–426.

9. Ritchey ML, Norbeck J, Huang C, et al. Urologic manifestations of Goldenhar syndrome. *Urology.* 1994;43:88–91.

HELLP SYNDROME

Definition. HELLP syndrome is an acronym for a severe variant of preeclampsia, characterized by **h**emolysis, **e**levated **l**iver **e**nzymes, and **l**ow **p**latelets.[1] This condition is life threatening for both mother and fetus. Sonographic signs of fetal compromise include IUGR, decreased tonus, decreased movement, and abnormal Doppler of the umbilical and cerebral arteries.

Incidence. HELLP syndrome affects 2 to 12% of the patients who develop preeclampsia,[2] and European-American women seem to be more affected than African-American women.[3]

Etiology. HELLP syndrome is a situation specific to pregnancies complicated by severe preeclampsia.

Recurrence Risk. Although the risk of recurrence is not precisely known, every patient affected by HELLP syndrome should be followed in a subsequent pregnancy as a patient at increased risk.[4]

Diagnosis. The maternal diagnosis is made by laboratory studies (hemolysis, elevated liver enzymes, and thrombocytopenia: platelets below 100,000 is the most consistent finding) and clinical signs and symptoms (edema, hypertension, nausea, and abdominal pain due to hepatic hemorrhage or rupture). The fetal findings include IUGR and reduced amniotic fluid volume, which are fetal responses to the chronic process of decreased placental blood supply, resulting from the maternal hypertension. In a more severe situation, with diminished fetal oxygen reserve, signs of distress may be found, such as decreased tonus, movement, respiratory movement, and abnormal Doppler velocimetry. Fetal demise and neonatal death are not uncommon in severe cases.

Associated Anomalies. A very important and dangerous condition that may be associated with HELLP syndrome is disseminated intravascular coagulation (DIC).[5]

Differential Diagnosis. Disorders that can develop are liver dysfunction or anemia, such as thrombocytopenic purpura, thrombotic thrombocytopenic purpura, hemolytic uremic syndrome, gallbladder disease, viral hepatitis, and acute fatty liver of pregnancy.

Prognosis. The prognosis is variable, according to the severity of both maternal and fetal status. Maternal morbidity and mortality are proportionate to the severity of systemic disease, whereas fetal morbidity and mortality are gestational age dependent in the majority of cases.[2]

Management. Patients with HELLP should be considered as having severe preeclampsia. Referral to a tertiary center and delivery of term pregnancies are recommended. Cases remote from term of pregnancy should be managed conservatively, with intensive monitoring of both maternal and fetal well-being. Delivery should be accomplished as soon as pulmonary maturity is reached.

REFERENCES

1. Weinstein L. Syndrome of hemolysis, elevated liver enzymes, and low platelet count: A severe consequence of hypertension in pregnancy. *Am J Obstet Gynecol.* 1982;142:159.
2. Sibai BM, Taslimi MM, El-Nazer A, et al. Maternal perinatal outcome associated with the syndrome of hemolysis, elevated liver enzymes, and low platelets in severe preeclampsia–eclampsia. *Am J Obstet Gynecol.* 1986;155:501.
3. Goodlin RC. Beware the great imitator—Severe preeclampsia. *Contemp Obstet Gynecol.* 1984;20:215.
4. Fairlie FM, Sibai BM. Hypertensive diseases in pregnancy. In: Reece EA, Hobbins JC, Mahoney MJ, Petrie RH, eds. *Medicine of the Fetus and Mother, vol. 58.* Philadelphia: JB Lippincott; 1992;58:925–942.
5. Van Dam PA, Renier M, Baekelandt M, et al. Disseminated intravascular coagulation and the syndrome of hemolysis, elevated liver enzymes, and low platelets in severe preeclampsia. *Obstet Gynecol.* 1989;73:97.

HERPES SIMPLEX INFECTION

Definition. Prenatal infection occurs with Herpes simplex virus type II,[1] rarely with type I.

Synonyms. None.

Incidence. Unknown.

Etiology and Pathogenesis. Transplacental or transcervical passage of the virus. Neonatal infection is usually acquired from maternal genital herpes, which is asymptomatic or unrecognized in 60 to 80% of women. The *Herpes simplex* type I transforms the HB-1 human cell line by association with the human gene for adenylate kinase 1 (on chromosome 9).[2]

Recurrence Risk. Unknown; no sibs have been reported to have been infected.

Diagnosis. Growth retardation, microcephaly, hydranencephaly, cerebellar necrosis, chorioretinitis, cataract, and microphthalmia. Hepatosplenomegaly may also be present.[3]

Genetic Anomaly. None.

Associated Anomalies. Inguinal hernias and aplasia cutis.

Differential Diagnosis. Other TORCH infections.

Prognosis. Most of these babies are born prematurely.

Management. Isolation of the virus in amniotic fluid culture does not necessarily indicate infection of the fetus. Treatment with acyclovir and vidarabine may be attempted.[4,5]

REFERENCES

1. Overall JC Jr. Herpes simplex virus infection of the fetus and newborn. *Pediatr Ann.* 1994;23:131–136.
2. Wilson DE, McKinlay MA, Staczek J, et al. Association of the herpes simplex-1 viral gene for thymidine kinase with the human gene for adenylate kinase-1 in biochemically transformed cells. *Biochem Genet.* 1980;18:981–1001.
3. Lanouette JM, Duquette DA, Jacques SM, et al. Prenatal diagnosis of fetal herpes simplex infection. *Fetal Diagn Ther.* 1996; 11:414–416.
4. Scott LL, Alexander J. Cost-effectiveness of acyclovir suppression to prevent recurrent genital herpes in term pregnancy. *Am J Perinatol.* 1998;15:57–62.
5. Scott LL, Sanchez PJ, Jackson GL, et al. Acyclovir suppression to prevent cesarean delivery after first-episode genital herpes. *Obstet Gynecol.* 1996;87:69–73.

HOLOPROSENCEPHALY

Definition. The association of midfacial anomalies and brain malformation results from partial development of the telencephalon. In the alobar form, the ventricle is continuous; in the lobar form, an attempt to form occipital horns and abnormal frontal horns are present. Because of a mechanism of reciprocal induction between the brain and the skull, the facial structures are also abnormal. The severity of the facial malformation reflects the severity of the intracranial anomalies.[1]

Synonyms. The following are parts of the holoprosencephaly complex: arhinencephaly, cebocephaly, ethmocephaly, and cyclopia.

Incidence. From 6 to 12 per 10,000 among liveborn infants but 40 per 10,000 among embryos; 50% are associated with trisomy 13.

Etiology. Autosomal dominant, recessive, and monogenic inheritance and infectious (CMV, toxoplasmosis), toxic (hydantoin), and maternal condition such as gestational diabetes[2] have all been reported.

Recurrence Risk. The proportion of sporadic cases is estimated to be 68%, with a 6% recurrence rate for sporadic, nonchromosomal forms. In the autosomal dominant form, the penetrance is estimated to be 82% for major types (alobar, semilobar, lobar) and 88% when major and minor types (atypical) are included. Thus, the recurrence risk after an isolated case is 13% for major types and 14% when minor types are included.[3]

Diagnosis. The diagnosis is suggested by numerous findings such as cyclopia (Figs. 21–43 and 21–44), cebocephaly, ethmocephaly, hypotelorism, proboscis, median cleft lip, single ventricular cavity, thalami fusion, absence of median structures, and microcephaly.[4]

Pathogenesis. Failure of sagittal cleavage of the telencephalon results in the presence of a midline single ventricle with variable degrees of separation (Fig. 21–45). This is probably due to mutations in the gene for the Sonic hedgehog morphogen and genes that encode its downstream intracellular signaling pathway.[5] There is also some evidence for a defect in cholesterol biosynthesis.[6,7]

Genetic Anomaly. Possibly located on the short arm of chromosome 3,[8] the long arm of chromosome 7,[9–11] or the long arm of chromosome 14.[12]

Associated Anomalies. Median cleft lip, proboscis, arhinencephaly, cebocephaly, ethmocephaly, and cyclopia.

Differential Diagnosis. The associated aneuploidies (trisomies 13 and 18) should be excluded by karyotype.

Prognosis. Depends on the form. The severe forms are usually associated with neonatal death. Some of the mildest forms

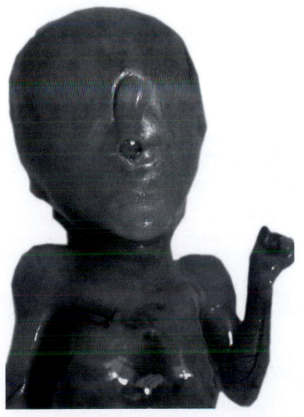
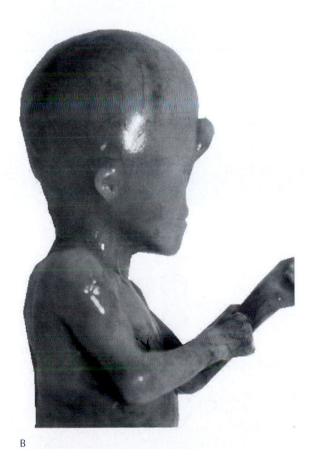

A   B

Figure 21–43. **(A** and **B)** The appearance of cyclopia at 16 weeks of gestation. Note the proboscis above the fused eye and the midfacial hypoplasia.

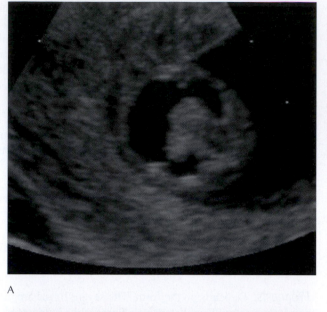

A

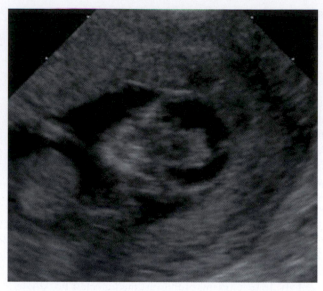

B

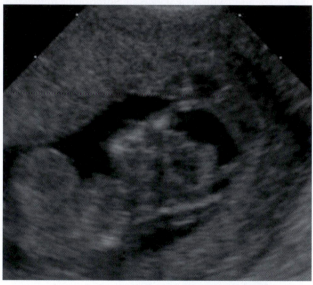

C

Figure 21–44. (A through **C)** Axial coronal and sagittal views of a lobar holoprosencephaly at 10 weeks of gestation. The lack of cleavage of the telencephalon has resulted in an undivided midline cavity that extends rostrally in a balloon shape (trisomy 18).

(single front incisor[13]) may demonstrate mild to moderate mental retardation and are at risk for pituitary dysfunction.

Management. Termination of pregnancy can be offered for the severe cases (semilobar, alobar).

Normal ventral induction

CLEAVAGE → INWARD ROTATION →

Holoprosencephaly

FAILURE OF CLEAVAGE → dorsal sac / single ventricle / FAILURE OF ROTATION →

Figure 21–45. Schematic drawing of normal and abnormal brain development leading to holoprosencephaly.

REFERENCES

1. Peebles DM. Holoprosencephaly. *Prenat Diagn.* 1998;18:477–480.
2. Martinez-Frias ML, Bermejo E, Rodriguez-Pinilla E, et al. Epidemiological analysis of outcomes of pregnancy in gestational diabetic mothers. *Am J Med Genet.* 1998;78:140–145.

3. Odent S, Le Marec B, Munnich A, et al. Segregation analysis in nonsyndromic holoprosencephaly. *Am J Med Genet.* 1998;77:139–143.

4. Parant O, Sarramon MF, Delisle MB, Fournie A. Prenatal diagnosis of holoprosencephaly. A series of twelve cases. *J Gynecol Obstet Biol Reprod (Paris).* 1997;26:687–696.

5. Ming JE, Roessler E, Muenke M. Human developmental disorders and the Sonic hedgehog pathway. *Mol Med Today.* 1998;4:343–349.

6. Roessler E, Muenke M. Holoprosencephaly: A paradigm for the complex genetics of brain development. *J Inherit Metab Dis.* 1998;21:481–497.

7. Lange Y, Steck TL. Four cholesterol-sensing proteins. *Curr Opin Struct Biol.* 1998;8:435–439.

8. Petek E, Kroisel PM, Wagner K. Isolation of a 370 kb YAC fragment spanning a translocation breakpoint at 3p14.1 associated with holoprosencephaly. *Clin Genet.* 1998;54:406–412.

9. Fryns JP. Another holoprosencephaly locus at 7q21.2? *J Med Genet.* 1998;35:614–615.

10. Frints SG, Schrander-Stumpel CT, Schoenmakers EF, et al. Strong variable clinical presentation in 3 patients with 7q terminal deletion. *Genet Couns.* 1998;9:5–14.

11. Vance GH, Nickerson C, Sarnat L, et al. Molecular cytogenetic analysis of patients with holoprosencephaly and structural rearrangements of 7q. *Am J Med Genet.* 1998;76:51–57.

12. Devriendt K, Fryns JP, Chen CP. Holoprosencephaly in deletions of proximal chromosome 14q. *J Med Genet.* 1998;35: 612.

13. Hall RK, Bankier A, Aldred MJ, et al. Solitary median maxillary central incisor, short stature, choanal atresia/midnasal stenosis (SMMCI) syndrome. *Oral Surg Oral Med Oral Pathol Oral Radiol Endo.* 1997;84:651–662.

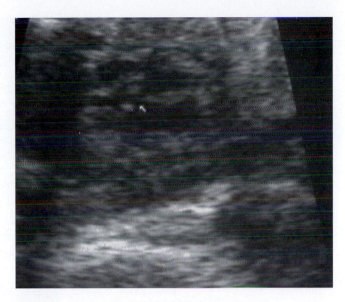

Figure 21–46. Ventricular septal defect, 1.3 mm long.

HOLT-ORAM SYNDROME

Definition. Holt-Oram syndrome consists of congenital heart disease and anomalies of the upper limb (phocomelia, 4.5%; radial ray aplasia; triphalangeal thumb; clinodactyly).[1]

Synonyms. Heart–hand syndrome (this syndrome appears genetically distinct from heart–hand syndrome types II and III).

Incidence. Uncommon.

Etiology. Autosomal dominant, with 100% penetrance and no evidence of reduced fitness. Increasing severity occurs in succeeding generations, consistent with anticipation.[1]

Recurrence Risk. Fifty percent.

Diagnosis. The cardiac lesions include atrial (30 to 60%) and ventricular septal defects (Fig. 21–46), patent ductus arteriosus, endocardial cushion defect, hypoplasia of the left ventricle, and conduction disturbances: 17% have complex cardiac anomalies.[2] The radial ray aplasia differs, from a difficult-to-diagnose triphalangeal thumb to more obvious club hand.[3] The absence of the thumb can also be recognized (Figs. 21–47 to 21–49).

Pathogenesis. Probable cardiomelic developmental field.[4]

Genetic Anomaly. Mutations in two of the T-box genes (TBX5 and TBX3) on chromosome 12q24.1[5] have been shown to be responsible for the congenital abnormalities associated with Holt–Oram syndrome.[6–8] TBX5 is only involved in anterior limb development.

Associated Anomalies. See Definition. A few inconstant anomalies such as renal anomalies also have been reported.

Differential Diagnosis. The differential diagnosis is usually radial ray aplasia and could include the TAR syndrome, Fanconi anemia, VACTERL association, and radial ray–choanal atresia.

Prognosis. Mainly related to the severity of the cardiac and orthopedic handicap.

Management. Usually no alteration of prenatal care is needed. Great orthopedic progress at pollicisation of the index finger to provide opposition have decreased the handicap of some of these children.[9]

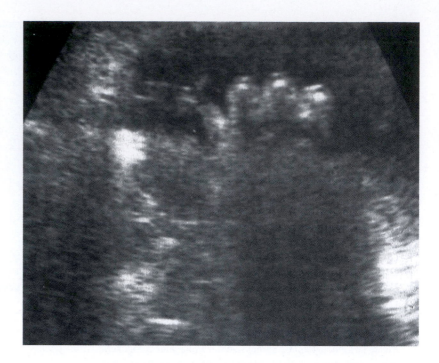

Figure 21–47. Coronal view of the four-digit hand.

REFERENCES

1. Newbury-Ecob RA, Leanage R, Raeburn JA, Young ID. Holt–Oram syndrome: A clinical genetic study. *J Med Genet.* 1996;33: 300–307.
2. Sletten LJ, Pierpont ME. Variation in severity of cardiac disease in Holt–Oram syndrome. *Am J Med Genet.* 1996;65: 128–132.
3. Brons JT, van Geijn HP, Wladimiroff JW, et al. Prenatal ultrasound diagnosis of the Holt–Oram syndrome. *Prenat Diagn.* 1988;8:175–181.
4. Wilson GN. Correlated heart/limb anomalies in mendelian syndromes provide evidence for a cardiomelic developmental field. *Am J Med Genet.* 1998;76:297–305.
5. Bonnet D, Terrett J, Pequignot-Viegas E, et al. Gene localization in 12q12 in Holt–Oram atrio-digital syndrome. *Arch Mal Coeur Vaiss.* 1995;88:661–666.
6. Campbell CE, Casey G, Goodrich K. Genomic structure of TBX2 indicates conservation with distantly related T-box genes. *Mamm Genome.* 1998;9:70–73.

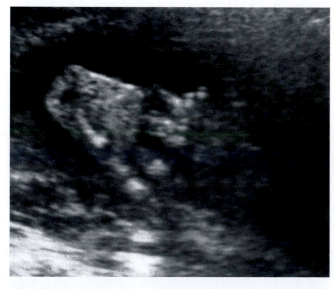

Figure 21–48. The four digits of the hand are seen. The radial side is clearly visible (lower left side of the image) and the thumb is clearly absent.

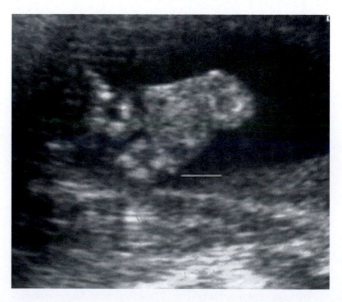

Figure 21–49. A small skin tag is seen in place of the thumb.

7. Smith J. Brachyury and the T-box genes. *Curr Opin Genet Dev.* 1997;7:474–480.
8. Li QY, Newbury-Ecob RA, Terrett JA, et al. Holt–Oram syndrome is caused by mutations in TBX5, a member of the Brachyury (T) gene family. *Nat Genet.* 1997;15:21–29.
9. Weber M, Wenz W, van Riel A, et al. The Holt–Oram syndrome. Review of the literature and current orthopedic treatment concepts. *Z Orthop Ihre Grenzgeb.* 1997;135:368–375.

HYDROLETHALUS SYNDROME

Definition. This syndrome associates polydactyly (postaxial in the hands and preaxial in the feet) and CNS malformations such as hydrocephalus.[1–4]

Synonyms. Salonen-Herva-Norio syndrome.

Incidence. Parents often have some ancestry in an eastern region of Finland, where the disorder can be as frequent as 0.5 per 10,000 births.[5] Outside of this subgroup, the incidence is very rare.

Etiology. Unknown.

Diagnosis. The findings of massive hydrocephalus, micrognathia, polydactyly (in particular a duplicated big toe), club feet, and hydramnios are very suggestive of the diagnosis. Other findings include cleft lip or palate, lung hypoplasia, and endocardial cushion defects.

Genetic Anomalies. Unknown.

Differential Diagnosis. Meckel's syndrome that also has polydactyly, CNS anomalies (cephalocele instead of hydrocephaly), and cystic kidneys.

Prognosis. Aside from an anecdotal survival of more than a few months,[6] neonatal death is the rule.

Management. Termination of pregnancy can be offered before viability. Standard prenatal care is not altered when continuation of the pregnancy is decided.

REFERENCES

1. Salonen R, Herva R, Norio R. The hydrolethalus syndrome: Delineation of a 'new' lethal malformation syndrome, based on 28 patients. *Clin Genet.* 1981;19:321–330.
2. Anyane-Yeboa K, Collins M, Kupsky W, et al. Hydrolethalus (Salonen–Herva–Norio) syndrome: Further clinicopathological delineation. *Am J Med Genet.* 1987;26:899–907.
3. Bachman H, Clark RD, Salahi W. Holoprosencephaly and polydactyly: A possible expression of the hydrolethalus syndrome. *J Med Genet.* 1990;27:50–52.
4. Pryde PG, Qureshi F, Hallak M, et al. Two consecutive hydrolethalus syndrome–affected pregnancies in a nonconsanguineous black couple: Discussion of problems in prenatal differential diagnosis of midline malformation syndromes. *Am J Med Genet.* 1993;46:537–541.
5. Salonen R, Herva R. Hydrolethalus syndrome. *J Med Genet.* 1990;27:756–759.
6. Aughton DJ, Cassidy SB. Hydrolethalus syndrome: Report of an apparent mild case, literature review, and differential diagnosis. *Am J Med Genet.* 1987;27:935–942.

HYPOPHOSPHATASIA

Definition. Anomaly is caused by defective bone mineralization and deficiency of serum and tissue liver/bone/kidney alkaline phosphatase, with three subtypes: *type 1* is lethal, with prenatal manifestations of short demineralized long bones, craniosynostosis, and neonatal hypercalcemia; *type 2* is demonstrated by ricketslike skeletal changes, fractures, and premature loss of teeth; and *type 3* demonstrates only metabolic anomalies detected on biochemical screening.

Synonyms. Phosphoethanolaminuria.

Incidence. Rare.

Etiology. Autosomal recessive. Carriers can be recognized by their low levels of serum alkaline phosphatase[1] and urinary phosphoethanolamine.

Recurrence Risk. Twenty-five percent.

Diagnosis. The diagnosis should be suspected in fetus with micromelia and demineralization of the bones. Spurs have been diagnosed postnatally that may be typical. These occur along the midshaft of long bones and at the knees and elbows.[2–4]

Pathogenesis. Anomaly of the tissue-nonspecific alkaline phosphatase (TNSALP) gene.

Genetic Anomaly. Types 1 and 2 are different disorders. There are numerous variant tissue-nonspecific alkaline phosphatase genes.[5]

Associated Anomalies. See Definition.

Differential Diagnosis. Hypophosphatasia is probably indistinguishable by ultrasound criteria only from OI type II and achondrogenesis type IA.

Prognosis. Lethal for the type 1.

Management. In a suspected fetus (25% recurrence risk) termination of the pregnancy can be offered.

REFERENCES

1. Rathbun JC, MacDonald JW, Robinson HMC, Wanklin JM. Hypophosphatasia: A genetic study. *Arch Dis Child.* 1961;36:540–542.
2. Goldstein DJ, Nichols WC, Mirkin LD. Short-limbed osteochondrodysplasia with osteochondral spurs of knee and elbow joints (spur-limbed dwarfism). *Dysmorph Clin Genet.* 1987;1:12–16.
3. Spranger J. 'Spur-limbed' dwarfism identified as hypophosphatasia (letter). *Dysmorph Clin Genet.* 1988;2:123.
4. Vandevijver N, De Die-Smulders CEM, Offermans JPM, et al. Lethal hypophosphatasia, spur type: Case report and fetopathological study. *Genet Counsel.* 1998;9:205–209.
5. Mornet E, Taillandier A, Peyramaure S, et al. Identification of fifteen novel mutations in the tissue-nonspecific alkaline phosphatase (TNSALP) gene in European patients with severe hypophosphatasia. *Eur J Hum Genet.* 1998;6:308–314.

HYPOPLASTIC LEFT HEART SYNDROME

Definition. Hypoplastic left heart syndrome (HLHS) is a congenital cardiac anomaly characterized by the association of a small left ventricle with aortic atresia or mitral hypoplasia or atresia.

Synonyms. Aortic atresia.[1]

Incidence. Hypoplastic left heart syndrome comprises 10 to 15% of prenatally detected congenital heart diseases[2] and affects 1.6 per 10,000 live births.[3]

Etiology. The etiology of HLHS is not precisely known. Autosomal recessive, autosomal dominant, and polygenic inheritances have been suggested.[3,4] Multifactorial is the more likely form of transmission.[3,5]

Recurrence Risk. The recurrence risk depends on the etiology and differs between 0.5 and 25%, with approximately 2% reported in most of the cases.[3] According to Norwood et al., the recurrence risk is 4% for those families with one affected child and 25% for those with two or more affected children.[6]

Diagnosis. The typical findings seen on four-chamber view include a small, thick-walled, and hyperechoic left ventricle (Figs. 21–50 and 21–51), with weak contractility. Aortic valve atresia, variable degree of hypoplasia of the ascending aorta (Figs. 21–52 and 21–53), and poor mitral valve motion are also expected.[2] The presence of an echogenic bundle where the atrial-ventricular (AV) valve should have been is a typical finding of mitral or tricuspid atresias. In HLHS, the

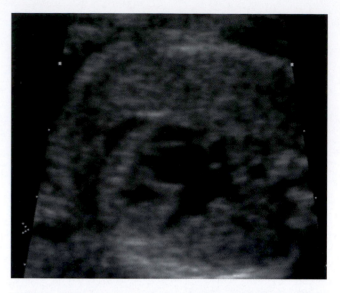

Figure 21–50. Four-chamber view. The left ventricle is posterior and to the right of the image. Note how much smaller it is than the right ventricle. There is also a small pericardial effusion in the atrioventricular groove on the right side of the heart.

aorta is small or not visible; in hypoplastic right heart syndrome, the pulmonary artery is hypoplastic or missing. The identification of a small amount of flow (usually only feasible with color Doppler) is important. If the flow is retrograde, the

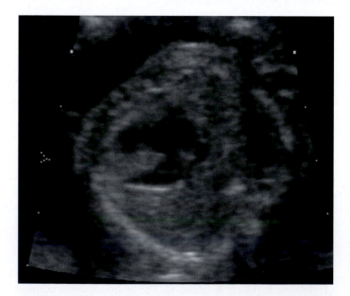

Figure 21–51. A ventricular septal defect connects the hypoplastic left ventricle with the right ventricle. This image could be confused with a similar image of endocardial cushion defect. However, in a complete form of endocardial cushion defect the AV valve would be seen to bridge the crux of the heart, whereas in hypoplastic left heart syndrome (HLHS) the atrioventricular is either normally implanted (if the HLHS results from aortic obstruction) or will appear as a thick echogenic band if the HLHS results from an inflow obstruction.

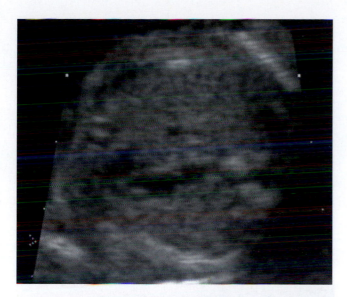

Figure 21–52. In the "three-vessel" view, the "line–dot–dot" configuration of the pulmonary artery, the ascending aorta, and the superior vena cava is incomplete. The hypoplastic ascending aorta is missing between the pulmonary artery and the superior vena cava.

septum is usually intact and the prognosis is poor. The presence of anterograde flow signals the presence of a ventricular septal defect.

Pathogenesis. Unknown.

Genetic Anomaly. A defect at 11q23.3 has been suggested.[7]

Associated Anomalies. In addition to the cardiac anomalies, extracardiac defects are frequently seen associated with HLHS, and the most common are the two-vessel cord, craniofacial, gastrointestinal, genitourinary, and CNS abnormalities.[3]

Differential Diagnosis. The single ventricles, hypoplastic right ventricles, and the severe forms of endocardial cushion defect all may appear similar on the four-chamber view. A careful observation of the position of the atria, AV valves, and great vessels often allows the correct diagnosis.

Prognosis. Hypoplastic left heart syndrome is responsible for 25% of cardiac deaths in the first week of life.[1] Almost all of the affected infants die within 6 weeks if they are not treated.[8] Several palliative procedures, including atrial septectomy,[9] banding of the pulmonary artery,[10] and creation of an aortopulmonary shunt,[11] have been used. Patients undergoing these procedures either died some time after the operation or have been followed for a very limited period. Thus far, Norwood reconstruction and cardiac transplantation are the most successful techniques, but the success rate is still very low.

Management. When the diagnosis is made before viability, the option of pregnancy termination should be offered. After viability, delivery in a tertiary center should be recommended, where a cardiovascular team is prepared to undertake surgical care of the infant.

REFERENCES

1. Hata T, Hata K, Makihara K, et al. Hypoplastic left heart syndrome: Color Doppler flow mapping. *Fetus.* 1991;467: 1–3.
2. Anderson NG, Brown J. Normal size left ventricle on antenatal scan in lethal hypoplastic left heart syndrome. *Pediatr Radiol.* 1991;21:436–437.
3. Grobman W, Pergament E. Isolated hypoplastic left heart syndrome in three siblings. *Obstet Gynecol.* 1996;88:673–675.
4. Shokeir MH. Hypoplastic left heart syndrome: An autosomal recessive disorder. *Clin Genet.* 1971;2:7–14.
5. Holmes LB, Rose V, Child AH, et al. Commentary on the inheritance of the hypoplastic left heart syndrome. *Birth Defects Original Article Series.* 1974;228–230.
6. Norwood WI, Lang P, Hansen DD. Physiologic repair of aortic atresia—Hypoplastic left heart syndrome. *N Engl J Med.* 1983;308:23.
7. Guenthard J, Bueler E, Jaeggi E, Wyler F. Possible genes for left heart formation on 11q23.3. *Ann Genet.* 1994;37:143–146.
8. Doty DB, Aortic atresia. *J Thorac Cardiovasc Surg.* 1980;79: 462–463.
9. Moodie DS, Gallen WJ, Friedberg DZ. Congenital aortic atresia. Report of long survival and some speculations about surgical approaches. *J Thorac Cardiovasc Surg.* 1972;63:726–731.

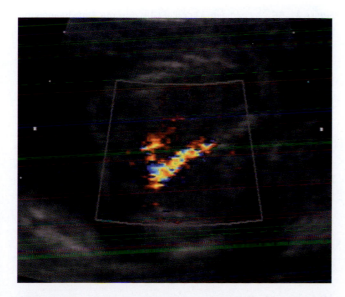

Figure 21–53. Color Doppler confirms the absence of the ascending aorta (in spite of a large ventricular septal defect in this case). This configuration may occur with progressive aortic obstruction (aortic stenosis), leading to aortic atresia at birth.

10. Doty DB, Knott HW. Hypoplastic left heart syndrome. Experience with an operation to establish functionally normal circulation. *J Thorac Cardiovasc Surg.* 1977;74:624–630.
11. Behrendt DM, Rochini A. An operation for the hypoplastic left heart syndrome: Preliminary report. *Ann Thorac Surg.* 1981;32:284–288.

KLIPPEL–FEIL SYNDROME

Definition. This syndrome is manifested by cervical vertebral fusion anomalies that cause a short neck with decreased mobility.[1,2] It is sometimes associated with congenital heart defects, renal anomalies (renal agenesis), genital anomalies, and ocular malformations. Type I comprises fusion of many cervical and upper thoracic vertebrae into bony blocks; type II comprises fusion at only one or two vertebrae (and may associate hemivertebrae and fusion of the occipitoatlantoic joint); and type III comprises both cervical fusion and lower thoracic or lumber fusion.[3,4]

Synonyms. None.

Incidence. Every 0.25 per 10,000 births, which may be an underestimate because some mild forms may be underreported.

Etiology and Pathology. Anomalies of segmentation of the somites in the 4th to 8th weeks.

Diagnosis. The short neck may be associated with opisthotonos (retroflexion of the head; Figs. 21–54 and 21–55) and the disorganization of the cervical vertebrae is potentially recognizable.

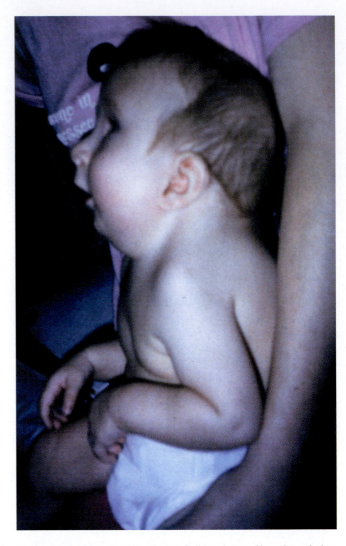

Figure 21–55. A child with Klippel–Feil syndrome. Note the opisthotonotic position, low-set ears, and micrognathia.

Genetic Anomalies. Dominant inheritance with reduced penetrance and variable expression of a defective gene on the long arm of chromosome 8 at locus 22.2.[5]

Differential Diagnosis. Iniencephaly presents with similar opisthotonos but appears more severe (cervical spina bifida). Dyssegmental dysplasia presents with similar vertebral findings but also demonstrates short limbs and cephaloceles.

Prognosis. The complications result from the vertebral fusion and include cord compression syndrome, cervical instability, and motility impairment.

Management. Termination of pregnancy can be offered before viability. Standard prenatal care is not altered when continuation of the pregnancy is decided. Confirmation of diagnosis after birth is important for genetic counseling.

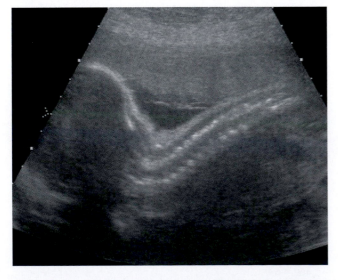

Figure 21–54. The opisthotonotic position should not be maintained for long periods of time. If the position continues to be held after stimulation, the diagnosis of Klippel–Feil syndrome should be suspected.

REFERENCES

1. Bauman GL. Absence of the cervical spine: Klippel–Feil syndrome. *JAMA*. 1932;98:129–132.
2. Bizarro AH. Brevicollis. *Lancet*. 1938;II:828–829.
3. Gunderson CH, Greenspan RH, Glaser GH, Lubs HA. The Klippel–Feil syndrome: Genetic and clinical reevaluation of cervical fusion. *Medicine*. 1967;46:491–512.
4. Raas-Rothschild A, Goodman RM, Grunbaum M, et al. Klippel–Feil anomaly with sacral agenesis: An additional subtype, type IV. *J Craniofac Genet Dev Biol*. 1988;8:297–301.
5. Clarke RA, Singh S, McKenzie H, et al. Familial Klippel–Feil syndrome and paracentric inversion inv(8)(q22.2q23.3). *Am J Hum Genet*. 1995;57:1364–1370.

KLIPPEL–TRENAUNAY–WEBER SYNDROME

Definition. This syndrome associates large cutaneous hemangiomata with hypertrophy of the related bones and soft tissues.[1,2]

Synonyms. Klippel–Trenaunay syndrome and angioosteohypertrophy syndrome.

Incidence. Rare.

Etiology. Happle suggested that a paradominant inheritance most satisfactorily explains the findings.[3] Heterozygous individuals for a single gene defect are phenotypically normal. The trait is only expressed when a somatic mutation occurs in the normal allele at an early stage of embryogenesis. The embryo is then a mosaic of homozygous or heterozygous cell

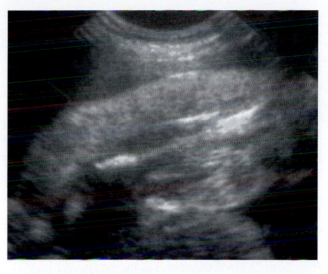

Figure 21–56. A large shell of soft tissue encompasses the thigh. The contralateral thigh is normal.

lines for the mutation. This explains the patchy distribution of the defect.[3]

Recurrence Risk. Probably none, although some cases have raised the possibility of autosomal dominance.[4,5]

Diagnosis. These may include hydrops fetalis (from high output cardiac failure) with limbs edema and hypertrophy (more girth then length; Fig. 21–56), ascites, abnormal abdominal hemangiomatous masses (Fig. 21–57A and B), and hepatomegaly.[6,7] A beautiful three-dimensional diagnosis was made recently.[8]

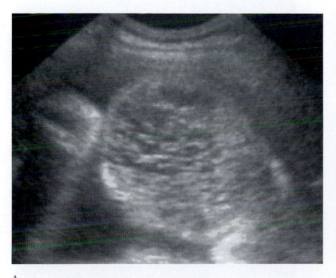

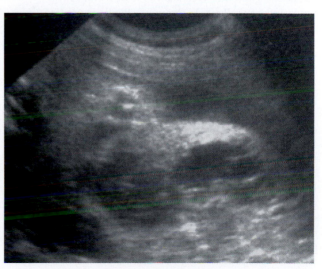

A   B

Figure 21–57. Two cross-sections at the level of the abdomen. Note the multicystic irregular **(A)** and poorly defined **(B)** masses.

Pathogenesis. Capillary malformations, atypical varicosities, and venous malformations, leading to localized masses.

Genetic Anomaly. This may be due to a single gene defect on chromosome 5q or p11.[9]

Associated Anomalies. Kasabach–Merritt syndrome of thrombocytopenia due to platelet consumption within the hemangioma and high output cardiac failure may complicate the outcome.

Differential Diagnosis. Lymphangioma and Proteus syndrome.

Prognosis. When detected prenatally, the disorder is usually more severe, and the prognosis is poor when associated with cardiac insufficiency.

Management. Termination of pregnancy can be offered in the severe forms; otherwise, no alteration of management is expected.

REFERENCES

1. Berry SA, Peterson C, Mize W, et al. Klippel–Trenaunay syndrome. *Am J Med Genet.* 1998;79:319–326.
2. Jacob AG, Driscoll DJ, Shaughnessy WJ, et al. Klippel–Trenaunay syndrome: Spectrum and management. *Mayo Clin Proc.* 1998;73:28–36.
3. Happle R. Mosaicism in human skin. Understanding the patterns and mechanisms. *Arch Dermatol.* 1993;129:1460–1470.
4. Lorda-Sanchez I, Prieto L, Rodriguez-Pinilla E, Martinez-Frias MI. Increased parental age and number of pregnancies in Klippel–Trenaunay–Weber syndrome. *Ann Hum Genet.* 1998; 62(Pt 3):235–239.
5. Ceballos-Quintal JM, Pinto-Escalante D, Castillo-Zapata I. A new case of Klippel–Trenaunay–Weber (KTW) syndrome: Evidence of autosomal dominant inheritance. *Am J Med Genet.* 1996;63:426–427.
6. Christenson L, Yankowitz J, Robinson R. Prenatal diagnosis of Klippel–Trenaunay–Weber syndrome as a cause for in utero heart failure and severe postnatal sequelae. *Prenatal Diag.* 1997;17: 1176–1180.
7. Paladini D, Lamberti A, Teodoro A, et al. Prenatal diagnosis and hemodynamic evaluation of Klippel–Trenaunay–Weber syndrome. *Ultrasound Obstet Gynecol.* 1998;12:215–217.
8. Shih JC, Shyu MK, Chang CY, et al. Application of the surface rendering technique of three-dimensional ultrasound in prenatal diagnosis and counseling of Klippel–Trenaunay–Weber syndrome. *Prenat Diagn.* 1998;18:298–302.
9. Whelan AJ, Watson MS, Porter FD, Steiner RD. Klippel–Trenaunay–Weber syndrome associated with a 5:11 balanced translocation. *Am J Med Genet.* 1995;59:492–494.

LARSEN'S SYNDROME

Definition. This syndrome associates short stature, multiple congenital joint dislocations, and abnormal facial features. There are two forms of the syndrome: lethal and nonlethal. The lethal form usually is fatal due to pulmonary hypoplasia.

Synonyms. None.

Incidence. Rare.

Etiology. Anomaly of the collagen due to a decreased α-1/α-2 chain ratio in type I collagen.

Diagnosis. The abnormal joint with dislocations (hip dislocation; genu recurvatum, Fig. 21–58; club hands from accessory carpal bones; club feet; etc.) can be associated with rhizomelic shortening of the upper extremities and hypoplastic fibula. A coronal cleft in the vertebral body can also be

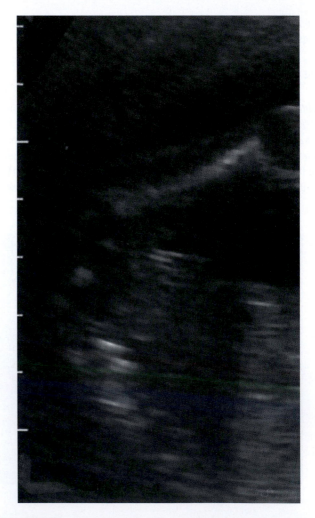

Figure 21–58. Genu recurvatum in a fetus with Larsen's syndrome. *(Courtesy of Dr. Peter Twinning, Nottingham, UK.)*

recognized. At the level of the face, a low nasal bridge, frontal bossing, and hypertelorism can be observed.[1,2]

Genetic Anomalies. Both autosomal dominant and recessive patterns of inheritance have been reported. The gene locus is at 3p21.1–p14.1.[3]

Differential Diagnosis. In the absence of familial history, these patients are usually identified as arthrogryposis.

Prognosis. When recognized, the management of the tracheomalacia, pulmonary insufficiency, and vertebral instability (cervical kyphosis from marked hypoplasia of one or two vertebral bodies—usually the fourth or fifth cervical vertebra) can improve the prognosis but probably only for the nonlethal form.

Management. Termination of pregnancy can be offered before viability. Standard prenatal care is not altered when continuation of the pregnancy is decided. Confirmation of diagnosis after birth is important for genetic counseling.

REFERENCES

1. Rochelson B, Petrikovsky B, Shmoys S. Prenatal diagnosis and obstetric management of Larsen syndrome. *Obstet Gynecol.* 1993;81(5, Pt 2):845–857.
2. Mostello D, Hoechstetter L, Bendon RW, Prenatal diagnosis of recurrent Larsen syndrome: Further definition of a lethal variant. *Prenat Diagn.* 1991;11:215–225.
3. Vujic M, Hallstensson K, Wahlstrom J, et al. Localization of a gene for autosomal dominant Larsen syndrome to chromosome region 3p21.1-14.1 in the proximity of, but distinct from, the COL7A1 locus. *Am J Hum Genet.* 1995;57:1104–1113.

LETHAL MULTIPLE PTERYGIUM SYNDROME

Definition. Massive and early hydrops with cystic hygroma and joint contractions.[1,2]

Synonyms. None.

Incidence. Unknown but not rare in the first trimester.

Etiology. Autosomal recessive, with a few cases suggesting an X-linked transmission.

Diagnosis. In the first trimester, the appearance of a thickened nuchal lucency extending around the whole body and, to a lesser, extending the limbs is characteristic.[3,4] These fetuses have hydrops and bob along in the fluid when shaken. Occasionally the diagnosis is not made until later in the preg-

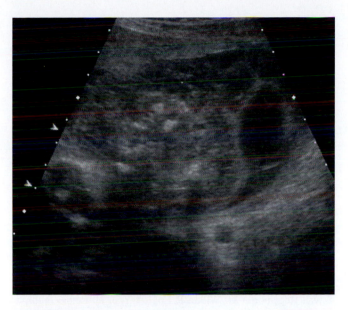

Figure 21–59. Section through the neck of a twin with lethal pterygium. Note the thickened soft tissues and the cystic hygroma.

nancy (Fig. 21–59) at a time when the joint contractions and the pterygia are more visible.[5]

Genetic Anomalies. Unknown.

Differential Diagnosis. Some of the severe aneuploidies may also present early with hydrops.[6] Arthrogryposes (fetal akinesia sequence) and Pena–Shokeir syndrome also present with joint contractions, but the most obvious ultrasound finding in lethal multiple pterygium syndrome is not the contractions but the hydrops. Limited pterygia of the popliteal regions can also been seen in fetuses with caudal regression syndrome. Noonan's syndrome also presents with cystic hygroma.[7]

Associated Anomalies. Some vertebral and other bony anomalies can be present.[8]

Prognosis. Lethal.

Management. Termination of pregnancy can be offered before viability. Standard prenatal care is not altered when continuation of the pregnancy is decided. Confirmation of diagnosis after birth is important for genetic counseling.

REFERENCES

1. Chen H, Immken L, Lachman R, et al. Syndrome of multiple pterygia, camptodactyly, facial anomalies, hypoplastic lungs and heart, cystic hygroma, and skeletal anomalies: Delineation of a new entity and review of lethal forms of multiple pterygium syndrome. *Am J Med Genet.* 1984;17:809–826.

2. Hall JG. The lethal multiple pterygium syndromes. *Am J Med Genet.* 1984;17:803–807.

3. de Die-Smulders CE, Vonsee HJ, Zandvoort JA, Fryns JP. The lethal multiple pterygium syndrome: Prenatal ultrasonographic and postmortem findings, a case report. *Eur J Obstet Gynecol Reprod Biol.* 1990;35:283–289.

4. Lockwood C, Irons M, Troiani J, et al. The prenatal sonographic diagnosis of lethal multiple pterygium syndrome: A heritable cause of recurrent abortion. *Am J Obstet Gynecol.* 1988;159:474–476.

5. Entezami M, Runkel S, Kunze J, et al. Prenatal diagnosis of a lethal multiple pterygium syndrome type II. Case report. *Fetal Diagn Ther.* 1998;13:35–38.

6. Azar GB, Snijders RJ, Gosden C, Nicolaides KH. Fetal nuchal cystic hygromata: Associated malformations and chromosomal defects. *Fetal Diagn Ther.* 1991;6:46–57.

7. Donnenfeld AE, Nazir MA, Sindoni F, Librizzi RJ. Prenatal sonographic documentation of cystic hygroma regression in Noonan syndrome. *Am J Med Genet.* 1991;39:461–465.

8. van Regemorter N, Wilkin P, Englert Y, et al. Lethal multiple pterygium syndrome. *Am J Med Genet.* 1984;17:827–834.

LISSENCEPHALY (TYPE I)

Definition. Lissencephaly is a cerebral developmental disorder, with agyria of the brain, accompanied or not by pachygyria, minimal or no hydrocephalus, a wide cortical mantle, and characteristic dysmorphic features.[1] Miller in 1963[2] and Dieker et al. in 1969[3] published the first descriptions.

Synonyms. Lissencephaly type I, Miller–Dieker syndrome (MDS), chromosome 17p13 syndrome, and chromosomal deletion 17p13.[1]

Prevalence. Unknown but rare, with a male-to-female ratio of 1 to 2.25.[1]

Etiology. Monosomy for the terminal segment of the short arm of chromosome 17, especially band 17p13. It may be discrete.[4]

Recurrence Risk. If it is *de novo* deletion or translocation, the recurrence risk is low. If the translocation is inherited from one parent (who has a balanced translocation), the recurrence risk may be as high as 25%. Affected children will not grow up to reproductive age.[1]

Diagnosis. Sonographic diagnosis in general is not accomplished earlier than late in the second trimester, when the characteristic cerebral anomalies can be noted (Figs. 21–60 through 21–62). The progressive microcephaly and failure of development of both sulci and gyri (which in normal conditions is well defined between 26 and 28 weeks[5]) are suggestive of lissencephaly. The occurrence of polyhydramnios associated with IUGR is an expected finding in the third

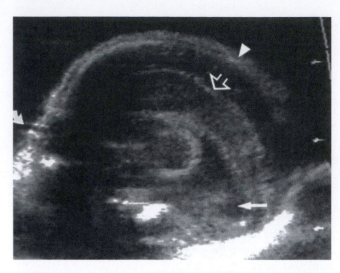

Figure 21–60. Parasagittal section of a head at 27 weeks of gestation. Section through the hemisphere shows a smooth surface *(open arrow)*. The cranium is a remarkable distance from the brain surface *(triangle)*. Posterior dilated portion of the lateral ventricle *(long arrow)*. *(Reproduced with permission from Harm-Gerd B, Eik-Nes S, Kiserud T, et al. The Fetus. 1991;2:7422.)*

trimester. Facial dysmorphism is characterized by prominent forehead, short nose, broad and flat nasal bridge, and protuberant upper lip.

Genetic Anomaly. Deletion at the 17p13.3 locus.

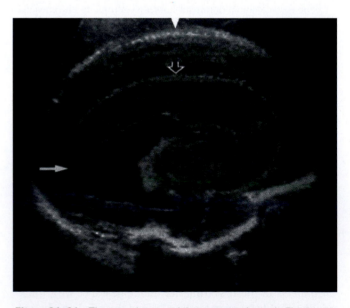

Figure 21–61. The same intracranial structures shown in Fig. 21–60 are visualized by transvaginal ultrasound. *(Reproduced with permission from Harm-Gerd B, Eik-Nes S, Kiserud T, et al. The Fetus. 1991;2:7422.)*

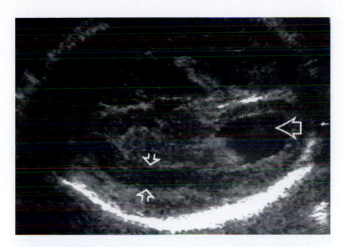

Figure 21–62. Transverse section through the lateral hemisphere at 31 weeks of gestation. The *small arrows* indicate the smooth narrow cortex. The *large arrows* point to the dilated posterior part of the lateral ventricle. *(Reproduced with permission from Harm-Gerd B, Eik-Nes S, Kiserud T, et al. The Fetus. 1991;2:7422.)*

Pathogenesis. Defective neuronal migration with four, rather than six, layers in the cortex.

Associated Anomalies. Duodenal atresia, urinary tract abnormalities, congenital heart defects, cryptorchidism, inguinal hernia, clinodactyly, polydactyly, and ear anomalies may be found.

Differential Diagnosis. Isolated lissencephaly sequence, Norman–Roberts syndrome, lissencephaly syndromes type II such as HARD+/−E (Walker–Walburg) syndrome and COM syndrome, and Neu-Laxova syndrome as a third lissencephaly type. All syndromes that may develop microcephaly should be suspected.

Prognosis. Usually, severe mental retardation affects these patients. Failure to thrive, infantile spasms, and seizures are also expected. The prognosis is poor, and death occurs usually within the first 2 years of life.[6]

Management. Karyotyping is recommended to detect the chromosomal defect. Differentiation from lissencephaly type II is important for genetic counseling purposes because type II has an autosomal recessive pattern of transmission. No causal treatment is available at this time. Usually, the ultrasound diagnosis is made during the third trimester, and termination is not an option. Standard prenatal care is not altered.

REFERENCES

1. Harm-Gerd B, Eik-Nes S, Kiserud T, et al. Lissencephaly, type I. *Fetus*. 1991;2:7422.

2. Miller JQ. Lissencephaly in two siblings. *Neurology*. 1963;13: 841.
3. Dieker H, Edwards RH, Zurhein G, et al. The lissencephaly syndrome. *Birth Defects*. 1969;5:53.
4. Dobyns WB, Stratton RF, Parke JT, et al. Miller–Dieker syndrome: Lissencephaly and monosomy 17p. *J Pediatr*. 1983;102: 552–558.
5. England MA. Normal development of the central nervous system. In: Levene MI, Bennett MJ, Punt J, eds. *Fetal and Neonatal Neurology and Neurosurgery*. Edinburgh: Churchill Livingstone; 1988:13–27.
6. Benacerraf BR. Miller–Dieker syndrome. In: Benacerraf BR, ed. *Ultrasound of Fetal Anomalies*. New York: Churchill Livingstone; 1998:130–132.

MECKEL'S SYNDROME

Definition. Meckel's syndrome is a rare and lethal syndrome characterized by occipital cephalocele, postaxial polydactyly, and dysplastic cystic kidneys. It can be associated with many other conditions, and fibrotic lesion of the liver is one of the most common associations.

Synonyms. Dysencephalia splanchnocystica and Meckel's syndrome (used in the English-language literature). *Meckel's syndrome* is the preferred appellation and is used by both Medline's Medical Subject Heading and the *Birth Defect Encyclopedia*[1]; other terms are Gruber syndrome (used in the European literature)[2] and Meckel–Gruber syndrome.

Incidence. Not precisely known, but investigators agree that this is a very rare condition. According to Bergsma, the incidence of Meckel's syndrome is 0.2 per 10,000 live births.[3] Salonen and Norio stated that the incidence of Meckel's syndrome at birth varies from 0.07 to 0.7 per 10,000 births. In Finland, the disorder is unusually frequent and reaches 1.1 per 10,000 births.[4] It is also estimated that this syndrome corresponds to 5% of all neural tube defects.[5]

Etiology. Autosomal recessive inheritance.

Recurrence Risk. A 25% recurrence risk is involved.

Genetic Anomaly. The locus for Meckel's syndrome is on chromosome 17, long arm, region 2, bands 1 through 4.[6] Phenotype variability and cases that did not have confirmed linkage to 17q suggest that there is some degree of locus heterogeneity.

Diagnosis. In 1981, Fraser and Lytwyn suggested that cystic dysplastic kidneys are a constant anomaly in Meckel's syndrome and therefore must be present in addition to at least two minor defects to make the diagnosis.[7] This concept is still discussed, and the reported incidence of renal disorder

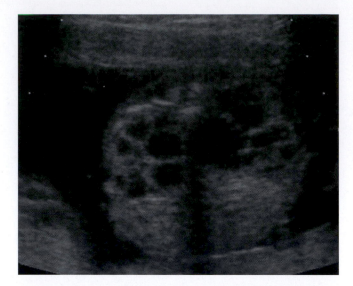

Figure 21–63. Large bilateral cystic kidneys that resemble multicystic kidneys. The amniotic fluid is normal, which is atypical.

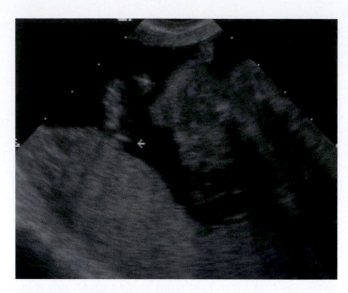

Figure 21–65. Postaxial polydactyly.

in this syndrome differs, from 95 to 100%. The kidneys initially have microscopic cysts that develop, destroying the parenchyma and enlarging the organ up to 10 or 20 times[5] (Fig. 21–63). The first sonographic finding in most cases is oligohydramnios due to renal dysfunction, and it develops early in the second trimester when the kidneys replace extracellular diffusion as the main source of amniotic fluid. However, some cases of Meckel's syndrome have normal amniotic fluid (see Fig. 21–63), and thus the presence of normal fluid does not exclude the diagnosis. Sometimes absence of the bladder can also be recognized. An early sonogram,

with normal aspect, in a family at risk for recurrence, does not exclude Meckel's syndrome, and a follow-up at 20 weeks of gestation is recommended.[5]

Occipital cephalocele is present in 60 to 80% of cases (Fig. 21–64A and B). Maternal serum or amniotic fluid α-fetoprotein levels may be normal because a membrane may cover the cephalocele. Postaxial polydactyly is present in 55 to 75% of cases (Fig. 21–65). Other limb anomalies such bowing and shortening may also be present. Finding at least two of the three features of the classic triad in the presence of a normal karyotype establishes the diagnosis (Fig. 21–66).

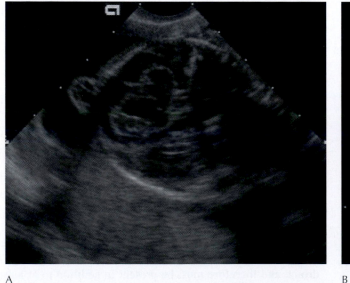

A
B

Figure 21–64. An 8-mm posterior cephalocele in axial **(A)** and sagittal **(B)** views.

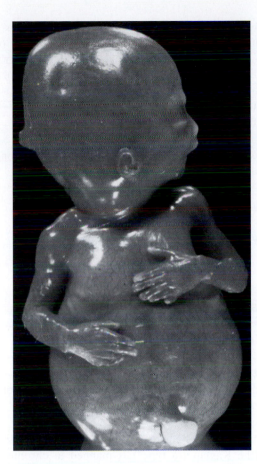

Figure 21–66. Autopsy specimen. Note the small posterior cephalocele and the large abdominal distention due to the bilateral cystic kidneys and the postaxial polydactyly.

Differential Diagnosis. The differential diagnosis will depend on the type of the associated anomalies. Due to several sonographic similarities between these conditions, trisomy 13 must be excluded by karyotype analysis. Another possible differential diagnosis is autosomal dominant polycystic kidney disease.[10]

Associated Anomalies. The constellation of possible anomalies associated with this syndrome is extensive (Table 21–2). In some situations, such a wide phenotypic variation makes the recognition of the disease more difficult.

Prognosis. Meckel's syndrome is a lethal disorder. Most infants are stillborn or die hours or days after birth. A few sometimes survive a few months, with poor quality of life. According to Ramadani and Nasrat, there has been one report of a survivor who died at the age of 28 months.[10] In 1997, Paavola et al. reported another atypical case of a survivor who died at age 18 months.[6]

Management. A karyotype study should be obtained when Meckel's syndrome is suspected to exclude chromosomal

TABLE 21–2. ANOMALIES ASSOCIATED WITH MECKEL'S SYNDROME

Central nervous system
    Occipital cephalocele
    Microcephaly
    Holoprosencephaly
    Cerebral and cerebellar hypoplasia
    Hypoplasia of pituitary gland
    Dandy–Walker malformation
Face
    Cleft lip and palate
    Micrognathia
    Ear anomalies
    Microphthalmia[10]
    Epicanthal folds
    Nasal anomalies
    Hypotelorism or hypertelorism
Mouth
    Lobulated tongue
    Cleft epiglottis
    Neonatal teeth
Skeletal
    Polydactyly
    Short limbs
    Talipes
    Bell-shaped thorax
    Syndactyly
    Clubfoot[5]
    Clinodactyly[5]
Renal
    Polycystic kidneys
    Renal agenesis
    Renal hypoplasia
    Horseshoe kidneys
    Double ureter
Hepatic
    Hepatic fibrosis
    Ductal agenesis
    Portal fibrosis
Genitalia
    Hypoplasia
    Ambiguous genitalia[10]
    Hermaphrodites[4]
    Cryptorchidism
Cardiac
    Ventricular or atrial defects[5]
    Aortic hypoplasia or coarctation[5]
    Aortic valvular stenosis[5]
    Rotational anomalies[5]
    Pulmonary stenosis

(Continued)

TABLE 21–2. *(continued)*

Lungs
  Hypoplasia of the lungs
Others
  Growth restriction
  Short webbed neck
  Malrotation of the guts
  Accessory spleen
  Adrenal agenesis
  Omphalocele
  Hypoplasia or absent bladder
  Imperforate anus
  Enlarged placenta
  Single umbilical artery

disorders. If the diagnosis is made before viability, termination can be offered. When the family decides to continue the pregnancy or if the diagnosis is made after viability, the standard obstetric management is not altered.

REFERENCES

1. Buyse ML, ed. *Birth Defects Encyclopedia.* Cambridge, MA: Blackwell Scientific; 1990.
2. Altmann P, Wagenbichler P, Schaller A. A casuistic report on the Gruber or Meckel syndrome. *Hum Genet.* 1977;38:357–362.
3. Bergsma D. Birth defects. In: *Atlas and Compendium. National Foundation—March of Dimes.* London: Macmillan Press; 1979:78.
4. Salonen R, Norio R. The Meckel syndrome: Clinicopathological findings in 67 patients. *Am J Med Genet.* 1984;18:671–689.
5. Nyberg DA, Hallesy D, Mahony BS, et al. Meckel–Gruber syndrome: Importance of prenatal diagnosis. *J Ultrasound Med.* 1990;9:691–696.
6. Paavola P, Salonen R, Weissenbach J, Peltonen L. The locus for Meckel syndrome with multiple congenital anomalies maps to chromosome 17q21–q24. *Nat Genet.* 1995;11:213–215.
7. Fraser FC, Lytwyn A. Spectrum of anomalies in the Mercilel syndrome, or maybe there is a malformation syndrome with at least one constant anomaly. *Am J Med Genet.* 1981;9:67–73.
8. Farag TI, Usha R, Mady SA, et al. Phenotypic variation in Meckel–Gruber syndrome. *Clin Genet.* 1990;38:176–179.
9. Weinstein BJ, Benacerraf BR. Meckel syndrome, first trimester diagnosis. *Fetus.* 1999;4:4–5.
10. Ramadani HM, Nasrat HA. Prenatal diagnosis of recurrent Meckel syndrome. *Int J Gynecol Obstet.* 1992;39:327–332.

MESOMELIC DYSPLASIA

Definition. As implied by its name, mesomelic dysplasia is a skeletal disorder with anomalies of the ulna and radius and of the tibia and fibula. These anomalies are predominantly hypoplasic and shortening, but these bones can also be malformed or fused. A large number of associated anomalies exist such as hypoplasia of the mandible, ulnar deviation of hands, talipes equinovarus, distal tapering of the humeri, and hypoplastic fibulae, radii, and ulnae,[1] bony spurs of the diaphyses,[2] carpal and tarsal synostosis, and dorsolateral foot deviation.[3,4] The most typical form (Langer type) is considered to be the homozygote form of the Leri–Weill dyschondrosteosis.[4,5]

Synonyms. Langer-type mesomelic dwarfism, dyschondrosteosis, and homozygous.

Incidence. Rare.

Etiology. Autosomal recessive inheritance.

Recurrence Risk. Twenty-five percent.

Diagnosis. The mesomelic findings have been recognized as early as the first trimester in an at-risk propositus[6] and in a routine examination in the second trimester.[7,8]

Pathogenesis. Nonsense mutation of the gene for the short stature homeobox (SHOX), which is involved in idiopathic growth retardation and possibly Turner short stature.[9]

Genetic Anomaly. The gene for one form of mesomelic dysplasia (the Kantaputra type[3]) is mapped to chromosomes 2q24–q32.[4] Leri–Weill dyschondrosteosis has been linked to the marker DXYS6814 in the pseudoautosomal region (PAR1) of the X and Y chromosomes (more severe in females)[4] and to the DCS gene of a microsatellite DNA marker at the DXYS233 locus.[9]

Associated Anomalies. See Definition. Aside from the mesomelic dysplasia, most other anomalies are skeletal and the most striking is micrognathia.

Differential Diagnosis. Many other skeletal dysplasias present with mesomelic anomalies and these would include chondrodysplasia punctata (look for stippled calcifications in the sacrum),[10] brachymesomelia,[11] and chondroectodermal dysplasia,[12] among many.

Prognosis. Disproportionate short stature. Some forms have normal intellectual capacity.

Management. When recognized prenatally, termination of pregnancy can be offered.

REFERENCES

1. Brodie SG, Lachman RS, Crandall BF, et al. Radiographic and morphologic findings in a previously undescribed type of

mesomelic dysplasia resembling atelosteogenesis type II. *Am J Med Genet.* 1998;80:247–251.

2. Kerner B, Rimoin DL, Lachman RS. Mesomelic shortening of the upper extremities with spur formation and cutaneous dimpling. *Pediatr Radiol.* 1998;28:794–797.

3. Kantaputra PN, Gorlin RJ, Langer LO Jr. Dominant mesomelic dysplasia, ankle, carpal, and tarsal synostosis type: A new autosomal dominant bone disorder. *Am J Med Genet.* 1992;44:730–737.

4. Fujimoto M, Kantaputra PN, Ikegawa S, et al. The gene for mesomelic dysplasia Kantaputra type is mapped to chromosome 2q24–q32. *J Hum Genet.* 1998;43:32–36.

5. Shears DJ, Vassal HJ, Goodman FR, et al. Mutation and deletion of the pseudoautosomal gene SHOX cause Leri–Weill dyschondrosteosis. *Nat Genet.* 1998;19:70–73.

6. den Hollander NS, van der Harten HJ, Vermeij-Keers C, et al. First-trimester diagnosis of Blomstrand lethal osteochondrodysplasia. *Am J Med Genet.* 1997;73:345–350.

7. Roth P, Agnani G, Arbez-Gindre F, et al. Langer mesomelic dwarfism: Ultrasonographic diagnosis of two cases in early midtrimester. *Prenat Diagn.* 1996;16:247–251.

8. Evans MI, Zador IE, Qureshi F, et al. Ultrasonographic prenatal diagnosis and fetal pathology of Langer mesomelic dwarfism. *Am J Med Genet.* 1988;31:915–920.

9. Belin V, Cusin V, Viot G, et al. SHOX mutations in dyschondrosteosis (Leri–Weill syndrome). *Nat Genet.* 1998;19:67–69.

10. Argo KM, Toriello HV, Jelsema RD, Zuidema LJ. Prenatal findings in chondrodysplasia punctata, tibia–metacarpal type. *Ultrasound Obstet Gynecol.* 1996;8:350–354.

11. Kivlin JD, Carey JC, Richey MA. Brachymesomelia and Peters anomaly: A new syndrome. *Am J Med Genet.* 1993;45:416–419.

12. Qureshi F, Jacques SM, Evans MI, et al. Skeletal histopathology in fetuses with chondroectodermal dysplasia (Ellis–van Creveld syndrome). *Am J Med Genet.* 1993;45:471–476.

MICROCEPHALIC OSTEODYSPLASTIC PRIMORDIAL DWARFISM (TYPES I THROUGH III)

Definition. These syndromes associate growth retardation with microcephaly and various facial anomalies.[1–6] The number of reported case is small, and the difference between the subtypes is probably not identifiable by prenatal ultrasound, which is the reason these syndromes are described together.

Synonyms. Osteodysplastic primordial dwarfism type I, brachymelic primordial dwarfism, Taybi–Linder syndrome, cephaloskeletal dysplasia, and low-birth-weight dwarfism with skeletal dysplasia.

Incidence. Fewer than 50 cases have been reported.

Etiology. Sporadic, with possible autosomal recessive inheritance.[2]

Recurrence Risk. Unknown.

Diagnosis. The findings include growth retardation with microcephaly, micrencephaly, lissencephaly, micrognathia, and moderately short limbs.[7] Types II and III may show platyspondyly.

Pathogenesis. Unknown.

Genetic Anomaly. Unknown.

Associated Anomalies. Beaked nose, large eyes, dysplastic ears, clinodactyly, dysgenesis of the corpus callosum, focal renal medullary dysplasia, small iliac wings with flat acetabular angles, coxa vara, V-shaped distal femoral metaphyses, triangular distal femoral epiphyses, pseudoepiphyses of metacarpals, short first metacarpals, and brachymesophalangy of the fifth digit.[8,9]

Differential Diagnosis. Aneuploidies (trisomies 13 and 18).

Prognosis. Not known. Most children die within the first year.

Management. Termination of pregnancy can be offered before viability; otherwise, no alteration of prenatal care is suggested.

REFERENCES

1. Majewski F, Goecke TO. Microcephalic osteodysplastic primordial dwarfism type II: Report of three cases and review. *Am J Med Genet.* 1998;80:25–31.

2. Sigaudy S, Toutain A, Moncla A, et al. Microcephalic osteodysplastic primordial dwarfism Taybi–Linder type: Report of four cases and review of the literature. *Am J Med Genet.* 1998;80:16–24.

3. al Gazali LI, Hamada M, Lytle W. Microcephalic osteodysplastic primordial dwarfism type II. *Clin Dysmorphol.* 1995;4:234–238.

4. Haan EA, Furness ME, Knowles S, et al. Osteodysplastic primordial dwarfism: Report of a further case with manifestations similar to those of types I and III. *Am J Med Genet.* 1989;33:224–227.

5. Majewski F, Stoeckenius M, Kemperdick H. Studies of microcephalic primordial dwarfism III: An intrauterine dwarf with platyspondyly and anomalies of pelvis and clavicles—Osteodysplastic primordial dwarfism type III. *Am J Med Genet.* 1982;12:37–42.

6. Majewski F, Ranke M, Schinzel A. Studies of microcephalic primordial dwarfism II: The osteodysplastic type II of primordial dwarfism. *Am J Med Genet.* 1982;12:23–35.

7. Kozlowski K, Donovan T, Masel J, Wright RG. Microcephalic, osteodysplastic, primordial dwarfism. *Australas Radiol.* 1993;37:111–114.

8. Berger A, Haschke N, Kohlhauser C, et al. Neonatal cholestasis and focal medullary dysplasia of the kidneys in a case of microcephalic osteodysplastic primordial dwarfism. *J Med Genet*. 1998;35:61–64.
9. Spranger S, Tariverdian G, Albert FK, et al. Case report. Microcephalic osteodysplastic primordial dwarfism type II: A child with unusual symptoms and clinical course. *Eur J Pediatr*. 1996; 155:796–799.

NEU-LAXOVA SYNDROMES

Definition. Neu-Laxova is a rare lethal syndrome characterized by ichthyosis, IUGR, microcephaly, short neck, CNS abnormalities, hypoplastic or atelectasia of the lungs, limb deformities, edema, polyhydramnios, and short umbilical cord.[1]

Synonyms. None.

Incidence. Rare.

Etiology. Unknown.

Diagnosis. Ultrasonographic findings may include receding forehead, hypertelorism, cataract, severe ectropion, proptosis, prominent eyes, malformed ears, flat nose, micrognathia, severe microcephaly, lissencephaly, dysgenesis of the corpus callosum, hypoplasia of the cerebellum, Dandy–Walker anomaly, choroid plexus cysts, unilateral renal agenesis, abnormal external genitalia (curved penis, cryptorchidism), hypoechoic skeletal structures, kyphosis, contractures of limbs, swelling and webbing of the knee and elbow joints, and severe edema of the hands and feet, giving the impression of absent digits, edema, polyhydramnios, IUGR, retardation and feeble fetal activity.[2–12]

Genetic Anomalies. Autosomal recessive. Many cases have been in consanguineous parents. In view of the 25% recurrence rate, at-risk pregnancies should be carefully monitored by ultrasonography for accurate dating, fetal limb activity, facial and skeletal anomalies, the detection of IUGR, and polyhydramnios.

Differential Diagnosis. Lissencephaly, cerebrooculofacioskeletal syndrome, and arthrogryposis.

Prognosis. Lethal.

Management. Termination of pregnancy can be offered before viability. Standard prenatal care is not altered when continuation of the pregnancy is decided. Confirmation of diagnosis after birth is important for genetic counseling.

REFERENCES

1. Lazjuk GI, Lurie IW, Ostrowskaja TI, et al. Brief clinical observations: The Neu-Laxova syndrome—A distinct entity. *Am J Med Genet*. 1979;3:261–267.
2. King JA, Gardner V, Chen H, Blackburn W. Neu-Laxova syndrome: Pathological evaluation of a fetus and review of the literature. *Pediatr Pathol Lab Med*. 1995;15:57–79.
3. Gulmezoglu AM, Ekici E. Sonographic diagnosis of Neu-Laxova syndrome. *J Clin Ultrasound*. 1994;22:48–51.
4. Bronshtein M, Blumenfeld I, Cohen I, Blumenfeld Z. Fetal ultrasonographic detection of hypodontia in the Neu-Laxova syndrome. *J Clin Ultrasound*. 1993;21:648–650.
5. Shapiro I, Borochowitz Z, Degani S, et al. Neu-Laxova syndrome: Prenatal ultrasonographic diagnosis, clinical and pathological studies, and new manifestations. *Am J Med Genet*. 1992;43:602–605.
6. Monaco R, Stabile M, Guida F, Sirimarco E. Echographic, radiological and anatomo–pathological evaluation of a fetus with Neu-Laxova syndrome. *Australas Radiol*. 1992;36: 51–53.
7. Naveed Manjunath CS, Sreenivas V. New manifestations of Neu-Laxova syndrome. *Am J Med Genet*. 1990;35:55–59.
8. Russo R, D'Armiento M, Martinelli P, Ventruto V. Neu-Laxova syndrome: Pathological, radiological, and prenatal findings in a stillborn female. *Am J Med Genet*. 1989;32:136–139.
9. Ostrovskaya TI, Lazjuk GI. Cerebral abnormalities in the Neu-Laxova syndrome. *Am J Med Genet*. 1988;30:747–756.
10. Tolmie JL, Mortimer G, Doyle D, et al. The Neu-Laxova syndrome in female sibs: Clinical and pathological features with prenatal diagnosis in the second sib. *Am J Med Genet*. 1987;27:175–182.
11. Muller LM, de Jong G, Mouton SC, et al. A case of the Neu-Laxova syndrome: Prenatal ultrasonographic monitoring in the third trimester and the histopathological findings. *Am J Med Genet*. 1987;26:421–429.
12. Ejeckam GG, Wadhwa JK, Williams JP, Lacson AG. Neu-Laxova syndrome: Report of two cases. *Pediatr Pathol*. 1986;5: 295–306.

NOONAN'S SYNDROME

Definition. In 1968, Noonan[1] described 19 cases of a syndrome very similar to the disorder described by Turner.[2] Among her patients, 17 had pulmonary stenosis and 2 had patent ductus arteriosus (12 males and 7 were females). Other anomalies include lymphedema, pterygium colli, deformity of the sternum with precocious closure of sutures resulting in a pectus carinatum superiorly and a pectus excavatum inferiorly, coarctation of the aorta, cryptorchidism, and thrombocytopenia. In addition to the fact that this syndrome occurs in both sexes, there is a large phenotypic overlap with Turner syndrome.

Synonyms. Turner syndrome with normal XX, pseudo-Turner, male-Turner syndrome, and Ullrich syndrome.

Incidence. Between 0.25 and 1 per 10,000 deliveries.

Etiology. Autosomal dominant, with sporadic new mutations.

Diagnosis. The initial anomaly most likely to be observed is a posterior nuchal cystic hygroma[3] that may regress later in gestation into a nuchal fold redundancy or pterygium colli.[4,5] Other anomalies have been suspected because of congenital heart disease,[6] pleural effusions, and hydrops.[7] Some fetuses also have been identified by triple marker screening.[8]

Genetic Anomalies. X-linked dominant inheritance of either a single mutant gene or a submicroscopic deletion was originally suspected,[9,10] but it is now recognized that one of the genes for Noonan's syndrome is located on chromosome 12 in the 12q24.2–q24.31 region.[11–13]

Differential Diagnosis. Turner's syndrome (excluded in males or by karyotype) is also unlikely to be familial, whereas Noonan's syndrome has a strong familial predilection. Other diagnoses include trisomy 21 and Escobar's syndrome.

Prognosis. Fairly normal life expectancy for those without major complications of heart disease.

Management. Termination of pregnancy can be offered before viability. Standard prenatal care is not altered when continuation of the pregnancy is decided.

REFERENCES

1. Noonan JA. Hypertelorism with Turner phenotype. A new syndrome with associated congenital heart disease. *Am J Dis Child.* 1968;116:373–383.
2. Turner HH. A syndrome of infantilism, congenital webbed necil, and cubitus valgus. *Endocrinology.* 1938;23:566.
3. Reynders CS, Pauker SP, Benacerraf BR. First trimester isolated fetal nuchal lucency: Significance and outcome. *J Ultrasound Med.* 1997;16:101–105.
4. Izquierdo L, Kushnir O, Sanchez D, et al. Prenatal diagnosis of Noonan's syndrome in a female infant with spontaneous resolution of cystic hygroma and hydrops. *West J Med.* 1990;152:418–421.
5. Donnenfeld AE, Nazir MA, Sindoni F, Librizzi RJ. Prenatal sonographic documentation of cystic hygroma regression in Noonan syndrome. *Am J Med Genet.* 1991;39:461–465.
6. Sonesson SE, Fouron JC, Lessard M. Intrauterine diagnosis and evolution of a cardiomyopathy in a fetus with Noonan's syndrome. *Acta Paediatr.* 1992;81:368–370.
7. Benacerraf BR, Greene MF, Holmes LB. The prenatal sonographic features of Noonan's syndrome. *J Ultrasound Med.* 1989;8:59–63.
8. Aranguren G, Garcia-Minaur S, Loridan L, et al. Multiple-marker screen positive results in Noonan syndrome. *Prenat Diagn.* 1996;16:183–184.
9. Nora JJ, Nora AH, Sinha AK, et al. The Ullrich–Noonan syndrome (Turner phenotype). *Am J Dis Child.* 1974;127:48–55.
10. Bolton MR, Pugh DM, Mattioli LF, et al. The Noonan syndrome: A family study. *Ann Intern Med.* 1974;80:626–629.
11. van der Burgt I, Berends E, Lommen E, et al. Clinical and molecular studies in a large Dutch family with Noonan syndrome. *Am J Med Genet.* 1994;53:187–191.
12. Brady AF, Jamieson CR, van der Burgt I, et al. Further delineation of the critical region for Noonan syndrome on the long arm of chromosome 12. *Eur J Hum Genet.* 1997;5:336–337.
13. Legius E, Schollen E, Matthijs G, Fryns J-P. Fine mapping of Noonan/cardio-facio cutaneous syndrome in a large family. *Eur J Hum Genet.* 1998;6:32–37.

OLIGOHYDRAMNIOS SEQUENCE

The oligohydramnios sequence is a set of related conditions resulting from a marked decrease in amniotic fluid. This typically results from bilateral renal agenesis (34%) (Fig. 21–67) or chronic leakage of fluid. Other conditions such as bilateral multicystic renal dysplasia (34%), unilateral renal agenesis and contralateral multicystic renal dysplasia (9%), renal tubular dysgenesis, autosomal recessive (infantile) polycystic disease, nonfunctioning but morphologically normal renal tracts (3%), and aberrant placental implantation (on a uterine septum, for instance) can lead to the same set of findings.[1]

Fifty percent of these fetuses have anomalies that are not part of the oligohydramnios sequence (VACTERL, Meckel, Smith–Lemli–Opitz).

In the oligohydramnios sequence, the decrease of fluid causes lung hypoplasia and fetal compression. The fetal compression results in abnormal limb positions with dislocations and an abnormal face (flat with low set ears). After delivery, these newborns die of pulmonary insufficiency (through the pneumothoraces).

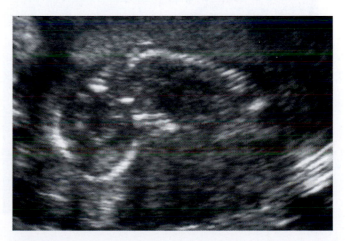

Figure 21–67. Oligohydramnios (anhydramnios) in an early second-trimester fetus with bilateral renal agenesis.

REFERENCE

1. Newbould MJ, Lendon M, Barson AJ. Oligohydramnios sequence: The spectrum of renal malformations. *Br J Obstet Gynaecol.* 1994;101:598–604.

OSTEOGENESIS IMPERFECTA

Definition. This heterogeneous group of genetic disorders (divided into four types assessed by Sillence: I, II or congenital, III, and IV) is characterized by severe bone fragility, leading to abnormal ossification and multiple fractures.[1] There are four types.

- *Type I* does not present prenatal deformities, and the diagnosis is made after birth when the limb deformities start to develop.
- *Type II* is the most severe form. It presents with multiple skeletal malformations, such as bone shortening and angulation, due to multiple fractures, demineralization of the skull, narrow and bell-shaped chest caused by fractures of the ribs, decreased fetal movement, and wrinkling of the surface of the bones due to multiple fractures.
- *Type III* is less severe than type II and usually presents as multiple fractures at birth, with development of progressive bone deformities from the neonatal period to adolescence. It is detectable as early as the second trimester in *type IIIc*.

- *Type IV* is the mildest presentation of the disorder and is not detectable prenatally. It usually involves premature osteoporosis in the 4th to 5th decades of life.

Synonyms. Osteogenesis imperfecta congenital, Van der Hoeve's syndrome, Lobstein's disease, trias fragilitas osseum, brittle bone disease, and Vrolik's disease.[2]

Incidence. Every 0.4 per 10,000 live births and about half (0.19 per 10,000) represents type II.[3]

Etiology. In the majority of cases of types I and IV, an autosomal dominant pattern is involved. Type II is a de novo dominant mutation (with a few reports of autosomal recessive pattern), and type III is autosomal recessive or dominant.[4]

Recurrence Risk. Depends on the form of transmission. In general, it ranges from 2 to 5% for type II, if it is not caused by a spontaneous mutation.[1]

Diagnosis. The sonographic findings that may be present (in particular, in type II) include broad, short, fractured long bones (Fig. 21–68A and B), with a wrinkled appearance caused by callus formation, decreased ossification of the skull (Fig. 21–69), with increased visualization of the intracranial structures, small bell-shaped chest (Figs. 21–70 and 21–71), abnormal skull shape, broad irregular ribs, angulation of the long bones, and abnormal face. A typical finding of OI type II

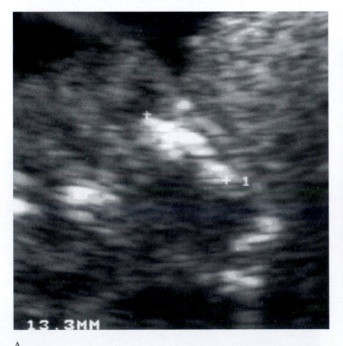

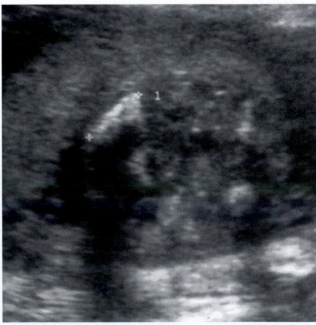

A　　　　　　　　　　　　　　　　　　　　　　　B

Figure 21–68. (A and **B)** The humerus measures 13 mm and the femur measures 14 mm (below the 5th centile).

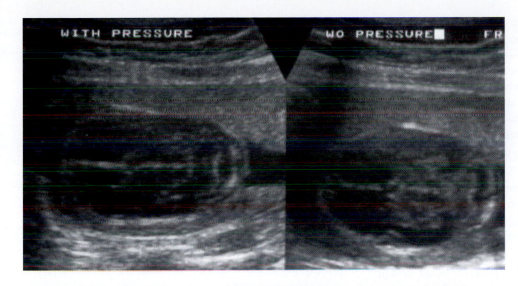

Figure 21–69. The skull demonstrates markedly decreased echogenicity and is readily compressible even with moderate transducer pressure *(left)*.

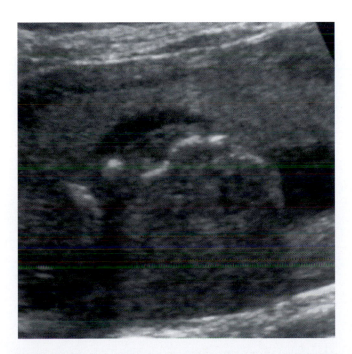

Figure 21–70. The ribs are soft, and the chest has a bell-shaped configuration.

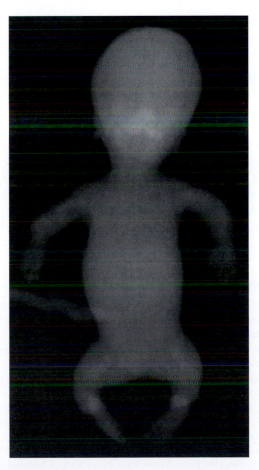

Figure 21–71. Frontal radiographs of the fetus show the poor mineralization and the numerous fractures.

is the ability to see both corticals of a bone. Normally, the distal cortical is shadowed by the proximal, but not with the severe demineralization of OI (achondrogenesis and hypophosphatasia may present the same finding). Most of the anomalies can be detected *in utero* by ultrasound early in the second trimester. A normal ultrasound for a high-risk patient does not exclude the disorder. In general, if the fractures do not occur *in utero,* the diagnosis is made only after birth.[1,5]

Genetic Anomaly. A disorder in one of the two genes responsible for type I collagen production (COLIA1 and COLIA2) is the cause of the disease.[6]

Pathogenes. A defect of formation, organization, and chemical composition in type I collagen (which is found in skin, ligaments, tendons, demineralized bone, and dentine) is responsible for decreased mineralization and bone fragility.[6]

Associated Anomalies. Kyphoscoliosis, deafness, hypotonia, inguinal hernias, hydrocephalus, hydrops, and prenatal growth deficiency.[4]

Differential Diagnosis. Hypophosphatasia (infantile form), achondrogenesis, and other short-limbed dwarfisms.[1]

Prognosis. Type II OI is uniformly lethal, and the most frequents causes are cerebral hemorrhage and respiratory failure. The other forms develop after birth, including progressive deformities of the long bones and short stature.[1,5]

Management. Due to the uniformly fatal outcome, termination of pregnancy could be offered at any stage of gestation when type II is diagnosed. For the other forms, termination could be offered before viability. If continuing the pregnancy is preferred, standard prenatal care should not be altered.

REFERENCES

1. Kennon JC, Vitsky JL, Tiller GE, Jeanty P. Osteogenesis imperfecta. *Fetus.* 1994;4:11–14.
2. Hale AV, Medford E, Izquierdo LA, Curet L. Osteogenesis imperfecta. *Fetus.* 1992;2:5–10.
3. Romero R, Pilu GL, Jeanty P. *Prenatal Diagnosis of Congenital Anomalies.* Norwalk, CT: Appleton & Lange; 1988.
4. Jones KL. Osteogenesis imperfecta syndrome, type I. In: Jones KL, ed. *Smith's Recognizable Patterns of Human Malformation.* Philadelphia: WB Saunders; 1997:486–487.
5. Benacerraf BR. Osteogenesis imperfecta. In: Benacerraf BR, ed. *Ultrasound of Fetal Syndromes.* New York: Churchill Livingstone; 1998:229–235.
6. Prockop DJ. Mutations in collagen genes as a cause of connective tissue diseases. *N Engl J Med.* 1992;326:8.

PENA–SHOKEIR SYNDROME

Definition. Pena–Shokeir syndrome is an inherited disorder and was first described by Pena and Shokeir in 1974.[1] It is characterized by arthrogryposis and dysmorphic features, resulting from fetal akinesia.

Synonym. Fetal akinesia/hypokinesia sequence and fetal akinesia deformation sequence.

Etiology. Autosomal recessive is the most common pattern of transmission. Several descriptions of unusual presentations suggest a heterogenic etiology.[2]

Recurrence Risk. The prediction of the recurrence risk is imprecise due to the multifactorial etiology. In most cases, it varies from 0 to 25%.[3]

Incidence. Unknown.

Pathophisyology. Active fetal movement starts in the mid–first trimester and is of major importance for the normal development of the joints and contiguous tissues. Absent or reduced fetal movement leads to stiff joints, pterygia, and abnormal neuromuscular function with decreased fetal swallowing, which causes pulmonary hypoplasia and polyhydramnios.[2]

Diagnosis. The combination of abnormal limb position, restrictive fetal movement with reduced or absent response to acoustic stimulation, growth retardation, polyhydramnios, and pulmonary hypoplasia establishes the diagnosis. Low-set malformed ears, hypertelorism, short neck, cleft palate, scalp edema, thoracic deformities, camptodactyly, and micrognathia may also be found.[3,4] Anomalies less frequently described in association with Pena–Shokeir syndrome include diaphragmatic hernia, gastroschisis, and microcephaly.

Differential Diagnosis. Trisomy 18 may present features that overlap with those of Pena–Shokeir syndrome, in particular craniofacial, limbs and intrathoracic abnormalities. Karyotype analysis establishes the differential diagnosis.[3,5] Nonlethal forms of arthrogryposis present the same set of findings, except for the pulmonary hypoplasia.[4]

Prognosis. Pena–Shokeir syndrome is a lethal condition. A significant number of the affected fetuses are born prematurely. Thirty percent of those born at term are stillborn. Among the survivors, the majority dies within few weeks of life.[5] Pulmonary complication is the main cause of death.

Management. Termination of pregnancy can be offered before viability. Standard prenatal care should be changed throughout the pregnancy only for maternal indications.

REFERENCES

1. Pena SDJ, Shokeir MHK. Syndrome of camptodactyly, multiple ankyloses facial anomalies and pulmonary hypoplasia: A lethal condition. *J Pediatr.* 1974;85:373–375.
2. Ajayi RA, Keen CE, Knott PD. Ultrasound diagnosis of the Pena Shokeir phenotype at 14 weeks of pregnancy. *Prenat Diagn.* 1995;15:762–764.
3. Jones KL. Pena–Shokeir phenotype. In: Jones KL, ed. *Smith's Recognizable Patterns of Human Malformation.* Philadelphia: WB Saunders; 1997:174–175.
4. Ohlsson A, Fong KW, Rose TH, Moore DC. Prenatal sonographic diagnosis of Pena–Shokeir syndrome type I, or fetal akinesia deformation sequence. *Am J Med Genet.* 1988;29:59–65.
5. Muller LM, de Jong G. Prenatal ultrasonographic features of the Pena–Shokeir I syndrome and the trisomy 18 syndrome. *Am J Med Genet.* 1986;25:119–129.

PENTALOGY OF CANTRELL

Definition. This congenital disorder is characterized by two major defects: *ectopia cordis* and an *abdominal wall defect* (most commonly an omphalocele, but gastroschisis may also be present) associated with disruption of three interposing structures: the distal sternum, anterior diaphragm, and diaphragmatic pericardium.[1] Variants of the classic form, such as incomplete expressions, have also been reported.

Synonyms. Thoraco-abdominal ectopia cordis, ectopia cordis, Cantrell–Heller–Ravitch syndrome; pentalogy syndrome, and peritoneopericardial diaphragmatic hernia.

Incidence. Very rare. Approximately 90 cases have been reported in the literature, and even fewer have had the complete syndrome confirmed.[2]

Etiology. Unknown. Sometimes it can be associated with chromosomal abnormalities.

Recurrence Risk. Unknown. No recurrence has been recorded. One set of monozygotic twins concordant for the syndrome has been reported.[3]

Diagnosis. Presence of complete disruption of the anterior chest and abdominal walls, causing the five defects as described by Cantrell et al., is the classic form and may be detected as early as the mid–second trimester. The typical finding of cardiac activity outside the chest in association with an omphalocele establishes the diagnosis (Fig. 21–72) Karyotype analysis is recommended to exclude chromosomal anomalies. Ascites and pleural effusion may occur due to compression of the contents of both the chest and the abdomen.

Genetic Anomaly. Unknown.

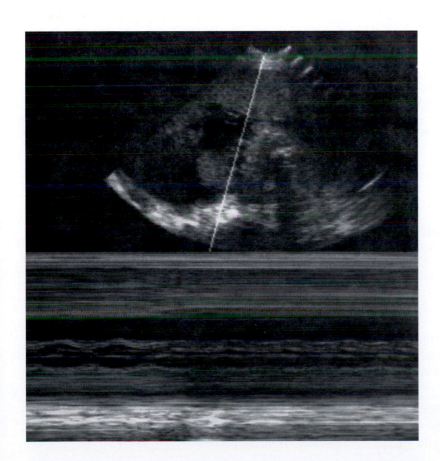

Figure 21–72. M-mode recording demonstrates the heart outside the chest of a 15-week fetus. The omphalocele is seen farther to the left.

Pathogenesis. Developmental failure of a segment of the lateral mesoderm between 14 and 18 days after conception, resulting in failure of the ventral wall closure and incomplete external primordial bands fusion.[2]

Associated Anomalies. Intracardiac anomalies [i.e., tetralogy of Fallot, ventricular septal defect (VSD)] are the rule. Others include cranial and facial anomalies, chromosomal abnormalities, clubfeet, and malrotation of the colon, hydrocephalus, and anencephaly.[4,5]

Differential Diagnosis. Isolated thoracic cardiac ectopy, ectopia cordis associated with amniotic band syndrome, body stalk abnormality, isolated omphalocele, Beckwith–Wiedeman syndrome, and chromosomal abnormalities.

Prognosis. Survival is exceptional and depends on the size of the abdominal wall defect, the extent of the cardiac defect, and the presence of associated anomalies. Rare milder forms may be surgically corrected. Cases presenting a complete extrusion of the heart and abdominal contents have an extremely poor prognosis.[2,5]

Management. Termination of pregnancy can be offered before viability. After viability, periodic ultrasonographic evaluation of the lesions, fetal growth, and delivery in a tertiary center are recommended.

REFERENCES

1. Cantrell JR, Haller JA, Ravitch MM. A syndrome of congenital defects involving the abdominal wall, sternum, diaphragm, pericardium, and heart. *Surg Gynecol Obstet.* 1958;107:602–614.
2. Craigo SD, Gillieson MS, Cetrulo CL. Pentalogy of Cantrell. *Fetus.* 1992;2:1–4.
3. Baker ME, Rosenberg ER, Trofatter KF, et al. The in utero findings in twin pentalogy of Cantrell. *J Ultrasound Med.* 1984;3: 525–527.
4. Toyama WM. Combined congenital defects of the anterior abdominal wall, sternum, diaphragm, pericardium, and heart: A case report and review of the syndrome. *Pediatrics.* 1972;50: 778–792.
5. Benacerraf BR. Pentallogy of Cantrell. In: Benacerraf BR, ed. *Ultrasound of Fetal Syndromes.* New York: Churchill Livingstone; 1998:267–269.

PFEIFFER'S SYNDROME

Definition. This congenital disorder, described by Pfeiffer in 1964,[1] is characterized by acrocephalic skull, syndactyly of hands and feet, and enlarged thumbs. It is divided into three types:

- type I: characterized by the classic appearance of craniosynostosis, broad thumbs, syndactyly, and normal intelligence; this form is compatible with life

- type II: cloverleaf skull, ocular proptosis, broad thumbs, variable visceral anomalies, elbow ankylosis, and severe compromise of the CNS; usually results in early death
- type III: craniosynostosis, severe ocular proptosis without cloverleaf skull, elbow ankylosis, and variable visceral anomalies; affected fetuses have severe neurologic compromise, with poor prognosis and early death.

Incidence. Unknown. Since the first description was published, approximately 30 cases have been reported.[2]

Etiology. Type I: autosomal dominant or fresh mutations; types II and III: sporadic.

Recurrence Risk. Variable, depending on the etiology. When the transmission has an autosomal dominant pattern, the recurrence risk is 50%. If caused by fresh mutations, the risk of recurrence is very low.

Diagnosis. Sonographic signs of Pfeiffer's syndrome include craniofacial anomalies (brachycephaly, acrocephaly, craniosynostosis of the coronal suture, hypertelorism, small nose, and low nasal bridge) and hand and foot anomalies (partial syndactyly of second and third fingers, second third and fourth toes, and broad thumb and big toe).[2]

Genetic Anomaly. Pfeiffer's syndrome is genetically heterogeneous. Some cases are linked to mutations at the FGFR1 gene at chromosome 8p11.22–p12.[3] Mutations at the FGFR2 gene, which map at chromosome 10q25–q26, also have been reported.[4]

Associated Anomalies. Cloanal atresia, tracheo and bronchomalacia, cloverleaf skull, fused vertebra, Arnold–Chiari malformation, hydrocephalus, and imperforate anus. After birth, seizures and mental retardation may develop.

Differential Diagnosis. The main differential diagnosis includes the syndromes that are characterized by craniosynostosis (Apert, Carpenter, Crouzon, Kleeblattschadel anomaly, and thanatophoric dysplasia).

Prognosis. The prognosis depends on the severity of associated anomalies, in particular on the severity of the CNS compromise. Type I has in general a good prognosis. Types II and III are not compatible with life, and death occurs early.

Management. Termination of pregnancy can be offered before viability. If continuing the pregnancy is decided, periodic sonographic evaluation of the anomalies (in particular CNS anomalies) is recommended.

REFERENCES

1. Pfeiffer R. Dominant erbliche Akrocephalosyndactylie. *Z Kinderheilkd*. 1964;90:301.
2. Jones KL. Pfeiffer syndrome. In: Jones KL, ed. *Smith's Recognizable Patterns of Human Malformation*. Philadelphia: WB Saunders; 1997:416–417.
3. Muenke M, Schell U, Hehr A, et al. A common mutation in the fibroblast growth factor receptor 1 gene in Pfeiffer syndrome. *Nat Genet*. 1994;8:268.
4. Rutland P, Pulleyn LJ, Reardon W, et al. Identical mutations in FGFR2 gene cause both Pfeiffer and Crouzon syndrome phenotypes. *Nat Genet*. 1995;9:173–176.

POLAND'S SYNDROME

Definition. Unilateral symbrachydactyly and ipsilateral aplasia of the sternal head of the pectoralis major muscle. Ispilateral aplasia of the breast exists in females. Dextrocardia has been reported in several cases.[1,2]

Synonyms. Poland–Moebius syndrome and subclavian artery supply disruption sequence.

Incidence. Every 0.2 per 10,000 births.[3]

Etiology. Sporadic interruption of the early embryonic blood supply in the subclavian arteries.[4] Several familial cases have been described.

Diagnosis. The chest asymmetry and symbrachydactyly can be recognized, but the long bones are probably too normal to be recognized.[5,6]

Genetic Anomalies. Not established.

Differential Diagnosis. When the unilaterality of the anomalies is recognized, few differential diagnoses exist.

Prognosis. Aside from the anomalies of the extremity, the prognosis is excellent.

Management. Standard prenatal care is not altered. Confirmation of diagnosis after birth is important for genetic counseling.

REFERENCES

1. Hazir T, Malik MS. Poland anomaly with dextrocardia: A case report. *J Pak Med Assoc*. 1996;46:181–182.
2. Burkhardt H, Buss J. Dextrocardia and Poland syndrome in a 59-year-old patient. *Z Kardiol*. 1997;86:639–643.
3. Czeizel A, Vitez M, Lenz W. Birth prevalence of Poland sequence and proportion of its familial cases (letter). *Am J Med Genet*. 1990;36:524.

4. Bouwes Bavinck JN, Weaver DD. Subclavian artery supply disruption sequence: Hypothesis of a vascular etiology for Poland, Klippel–Feil, and Moebius anomalies. *Am J Med Genet*. 1986;23:903–918.
5. Sferlazza SJ, Cohen MA. Poland's syndrome: A sonographic sign. *AJR*. 1996;167:1597.
6. Risseeuw GA, Janevski B, Meradji M, et al. Poland's syndrome, including ultrasonography of the pectoralis muscle as a new diagnostic modality. *J Belge Radiol*. 1985;68:231–236.

POTTER SEQUENCE

Several entities use the eponym *Potter:*

1. Potter syndrome, now called either *oligohydramnios sequence* or *bilateral renal agenesis* (BRA) depending on whether the cause of the syndrome (BRA) or the mechanism is referred to.
2. Potter syndrome type I is now referred to as *autosomal recessive polycystic kidney disease.*
3. Potter syndrome type II is now referred to as *renal dysplasia.*
4. Potter syndrome type III is now referred to as *autosomal dominant polycystic kidney disease.*

PRUNE BELLY SYNDROME

Definition. Prune belly syndrome is a rare congenital disorder, more common in males, consisting of deficiency of abdominal wall muscles (absent or hypoplastic), cryptorchidism, and genitourinary malformations.

Synonym. Eagle–Barret syndrome.[1]

Etiology. Many theories have been proposed to explain the pathogenesis of this anomaly:

- *abnormal mesodermal development:* developmental arrest of the mesodermal elements would lead to severe abdominal laxity and defective development of the urinary tract[2]
- *primary obstructive urinary anomaly:* the bladder outlet obstruction due to urethral obstruction distends the abdominal wall causing the prune belly syndrome[3,4]
- *genetic defect:* this is suspected because of the predominance in males and few familial cases[5,6]
- *abdominal distension caused by multiple factors*[7]

Recurrence Risk. Unknown, but low.

Incidence. From 0.25 to 0.3 per 10,000 live births, almost exclusively in males.[8]

Diagnosis. The diagnosis should be suspected in fetuses with very large abdominal masses. These are typically bladder

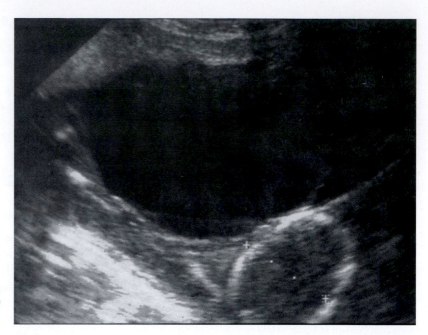

Figure 21–73. A massively distended bladder, as in this case of urethral agenesis, is the main cause of prune belly syndrome.

obstruction (urethral valves, urethral agenesis, Fig. 21–73), but other large abdominal masses such as ovarian cyst and hydrometrocolpos can also be the cause. The detection of cryptorchidism is usually not possible due to the oligohydramnios.

Differential Diagnosis. Urinary tract anomalies such as megacystis megaureter, urethral obstruction, and primary vesicourethral reflux are differential diagnoses.[1] Neurogenic bladder and megacystis microcolon intestinal hypoperistalsis syndrome may also be considered, although the latter presents with normal amniotic fluid.

Prognosis. The prognosis depends on the degree of renal function compromise. The early urinary obstruction, present in the majority of cases, leads to renal failure, pulmonary hypoplasia, and death in the neonatal period. Early decompression of severe bladder obstruction by vesico-amniotic shunt may prevent or attenuate these complications, thus improving the prognosis. Fetuses who develop mild urinary tract distention have a better prognosis. Mild hydronephrosis and megalourethra may be the only manifestations in these cases.[1]

Management. Termination of pregnancy can be offered before viability. Sonographic monitoring of the urinary tract and amniotic fluid volume is required throughout the pregnancy. Early vesical decompression in selected cases has been proposed to improve renal and pulmonary function when early or severe distention of the urinary tract is observed.[9] Renal transplantation may be required after birth in severe cases.[10]

REFERENCES

1. Benacerraf BR. Prune-belly syndrome. In: Benacerraf BR, ed. *Ultrasound of Fetal Syndromes.* New York: Churchill Livingstone; 1998:269–271.
2. Ives EJ. The abdominal muscle deficiency triad syndrome: Experience with ten cases. *Birth Defects.* 1974;10:127–135.
3. Pagon RA, Smith DW, Shepard TH. Urethral obstruction malformation complex: A cause of abdominal muscle deficiency and the prune-belly. *J Pediatr.* 1979;94:900–906.
4. Greskovich FJ III, Nyberg LM Jr. The prune-belly syndrome: A review of its etiology, defects, treatment and prognosis. *J Urol.* 1988;140:707–712.
5. Adeyokunnu AA, Familusi JB. Prune-belly syndrome in two siblings and a first cousin. *AJDC.* 1982;136:23–25.
6. Petersen DS, Fish L, Cass AS. Twins with congenital deficiency of abdominal musculature. *J Urol.* 1972;107:670–672.
7. Nakayama DK, Harrison MR, Chinn DH, Lorimier AA. The pathogenesis of prune-belly. *AJDC.* 1984;138:834–836.
8. Shih WJ, Grenbaum LD, Baro C. In utero sonogram in prune-belly syndrome. *Urology.* 1982;20:102–105.
9. Diamond DA, Sanders R, Jeffs RD. Fetal hydronephrosis: Considerations regarding urological intervention. *J Urol.* 1984;131:1155–1159.
10. Kobata R, Tsukahara H, Takeuchi M, et al. Early detection of prune belly syndrome in utero by ultrasonography. *Acta Paediatr Japan.* 1997;39:705–709.

ROBERTS–SC PHOCOMELIA SYNDROME

Definition. Roberts' syndrome is a rare developmental disorder characterized by multiple malformations, in particular symmetrical limb reduction, craniofacial anomalies such as bilateral cleft lip and palate, nose and ear anomalies, and severe mental and growth retardation. It was initially described by Roberts in 1919[1] and more recently reviewed by Appelt et al.[2] In 1974, Herrmann et al. described cases of a very similar entity called pseudothalidomide, or SC, syndrome.[3] SC are the initials of the two families that were originally described. Roberts' syndrome and SC phocomelia are now considered a single genetic entity, with a wide phenotypic variation.[4]

Incidence. Unknown.

Etiology. This disorder has an autosomal recessive transmission with marked variability of phenotypic expression. The unique cytogenetic abnormality, called *premature centromere separation,* which disrupts the process of chromatid pairing, is responsible for the development of multiple structural anomalies found in Roberts' syndrome.[5]

Recurrence Risk. The recurrence risk for couples with positive family history is 25%.

Diagnosis. The presence of midfacial clefts (lip and palate), nose and ear abnormalities, facial hemangioma, hypertelorism, microcephaly, curly silvery blond hair, tetraphocomelia, severe growth, and mental retardation is very suggestive of Roberts' syndrome.[6-8] Less common findings include oligodactyly, cryptorchidism, enlarged phallus (compared with the rest of the body), oligohydramnios, renal anomalies (polycystic or dysplastic kidneys), heart defects (in particular atrial septal defect and patent ductus arteriosus), and gastrointestinal abnormalities (obstructions). Sonographic detection of those features is highly indicative of Roberts syndrome. Clinical findings and cytogenetic studies make the diagnosis after birth.

Genetic Anomaly. Cytogenic analysis of fetal cells, obtained from chorionic villi sample during the first trimester, and amniocentesis or cordocentesis during the second and third trimesters, are required to confirm the diagnosis prenatally. The presence of premature centromere separation establishes the diagnosis. One negative cytogenetic analysis does not exclude Roberts' syndrome. A second analysis using a different type of fetal tissue is required.

Prognosis. Most patients born at term with less than 37 cm of birth length and severe facial and limb defects have been stillborn or have died early in childhood. Patients born with more than 37 cm of birth length and less severe defects have a better prognosis.[4] However, survival beyond the infancy is infrequent.

Management. When detected before viability, termination of pregnancy can be offered. After viability, standard obstetric management is not altered. For those families previously affected, chorionic villi sample for cytogenetic studies during the first trimester must be offered.

REFERENCES

1. Roberts JB. A child with double cleft of lip and palate, protrusion of the intermaxillary portion of the upper jaw and imperfect development of the bones of the four extremities. *Ann Surg.* 1919;70:252.
2. Appelt H, Gerken H, Lenz W. Tetraphokomelie mit Lippen-Kiefer-Gaumenspalte und Clitorishypertrophie—Ein Syndrom. *Paediatr Paedol.* 1966;2:119.
3. Herrmann J. A familial dysmorphogenetic syndrome of limb deformities, characteristic facial appearance and associated anomalies: The pseudothalidomide or SC-syndrome. *Birth Defects.* 1969;5:81.
4. Jones KL, Roberts SC. Phocomelia. In: Jones KL, ed. *Smith's Recognizable Patterns of Human Malformation.* Philadelphia: WB Saunders; 1997:298–299.
5. German J. Roberts syndrome 1. Cytological evidence for a disturbance in chromatid pairing. *Clin Genet.* 1979;16:441–447.
6. Robins DB, Ladda RL, Thieme GA, et al. Prenatal detection of Roberts–SC phocomelia syndrome: Report of 2 sibs with characteristic manifestations. *Am J Med Genet.* 1989;32:390–394.
7. Stioui S, Privitera O, Brambati B, et al. First-trimester prenatal diagnosis of Roberts syndrome. *Prenat Diagn.* 1992;12:145–149.
8. Palladini D, Palmieri S, Lecora M, et al. Prenatal ultrasound diagnosis of Roberts syndrome in a family with negative history. *Ultrasound Obstet Gynecol.* 1996;7:208–210.

ROBIN SEQUENCE

Definition. This syndrome is associated with micrognathia, glossoptosis, and a cleft palate.

Synonyms. Cleft palate–micrognathia–glossoptosis, Pierre Robin syndrome, and Robin anomalad.

Incidence. Uncommon.

Etiology. Autosomal recessive, with a few X-linked cases.

Diagnosis. It is easiest is to obtain a sagittal section of the face, in which the micrognathia is most visible. Another important clue is often the polyhydramnios resulting from the failure to swallow properly due to the macroretroglossia.[1,2]

Genetic Anomalies. Unknown (this is a heterogeneous group of conditions).

Differential Diagnosis. Agnathia–microstomia–synotia syndrome (otocephaly) resembles a severe form of Pierre–Robin syndrome. Other causes of micrognathia include trisomies 13 and 18.

Associated Anomalies. May be associated with trisomy 18, Stickler's syndrome, and other syndromes.

Prognosis. Upper airway obstruction, neonatal respiratory distress, and feeding problems.

Management. Termination of pregnancy can be offered before viability. Standard prenatal care is not altered when continuation of the pregnancy is decided. Confirmation of diagnosis after birth is important for genetic counseling.

REFERENCES

1. Pilu G, Romero R, Reece EA, et al. The prenatal diagnosis of Robin anomalad. *Am J Obstet Gynecol.* 1986;154:630–632.
2. Bromley B, Benacerraf BR. Fetal micrognathia: Associated anomalies and outcome. *J Ultrasound Med.* 1994;13:529–533.

SEPTO-OPTIC DYSPLASIA

Definition. Septo-optic dysplasia (SOD) is a syndrome characterized by anomalies of cerebral midline structures such as absence of the septum pellucidum, congenital optic nerve dysplasia, and panhypopituitarism, leading to multiple endocrine defects [diabetes insipidus, hypogonadotropic hypogonadism, hypothyroidism, adrenal insufficiency, abnormal thyrotropin releasing hormone (TRH) test, gonadotropin releasing hormone (GnRH) test, and GH releasing hormone (GHRH)]. Septo-optic dysplasia may represent a mild form of holoprosencephaly.

Synonyms. Morsier syndrome.

Incidence. Unknown but rare.

Etiology and Pathology. Although a vascular disruption sequence has been postulated[1–3] more recent genetic anomalies seem to explain the findings (see Genetic Anomalies). A possible Mendelian inheritance (autosomal recessive) also has been postulated.[4,5]

Diagnosis. Absence of the septum pellucidum is probably the most typical finding.[6] Hypotelorism, enlarged cerebral ventricles, communicating lateral ventricles, and bilateral cleft lip and palate have also been recognized prenatally.[7]

Genetic Anomalies. An Arg53Cys missense mutation was found in two children within the HESX1 homeodomain,

which destroyed its ability to bind target DNA. Mice deficient of the HESX1 homeobox gene present with neural defects similar to those of SOD.[8]

Differential Diagnosis. Several variants associated with schizencephaly, dysgenesis of the corpus callosum, microphthalmos, and incomplete forms have been described. Lobar holoprosencephaly may also resemble SOD.

Prognosis. The variable degree of mental deficiency (from minimal to severe) and the presence of multiple endocrine dysfunction will affect the prognosis for each infant. Prevention of hyperthermia (in case of fever), dehydration (fever and diabetes insipidus), and other endocrine dysfunctions should be sought and corrected.

Management. Termination of pregnancy can be offered before viability. Standard prenatal care is not altered when continuation of the pregnancy is decided. Confirmation of diagnosis after birth is important for genetic counseling.

REFERENCES

1. Brodsky MC. Hypothesis: Septo-optic dysplasia is a vascular disruption sequence. *Surv Ophthalmol.* 1998;42:489–490.
2. Lubinsky MS. Association of prenatal vascular disruptions with decreased maternal age. *Am J Med Genet.* 1997;69:237–239.
3. Lubinsky MS. Hypothesis: Septo-optic dysplasia is a vascular disruption sequence. *Am J Med Genet.* 1997;69:235–236.
4. Wales JK, Quarrell OW. Evidence for possible mendelian inheritance of septo-optic dysplasia. *Acta Paediatr.* 1996;85: 391–392.
5. Benner JD, Preslan MW, Gratz E, et al. Septo-optic dysplasia in two siblings. *Am J Ophthalmol.* 1990;109:632–637.
6. Schmidt-Riese U, Zieger M. Ultrasound diagnosis of isolated aplasia of the septum pellucidum. *Ultraschall Med.* 1994;15: 286–292.
7. Pilu G, Sandri F, Cerisoli M, et al. Sonographic findings in septo-optic dysplasia in the fetus and newborn infant. *Am J Perinatol.* 1990;7:337–339.
8. Dattani MT, Martinez-Barbera JP, Thomas PQ, et al. Mutations in the homeobox gene HESX1/Hesx1 associated with septo-optic dysplasia in human and mouse. *Nat Genet.* 1998;19:125–133.

SHORT RIB POLYDACTYLY SYNDROMES

Definition. Short rib polydactyly syndromes are lethal forms of skeletal dysplasia, characterized by thoracic hypoplasia, polydactyly, and shortening of the long bones. Three types of the disorder have been described: type I was described by Saldino and Noonan in 1972,[1] type II was described by Majewski et al. in 1971,[2] and type III was described by Naumoff et al. in 1977.[3] Clinical, radiographic, and morphologic studies suggest that types I and III represent phenotypic variations of the same disorder.

Incidence. Because of the rarity of the condition, the incidence is not precisely known. No sex preference has been observed.[4]

Etiology. The disorder has an autosomal recessive transmission; thus, the recurrence risk is 25%.[4]

Diagnosis. Prenatal diagnosis by ultrasound can be accomplished by finding the characteristic triad, which includes micromelic dwarfism, short and horizontal ribs with narrow thorax (what leads to hypoplasia of the lungs), and polydactyly.

Some typical features, more frequently seen after birth, differentiate type I from type II. *Type I* (Saldino–Noonan) presents with short stature, postaxial polydactyly of hands or feet, syndactyly, underossified phalanges, notchlike ossification defect of vertebral bodies, small iliac bones, and triangular ossification defects above the acetabulum. Cardiac, gastrointestinal, and urogenital malformations can also be found. Occasionally, preaxial polydactyly and sex reversal (46,XY with female phenotype) can occur.[5] *Type II* (Majewski) presents with short stature with extremely short limbs, midline cleft lip, cleft palate, short flat nose, low-set and malformed ears, preaxial and postaxial polysyndactyly of hands and feet, premature ossification of proximal epiphyses of the femur, humerus, and lateral cuboids, underossified phalanges, high clavicles, and ambiguous genitalia. Less frequently, hydrops and polyhydramnios can also be found.[6]

Genetic Anomalies. Probable gene anomaly of either 4q13 or 4p16.

Differntial Diagnosis. The differential diagnosis includes all skeletal dysplasias associated with micromelia and short ribs such as thanatophoric dwarfism, chondrodysplasia punctata, osteogenesis imperfecta, and camptomelic dysplasia.[7] Orofacial-digital syndrome type II is another differential diagnosis of the Majewski type.[6] Most of these conditions are excluded only after birth, by radiographic and morphologic studies.

Prognosis. Short rib polydactyly syndromes are lethal conditions. Affected neonates usually die few hours after birth from respiratory insufficiency, due to severe pulmonary hypoplasia.[5,6]

Management. Termination of pregnancy can be offered before viability. Standard prenatal care is not changed when continuing the pregnancy is decided. Confirmation of diagnosis after birth is important for genetic counseling.

REFERENCES

1. Saldino RM, Noonan CD. Severe thoracic dystrophy with striking micromelia, abnormal osseous development, including the spine, and multiple visceral anomalies. *AJR.* 1972;114:257–263.
2. Majewski F, Pfeiffer RA, Lenz W, et al. Polydactyly, short limbs, and genital malformations—A new syndrome? *Z Kinderheilkd.* 1971;111:118–138.
3. Naumoff P, Young LW, Maser J, Amortegui AJ. Short rib polydactyly syndrome type 3. *Radiology.* 1977;122:443–447.
4. Meng HW, Pao LK, Shio JL. Prenatal diagnosis of recurrence of short rib polydactyly syndrome. *Am J Med Genet.* 1995;55:279–284.
5. Jones KL. Short rib polydactyly syndrome type I (Saldino-Noonan type). In: Jones KL, ed. *Smith's Recognizable Patterns of Human Malformation,* 5th ed. Philadelphia: WB Saunders; 1997.
6. Jones KL. Short rib polydactyly syndrome type II (Majewski type). In: Jones KL, ed. *Smith's Recognizable Patterns of Human Malformation,* 5th ed. Philadelphia: WB Saunders; 1997.
7. Gembruch U, Hansmann M, Fodisch HJ. Early prenatal diagnosis of short rib polydactyly (SRP) syndrome type I (Majewski) by ultrasound in a case at risk. *Prenat Diagn.* 1985;5:357–362.

SIRENOMELIA

Definition. This is a congenital anomaly, caused by a disruptive vascular defect, characterized by fusion of the lower extremities, associated with renal agenesis, absence of the sacrum, rectum, and bladder. It was previously considered to represent a severe form of caudal regression syndrome.

Synonyms. Mermaid syndrome and sirenomelia sequence.

Etiology. Although the etiology is unknown, sirenomelia is not thought to be hereditary.

Recurrence Risk. Unknown.

Diagnosis. The diagnosis of sirenomelia is based on the presence of fusion of the lower extremities (Fig. 21–74), associated with other skeletal and lumbar spine deformities, bilateral renal agenesis (which leads to severe oligohydramnios and lungs hypoplasia), and heart and abdominal wall defects.[1,2] The defect varies from simple cutaneous fusion of the limbs to absence of all long bones but one femur. The defect of the feet is proportional with the defect of the long bones, with cutaneous defect commonly presenting with a double fused foot with 10 toes and more a severe defect presenting with a more rudimentary foot and ectromelia. Because the legs are fused, the rotation of the legs does not occur and they remain in their fetal position. Thus, the fibulae, when present, are between the tibia and the sole of the foot, which is oriented "ventrally" instead of "dorsally."

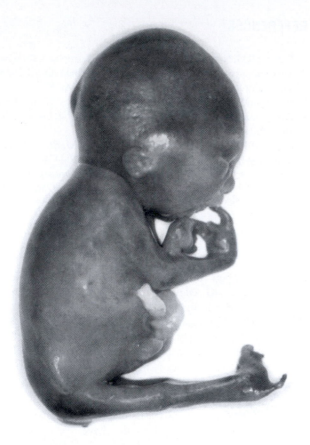

Figure 21–74. The fetal extremity and the flipperlike deformity of the foot are characteristic of sirenomelia.

Pathogenesis. An alteration in early vascular development leads to a "vitelline arterial steal" in which blood flow is diverted from the caudal region of the embryo to the placenta, resulting in multiple defects of the lower extremities.[3] Many of these fetuses have an aberrant vasculature, with the umbilical arteries connected to the old viteline arteries (the superior mesenteric arteries).

Genetic Anomaly. Unknown.

Associated Anomalies. Cardiac, renal, abdominal wall, chest, and lower spine defects are frequently seen. Single umbilical artery, imperforate anus, and absence of the genitals are commonly found.

Differential Diagnosis. Caudal regression syndrome is the main differential diagnosis, and it usually presents with deformities milder than sirenomelia and normal amniotic fluid volume. Due to the bilateral renal agenesis, fetuses affected by sirenomela frequently have Potter facies. The fusion of the lower extremities, present in sirenomelia, establishes the differential diagnosis. Other conditions that should be excluded are Fraser's and VATER syndromes.[1]

Prognosis. This is a lethal condition because of the associated renal agenesis and its complications. Exceptional cases present without renal agenesis and may survive.

Management. Termination of pregnancy can be offered before viability. Standard prenatal care is not altered throughout the pregnancy if continuation is decided.

REFERENCES

1. Benacerraf BR. Caudal regression syndrome and sirenomelia. In: Benacerraf BR, ed. *Ultrasound of Fetal Syndromes*. New York: Churchill Livingstone; 1998;250–254.
2. Jones KL. Sirenomelia sequence. In: Jones KL, ed. *Smith's Recognizable Patterns of Human Malformation*. Philadelphia: WB Saunders; 1998:634.
3. Stevenson RE, Jones KL, Phelan MC, et al. Vascular steal: The pathogenic mechanism producing sirenomelia and associated defects of the viscera and soft tissues. *Pediatrics*. 1986;78:451–457.

THANATOPHORIC DYSPLASIA

Definition. Thanatophoric dysplasia is a lethal congenital form of short-limbed chondrodysplasia and is divided into two subtypes.[1]

- *Type I* is characterized by extreme rhizomelia, bowed long bones, narrow thorax, a relatively large head, normal trunk length, and absent cloverleaf skull. The spine shows platyspondyly, the cranium has a short base, and, frequently, the foramen magnum is decreased in size. The forehead is prominent, and hypertelorism and a saddle nose may be present. Hands and feet are normal, but fingers are short.
- *Type II* is characterized by short, straight long bones and cloverleaf skull.[2]

Synonyms. Thanatophoric dwarfism.

Incidence. Every 0.69 per 10,000 births; the male-to-female ratio is 2 to 1.[3]

Etiology. Possibly autosomal dominant but the majority of cases results from new mutations of FGFR3.[4]

Recurrence Risk. A general empiric risk has been estimated as 2%.[5]

Diagnosis. The sonographic diagnosis can be made in the presence of short-limbed dwarfism (Fig. 21–75), hypoplastic thorax (Fig. 21–76), cloverleaf skull, frontal bossing (Fig. 21–77), and simian crease. Femur bowing, narrow thorax, large head size even without ventriculomegaly, and redundant soft tissues are features that become more

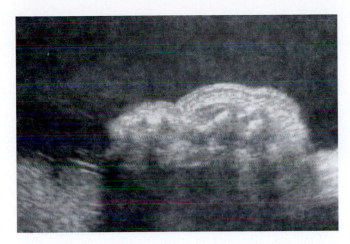

Figure 21–75. A very short arm with redundant soft tissue. The hand *(left)* is about as wide as the forearm.

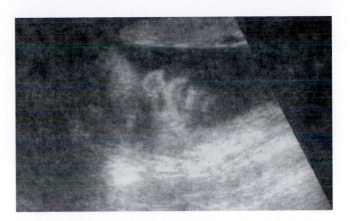

Figure 21–77. Frontal bossing.

pronounced with advancing gestation but may not be present in midtrimester. In 70% of cases, thanatophoric dysplasia is associated with polyhydramnios, which may be massive and lead to premature labor. Fetal movements do not seem to be affected by the disease, but a decrease in motion during the third trimester has been reported. Decreased hand flexure is probably responsible for the presence of simian crease. In the absence of cloverleaf skull, the disease should be suspected when severe rhizomelic dwarfism and a narrow thorax are detected.[1] Sonographic measurement of fetal femur length, especially when correlated with biparietal diameter, is a reliable method in the identification of certain forms of short-limbed skeletal dysplasias and of thanatophoric dysplasia.[6]

Pathogenesis. Characteristic generalized disruption of growth plate with persistent mesenchymal-like tissue.[7]

Associated Anomalies. Cloverleaf skull (just in type II), horseshoe kidney, hydronephrosis, atrial septal defect, defective tricuspid valve, imperforate anus, and radioulnar synostosis.

Differential Diagnosis. Chondroectodermal dysplasia (Ellis–van Creveld syndrome), asphyxiating thoracic dysplasia, short rib polydactyly syndromes, and homozygous achondroplasia.[3] All short-limbed dwarfism should be considered. If type II is suspected, conditions that have association with craniosynostosis and cloverleaf skull should be excluded (Apert, Crouzon, Pfeiffer, Carpenter, and Kleeblattschadel syndromes).

Prognosis. This is a uniformly lethal condition and in general the affected die shortly after birth.[3,7] The cause of death is respiratory failure due to hypoplastic lungs.

Management. The option of pregnancy termination should be offered before viability. Sonographic evaluation of hydrocephalus is recommended, considering that it may cause malpresentation and difficult delivery. If massive hydrocephalus is developed, cephalocentesis or elective cesarean section should be considered to avoid maternal trauma.[1]

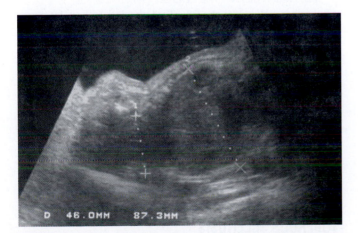

Figure 21–76. The chest is small compared with the abdomen; its diameter is approximately as large as the abdomen. This results from the short ribs and is the cause of pulmonary hypoplasia.

REFERENCES

1. Norris CD, Tiller G, Jeanty P, Malini S. Thanatophoric dysplasia in monozygotic twins. *Fetus.* 1994;4:27–32.
2. Fleischer AC, Romero R, Manning FA, et al. *The Principles and Practice of Ultrasonography in Obstetrics and Gynecology,* 5th ed. Norwalk, CT: Appleton & Lange; 1995:295–297.
3. Romero R, Pilu GL, Jeanty P. *Prenatal Diagnosis of Congenital Anomalies.* Norwalk, CT: Appleton & Lange; 1988:335–339.
4. Tavormina PL, Shiang R, Thompson LM, et al. Thanatophoric dysplasia (types I and II) caused by distinct mutations in fibroblast growth factor receptor 3. *Nat Genet.* 1995;9:321–328.

5. Chemke J, Graff G, Lancet M. Familial thanatophoric dwarfism. *Lancet.* 1971;1:1358.

6. Burrows PE, Stannard MW, Pearrow J, et al. Early antenatal sonographic recognition of thanatophoric dysplasia with clover-leaf skull deformity. *AJR.* 1984;143:841–843.

7. Buyse ML. *Birth Defects Encyclopedia.* Cambridge; MA: Blackwell Scientific Medical Publications; 1990:1661–1662.

THROMBOCYTOPENIA–ABSENT RADIUS SYNDROMES

Definition. This congenital disorder was described by Gross et al. in 1956[1] and is characterized by bilateral radial aplasia with normal thumbs and thrombocytopenia at a level lower than 100,000 per microliter.

Synonyms. TAR syndrome, megakaryocytopenia-absent radius, and radial aplasia–thrombocytopenia syndrome.

Incidence. Uncommon.

Etiology. Autosomal recessive disorder.

Recurrence Risk. The recurrence risk is 25%.

Diagnosis. The major finding is that of bilateral club hand due to the missing radii. In some cases, the abnormal position of the hands has been detected in the first trimester.[2] A fetal blood sampling is performed to assess the level of platelets and the number of megakaryocytes.[3,4] When cardiac and renal anomalies are present, oligohydramnios may develop during the second trimester, making the evaluation of the limbs more difficult. In such a case, both amnioinfusion and fetoscopy have been proposed.[5]

Genetic Anomalies. Not known. Radial ray aplasia may result from chromosomal, teratogenic, genetic, and multifactorial causes.

Differential Diagnosis. The most common differential diagnoses include trisomy 18 and Holt–Oram syndrome. Other differential diagnoses include other limb reduction abnormalities, in particular those that may present associated thrombocytopenia (Fanconi's pancytopenia: usually presents with aplasia of the thumbs and chromosome fragility, Roberts–SC syndrome: usually presents with cleft lip and palate and premature separation of centromeric heterochromatin; Aase's syndrome: usually present in mild forms of skeletal deformities).[6]

Associated Anomalies. The following anomalies may be incidentally associated with thrombocytopenia–absent radius: anemia, eosinophilia, and skeletal defects of upper and lower extremities such as ulnar, humeral, and femoral hypoplasia, congenital hip dislocation, toe syndactyly, talipes equino-varus, and genu varum.[7] Cardiac (30% of cases) and renal defects may be found. An increased susceptibility to infections is also observed.

Prognosis. Forty percent of affected infants die during early infancy.[8] Hemorrhage and heart disease are the main causes of death. Seven percent have mental impairment. Motor and developmental retardation is expected because of the skeletal defects. Hematologic profile improves with age.[6] The prognosis improves after the first year of life.

Management. Termination of pregnancy can be offered before viability. The infusion of platelets has been advocated before delivery to prevent hemorrhage during delivery.[9] Postnatal transplantation of allogeneic bone marrow from a histocompatible sibling may correct a persistently low platelet count.[10]

REFERENCES

1. Gross H, Groh C, Weippl G. Congenitale hypoplastische thrombopenie mit radialaplasie. *Neue Osterr Z Kinderheilkd.* 1956;1:574.

2. Boute O, Depret-Mosser S, Vinatier D, et al. Prenatal diagnosis of thrombocytopenia-absent radius syndrome. *Fetal Diagn Ther.* 1996;11:224–230.

3. Ergur Ar, Yergok YZ, Ertekin A, et al. Prenatal diagnosis of an uncommon syndrome: Thrombocytopenia absent radius (TAR). *Zentralbl Gynakol.* 1998;120:75–78.

4. Donnenfeld AE, Wiseman B, Lavi E, Weiner S. Prenatal diagnosis of thrombocytopenia absent radius syndrome by ultrasound and cordocentesis. *Prenat Diagn.* 1990;10:29–35.

5. Filkins K, Russo J, Bilinki I, et al. Prenatal diagnosis of thrombocytopenia absent radius syndrome using ultrasound and fetoscopy. *Prenat Diagn.* 1984;4:139–142.

6. Donnenfeld AE, Wiseman B, Lavi E, Weiner S. Prenatal diagnosis of thrombocytopenia absent radius syndrome by ultrasound and cordocentesis. *Prenat Diagn.* 1990;10:29–35.

7. Hedberg VA, Lipton JM. Thrombocytopenia with absent radii. A review of 100 cases. *Am J Pediatr Hematol Oncol.* 1988;10:51–64.

8. Jones KL. Radial aplasia–thrombocytopenia syndrome. In: Jones KL, ed. *Smith's Recognizable Patterns of Human Malformation.* Philadelphia: WB Saunders; 1998;322–323.

9. Weinblatt M, Petrikovsky B, Bialer M, et al. Prenatal evaluation and in utero platelet transfusion for thrombocytopenia absent radii syndrome. *Prenat Diagn.* 1994;14:892–896.

10. Brochstein JA, Shank B, Kernan NA, et al. Marrow transplantation for thrombocytopenia–absent radii syndrome. *J Pediatr.* 1992;121:587–589.

TUBEROUS SCLEROSIS

Definition. This syndrome is associated with facial angiofibroma (often incorrectly called *adenoma sebaceum*), epilepsy,

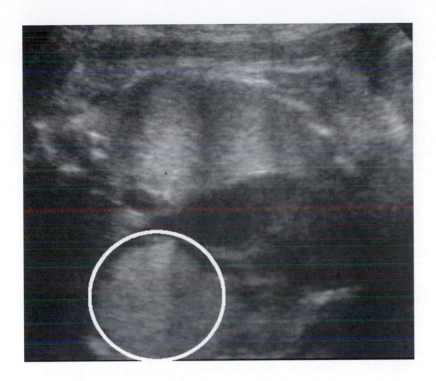

Figure 21–78. The typical café-au-lait spot of tuberous sclerosis.

mental retardation, renal cysts, multiple and bilateral angiofibroma of the kidney,[1] and rhabdomyoma of the heart. Diverse cutaneous manifestation such as hypochromic patches (visible under Wood light) and "café au lait" patches (light brown areas; Fig. 21–78) are also typical of the syndrome.[2] Brain tumors such as ependymoma of the third ventricle and astrocytoma may also be present.

Synonyms. Bourneville's sclerosis.

Incidence. From 0.3 to 1 per 10,000 births.[3]

Etiology. Autosomal dominant inheritance, with a large proportion of fresh mutations (sporadic cases). The expression is highly variable.

Recurrence Risk. Low in cases of new mutation, higher in cases of gonadal mosaicism, and 50% in cases of parental involvement.

Diagnosis. The diagnosis is usually suggested by the discovery of cardiac tumors[4] (Fig. 21–79) that resemble small uterine fibroids (round usually well-delineated homogeneous

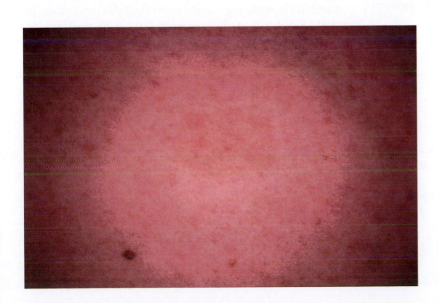

Figure 21–79. A large rhabdomyoma.

masses). Between 51 and 86% of cardiac rhabdomyomas are associated with tuberous sclerosis.[5] Occasionally, the finding of a rhabdo during routine second-trimester ultrasound examination may lead to the recognition that the mother is affected (this was the case in the patient in Fig. 21–78 when the lesion shown in Fig. 21–79 was recognized).[6] Cardiac rhabdomyomata increase prenatally, may regress in early infancy, remain unchanged during childhood, and regress in adolescence.[7] The rhabdos may cause rhythm disruptions (Wolff-Parkinson-White syndrome, supraventricular tachycardia, and paroxysmal arrhythmias) and obstructions or regurgitation. Renal angiofibromas have not been recognized prenatally, although this may simply be a matter of time. Some recent unpublished reports have demonstrated that the periventricular subependymal nodules may also be detected.[8]

Pathogenesis. There is an abnormal gene code for abnormal hamartin and tuberin, proteins that may have a role in the metabolism of GTP.

Genetic Anomaly. Two loci exist for tuberous sclerosis: one on chromosome 9q and the other elsewhere, perhaps on 11q.[9,10]

Associated Anomalies. See Definition.

Differential Diagnosis. The predominant prenatal finding is that of the rhabdos. Other cardiac tumors such as fibroma should also be considered.

Prognosis. When no hydrops result from the presence of the rhabdos, the prognosis depends on the other complications of the disorder. Because of the great variability of expression, an accurate prediction of the status of the child is difficult to infer from the status of the parent. Further, new genetic evidence seems to indicate that the mental prognosis changes with the locus of the defective gene, which may influence the decision about the pregnancy in the future.

Management. Termination of the pregnancy may be offered before viability.

REFERENCES

1. Cook JA, Oliver K, Mueller RF, Sampson J. A cross sectional study of renal involvement in tuberous sclerosis. *J Med Genet.* 1996;33:480–484.
2. Webb DW, Clarke A, Fryer A, Osborne JP. The cutaneous features of tuberous sclerosis: A population study. *Br J Dermatol.* 1996;135:1–5.
3. Hunt A, Lindenbaum RH. Tuberous sclerosis: A new estimate of prevalence within the Oxford region. *J Med Genet.* 1984;21:272–277.
4. Gushiken BJ, Callen PW, Silverman NH. Prenatal diagnosis of

tuberous sclerosis in monozygotic twins with cardiac masses. *J Ultrasound Med.* 1999;18:165–168.
5. Harding CO, Pagon RA. Incidence of tuberous sclerosis in patients with cardiac rhabdomyoma. *Am J Med Genet.* 1990;37:443–446.
6. Journel H, Roussey M, Plais MH, et al. Prenatal diagnosis of familial tuberous sclerosis following detection of cardiac rhabdomyoma by ultrasound. *Prenatal Diag.* 1986;6:283–289.
7. Smith HC, Watson GH, Patel RG, Super M. Cardiac rhabdomyomata in tuberous sclerosis: Their course and diagnostic value. *Arch Dis Child.* 1989;64:196–200.
8. Euroson Tours, 1998.
9. Northrup H, Kwiatkowski DJ, Roach ES, et al. Evidence for genetic heterogeneity in tuberous sclerosis: One locus on chromosome 9 and at least one locus elsewhere. *Am J Hum Genet.* 1992;51:709–720.
10. Haines JL, Short MP, Kwiatkowski DJ, et al. Localization of one gene for tuberous sclerosis within 9q32–9q34, and further evidence for heterogeneity. *Am J Hum Genet.* 1991;49:764–772.

TURNER'S (MONOSOMY X) SYNDROME

Definition. This chromosomal disorder of female patients was described by Turner in 1938[1] and is characterized by the absence of one X chromosome (45,X0).

Synonym. Monosomy X and Ullrich–Turner syndrome.[2]

Incidence. From 2.5 to 5.5 per 10,000 liveborn females in the Caucasian population. In the Japanese population, it has been estimated to be between 7 and 21 per 10,000 liveborn females.[3] The incidence in all pregnancies, however, is considered much higher because Turner's syndrome accounts for one-fourth of the spontaneous abortions caused by chromosomal anomalies.[4]

Etiology. Absence of one sex chromosome, in general the paternal chromosome, occurs sporadically in most cases; between 8 and 16% of all cases are mosaic. Advanced maternal age is not associated with this aneuploidy.

Recurrence Risk. Considering that Turner's syndrome is a sporadic event in the majority of the cases, chances of recurrence are extremely low, although not precisely known.

Diagnosis. Cystic hygroma is the most characteristic prenatal feature in this syndrome. In general, the finding is consistent with a large septated cystic mass posterior to the neck (Fig. 21–80A and B), connections of the lymphatic circulation. Spontaneous remission of the cyst may occur, resulting, in many cases, in webbing of the neck. Other common findings include lymphedema, in particular of the dorsum of hands and feet, or, in the more severe cases, anasarca, hydrops, short cervical spine, IUGR, short neck, prominent auricles, horseshoe kidney, heart defects (coarctation and

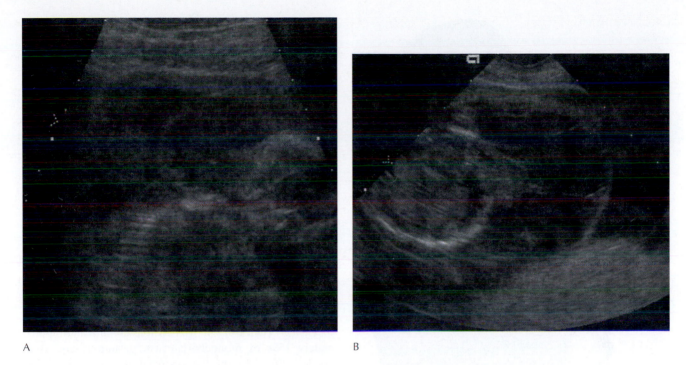

A   B

Figure 21–80. Sagittal **(A)** and axial **(B)** views of the neck demonstrate large septated masses.

bicuspid aortic valve), bone dysplasia, and short stature (Fig. 21–81). Dysgenesis of the ovaries occurs in 90% of cases, causing absent menses and infertility in adult life. Variable degrees of mental and developmental retardation are also frequently seen.[5] Elevated maternal serum beta-hCG has been reported in association with Turner's syndrome.[6]

Differential Diagnosis. Head and neck cystic masses such as cephalocele and meningocele must be excluded. Usually these conditions are associated with hydrocephalus, cranial, and spine defects. Often the angle of junction of the cystic mass with skin can be used in the differential diagnosis. Cystic hygromas that lift the subcutaneous tissues tend to have smooth junction angle, whereas cephaloceles that herniate through the skin tend to have acute angle of junction. Cystic hygroma may occasionally be present in Robert's syndrome and other autosomal recessive disorders.[2,7] Chromosomal analysis can exclude these conditions.

Genetic Anomaly. Absence or structural abnormalities of one X chromosome, such as deletion of the sex-determining region (XY Yp deletion) or mosaicism (45,X/46,XX or 45X/46XY), can also be responsible for this condition.[3]

Prognosis. Intrauterine demise occurs in many cases, in general caused by hydrops, which is the major intrauterine complication. Among survivors, the prognosis will depend ba-

sically on the severity of the associated anomalies. Mosaics tend to have a better prognosis, and some cases with discrete manifestations the syndrome remains undiagnosed for years.[8]

Management. A karyotype is recommended when Turner's syndrome is suspected. Termination of pregnancy can be offered before viability. After viability, standard prenatal care is not altered.

REFERENCES

1. Turner HH. A syndrome of infantilism, congenital webbed neck, and cubitus valgus. *Endocrinology.* 1938;23:566.
2. Blagowidow N, Page DC, Huff D, Mennuti MT. Ullrich–Turner syndrome in an XY female fetus with deletion of the sex-determining portion of the Y chromosome. *Am J Med Genet.* 1989;34:159–162.
3. Gravholr CH, Juul S, Naeraa RW, Hansen J. Prenatal and postnatal prevalence of Turner's syndrome: A registry study. *B Med J.* 1996;312:16–21.
4. Robinow M, Spisso K, Buschi AJ, Brenbridge ANAG. Turner syndrome: Sonography showing fetal hydrops simulating hydramnios. *AJR.* 1980;135:846–848.
5. Jones KL. X0 syndrome (Turner syndrome). In: Jones KL, ed. *Smith's Recognizable Patterns of Human Malformation.* Philadelphia: WB Saunders; 1997:81–87.

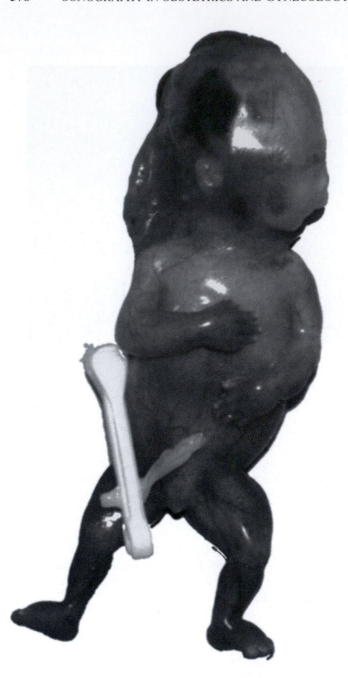

Figure 21–81. The fetus at autopsy.

6. Laundon CH, Spencer K, Macri JN, et al. Free beta hCG screening of hydropic and non-hydropic Turner syndrome pregnancies. *Prenat Diagn*. 1996;16:853–856.

7. Brown BSJ, Thompson DL. Ultrasonographic features of the fetal Turner syndrome. *J Can Assoc Radiol*. 1984;35:40–46.

8. Koeberl DD, McGillivray B, Sybert VP. Prenatal diagnosis of 45,X/46XX mosaicism and 45,X: Implications for postnatal outcome. *Am J Hum Genet*. 1995;57:661–666.

TWIN-TO-TWIN TRANSFUSION SYNDROME

Definition. Twin-to-twin transfusion syndrome is a congenital entity unique to monochorionic diamniotic twin pregnancies and is characterized by an imbalanced blood exchange between the twins' circulation, which occurs through interplacental anastomosis, and may cause fetal compromise, from growth discordance to death of both fetuses. The syndrome was first described by Schatz in 1875.[1]

Synonym. Stuck twin.

Etiology. Vascular anastomosis.

Recurrence Risk. Unknown, but very low, considering the small chance of developing a second monochorionic–diamniotic twin pregnancy.

Incidence. Twin-to-twin transfusion complicates approximately 15% of monochorial twin gestations and is responsible for 17% of the perinatal mortality in multiple pregnancies.

Diagnosis. Ultrasonographic criteria for the diagnosis of twin-to-twin transfusion syndrome include monochorionic placentation, with visualization of a separating membrane, fetus of the same sex, midpregnancy polyhydramnios–oligohydramnios sequence (polyhydramnios at the recipient's sac and oligohydramnios at the donor's sac), in the absence of other causes of abnormal amniotic fluid volume, and marked growth discordance.[2] Significant weight discordance is considered a difference of 20% or more between the twins' sizes. Other findings that may be observed include nonvisualization of the donor's bladder with enlarged recipient's bladder, abnormal Doppler systole/diastole (S/D) ratio at the umbilical cord, hydrops, or evidence of congestive heart failure of either twin (more commonly found in the recipient twin). Milder forms of the disease are more difficult to diagnose because of the lack of uniform criteria; however, one should suspect twin-to-twin transfusion in the presence of amniotic fluid discrepancy between the cavities.

Pathogenesis. If embryonic splitting occurs before day 3 after fertilization, two independent fetuses with separate placentas will result. A single placenta with two amniotic cavities occurs if splitting takes place between days 4 and 7. If division of the embryoblast occurs after about 8 days, the twins share a single placenta and amniotic cavity (monochorionic–monoamniotic twins). Division beyond day 12 results in conjoint twins. When two fetuses share the same placenta, vascular anastomoses develop between their circulation systems. These anastomoses can be of three types: vein to vein, artery to artery, and artery to vein. Even when there are multiple vascular connections within a single placenta, no transfusion should occur, provided the anastomoses are balanced.

Placentas from pregnancies with twin-to-twin transfusion syndrome have fewer anastomoses, which are more likely to be solitary and of the deep arteriovenous type than those without twin-to-twin transfusion syndrome. Provided transfusion occurs, the donor, or "pump," twin becomes hypovolemic due to blood loss. Hypoxia develops because of placental insufficiency, which is also responsible for IUGR. Poor renal perfusion leads to oligohydramnios. This latter feature, when severe, is responsible for the classic appearance of the stuck twin: the amniotic sac becomes too small, the amniotic membrane comes in close contact with the body of the "pump" twin, and the fetus appears trapped to the uterine wall. Hypervolemia with increased renal perfusion leads to polyhydramnios in the sac of the recipient twin. Because there is no loss of protein or cellular components from its circulation, colloid osmotic pressure draws water from the maternal compartment across the placenta, establishing a vicious cycle of hypervolemia, polyuria, and hyperosmolarity, leading to high output cardiac failure, hydrops, and polyhydramnios.

In the most severe forms, the diagnosis should not be difficult: a single placenta, massive polyhydramnios in the sac of the recipient twin, a stuck donor twin attached to the uterine wall with poor mobility, and obvious growth discordance. Milder forms of the disease are more difficult to diagnose because of the lack of uniform criteria; however, one should suspect twin-to-twin transfusion in the presence of amniotic fluid discrepancy between the cavities, regardless of the amount of weight discordance between the twins. An intertwin hemoglobin difference greater than 2.4g/dL in fetal blood obtained by cordocentesis has been shown to be consistent with stuck twin syndrome.

Associated Anomalies. The overdistention of the uterus caused by the polyhydramnios can causes preterm labor, amniorrhexis, abruptio placentae, and respiratory and abdominal discomfort. Death of one twin can cause embolic phenomena (twin embolization syndrome) and coagulation problems in the remaining twin, and sequelae such as neurologic, cardiac, and renal diseases are common among survivors.

Differential Diagnosis. Differential diagnosis should be mainly concerned with twins of discordant size without transfusion as the underlying pathophysiologic mechanism for the problem. Some investigators have proposed a new entity called *twin oligohydramnios–polyhydramnios sequence,* in which twin-to-twin transfusion is included.[3] Histopathologic studies of the placenta are required to differentiate twin-to-twin transfusion from the other conditions included in twin oligohydramnios–polyhydramnios sequence. Isolated IUGR can be considered if the growth discrepancy is minimal (less than 15%) and the other features of the syndrome are not present. Dichorionic twin pregnancy with fused placentas and growth restriction of one of the fetuses is another condition that can lead to misdiagnosis. This can be excluded if the twins have different sexes or, after birth, by histopathologic analysis of the placenta.

Prognosis. When the disease manifests during the second trimester, there is a higher risk of perinatal morbidity and mortality. Intrauterine hypoxia, preterm delivery, and death of one fetus (usually the donor) with subsequent death or hypoxic-ischemic sequelae (see twin embolization syndrome, above) in the surviving twin are the most common complications to watch for in these pregnancies. The absent end diastolic flow in the donor's umbilical artery accompanied by venous pulsation in the recipient's umbilical vein are usually associated with a poor prognosis. Hydrops or evidence of congestive heart failure of either twin are also associated with ominous prognosis. These signs are found more commonly in the recipient twin.

Management. Although efficacy of the therapies available is still controversial, the elevated mortalitility rate (which can be as high as 100%) when expectant management is decided imposes the necessity of invasive therapy. Treatment includes serial amniocentesis to drain polyhydramnios in the sac of the recipient twin[4] and, more recently, ablation of communicating vessels on the placental surface by neodimium: YAG laser guided by fetoscopy[5] and umbilical cord ligation.[6] Intensive monitoring with weekly nonstress test, alternating with biophysical profiles is recommended from the time of diagnosis to delivery.

REFERENCES

1. Schatz F. *Arch Gynaekol.* 1875;7:336.
2. Wittmann BK, Baldwin VJ, Nichol B. Antenatal diagnosis of twin transfusion syndrome by ultrasound. *Obstet Gynecol.* 1981;58:123–127.
3. Bruner JP, Anderson TL, Rosemono RL, et al. Placental pathophysiology of the twin oligohydramnios-polyhydramnios sequence and the twin–twin transfusion syndrome. *Placenta.* 1998;19:81–86.
4. Saunders NJ, Snijders RJM, Nicolaides KH. Therapeutic amniocantesis in twin–twin transfusion syndrome appearing in the second trimester of pregnancy. *Am J Obstet Gynecol.* 1992:820–824.
5. De Lia JE, Cruikshank DP, Keye WR. Fetoscopic neodymium: YAG laser occlusion of placental vessels in severe twin–twin transfusion syndrome. *Obstet Gynecol.* 1990;75:1046–1053.
6. Quintero RA, Romero R, Reich H, et al. In utero percutaneous umbilical cord ligation in the management of complicated monochorionic multiple gestations. *Ultrasound Obstet Gynecol.* 1996;8:16–22.

VACTERL ASSOCIATION

Definition. VACTERL is an acronym for a nonrandom association of malformations including *v*ertebral anomalies, *a*nal atresia, *c*ardiac anomalies, *t*racheoesophageal fistula or *e*sophageal atresia, *r*enal and urinary anomalies, and *l*imb defect. Three of the anomalies must be present to recognize the syndrome, but 7 to 8 are not uncommon.[1,2]

Synonyms. VATER sequence, VATER association, and VACTERL syndrome.

Incidence. Uncommon; approximately 300 cases have been reported.

Etiology. Sporadic. Although VACTERL syndrome occurs as a sporadic event in the majority of cases, a high frequency among offspring of diabetic mothers has been observed.[3]

Recurrence Risk. Varies from 1 to 50%.

Pathogenesis. Defective mesodermal development of unknown origin, possibly a mitochondrial disorder.[4]

Diagnosis. The association of vertebral anomalies [in particular at the lumbosacral level; (Fig. 21–82)] and renal, heart, and radial defects constitute the classic manifestations of VACTERL syndrome. It is well known, however, that some affected fetuses will not present all typical findings.[5] The diagnosis can also be suspected because of polyhydramnios in the presence of a small or absent fetal stomach (the tracheoesophageal fistula) hemivertebrae or scoliosis, limb (and in particular radius anomalies, club hand, reduction defects, and polydactylies), and renal and cardiac defects. The presence of supernumary rib (13 and 14 pairs thoracic, 6 to 7 lumbar) may be recognized especially with three-dimensional rendering. The ultrasound diagnosis of VACTERL syndrome may be accomplished early in the second trimester, if the fetus is severely affected.[5]

Genetic Anomalies. Unknown.

Differential Diagnosis. Nearly half of patients with tracheoesophageal fistula will exhibit other VACTERL malformations.[6] Towne's syndrome has many similar features. Because VACTERL syndrome is constituted by anomalies of multiple systems, chromosomal disorders such as trisomies 18 and 13 must be excluded by karyotype study. Disorders characterized by the presence of vertebral, renal, or radial defects (such as TAR syndrome, Fanconi's anemia, Roberts's syndrome, Holt–Oram syndrome, Nager's syndrome, caudal regression syndrome, sirenomelia, MURCS association, electrodactyly–ectodermal dysplasia syndrome, and Jarcho–Levin syndrome) should be considered.[5]

Associated Anomalies. Numerous. Hydrocephalus is commonly associated.[7]

Prognosis. Overall poor, but depends on the particular association of anomalies.

Management. Termination of pregnancy can be offered before viability. Monthly sonographic monitoring of fetal growth and evaluation of the structural defects are recommended. Delivery in a tertiary center is required for prompt surgical repair and rehabilitation.

Figure 21–82. The presence of a hemivertebra should raise the possibility of VACTERL association.

REFERENCES

1. Khoury MJ, Cordero JF, Greenberg F, et al. A population study of the VACTERL association: Evidence for its etiologic heterogeneity. *Pediatrics.* 1983;71:815–820.
2. Rittler M, Paz JE, Castilla EE. VACTERL association, epidemiologic definition and delineation. *Am J Med Genet.* 1996; 63:529–536.
3. Jones KL. Vater association. In: Jones KL, ed. *Smith's Recognizable Patterns of Human Malformation.* Philadelphia: WB Saunders; 1998:664–665.
4. Damian MS, Seibel P, Schachenmayr W, et al. VACTERL with the mitochondrial np 3243 point mutation. *Am J Med Genet.* 1996;62:398–403.
5. Benacerraf BR. VATER association. In: Benacerraf BR, ed. *Ultrasound of Fetal Syndromes.* New York: Churchill Livingstone; 1998:285–287.
6. McMullen KP, Karnes PS, Moir CR, Michels VV. Familial recurrence of tracheoesophageal fistula and associated malformations. *Am J Med Genet.* 1996;63:525–528.

7. Froster UG, Wallner SJ, Reusche E, et al. VACTERL with hydrocephalus and branchial arch defects: Prenatal, clinical, and autopsy findings in two brothers. *Am J Med Genet.* 1996;62: 169–172.

WALKER–WARBURG SYNDROME

Definition. Walker–Walburg syndrome is a genetic disorder characterized by retinal detachment, cataract, microophthalmia, muscle and skeletal, and CNS anomalies (hydrocephalus, lissencephaly, cephalocele) associated with mental retardation. It was first reported by Walker in 1942[1] and reviewed by Warburg in 1971.[2]

Synonyms. Lissencephaly type II, HARDE syndrome (hydrocephalus, agyria, retinal dysplasia, and encephalocele), muscle–eye–brain disease, cerebro-oculo-muscular syndrome, cerebrocular dysplasia and muscular dystrophy, Walburg's syndrome, Walker's lissencephaly, encephalophthalmic dysplasia, and oculocerebral malformation.[3,4]

Incidence. Unknown.

Etiology. Autosomal recessive.[5]

Recurrence Risk. The recurrence risk for couples with previously affected children is 25%.

Diagnosis. Dobyns et al. reviewed 63 cases in 1989 and established the diagnostic criteria, which include type II lissencephaly, cerebellar malformations, retinal malformation (in general retinal nonattachment), and congenital muscular dystrophy.[4] Congenital muscular dystrophy is present in 100% of cases. However, a wide variability of eyes and cerebral manifestation has been reported, in addition to the main anomalies, including microphthalmia, buphthalmus, congenital glaucoma, cataract, optic nerve hypoplasia, persistent hyaloid artery, cataract, Dandy–Walker malformation, hydrocephalus, cephalocele (Fig. 21–83) microcephaly, and agenesis of the corpus calosum.[6] Based on this wide spectrum of defects, the association of any type of eye with cerebral malformations should raise the suspicion of Walker–Walburg syndrome. The finding of a concentric ring inside the vitreous body (the detached retina) or the presence of lipoma of the corpus calosum are findings very suggestive of the diagnosis. When prenatal sonographic findings are inconclusive, magnetic resonance imaging, computed tomography, electromyography, and autopsy studies are indicated after birth to provide accurate genetic counseling to the family.

Genetic Anomaly. Defect of 9q31.

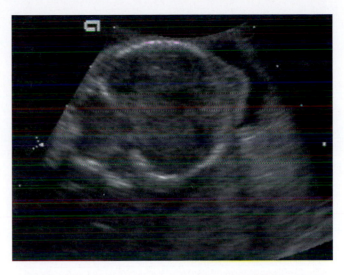

Figure 21–83. A small omphalocele in a fetus with Walker–Warburg syndrome. The previous child of this family was similarly affected.

Associated Anomalies. Cleft lip and genital malformations may be occasionally found.

Differential Diagnosis. Anomalies associated with lissencephaly such as Miller–Dieker and Neu-Laxova are major differential diagnoses. Other disorders that should be excluded are Meckel's syndrome, Fryns' syndrome, trisomies 18 and 13, and maternal viral infections.

Prognosis. Most of the newborns affected by Walker–Warburg syndrome die within the first year of life. Of those few who survive until 5 years of age, the majority has severe mental and developmental retardation.[7]

Management. When detected before viability, termination of pregnancy can be offered. After viability, standard prenatal care is not altered.

Acknowledgments
The authors would like to express their gratitude to Dr. Gisele Duboc for her assistance in the review and references of the AIDS embryopathy study.

REFERENCES

1. Walker AE. Lissencephaly. *Arch Neurol Psychiatry.* 1942;48: 13–29.
2. Warburg M. The heterogeneity of microphthalmia in the mentally retarded. *Birth Defects.* 1971;VII:136–152.
3. Crowe C, Jassani M, Dickerman L. The prenatal diagnosis of the Walker–Walburg syndrome. *Prenat Diagn.* 1986;6:177–185.

4. Dobyns WB, Pagon RA, Armstrong D, et al. Diagnostic criteria for Walker–Walburg syndrome. *Am J Med Genet*. 1989;32:195–210.

5. Chemke J, Czernobilsky B, Mundel G, Barishak YR. A familial syndrome of central nervous system and ocular malformations. *Clin Genet*. 1975;7:1–7.

6. Chitayat D, Toi A, Babul R, et al. Prenatal diagnosis of retinal nonattachment in the Walker–Walburg syndrome. *Am J Med Genet*. 1995;56:351–358.

7. Jones KL. Walker–Warburg syndrome. In: Jones KL, ed. *Smith's Recognizable Patterns of Human Malformation*. Philadelphia: WB Saunders; 1997:192–193.

22

Ultrasound Detection of Chromosomal Anomalies[*]

Philippe Jeanty • Werther Adrian Clavelli •
Silvia Susana Romaris

In Chapter 21 (Fetal Syndromes), several syndromes, the majority of which could be traced to genetic anomalies, were reviewed. In this chapter, syndromes and associated findings that can be traced to chromosomal anomalies are reviewed. Many standard textbooks[1–7] and other sources[8,9] have been used to write this chapter; hence, specific points have not been cited; these are considered basic sources and should be part of every library.

Figure 22–1 shows the increase in frequency of aneuploidy with advancing maternal age.[10,11] After 35 years of age, the risk increases steeply, not only for trisomy 21 but also for other aneuploidies in general. Some chromosomal anomalies are increased with the maternal age, and these include trisomies 13, 18, and 21, but not all chromosomal anomalies are increased with maternal age; in particular, triploidy and most of the sex chromosomal aneuploidies do not increase with maternal age.

Fetuses that have structural anomalies often also have chromosomal anomalies (Fig. 22–2). Wladimiroff et al.[12] and Palmer et al.[13] demonstrated that between 10 and 30% of fetuses that have structural anomalies also have chromosomal anomalies. In their studies, approximately half of the fetuses had a trisomy, one-fourth had a monosomy, approximately 10 to 15% had a mosaic, and the remainder had a few triploidies and miscellaneous aneuploidies.

In addition, Nicolaides et al.[14] showed that babies who have more than one anomaly are more likely to have chromosomal anomalies, and the graph from their study clearly demonstrates this association.

Plachot et al.[15] conducted a very interesting study in which eggs fertilized *in vitro* were used to assess the frequency of chromosomal anomalies in the fertilized eggs. In those experiments, 38% of the fertilized eggs demonstrated an aneuploidy (26% due to aneuploid oocytes, 8% to aneuploid sperm, 2% to polyploidy, and 6% to parthenogenesis). However, in practice, 38% of embryos do not demonstrate aneuploidies because approximately one-fourth of the embryos disappear and are not able to implant and, among those that are implanted, approximately one-half survive into the first trimester. Further, during the first trimester, the majority of these embryos are lost to miscarriages, and the number of aneuploidies decreases to approximately 1% in the second and third trimesters.

[*]Adapted from *The Ultrasound Detection of Chromosomal Anomalies—A Multimedia Lecture* by Philippe Jeanty. ISBN (0-9667878-0-3). Available from: http://www.prenataldiagnosis.com and http://www.TheFetus.net. (*Reprinted with permission from http://www.TheFetus.net.*)

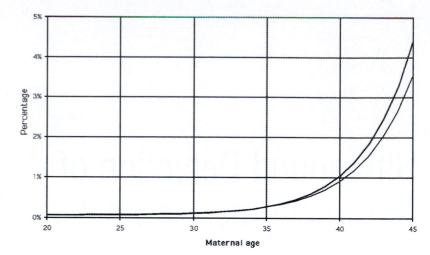

Figure 22–1. Frequency of aneuploidy per 10,000 deliveries according to maternal age at delivery. *(Adapted from Hecht CA, Hook EB. Prenat Diagn. 1994;14: 729–738; Bray I, Wright DE, Davies C, Hook EB. Prenat Diagn. 1998;18:9–20.)*

COMPLEMENTARY INVESTIGATIONS

The usual aneuploid findings include biochemical alterations, structural anomalies, and growth restriction, which are reviewed in the following section. When a fetus is suspected to have an aneuploidy, a karyotype is obtained by chorionic villus sampling, amniocentesis, or fetal blood sampling. Echocardiography was performed previously on these fetuses, but echocardiography is presently preferred as part of the normal examination.

Triple Screen

Biochemical alterations are commonly evaluated with a test called the *triple screen*. This is a maternal blood test in which maternal serum values are assessed and expressed as a multiple of the median. The triple screen tests three components: α-fetoprotein, beta–human chorionic gonadotropin (β-hCG), and unconjugated estriol. Abnormal combinations of these three values have predictive value in the detection of trisomies 21 and 18 (Fig. 22–3).

There are other markers that are being investigated, for instance, free β-hCG, α-hCG, and the pregnancy-associated plasma protein A. Other investigators are also investigating urine tests versus blood tests. Thus, some studies may describe quadruple tests rather than triple tests or some other combination. Approximately 5% of triple screen tests are positive, 95% of which are falsely positive.[16] The triple screen test detects trisomy 21 in approximately 60% of pregnancies in women younger than 35 years and in almost 100% of pregnancies in women older than 35 years, trisomy 18 in 40%, neural tube defects in 85%, and abdominal wall defects in 75%. Thus, this simple blood test can reveal valuable information with regard to the pregnancy. An important question that referring clinicians and patients will have is, To what degree does a normal ultrasound decrease the risk of the triple screen? Unfortunately, there is no consistent data in the literature; Nyberg et al.[17] reported a decrease in risk of approximately 45%, whereas Bahado-Singh et al.[18] reported a decrease of approximately 800%. As physicians, we use the Nyberg value when speaking with our patients; therefore, a risk of 1 in 180 decreases to 1 in 270.

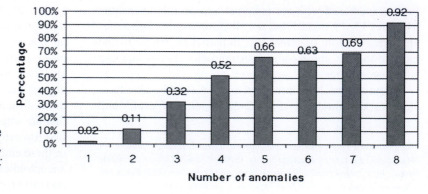

Figure 22–2. Frequency of aneuploidies versus the number of anomalies. *(Adapted from Nicolaides KH, Brizot ML, Snijders RJ. Br J Obstet Gynaecol. 1994;10: 782–786.)*

	Trisomy 21	Trisomy 18
α-fetoprotein	< 0.7 MoM	≤ 0.75 MoM
β-human-Chorionic Gonadotropin	≥ 2	≤ 0.6
Unconjugated Estriol	≤ 0.6	≤ 0.55

Figure 22–3. Abnormal combinations of the components of the triple screen have predictive value in the detection of trisomies 18 and 21.

REVIEW OF THE GENETIC CONCEPTS AND TERMINOLOGY

A *chromosome* is a linear structure with a short arm *p,* a centromere that attaches the short arm and long arm, and a long arm *q,* which follows the letter *p* in the alphabet (Fig. 22–4).

A cell that contains the normal number of sets of chromosomes is called *euploid.* Therefore, in the gamete (ovum or sperm), which contain 23 chromosomes, a cell with one set of chromosomes is called *haploid.* Other cells in the body contain two sets of chromosome, and these cells are called *diploid.*

Chromosomes are displayed in a karyotype by order of decreasing size, with the small arm p on top and the longer arm q on the bottom. The sex chromosomes are displayed as the last pair in a karyotype. The other 22 pairs of chromosomes are called *autosomes.*

Fluorescence in situ hybridization is a technique by which chromosomes are recognized by being labeled with fluorescent probes. This technique allows very rapids results, usually within hours rather than days for amniocentesis, but it provides information concerning only selected portions of chromosomes.

Mitosis

One of the important forms of cell division is *mitosis,* which results in two daughter cells that are identical to the parent cell. The cell contains DNA that organizes itself into chromatids before division. Each cell contains one chromosome from the mother and one chromosome from the father, and these are called *homologue chromosomes.* In human cells, there are 23 pairs of chromosomes and thus 46 chromosomes. In the early stage of cell division, the chromatids replicate into identical copies called *sister chromatids.* The sister chromatids then separate from each other and migrate into each daughter cell. At the end of the division, two cells identical to the parent cell are produced.

Meiosis

Meiosis is the other form of cell division that occurs in the germ cells and results in two daughter cells containing half of the genetic material of the parent cell. The difference between meiosis and mitosis is that, during the first phase of the meiosis, the gametocytes (either the oocyte or the spermatocyte) divide into secondary gametocytes that contain undivided chromosomes. During the first phase of meiosis, the homologue chromosomes pair and exchange segments during two events called *synapsis* and *recombination,* so that segments of one chromosome are transferred onto the homologue chromosome. In contrast, during the first phase of meiosis, the sister chromatids do not separate but migrate toward the daughter cells, so that each daughter cell receives one chromosome and each chromosome is a double chromatid chromosome. In the second phase of meiosis, the two secondary gametocytes that were just produced divide, and each daughter cell receives one chromatid from the parent cell. Thus, at the end of the second division of meiosis, four cells are produced, which may be four spermatids, which are equal in size, or one mature ovum and three polar bodies, which are unequal in size.

Chromosomal Anomalies

Aneuploidy. A cell that contains an uneven number of chromosomes is called *aneuploid.* A common example is *trisomy,* which presents with an extra chromosome. Another example is *monosomy,* a condition in which a chromosome is absent. Monosomy is less common than trisomy because the absence of a chromosome is more lethal than the presence of an extra one unless the missing chromosome is a sex chromosome.

When a cell contains three sets of chromosomes, it is called *triploid.* The most common form of triploidy results from the fertilization of a normal egg by two normal sperm, a condition called *dispermy.* Less frequently, an abnormal

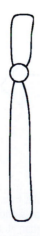

Figure 22–4. Sketch of the linear structure of a chromosome.

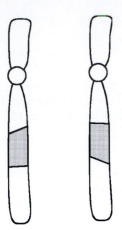

Figure 22–5. A segment of the chromosome has been inverted, without deletion of material.

sperm that contains two sets of chromosomes can fertilize a normal egg, or a normal sperm can fertilize an abnormal egg that contains two sets of chromosomes. A cell that contains four sets of chromosomes is called *tetraploid*.

Inversion. An *inversion* results from a double break in an arm of a chromosome, with the segment between the two breaks being reinserted upside-down (Fig. 22–5). This condition is usually fairly benign. For instance, the notation INV(11)(q13-q22) represents an inversion of the segment between band 13 and band 22 of the long arm of chromosome 11.

Isochromosomes. An *isochromosome* results from an aberrant equatorial rather than a longitudinal division of the sister chromatid. One chromosome receives both short (p) arms, and another receives both long (q) arms (Fig. 22–6).

Uniparental Disomy. *Uniparental disomy* is a condition that results from gametocytes with an abnormal number of chromosomes. The association of a normal gamete with a disomic gamete will produce a trisomic embryo, and all the cells of that embryo will be trisomic. The union of a normal gamete with a nullisomic gamete will produce a monosomy. The union of two nullisomic gametes will produce an embryo with a double monosomy, and such embryos are not expected to survive. The association of a disomic gamete with a nullisomic gamete or, more commonly, the rescue of a trisomic gamete by loss of a chromosome may produce a gamete that has two chromosomes, the normal number, but both homologue chromosomes of a certain pair come from one parent rather than each homologue coming from different parents.

Deletions. There are two forms of deletions. *Terminal deletions* result from loss of terminal material in the chromosome, and *interstitial deletions* result from loss of the middle material.

Duplications. Duplications result from an unequal transfer between sister chromatid during synapsis and recombination, so that one arm receives more material than it should, leading to partial trisomy or monosomy of the affected segments (Fig. 22–7).

Ring Chromosome. A ring chromosome is produced by the fusion, usually with loss of the distal material, of the small arm with the long arm.

Reciprocal Translocation. A reciprocal translocation results from exchange of material between two nonhomologous chromosomes; instead of these two chromosomes being part of a pair, they are part of different pairs (e.g., 1 and 9; Fig. 22–8). If a reciprocal translocation of the distal end of chromosomes 1 and 9 has occurred, the parent may transfer a set of perfectly normal chromosomes to the child, a balanced set in which the right amount of material is transmitted on the wrong set

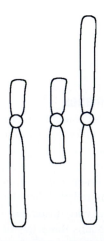

Figure 22–6. The division of the left most chromosome has resulted in one chromosome that received both short (p) arms *(middle)* and one chromosome that received both long (q) arms *(right).*

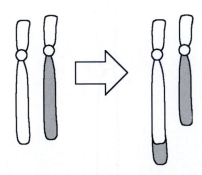

Figure 22–7. Duplication results from an unequal transfer between sister chromatids during synapsis and recombinations, so that one arm receives more material than it has given, leading to partial trisomy or monosomy of the affected segments.

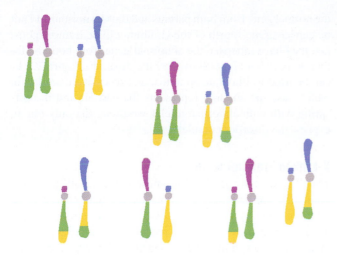

Figure 22–8. The two pairs of chromosomes in the *top row* divided and resulted in a balanced translocation *(middle row)*. Thus, the parent can transfer to its offspring a balanced set in which the correct amount of material is transmitted to the wrong set of chromosomes *(bottom row, first set)*, a set of perfectly normal chromosomes *(bottom row, second set)*, or an imbalanced set with duplication of one portion of a chromosome and deletion of the equivalent portion of the other chromosome *(bottom row, third and fourth sets)*.

of chromosomes, or an imbalanced set with duplication of one portion of a chromosome and deletion of the equivalent portion of the other chromosome.

Robertsonian Translocation. The fusion of two acrocentric chromosomes, which are chromosomes with very short p arms, results in a composite chromosome in which the long arms of both original chromosomes are retained (Fig. 22–9). This is called a *Robertsonian translocation* in honor of the entomologist who, at the beginning of the 20th century, described the phenomenon in insects. It occurs with the acrocentric chromosomes, which are chromosomes 13, 14, 15, 21, and 22.

Dominant and Recessive Alleles

For each pair of chromosomes, one is inherited from the mother and one from the father, and these are called *homologue chromosomes*. Similar genes exist on homologue chromosomes and they are called *alleles*. When both alleles are identical, the individual is called *homozygous*. When both alleles are different, the individual is referred to as *heterozygous*.

When both alleles are different and the altered or "mutant" allele is expressed, the disorder is said to be *dominant*. When both alleles are different and the function of the normal allele masks the expression of the altered or "mutant" allele, the disorder is said to be *recessive*. Both alleles of a recessive disorder must be altered or "mutant" for the disorder to be manifest.

Autosomal Dominant

Knowledge of the transmission of autosomal dominant and recessive disorders is an important topic for those who perform prenatal diagnoses by ultrasound. Autosomal dominant disorders are usually manifested in the heterozygous form. They affect males and females equally. They have variable degree of expression, and may have an age-dependent expression. Autosomal dominant disorders are usually due to the production of a defective protein or developmental morphogenesis. One allele codes for the correct protein, and the mutant allele codes for the defective protein.

Figure 22–10 illustrates what would happen in an autosomal dominant disorder. As an example, assume that the father is carrier of the gene and, because this is an autosomal dominant disorder, that the father is affected. Half of his children will have the abnormal gene and half of his children will have the normal gene. The mother transmits normal genes to

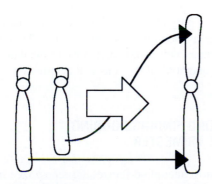

Figure 22–9. The fusion of two acrocentric chromosomes, which are chromosomes with very short arms, results in a composite chromosome in which the long arm of both original chromosomes are retained.

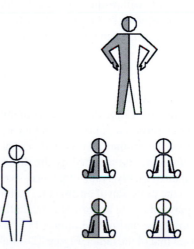

Figure 22–10. In an autosomal dominant disorder in which the father is affected *(shading)*, half of his children will have the abnormal gene and half will have the normal gene. The mother transmits normal genes to all her children. Therefore, 50% of the offspring will have the abnormal gene and be affected and 50% will be normal.

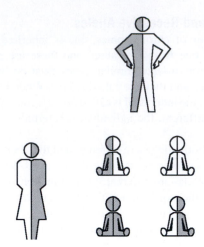

Figure 22–11. The father will transmit the abnormal gene to half of his children, as will the mother. Therefore, half of the children will be affected. One-fourth of the children will receive the abnormal gene from both the mother and the father and thus will be homozygous for the abnormal gene.

all of her children. Therefore, 50% of the children will have the abnormal gene and be affected and half of the children will be normal.

In a less common scenario, both parents are affected by the autosomal dominant disorder, and an example is the union of two parents with achondroplasia (Fig. 22–11). In this case, the father will transmit the abnormal gene to half of his children, as will the mother. Therefore, half of the children will be affected. One-fourth of the children will receive the abnormal gene from both the mother and the father and thus will be homozygous for the abnormal gene, and this is often a lethal condition. In the example of parents with achondroplasia, this will result in a fetus that has a condition similar to achondrogenesis. One-fourth of the children will receive the normal gene from both father and mother and will be perfectly normal.

Autosomal Recessive

An autosomal recessive disorder is usually manifested only in the homozygous form, i.e., in babies that have the abnormal gene from both the mother and the father. The mother and the father usually are not affected by the disorder. It affects males and females equally. Autosomal recessive disorders are usually due to the omission of an enzyme, factor, or receptor. If only one parent has the abnormal gene, half the offspring will inherit the gene and not be affected but have the same carrier status as that of the father. Figure 22–11 also illustrates this point, but the shading would represent the carrier rather than the affected member.

If both parents carry the recessive gene, half of the children will inherit the abnormal gene from either the father or the mother and will simply be carrier. One-fourth will inherit

the normal gene from both parents and thus be normal and not be carriers. One-fourth of the children will be homozygous, i.e., they have inherited the abnormal gene from both the father and mother and will express the disorder. Figure 22–11 can be used to illustrate an autosomal recessive disorder, in which case the shading represents the carrier, and the offspring with both abnormal alleles would be the only one to express the disorder completely.

X-Linked Transmission

Thus far, we have dealt with autosomal anomalies. At this point, it is worth noting the anomalies associated with the sex chromosomes, in particular the X-linked disorders. X-linked disorders can be dominant or recessive in heterozygous females and are usually manifested in males who are called *hemizygous* because they have only one chromosome. In X-linked dominant disorders, if the mother is affected, half of the children will be affected, and this is the usual transmission; however, if the father is affected, then all of his daughters but none of his sons will be affected. Let us begin with an X-linked dominant disorders in which the mother is affected. Because the father does not have the abnormal gene, he will transmit only normal genes to his children. The mother will transmit the affected X chromosome to half of her children. There is nothing unusual aside from the fact that the X chromosome is affected. The situation is more unusual when the father carries the abnormal gene, in which case the father is affected because he has inherited a dominant disorder. The father will transmit his abnormal X chromosome to all his daughters but will not transmit the X chromosome to his sons (he only passes the Y chromosome to his sons). Therefore, all the daughters but none of the sons of the affected father will be affected.

In X-linked recessive disorders, it is usually only the males that are affected, and they are affected from their carrier mother. If the mother is affected, half of the sons will be affected, and half of the daughters will be carriers. If the father is affected, all the sons will be normal, and all the daughters will be carriers. In the unusual case in which both the mother and the father have an abnormal X-linked recessive disorder, the father has only one X chromosome and thus will be affected, whereas the mother is only a carrier. Therefore, 50% of the daughters will be affected, 50% of the daughters will be carriers, and 50% of the sons will be affected.

ULTRASOUND FINDINGS DURING THE FIRST TRIMESTER

Although most aneuploid fetuses are recognized in the first trimester, they usually present as failed pregnancies and impending miscarriages. Nevertheless, several observations should raise the suspicion of aneuploidy during the first trimester.

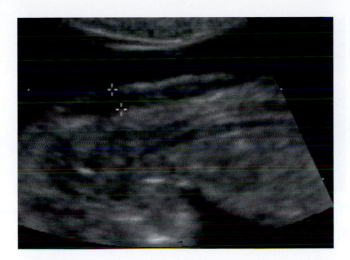

Figure 22–12. A small nuchal lucency. The size is obtained by measuring the distance between the white lines.

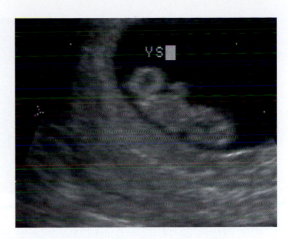

Figure 22–13. The amnion is very tightly apposed around this embryo. The embryo subsequently aborted and was identified as having trisomy 16.

Nuchal Edema

A small black space under the skin of the fetus behind the neck is called a *nuchal lucency* between 10 and 14 weeks and a *nuchal fold* between 15 and 22 weeks (Fig. 22–12). This is different from cystic hygroma, in which a major amount of fluid accumulates under the skin behind the neck. A nuchal lucency is usually considered abnormal if it is greater than 2.5 mm between 10 and 14 weeks (upper limit of 2 mm for embryos with a crown–rump length of 35 mm and 2.5 mm for embryos with a crown–rump length of 85 mm).[19] In practice, however, this difference is not significant and 3 mm is a good cutoff value. The easiest way to obtain the measurement is to perform a transvaginal examination and obtain a view of the back of the neck of the fetus.

The calipers should be placed on the white lines surrounding the nuchal lucency. The suspicion is that the nuchal lucency is due to overperfusion of the cephalic end of the fetus due to narrowing of the isthmus, which increases the size of the aorta over the ductus and increases the perfusion of the cephalic end.[20] Further, these embryos often present with some early cardiac failure, which is manifested by an abnormal ductus venosus tracing.[21] Overall, approximately 30% of fetuses that have a nuchal lucency will have an aneuploidy, and the most common aneuploidies are trisomies 21 and 18 and monosomy X. Several studies have also demonstrated that the risk of aneuploidy increases with the thickness of the nuchal lucency.[22–24] In fetuses in which the karyotype is normal despite the nuchal lucency, the nuchal lucency can also be a marker for a nonchromosomal disorder in approximately 4% of cases. Such disorders include Noonan's syndrome, cystic hygroma, hydrops, omphalocele, obstructive uropathy, genetic syndromes, and many others that are constantly being described. There is also a tendency for fetuses with a thick nuchal lucency to have a poor outcome and decreased survival rate compared with those with a thin nuchal fold. In general, the nuchal lucency spontaneously regresses and is rarely seen after 20 weeks.

Tight Amnion

When the amnion is too close to the fetus, e.g., when the gestational sac is occupied predominantly by the extraamniotic coelom or when the amniotic cavity is tightly wrapped around the fetus, that fetus is often at risk for trisomy 16 or triploidy (Fig. 22–13).

Two-Vessel Cord

The presence of a two-vessel cord can be a marker for aneuploidy. This is not typically sought in the first trimester but, as Figure 22–14 demonstrates, the finding can be recognized in a 10-week fetus.

One would look for a two-vessel cord if the fetus has other findings such as a thick nuchal lucency. Between 0.2 and 1% of pregnancies present with a two-vessel cord. Of these, approximately 1 to 10% have an aneuploidy, including trisomies 18 and 13, triploidy, and monosomy X.

Yolk Sac Anomalies

Levi and colleagues have published several studies in which they demonstrate that an irregular yolk sac and a yolk sac that is too large are predictors of pregnancies that will spontaneously abort during the first trimester.[25–27]

Major Structural Anomalies

The presence of certain major anomalies should also prompt a karyotypic analysis. Figures 22–15 through 22–17 show three fetuses at 9 and 10 weeks. One appeared to have an omphalocele (greater than the normal physiologic herniation of the guts[28]) and had trisomy 18, the other had a large obstructed bladder and a small omphalocele and had trisomy 13, and the other had alobar holoprosencephaly and trisomy 18.

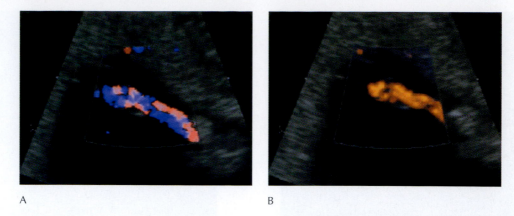

A

B

Figure 22–14. Color Doppler **(A)** and energy Doppler **(B)** demonstrate a two-vessel cord in a 10-week fetus.

Thus, in the presence of major anomalies during the first trimester, a karyotype is indicated.

Shapeless Embryo

A shapeless embryo is an embryo with no distinctive head and body at a time when these findings should be recognized. This can be a sign of various trisomies, usually very lethal trisomies such as 8 and 16, and triploidy.

SECOND-TRIMESTER FINDINGS

In this section, the sonographic markers that can be used in second- and third-trimester fetuses are reviewed.

Central Nervous System

Ventriculomegaly is a common finding that occurs in 5 to 25 per 10,000 deliveries (Fig. 22–18). The normal measurement of the atrium should be less than 10 mm at any time during gestation. When it is between 10 and 15 mm (the gray zone), it is suspicious for aneuploidy; when it is greater than 15 mm,

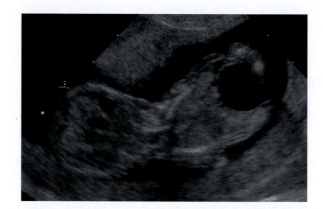

Figure 22–16. Posterior urethral valves in trisomy 13.

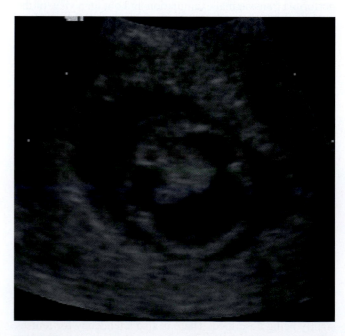

Figure 22–17. Alobar holoprosencephaly at 10 weeks, indicating trisomy 18.

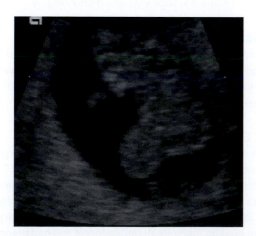

Figure 22–15. Omplalocele at 9 weeks, indicating trisomy 18.

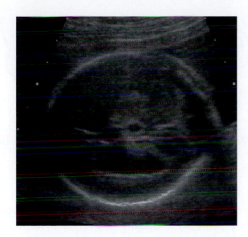

Figure 22–18. Mild ventriculomegaly may be sign of aneuploidy.

it is more likely to represent hydrocephalus. Approximately 15% of fetuses with ventriculomegaly will have an aneuploidy, only 2% if the hydrocephalus is isolated, but 17% if other findings are noted. Ventriculomegaly is not a predictor of a particular type of aneuploidy.

Choroid plexus cysts (CPCs) occur in 1% of the normal population (Fig. 22–19). According to the literature, approximately 30 to 60% of fetuses with trisomy 18 have CPCs. Further, approximately 97% of fetuses that have trisomy 18 and CPCs have associated anomalies.

The issue of whether an amniocentesis should be performed for fetuses with CPC has been debated. The following example may decide the debate.[29] Assume a population of 1 million fetuses. Because the incidence of CPC is 1% in midtrimester fetuses, among 1 million fetuses 10,000 will have CPC and be normal. Because the incidence of trisomy 18 is 3 per 10,000, 300 fetuses will have trisomy 18. Because the prevalence of CPC in trisomy 18 is 30%, the fetuses with trisomy 18 will be comprise 100 cases of CPCs. Because the sensitivity of ultrasound in detecting trisomy 18

is 75%, of those 100 fetuses that have trisomy 18 and CPCs, 25 would be missed by a normal ultrasound alone. Therefore, 25 fetuses with trisomy 18 and CPCs would be missed out of 10,075 fetuses that have CPC and correctly identified as either normal or having trisomy 18. This is roughly a miss of 1 in 400 fetuses with only CPC and trisomy 18, and this is the reason that performing amniocentesis in fetuses that have only CPC and no other finding is probably not worthwhile because, to detect that fetus with trisomy 18, one would have to perform amniocentesis in 400 normal fetuses. If one assumes that the risk of miscarriage after amniocentesis is 1 in 200 or even 1 in 400, amniocentesis would endanger the lives of 1 to 2 normal fetuses to detect 1 fetus with trisomy 18, whose outcome is dismal in any case.

Dysgenesis of the corpus callosum may be an isolated finding of little significance but may also be associated with trisomies 13 and 18, in which case it is rarely an isolated finding. Ultrasound findings include widening of the interhemispheric fissure, the teardrop-shaped lateral ventricles, and colpocephaly (Fig. 22–20).

The presence of an enlarged cisterna magna or a Dandy–Walker malformation, either with a blocked fourth ventricle or a communicating fourth ventricle, may also be an indicator of aneuploidy. Isolated Dandy–Walker cysts do not indicate great risk; however, when associated anomalies are present, the risk increase to approximately 50%, predominantly for trisomies 13 and trisomy 18.

Holoprosencephaly occurs in 1 per 10,000 deliveries. Fetuses with holoprosencephaly have a higher risk of aneuploidies than do those with simple ventriculomegaly. Approximately one-third will have an aneuploidy, if holoprosencephaly is isolated; if other anomalies are noted, almost 40% will have an aneuploidy. Thus, this is a very significant finding, and trisomies 13 and 18 will be the most likely aneuploidies.

Microcephaly occurs in 10 per 10,000 deliveries. This is a difficult diagnosis to make. The commonly used criteria include a biparietal diameter (BPD) below the first percentile

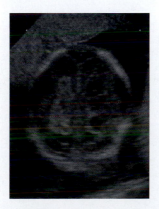

Figure 22–19. Choroid plexus cysts in a fetus with trisomy 18. The cysts are indistinguishable from those of a normal fetus.

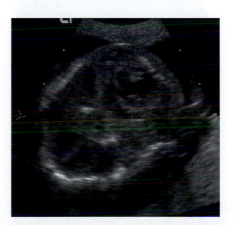

Figure 22–20. Dandy–Walker variant in trisomy 13.

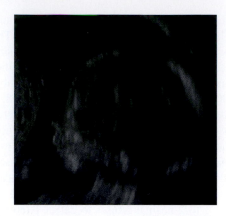

Figure 22–21. Micrognathia. Note the small chin and compare it with the postnatal appearance (Fig. 22–22) in this fetus with trisomy 18.

or a head perimeter greater to femur length below the 2.5 percentile.[30,31] The BPD is a difficult criterion to use the because it is not much affected by microcephaly. What is affected is the size of the cranial vault in relation to the size of the face, which is easier to determine in a sagittal view of the head. Twenty percent of fetuses with microcephaly have an aneuploidy.

Head and Neck

Facial clefts occur in 14 per 10,000 deliveries, and they are associated with several aneuploidies such as trisomies 13 and 18, but others such as 4p syndrome may also have clefts.

Micrognathia is a nonspecific finding but may associated with trisomies 18 and 13 and triploidy. This finding is easier to determine in a sagittal view of the face. Figures 22–21 and 22–22 show two normal sagittal views of the profile; note the

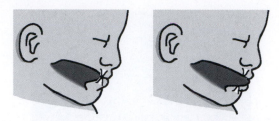

Figure 22–23. In macroglossia, the tongue extends past the tooth buds.

position of the chin in relation to the middle section, which indicates a fetus with trisomy 18, on both the ultrasound image and the postdelivery image.

Macroglossia is the presence of a tongue that is too large and is a finding typical of trisomy 21 and Beckwith–Wiedeman syndrome. Normally, the tongue should not pass the alveolar ridge of the teeth, but in cases of macroglossia the tongue extends pass the tooth buds (Figs. 22–23 and 22–24).

A nuchal fold is usually considered abnormal if it is greater than 6 mm between 15 and 22 weeks. Although the measurement can be obtained in a sagittal section of the hand and neck, it is more typically obtained in the axial section of the head through the cerebellum. Even an isolated nuchal fold is a significant finding, mainly as a predictor for trisomy 21.

Cystic hygroma is a very common finding, occurring in 0.5% of all spontaneous abortions. It is also associated with hydrops in 40 to 100% of cases, with congenital heart defect in 0 to 92% of cases, and with aneuploidy in 46 to 90% of cases. Cystic hygroma can be localized in the back of the neck or may extend farther down the back of the embryo or fetus (Fig. 22–25).

Ears that are too small or too round or have a malformed helix may be associated with trisomies 13, 18, and 21; monosomy X; and several other translocations. Therefore, in the

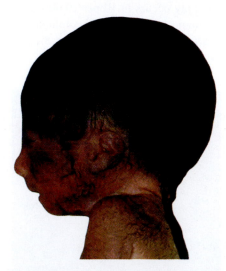

Figure 22–22. Micrognathia. Note the small chin and compare it with the ultrasound appearance (Fig. 22–21) in this fetus with trisomy 18.

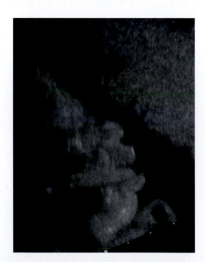

Figure 22–24. Macroglossia.

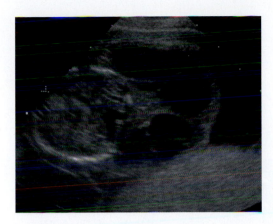

Figure 22–25. This is a large cystic hygroma in a fetus with monosomy X, or Turner's syndrome. What appears to be amniotic fluid behind the neck of the fetus is in fact a large cystic hygroma. Note not only the large cysts but also the large septations that separate the cysts. These septations differentiate this condition from cephaloceles.

proper context, the finding of an abnormal ear may suggest the need for a karyotype.

Microphtalmia is a condition in which the eyes that too small, and it is often associated with hypotelorism. Microphtalmia is associated with several aneuploidies. In Figure 22–26, the eyes are also a bit more echogenic than they would normally appear.

A cataract, which is an opacification of the lens of the eye, is a finding that may be associated with aneuploidy. It is associated with other conditions such as TORCH infections, but it may also be associated with aneuploidy. The way to observe a cataract is to make a section through the eye and observe echoes of low level intensity inside the lens.

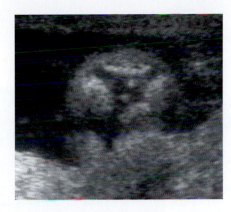

Figure 22–27. Two small wormian bones appear in the posterior fontanel.

The finding of hypotelorism should suggest that the fetus has cyclopia and proboscis, which are typical of holoprosencephaly and thus are associated with trisomy 13. Hypotelorism is a decrease of the interocular distance, and fetuses will have an interocular distance less than one-third the binocular distance.

Wormian bones, described by Olaus Worm, a Danish anatomist living in the 16th century, are little bones that occur in the fontanels and sutures (Fig. 22–27). They are also called *Inca bones*. They may occur in several disorders including trisomy 21, cleidocranial dysplasia, osteogenesis imperfecta, hypothyroidism, pycnodysostosis, and progeria.

Hypoplasia of the nose is a typical finding in trisomy 18.

A low nasal bridge is a common finding in many aneuploidies, but it is also common in other conditions such as skeletal dysplasias (Fig. 22–28). The portion that is hypoplastic is the nasal spine; and when it is too small, it appears as if the nose base is too low. This is seen by ultrasound as a continuous dark echo between the eyes of the fetus.

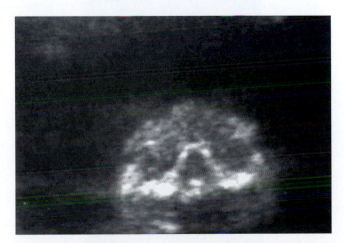

Figure 22–26. Microphtalmia is associated with several aneuploidies. Note that the eyes are also more echogenic than they would normally appear.

Figure 22–28. Low nasal bridge in a fetus with trisomy 21.

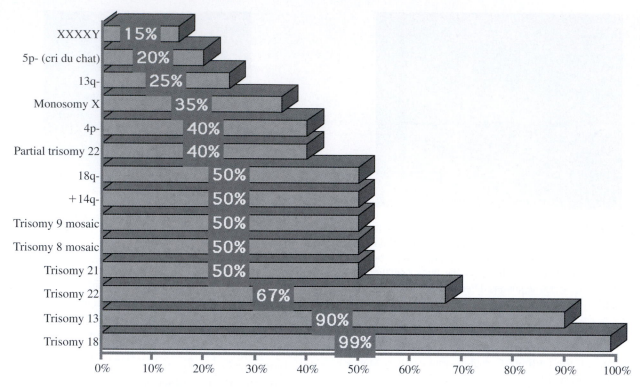

Figure 22–29. Frequency of cardiac anomalies in several aneuploidies.

Cardiovascular Anomalies

Cardiac anomalies are very common: 85 per 10,000 newborns will have a cardiac anomaly. However, among fetuses with an aneuploidy, the association is even more dramatic: 99% of fetuses with trisomy 18 have a cardiac anomaly, 90% trisomy 13, and 50% trisomy 21. Therefore, there is a great association between the finding of a cardiac anomaly and an aneuploidy. Overall, 29% of fetuses with a cardiac anomaly also have an aneuploidy, and 16% of fetuses that have an isolated cardiac anomaly have an aneuploidy; and when the cardiac anomaly is associated with other anomalies, 66% of these fetuses will have an aneuploidy. Overall, the finding of a cardiac anomaly is related more to trisomies 18 and 21 because they are so common and less to the other aneuploidies (Fig. 22–29).

Echogenic Focus in the Heart. Brown et al. were the first to describe the association between echogenic foci and trisomy 21.[32] Subsequent studies have demonstrated that approximately 5% of midtrimester pregnancies have an echogenic foci in the heart. Different investigators have reported an association of 0 to 3% with trisomy 21.[33–39] The issue of one or more echogenic foci or whether the foci are on the right or left side is more predictive of aneuploidy has not been settled at the current time. Figures 22–30 and 22–31 show an echogenic focus in a normal fetus and a fetus with

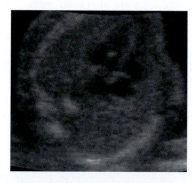

Figure 22–30. Echogenic focus in the left ventricle of a normal fetus.

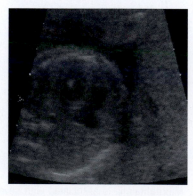

Figure 22–31. Echogenic focus in the left ventricle of a fetus with trisomy 21.

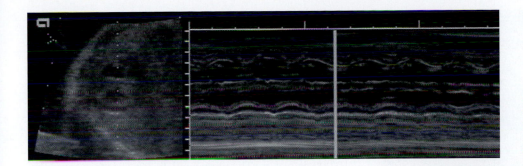

Figure 22–32. The presence of a small amount of pericardial fluid is often a normal finding, but pericardial fluid may be an indicator of an aneuploidy, in particular trisomy 21.

trisomy 21, respectively; there are no criteria for distinguishing the echogenic foci of normal fetuses from those of fetuses with aneuploidies.

The presence of a small layer of pericardial fluid is a common finding (Fig. 22–32). Up to 2 mm is usually considered normal[40]; when the layer is greater than 2 mm, one can consider a pericardial effusion. Pericardial effusions are associated with some aneuploidies, in particular trisomy 21, and with TORCH infections.

Hydrops is a fairly common finding at delivery, 10 per 10,000, and 12 to 16% of nonimmune hydrops may be associated with aneuploidy.

Chest

Most of the other findings that are present in the chest are discussed in sections concerning the heart, gastrointestinal, and skeletal systems. Approximately 5% of fetuses with a pleural effusion will have an aneuploidy, usually trisomies 21 and 13 and monosomy X.

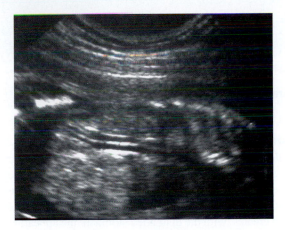

Figure 22–33. Sometimes the easiest way to identify a two-vessel cord is to look at the aortic bifurcation rather than the cord in amniotic fluid. In this image, one iliac is larger than the other because the larger one transports blood to the umbilical artery and the smaller one transports blood to half of the pelvis and other leg.

Two-Vessel Cord

Between 0.2 and 1% of pregnancies present with a two-vessel cord (Fig. 22–33). Among these, approximately 1 to 10% have an aneuploidy, including trisomies 18 and 13, triploidy, and monosomy X.[41–52]

Cord Cysts

Although most cord cysts are benign, they may be present in fetuses with aneuploidy, in particular trisomies 13 and 18 (Fig. 22–34).

Swiss-Cheese Placenta

The typical appearance of a Swiss-cheese placenta is that of a placenta that contains innumerable, small, round vesicles that are quite different from bleeding or blood accumulated in the cotyledons (Fig. 22–35). These are much smaller and much rounder. The Swiss-cheese placenta is very typical of triploidy, but it may also occur in trisomy 18.

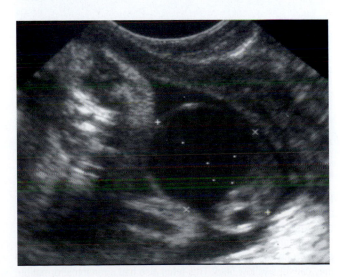

Figure 22–34. Fetus with trisomy 13: has a cyst at the base of the cord.

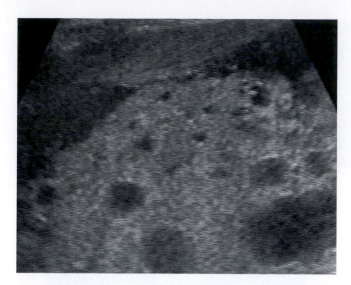

Figure 22–35. Placental vessicles in triploidy.

Gastrointestinal Findings

Duodenal Atresia. Duodenal atresia occurs in 1 per 10,000 deliveries (Fig. 22–36). It is due to a failure of the recanalization of the gut distal to the ampulla of Vater. Because of the obstruction, the proximal portion the duodenum distends, which creates, with the distended stomach, the appearance of a double bubble. Another consequence of the obstruction is that content does not pass through the proximal jejunum and

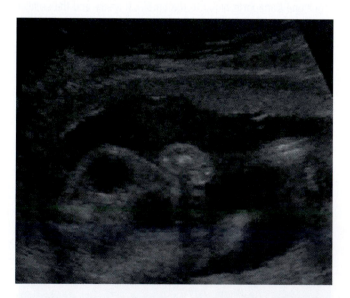

Figure 22–36. Image shows a double bubble in a fetus with duodenal atresia and triploidy. The distended stomach and large bubble that compose the proximal portion of the diodenum are clearly visible. Interestingly, this fetus does not have polyhydramnios, although polyhydramnios is expected in fetuses with duodenal atresia because they cannot swallow fluid. This fetus also had a renal malformation; thus, it could not swallow fluid properly or produce an adequate amount of fluid.

thus the jejunum thins down; this condition is called a *disused jejunum*.

Forty percent of fetuses that have an isolated duodenal atresia will have an aneuploidy; however, if other associated anomalies are present, the percentage rises to 66. Duodenal atresia is mostly a marker for trisomy 21.

Esophageal Atresia or Tracheoesophageal Fistulas. Esophageal atresia or tracheoesophageal fistulas occur in 2 per 10,000 deliveries. The ultrasound diagnosis is fairly straightforward: the stomach too small for its gestational age and there is an increase in amniotic fluid in the third trimester. A stomach that is too small is not much larger than the gallbladder. However, there are many conditions that present with the same findings. Esophageal atresia or tracheoesophageal fistulas are classified into five groups (Fig. 22–37). A small stomach will be present only in cases of types B and C, and more than 95% of fetuses have an associated fistula. Therefore, the absence of a stomach is rare on ultrasound, and polyhydramnios develops only in the third trimester.

A recent study has addressed the association of tracheoesophageal fistula and aneuploidy.[53] In the presence of esophageal atresia combined with tracheoesophageal fistula, 7% of these fetuses will have an aneuploidy. If there is only a tracheoesophageal fistula, the number differs between 3 and 10%. However, in cases of pure esophageal atresia without associated tracheoesophageal fistula, 20 to 25% of these fetuses will have an aneuploidy and the most likely one is trisomy 18 (Fig. 22–38).

Omphalocele. Omphaloceles occur in 1 per 10,000 deliveries, and 20 to 60% of these fetuses will have an aneuploidy (Fig. 22–39). The risk of aneuploidy increases if the fetus has either oligohydramnios or polyhydramnios. Nyberg et al. demonstrated that the risk of aneuploidy is 16% if the omphalocele contains the liver and bowel and increases to 66% if only bowel is present.[54] Thirteen percent of fetuses that have just an omphalocele have an aneuploidy, but with an associated anomaly the risk increases to 46%. Trisomies 18 and 13 are the most likely aneuploidies.

Diaphragmatic hernia occurs in 3 to 4 per 10,000 deliveries. This is a fairly easy diagnosis by ultrasound because the position of the stomach alongside the heart is characteristic (Fig. 22–40). Although an isolated diaphragmatic hernia is seldom associated with aneuploidy, the presence of a diaphragmatic hernia and associated anomalies is associated with aneuploidy in approximately 30% of cases, and the most likely aneuploidy is trisomy 18.

Hyperechoic bowel is a common finding and occurs in approximately 0.5% of pregnancies during the second trimester. To be considered hyperechoic, the bowel has to be whiter than the other abdominal structures and it is usually as white as bone but without the shadowing. The reason for this occurrence is unknown; it may be a normal variant,

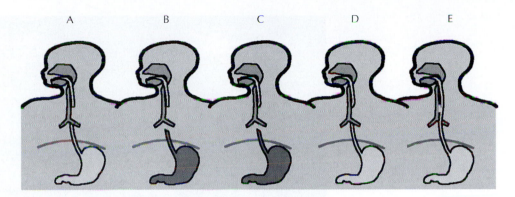

Figure 22–37. Type A, esophageal atresia, which is the most common type, occurs in 85 to 93% of cases. In type A, the proximal esophagus terminates in a blind pouch. However, the distal esophagus is connected to the tracheobronchial tree, so some fluid will pass into the stomach. Type B is second most common type and occurs in 3 to 10% of cases. The proximal esophagus terminates in a blind pouch. However, the distal esophagus is not connected to the tracheobronchial tree, so not fluid will pass into the stomach, and the stomach will appear too small. In type C, there is a connection of the distal part of the proximal portion of the esophagus, but there is no connection to the distal portion; therefore, no fluid can pass into the stomach, and the stomach will not be full. Type D occurs in 1 to 1.5% of cases. Both the proximal and distal portions of the esophagus are connected to the tracheobronchial tree; thus, the ultrasound appearance of the stomach is essentially normal. Type E occurs in 1.8 to 4% of cases. The esophagus is continuous but has an H connection to the tracheobronchial tree; thus, the stomach will appear normal.

it may represent swallowed blood that persists undigested in the gut of the fetus, later in gestation it may represent either meconium ileus or meconium peritonitis (this is rarely the case early in the second trimester), it may represent varicella infection, or it may be a marker for trisomy 21.

The difficulty with the echogenic bowel is that this is a poorly defined criteria (Fig. 22–41). In addition, there is marked a variability between ultrasound manufacturers and between transducers. Some scanners can demonstrate an echogenic bowel, whereas others cannot.

To Karyotype or not to Karyotype? We do not consider a hyperechoic bowel with no associated findings a justification for amniocentesis. The indication, when it exists, is usually related to other findings, and the hyperechoic bowel rarely affects the decision one way or another. Some investigators disagree and recommend amniocentesis on the sole finding of hyperechoic bowel,[55–60] whereas others do not recommend karyotyping.[61–63]

Malrotation of the bowel is another nonspecific finding that may be part of many aneuploidies.[64–71]

Bowel Obstructions. Although bowel obstructions are seldom associated with aneuploidies, approximately 1% of fetuses with trisomy 21 will present with bowel obstruction.[72,73]

Urinary Tract Anomalies

Urinary tract anomalies are common and occurred in 20 to 30 per 10,000 deliveries. The presence of mild hydronephrosis (greater than 4 mm) is suggestive in some cases of trisomy 21 (Fig. 22–42). When the hydronephrosis is moderate to severe, it may be associated with trisomy 13 or 18. Multicystic dysplasia is also associated with trisomies 13 and 18, as is renal agenesis.

The risk of aneuploidy seldom depends on the type of urinary tract anomaly, by whether the anomaly is unilateral or bilateral, or by the level of amniotic fluid. When associated

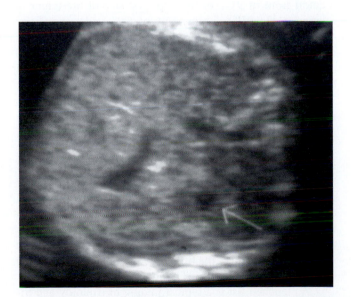

Figure 22–38. This fetus has a Klinefelter and trisomy 18 mosaic and presents with a tracheoesophageal fistula and a small stomach.

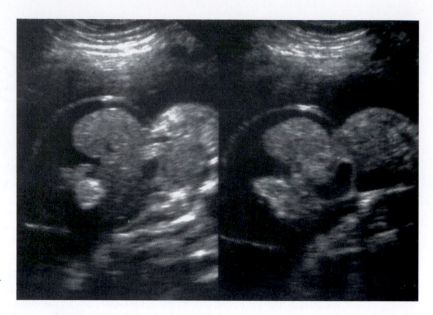

Figure 22–39. Large omphalocele in a fetus with trisomy 18.

anomalies are present, only 25% of these fetuses will have an aneuploidy.

Genital Findings

Ambiguous genitalia or clitoromegaly (Fig. 22–43) is common in triploidy and in many other sex chromosomal anomalies such as XXY, XXYY, XYYY. They may also be present in trisomy 18, 4p deletion, and many other conditions.

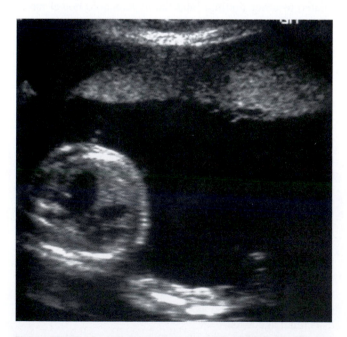

Figure 22–40. Typical appearance of diaphragmatic hernia, with the stomach alongside the heart, the shift of the heart, and polyhydramnios.

Skeletal Findings

In this section, the many skeletal findings that could be markers for aneuploidies are reviewed. These include shortening of the limbs, clinodactyly, syndactyly, simian crease, radial ray aplasia, clubfoot, rockerbottom foot, and sandal gap. In addition, other skeletal findings such as 11 pairs of ribs, hypoplasia of the clavicle, double ossification center of the manubrium, and wide angle of the iliac wings are reviewed.

Limb Shortening. It has long been known that children with Down's syndrome have shorter limbs than do normal children. In their study population, Benacceraf et al. observed a cutoff limit of 91% of the expected size of the femur in relation to the BPD, a sensitivity of 68% and a specificity of 98% in detecting fetuses with trisomy 21.[74] These rates were not confirmed in other studies,[75,76] although the trend clearly exists and has been extended to the finding of a short humerus.[77]

Brachymesophalangia of the fifth digit results from a too-small middle phalanx of the fifth digit, which occurs in 68% of cases with trisomy 21 (Fig. 22–44). Benacceraf et al. studied the predictive value of this finding and found that, if the middle phalanx of the fifth digit is less than 70% of the middle phalanx of the fourth digit, there is a 70% chance of trisomy 21.[78,79] Although few would make major clinical decisions based on this finding, a hypoplastic middle phalanx is an important observation. Another anomaly commonly associated with brachymesophalangia is clinodactyly, in which the distal end of the fifth finger is bent toward the hand because of the deformed and hypoplastic middle phalanx.

A clenched fist is a typical finding of triploidy and trisomy 18 (Fig. 22–45). The overlapping of the finger gives the impression of a clenched fist that does not change during

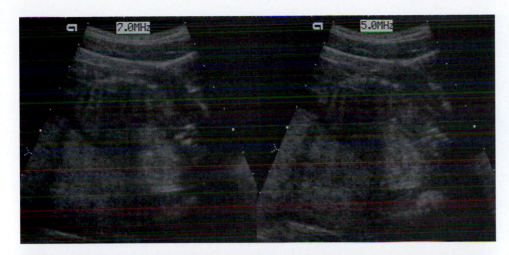

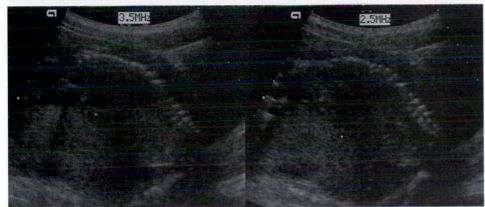

Figure 22–41. This is a series of four images taken a few seconds apart. The first image *(upper left)* was obtained at 7 MHz, and the bowel is hyperechogenic. The second image *(upper right)* was obtained at 5 MHz; the echogeneity is still clearly noticeable but not as brilliant. The third image *(lower left)* was obtained at 3.5 MHz, and the bowel is not as hyperechogenic. Compare the echogeneity of the bowel with that of the placenta, which is adjacent to the fetus, and observe the difference between in the images taken at 7 and 3.5 MHz. The fourth image *(lower right)* was obtained at 2.5 MHz, and the hyperechogeneity has completely disappeared. Because of the variability, basing a clinical decision on an echogenic bowel is not recommended.

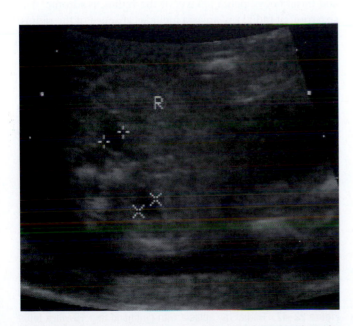

Figure 22–42. Fetus with trisomy 21 and mild bilateral pyelectasis.

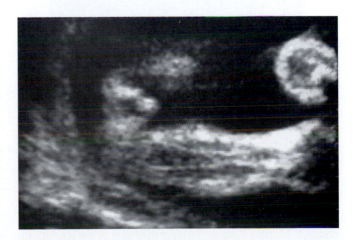

Figure 22–43. Clitoromegaly in a fetus with trisomy 18.

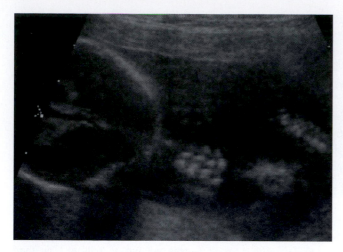

Figure 22–44. In this image, the middle phalanx of the fifth digit is too short.

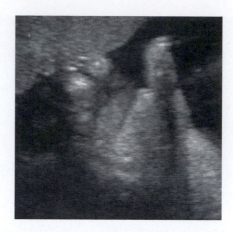

Figure 22–46. Fetus with a clearly visible simian crease.

the examination. The typical finding is the overlapping of the third digit by the second digit and of the fourth digit by the fifth digit.

Simian Crease. There are two normal transverse palmar creases: the proximal palmar crease and the distal palmar crease. In fetuses that do not open and close their hands often enough during early gestation, only one crease, called the *simian crease*, develops (Fig. 22–46).[80] Simian creases are present in 4% of the normal population in one hand and in 1% of the normal population in both hands. These creases are interesting because they are present in 45% of the fetuses with trisomy 21.[3,81] They also occur in cases of trisomies 18 and 13 and in many conditions associated with decreased flexion

of the hands such as skeletal dysplasias. Although searching for a simian crease prenatally may seem very difficult, this is in fact fairly easy to do under the right conditions (amniotic fluid and semi-open hand).

What is the risk of trisomy 21 when a simian crease is found? To answer that question, assume a population of 10,000 fetuses. Because 4% of the normal population has a simian crease, there will be 400 cases. Further, because trisomy 21 occurs at a rate of 13 per 10,000 and because 45% of fetuses with trisomy 21 have a simian crease, 6 of those 13 fetuses will have a simian crease. Therefore, the number of simian creases will be 406 (400 plus 6), and the likelihood of trisomy 21 when a simian crease is found is 6 of 406, which is roughly 1.5%.

Radial ray aplasia is a typical finding in trisomy 18, with very few differential diagnoses such as Holt–Oram syndrome and thrombocytopenia aplasia of the radius syndrome. The spectrum of radial ray aplasia includes absence of the radius, absence of the radius and thumb, or absence of the radius and the whole hand (Fig. 22–47).

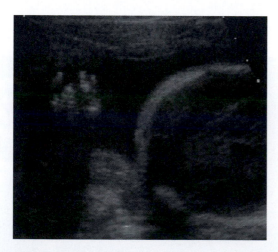

Figure 22–45. Hand in a fetus with trisomy 18 shows the typical clenched fist. Note the overlapping of third digit by the second digit and of the fourth digit by the fifth digit.

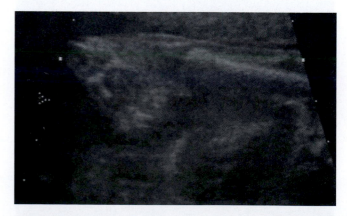

Figure 22–47. Radial ray aplasia with clubhand in a 19-week fetus with trisomy 18.

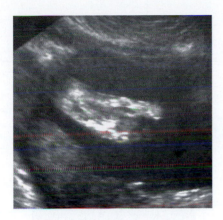

Figure 22–48. Elevation of the first toe in a fetus with trisomy 21.

Another finding of trisomy 21 is elevation of the first toe. This can be seen by ultrasound because the first toe is no longer in the same plane as the other toes (Fig. 22–48). In a sagittal section, one can see the angle between the big toe and the rest of the foot.[82]

A rockerbottom foot is a foot that has a convex rather than a concave sole because of malpositioning of the calcaneus and talus. It is typically associated with trisomy 18.

A sandal gap is a slight interspace between the first and second toes, and this is a risk factor for trisomy 21 (Fig. 22–49).[83]

Findings Related to Anomalies of the Skull and Skull Shape. Brachycephaly is a deformity of the head in which the skull appears too round, and this is manifested by a short occip-

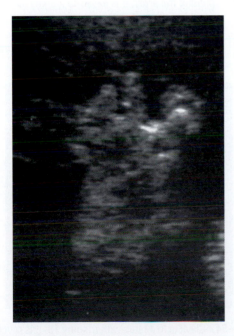

Figure 22–49. Sandal gap in a 30-week fetus with trisomy 21.

itofrontal distance (Fig. 22–50). This is measured by the cephalic index, which is the ratio of the biparietal diameter to the occipital frontal diameter, and normal values should be between 75 and 85%. If the cephalic index is greater than 85%, the fetus has brachycephaly (Fig. 22–51). If the head is too flat from side to side, the condition is referred to as *scaphocephaly*, a finding in fetuses that have *in utero* crowding or premature rupture of the membranes, for instance. This finding is not related to aneuploidy. Brachycephaly is a reliable indicator in children with trisomy 21 but a less reliable criterion in fetuses.

A strawberry head is a deformed head with narrowing of the frontal region and flattening of the occipital region. This is a marker for trisomy 18, and it has not been found without other associated anomalies (Fig. 22–52).

Eleven Pairs of Ribs. The presence of 11 pairs of ribs may be an indicator of aneuploidy. Five percent of the normal population has 11 pairs of ribs. This finding is interesting because it occurs in one-third of fetuses with trisomy 21 and in fetuses with trisomy 18. It is also present in some skeletal dysplasias such as camptomelic dysplasia and cleidocranial dysplasia.[83–85] Counting 11 pairs of ribs used to be very tedious: one used to have to take a single section that would include all pairs of ribs and not omit any. With the advent of the cineloop, it has become easier to take a sweep through the rib cage and then to go back and forth through the ribs in each frame. With the introduction of three-dimensional ultrasound, counting ribs has become even easier because a single reconstruction demonstrates all the ribs (Fig. 22–53).

Hypoplasia of the clavicle is a common finding in trisomy 18 (Fig. 22–54). The length of the clavicle, expressed in millimeters, should be approximately equal to the gestational age, expressed in weeks. Therefore, a 22-week fetus should have a clavicle that measures approximately 22 mm.

Iliac Wing Angle. Borg et al. recently demonstrated that the increase in the angle between the iliac wings, which has been a staple of the radiologic diagnosis of trisomy 21 for many years, can also be recognized prenatally by ultrasound (Fig. 22–55).[86] In their nomogram, in an axial view of the pelvis, the normal angle between the iliac wings should be smaller than 70° ± 15. In their studies, fetuses with trisomy 21 had iliac wing angles larger than 100° ± 10.

A double ossification center of the manubrium is another marker for aneuploidy (Fig. 22–56). One would look for two ossification centers in a craniocaudal alignment, which distinguishes the ossification center of the manubrium from the ossification centers of the sternebrae, which are side by side (Fig. 22–57). Ossification of the manubrium starts in the fifth month of pregnancy. The manubrium first appears as a hypoechoic center and then it becomes hyperechoic as it ossifies. A double ossification center of the manubrium is present in

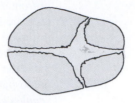
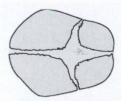
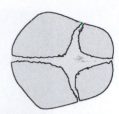

Figure 22–50. The left-most skull is too flat from side to side, a condition known as *scaphocephaly*, which is not associated with aneuploidies. The middle skull is normal. The right-most skull demonstrates brachycephaly.

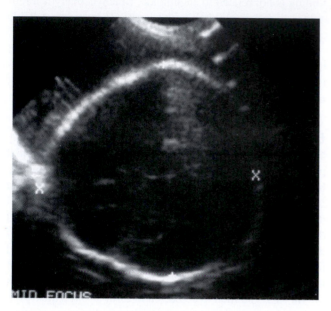

Figure 22–51. Example of obvious brachycephaly: the cephalic index does not need to be measured in such obvious cases.

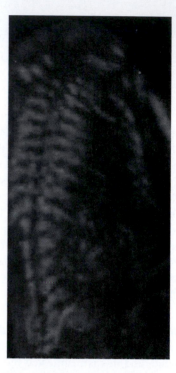

Figure 22–53. Three-dimensional reconstruction of the spine and rib cage. By spinning the array, it is easier to identify all the ribs.

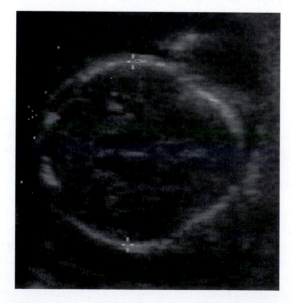

Figure 22–52. Typical appearance of strawberry head in a fetus with trisomy 18.

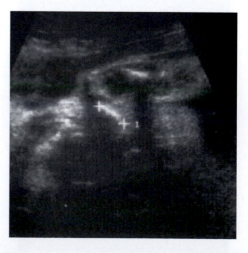

Figure 22–54. Clavicle in a fetus with trisomy 18. It is much shorter than expected for its gestational age.

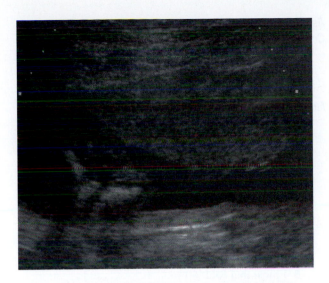

Figure 22–55. Widened iliac wing in a fetus with trisomy 21.

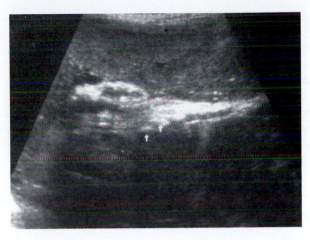

Figure 22–57. Sagittal section of a fetus with trisomy 21 in the third trimester *(head to the left)* shows the double ossification center of the manubrium *(arrows)* and the ossification centers of several sternebrae.

10% of the normal population, but it is also present in 33 to 80% of cases with trisomy 21 and in 25% of cases with monosomy X.

Growth Restriction

Fewer than 1% of fetuses that suffer from intrauterine growth restriction (IUGR) have an aneuploidy. Growth restriction is most typical of triploidy and trisomies 13 and 18. The association between IUGR and aneuploidy is more likely if the IUGR is detected in the second trimester. A very typical finding of triploidy is a very large disproportion between the head and the abdomen, in which the size abdomen is much smaller than the size of the head.

SCORING SYSTEMS

Schneider and Nicolaides[1] developed a very elaborate and well-conceived scoring system that considers the age of the patient and the different findings, and the risk factor is presented to the patient in the form of 1 in XXX. The interested

reader is referred to their work, which contains numerous tables.

The scoring systems that Benacerraf et al. designed uses minor and major criteria.[87–89] Major criteria include major anomalies (such as endocardial cushion defect and omphaloceles), a nuchal fold, a short femur, a short humerus, pyelectasis greater than 4 mm, or a maternal age older than 40 years. The minor criteria include echogenic bowel, echogenic cardiac focus, or a maternal age between 35 and 40 years. Major criteria have a score of 2 and minor criteria a score of 1. In their population, a score greater than 2 is associated with a 75% risk of trisomy 21, with only a 5 to 10% false positive rate. This scoring system is useful because it is simple to use and does not requires tables; however, it only predicts for trisomy 21.

Our scoring system is even simpler. If the fetus has major anomalies such as an endocardial cushion defect, omphalocele, or any other anomalies with an intrinsic risk greater than 1% in association with aneuploidy, we offer amniocentesis. If the fetus has only one small anomaly, such as an echogenic focus in the heart, CPC, and pyelectasis, the triple screen is

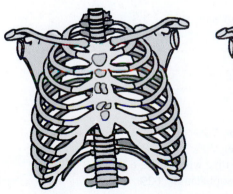
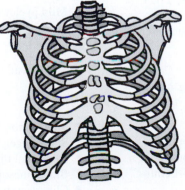

Figure 22–56. Double ossification center of the manubrium presents as two ossification centers in a craniocaudal alignment, which distinguishes the ossification center of the manubrium from those of the sternebrae, which are side by side *(normal is shown at left, abnormal at right)*.

normal, and the mother is younger than 35 years, then we typically do not recommend an amniocentesis unless the patient is very anxious about the finding. Most of these patients do not have amniocentesis. In the occasional fetus with two small findings, such as a single umbilical artery, CPC, pyelectasis, a simian crease, maternal age older than 35 years, abnormal triple screen, or any of the small findings in combination, we tend to recommend a karyotype because these fetuses are not very common, and the likelihood of aneuploidy is probably greater than 1% in this group.

DIFFERENTIAL DIAGNOSES

An occasional finding with normal amniocentesis is a fetus with multiple anomalies. There are some syndromes that may resemble aneuploidies such as Smith–Lemli–Optiz syndrome, Meckel's syndrome, iniencephaly, the cardiosplenic syndromes, and the TORCH infections. These should occasionally be included in the differential diagnosis of aneuploidies.

TRISOMY 21

Synonyms. Down's syndrome, Mongolism (do not use!).

Definition. Multiple malformation syndromes, with a trisomy for all of or a large part of chromosome 21.[3]

Prevalence. Every 13 per 10,000 live births, with a maternal age effect.

Etiology. Presence of an extra chromosome 21 or a long arm including the q22.1 band in all or some (mosaic) cells:[1]

- 93% are free trisomies due to meiotic nondisjunction in one parent; 60% are maternal during the first meiotic division and 20% are paternal nondisjunction during the first or second meiotic division
- 5% are Roberstsonian translocations (14/21, 21/21, or 21/22) either de novo or parental
- 2% are mosaic (postzygotic event) and have a variable phenotype

Pathogenesis. Unknown; increases with advancing maternal age.

Differential Diagnosis. Multiple malformation syndromes, including severe IUGR and polyhydramnios, and congenital heart disease such as trisomies 18 and 13, Smith–Lemli–Optiz, or individual anomalies.

Associated Anomalies
Central Nervous System

- Mild ventriculomegaly (less than 15 mm)

Face, Neck, and Skull

- Flattened face, 90%
- Nuchal fold
- Nuchal translucency
- Oblique palpebral fissure, 80%
- Flat occiput, 78%
- Brachycephaly, 75%
- High arch palate, 70%
- Low nasal bridge, 60%
- Ear anomalies, 50%
- Epicanthal fold, 40%
- Cataract, 3%
- Low-set ears
- Macroglossia
- Small nose
- Mild microcephaly

Cardiovascular (40 to 60%)

- Endocardial cushion defect
- Ventricular septal defect
- Atrial septal defect
- Aberrant subclavian artery
- Tetralogy of Fallot (pericardial effusion)

Gastrointestinal

- Duodenal atresia, 30%
- Tracheoesophageal fistula
- Omphalocele
- Pyloric stenosis
- Annular pancreas
- Hirschprung's disease
- Imperforate anus
- "Bright bowel"

Urinary Tract

- Mild pyelectasis

Reproductive Tract

- Small penis

Skeletal

- Short limbs, 70%
- Short finger, 70%
- Abnormal iliac wing angle, 67%
- Brachymesophalangia, 62%
- Clinodactyly, 50%

- Simian crease, 50%
- Sandal gap, 45%
- Plantar crease between first and second toes, 28%
- Single flexion crease of fifth phalangeal joint, 20%
- 11 Pairs of ribs
- Instability of atlas–axis joint
- Double ossification of the manubrium
- Funnel or pigeon breast
- Hip anomalies

Other Findings and Anomalies

- Hypotonia, 20 to 80%
- Goiter
- Leukemia, 1%

Prognosis. Approximately two-thirds of fetuses with trisomy 21 die before delivery. Approximately one-third of survivors die during the first year, and half die before the age of 4 years. The life expectancy of the remaining survivors is brief. Mental retardation (moderate to severe) is the rule, but in some mosaic cases intelligence may be almost normal. There is decreased muscle tone. Some anomalies will need corrective surgery (heart defects, duodenal atresia).

Recurrence Risk. For free trisomy in young mothers, the risk is 1 to 2%; the risk in older mothers depends on the maternal age. With Robertsonian translocation, all offspring are either mono- or trisomic for 14/21 or 21/22; the risk from the mother is 16% and the risk from the father is 5%. For the proband's offspring, the risk is 50%.

Management. When ultrasound findings are consistent with trisomy 21, prenatal karyotyping should be undertaken. Pregnancy termination can be offered before viability. No alterations of prenatal care are necessary should the pregnancy be allowed to go to term.

TRISOMY 18

Synonyms. Edwards' syndrome, trisomy E.

Definition. Multiple malformation syndromes with a trisomy for all of or a large part of chromosome 18.

Prevalence. Every 3 per 10,000 live births, with a maternal age effect.

Etiology. Parental nondisjunction, rarely parental translocation. Approximately 80% of parents have a straight trisomy, another 10% are mosaics, whereas the rest either are double trisomies for another chromosome or have a translocation. Pericentric inversion in chromosomes has been described to recombine during meiosis and cause unbalanced offspring phenotypically similar to those fetuses with trisomy 18.

Pathogenesis. Trisomy 18 results from a faulty chromosomal distribution, which is mostly likely to occur in the older gravida age. Advanced maternal age is a risk factor, and the parental origin of an extra chromosome is maternal age in 96% of cases in whom chromosomal origin could be determined.

Differential Diagnosis. Multiple malformation syndromes, which include severe IUGR and polyhydramnios, and congenital heart disease such as, trisomy 13, triploidy, Pena–Shokeir syndrome should also be included in the differential diagnosis.

Prognosis. Although trisomy 18 is less common than trisomy 21, it is more lethal: 96% of liveborn infants with trisomy 18 die in the first month, 50% within 2 months, and only 10% survive the first year and are profoundly mentally retarded. Approximately 68% of the fetuses with an *in utero* diagnosis of trisomy 18 die before delivery.

Recurrence Risk. For full trisomy 18, the recurrence risk is lower than the 1% for full trisomy 21 syndrome. A carrier of pericentric inversion in chromosome 18 may produce affected offspring in 6% of pregnancies and carrier offspring in 53% of such pregnancies.

Management. When ultrasound findings are consistent with trisomy 18, prenatal karyotyping should be undertaken. Pregnancy termination can be offered before viability. No alterations of prenatal care are necessary should the pregnancy be allowed to go to term. Tocolysis for preterm labor and cesarean section should be avoided.

Associated Anomalies
Central Nervous System

- Meningomyelocele, 16%
- Arnold–Chiari malformation, 13%
- Abnormal gyration, 13%
- Heterotopics, 13%
- Abnormal olivary nuclei, 10%
- Arachnoid cyst, 3%
- Hypoplastic cerebellar vermis, 3%
- Alobar holoprosencephaly, 3%

Face, Neck, and Skull

- Low-set ears, 58%
- Micrognathia, 48%
- Small face, 35%
- Abnormal ears, 35%
- Small eyes, 26%
- Small mouth, 16%

- Microcephaly, 16%
- Large anterior fontanelle, 13%
- Hypertelorism, 6%
- Choanal atresia, 6%
- Preauricular tag, 6%
- High arcade palate, 6%
- Cleft palate, 3%
- Small anterior fontanelle, 3%
- Third fontanelle, 3%
- Low hair line, 3%

Cardiovascular

- Ventricular septal defect, 81%
- Polyvalvular dysplasia, 65%
- Bicuspid aortic valve, 45%
- Bicuspid pulmonary valve, 42%
- Coarctation of the aorta, 35%
- Atrial septal defect, 10%
- Endocardial cushion defect, 10%
- Mitral atresia, 6%
- Double right ventricle, 6%
- Dextrocardia, 6%
- Transposition of great vessels, 6%
- Retroesophageal subclavian vein, 6%
- Tetralogy of Fallot, 3%
- Hypolastic left ventricle, 3%
- Common atrium, 3%
- Anomalous pulmonary venous return, 6%
- Single coronary ostium, 3%

Gastrointestinal

- Omphalocele, 29%
- Meckel's diverticulum, 26%
- Malrotation of intestine, 23%
- Diaphragmatic hernia, 19%
- Ectopic pancreas, 16%
- Tracheoesophageal fistula, 10%
- Diaphragmatic hernia, 10%
- Ectopic gastric tissue, 6%
- Ileal atresia, 3%
- Imperforate anus, 3%
- Absent gallbladder, 3%
- Absent appendix, 3%
- Inguinal hernia, 3%
- Anomalies of the pancreas, 6%
- Accessory spleen, 3%

Urinary Tract

- Horseshoe kidney, 23%
- Hydroureter, 16%
- Duplicated ureter, 13%
- Renal microcysts, 6%
- Renal cystic dysplasia, 6%

- Bladder diverticulum, 3%
- Bladder outlet obstruction, 3%

Reproductive Tract

- Cryptorchidism, 26%
- Dysplastic ovaries, 16%
- Bicornuate uterus, 10%
- Hypospadias, 3%
- Septate uterus, 3%
- Abnormal external genitalia, 3%

Skeletal

- Overlapping fingers, 71%
- Rockerbottom feet, 39%
- Clubfeet, 32%
- Single palmar crease, 23%
- Hypoplastic nails, 19%
- Short sternum, 13%
- Clinodactyly, 13%
- Syndactyly, 10%
- Abnormal ribs, 10%
- Hip dislocation, 6%
- Deviation of hands, 6%
- Small pelvis, 6%
- Hemivertebrae, 3%
- Redundant skin, 3%
- Cleft in hand, 3%
- Small great toe, 3%

Other Findings and Anomalies

- Body: IUGR, 87%; thin body habitus, 13%; hydrops, 10%; cystic hygroma, 3%; redundant skin, 3
- Respiratory system: pulmonary hypoplasia, 58%
- Other findings: extramedullary hematopoiesis, 23%; adrenal hypoplasia, 23%
- Placenta and cord: two-vessel cord, 29%; polyhydramnios, 29%; villitis, 13%; chorioamnionitis, 6%, trophoblastic inclusions, 3%

TRISOMY 13

Synonyms. Patau's syndrome and D trisomy.

Definition. Multiple malformation syndromes with trisomy for all of or a large part of chromosome 13.

Etiology. Presence of an extra chromosome 13 or part of the long arm [proximal segment 13pter(q14) or distal segment 13q14(qter)]. The majority is free trisomy due to meiotic nondisjunction in one parent. A few are mosaic (postzygotic event) and have a variable phenotype. The rare Robertsonian translocations (13/14, 13/15) are either de novo or parental.

Pathogenesis. Unknown; increases with advancing maternal age.

Differential Diagnosis. Multiple malformation syndromes, which include severe IUGR, polyhydramnios, and congenital heart disease such as trisomy 18, or individual anomalies.

Prognosis. Most fetuses with trisomy 13 die before delivery or are stillborn. Of those that survive, 80% die during the first month and 95% before 6 months.

Recurrence Risk. The risk for the trisomy is not increased; for Robertsonian translocation, the risk is 2%.

Management. When ultrasound findings are consistent with trisomy 13, prenatal karyotyping should be undertaken. Pregnancy termination can be offered before viability. No alterations of prenatal care are necessary should the pregnancy be allowed to go to term.

Associated Anomalies
Central Nervous System

- Holoprosencephaly
- Deafness
- Dysgenesis of the corpus callosum
- Hydrocephaly
- Cerebellar hypoplasia
- Meningomyelocele

Face, Neck, and Skull

- Cleft lip and palate, 60 to 80%
- Hypo- and hypertelorism
- Anophthalmia
- Microphthalmia
- Retinal dysplasia
- Cataract
- Corneal opacities
- Intraocular cartilage
- Microcephaly
- Wide sutures and fontanelles
- Abnormal ears
- Nuchal fold
- Cleft tongue
- Absence of the philtrum
- Micrognathia

Cardiovascular (80%)

- Ventricular septal defect, 50 to 60%
- Atrial septal defect, 40 to 50%
- Dextroposition, 20 to 50%

- Coarctation
- Anomalous pulmonary venous return
- Overriding aorta
- Pulmonary stenosis
- Hypoplasia aorta
- Mitral atresia
- Aortic atresia bicuspid aortic valve

Gastrointestinal (50 to 80%)

- Umbilical hernia
- Omphalocele
- Heterotopic pancreas
- Malrotation, 20 to 30%
- Diaphragmatic hernia
- Elongated gallbladder
- Accessory spleen

Urinary Tract

- Mild pyelectasis

Reproductive Tract (80%)

- Cystic kidneys, 40 to 50%
- Hydronephrosis, 10 to 20%
- Horseshoe kidney
- Multiple renal arteries
- Duplication of the renal pelvis, 10 to 20%

Reproductive Tract (50 to 100%)

- Cryptorchidism
- Hypospadias
- Abnormal scrotum
- Bicornuate uterus, 50 to 80%

Skeletal

- Simian crease
- Clenched fist
- Camptodactyly
- Syndactyly
- Polydactyly
- Club-hand with ulnar deviation
- Radial aplasia
- Sandal gap
- Club-feet
- Elevation of the big toe, 10 to 50%
- 11 pairs of ribs
- Abnormal iliac wings

Other Findings and Anomalies

- Two-vessel cord
- Situs inversus
- IUGR

TRISOMY 8

Synonyms. Warkanys syndrome.

Definition. Predominantly final malformations syndrome with a trisomy for all of or a large part of chromosome 8.

Prevalence. Fewer than 100 cases have been reported.

Etiology. Presence of an extra chromosome 8 or part of the short arm.

Pathogenesis. Unknown.

Differential Diagnosis. Other aneuploidies.

Prognosis. The survival rates are better than with other trisomies; some reasonably healthy adults exist.

Recurrence Risk. Unknown.

Management. When ultrasound findings are consistent with trisomy 8, prenatal karyotyping should be undertaken. Pregnancy termination can be offered before viability. No alterations of prenatal care are necessary should the pregnancy be allowed to go to term.

Associated Anomalies
Central Nervous System

- Agenesis of the corpus callosum
- Hydrocephalus

Face, Neck, and Skull

- Everted lips
- Large dysplastic ears
- Prominent forehead
- Broad nose
- Microphtalmia
- Cataract

Cardiovascular (40 to 60%)

- Ventricular septal defect
- Atrial septal defect
- Great vessel anomalies

Gastrointestinal

- Diaphragmatic hernia
- Esophageal atresia
- Absence of the gallbladder

Urinary Tract

- Hydronephrosis
- Reflux

Reproductive Tract

- Cryptorchidism

Skeletal

- Vertebral anomalies (hemivertebrae, spina bifida, kyphoscoliosis)
- Joint contractures
- Abnormal metacarpals and metatarsals
- Simian crease
- Deep longitudinal plantar crease

Other Findings and Anomalies

- Associated malignancy
- May be related to advanced parental age

TRISOMY 9

Synonyms. None.

Definition. Trisomy for all of or a large part of chromosome 9. Most cases are mosaic, with 2 to 97% abnormal cells.

Prevalence. Fewer than 30 cases have been reported.

Etiology. Not associated with parental age.

Pathogenesis. Unknown.

Differential Diagnosis. Other aneuploidies.

Prognosis. Very lethal trisomy; most newborns die and very few survive beyond 4 months.

Recurrence Risk. Unknown.

Management. When ultrasound findings are consistent with trisomy 9, prenatal karyotyping should be undertaken. Pregnancy termination can be offered before viability. No alterations of prenatal care are necessary should the pregnancy be allowed to go to term. Tocolysis for preterm labor and cesarean section should be avoided.

Associated Anomalies
Central Nervous System

- Dysgenesis of the corpus callosum

Face, Neck, and Skull

- Abnormal and low-set ears
- Micrognathia
- Small palpebral fissure

- Microcephaly
- Broad nose
- Wide sutures: craniosynostosis
- Cleft and high arched palate
- Short neck

Cardiovascular

- Atrial or ventricular septal defect
- Persistent left superior vena cava
- Single umbilical artery

Gastrointestinal

- Malrotation
- Diaphragmatic hernia
- Omphalocele, 29%

Reproductive Tract

- Cryptorchidism
- Small penis
- Hypoplastic scrotum

Skeletal

- Hypoplastic bones
- Hand anomalies (abnormal fingers, overlapping, hypoplastic phalanges)
- Simian crease
- Rockerbottom feet
- Deep palmar furrow

Other Findings and Anomalies

- IUGR

4p-SYNDROME

Synonyms. Monosomy 4p, partial deletion of chromosome 4, and Wolf's syndrome.

Definition. Absence of part of the short arm of chromosome 4; 87% of cases are due to de novo deletions (predominantly paternal in origin) and 13% are inherited from parents with balanced translocations (predominantly maternal).

Prevalence. More than 100 cases have been reported.

Etiology. Abnormal chromosome breakage during synapsis and recombination.

Pathogenesis. Unknown.

Differential Diagnosis. Other aneuploidies, in particular trisomy 13.

Prognosis. Lethal; most newborns die and very few surviving beyond 1 year.

Recurrence risk. Unknown.

Management. When ultrasound findings are consistent with partial deletion of chromosome 4, prenatal karyotyping should be undertaken. Pregnancy termination can be offered before viability. No alterations of prenatal care are necessary should the pregnancy be allowed to go to term. Tocolysis for preterm labor and cesarean section should be avoided.

Associated Anomalies
Central Nervous System

- Absence of the cavum septum pelludidum
- Interventricular cysts
- Unspecified

Cardiovascular (80%)

- Atrial septal defect
- Unspecified

Gastrointestinal (50 to 80%)

- Malrotation
- Unspecified

Urinary Tract

- Hypoplastic kidney
- Reflux
- Various

Reproductive Tract

- Hypospadias

Skeletal

- Simian crease
- Scoliosis
- Abnormal ossification of the sternum
- Unspecified

Other Findings and Anomalies

- IUGR
- Decreased fetal movements
- Weak cry after birth

TRIPLOIDY

Synonyms. Incomplete molar gestation, partial triploid mole.

Definition. Presence of three sets of chromosomes, resulting in focal hydropic swelling of chorionic villi with throphoblastic hyperplasia and identifiable embryonic or fetal tissues.

Prevalence. In 1% of conceptuses but in 0.1 to 1 per 10,000 pregnancies.

Etiology. Abnormal fertilization.

Pathogenesis. Fertilization of a normal (haploid) ovum by two normal (haploid) sperm or fertilization of a normal ovum by an abnormal (diploid) sperm. All configurations (XXX; XXY; XYY) have been found.

Differential Diagnosis. Twin gestation with one fertilized ovum undergoing molar degeneration and hydropic changes in a missed abortion.

Prognosis. Most die *in utero* during the first trimester or early in the second trimester; if born alive, infants die within a few hours.

Recurrence Risk. Unknown, but probably none.

Management. When ultrasound findings are consistent with triploidy, prenatal karyotyping should be undertaken. Pregnancy termination can be offered before viability. No alterations of prenatal care are necessary should the pregnancy be allowed to go to term. Tocolysis for preterm labor and cesarean section should be avoided.

Associated Anomalies
Central Nervous System

- Relative macrocephaly
- Agenesis of corpus callosum
- Dandy–Walker malformation
- Holoprosencephaly
- Arnold–Chiari malformation
- Spina bifida
- Meningomyelocele
- Hydrocephalus
- Central and cerebellar hypoplasia

Face, Neck, and Skull

- Cleft lip
- Low-set ears
- Micrognathia
- Hypertelorism
- Cystic hygroma

Cardiovascular (40 to 60%)

- Ventricular septal defect
- Atrial septal defect
- Many others

Gastrointestinal

- Omphalocele
- Unspecified

Urinary Tract

- Hydronephrosis
- Dysgenesis of kidneys
- Multicystic kidneys

Reproductive Tract

- Hypospadias
- Ambiguity of external genitalia
- Cryptorchidism

Skeletal

- Skeletal dysplasias
- Syndactyly of third and fourth toes and fingers
- Short hallux
- Clubfoot
- Rockerbottom foot
- Unspecified

Other Findings and Anomalies

- IUGR
- Decreased fetal movement
- Lung hypoplasia

MONOSOMY X

Synonyms. Turner's syndrome and 45,X0.

Definition. Absence of one X chromosome, either in all cells or as a mosaic (45,X0 or 46,XX). Absence of the short arm results in the Turner phenotype. Absence of the short arm up to Xp11 or of the long arm up to Xq21 results in gonadal dysgenesis.

Prevalence. Every 2 per 10,000 live births.

Etiology. Complete monosomy (57%), presence of an abnormal X chromosome (ring chromosome, 10%; isochromosome, 17%), or mosaic with 46,XX or 46,XY. Mosaic 45X0 or 46,XY may span the range between phenotypical Turner's syndrome, ambiguous genitalia, and hermaphroditic and almost normal male genitalia.

Pathogenesis. Meiotic nondisjunction during gametogenesis (complete monosomy) or mitotic error. The missing X is of paternal origin. Risk does not increase with advancing maternal age.

Differential Diagnosis. Hydrops fetalis.

Prognosis. Most (95%) die *in utero;* those who survive may have a normal life span but be infertile (99%) or have early menopause.

Recurrence Risk. Not known, but probably low.

Management. When ultrasound findings are consistent with monosomy X, prenatal karyotyping should be undertaken. Pregnancy termination can be offered before viability. No alterations of prenatal care are necessary should the pregnancy be allowed to go to term. Tocolysis for preterm labor and cesarean section should be avoided.

Associated Anomalies
Central Nervous System

- Nothing in particular

Face, Neck, and Skull

- Cystic hygroma, above 80%
- Ear anomalies, 80%
- Short neck, 80%
- Narrow palate, 80%
- Micrognathia, above 70%
- Increased nuchal thickness, 50%
- Short metacarpal of the fourth digit, 50%
- Short metatarsal of the fourth digit, 50%
- Hypertelorism

Cardiovascular (40 to 60%)

- Bicuspid aorta valve
- Coarctation of the aorta
- Dilatation of the aorta
- Hypoplastic left heart syndrome
- Cardiac anomalies are more likely if there is a nuchal thickening[35]

Gastrointestinal

- Nothing in particular

Urinary Tract

- Horseshoe kidneys
- Duplicated renal pelvis

Reproductive Tract

- Nothing in particular prenatally
- Primary or secondary amenorrhea at puberty

Skeletal

- Simian crease
- Cubitus valgus (not detected prenatally)
- Short stature (probably not detected prenatally)

Other Findings and Anomalies

- Broad chest
- Pectus excavatum
- IUGR

REFERENCES

1. Snijders R, Nicolaides K. *Ultrasound Markers for Fetal Chromosomal Defects.* London: Parthenon Publishing; 1996.
2. Dimmick DE, Kalousek DK. *Developmental Pathology of the Embryo and Fetus.* Philadelphia, JB Lippincott; 1992.
3. Jones KL. *Smith's Recognizable Patterns of Human Malformations,* 5th ed. Philadelphia: WB Saunders; 1997.
4. Gardner A, Sutherland TV. *Chromosome Abnormalities and Genetic Counseling.* Oxford: Oxford University Press; 1996.
5. Benacerraf BR. *Ultrasound of Fetal Syndromes.* New York: Churchill Livingstone; 1998.
6. Buyse ML. *Birth Defects Encyclopedia.* Cambridge, MA: Blackwell Scientific Publications; 1990.
7. Wigglesworth B, Singer EV. *Textbook of Fetal and Perinatal Pathology.* Cambridge, MA: Blackwell Scientific Publications; 1991.
8. McKusick VA, et al. *On-Line Mendelian Inheritance in Man.* Available from: http://www.ncbi.nlm.nih.gov/Omim/searchomim.html.
9. National Institute of Health. *Medline.* Available from: http://www.ncbi.nlm.nih.gov/pubmed.
10. Hecht CA, Hook EB. The imprecision in rates of Down syndrome by 1-year maternal age intervals: A critical analysis of rates used in biochemical screening. *Prenat Diagn.* 1994;14:729–738.
11. Bray I, Wright DE, Davies C, Hook EB. Joint estimation of Down syndrome risk and ascertainment rates: A meta-analysis of nine published data sets. *Prenat Diagn.* 1998;18:9–20.
12. Wladimiroff JW, Sachs ES, Reuss A, et al. Prenatal diagnosis of chromosome abnormalities in the presence of fetal structural defects. *Am J Med Genet.* 1988;29:289–291.
13. Palmer CG, Miles JH, Howard-Peebles PN, et al. Fetal karyotype following ascertainment of fetal anomalies by ultrasound. *Prenat Diagn.* 1987;7:551–555.
14. Nicolaides KH, Snijders RJ, Gosden CM, et al. Ultrasonographically detectable markers of fetal chromosomal abnormalities. *Lancet.* 1992;340(8821):704–707.
15. Plachot M, De Grouchy J, Junca AM, et al. Chromosome analysis of ovocytes and human embryos collected after fertilization in vitro. A model of natural selection against aneuploidy. *Rev Fr Gynecol Obstet.* 1988;83:613–617.
16. Benn PA, Horne D, Craffey A, et al. Maternal serum screening for birth defects: Results of a Connecticut regional program. *Conn Med.* 1996;60:323–327.
17. Nyberg DA, Luthy DA, Cheng EY, et al. Role of prenatal ultrasonography in women with positive screen for Down syndrome on the basis of maternal serum markers. *Am J Obstet Gynecol.* 1995;173:1030–1035.
18. Bahado-Singh RO, Tan A, Deren O, et al. Risk of Down syndrome and any clinically significant chromosome defect in pregnancies with abnormal triple-screen and normal targeted

ultrasonographic results. *Am J Obstet Gynecol.* 1996;175(4, Pt 1):824–829.

19. Nicolaides KH, Brizot ML, Snijders RJ. Fetal nuchal translucency: Ultrasound screening for fetal trisomy in the first trimester of pregnancy. *Br J Obstet Gynaecol.* 1994;101: 782–786.

20. Hyett J, Moscoso G, Nicolaides K. Increased nuchal translucency in trisomy 21 fetuses: Relationship to narrowing of the aortic isthmus. *Hum Reprod.* 1995;10:3049–3051.

21. Montenegro N, Matias A, Areias JC, et al. Increased fetal nuchal translucency: Possible involvement of early cardiac failure. *Ultrasound Obstet Gynecol.* 1997;10:265–268.

22. Nicolaides KH, Brizot ML, Snijders RJ. Fetal nuchal translucency: Ultrasound screening for fetal trisomy in the first trimester of pregnancy. *Br J Obstet Gynaecol.* 1994;101:782–786.

23. Pandya PP, Brizot ML, Kuhn P, et al. First-trimester fetal nuchal translucency thickness and risk for trisomies. *Obstet Gynecol.* 1994;84:420–423.

24. Pandya PP, Kondylios A, Hilbert L, et al. Chromosomal defects and outcome in 1015 fetuses with increased nuchal translucency. *Ultrasound Obstet Gynecol.* 1995;5:15–19.

25. Levi CS, Lyons EA, Lindsay DJ. Ultrasound in the first trimester of pregnancy. *Radiol Clin North Am.* 1990;28:19–38.

26. Levi CS, Lyons EA, Lindsay DJ. Early diagnosis of nonviable pregnancy with endovaginal US. *Radiology.* 1988;167: 383–385.

27. Lyons EA, Levi CS. Ultrasound in the first trimester of pregnancy. *Radiol Clin North Am.* 1982;20:259–270.

28. van Zalen-Sprock RM, Vugt JM, van Geijn HP. First-trimester sonography of physiological midgut herniation and early diagnosis of omphalocele. *Prenat Diagn.* 1997;17:511–518.

29. Benacerraf BR, Harlow B, Frigoletto FD Jr. Are choroid plexus cysts an indication for second-trimester amniocentesis? *Am J Obstet Gynecol.* 1990;162:1001–1006.

30. Chervenak FA, Jeanty P, Cantraine F, et al. The diagnosis of fetal microcephaly. *Am J Obstet Gynecol.* 1984;149:512–517.

31. Chervenak FA, Rosenberg J, Brightman RC, et al. A prospective study of the accuracy of ultrasound in predicting fetal microcephaly. *Obstet Gynecol.* 1987;69:908–910.

32. Brown DL, Roberts DJ, Miller WA. Left ventricular echogenic focus in the fetal heart: Pathologic correlation. *J Ultrasound Med.* 1994;13:613–616.

33. Bromley B, Lieberman E, Laboda L, Benacerraf BR. Echogenic intracardiac focus: A sonographic sign for fetal Down syndrome. *Obstet Gynecol.* 1995;86:998–1001.

34. Bronshtein M, Jakobi P, Ofir C. Multiple fetal intracardiac echogenic foci: Not always a benign sonographic finding. *Prenat Diagn.* 1996;16:131–135.

35. Dildy GA, Judd VE, Clark SL. Prospective evaluation of the antenatal incidence and postnatal significance of the fetal echogenic cardiac focus: A case-control study. *Am J Obstet Gynecol.* 1996;175(4, Pt 1):1008–1012.

36. Simpson JM, Cook A, Sharland G. The significance of echogenic foci in the fetal heart: A prospective study of 228 cases. *Ultrasound Obstet Gynecol.* 1996;8:225–228.

37. Petrikovsky B, Challenger M, Gross B. Unusual appearances of echogenic foci within the fetal heart: Are they benign? *Ultrasound Obstet Gynecol.* 1996;8:229–231.

38. Bromley B, Lieberman E, Benacerraf BR. The incorporation of maternal age into the sonographic scoring index for the detection at 14–20 weeks of fetuses with Down's syndrome. *Ultrasound Obstet Gynecol.* 1997;10:321–324.

39. Bromley B, Lieberman E, Shipp TD, et al. Significance of an echogenic intracardiac focus in fetuses at high and low risk for aneuploidy. *J Ultrasound Med.* 1998;17:127–131.

40. Jeanty P, Romero R, Hobbins JC. Fetal pericardial fluid: A normal finding of the second half of gestation. *Am J Obstet Gynecol.* 1984;149:529–532.

41. Leschot NJ, De Nef JJ, Geraedts JP, et al. Five familial cases with a trisomy 16p syndrome due to translocation. *Clin Genet.* 1979;16:205–214.

42. Canki N, Warburton D, Byrne J. Morphological characteristics of monosomy X in spontaneous abortions. *Ann Genet.* 1988;31: 4–13.

43. Saller DN Jr, Keene CL, Sun CC, Schwartz S. The association of single umbilical artery with cytogenetically abnormal pregnancies. *Am J Obstet Gynecol.* 1990;163:922–925.

44. Khong TY, George K. Chromosomal abnormalities associated with a single umbilical artery. *Prenat Diagn.* 1992;12: 965–968.

45. Catanzarite VA, Hendricks SK, Maida C, et al. Prenatal diagnosis of the two-vessel cord: Implications for patient counselling and obstetric management. *Ultrasound Obstet Gynecol.* 1995;5: 98–105.

46. Gonen R, Dar H, Degani S. The karyotype of fetuses with anomalies detected by second trimester ultrasonography. *Eur J Obstet Gynecol Reprod Biol.* 1995;58:153–155.

47. Chen CP, Jan SW, Liu FF, et al. Prenatal diagnosis of omphalocele associated with umbilical cord cyst. *Acta Obstet Gynecol Scand.* 1995;74:832–835.

48. Chen CP, Liu FF, Jan SW, et al. Prenatal diagnosis of partial monosomy 3p and partial trisomy 2p in a fetus associated with shortening of the long bones and a single umbilical artery. *Prenat Diagn.* 1996;16:270–275.

49. Carrasco Juan JL, Cigudosa JC, Otero Gomez A, et al. De novo trisomy 16p. *Am J Med Genet.* 1997;68:219–221.

50. Sanchez JM, Lopez De Diaz S, Panal MJ, et al. Severe fetal malformations associated with trisomy 16 confined to the placenta. *Prenat Diagn.* 1997;17:777–779.

51. Entezami M, Coumbos A, Runkel S, et al. Combined partial trisomy 3p/monosomy 5p resulting in sonographic abnormalities. *Clin Genet.* 1997;52:96–99.

52. Chung YP, Hwa HL, Tseng LH, et al. Prenatal diagnosis of monosomy 10q25 associated with single umbilical artery and sex reversal: Report of a case. *Prenat Diagn.* 1998;18:73–77.

53. Torfs CP, Curry CJ, Bateson TF. Population-based study of tracheoesophageal fistula and esophageal atresia. *Teratology.* 1995;52:220–232.

54. Nyberg DA, Fitzsimmons J, Mack LA, et al. Chromosomal abnormalities in fetuses with omphalocele. Significance of omphalocele contents. *J Ultrasound Med.* 1989;8:299–308.

55. Hamada H, Okuno S, Fujiki Y, et al. Echogenic fetal bowel in the third trimester associated with trisomy 18. *Eur J Obstet Gynecol Reprod Biol.* 1996;67:65–67.

56. Slotnick RN, Abuhamad AZ. Prognostic implications of fetal echogenic bowel. *Lancet.* 1996;347(8994):85–87.

57. MacGregor SN, Tamura R, Sabbagha R, et al. Isolated hyperechoic fetal bowel: Significance and implications for management. *Am J Obstet Gynecol.* 1995;17:1254–1258.

58. Seoud MA, Alley DC, Smith DL, Levy DL. Prenatal sonographic findings in trisomy 13, 18, 21 and 22. A review of 46 cases. *J Reprod Med.* 1994;39:781–787.

59. Bromley B, Doubilet P, Frigoletto FD Jr, et al. Is fetal hyperechoic bowel on second-trimester sonogram an indication for amniocentesis? *Obstet Gynecol.* 1994;83(5, Pt 1): 647–651.

60. Scioscia AL, Pretorius DH, Budorick NE, et al. Second-trimester echogenic bowel and chromosomal abnormalities. *Am J Obstet Gynecol.* 1992;167(4, Pt 1):889–894.

61. Bahado-Singh R, Morotti R, Copel JA, Mahoney MJ. Hyperechoic fetal bowel: The perinatal consequences. *Prenat Diagn.* 1994;14:981–987.

62. Sipes SL, Weiner CP, Wenstrom KD, et al. Fetal echogenic bowel on ultrasound: Is there clinical significance? *Fetal Diagn Ther.* 1994;9:38–43.

63. Dicke JM, Crane JP. Sonographically detected hyperechoic fetal bowel: Significance and implications for pregnancy management. *Obstet Gynecol.* 1992;80:778–782.

64. Rao VV, Carpenter NJ, Gucsavas M, et al. Partial trisomy 13q identified by sequential fluorescence in situ hybridization. *Am J Med Genet.* 1995;58:50–53.

65. Ariel I, Anteby E, Soffer D, et al. Monosomy 8q: Prenatal diagnosis and autopsy findings. *Prenat Diagn.* 1994;14: 640–643.

66. Butt AM, Mehta D, Goodeve JA, Flinter FA. Probable de novo 17q duplication (q11.2–q21.1): A newly recognised chromosomal syndrome in a child with Klinefelter's syndrome. *J Med Genet.* 1993;30:436–437.

67. Delicado A, Escribano E, Lopez Pajares I, et al. A malformed child with a recombinant chromosome 7, rec(7) dup p, derived from a maternal pericentric inversion inv(7)(p15q36). *J Med Genet.* 1991;28:126–127.

68. Fryns JP, Kleczkowska A, Moerman F, et al. Partial distal 6p trisomy in a malformed fetus. *Ann Genet.* 1986;29:53–54.

69. Dammert W, Currarino G. Mesourachus and colon obstruction. *J Pediatr Surg.* 1983;18:308–310.

70. Schinzel A, Schmid W, Fraccaro M, et al. The "cat eye syndrome": Dicentric small marker chromosome probably derived from a no. 22 (tetrasomy 22pter to q11) associated with a characteristic phenotype. Report of 11 patients and delineation of the clinical picture. *Hum Genet.* 1981;57:148–158.

71. Ngai RL, Chan AK, Lee JP, Mak CK. Segmental colonic dilatation in a neonate. *J Pediatr Surg.* 1992;27:506–508.

72. Dammert W, Currarino G. Mesourachus and colon obstruction. *J Pediatr Surg.* 1983;18:308–310.

73. Ngai RL, Chan AK, Lee JP, Mak CK. Segmental colonic dilatation in a neonate. *J Pediatr Surg.* 1992;27:506–508.

74. Benacerraf BR, Gelman R, Frigoletto FD Jr. Sonographic identification of second-trimester fetuses with Down's syndrome. *N Engl J Med.* 1987;317:1371–1376.

75. Rodis JF, Vintzileos AM, Fleming AD, et al. Comparison of humerus length with femur length in fetuses with Down syndrome. *Am J Obstet Gynecol.* 1991;165(4, Pt 1):1051–1056.

76. Twining P, Whalley DR, Lewin E, Foulkes K. Is a short femur length a useful ultrasound marker for Down's syndrome? *Br J Radiol.* 1991;64:990–992.

77. Benacerraf BR, Neuberg D, Frigoletto FD Jr. Humeral shortening in second-trimester fetuses with Down syndrome. *Obstet Gynecol.* 1991;77:223–227.

78. Benacerraf BR, Harlow BL, Frigoletto FD Jr. Hypoplasia of the middle phalanx of the fifth digit. A feature of the second trimester fetus with Down's syndrome. *J Ultrasound Med.* 1990; 9:389–394.

79. Benacerraf BR, Osathanondh R, Frigoletto FD. Sonographic demonstration of hypoplasia of the middle phalanx of the fifth digit: A finding associated with Down syndrome. *Am J Obstet Gynecol.* 1988;159:181–183.

80. Jeanty P. Prenatal detection of simian crease. *J Ultrasound Med.* 1990;9:131–136.

81. Willich E, Fuhr U, Kroll W. Skeletal changes in Down's syndrome. A correlation between radiological and cytogenetic findings. *ROFO Fortschr Geb Rontgenstr Nuklearmed.* 1977;127: 135–142.

82. Wilkins I. Separation of the great toe in fetuses with Down syndrome. *J Ultrasound Med.* 1994;13:229–231.

83. Ho NK. Eleven pairs of ribs of trisomy 18. *J Pediatr.* 1989;114: 902.

84. Bruni L, Tozzi MC, Colloridi F, et al. Trisomy 18 with unusual clinical and chromosome features. *Pediatr Med Chir.* 1995;17: 85–87.

85. Edwards DK 3d, Berry CC, Hilton SW. Trisomy 21 in newborn infants: Chest radiographic diagnosis. *Radiology.* 1988;167: 317–318.

86. Bork MD, Egan JF, Cusick W, et al. Iliac wing angle as a marker for trisomy 21 in the second trimester. *Obstet Gynecol.* 1997;89(5, Pt 1):734–737.

87. Benacerraf BR, Neuberg D, Bromley B, Frigoletto FD Jr. Sonographic scoring index for prenatal detection of chromosomal abnormalities. *J Ultrasound Med.* 1992;11:449–458.

88. Nadel AS, Bromley B, Frigoletto FD Jr, Benacerraf BR. Can the presumed risk of autosomal trisomy be decreased in fetuses of older women following a normal sonogram? *J Ultrasound Med.* 1995;14:297–302.

89. Bromley B, Lieberman E, Benacerraf BR. The incorporation of maternal age into the sonographic scoring index for the detection at 14–20 weeks of fetuses with Down's syndrome. *Ultrasound Obstet Gynecol.* 1997;10:321–324.

23

Intrauterine Growth Restriction

Diagnosis, Prognostication, and Management Based on Ultrasound Methods

Frank A. Manning

Intrauterine growth restriction (IUGR) continues to be among the most commonly recognized abnormalities of the fetal condition and is known to be a compounding factor in 26% or more of stillbirths.[1] When present, it carries up to a sevenfold increased risk of perinatal mortality and is particularly dramatic in the increased risk of significant perinatal morbidity.[2,3] Recognition of serious perinatal risks associated with IUGR has vaulted it to a position of diagnostic prominence among fetal imagers and perinatologists. Intense interest in ultrasound-based diagnostic modalities and clinical management protocols has resulted. Contemporary ultrasound literature offers clear insight into unraveling this often complex diagnostic dilemma, as well as rational perinatal management protocols based on ultrasound data.

Intrauterine growth restriction refers to a subset of neonates whose birth weight falls below an arbitrarily defined lower limit. The limit is derived from weight-to-age distribution curves corrected for sex and derived from an analogous population. The definition is based on the assumption of a gaussian distribution of weight and age, although the latter is known to be erroneous. As a perinatal diagnosis, IUGR reflects extrapolation of neonatal curves to the fetus, substituting either estimates of fetal weight or select fetal biometric indices (e.g., abdominal circumference). Several aspects of this definition warrant further comment.

DEFINITION AND INCIDENCE OF INTRAUTERINE GROWTH RESTRICTION

The incidence of IUGR will change with the defined "cutoff" point. Using the common definition of below the 10th percentile, the incidence of IUGR with a referred population is approximately 7%. The discrepancy is a reflection of a nonuniform distribution of birth weights against age. A stricter definition, more than 2 standard deviations below the mean (approximately below the third percentile), will yield substantially fewer cases. The incidence of serious perinatal sequelae, including death, differs with the defined cutoff point. Streeter and associates,[2] in a study of neonatal morbidity among 134 proven IUGR neonates, demonstrated a progressive rise in the incidence of serious morbidity as the birth weight percentile ranking fell. Subsequently the inverse relation between birth weight percentile and perinatal morbidity and mortality has been confirmed in 1560 perinates with birth weight at or below the 10th percentile evaluated in

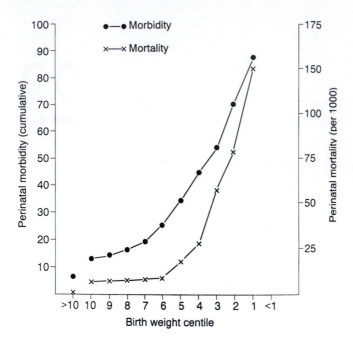

Figure 23–1. The relation between birth weight percentile and perinatal mortality and morbidity in 1560 small-for-gestational age fetuses observed in the Fetal Assessment Program at the University of Manitoba (1987–1993 inclusive). A progressive increase in both mortality and morbidity is observed as birth weight percentile falls. It is evident from these data that there is no exact percentile cutoff to predict adverse outcome.

our Fetal Assessment Program at the University of Manitoba[3] (Fig. 23–1). This distribution characteristic is of considerable clinical importance to ultrasonographers and obstetricians, because diagnosis of IUGR frequently prompts intervention. Based on these data, it is recommended that IUGR be defined as a percentile ranking equal to or less than the fifth percentile for gestational age and sex. It follows that the distribution curves used for setting this diagnosis should be appropriate for the study population. For example, it is inappropriate to use high-altitude curves, such as the Denver curve,[4] for a sea level population because this curve will underestimate the true incidence of IUGR by as much as 50%.[5]

Accuracy of Age Estimate

Assignment of weight percentile depends critically on the accuracy of gestational age estimates. The methods for fetal age determination by ultrasound morphometrics are discussed in detail in Chap. 7, but some additional comments in the context of IUGR recognition are warranted. Determination of gestational (fetal) age and its correlate, the estimated date of confinement, is standard obstetric practice. These estimates are not only considered essential by the patient, but they also form the critical base from which pathologic deviation from the normal is recognized.

Originally, gestational age estimates were considered most important in later pregnancy for determination of fe-

tal viability when premature delivery, either spontaneous or induced, was likely, for recognition of IUGR and for identification of prolonged pregnancy. Accuracy of the age estimate is not only critical in planning appropriate management for such conditions, but it also may alter profoundly the incidence of suspected high-risk factors in a population. Consider, for example, the incidence of IUGR in a given population. The incidence of suspected disease is as high as 20% when gestational age is based on menstrual history and as low as 5% when based on ultrasound-derived dates.[6] Similarly, the incidence of prolonged or postdate pregnancy (>294 completed days) is 9% using menstrual dates but only 3% using ultrasound-derived dates.[7]

Although there is no doubt that an accurate fix on gestational age is a key step in perinatal management, this is especially true in a high-risk pregnancy. Traditionally, the method used to estimate fetal age was the cessation of menses due to fetal hormonal override beginning near conception. Considering the vagaries of the menstrual cycle and its response to intrinsic and extrinsic modulation, however, it is not surprising that this method is not a very precise measure of fetal age. The range of estimate of gestational age by last normal menstrual period (LNMP) is relatively wide: Among 77,300 studied pregnancies, the range of estimate (2 standard deviations) between actual and calculated delivery dates was 25.75 days.[8] Even in women described as having "impeccable" dates and early assessment, almost 14% delivered more than 2 weeks outside the predicted date.[9] The reliability of ancillary methods, such as date of quickening and detection (auscultation) of the fetal heart, is so variable as to be of little real clinical value.

Estimation of gestational age by ultrasound is based on a different principle, that is, the known relation between fetal age and fetal size, in part and in whole. Because contemporary ultrasound methods accurately measure a wide range of fetal physical parameters, it is possible to construct distribution plots (nomograms) of given measurements against gestational age. From such nomograms, mean fetal age and range of estimate can be calculated. Interestingly, virtually all such nomograms yield estimate accuracy at least comparable to LNMP, and the majority yield substantially better estimate accuracy. The ultrasound method for fetal age determination has several other inherent advantages. Among these are the opportunity to select the most accurate variable for a given fetal age range (e.g., crown–rump length versus biparietal diameter [BPD]), to combine variables to refine predictive accuracy (e.g., BPD and femur length), and to measure variables sequentially (growth velocity).

Basic Principles of Age Estimate. The selection of the optimal method(s) and the interpretation of predictive accuracy are dependent on five basic principles, which have remained constant despite the advances in imaging quality and the emergence of alternate fetal morphometric variables and accompanying nomograms.

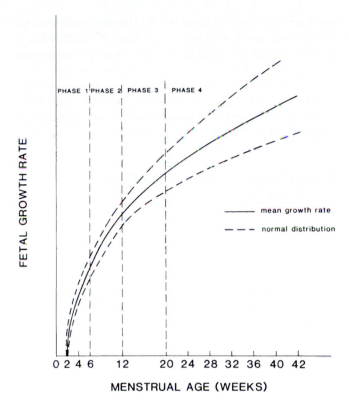

Figure 23–2. A schematic of fetal growth rate of a given physical parameter. In early pregnancy, growth is exponential, slowing toward linearity as fetal age advances. The normal distribution of measurements widens as age increases and growth rate slows. Therefore, accuracy of a single measure in estimating age is inversely proportional to true age. *(Reproduced with permission from Creasy R, ed. Maternal–Fetal Medicine. London: Churchill Livingstone, 1986.)*

The Accuracy of Ultrasound Estimate of Fetal Age Is Inversely Related to Fetal Age. The rate at which a fetus grows is not constant, but it shows a progressive and sustained transition from the exponential rates evident at conception to the linear rate evident at late pregnancy (Fig. 23–2). The more rapid the growth rate, the more pronounced the incremental change in a given physical parameter per unit of time. Fetal growth is the net result of the interaction between intrinsic growth potential and environmental factors that can enhance or inhibit growth. The influence of environmental factors becomes progressively more apparent as gestational age advances. Hence, the distribution of physical measurements for a population of fetuses of the same age will widen as age advances. Therefore, *the accuracy of a physical measurement parameter in predicting gestational age is inversely proportional to gestational age.* This important clinical phenomenon has been observed for virtually every physical determinant of fetal age that can be measured by ultrasound. This observation is also of considerable importance in the recognition and classification of IUGR because it implies that, with an intrinsic etiology (e.g., aneuploidy), the disease process is evident early and uniformly, whereas with extrinsic disease the manifesta-

tion of clinical features is of later onset and more diverse in character.

The Optimal Method for Ultrasound Determination of Fetal Age Depends on Gestational Age. In our clinical laboratory, a gestational sac, signaling intrauterine pregnancy, has been identified as early as the 25th day after the first day of the LNMP (conceptual age 10 days). The developing embryo has been visualized as early as the 34th day after LNMP (conceptual age 20 days), and fetal heart motion has been seen as early as the 38th day after LNMP (conceptual age 24 days). Although gestational sac volume can be used to estimate gestational age from as early as 4 weeks from LNMP, crown–rump length determination is the most practical early measure used. Crown–rump length can be determined from as early as 5 weeks to 12 weeks of gestation, and remains one of the most accurate methods of fetal age determination. The range of error of estimate with crown–rump length is ±3 days,[10] and it is substantially more accurate than estimates based on menstrual history. From about the 12th week onward, crown–rump length determination becomes more difficult because of deflexion and variable position of the developing fetal head. From about 10 to 12 weeks, the fetal head may be well visualized and intracranial anatomic landmarks identified. The BPD can be measured from about 12 weeks. Between the 12th and 20th weeks, this measurement yields an estimate error of less than 7 days.[11] In an ongoing study in our institution, we have been unable to show a significant difference in estimate error between crown–rump measurement done between 6 and 12 weeks and BPD measurements done between 12 and 20 weeks. Both yield estimate errors substantially less than those associated with dating by menstrual history.[12] Although fetal long bone structure (humerus and femur) is seen as early as 10 weeks of gestation, accurate measurement of length is difficult before about 14 weeks of gestation. Fetal long bone measurements are technically possible from about 14 to 16 weeks of gestation.

The Technical Error of Measurement Is Relatively Constant. The axial resolution of a given ultrasound line can be as high as 0.2 mm; this axial resolution does not differ with absolute target size. Therefore, assuming that the target insonation angle is appropriate and the guiding landmarks are seen, the error of estimate due to axial resolution is constant and minimal; however, as ultrasound resolution has increased, the selection of the start and endpoints for a given measurement has become more difficult. For example, BPD measurement by the older bistable B-mode methods was relatively simple because only the bone table of the calvarium produced a recognizable signal. With modern equipment, not only is the bone of the calvarium seen, but so are hair, skin, and subcutaneous tissue. Therefore, it becomes essential to assume that the beginning point of measurement is set at the calvarium surface and not at the scalp surface.

The Accuracy of Gestational Age Estimates by Ultrasound Increases as More Variables Are Measured. There is no doubt concerning a relation between a growing fetal physical parameter and gestational age. In the early days of ultrasound determination of fetal age, dimensions of the fetal head were the only fetal landmarks that could be measured in a reproducible and certain manner. These dimensions, especially the BPD, became the mainstay of fetal age estimates. With high-resolution ultrasound, we now have a broad spectrum of fetal physical parameters that can be measured simply and accurately. To date, all such parameters have been shown to be subject to the vicissitudes of the inherent population variability that is characteristic of later pregnancy. No single variable has shown an appreciable advantage in predictive accuracy.

This inherent variability in a fetal population of equal age is not constant across physical variables, however, it changes for each individual parameter. This principle is of considerable clinical importance because the error of estimate for the mean of composite variables will always be less than the error for any single variable. For example, Hadlock and colleagues,[13] using a composite estimate of BPD, abdominal circumference, head circumference, and femur length, showed 8% improvement in predictive accuracy in early pregnancy (12 to 18 weeks), and up to 28% improvement in late pregnancy (36 to 42 weeks). Thus, it seems reasonable to conclude that all ultrasound estimates of fetal age beyond the crown–rump measurement stage should be based on several variables. Which variables and how many should be included in the composite estimate is currently an area of active research. It seems obvious that there will be a point of diminishing return at which the addition of other variables will no longer refine accuracy, but this point is still undefined. In our practice, we use a composite of BPD, femur length, and abdominal circumference to estimate fetal age. Estimates of fetal age based on a single variable, such as BPD, should and will disappear from clinical practice.

In Late Gestation the Accuracy of Fetal Age Determination Is Enhanced by Serial Measurements. For reasons cited previously, determination of fetal age in late pregnancy (>20 weeks) based on a single ultrasound examination can be fraught with considerable error; the magnitude increases as gestational age advances (Fig. 23–2). The clinical dilemma this presents is common and usually occurs in the patient with an unknown or uncertain menstrual history who enters the medical system late in pregnancy. Because it is uncommon for dates to be underestimated by available menstrual data, patients such as these are frequently suspected to have IUGR. Determination of fetal growth velocity, derived from biweekly interval morphometric variables, coupled with functional assessment (amniotic fluid volume, biophysical profile score) and intrafetal proportions, is the method of choice for evaluation and management of pregnancies of uncertain dates and suspected IUGR. The observation of normal interval growth and objective evidence of fetal wellbeing virtually exclude the possibility of pathologic growth restraint (Fig. 23–3A). In contrast, a reduction in growth velocity is evidence of pathologic growth restraint regardless of whether or not fetal age is known with certainty. In such cases, functional signs of fetal health may be used to time intervention effectively (Fig. 23–3B).

INTRAUTERINE GROWTH RESTRICTION CLASSIFICATION BY ETIOLOGY

Intrauterine growth restriction, defined by a birth weight below a given percentile (usually the 10th percentile for gestational age and sex), does not invariably connote pathology, nor does a normal weight percentile exclude pathologic growth restraint. The net fetal mass (weight) is a result of a complex interaction between the intrinsic inherited growth potential and the supporting environment (Fig. 23–4). The IUGR population selected by ultrasound morphometric methods is heterogeneous. The majority of these IUGR fetuses (75 to 80%) are normal infants without extrinsic growth restriction, merely manifesting a genetic predisposition toward the lower end of the growth spectrum. Such fetuses are not at increased perinatal risk, and there is no need of obstetric intervention for fetal indications.

Within a population of IUGR perinates, as defined by weight/age percentile rank, 20 to 25% will exhibit growth restraint due to pathologic influences. This abnormal subpopulation is composed mostly (approximately 75 to 80%) of perinates suffering from uteroplacental dysfunction of diverse etiology. This subset, representing some 15 to 20% of the entire IUGR population, is at very exaggerated risk for perinatal compromise and death. Accurate recognition of this subgroup by ultrasound-based techniques, coupled with intensive monitoring of fetal growth and well-being and timely interventional strategies, has been the key to substantial reduction in morbid outcome. The remaining subgroup of IUGR fetuses, representing 5 to 10% of the total IUGR population, suffers growth restraint due to pathologic impairment of intrinsic growth potential. Impairment is the result of chromosomal aberrations (e.g., trisomy 18 or 21), intrinsic disruption of organ differentiation (e.g., renal digenesis) or development (e.g., short limb dystrophies), or severe insult of diverse nature (e.g., rubella) in early embryonic and fetal stages. In such fetuses, because the prognosis is usually fixed by the time of diagnosis and is beyond a stage where effective therapies exist, the key ultrasound-based diagnostic step is the recognition of etiology to avoid iatrogenic complications for the mother. The heterogeneity of the IUGR population dictates two loosely defined management schemes: timed intervention for the subset with extrinsic restraints on growth (15 to 20% of the population) and conservatism for the remainder (75 to 80% of

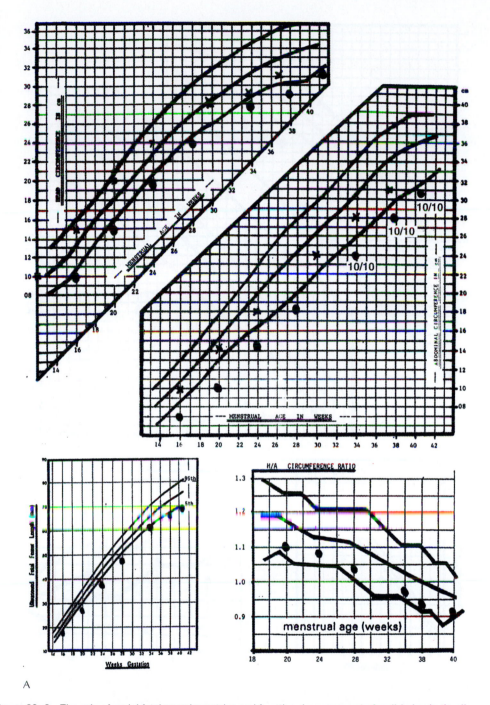

Figure 23–3. The role of serial fetal morphometrics and functional assessment of well-being in the diagnosis and management of intrauterine growth restriction. One fetus **(A)** presents with a discrepancy of 4 weeks between fetal age by menstrual history (•) and, at initial ultrasound, morphometrics (★). Fetal growth velocity, intrafetal proportions, and functional parameters are consistently normal. H/A, head/abdomen. *(Figure continued.)*

the population). It follows that there must be a coupling of ultrasound-based diagnostic information to recognize the population at risk and to differentiate this subpopulation by etiology and specific risk. The failure to attend to this second component of the diagnostic process denigrates the value of ultrasound.

ADAPTATION AND COMPENSATION BY THE FETUS

It is becoming increasingly evident that the human fetus possesses inherent and remarkable reflex and adaptive processes by which it can compensate for the consequences of reduced growth potential. Such adaptation accounts for a myriad of

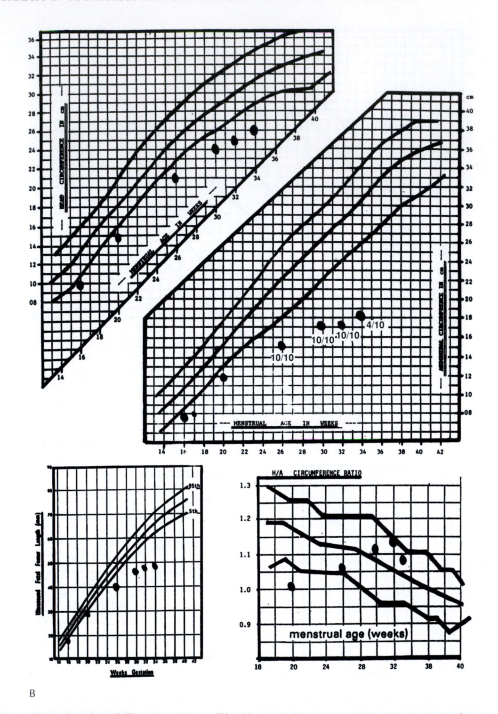

B

Figure 23–3. *(continued)* The second fetus **(B)** with uncertain menstrual dates demonstrates late onset (26 weeks), diminished growth velocity, progressive change in intrafetal proportions, and at 34 weeks developed evidence of functional compromise (biophysical profile score 4/10, oligohydramnios).

ultrasound signs that may be used to determine the severity and possible etiology of the IUGR process and to provide crucial information about relative fetal risk. Included in methods of adaptation are hypoxemic reflex redistribution of cardiac output with selective reduction in perfusion of kidney and lung, manifested by diminished amniotic fluid production and ultimately oligohydramnios, and sustained cerebral blood flow manifested by increased carotid-to-aortic (umbilical artery) blood flow velocity ratio. Over a longer time span, these reflex redistributions in blood flow probably account for the "head sparing" phenomenon of extrinsic IUGR, which is manifested by an altered cranial-to-abdominal circumference.[14] Endocrine responses are complex, but include a rise in circulating arginine vasopressin, an aggravating factor in the

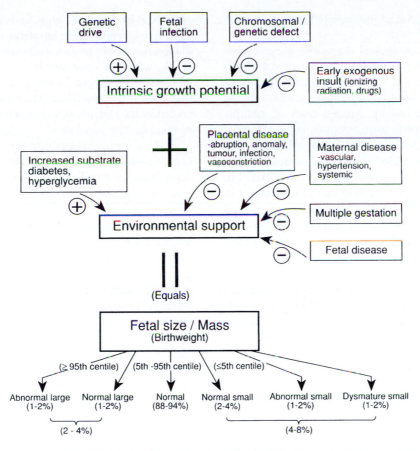

Figure 23–4. A schematic of the factors determining fetal growth. The ultimate fetal mass (weight) is the net result of the interaction between the intrinsic growth potential and the environmental support. Both growth regulations are subject to modulation by intrinsic (e.g., genetic drive) and extrinsic (e.g., placental disease) factors. About 4 to 8% of perinates will fail to grow to a mass at or above the 10th percentile.

development of oligohydramnios[15]; a rise in circulating catecholamines, resulting in loss of glycogen and thus reducing liver and muscle mass; and a reduction in fat stores. Central nervous system–mediated adaptive responses include a reduction or cessation of skeletal muscle movement including respiratory movement, a response known to reduce oxygen consumption by up to 17%.[16] The absence of breathing and movement over a sustained period of time in the growth-restricted fetus is suggestive of severe compromise and impending death.[17] Including these more indirect ultrasound-based signs with weight/age percentile estimates is very useful in refining diagnostic acuity, etiology, and prognostication for management strategies.

PRINCIPLES OF DIAGNOSIS OF INTRAUTERINE GROWTH RESTRICTION

Because IUGR is a common condition (5 to 10% of pregnancies) and a common finding among stillbirths (26%), accurate prenatal recognition is of considerable clinical importance.

The algorithm for ultrasound diagnosis of IUGR and for plotting rational management rests on several key principles.

1. The population of fetuses with growth impairment is heterogeneous by etiology and by prognosis.
2. Accurate diagnosis depends on consideration of fetal morphometric, morphologic, and functional data as derived from ultrasound methods.
3. The accuracy of diagnosis and implementation of management strategies will directly depend on the certainty of the fetal age estimate.
4. Accurate diagnosis and selective management can result in significant reduction in mortality and morbidity associated with IUGR.

The most common entry mode of the patient with suspected IUGR into the ultrasound diagnostic schemata occurs as a result of a clinical diagnosis of a discrepancy between uterine size and gestational age. Uterine size can be measured objectively by symphysis-to-fundal height ratios or subjectively by an impression of reduced uterine volume. The predictive accuracy of clinical parameters for the diagnosis of IUGR is poor.

These parameters of clinical diagnostic accuracy become further compromised among patients in whom the menstrual history is unknown or uncertain or in whom clinical examination is difficult because of uterine anomaly, uterine fibroids, multiparity, or obesity. Among cases of multiple pregnancy, in which growth impairment of one or more of the fetuses is common, detection of IUGR by clinical assessment is inaccurate. In separate British and American clinical studies, experienced clinicians recognized existing IUGR in about two-thirds of cases and overdiagnosed the condition in up to 40% of instances.[18,19] It follows that a more precise and objective diagnostic measure must be employed to assess the fetus(es) with suspected IUGR. All existing evidence points to ultrasound as this objective modality.

Ultrasound methods are applied to the diagnosis of IUGR in two general ways. First, it is used to recognize a discrepancy between expected and observed fetal mass (volume) for a given gestational age. Second, it is employed to determine the etiology, severity, and prognosis for the observed discrepancy.

RECOGNITION OF GROWTH IMPAIRMENT

The first step in diagnosis of IUGR involves calculation of fetal mass and gestational age, both of which may be estimated from discrete fetal measurements. Determination of fetal age from ultrasound-derived fetal morphometrics has been briefly referenced in this text and is described in detail elsewhere. Estimation of fetal mass (weight) is also derived from fetal morphometrics and is based on the assumption of a constant reproducible relation between select fetal parameters and fetal volume. This method assumes a constant density of the fetus across a range of volumes and among healthy and compromised fetuses. Several aspects of this presumed relation warrant further comment, because the accuracy of diagnosis (and hence management) may depend critically on these assumptions.

Calculation of density (grams per milliliter) using a water displacement method for calculation of volume indicates there is significant variation in density among the population of perinates and within different organ structures in the individual fetus.[20] The average density of the perinate is slightly less than water (0.919 ± 0.07 g/mL) but may vary from 0.833 to 1.012 g/mL (range of variation 21.5%). It may be calculated from these data that, among a population of perinates of known volume, the average error of weight (mass) estimate will be approximately 8%, but in some fetuses the average error may be as high as 21%. The density distribution among IUGR fetuses, a population in whom a reduction in body fat may be expected, is unknown and needs further study. Further, within the individual fetus the density of various structures is known to differ. For example, the mean density

of the fetal head is 0.571 g/mL and of the body is 1.118 g/mL. Failure to consider these intrafetal variations can compound diagnostic error in fetuses with such conditions as dysmature IUGR, which in some instances are known to cause differential effects on organ growth (e.g., head sparing). It follows that, even if fetal morphometries were known with absolute precision, the weight estimate error will always exist because of these density variations.

The clinician ultrasonographer is presented with a number of formulas that use fetal morphometrics to calculate fetal mass. These methods are generally derived from an equation defining either a linear or exponential line of best fit of fetal morphometrics to recorded birth weight. Most formulas are derived from a relatively small population of uneven weight distribution, with variable intervals between measurement and delivery, and do not account for a change in relative density due to lung expansion. Considering these sources of error of mensuration of fetal parameter, it is not surprising that there is considerable range of error between estimated (fetal) and measured (neonatal) weight. When volume is known with certainty (by water displacement method), the error of estimate is $\pm 7.2\%$ (2 standard deviations).[19] Detailed, highly accurate measurement of neonatal physical dimension yields an estimate error of calculated weight of $\pm 8.2\%$, the slight increase in estimate error presumed due to measurement error.[19]

The most exact estimate of fetal volume is based on a static ultrasound method of serial cross-sectioned scan with computer reconstruction to calculate volume. This method, reported by McCallum and coworkers in 1979,[21] is time consuming and cumbersome but yields an estimate error comparable to that of direct displacement methods. Unfortunately, the method has not been reliably reproduced using dynamic ultrasound methods and hence is rarely employed. The most commonly used methods today are based on selective variables. Initially, fetal BPD was used to estimate fetal mass but, because the fetal head represents only 20% of total fetal volume, it is not surprising this method proved so inaccurate as to be of no clinical value. Combining fetal head measurements (BPD or head circumference) with abdominal circumference measurements has been reported as a method for estimating fetal mass.[22] The method has several inherent disadvantages. Harman and coworkers[23] studied the method among 198 fetuses and outlined some of these disadvantages. They noted that in more than 20% (35 fetuses) the variance between estimated and observed weight exceeded 10%, that in 22% of cases BPD could not be reliably measured, and that the relation between abdominal circumference and BPD in the growth-restricted fetus did not conform to the Shepard equation. Hadlock and associates[24,25] reported a method of fetal weight estimation based on composite measurements of head circumference, abdominal circumference, and femur length that yields an estimate of error of $\pm 15\%$ (2 standard deviations).[24,25] Abdominal circumference as a sole measure to estimate fetal weight yields an estimate of error of $\pm 15\%$ (Fig. 23–5).[26] By such methods, IUGR is diagnosed

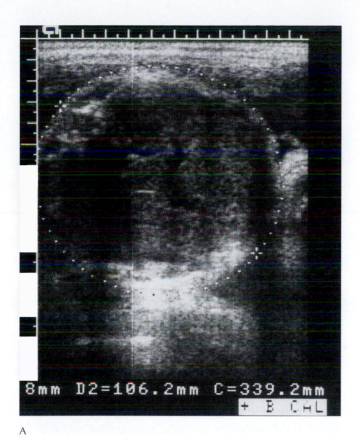

`8mm  D2=106.2mm  C=339.2mm`

A

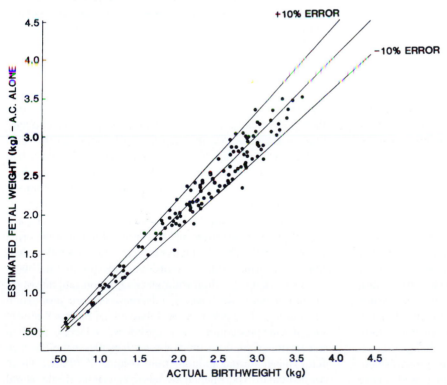

B

Figure 23–5. Ultrasound estimation of fetal mass. Abdominal circumference is measured at the level of the fetal liver **(A)**. Because the upper fetal abdomen is cylindrical in shape, there is little variation in measured circumference provided fetal liver and major hepatic veins are present. Abdominal circumference (A.C.) gives an estimate of fetal weight to within a 15% error in nearly all instances and to within ±10% in the majority of instances **(B)**.

when the estimated weight falls below the 10th percentile for gestational age. Whereas the neonatal curves of weight to age include sex correction, described fetal curves usually do not consider sex differences due to potential error in sex assignment. Converting abdominal circumference measurement into fetal weight introduces further potential for error and conveys no clinical advantage.

Serial assessment of fetal growth parameters (see Figs. 23–3A and B), either derived (fetal weight estimates) or direct, is of considerable value in establishing the diagnosis of IUGR, in determining rate of progression and often in determining etiology. With the exception of the fetus with extreme IUGR (below the third percentile) or the fetus with overt functional signs of compromise (see the following discussion), serial estimates of growth parameters are recommended for all fetuses with proven or suspected IUGR. The interval between examinations is not constant but may change inversely with the gestational age at diagnosis, the presumed severity of disease at initial diagnosis, fetal well-being at diagnosis, maternal condition (e.g., severity of hypertension), and the results of previous examination. The interval may change directly with the uncertainty of menstrual dates and the suspicion of normal small fetus. Because the diagnosis and management of IUGR depend on other factors in addition to fetal growth parameters, it is essential to ensure confirmation of fetal well-being by antepartum testing in addition to such studies.

When fetal biophysical profile scoring is used for determination of well-being, growth parameters are usually measured weekly. When antepartum fetal heart rate testing methods are used to confirm fetal well-being, growth parameter determination may be extended to biweekly intervals. An interval of 2 weeks is recommended for comparison of growth parameters, because comparison at shorter intervals precludes differentiation of change because of measurement error. The potential for confusion is even greater when derived growth estimates (fetal weight) are used. Serial estimates done at biweekly intervals will generally yield one of the following patterns. The growth velocity (change in measured parameters over time) may parallel the normal distribution curve, but it will remain below the 10th percentile. In such fetuses the diagnosis of a normal small fetus is most likely, although mistaken dates cannot be excluded with certainty. Such fetuses, in the absence of functional signs of compromise, require serial biweekly assessment to confirm continuing normal growth velocity. It is uncommon for such fetuses to develop subsequent aggravated growth restraint, and the perinatal prognosis is excellent. The second pattern observed is a flattened growth velocity in which interval testing reveals a widening variance from expected growth velocity (see Fig. 23–3B). Such fetuses may be considered to have dysmature IUGR until proven otherwise, and they need intensive monitoring for functional signs of IUGR and a change in fetal condition. A variant may be observed in the fetus whose initial growth parameters are above the lower limit but subsequently fall through the percentiles. Such fetuses can exhibit all the functional signs of dysmature IUGR and may die before the growth parameters ever fall below the lower limit of distribution.

Functional Evaluation of Intrauterine Growth Restriction

Estimation of fetal growth parameters may be the method for initial recognition of IUGR, but it is ultrasound assessment of the functional signs that leads to the specific diagnosis, presumed etiology, and appropriate management. This evolution from recognition to specific assessment of fetal signs is a key step in reducing perinatal morbidity and mortality and iatrogenic complications for the mother.

The functional signs of IUGR may be loosely classified into "hard" (objective) signs and "soft" (subjective) signs. The hard signs are measurable and reproducible and are of major value in assigning etiology and prognosis. Four hard signs are described in the following sections.

Amniotic Fluid Volume and Intrauterine Growth Restriction

Whereas in earlier gestation amniotic fluid may be derived from nonrenal sources at the gestational age threshold at which IUGR becomes a clinical management problem (at the time of writing about 24 weeks of gestation and beyond), the major source of amniotic fluid is the fetal kidney, with the fetal lung contributing to a lesser degree. The egress of the fluid is controlled by fetal swallowing, with absorption from the gastrointestinal tract and clearance by the placenta. Oligohydramnios in the presence of intact membranes may, therefore, be a result of either increased elimination or decreased production of fluid or some combination thereof. Decreased production is the most probable explanation for the reduction in amniotic fluid volume in the fetus with growth restraint. Decreased renal perfusion is known to occur as part of the adaptive cardiac output redistribution reflex stimulated by fetal hypoxemia and acidemia.[27] Further, fetal hypoxemia also results in release of fetal hormones, including arginine vasopressin,[15] which enhances the reabsorption of glomerular filtrate and causes a reduction in the urine production rate. The cumulative effects of even a subtle reduction in fetal urine production can, over time, produce dramatic changes in amniotic fluid volume: Given a constant rate of fetal elimination (swallowing), a decrease of urine production of as little as 1 cc per hour (less than 3% of the usual hourly rate of urine production) can in the course of 3 weeks result in a reduction of amniotic fluid of more than 50% in the 28-week fetus (mean normal amniotic fluid volume of 800 cc). There are no human experimental models to determine the threshold rate of amniotic fluid volume reduction that can be detected by high-resolution ultrasound methods. Conversely, the threshold for ultrasound detection of increases in volume is known. In the human fetus with oligohydramnios, an infusion of

TABLE 23–1. DIAGNOSIS OF INTRAUTERINE GROWTH RESTRICTION PREDICTIVE ACCURACY PARAMETERS OF AMNIOTIC FLUID VOLUME ASSESSMENT BY ULTRASOUND

Study	No. of Cases	Prevalence of IUGR (%)	Sensitivity (%)	Specificity (%)	Positive Predictive Accuracy (%)	Negative Predictive Accuracy (%)	False-Positive Rate (%)	False-Negative Rate (%)
Manning et al., 1981[32]	120	26	84	97	90	95	3	16
Phillipson et al., 1983[35]	192	24	83	60	40	92	40	17
Hill et al., 1983[36]	317	2	50	100	—	—	—	50
Chamberlain et al., 1984[37]	7298	5.5	13	97.7	25	97.7	—	—
Hoddick et al., 1984[38]	125	100	4	—	—	50	—	—
Manning, 1992[44]	2270	100	35	97	33	97	—	—

All studies use the broadest definitions of intrauterine growth restriction (IUGR) ($\leq$10th percentile) without reference to the etiologic category. Predictive accuracy parameters for dysmature IUGR are likely enhanced.

at least 50 cc is required before a change can be detected. In the human fetus with dysmature IUGR, the presence of hypoxemia and acidemia has been detected by umbilical blood analysis,[28] and a reduction of fetal urine production has been measured by ultrasound monitoring of fetal bladder volume.[29,30] It is assumed, therefore, that an association of oligohydramnios and dysmature IUGR occurs as a result of altered fetal renal function secondary to episodes of fetal hypoxemia. A correlation between fetal urine production rates and PO_2 as measured antenatally has been reported.[31]

The major problem in using amniotic fluid volume in the diagnosis, assessment, and management of IUGR remains the difficulty in obtaining an accurate measure of absolute volume: There are at present no practical reliable means of determination of absolute volume, and accordingly clinical application of amniotic fluid volume in the fetus at risk for IUGR is based on a statistical association between the pocket sizes (distribution of fluid) and the incidence of IUGR. Two semiquantitative methods are reported: the largest vertical pocket method[32] and the amniotic fluid index.[33] Comparative studies of the predictive accuracy of the two methods have yielded conflicting results.[34] The reasonable conclusion seems to be that the tests are interchangeable and the choice of testing method is a personal preference.

Largest Vertical Pocket. The original method for assessment of amniotic fluid volume is based on measurement of the vertical depth of the largest pocket of fluid visualized.[32] According to this method, a general scan of the uterus is done to determine the distribution of the amniotic fluid and to identify the pocket to be measured. The largest pocket is identified and measured in the vertical plane.

Amniotic Fluid Index. This method, reported by Phelan et al.,[33] is an expanded modification of the single pocket method by which the uterus is divided into four quadrants, the vertical depth of the maximal pocket in each quadrant is measured, and the sum of the measures for each quadrant is reported as an amniotic fluid index.

Amniotic Fluid Volume: Predictive Accuracy in Intrauterine Growth Restricted Fetuses (Table 23–1)

The predictive accuracy of amniotic fluid volume determination differs directly by the etiology of small-for-gestational age (SGA) size and, therefore, will differ by the composition of the clinical population studied. Pathologic decreases in amniotic fluid volume in the normal small fetus are rare and unrelated to the etiology of the IUGR. Similarly, in the fetus with IUGR secondary to fetal anomaly, decreased fluid volume is not expected, although, in some instances, such as obstructive uropathies, renal dysgenesis/agenesis syndromes, skeletal dysplasias (in particular thanatophoric dwarfism), and in some karyotypic abnormalities (triploidy and trisomy 18), oligohydramnios may occur in association with the severe degrees of IUGR. In addition, the abnormal fetus may be subject to other causes of placental dysfunction (e.g., preeclampsia) and therefore may have a dual etiology for the growth restraint; in such cases, these anomalous fetuses may exhibit other signs of dysmature IUGR including oligohydramnios. As a general and very useful clinical rule, *the value of screening for decreased amniotic fluid volume in the SGA fetus is restricted primarily to the fetus with dysmature IUGR.* The original report on the relation between amniotic fluid volume and IUGR was from a population of 120 fetuses referred because of a marked discrepancy between clinical size and gestational age as estimated from clinical parameters.[32] Of the 29 fetuses exhibiting oligohydramnios, defined in this study by the very stringent criteria of a maximal fluid pocket of less than 1 cm, 26 were IUGR (positive predictive accuracy 90%); and of the 91 fetuses with normal fluid, 86 were normal (negative predictive accuracy 95%). The method yielded a sensitivity of 84% and a specificity of 97%. Application of this method to the more general population has yielded generally lower but still clinically useful test accuracy parameters. Most studies of the method have reported high positive predictive accuracy (range 79 to 100%),[32,35–37,38–41] and the reported sensitivity (the proportion of IUGR fetuses in a given study that exhibit decreased fluid) is in the range of 60 to 80%. Not all clinical studies of the relation between amniotic fluid volume and the incidence of IUGR have yielded such encouraging results. Hoddick et al.,[42] in a retrospective study of 125 SGA fetuses, of whom 58 had birth weights between the fifth and tenth percentiles and 67 were at or below the fifth percentiles, found little relation between amniotic fluid and IUGR; only four had a largest pocket of less than 1 cm (8.17%), and only 18 had a largest fluid pocket of 3 cm or less (35%). These data remain difficult to reconcile with others' experience with the method and may be more a reflection of the etiologic composition of the IUGR fetuses than a refutation of the validity of amniotic fluid monitoring in the recognition and management of IUGR. Nicolaides and colleagues, in a study of 326 IUGR fetuses, reported the presence of severe oligohydramnios (<1 cm) in 106 cases (33%) and a subjective reduction in amniotic fluid was reported in 214 cases (66%).[43] Because this study population included 56 fetuses with a karyotypic anomaly, the frequency of decreased amniotic fluid volume among IUGR fetuses with a normal karyotype is likely to be higher. In a recent review of 157 fetuses with dysmature IUGR (as defined after delivery) from the referred population at the Fetal Assessment Program at the University of Manitoba, 130 (82%) had oligohydramnios as defined by a largest fluid pocket of 2 cm or less and 34 (22%) had severe oligohydramnios (largest pocket less than 1 cm).[44]

The cutoff value for pocket depth to define oligohydramnios is somewhat arbitrary and differs according to the acceptable ratio between positive predictive accuracy and sensitivity. Based on our reported experience with more than 5500 referred high-risk patients, the cutoff value of a maximal pocket of 2 cm seems reasonable and is recommended. The maximal rate of rise in the incidence of adverse perinatal outcome appears to begin at or near this value. Based on our experience of more than 145,000 observations of amniotic fluid volume in more than 75,000 referred high-risk pregnancies and including more than 10,000 patients referred with a clinical suspicion of IUGR, certain clinical axioms seem evident.

1. The presence of normal amniotic fluid volume does not exclude the diagnosis of any type of IUGR, but the probability of disease is sharply reduced in the presence of normal fluid volume.
2. In the fetus with morphometric evidence of IUGR, provided the fetal renal system is present and functional and provided the membranes are intact, the observation of oligohydramnios (maximal pocket less than 2 cm) is a very powerful indicator of a dysmature etiology of disease. This latter clinical observation has considerable significance in the development of rational management strategies because it implies intervention for the nonanomalous fetus for whom extrauterine survival is at least a consideration. In my experience, the working rule, that *the fetus with oligohydramnios always has dysmaturity*

until proven otherwise, has been reliable and extremely useful.
3. It is important to recognize that oligohydramnios secondary to placental dysfunction can also be seen in some forms of chromosomal anomalies, notably with trisomies 13 and 18.
4. It always remains essential to attempt to confirm that the fetal kidneys are present and can function because renal agenesis, a lethal fetal malformation, can present classically in the second half of pregnancy as severe IUGR and oligohydramnios.

The fetus with absent renal function due to primary bilateral parenchymal disease (agenesis or dysgenesis) presents a difficult diagnostic challenge. Such fetuses almost invariably present beyond 20 weeks of gestation with oligohydramnios and severe IUGR. Impaired visualization due to oligohydramnios can make recognition of renal parenchymal disorders extremely difficult. Differentiation from severe dysmature IUGR is of critical importance because the management strategies differ radically. The observation of urine within the fetal bladder and observed variation of bladder volume over time (hours) points directly to dysmature IUGR (assuming intact membranes). Administration of furosemide to the mother has been advocated in such circumstances with the expectation of transplacental passage and a fetal diuretic effect.[45] The theory, although intriguing, appears to be without substance because in the ovine fetus furosemide does not cross the placenta.[46] Administration to the dysmature fetus with subsequently proven intact renal function does not induce diuresis *in utero.*[47] The observation of a severely reduced thoracic-to-abdominal circumference ratio strongly suggests pulmonary hypoplasia,[48] a nearly uniform finding in fetuses with renal agenesis/dysgenesis. This diagnostic dilemma may be resolved by experimental methods, such as instillation of normal saline into the amniotic cavity to enhance visualization of the renal fossae, direct injection (intramuscular or intravenous) of a diuretic to the fetus, or intravascular injection to improve an intrauterine fetal glomerular filtration rate.

Fetal Vessel Doppler Velocimetry

Mensuration of the spectrum of blood flow velocities in fetal vessels using pulsed or continuous wave Doppler ultrasound methods is a useful adjunctive test in the diagnosis and evaluation of the IUGR fetus.[49] Increased placental vascular existence produces a range of abnormal velocimetry patterns in the umbilical artery, with the pattern changing directly with placental blood flow resistance. Initially, increased existence results in a shift to high-velocity flow during systole and reduced flow velocity in diastole. Comparison of these velocity envelopes in systole and diastole demonstrates an increase in ratio (elevated systole/diastole [S/D] ratio, elevated pulsatility index). With more advanced disease, diastolic flow velocity can become unmeasurable producing an infinite S/D ratio. With extreme increase in placental microvascular resistance, diastolic low velocities may reverse, perhaps because of a reverberation effect of the systolic injection force.

In the fetal lamb, occlusion of the fetal placental microcirculation by repetitive emboli infusion initially causes an increase in the peak systolic velocities (a rise in S/D ratio) and with progressive embolic occlusion the diastolic velocities decrease and then disappear (absent end-diastolic flow).[50] With further occlusion, diastolic velocities in the opposite direction to expected flow may appear (reverse end-diastolic flow). In the human fetus there is a correlation between the number and character of fetal vessels in a cross-section of placental specimens by light microscopy and the umbilical artery velocity waveform.[51]

Measurement of umbilical artery velocity waveform in the human fetus is not always easy and may be prone to a variety of measurement error.[52] The S/D ratio differs by sampling site, generally increasing as the sample site moves toward the umbilicus and may appear abnormal by standard nomograms if the sample site is at or very near the aortic origin of the artery.[53] The fetal heart rate may also affect the S/D ratio, with an increase in ratio as heart rate rises, but this effect, except at extremes of heart rate, introduces negligible and clinically insignificant error. There is a gradual reduction in the S/D ratio with advancing gestational age. This relation compounds the application of the method because an accurate fix on gestational age is needed.

The character umbilical artery flow velocity waveform in IUGR fetuses has been studied extensively,[54-60] demonstrating a high probability of abnormal flow patterns in the affected perinate. In these studies the positive predictive accuracy of an abnormal umbilical artery Doppler waveform ranged from 50 to 81%, the sensitivity ranged from 22 to 100%, the specificity ranged from 83 to 95%, and the negative predictive accuracy ranged from 68 to 100%. The test accuracy parameters improve as the degree of abnormality of the waveform analysis increases. Among fetuses with absent end-diastolic flow the incidence of IUGR is 94% and with reverse end-diastolic flow it is 100% (see Table 23–2).

TABLE 23–2. THE RELATIONSHIP BETWEEN ABNORMAL END-DIASTOLIC FLOW PATTERN IN THE UMBILICAL ARTERY AND PERINATAL OUTCOME: EXPERIENCE IN 94 CASES

Variable	AEDF	REDF	Total
No.	72	22	94
IUGR	67 (94%)	22 (100%)	89 (94.5%)
PNM	14 (19%)	6 (27.3%)	20 (21.3%)
cPNM	6 (83%)	3 (13.6%)	9 (9.6%)
ABN karyotype	—	—	6 (6.4%)

AEDF, absent end-diastolic flow; REDF, reverse end-diastolic flow; IUGR, intrauterine growth retardation; PNM, perinatal mortality; cPNM, PNM corrected for lethal anomalies; ABN, abnormal.
From Serra-Serra et al., 1994.[60]

The clinical value of Doppler flow velocity measurements in screening for IUGR has not been validated. One of the frequently recurring problems is diagnosis and management of IUGR in the patient with either an unknown or uncertain date; in these cases the S/D ratio, provided there remains a degree of diastolic flow, is not helpful. When applied as a screening test to the general population, umbilical artery velocity waveform analysis has yielded poor predictive accuracy. Beattie and Dornan[61] examined diagnostic accuracy among 2097 unselected singleton pregnancies. Umbilical artery velocity waveforms were recorded at 28, 34, and 38 weeks, and the pulsatility index was recorded. Management was not based on these results. The predictive accuracy was poor across all gestational ages at testing, with maximal sensitivity of only 32% (achieved at 34 weeks) and a maximal positive predictive accuracy of 12% (also achieved at 34 weeks). In 405 unselected fetuses Bruinse et al.[62] also demonstrated clinically unacceptable low predictive accuracy (maximal sensitivity 22% at 34 weeks). Sijmons and coworkers studied predictive accuracy of umbilical artery velocity waveform analysis, also done serially at 28 and 34 weeks, and reported a pulsatility index among 400 fetuses of high-risk pregnancies but not otherwise selected for a high incidence of IUGR.[63] The method yielded a maximal sensitivity of 22% (at 34 weeks) and a maximal positive predictive value of 53% (also at 34 weeks). Clearly these are levels of accuracy far below those that are likely to be of value to the clinician.

In practical clinical terms the use of umbilical artery velocity waveforms to detect or manage IUGR is of little clinical value. Recognition of IUGR solely on the basis of absent or reverse umbilical artery diastolic flow velocities is a clinical rarity. Most IUGR fetuses are recognized by morphometric and other variables long before these flow velocity abnormalities appear. Initially, it was hoped that the use of umbilical artery velocity waveforms might be of value in differentiating between the different types of IUGR. This clinical expectation is also unfulfilled. Abnormal waveform velocities are not specific to dysmature IUGR, but rather occur frequently (6.4%) in SGA fetuses with developmental anomalies[60] (see Table 23–2). The explanation for this association is unclear, but it is assumed to be a result of an associated defect in placental vascularization.

Flow velocity waveform may be measured in intrafetal vessels including the aorta,[64] internal carotid artery,[65] and renal artery.[66] In the highly selected population of fetuses with proven IUGR, a relation between flow velocity waveform abnormalities in intrafetal vessels and IUGR is observed, but at present the practical clinical utility of such measures in the diagnosis, categorization, and management is in doubt.

INTRAFETAL PROPORTIONS

Fetal proportions in IUGR fetuses are based on comparison of fetal head size to abdominal size, termed the head-to-abdomen ratio, as first described by Campbell.[14] In the normal fetus the head initially grows faster than the abdomen until about 36 weeks of gestation; thereafter, abdominal growth rate slightly exceeds head growth. In fetuses with growth restraint due to placental insufficiency (dysmature IUGR), liver size is reduced as a result of diminished glycogen deposition, whereas head size and growth are maintained ("brain sparing effect"). These protective adaptations are manifested by asymmetry of the head to abdomen, an effect that may be recognized and monitored by a standard nomogram.[14] Provided there are no overt fetal anomalies that may skew fetal measurements, an abnormal increase in the head-to-abdomen ratio in the IUGR fetus is highly suggestive of a dysmature etiology. Studies of the predictive value of this ratio have yielded differing results. In a highly select population of fetuses at risk for dysmature IUGR, Crane and Kopta[67] reported perfect predictive accuracy with this method: Of the 37 patients with a normal ratio (79%), none had IUGR, whereas of the remaining 10 patients (21%) with an elevated ratio, all had IUGR. In contrast, Divon and associates[68] studied an IUGR population of mixed etiologies and found much lower predictive accuracies. In this population the head-to-abdomen ratio yielded a sensitivity of 36%, a specificity of 90%, a positive predictive value of 67%, and a negative predictive value of 72%. Experience with 2200 IUGR fetuses studied at the Fetal Assessment Program at the University of Manitoba suggests that the predictive value of the head-to-abdomen ratio is strongly influenced by the type of IUGR considered, its severity, and the gestational age of the fetus at testing. In the older fetus (>28 weeks) with severe dysmature IUGR, the sensitivity of the measurement is high (>93%), but this sensitivity diminishes inversely with gestational age and disease severity. The very immature fetus (<26 weeks) with severe dysmature IUGR commonly exhibits paradoxical findings of symmetry of head to abdomen. The explanation for this phenomenon in the immature fetus is unknown but may be related to an immature cardiac output redistribution adaptive reflex. In the normal small fetus the head-to-abdomen ratio remains normal. The head-to-abdomen ratio cannot be used in assessment of anomalous fetuses with IUGR. As may be predicted by the pathophysiology adaptation of dysmature IUGR, intrafetal comparisons of biometric variables affected in a similar way by the cardiac redistribution adaptive reflexes are unlikely to function as discriminators of IUGR type. Hence, femur length-to-abdominal circumference ratio does not identify nor discriminate IUGR well.

Assessment of Fetal Well-being

Knowing that the fetus under study is at minimal risk of asphyxial complications in the near future greatly reduces clinical anxiety surrounding the diagnosis of IUGR and reduces the need for immediate intervention for fetal indication. The myriad of fetal biophysical activities observed by real-time ultrasound examination can yield this critical in-

formation. This is discussed in detail in another chapter (see Chap. 26), but additional comments are warranted with specific reference to management of IUGR.

In its purest and most simplistic form, the management of IUGR depends on recognition and delivery of the fetus at risk of asphyxial complications and observation and conservatism of the other fetuses. It may be argued that weight percentile ranking or growth velocity is of minimal significance provided the fetus is not exposed to conditions of asphyxia. The relation between biophysical variables, as combined in a fetal biophysical profile score, and the risk of asphyxial complications has been well described.[17] In the presence of normal variables, the risk of stillbirth within a week is less than 0.6 per 1000,[69] and as variables are lost, the risk rises so that when all variables are absent, the risk of asphyxial death reaches more than 600 per 1000.[17] Similar trends have been reported for perinatal morbidity.[70]

Application of these data to the management of IUGR has considerable clinical impact. In the immature IUGR fetus in whom the risk of prematurity-related mortality can be calculated and is known to be high, observation of a normal fetal biophysical profile score indicates the risks of sustained fetal life to be less than the risk of delivery. The balance may change until the neonatal risk becomes negligible and easy delivery can be accomplished. In contrast, in the fetus with a deteriorating score, intervention may be indicated even in the presence of considerable prematurity because the balance no longer favors continued fetal existence. This profile has been used in the management of more than 2625 perinates in our center, yielding a corrected perinatal mortality of 8.4 per 1000. Perinatal death in the structurally normal mature IUGR fetus (≥34 weeks) managed according to the fetal biophysical score is now very rare. In our most recent experience, there were no perinatal deaths in 731 structurally normal IUGR fetuses (corrected perinatal mortality 0 per 1000)[71] (Table 23–3).

TABLE 23–3. CORRECTED PERINATAL MORTALITY (PNM) RATIOS (EXCLUDES LETHAL ANOMALY) AMONG LOW-RISK AND HIGH-RISK (SCREENED/UNSCREENED) PREGNANCIES AND AMONG SMALL-FOR-GESTATIONAL AGE (SGA) FETUSES (SCREENED/UNSCREENED): MANITOBA EXPERIENCE[a]

Category	No. of Cases	Corrected PNM (per 1000 Live Births)
All cases	144,786	5.6
All low risk	101,350	3.8
All high risk	43,436	9.8
Screened high risk[a]	31,740	2.2
All SGA (7% total population)	10,135	27.8
Unscreened SGA	7,460	21.3
Screened SGA[a]	2,675	8.4
Screened mature (≥34 weeks) SGA[a]	731	0

[a]Management based on fetal biophysical profile score.

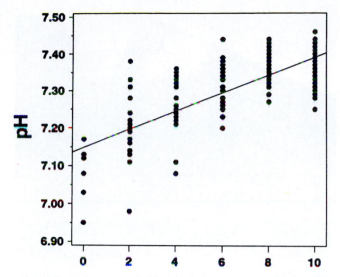

Figure 23–6. Biophysical profile score (BPS) and umbilical venous fetal pH in 389 high-risk fetuses, of which 104 were intrauterine growth restricted (≥2 SD below mean weight for gestational age). A highly significant linear relationship between BPS and pH was observed (pH = 7.132 + 0.248 × BPS) (R^{2}0.5173, $p < 0.001$). No fetus with a normal BPS (≥8) had a pH of less than 7.20, whereas all fetuses with a score of 0 out of 10 were acidotic.

Cordocentesis in Intrauterine Growth Restriction

Ultrasound-guided percutaneous fetal umbilical blood sampling (cordocentesis), first described by Daffos and coworkers,[72] is now a widely used investigative method in perinatal medicine. The role of cordocentesis in the diagnosis and management of the IUGR fetus remains an area of active investigation. This procedure is not without risk; fetal death as a direct consequence has been reported.[72,73] Fetal blood sampling is a rapid method for karyotype determination and is indicated in any IUGR fetus with proven or suspected structural anomalies; however, routine fetal karyotype determination in the structurally normal fetus does not appear to be warranted. Fetal blood sampling has provided insight into the frequency of hypoxemia and acidemia and metabolic abnormalities among IUGR fetuses.[74,75] The strong correlation between fetal umbilical venous pH and the fetal biophysical profile score (Fig. 23–6) obviates the need for cordocentesis for assessment of asphyxia in almost all cases.[76]

ANCILLARY ULTRASOUND SIGNS

There are several "soft" signs of IUGR that, although difficult to quantify, are nonetheless known to the experienced observer and offer some valuable insight into the type, progression, and severity of IUGR. Foremost among these subjective measures are the assessment of fetal fat layers and the distribution of fetal fat. After approximately 24 weeks of gestation, it is usual to see echolucent fat layering in the sub-

cutaneous tissue, best recognized in the area of the fetal thigh, in the posterior fetal neck and fetal scalp, and in the fetal malar region. Measurement of these fat layers is possible but difficult, and in my experience the measured results are neither reproducible nor of any obvious advantage over the subjective gradation. Assessment of fat distribution is of most use in differentiating the normal small fetus, in whom fat layers are usually seen, from the dysmature IUGR fetus, in whom fat layers are either lacking or appear reduced in thickness and are less widely distributed (Fig. 23–7). The impression of a lean or gaunt fetus, although difficult to quantitate, is often of clinical value and should not be ignored.

Changes in the ultrasound characteristics of the placenta may also offer insight into the etiology of IUGR, but the clinical value of these observations is limited.

The role of fetal echocardiography in the evaluation of the fetus with IUGR is as yet undetermined. DeVore[49] described dilation of the chambers of the right side of the heart as a finding in 72% of fetuses with asymmetric IUGR and suggested that these changes may be due to increased preload, the result of preferential shunting of umbilical vein blood flow past the hepatic circulation and directly to the right atrium. He reported an IUGR fetus that developed tricuspid valve incompetence that progressed from partial systolic regurgitation to holosystolic regurgitation.[49] Because the application of these ultrasound techniques to measure cardiac function is difficult and highly dependent on operator experience and interpretation, they are at present of limited value. In contrast, the use of these methods to detect structural cardiac defects is a valuable adjunct in the assessment of the growth-retarded fetus.

MANAGEMENT OF INTRAUTERINE GROWTH RESTRICTION INTEGRATION OF ULTRASOUND DATA

In view of extensive and diverse information that can be accumulated by ultrasound assessment, it has now become possible to recognize, categorize, and ultimately treat IUGR with ever-increasing clinical precision. Application of the principles described above can result in a significant and sustained reduction in the mortality and morbidity of the condition. From the outset it is necessary to recognize that delivery usually remains the only effective treatment. It follows that, after recognition of the condition, the remaining role of ultrasound evaluation is to provide input to balance the equation of fetal to neonatal risks. In this context, ultrasound data have moved beyond the recognition component to the management component. This shift, no doubt, accounts for the dramatic reduction in morbidity and mortality now being reported.

The algorithm for diagnosis and management of IUGR is complex and subject to variation by preference and experience. The algorithm used in our center is presented in graphic and descriptive terms (Fig. 23–8). The patient enters the diagnostic point from a variety of routes, most notably either

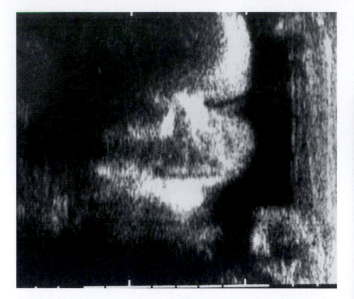

A

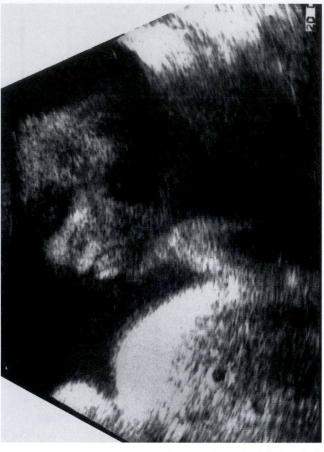

C

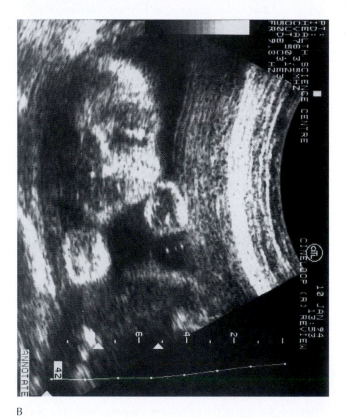

B

Figure 23–7. Facial characteristics in appropriate size for gestational age (AGA) and intrauterine growth-restricted (IUGR) fetuses. In the AGA fetus **(A)** a prominent malar fat pad is evident. With mild IUGR **(B)** the malar fat pad is present but less pronounced. In the severely affected dysmature IUGR fetus **(C),** the malar fat pad is absent and the facies assume an elfin characteristic. Fetal facial characteristics, although not diagnostic, offer some additional insight into the presence and severity of IUGR.

by clinical suspicion of IUGR or by recognition of suggestive signs in the course of ultrasound examination for other purposes. The multiple pregnancy represents a variant in entry to diagnosis because clinical detection of IUGR in one or both twins is very common.

At initial assessment, both morphometric and functional data are considered. The determination of IUGR at the outset is almost always based on fetal morphometric data. In the use of nonderived indices for morphometrics, usually abdominal circumference is recommended, although use of other indices, such as head-to-abdomen ratio, fetal mass estimation, or a ponderal index, may be substituted. A normal distribution plot of abdominal circumference to gestational age and normal functional signs virtually excludes the diagnosis of IUGR in fetuses of known gestational age. Repeat assessment would only be indicated if the maternal condition changes or

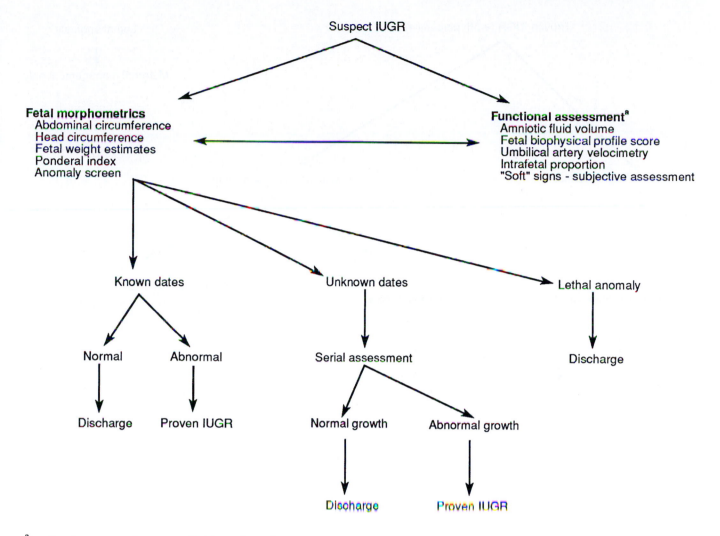

ᵃfunctional assessment occurs at all visits and modifies management.

Figure 23–8. Schematic for investigation of the fetus with suspected intrauterine growth restriction (IUGR) by dynamic ultrasound method. Fetal morphometrics and functional assessment are intimately interrelated in assigning etiology and prognosis and guiding management. The multifactional approach to diagnosis is a key step in developing national management strategies. Functional assessment occurs at all visits and modifies management, as per Figure 23–9.

the clinical impression of IUGR persists or exacerbates. In the patient with unknown menstrual dates, repeat assessment at an interval sufficient to measure fetal growth (or absence thereof), usually 2 weeks, is indicated. If at repeat assessment the functional signs remain normal and normal growth parameters are demonstrated, the patient may be safely assumed to have mistaken data and discharged from the algorithm with the previously cited provisos. If the selected growth rate is below the lower limit ascribed (fifth percentile) at first visit in a patient with unknown dates or at repeat visits in a patient with unknown dates, a diagnosis of IUGR is established and efforts are then directed toward determining etiology, severity, and prognosis (see Fig. 23–8). In such fetuses, ultrasound assessment should be done at least weekly, and conserva-

tive management continued, provided fetal growth is demonstrated and functional signs remain normal (see Fig. 23–3). Intervention in such fetuses may take place when fetal maturity is affirmed and delivery can be instituted with minimal difficulty.

In the fetus with a proven major anomaly, a decision toward total conservative management with a view to absolute minimization of maternal risk is the usual rule. In our center, a prompt delivery is indicated in an IUGR fetus regardless of gestational age by a confirmed abnormal biophysical profile score, isolated observation of oligohydramnios by defined criteria (<1 cm largest vertical pocket), or both in an IUGR fetus of at least 25 weeks' gestation. Umbilical artery velocimetry and intrafetal proportion are not used to

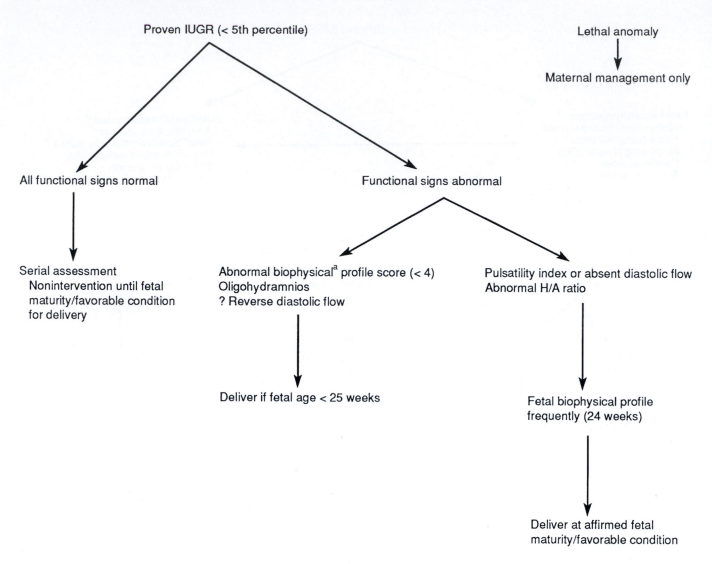

^aalternate fetal assessment methods may be substituted.

Figure 23–9. Proposed management of the fetus with proven intrauterine growth restriction (IUGR) as defined by morphometric indices at or below the fifth percentile for gestational age. Provided functional signs are normal, conservative management (observation) can be safely continued until low-risk delivery can be accomplished. In contrast, if functional signs are abnormal, intervention is recommended at any gestational age beyond which neonatal survival is possible. H/A, head/abdomen.

precipitate intervention, but rather to guide the frequency of fetal surveillance. In the presence of a distinctly abnormal pulsatility index or absent flow, fetal surveillance should be intensified. The finding of reverse diastolic flow to prompt delivery in the IUGR fetus remains inconclusive at present, but it seems likely that with further experience this finding will also be a signal to precipitate immediate delivery. In the dysmature IUGR fetus and in other types, it has been our policy to continue conservative management only until fetal maturity is affirmed and delivery can be accomplished with minimal maternal risk. This method of management has been applied to more than 1200 proven IUGR fetuses, yielding a corrected perinatal mortality (excluding fetuses with anomalies) of 12.5 per 1000. This represents a significant reduction from the expected rate among IUGR fetuses (from 60 to 80 deaths per 1000) (Fig. 23–9).

LONG-TERM CONSEQUENCES OF IUGR: THE ALPHA-OMEGA THEORY

The alpha-omega theory portends that fetal adaptation to intrauterine insult(s) may manifest as postnatal diseases across the lifespan of the individual.[77] The omega effect, that is, late onset adult disease secondary to residual effects of fetal adaptation, may be especially relevant to the IUGR fetus. Barker et al. presented provocative data demonstrating a powerful association between birth weight and late adult onset (50 years or older) hypertension, coronary artery disease, and lethal myocardial infaction.[78] More recently, in men of age 50 years or older, low birth weight has been linked with an increased risk of adult onset diabetes, insulin resistance, and peripheral vascular disease.[78,79] Although a direct association between growth restriction and these adult disease has not yet been described, given that in the study patients were all born in the late 1930s and 1940s when survival of premature infants was a fraction of today's expectations, it may be reasonably inferred that the low birth weight subjects demonstrating late onset adult disease were not premature at birth but were growth restricted. Although a theoretical concept at the time of this writing, it may be that intervention for recognized growth restriction may yield lifelong benefits to the individual.

REFERENCES

1. Morrison I, Olson J. Weight specific stillbirths and associated causes of death: An analysis of 765 consecutive stillbirths. *Am J Obstet Gynecol.* 1985;152:975.
2. Streeter H, Manning FA. Classification of neonatal morbidity and mortality by birth weight percentile in IUGR neonates (abstract). *Proc Soc Obstet Gynecol Can.* 1980.
3. Manning FA. IUGR: Etiology, pathophysiology, diagnosis and treatment. In: Manning FA, ed. *Aspects of Fetal Life,* Norwalk, CT: Appleton & Lange; 1995.
4. Lubchenco LO, Hansman C, Dressler M, et al. Intrauterine growth as estimated from liveborn birthweight data at 24–42 weeks of gestation. *Pediatrics.* 1963;32:793.
5. Creasy RK, Resnick R. Intrauterine growth retardation. In: Creasy RK, Resnick R, eds. *Maternal Fetal Medicine: Principles and Practice.* Philadelphia: Saunders; 1984:491ff.
6. Grennert L, Persson P, Gerrser G, et al. Benefits of ultrasound screening of a pregnant population. *Acta Obstet Gynecol Scand.* 1978;78(suppl):5.
7. Usher RH, Boyd ME, McLean FH, et al. Assessment of fetal risk in postdates pregnancies. *Am J Obstet Gynecol.* 1988;158:259.
8. Maternal physiology in pregnancy: Duration of pregnancy. In: Eastman WJ, Hellman LM, eds. *Williams Obstetrics.* New York: Appleton-Century-Crofts; 1966:218.
9. Campbell S. Fetal growth. *Clin Obstet Gynecol.* 1974;1:41.
10. Robinson HP. Sonar measurement of fetal crown-rump length as a means of assessing maturity in the first trimester of pregnancy. *Br Med J.* 1973;4:28.
11. Hadlock FP, Deter R, Harrist R, et al. Fetal biparietal diameter: A critical re-evaluation of the relation to menstrual age by means of realtime ultrasound. *J Ultrasound Med.* 1982;1:97.
12. Manning FA. Morrison I, Harman CR. Unpublished data. 1994.
13. Hadlock FP, Deter R, Harrist R, et al. Computer assisted analysis of fetal age in the third trimester using multiple fetal growth parameters. *J Clin Ultrasound.* 1983;11:313.
14. Campbell S. Ultrasound measurement of the fetal head to abdomen circumference ratio in assessment of growth retardation. *Br J Obstet Gynaecol.* 1977;84:165.
15. Towell ME, Figueroa J, Markowitz S, et al. The effect of mild hypoxemia maintained for 24 hours on maternal and fetal glucose, lactate, cortisol, and anginene vasopressin in pregnant sheep at 122 to 139 days' gestation. *Am J Obstet Gynecol.* 1987;157:1550.
16. Manning FA, Platt LD, Sipos L. Antepartum fetal evaluation: Development of a fetal biophysical profile. *Am J Obstet Gynecol.* 1980;136:787.
17. Manning FA, Morrison I, Lange IR, et al. Fetal assessment based on fetal biophysical profile scoring: Experience in 12,620 referred high risk pregnancies. I: Perinatal mortality by frequency and etiology. *Am J Obstet Gynecol.* 1985;151:343–350.
18. Campbell S. The assessment of fetal growth by diagnostic ultrasound. *Clin Perinatol.* 1974;1:507.
19. Chattingers S, Axelsson O, Lindre C. The clinical value of measurement of symphysis fundal distance and ultrasound measurement in the diagnosis of IUGR. *J Perinat Med.* 1985;13:227–232.
20. Thompson TE, Manning FA, Morrison I. Determination of fetal volume in utero by an ultrasound method correlation with neonatal birth weight. *J Ultrasound Med.* 1983;2:113.
21. McCallum WE, Brinkley TF. Estimation of fetal weight from ultrasound measurement. *Am J Obstet Gynecol.* 1979;133:195.
22. Shepard MJ, Richards VA, Berkowitz RL, et al. An evaluation of two equations for predicting fetal weight by ultrasound. *Am J Obstet Gynecol.* 1982;152:47.
23. Harman CR, Holme S, Gardiner R, et al. Ultrasonic weight estimation in the "clinically small" fetus: A prospective comparison of two methods (abstract). *Proc Soc Obstet Gynecol Can* 1984.
24. Hadlock FP, Deter R, Harrist R, et al. Fetal abdominal circumference: Relation to menstrual age. *AJR.* 1982;139:367.
25. Hadlock FP, Deter R, Harrist R, et al. A date-independent predictor of intrauterine growth retardation: Femur length/abdominal circumference ratio. *AJR.* 1983;141:979.
26. Campbell S, Wilkin P. Ultrasonic measurement of fetal abdominal circumference in the estimation of fetal weight. *Br J Obstet Gynaecol.* 1975;82:689.
27. Cohn HE, Sacks ET, Heyman MA, et al. Cardiovascular responses to hypoxemia and acidemia in fetal lambs. *Am J Obstet Gynecol.* 1974;120:817.
28. Manning FA, Snijders RL, Harman CR, et al. Fetal biophysical profile scoring. VI: Correlation with antepartum umbilical venous pH. *Am J Obstet Gynecol.* 1993;169:755.
29. Wladimiroff JW, Campbell S. Fetal urine production in normal and complicated pregnancy. *Lancet.* 1974;1:151–154.
30. Kurjak A, Kirkinen P, Latin V, et al. Ultrasound assessment of renal function in normal and complicated pregnancies. *Am J Obstet Gynecol.* 1981;141:266–270.
31. Nicolaides KH, Peters MT, Vyas S, et al. Relation of the rate of fetal urine production to oxygen tension in small-for-gestational age fetuses. *Am J Obstet Gynecol.* 1990;162:387–391.
32. Manning FA, Hill LM, Platt LD. Qualitative amniotic fluid volume determination by ultrasound: Antepartum detection

of intrauterine growth retardation. *Am J Obstet Gynecol.* 1981;139:254–258.

33. Phelan JP, Platt LD, Yeh S. The role of ultrasound assessment of amniotic fluid volume in the management of the postdate pregnancy. *Am J Obstet Gynecol.* 1985;151:304.

34. Magann EF, Morton ML, Nolan TE, et al. Comparative efficacy of two sonographic measurements for the detection of aberrations in amniotic fluid volume (abstract 151). *Proc Soc Gynecol Invest.* 1993.

35. Phillipson EH, Sokol RJ, Williams T. Oligohydramnios: Clinical association and predictive accuracy for intrauterine growth retardation. *Am J Obstet Gynecol.* 1983;146:271.

36. Hill LM, Brickle R, Wolfgram KR, et al. Oligohydramnios: Ultrasonically detected incidence and subsequent outcome. *Am J Obstet Gynecol.* 1983;147:407.

37. Chamberlain PFC, Manning FA, Morrison I, et al. Ultrasound evaluation of amniotic fluid volume. I: The relationship of marginal and decreased amniotic fluid volume to perinatal outcome. *Am J Obstet Gynecol.* 1984;150:245.

38. Manning FA. Unpublished data, 1992.

39. Patterson RM, Prihoda TJ, Pouliot MR. Sonographic amniotic fluid measurement and IUGR: A reappraisal. *Am J Obstet Gynecol.* 1984;157:440–446.

40. Gross TL, Sokol RJ, Wilson M, et al. Using ultrasound and amniotic fluid volume to diagnose IUGR before birth: A clinical model. *Am J Obstet Gynecol.* 1982;143:265.

41. Divon MY, Chamberlain PF, Sipos L, et al. Identification of the small for gestational age fetus with the use of gestational-age independent indices of fetal growth. *Am J Obstet Gynecol.* 1985;155:1197.

42. Hoddick WK, Callen PW, Filly RA, et al. Ultrasound determination of qualitative amniotic fluid volume in intrauterine growth retardation: Appraisal of the 1 cm rule. *Am J Obstet Gynecol.* 1984;149:758.

43. Nicolaides KH, Snijders RJM, Noble P. Cordocentesis in the study of growth-retarded fetuses. In: Divon MY, ed. *Abnormal Fetal Growth.* New York: Elsevier; 1991:166ff.

44. Manning FA. Unpublished data, 1994.

45. Barret RJ, Rayburn WF, Barr MJ Jr. Furosemide (Lasix) challenge test in assessment bilateral fetal hydronephrosis. *Am J Obstet Gynecol.* 1983;147:846.

46. Chamberlain PF, Cumming M, Torchia M, et al. Ovine fetal urine production following maternal intravenous furosemide administration. *Am J Obstet Gynecol.* 1985;151:815.

47. Harman CR. Maternal furosemide may not provoke urine production in the compromised fetus. *Am J Obstet Gynecol.* 1984;150:322.

48. Nimrod C, Nicholson S, Davies D, et al. Pulmonary hypoplasia testing in clinical obstetrics. *Am J Obstet Gynecol.* 1988;158:277.

49. DeVore GR. Fetal echocardiography: Its use in the fetus with growth disturbance. In: Divon MY, ed. *Abnormal Fetal Growth.* New York: Elsevier; 1991:266ff.

50. Morrow RJ, Adamson SL, Bull SB, et al. Effect of placental embolization on the umbilical artery velocity waveform in sheep. *Am J Obstet Gynecol.* 1989;161:1055.

51. Giles WB, Trudinger BJ, Baird P. Fetal umbilical artery velocity waveforms and placental resistance: Pathological correlation. *Br J Obstet Gynecol.* 1985;92:31.

52. Kay HH, Carroll BA, Bowie JD, et al. "Non-uniformity" of

fetal umbilical systolic/diastolic ratios as determined by duplex Doppler sonography. *J Ultrasound Med.* 1989;8:417.

53. Mahalek KE, Rosenberg J, Berkowitz GS, et al. Umbilical and uterine artery flow velocity wave-forms. Effects of the sampling site on Doppler ratios. *J Ultrasound Med.* 1989;8: 171–176.

54. Fleischer A, Schulman H, Farmakides G, et al. Umbilical artery velocity waveforms and intrauterine growth retardation. *Am J Obstet Gynecol.* 1985;151:502–505.

55. Mulders LG, Wijn PF, Jongsma HW, et al. A comparative study of three indices of umbilical blood flow in relation to prediction of growth retardation. *J Perinat Med.* 1987;15:3–12.

56. Divon MY, Guidetti DA, Braverman JJ, et al. Intrauterine growth retardation. A prospective study of the diagnostic value of real-time sonography combined with umbilical artery flow velocimetry. *Obstet Gynecol.* 1988;72:611–614.

57. Berkowitz GS, Chitkara U, Rosenberg J, et al. Sonographic estimation of fetal weight and Doppler analysis of umbilical artery velocimetry in the prediction of intrauterine growth retardation: A prospective study. *Am J Obstet Gynecol.* 1988;158:1149–1153.

58. Dempster J, Mires GJ, Patel N, et al. Umbilical artery velocity waveforms: Poor association with small-for-gestational-age babies. *Br J Obstet Gynaecol.* 1989;96:692–696.

59. Arduni D, Rizzo G, Romanini C, et al. Fetal blood flow velocity waveforms as predictors of growth retardation. *Obstet Gynecol.* 1987;70:7–10.

60. Serra-Serra V, Redman CR, Manning FA, et al. Unpublished data, 1994.

61. Beattie RB, Dornan JC. Antenatal screening for intrauterine growth retardation with umbilical artery Doppler ultrasonography. *Br Med J.* 1989;298:631–635.

62. Bruinse HW, Sijmons EA, Reuwar PJ. Clinical value of screening for IUGR by Doppler ultrasound. *J Ultrasound Med.* 1989;8:207–209.

63. Sijmons EA, Reuwer PJ, van Beek E, et al. The validity of screening for small-for-gestational-age and low-weight-for-length infants by Doppler ultrasound. *Br J Obstet Gynaecol.* 1989;96:557–561.

64. Jouppila P, Kirkinen P. Non-invasive assessment of fetal aortic blood flow in normal and abnormal pregnancy. *Clin Obstet Gynecol.* 1989;32:702–709.

65. Veille JC, Cohen I. Middle cerebral artery blood flow in normal and growth retarded fetuses. *Am J Obstet Gynecol.* 1990;162:391–396.

66. Veille JC, Kanaan C. Duplex Doppler ultrasonographic evaluation of the fetal renal artery in normal and abnormal fetuses. *Am J Obstet Gynecol.* 1989;161:1502–1507.

67. Crane JP, Kopta MM. Prediction of intrauterine growth retardation via ultrasonically measured head/abdomen circumference ratios. *Obstet Gynecol.* 1979;54:597.

68. Divon MY, Guidetti DA, Braverman JJ, et al. Intrauterine growth retardation: A prospective study of the diagnostic value of real-time sonography combined with umbilical artery flow velicometry. *Obstet Gynecol.* 1988;72:611.

69. Manning FA, Morrison I, Harman CR, et al. Fetal assessment by fetal BPS: Experience in 19,221 referred high risk pregnancies. II: The false negative rate by frequency and etiology. *Am J Obstet Gynecol.* 1987;154:880.

70. Manning FA, Morrison I, Harman CR, et al. Fetal assessment

by fetal biophysical profile score. III: Positive predictive accuracy of the very abnormal test. *Am J Obstet Gynecol.* 1990;162: 398.

71. Morrison I, Manning FA, Harman CR, et al. Perinatal outcome in mature (≥34 week) fetuses with IUGR. *J Mat Fetal Med.* 1994;3:75.

72. Daffos F, Capella-Pavlovsky M, Forestier F. Fetal blood sampling during pregnancy with use of a needle guided by ultrasound: A study of 606 consecutive cases. *Am J Obstet Gynecol.* 1985;153:655.

73. Nicolaides KH. Cordocentesis. *Clin Obstet Gynecol.* 1988;31: 123.

74. Nicolaides KH, Economides DL, Soothill PW. Blood gases, pH, and lactate in appropriate and small for gestational age fetuses. *Am J Obstet Gynecol.* 1989;161:966.

75. Economides DL, Nicolaides KH, Gahl W, et al. Cordocentesis in the diagnosis of intrauterine starvation. *Am J Obstet Gynecol.* 1989;161:1004–1008.

76. Manning FA, Snijders RL, Nicolaides KH, et al. Fetal biophysical profile score. VI: Correlation with antepartum umbilical venous fetal pH. *Am J Obstet Gynecol.* 1993;169:755.

77. Manning FA, Harman CR, Merticoglou S, et al. The alpha-omega theory: Evidence for the alpha effect. *Am J Obstet Gynecol.* 2000;182:39.

78. Barker DJP, Osmond C, Golding J, et al. Growth in utero, blood pressure in childhood and adult life and mortality for cardiovascular disease. *Br Med J.* 1989;298:564.

79. Martyn CN, Gale CR, Jespersen S, Sherriff SB. Impaired fetal growth and atherosclerosis of carotid and peripheral arteries. *Lancet.* 1998;352:173.

24

Sonography of Multiple Gestations*

*Jacqueline Reyes • Luís F. Gonçalves • Sandra Rejane Silva •
Philippe Jeanty*

Multiple gestations account for 1 to 2% of all births[1] and represent 10 to 14% of the overall perinatal mortality, a rate 5 to 10 times higher than that of singletons. Because of the increased use of assisted reproductive technologies, the number of high-order pregnancies has steeply increased over the past 20 years. The aim of early diagnosis of multiple gestations and their associated complications is the reduction of perinatal morbidity and mortality. Sonography allows determination of zygosity, chorionicity, amnionicity, placental location, and fetal presentation and the detection of complications such as growth discrepancy, abnormal vascular anastomoses, amniotic fluid volume imbalance, and cord entanglement.[2] In this chapter, we discuss the ultrasonographic evaluation, most common complications, and the role of invasive procedures in the management of multiple pregnancies.

EMBRYOLOGY

Two mechanisms may lead to a multiple pregnancy: fertilization of two or more oocytes or early embryonic splitting of a single ovum. The most common mechanism is fertilization of several oocytes in a single menstrual cycle (two-thirds of cases). This type of twinning results in genetically different individuals (also known as polyzygotic, non-identical, or fraternal twins) and has a hereditary tendency. It is associated with a recurrence risk three times higher than that of the general population.[3] Each zygote develops its own chorion, placenta, and amniotic cavity. Every fetal–placental–amniotic compartment is individualized, and there are no (or are very rare) vascular communications between them. Circulatory complications are thus rare, unless the placentas become fused during pregnancy. The incidence of dizygotic twin differs in different populations, whereas the incidence of monozygotic twins is fairly constant (Fig. 24–1).

In one-third of cases, early embryonic splitting of a single ovum is the mechanism of twinning. Four situations may arise as a result of this process: dichorionic–diamniotic placentation (one-third of cases), monochorionic–diamniotic placentation, monochorionic–monoamniotic placentation, and conjoined twins. If early embryonic splitting occurs before day 3 after fertilization (during the two- to eight-cell stage), two independent fetuses with separate placentas will result. A single placenta with two amniotic cavities occurs if splitting takes place between days 4 and 7 (blastocyst stage). If division of the embryoblast occurs after about 8 days, the twins share a single placenta and amniotic cavity (monochorionic–monoamniotic twins). Division beyond day 13 results in conjoined twins (Fig. 24–2).

*Originally published on *www.TheFetus.net* (© 2000 Philippe Jeanty, MD, PhD, Jacqueline Reyes, MD, Luís Flávio de Andrade Gonçalves, MD, Sandra Rejane Silva, MD). Some images courtesy Gianluigi Pilu, MD. A few drawings were adapted from Lifeart by the Techpool studio.

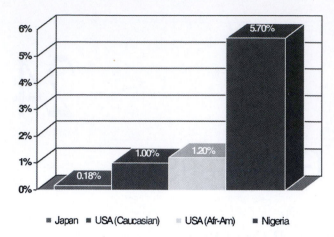

Figure 24–1. The incidence of dizygotic twin differs in different populations. From *left* to *right:* Japan, European-American population, African-American population, and Nigeria.

Less frequently, monozygotic and dizygotic twinning may occur simultaneously in a pregnancy with three or more embryos (Fig. 24–3).

CLINICAL IMPLICATIONS OF ZYGOSITY AND CHORIONICITY

Improving the outcome of multiple pregnancies is a major challenge for prenatal care. The mortality rate for twins is 4 to 11 times higher than that for singletons. Stillbirths account for approximately one-third of the perinatal deaths. The remaining two-thirds occur during the neonatal period, mainly as a result of prematurity (Figs. 24–4 to 24–6).

The different types of twins are listed in Table 24–1 (further details are in the text). The table is organized from

Figure 24–2. Schematic drawing demonstrating the outcome of twinning at different stages of early embryonic life. *(Top)* Fission before the formation of the inner cell mass and any differentiation will produce two embryos with two separate chorions, amnions and placentas. *(Middle)* Twinning at the early blastocyst stage, after formation of the inner cell mass, will cause the development of two embryos, with one placenta and one chorion but two separate amnions. *(Bottom)* If separation occurs after the formation of the embryonic disc, the amnion has already formed and will lead to a monoamniotic–monochorionic pregnancy. Incomplete fission at this stage or later will result in conjoined twins.

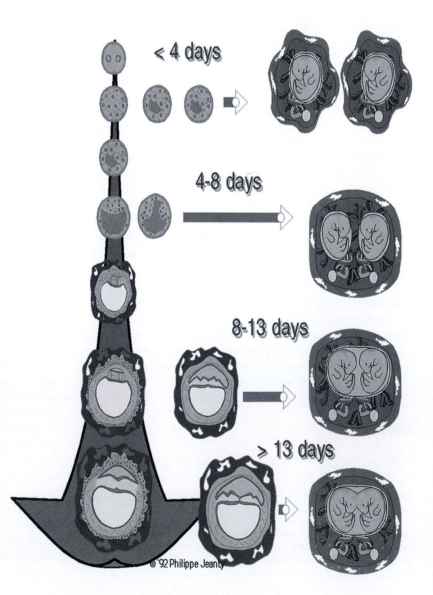

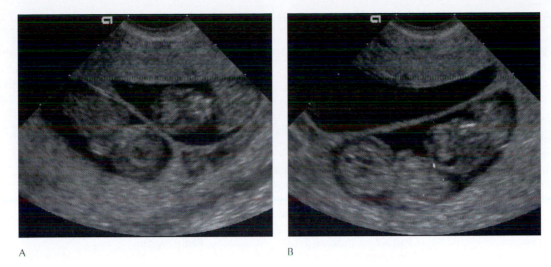

A   B

Figure 24–3. Dichorionic–triamniotic pregnancy in an assisted pregnancy. **(A)** There is a thick septum between the two embryos. **(B)** The septation, is barely visible.

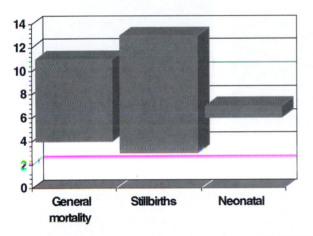

Figure 24–4. Compared with singletons, the rate of mortality of twins is 4 to 11 higher, that of stillbirths 3 to 13 times higher, and that of neonatal death 6 to 7 times higher.

the most dissimilar on top to the most similar at the bottom (Figs. 24–7 and 24–8).

Precise determination of zygosity and chorionicity is the most important step for the proper management of multiple pregnancies. Monochorionic–monoamniotic pregnancies are associated with the highest mortality rate (50%), followed by monochorionic–diamniotic pregnancies (26%) and dichorionic–diamniotic pregnancies (9%). Mortality is even higher before 24 weeks of gestation.[4] The elevated mortality rate seen in monochorionic placentation is caused mainly by aberrant vascular communications in the placenta, leading to twin-to-twin transfusion syndrome. In monoamniotic twins, the risk is increased by the possibility of cord accidents. Thus, monochorionic twins are at a higher risk of prematurity, intrauterine death, and neurologic damage secondary to complications of twin-to-twin transfusion syndrome.

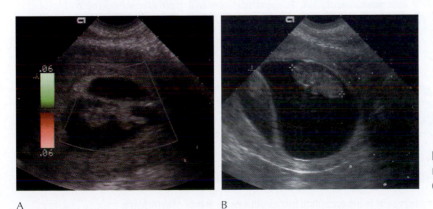

A   B

Figure 24–5. The increased mortality of twins is already apparent in the first trimester scan with dual demise.

TABLE 24–1. A CLASSIFICATION OF TWINS FROM MOST DISSIMILAR TO MOST IDENTICAL, FROM TOP TO BOTTOM

Dizygotic twins (1/90):		
Superfecondation	Not the same father	Many case reports in the literature of the 19th century
Superfetation	Not the same cycle	Historically these were misinterpretations of growth discordance, but recent DNA studies have demonstrated that the condition is occasionally possible, in particular with assisted reproductive techniques
Fraternal twins	Same father, same cycle	The usual twins
Monozygotic twins (1/250):		
Diamniotic dichorionic	Same zygote, 2 separate sacs	Early separation
Diamniotic monochorionic	Same zygote, 2 separate amnions	
Monoamniotic monochorionic	Same zygote, same sac	Late separation
Conjoint	Equally but incompletely divided	Incomplete separation
Duplicata incompleta	Incompletely duplicated	
Ectoparasitic twin	Partial fetus attached to sib	Partial division
Fetus-in-fetu	Embedded	

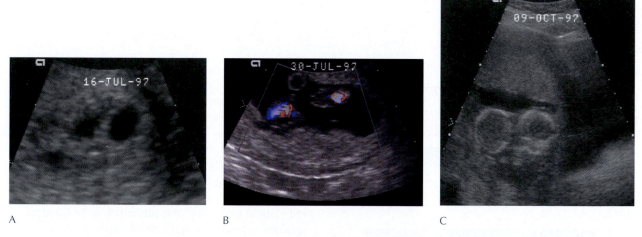

Figure 24–6. A normal dichorionic pregnancy **(A)** with appropriate early growth **(B)** (despite vaginal bleeding). The repeat examination demonstrates the demise of both twins **(C)**.

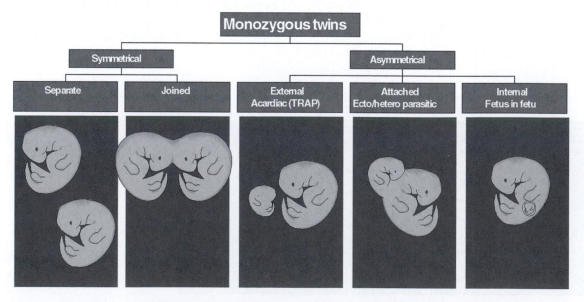

Figure 24–7. A classification of monozygous twins according to their symmetry or lack of symmetry.

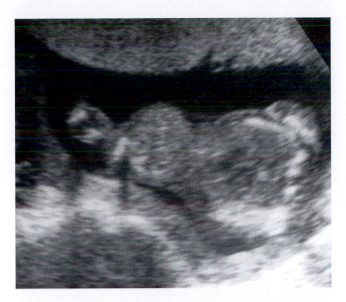

Figure 24–8. Ectoparasitic twins are parts of twins implanted in another fetus. In this case what appears to be an omphalocele on the left is a fetal abdomen, with lower legs on the extreme left. *(Courtesy Glynis Sack, MD, www.TheFetus.net)*

As illustrated from data from the Collaborative Perinatal Project (Figs. 24–9 and 24–10), the excess mortality in twins is due predominantly to the contribution of the monochorionic twins.

Also important is the determination of the number of viable fetuses: higher-order multiple fetuses have a greater risk of prematurity. A singleton gestation has an average length of 39 weeks versus 35 weeks for twins, 33 weeks for triplets, and 29 weeks for quadruplets. Early ultrasound evaluation at 9 to 12 weeks can precisely inform chorionicity, amnionicity, and the number of viable fetuses. This information is important for the development of appropriate methods of surveillance and intervention during the second trimester of pregnancy aimed at reducing the excess fetal loss in twins[5,6] (Fig. 24–11).

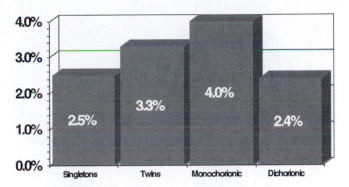

Figure 24–9. The excess mortality in twins is due predominantly to the contribution of the monochorionic twins.

The chorionicity and zygosity of twins is shown in Fig. 24–12 compiled from the Birmingham twin survey.[7] Sixty-five percent of twins have the same sex; of these, 28% are monozygotic and 37% are dizygotic. The figure also demonstrates that 80% of twins are diamniotic–dichorionic and that 90% of these diamniotic–dichorionic twins are also dizygotic. Further, 43% of same-sex twins are monozygotic. This helps answer the common question from patients: "If I have same-sex fetuses, what is the likelihood that they are identical?"

Dichorionic twins are easier to recognize than monochorionic twins in the first trimester. The criterion is simply that dichorionic twins have a thick membrane (actually some interposing tissue), whereas monochorionic twins have either a very thin or barely visible membrane. This is illustrated in Fig. 24–13.

Subsequently, dizygotic twins can be identified when they have a separate placenta or different sex (Fig. 24–14).

THE NAMING OF TWINS

In the days before ultrasound, when the obstetrician delivered a set of twins, it was traditional to call the first one out

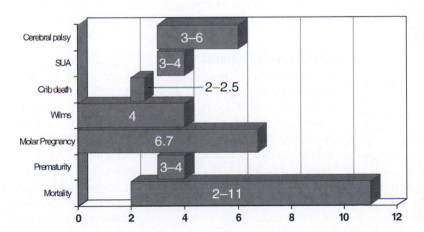

Figure 24–10. The relative risk of twins versus that of singletons affects not only mortality but also morbidity.

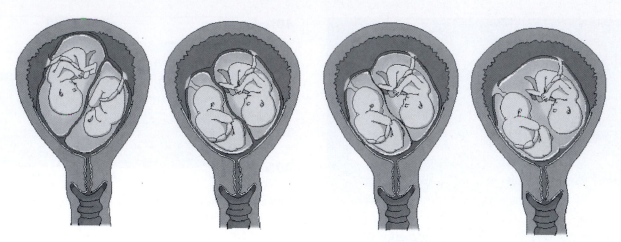

Figure 24–11. Frequency and mortality according to the types of placentation.[233]

'twin A' and the second one 'twin B' (Fig. 24–15). By some twisted extrapolation, this nomenclature has been applied to ultrasound, although we have observed that the presenting twin is not always the same one from examination to examination (see Fig. 24–15). A much better terminology, aside from the monoamniotic twins, is to describe the relative positions of the twins: left upper and right lower. One of the characteristics is bound to be constant from examination to

examination because the membrane prevents the twins from switching sides.

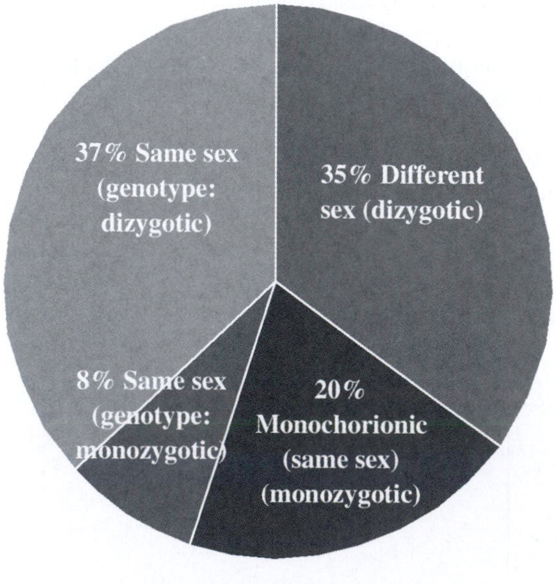

MONOCHORIONIC TWINS

Definition

Monochorionic twinning is a type of gestation in which the fetuses share a single chorion (the outer membrane) and may or may not share the amnion (the inner membrane). When the amnion is shared, the twins are called *monochorionic–monoamniotic* and the reader is referred to the specific section in this chapter (Fig. 24–16). When they do not share the amnion, the twins are called *monochorionic–diamniotic*. Independent of the number of amniotic sacs, all monochorionic twins are monozygotic.[8,9]

Monochorionic placentation occurs in two-thirds of monozygous twins and represents approximately 0.3% of all spontaneous conceptions.[10] It is highly associated with the overall adverse outcome in multiple gestations. Of all intrauterine deaths in twins, 73% are associated with monochorionic placentation,[11] and among livebirths, there is an elevated incidence of perinatal mortality, birth weight discrepancies, and intrauterine growth retardation (IUGR).[12,13]

Sonographic Features

Determination of chorionicity can be performed by transvaginal ultrasound as early as 5 weeks.[14,15] In early pregnancy, the separate sacs are clearly visible. In monochorionic twins, there is a single placental mass, with or without a dividing membrane. When there is a dividing membrane, it is composed of two layers representing the two layers of amnion. In contrast, the intertwin membrane of dichorionic twins is composed of a layer of chorion sandwiched between two layers of amnion. Therefore, the intertwin membrane in dichorionic twins is thicker, especially between 6 and

Figure 24–12. The chorionicity and zygosity of twins is expressed in the following chart compiled from the Birmingham twin survey.[8] 65% of twins are like sex. Of these 28% are monozygotic and 37% are dizygotic. The chart also demonstrates that 80% of twins are diamniotic-dichorionic and that 90% of these diamniotic-dichorionic are also dizygotic. Further 43% of like sex twins are monozygotic. This helps answer the common question from patients: "If I have like-sex fetuses, what is the likelihood that they are identical?."

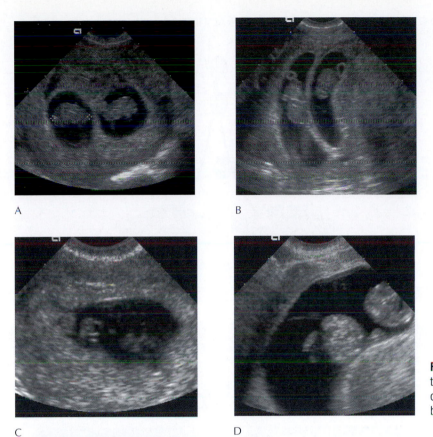

A

B

C

D

Figure 24–13. The two *top* images show dichorionic twins, which are easily recognized from the monochorionic twins on the two *bottom* images (first trimester) by the thick intervening membrane.

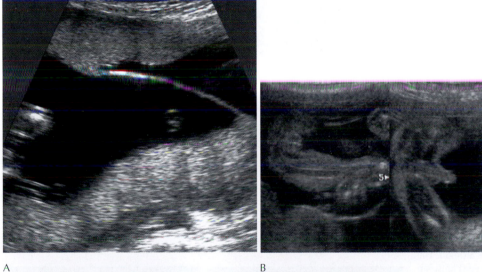

A

B

Figure 24–14. Dizygotic twins can be suspected or identified in the second trimester, when they have separate placenta or discordant sex.

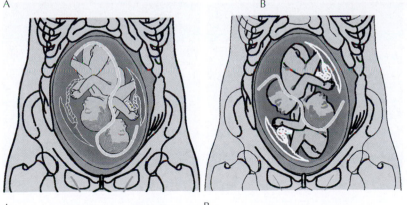

A

B

Figure 24–15. The vestigial convention of naming of twins **A** and **B** should be replaced by a description of the actual positions.

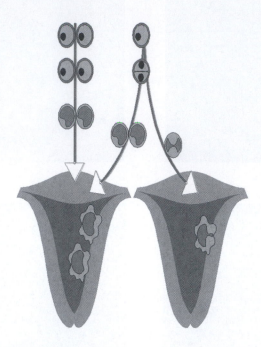

Dichorionic - Diamniotic

2 chorions

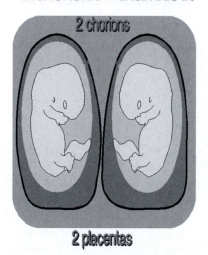

2 placentas

Monochorionic - Diamniotic

1 chorion

2 amnions

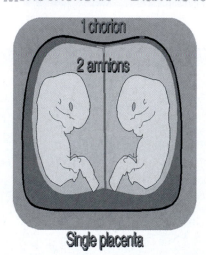

Single placenta

A

Figure 24–16. The implantation of two fertilized eggs (*left side* of the drawing) will result in two gestational sacs that share neither the chorion nor the amnion. The drawing illustrates how the placenta can insert between the two sacs, producing the lambda sign. On the *right side* of the drawing, a single egg can either split early (before 4 days) into two embryos and the two embryos will then resemble the previous condition, or the fertilized egg can split between the 4th and 8th days at a time when the chorion is no longer divisible. Both embryos will then share the chorion, the placenta will not be able to infiltrate between the two gestational sacs, and the membrane insertion will have the T appearance. The ultrasound images underneath the drawings illustrate the membrane insertion in both cases.

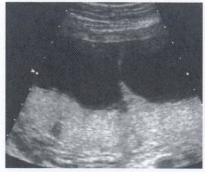

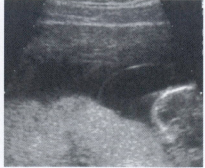

B   C

9 weeks, when a septum can be observed between the chorionic sacs. After 9 weeks, the septum becomes progressively thinner; however, it remains thick and relatively easy to identify at the insertion point into the placental mass as a triangular projection called the lambda or "twin-peak" sign.[16,17] Sepulveda et al.[18] studied 368 twin pregnancies at 10 to 14 weeks of gestation, classifying them as monochorionic if there was a single placental mass in the absence of the lambda sign at the intertwin membrane–placental junction and as dichorionic if there was a single placental mass but the lambda sign was present or the placentas were not adjacent to each other. In 81 (22%) of cases the pregnancies were classified as monochorionic, and in 287 (78%) of cases, the pregnancies were classified as dichorionic. All pregnancies classified as monochorionic resulted in the delivery of same-sex twins and all different-sex pairs were correctly classified as dichorionic.

Other investigators have suggested counting the number of layers of fetal membranes to determine chorionicity, but this strategy is not always possible and should be used in conjunction with other sonographic criteria.[19–24] Membrane thickness is also occasionally useful to predict the type of placentation. Thick membranes suggest dichorionic placentation, whereas thin membranes suggest monochorionic placentation.[25–27] Another important criterion of differential diagnosis is the sex of the fetuses.[28] If they are of different sex, the odds are that the fetuses are dichorionic. There is a small risk, however, of a cytogenetic change that could result in monozygotic twins presenting as a boy and a girl. The most common cause of this rare anomaly is the early loss (during the embryo stage) of a Y chromosome in a cell line that eventually becomes Turner's syndrome (Figs. 24–17 and 24–18).

Associated Syndromes

Monochorionic twins are at risk for twin-to-twin transfusion,[29–33] twin embolization syndrome, higher rates of con-

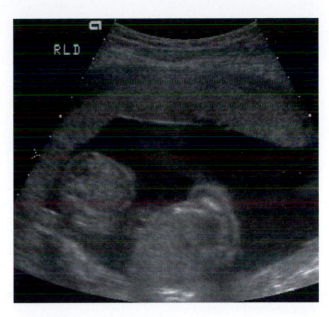

Figure 24–18. Very asymmetrical growth may occur in heterokaryotypic twins.

genital malformations,[34,35] growth restriction, and prematurity. Death of one twin may have serious implications for the survivor[36–43] because of the increased risk of preterm delivery and the risk of neurologic handicap secondary to hypotensive episodes caused by hemorrhage from the live fetus into the dead fetoplacental unit through vascular anastomoses.[44–47]

MONOAMNIOTIC TWINS

Definition

Monoamniotic twins are those that share not only the chorion (the outer membrane) but also the amnion (the inner membrane) and thus are in the same gestational sac[48] (Fig. 24–19).

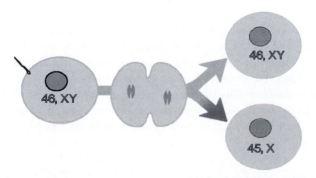

Figure 24–17. In rare instances, not only the primordial fertilized egg divides, but one of the two daughter cells also loses genetic material (and more commonly the Y chromosome), resulting in a heterokaryotypic monozygotic twin pregnancy consisting of a boy and a girl with Turner's syndrome.

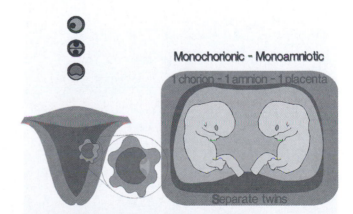

Figure 24–19. Monoamniotic twins share the chorion and the amnion and thus are in the same gestational sac.

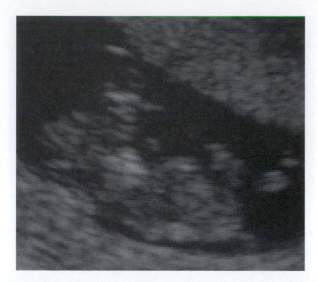

Figure 24–20. Absence of a dividing membrane between two fetuses that are intimately in contact.

They result from splitting between 7 and 13 days after fertilization[49,50] and represent 1% of twin pregnancies.[51–53]

Sonographic Features

Monoamniotic twins can be suspected if the following features are observed[55] (Figs. 24–20 to 24–22).

- single placenta and same-sex twins
- close approximation of the cord insertions
- entanglement of the cords
- normal and identical amniotic fluid volume around both fetuses
- unrestricted fetal movement

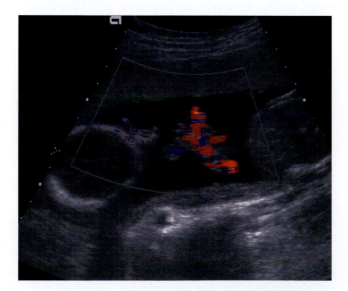

Figure 24–21. Close approximation of the cord insertions.

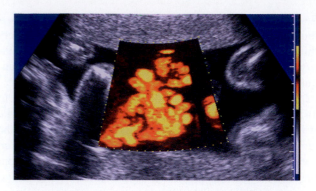

A

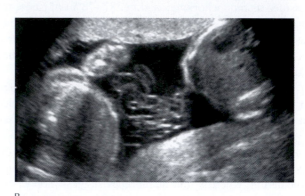

B

Figure 24–22. Cord entanglement (power Doppler on *top*, and gray scale on *bottom*). *(Courtesy of Dr. Luis Izquierdo).*

- absence of a dividing membrane demonstrated on two studies at least 12 to 15 h apart[55]
- a single yolk sac may be a normal finding[56]

Counting twins with different chorionicity by counting the number of gestational sacs is easier in the first trimester when thick layers of tissue separate the sacs. However, differentiating monochorionic–diamniotic from monochorionic–monoamniotic twins is not easy.[57] The amniotic membrane is very thin, and unless the ultrasound beam is perpendicular, it may be difficult to observe. A simple trick that is convincing when present is to roll the patient to the side and observe the passive motion of the embryos. If they both gravitate to the bottom of the gestational sac, no matter the decubitus position, the suspicion of monoamniotic twins is high. If they do not, a dividing membrane is suspected. The findings, however, can be equivocal.[58] This must be an accurate diagnosis because it identifies patients at higher risk for cord accidents.[59]

Differential Diagnosis

Monoamniotic twins can easily be confused with monochorionic–diamniotic twins, especially when there is twin-to-twin transfusion and one of the twins is stuck (see elsewhere in this chapter). A careful search for a membrane, in particular between the limbs and the body, is the only way to ascertain the diagnosis. The absence or reduced amniotic fluid around the stuck twin also should raise the suspicion of a diamniotic gestation.

Associated Syndromes

Monoamniotic twins may be affected by multiple pathologic conditions including twin-to-twin transfusion (although less commonly and less severe than in monochorionic–diamniotic twins),[60–62] tangled umbilical cords,[63–72] and increased risk of congenital anomalies (15 to 20%).[73–81] Cord entanglement occurs in 40 to 70% of monoamniotic twins because of their increased mobility in the second trimester. During the third trimester, the reduced space is usually no longer sufficient to allow the twins to move around.[82,83] Cord entanglement appears to be a pathognomonic sign of monoamnionicity[84] and can be seen as early as the first trimester. In cases of cord entanglement, despite apparent cord compression with absent end-diastolic velocities (AEDVs), some fetuses may grow appropriately.[85] The significance of AEDV in monoamniotic twins may thus be less predictive than in singletons. The presence of a notch in the umbilical artery velocity waveform may reflect hemodynamic alterations in the fetal–placental circulation secondary to narrowing of the umbilical vessels involved in cord entanglement. Because of these complications, the overall mortality for monoamniotic twins can be as high as 50 to 60%.[86–90]

FETAL GROWTH

Intrauterine growth restriction is a pathologic situation, caused in the majority of cases by placental insufficiency. Poor maternal–fetal exchange reduces the offer of nutrients to the fetus, which grows more slowly than normal. This condition is seen in 25% of twin gestations, a rate 10 times higher than that found in the general population. Growth rate in multiple gestations during the first and early second trimesters parallels the growth rate of singleton pregnancies, dropping off during the late second and third trimesters.

Serial growth assessment is the most accurate method to diagnose IUGR. Some controversy remains concerning the use of growth nomograms derived from the general population in multiple pregnancies (Fig. 24–23). The expected growth of head, limbs, and abdomen for twins is discussed below.

Head

Reece et al.[91] reported that the growth of the fetal head was not significantly different from that observed in singleton pregnancies. According to their findings, nomograms derived from singleton pregnancies remain useful for twin gestations.

Limbs

Another study conducted by Reece et al.[92] evaluated the growth of the long bones in multiple and singleton gesta-

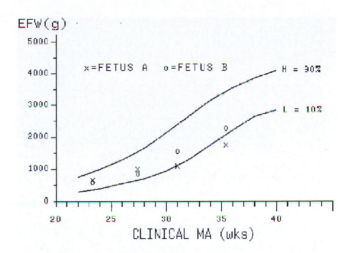

Figure 24–23. Twins commonly experience decreased growth after 26 to 28 weeks, and, as in this set, the effect may be more pronounced on the smaller of the twins.

tions. Although a difference in fetal growth between these two groups was found, the investigators concluded that it was not statistically significant to justify the generation of separate nomograms for twins.

Abdomen

Neonatal differences in abdominal circumference from the normal singleton population are frequently identified. It is still unclear whether these differences occur because of genetic differences in growth potential of twins or whether they are secondary to decrease supplies. Our personal impression is that it is better to consider twin growth with singleton measurement. Using special twin charts increases the risk that the nomograms are established on fetuses with less than adequate growth and thus mask the presence of growth restriction in the index fetus. Despite the controversies regarding the use of nomograms in twin gestations, concordant growth should be expected between fetuses (Fig. 24–24).

Growth Discrepancies

Definition. Anthony Vintzileos has pointed out that the term *growth discordance* was introduced many years ago when obstetricians had no ultrasound to estimate fetal weights or gestational ages. In these dark old days, they had only a scale, so they only could measure the weights after birth. Since then, the term has been used to underline the associated increased mortality and morbidity that only affects the small (IUGR) twin. It would be inappropriate to institute fetal surveillance in the setting of discordance when one twin has an estimated fetal weight at the 50% percentile and the other at the 90% percentile, because neither of these twins would have IUGR. The data have shown that there only is increased morbidity and mortality when discordance is associated with IUGR. Conversely, when both twins have IUGR, fetal surveillance is indicated because of the increased risk, despite the lack of

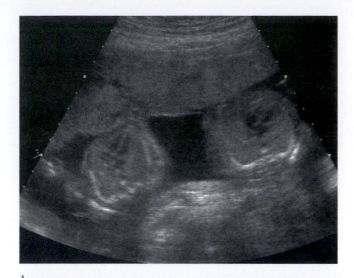

A

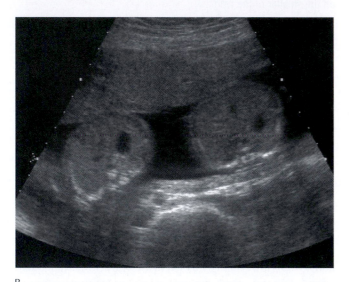

B

Figure 24–24. Appropriate growth of twins with similar sized chest **(A)** and abdominal areas **(B)**.

discordance. Thus, the term should be abandoned because it promulgates confusion and unnecessary testing.

Fetal growth discrepancy is defined as a greater than 20% difference in the intertwin estimated fetal weight. It is generally caused by placental insufficiency resulting in the growth restriction of one twin,[93–100] the death of one twin after the 16th week, or chromosomal abnormalities. The definition of growth discrepancy should be categorized with respect to gestational week because the level of discrepancy changes at different stages of pregnancy.[101] Most cases of growth discrepancy are diagnosed at the second half of the pregnancy. However, pathology can be present as early as the first trimester.[102,103]

Sonographic Features. The standard care for twin pregnancy includes serial sonographic evaluations to assess the

growth of each fetus.[104,105] Findings suggestive of growth discrepancy include:

- estimated fetal weights that are discordant by more than 20%[106–119]; discordance can be classified as mild (15 to 25%) or severe (>25%); cases of preterm twin gestations with severe discrepancy are associated with a higher morbidity rate[120–122]
- abdominal circumference diverging by 20 mm or more[123–126]
- difference in biparietal diameter greater than 6 mm, with the smaller biparietal diameter less than 2 standard deviations below the mean[127]
- head perimeter diverging by more than 5%
- umbilical artery systolic-to-diastolic ratios that are discordant by more than 15% and an elevated umbilical artery systolic-to-diastolic ratio (≥0.4) in one or both twins.[128–134]

Differential Diagnosis. Twin-to-twin transfusion syndrome is the main differential diagnosis.[135–138] Observation of discordant sexes or dichorionic placentation excludes this possibility.[139] In general, twin-to-twin transfusion syndrome is associated with the polyhydramnios–oligohydramnios and/ or anemia–polycythemia sequences.[140] Differences in genetic growth potential between the twins are another possibility: both twins would have normal growth but significant size discrepancy. These cases have adequate growth on serial sonographic analysis plotted in a growth chart, normal amniotic fluid volume, and birth weight usually above 2500 g. Females of different sex pairs are more likely to present growth discrepancy.[141]

Associated Syndromes. Growth discrepancy can be associated with low amniotic fluid volume in the sac of the growth-restricted fetus.[142] The smaller twin is at increased risk of perinatal morbidity and mortality as well as reduced physical and mental development later in life.[143,144] The association with prematurity also implies a high perinatal morbidity and mortality for the affected twin. When growth discrepancy is associated with the death of one of the twins, the presence of a fetus papyraceous is expected on subsequent scans. When the etiology of the condition is a chromosomal abnormality, fetal structural defects may be found at sonographic evaluation. Twin pregnancies resulting from *in vitro* fertilization or gamete intrafallopian transfer are more likely to result in birth weight discordance and in fetuses with high serum α-fetoprotein levels.[145,146]

Doppler Evaluation. Doppler assessment of uterine and umbilical blood flows may be used to evaluate fetal well-being in multiple gestations.[147] It has been demonstrated that fetuses with abnormal Doppler velocimetry have increased morbidity and mortality rates.[148] Some have found umbilical Doppler velocimetry useful in predicting discrepancy in twins[149]; it is certainly an important tool to diagnose congenital anomalies such as twin reversed arterial perfusion sequence, where a retrograde perfusion in the umbilical artery of the abnormal twin is found.[150] Other important applications of Doppler velocimetry are the demonstration of superficial anastomoses in twin–twin transfusion syndrome and identification of cord entanglement, which is a pathognomonic sign of monoamnionicity.[151–154]

CHROMOSOMAL ANOMALIES

Chromosomal abnormalities are more frequent in multiple pregnancies than in the general population. In dizygotic pregnancies, two oocytes are fertilized and each oocyte has an inherent risk of a chromosomal anomaly. The result is an increased rate of chromosomal abnormalities for any given maternal age. The genetic risk is calculated as 166% of the empiric maternal age risk. Rodis et al.[155] constructed a nomogram for the calculation of risk of chromosomal abnormalities in twin gestations. For example, in the United States, a 33-year-old mother with a twin gestation carries the same risk of chromosomal abnormalities as a 35-year-old woman with a singleton pregnancy. This concept has clinical implications in the management of twin gestations and the maternal age at which cytogenetic studies should be offered.

When karyotyping is recommended, chorionic villus sampling is an early and safe technique of prenatal diagnosis in multiple pregnancies.[156,157] If the invasive procedure is performed during the second trimester, amniocentesis should be the first choice.

Fetal sex assignment can be another useful bit of information, particularly in pregnancies at risk for severe sex-linked diseases and fetal disorders involving the genitalia.[158] It is worth mentioning that there have been reports of discordant sex in monozygous twins[159–164] (see Fig. 24–24).

Monozygotic twins are highly concordant for minor anomalies, tend to be concordant for rare congenital defects and malformations, and are predominantly discordant for more common major malformations. In general, the smaller twin is the more severely affected.[165] There are reports of discordant karyotype in identical twins, with the recommendation of sampling both sacs if one or both fetuses present ultrasound abnormalities, even if the scan is suggests a monochorionic pregnancy.[166] This technique must be performed carefully by making sure that each sample is properly attributed to the correspondent twin.

Klinefelter's syndrome with inversion of chromosome 13 in the co-twin,[167] trisomy 13,[168] aneuploidy,[169] and gonadal dysgenesis[170,171] are some of the discordant chromosomal abnormalities reported in twins.

CONGENITAL ANOMALIES

Multiple gestations have approximately twice as many congenital anomalies when compared with the expected rate for the general population. Major anomalies are seen in 2.1% of twins versus 1.2% of singletons, whereas minor anomalies are seen in 4.1% of twins versus 2.4% of singletons.

Some of the anomalies reported in multiple gestations are cloacal dysgenesis sequence,[172] cyclopia,[173] amniotic band disruption complex,[174] cystic hygroma,[175] cerebral and ocular abnormalities,[176] microcephaly,[177] and Russel–Silver syndrome,[178,179] among others.

According to the literature, the occurrence of malformations is higher in monozygotic than in dizygotic twins. The reported incidence of anomalies in monozygotic twins is approximately 16.7% for minor anomalies and an additional 16.7% for major anomalies. If a malformation is observed in one twin, the other has a high chance of being equally affected. Concordance, however, is seen in just 10 to 20% of monozygotic twins.

A careful anatomy survey is necessary to exclude a discordant anomaly, especially in monozygotic pairs. Three theories have been proposed to explain the etiology of structural anomalies in monozygotic twins.

1. The first theory postulates that the crowding of the uterine cavity may be associated with certain types of anomalies. This would explain the statistically significant concordance seen in musculoskeletal abnormalities in monozygotic twinning, predominantly clubfeet.
2. The second theory advocates the occurrence of an early defect in the process of splitting or a delay at the splitting of the embryo that should cause structural anomalies in the fetuses. The ultimate example of this theory is the conjoined twins.
3. The third theory associates fetal anomalies to a vascular compromise secondary to a shared placenta. Syndromes that relate to this etiology include twin reversed arterial perfusion, twin–twin transfusion syndrome, and twin embolization syndrome.

UNIQUE MONOZYGOTIC MONOCHORIONIC SYNDROMES

Twin–Twin Transfusion (Stuck Twin)

Definition. Twin–twin transfusion syndrome is a pathologic condition whereby a donor fetus bleeds into the circulation of a recipient fetus through the abnormal intertwin placental anastomoses. The donor twin becomes anemic, hypovolemic, growth restricted, and as a consequence has a reduced urinary production. Because swallowing of the fluid is not impaired, the amniotic fluid volume progressively decreases. The recipient twin becomes hypervolemic. Lacking a mechanism to remove blood, the recipient twin eliminates as much fluid as possible, thus becoming hypercytemic or even hydropic in

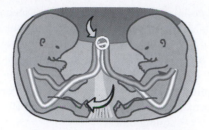

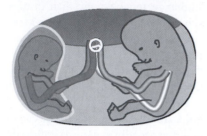

Figure 24–25. In twin–twin transfusion syndrome (*top drawing;* note the artery-to-vein connection), the donor twin *(at left)* becomes anemic, hypovolemic, growth restricted, and as a consequence has a reduced urinary production. Because swallowing of the fluid is not impaired, the amniotic fluid volume progressively decreases *(yellows lines represents the interamniotic membrane).* Conversely, the recipient twin *(at right)* becomes hypervolemic. The elevated urinary production from the recipient twin leads to polyhydramnios and an overdistention of the amniotic cavity, which compresses the donor and its vascular supply against the uterine wall, further decreasing perfusion to the donor fetus. The end condition is the "stuck twin" *(lower drawing).*

the more severe cases. The elevated urinary production from the recipient twin leads to polyhydramnios and an overdistention of the amniotic cavity, which compresses the donor and its vascular supply against the uterine wall, further decreasing perfusion to the donor fetus. The reduction in amniotic fluid on the donor side results in a close apposition of the intertwin membrane that fixes the donor fetus to the uterus, a condition known as "stuck twin"[180] (Fig. 24–25).

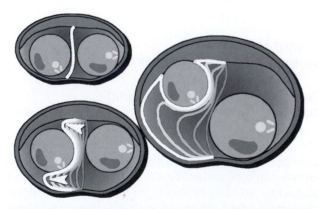

Figure 24–26. As the transfusion progresses, the donor twin loses more fluid and the recipient produces more. The net effect is that the membranes become closely apposed to the donor twin.

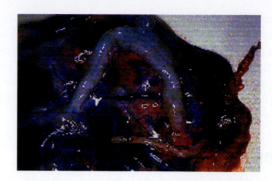

Figure 24–27. The difference in the size of the cord is clearly visible.

Sonographic Features. Commonly reported criteria for the diagnosis of twin-to-twin transfusion syndrome are (Figs. 24–26 to 24–31):

- monochorionic placentation, with visualization of a separating membrane
- same-sex fetuses
- mid-trimester polyhydramnios–oligohydramnios sequence (polyhydramnios at the recipient's sac and oligohydramnios at the donor's sac), in the absence of other causes of abnormal amniotic fluid volume
- size discordance, with the larger twin in the polyhydramniotic sac and the smaller stuck against the uterine wall (abdominal circumference difference or weight discrepancy >20%)[181–185]
- nonvisualization of the donor's bladder and enlarged recipient's bladder
- abnormal Doppler systolic/diastolic ratio at the umbilical cord (>0.4); the absent end-diastolic flow in the donor's umbilical artery and the venous pulsation in the recipient's umbilical vein are usually associated with a poor prognosis[186–192]

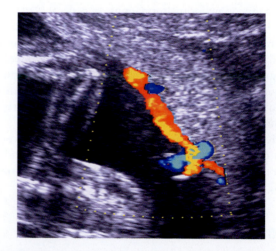

Figure 24–28. The anastomosis is occasionally visible. *(Courtesy of Dr. G. Pilu).*

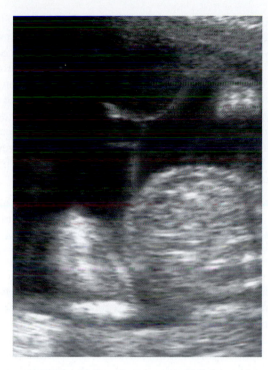

Figure 24–29. Before the donor twin becomes stuck, a typical intermediate stage is the "folding membrane" stage, where the redundant membrane progressively folds as it wraps itself around the donor.

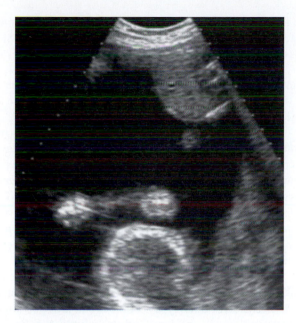

Figure 24–31. The typical appearance of the "stuck twin" immobilized in a portion of the uterus.

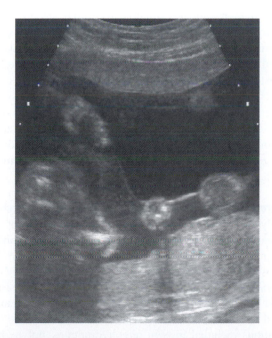

Figure 24–30. At some point, the "folding membrane" stage could resemble amniotic band syndrome. Awareness of the condition will prevent a misdiagnosis.

- hydrops or evidence of congestive heart failure of either twin (although more common in the recipient twin)[193–195]

The criteria used to select cases for the open multicentric randomized trial to evaluate serial amniodrainage versus endoscopic placental surgery in the treatment of twin-to-twin transfusion syndrome are[196]:

- Twin pregnancy diagnosed as monochorionic during a first-trimester scan and/or as having a single placental mass and concordant sex on the second-trimester scan.
- Polyhydramnios in one sac, with a deepest vertical pool of amniotic fluid of at least 6.0 cm at less than 20 weeks of gestation, 8.0 cm at 20 to 22 weeks, and 12.0 cm at 23 to 25 weeks. The polyhydramnios should be related to polyuria, with a distended fetal bladder during most of the examination period.
- Oligohydramnios (stuck twin) in the other sac, with a deepest vertical pool of amniotic fluid of at most 2.0 cm. The oligohydramnios should be likely related to fetal oliguria, with a collapsed bladder during most of the examination period.

In the most severe forms, the diagnosis should not be difficult: a single placenta, massive polyhydramnios in the sac of the recipient twin, and a stuck donor twin attached to the uterine wall with poor mobility and obvious growth discordance. Milder forms of the disease are more difficult to diagnose because of the lack of uniform criteria; however, one should suspect twin-to-twin transfusion in the presence of amniotic fluid discrepancy between the cavities, regardless of the percentage of weight discrepancy between the twins.

An intertwin hemoglobin difference of more than 2.4 gm/dL in fetal blood obtained by cordocentesis has been shown to be consistent with stuck twin syndrome.[197]

Prevalence. Twin-to-twin transfusion complicates about 15 to 35% of monochorial twin gestations and is responsible for 17% of the perinatal mortality in multiple pregnancies.[198,199]

Pathogenesis. If embryonic splitting occurs before day 3 after fertilization, two independent fetuses with separate placentas will result. A single placenta with two amniotic cavities occurs if splitting takes place between days 4 and 7. If division of the embryoblast occurs after about 8 days, the twins share a single placenta and amniotic cavity (monochorionic–monoamniotic twins). Division beyond day 12 results in conjoint twins.[200]

When two fetuses share the same placenta, vascular anastomoses develop between their circulations. These anastomoses can be of three types: vein to vein, artery to artery, and artery to vein. Even when there are multiple vascular connections within a single placenta, no transfusion should occur provided the anastomoses are balanced. Placentas from pregnancies with twin-to-twin transfusion syndrome have fewer anastomoses, which are more likely to be solitary and of deep arteriovenous type than those without twin-to-twin transfusion syndrome.[201–206] When the transfusion occurs, the donor, or "pump," twin becomes hypovolemic due to blood loss. Hypoxia develops because of placental insufficiency, which is also responsible for IUGR. Poor renal perfusion leads to oligohydramnios. This latter feature, when severe, is responsible for the classic appearance of the stuck twin: the amniotic sac becomes too small, the amniotic membrane comes in close contact with the body of the "pump" twin, and the fetus appears trapped to the uterine wall. Hypervolemia with increased renal perfusion leads to polyhydramnios in the sac of the recipient twin.[207] Because there is no loss of protein or cellular components from its circulation, colloid osmotic pressure draws water from the maternal compartment across the placenta, establishing a vicious cycle of hypervolemia, polyuria, and hyperosmolarity, leading to high output cardiac failure, hydrops, and polyhydramnios.[208]

Prognosis. Basically, the prognosis depends on the stage of the pregnancy at which the disease manifests and the severity of the circulatory imbalance. When signs of twin–twin transfusion syndrome are seen at mid-gestation, there is a higher risk of perinatal morbidity and mortality.[209–211] Intrauterine hypoxia, preterm delivery, and death of one fetus (usually the donor) with subsequent death or hypoxia ischemia in the surviving twin are the most common complications to watch for in these pregnancies.

Management. Aggressive treatment appears to be more successful than conservative medical management.[212] For many years, the most employed technique has been amniodrainage

of the recipient amniotic sac by serial amniocentesis.[213–220] The aim of amniodrainage is to restore the normal amniotic fluid volume and thereby decrease the pressure on the donor vasculature, improve its perfusion, and decrease the risk of polyhydramnios-induced preterm labor and thus prolong the pregnancy. The number of amniocentesis and volume of fluid drained differs, depending on the severity of the polyhydramnios, degree of fetal compromise, and maternal symptoms. Approximately 1 L of amniotic fluid should be removed for every 10 cm of amniotic fluid index elevation. Possible mechanisms of action for serial amniodrainage are:

- restoration of placental shape with realignment of maternal spiral artery entry points with placental lobules
- reopening of compensatory low-pressure venovenous anastomoses

Amniodrainage, however, only temporarily corrects the symptoms and multiple complications and does not alter or interrupt the pathologic chain of events responsible for the condition. Perinatal survival with amniodrainage is quoted as $61 \pm 22\%$. However, there remains a risk of serious chronic handicap in $19 \pm 5\%$ of the survivors.[221–234] More recently, ablation of communicating vessels on the placental surface by neodymium YAG laser guided by fetoscopy has been proposed.[235–251] The aim of this technique is to interrupt the abnormal placental vascular communications between the twins. Although the survival rate between amniodrainage and fetoscopy is similar, preliminary studies suggest a significant decrease in neurologic handicap among survivors submitted to fetoscopy (Table 24–2). A multicentric randomized trial is currently being conducted by the EUROFOETUS group to answer this question.[196]

Although some investigators have advocated intentional rupture of the intervening membrane (amniotic septostomy) to equalize the volume of fluid in both sacs,[252,253] it has been argued that artificial normalization of the fluid volumes with septostomy would not change the hemodynamic status of the fetuses and disruption of the membranes could lead to death of the fetuses from cord entanglement.[254] Ligation of the umbilical cord[255] of the donor twin and maternal treatment with indomethacin or digoxin[256,257] have also been proposed as therapeutic options in selected cases. Further information on treatment can be obtained at www.fetalmd.com.

Differential Diagnosis. The differential diagnosis should mainly include twins of discordant size that do not have the transfusion syndrome as the underlying pathophysiologic mechanism for the problem. Some investigators have proposed a new entity called *twin oligohydramnios–polyhydramnios sequence*[258,259] of which twin–twin transfusion would be part. Histopathologic studies of the placenta are required to differentiate twin–twin transfusion from the other conditions included in twin oligohydramnios–polyhydramnios sequence. Isolated IUGR can be considered if the growth discrepancy is less than 15% and the other features of the

TABLE 24–2. MANAGEMENT OF TWIN–TWIN TRANSFUSION SYNDROME BY LASER COAGULATION

				Outcome			
				Intact Survival of		Death of	Neurologic Handicap
Reference	Study Design	Cases	Technique	Both Twins	One Twin	Both Twins	in Survivors
De Lia et al.[249]	Case series	26	Nd:YAG laser coagulation of the placental vessels crossing the interamniotic membrane	34.6% (9/26)[1]	34.6% (9/26)	30.8% (8/26)	4% (27/28)
Ville et al.[237]	Case series	41	Nd:YAG laser coagulation of the placental vessels crossing the interamniotic membrane	36.5% (15/41)	41.5% (16/41)	22% (10/41)	6.5% (3/46)
Hecher et al.[250]	Comparative study	116	Nd:YAG laser coagulation of the placental vessels crossing the interamniotic membrane ($n = 73$; Hamburg)	42% (31/73) $p = 1.00$	37% (27/73) $p = 0.058$	3% (2/73) $p = 0.003$	6% (5/89) $p = 0.030$
			Serial amniocentesis ($n = 43$; Bonn)	42% (18/43)	19% (8/43)	19% (8/43)	18% (8/44)
De Lia et al.[248]	Case series	67	Nd:YAG laser coagulation of the placental vessels crossing the interamniotic membrane	56.7% (38/67)	25.4% (17/67)	17.9% (12/67)	4.3% (4/93)

[1] One triplet pregnancy.

syndrome are not present. Dichorionic twin pregnancy with fused placentas and growth restriction of one of the fetuses is another condition that can lead to misdiagnosis. This can be excluded if the twins have different sexes or after birth by histopathologic analysis of the placenta. Other differential diagnoses to be considered are TORCH infections restricted to one twin, asymmetric chorionic development, fetomaternal hemorrhage, abruption, agenesis of the ductus venosus, and bilateral renal agenesis.[260–262]

Associated Syndromes. The overdistention of the uterus caused by the polyhydramnios can cause preterm labor, amniorrhexis, abruptio placentae, and maternal respiratory and abdominal discomfort. Death of one twin is associated with at least a 25% risk of death or neurologic handicap of the surviving twin. Although the cause of neurologic handicap has been usually attributed to embolization,[263–268] currently accepted evidence indicates severe hypotension with hemorrhage from the live fetus into the dead fetoplacental unit as the causative factor.[44,45,269]

FETUS PAPYRACEOUS

Papyraceous fetus is characterized by a macerated fetus (Fig. 24–32) resulting from an early loss (second trimester) of one twin, and it may affect both mono- and dichorionic gestations. The nonviable fetus is compressed by the expanding sac of the co-twin and partially absorbed throughout the pregnancy.[270,271] The surviving twin often has sequelae of twin embolization syndrome such as aplasia cutis, a rare disorder characterized by localized absence of skin.[272,273]

TWIN EMBOLIZATION SYNDROME

Definition

Twin embolization syndrome is a complication of monozygotic twinning after *in utero* demise of the co-twin.[274] It results from the embolization of placentary and fetal thromboplastins or from the direct embolization of necrosed fragments of the placenta from the dead fetus and disseminated intravascular coagulation, causing embolization or even an endarteritis.[275,276] The emboli damages predominantly high vascularized organs such as the brain and kidneys but can affect almost all organ systems. In the central nervous system (CNS), these emboli can result in ventriculomegaly, porencephaly, cerebral atrophy, cystic encephalomalacia, or microcephaly.[277] Extracranial abnormalities include small bowel atresia, gastroschisis, hydrothorax, aplasia cutis, and renal cortical necrosis.[278,279]

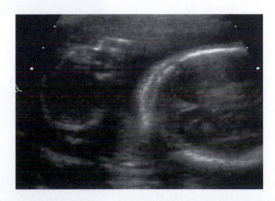

Figure 24–32. A macerated fetus next to the live co-twin.

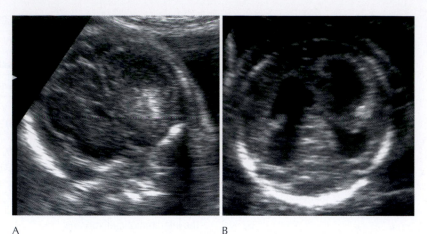

Figure 24–33. After the demise of a co-twin, the survivor developed an intraparenchymal hemorrhage in the brain **(A)** (echogenic area) that evolved into an area of porencephaly **(B)**.

A   B

Sonographic Features

Dead twin associated with a surviving twin affected by (Fig. 24–33):

- CNS anomalies: ventriculomegaly, porencephaly, cerebral atrophy, cystic encephalomalacia, microcephaly
- somatic anomalies
- small bowel atresia
- gastroschisis
- hydrothorax
- aplasia cutis
- renal cortical necrosis
- limb amputation

Differential Diagnosis

The presence of any of the above-mentioned anomalies in the surviving twin with a dead co-twin should raise the suspicion.[280] Only fetal death occurring during the second and third terms of pregnancy is considered.[281]

Associated Syndromes

If one fetus dies due to twin–twin transfusion syndrome, a retrograde blood flow carrying thromboplastic material from the dead twin may reach the blood stream of the survivor through the placental anastomosis, causing disseminated intravascular coagulation. Another possibility is the emboli itself from the dead twin reaches the survivor's circulation.

TWIN-REVERSED ARTERIAL PERFUSION SYNDROME (OR ACARDIAC TWIN)

Definition

Twin-reversed arterial perfusion (TRAP) sequence is a rare condition that has been reported at an incidence of 1% in monochorionic twin pregnancies (0.3 per 10,000 births), resulting in coexistence of a normal "pump" twin and an acardiac twin.[282–286]

Sonographic Features

The pathognomonic feature is the presence of reversed arterial perfusion on Doppler (Fig. 24–34). When imaging the

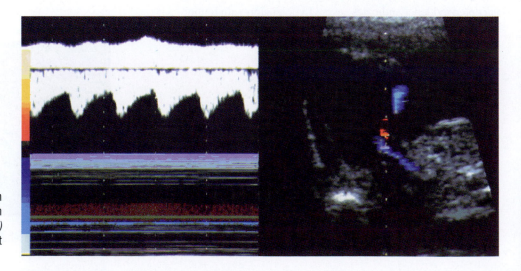

Figure 24–34. Reverse flow on pulsed color Doppler: arterial flow in the vessel goes in *(under the baseline)* and venous flow in the vessel goes out *(above the baseline).*

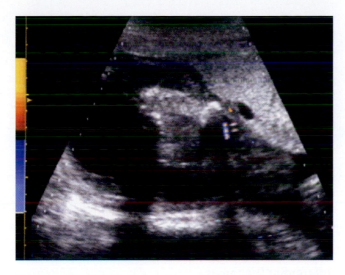

Figure 24–35. This large mass is an acardiac twin (large cystic hygroma on the *left*), and there are poorly defined body parts on the right.

umbilical cord with Doppler, arterial waveforms are observed from the placenta toward the acardiac twin. Venous blood flow goes in the opposite direction.[287–290] This finding results from the absence of a heart (pump) in the acardiac twin in association with artery-to-artery communications in the placenta, allowing the acardiac twin to get its blood supply from the normal twin.[291]

The abnormal fetus presents with impaired or absent development of cephalic pole, heart, upper limbs, and many viscera (Fig. 24–35). The lower limbs are relatively well pre-

served, although clubbing and abnormal toes are common. The appearance is so pathognomonic that the diagnosis has been made as early as 10 weeks.[292] A two-vessels cord is the rule (66%).[293] The membrane development between the twins is inconsistent and varies from full sac to strips of membrane. Occasionally, the umbilical artery of the acardiac twin connects to the superior mesenteric artery (instead of the iliac artery), which is the persistence of a "primitive" vitelline supply (Fig. 24–36).

Pathogenesis

The mechanism that has been proposed is the association of paired artery-to-artery and vein-to-vein anastomoses through the placenta combined with delayed cardiac function of one of the twins early in pregnancy.[294,295] Some investigators have also suggested that aneuploidies, which could lead the abnormal twin to have a slower development than the healthy twin, as a possible etiological factor.[296] Chromosomal abnormalities have been found in 33% of acardiac twins.[297–299] If one twin develops more slowly, the imbalance in the blood pressure of the twins will result in a retrograde transfer of blood from the healthy twin to the abnormal twin. The retrograde flow of poorly oxygenated blood through the developing heart of the abnormal twin interferes with the development of that twin's heart, which rarely goes beyond the stage of tubular heart, causing the "acardia." The upper half of the body of an acardiac twin is extremely poorly developed and, sometimes, not developed at all. Head, cervical spine, and upper limbs are usually absent. Edema and sonolucent areas in the upper body, consistent with cystic hygroma, are common. In contrast, the lower half of the body, although malformed, is better

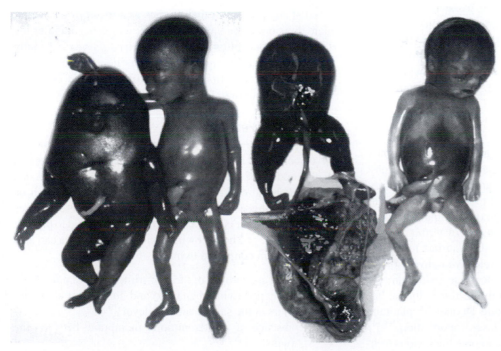

Figure 24–36. Two sets of acardiac twins demonstrate the range of development **(A)** (or absence of development, **B**) of the cephalic end.

A   B

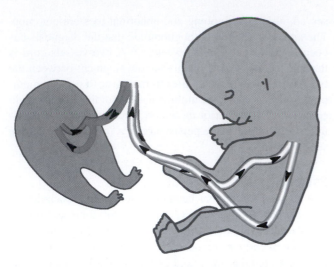

Figure 24–37. In twin-reversed arterial perfusion syndrome, the "acardiac" twin is perfused retrogradely with poorly oxygenated blood that should have gone to the placenta.

TABLE 24–3. VARIATIONS IN TWIN-REVERSED ARTERIAL PERFUSION SYNDROME

Name	Malformation
Acephalus	No cephalic structure present[311]
Anceps	Some cranial structure and neural tissue present[312]
Acormus	Cephalic structure but no truncal structures
Amorphus	No distinguishable rostral or caudal structure[313]

Nomenclature

Investigators have had a field day at creating a nomenclature for each variant (Table 24–3). This is of little significance, because the disorder is invariably fatal, and the only concern is the preservation of the pump twin.

Differential Diagnosis

Few entities can resemble an acardiac twin. Occasionally a twin-to-twin transfusion could resemble a TRAP. These entities can be differentiated by the recognition of a membrane (even in a stuck twin) and, of course, cardiac activity in the smaller fetus. A fetal demise in a twin pregnancy could also resemble acardius; however, there should be no Doppler signal in the dead fetus.

Associated Syndromes

There are no associated syndromes.

CONJOINED TWINS

Definition

Conjoined twins are monochorionic–monoamniotic twins fused at any portion of their bodies as a result of an incomplete division of the embryonic disk, which occurs after the 13th day of conception.[314–319] The term *conjoined* is actually a misnomer because most researchers consider the pathogenesis of the condition to result from failure of complete separation rather than from fusion of the twins.[320]

Sonographic Features

The minimal sonographic criterion for the prenatal diagnosis of conjoined twins is the visualization of fused portion of the bodies of monozygotic–monoamniotic twins. Aside from this basic criterion, several sonographic signs can be observed in this condition. Careful search for these features and serial scans for confirmation are recommended to prevent misdiagnosis.[321] The following sonographic criteria can also be observed in conjoined twins:

- bifid appearance of the first-trimester fetal pole (V- or Y-shaped twin pregnancy) and continuous skin contours at the same anatomic level[319]
- absence of a interamniotic membrane between the twins
- inability to separate fetal bodies

developed. This pattern of development may be explained by the mechanism of perfusion of the acardiac twin. Blood that enters the abdomen of the fetus is deoxygenated blood that left the normal twin. The morphologic abnormalities in the acardiac twin are consistent with perfusion of tissues supplied by the common iliac and lower branches of the aorta with deoxygenated blood. Most of the oxygen available is extracted when the blood enters the acardiac twin, allowing for some development of the lower body and extremities. Lower pressure in the retrogradely perfused upper half of the body and low oxygen saturation impair the development of this area.

The acardiac twin is thus a parasite.[300,301] It requires blood pumped from the normal twin to keep developing, putting the pump fetus at risk of high output cardiac failure[303] (Fig. 24–37). The risk is directly dependent on the size of the acardiac twin: the heavier the acardiac twin, the greater the risk of cardiac failure and death for the normal twin. Overall only 50% of pump twins survive, and the mortality for acardius is 100%.[303–305]

Management

Management includes conservative and invasive therapies. Conservative management includes serial cardiotocography, ultrasonography, echocardiography, and opportune delivery. Noninvasive therapies may be used to support the cardiac function of the pump twin with digoxin and indomethacin. The more invasive management consists of termination of pregnancy or interruption of flow to the acardiac fetus, surgical extraction (hysterotomy with selective delivery of the acardiac twin) and ligation of the acardiac twin's umbilical cord,[306,307] ultrasound-guided embolization of the cardiac twin's umbilical artery with absolute alcohol,[308] platinum coils or thrombogenic coils, and laser vaporization.[309,310] Large numbers are not available to compare the various techniques.

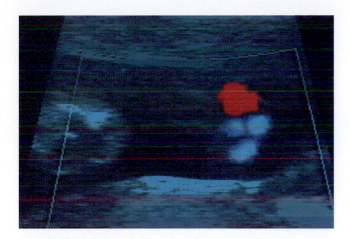

Figure 24–38. The presence of more than three vessels in a cord is a strong marker of conjoined twins.

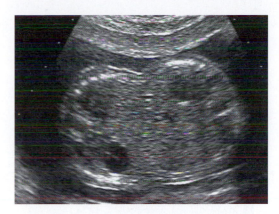

Figure 24–40. Conjoined abdomen in frontal position. Note the stomach bubbles in diagonal positions.

- presence of fetal anomalies
- abnormal number of vessels (more than three) in the umbilical cord (Fig. 24–38)
- the heads and bodies of both twins are seen at the same level[322] (Figs. 24–39 and 24–40)
- unusual extension of the spines
- unusual proximity of the extremities[319]
- fixed position of the fetuses relative one to another, even after external stimulation or maternal movement
- presence of a single heart (Fig. 24–41)

One unusual case of conjoined twins that only shared a part of the cord has also been described.[323]

The presence of these signs changes according to the different types of conjoined twins. These must be considered whenever a monochorionic and monoamniotic pregnancy is suspected. Discordant presentation does not exclude conjoined twins. Although the diagnosis of conjoined twins is easier during the first trimester, the type and severity of the condition is better achieved during the second trimester, when a more precise evaluation of the shared organs can be done.[324–326] Diagnosis with three-dimensional transvaginal sonography during the first trimester has also been described.[327,328] If diagnosis is made before viability, termination of pregnancy can be offered.[329–333]

Prevalence

This is a rare condition and the reported frequency differs from 0.1 to 0.35 per 10,000 births.[319] If stillborns are excluded, the estimate is 0.05 per 10,000 births. Females are more commonly affected, with a male-to-female ratio of 1.6–3 to 1. No association with maternal age, race, parity, or heredity has been observed. The recurrence risk is negligible.[319,334,335]

Prognosis

Most of the conjoined twins are born prematurely, 40% are stillborn, and 35% die within 24 h.[336] Among the survivors, the prognosis and attempts in surgical separation will depend on the type of conjunction, degree of involvement of the shared organs, and the presence of associated

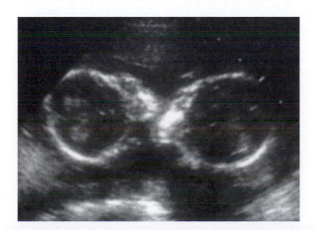

Figure 24–39. The heads are seen in an unnatural position at the same and constant level.

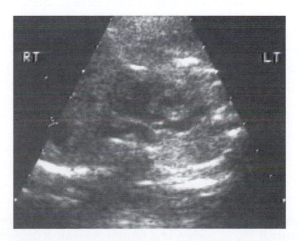

Figure 24–41. A shared heart is a sign of nonoperability.

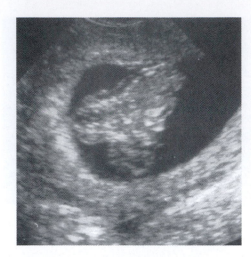

Figure 24–42. Duplicata incompleta. *(Adapted with permission from Romero R, Pila G, Jeanty P, et al. Prenatal Diagnosis of Congenital Anomalies, Norwalk, CT: Appleton;1989.)*

anomalies.[319,337] The most ominous prognosis is among those twins who share liver and or heart. Attempts of separation in cases of a common liver can be done as long as two biliary tracts are seen. In the presence of a shared heart, separation is only attempted if two normal hearts coexist in a single pericardium.[338,339]

Management

The method of choice for delivery is cesarean section to maximize survival and prevent maternal and fetal trauma.[340,341]

Classifications

Conjoined twins are classified according to the area of the bodies where the fusion takes place and the involvement of internal organs. The symmetrical and equal forms, in which the twins have equal or nearly equal duplication of structures, are called *duplicata completa*. When there is an unequal duplication of structures, the twins are called *duplicata incompleta,* and this category includes the most severe types of conjoined twins in which just a few organs systems are duplicated. The most frequent varieties of conjoined twins are thoracopagus (40 to 74%), omphalopagus (10 to 33%), pygopagus (18%), ischiopagus (6%), and craniopagus (1 to

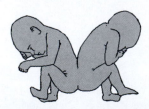

Figure 24–43. Terata catadidyma. *(Adapted with permission from Romero R, Pila G, Jeanty P, et al. Prenatal Diagnosis of Congenital Anomalies, Norwalk, CT: Appleton;1989.)*

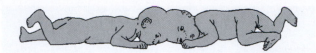

Figure 24–44. Terata anadidyma. *(Adapted with permission from Romero R, Pila G, Jeanty P, et al. Prenatal Diagnosis of Congenital Anomalies, Norwalk, CT: Appleton;1989.)*

6%). The classification of conjoined twins is described in Table 24–3.

Classification of Conjoined Twins

Duplicata Incompleta. Duplication occurring in only one part or region of the body (Fig. 24–42). Examples are diprosopus (one body, one head, and two faces[342,343]), dicephalus (one body and two heads), and dipygus (one head, thorax and abdomen with two pelvises, and/or external genitalia[344]).

Duplicata Completa. Two complete conjoined twins.

Terata Catadidyma. Conjunction in the lower part of the body (Fig. 24–43). Examples are ischiopagus (joined by the inferior portion of the coccyx and sacrum) and pygopagus (joined by the lateral and posterior portions of the coccyx and sacrum).

Terata Anadidyma. Conjunction in the upper part of the body (Fig. 24–44). Examples are syncephalus (joined by the face) and craniopagus (joined at the homologous portion of the cranial vault).

Terata Anacatadidyma. Conjunction at the midpart of the body (Fig. 24–45). Examples are thoracopagus (joined at the thoracic wall[319]), xiphopagus (joined at the xiphoid process[345]), omphalopagus (joined at the area between the xiphoid cartilage and the umbilicus[314]), and rachipagus (joined at the level of the spine above the sacrum).

In one attempt to universalize the current nomenclature, a new classification has been proposed based on the theoretical site of union.

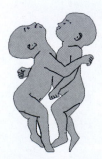

Figure 24–45. Terata anacatadidyma. *(Adapted with permission from Romero R, Pila G, Jeanty P, et al. Prenatal Diagnosis of Congenital Anomalies, Norwalk, CT: Appleton; 1989.)*

Ventral Union. Twins united along the ventral aspect.

Cephalopagus. The twins are fused from the top of the head down to the umbilicus. There are two rudimentary (fused) faces, four arms, and four legs. The lower abdomen and pelvis are separated.[346] The cephalothoracopagus Janiceps type is a rare variety of conjoined twins in which the fetuses are joined face to face, with the face of each fetus being split at the midline and in half turned outward, so that each observed face is made up of the right face of one fetus and the left face of the other. The name originates from Janus, in Roman mythology, the god of gates and doorways; his statue has two faces, facing east and west, representing the beginning and ending of the day, and one head.[347,348]

Thoracopagus. The twins are united face to face from the upper thorax down to the umbilicus; the heart is always involved. There are four arms, four legs, and two pelvises.

Omphalopagus. The twins are joined face to face primarily in the area of the umbilicus and sometimes involving the lower thorax, but two distinct hearts are always preserved. There is not even a cardiac vessel in common. There are two pelvises, four arms, and four legs.[349,350]

Ischiopagus. The twins are united ventrally from the umbilicus to a large conjoined pelvis with two sacrums and two symphyses pubises. They appear more frequently joined end to end, with the spine in a straight line, but they can also present face to face with a joined abdomen. There are four arms, four legs, and, in general, a common external genitalia and a common anus.

Lateral Union. Twins are joined side by side, with shared umbilicus, abdomen, and pelvis.

Parapagus. These twins share a conjoined pelvis, one symphysis pubis, and one or two sacrums. When the union is limited to the abdomen and pelvis (does not involve the thorax), it is called *dithoracic parapagus*. If there is one trunk with two heads, it is called *dicephalic parapagus*. If there is a single trunk and a single head with two faces, it is called *diprosopic parapagus*. There are two, three, or four arms and two or three legs.

Dorsal Union. Twins are joined at the dorsal aspect of the primitive embryonic disk. There is no involvement of the thorax and abdomen.

Craniopagus. Twins are united at any portion of the skull, except the face or foramen magnum. They share bones of the cranium, meninges, and occasionally brain surface. There are two trunks, four arms, and four legs.[351]

Pygopagus. Twins share dorsally the sacrococcygeal, perineal regions, and occasionally the spinal cord. There are one anus, two rectums, four arms, and four legs.

Rachipagus. Twins are fused dorsally above the sacrum, involving different segments of the column. This type is extremely rare.

Differential Diagnosis

Conjoined twins have a unique presentation and the few differential diagnoses could include lymphangioma, teratoma, or cystic hygroma.

Associated Syndromes

Congenital anomalies of organs other than the shared ones are present in 50% of cases of conjoined twins. Cardiac defects are the most common association (20 to 30%); thus, echocardiography is recommended in all cases. Neural tube defects and mid-line fusion defects, orofacial clefts, imperforate anus, and diaphragmatic hernia are also frequently seen. Polyhydramnios is observed in 50 to 75% of cases.

FETUS-IN-FETU

Definition

A fetus-in-fetu is an encapsulated, pedunculated vertebrate tumor. It represents a malformed monozygotic, monochorionic, diamniotic, parasitic twin included in a host (or autosite) twin (see Etiology, below). Characteristically, the fetus-in-fetu complex will be composed of a fibrous membrane (equivalent to the chorioamniotic complex) that contains some fluid (equivalent to the amniotic fluid) and a fetus suspended by a cord or pedicle. The presence of a rudimentary spinal architecture is used to differentiate a fetus-in-fetu from a teratoma because teratomas are not supposed to develop through the primitive streak stage (12 to 15 days). This last criterion has been considered too stringent by many investigators who regard a rudimentary body architecture (metameric segmentation, craniocaudal and lateral differentiation, body coelom, and "gestational sac") or the presence of an associated fetus-in-fetu as equivalent criteria. Although teratomas can achieve striking degrees of differentiation by the inductive effect of adjacent tissues on one another, they do not present the criteria mentioned above.

Synonyms

As for any unusual anomalies, several descriptive terms have been used. These include cryptodidymus ($\kappa \rho \iota \pi \tau o$ = hidden, $\delta \iota \delta \upsilon \mu o \varsigma$ = twin), dermocyme ($\delta \varepsilon \rho \mu \alpha$ = skin, $\kappa \upsilon \mu \alpha$ = fetus), double monster, endocyme fetus ($\varepsilon \nu \delta o \nu$ = inside, $\kappa \upsilon \mu \alpha$ = fetus) (note that the word *fetus* is redundant), fetiform teratoma, fetal inclusion, included heteropagus twin

($\varepsilon\tau\varepsilon\rho o\varsigma$ = other, $\pi\alpha\gamma o\varsigma$ = which is fixed), and suppressed twin.

Prevalence

The prevalence is unknown. About 70 cases[352–416] have been reported, but this number changes according to how strictly identification criteria are used (see Definition, above). Several cases have been formally recognized by some as fetus-in-fetu but categorically rejected by others. Seven cases have been detected *in utero*. An estimated frequency of 0.02 per 10,000 births is commonly reported in the literature, but this number is based on the unsubstantiated assumption that fetus-in-fetu represents 5% of conjoined twins. Further (see Etiology), the current trend is to consider that fetus-in-fetu does not represent a form of conjoined twins. The male-to-female ratio in the 39 reports that we reviewed was 1.3 males to 1 female. This is in contrast with conjoined twin, which occurs predominantly in girls.

Historical Review

Several cases of fetus-in-fetu were reported in the past, and no distinction from teratoma was made until the first quarter of the 20th century. For this reason, those reports that did not clearly identify the presence of a spine should be considered with caution. Further, because of possible confusion with abdominocyesis, cases in women of childbearing age should be interpreted cautiously. The most credible old cases are those reported by Young,[366] Highmore,[367] and Taylor.[369] Only the first two reports include figures. Young reported the case of an 18-week-old boy examined for vomiting.[366] On physical examination, a smooth, round tumor was palpated in the left upper quadrant. The patient was lost to follow-up but returned 5 months later, emaciated. The tumor had grown and extended to the scrobiculus cordis (the epigastric fossa), and the child poorly tolerated breast-feeding. Young described episodes of enlargement and decrease of the abdominal perimeter, which he attributed to accumulation of fluid in the cyst. The child died at 9 months. On autopsy, a large mass occupying most of the abdomen was found. Opening the cyst revealed the fetus-in-fetus. Young wrote a remarkably complete description of the findings.

The case reported by Highmore[367] is even more extraordinary in that it occurred in a teenaged boy (Fig. 24–46). This 15-year-old boy had a 7-year history of abdominal complaints and mass. As in the previous case, the child died of malnutrition. At autopsy, a large tumor containing a fetus was discovered.

Etiology

Several etiologies have been proposed.

A primordial organizer defect was once thought to explain dermoids, teratoma, and embryoma.

Another theory suggested that the fetus-in-fetu derived from germ cells from the host that evolved on their own. This

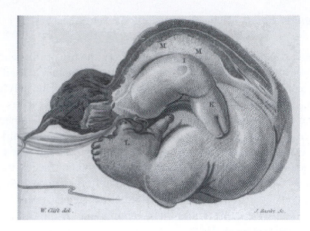

Figure 24–46. Drawing from the case reported by Highmore.[367]

appears to be supported by the occasional localization in an ectopic testicle. However, that localization can also result from migration of the fetus-in-fetu along with the germ cells, when the germ cells of the host return from the yolk sac into the retroperitoneal cavity on their way to the gonads.

A parthenogenetic origin has also been suspected. In this theory, germ cells from the retroperitoneal region (where they normally are located) are parthenogenetically stimulated and evolve into a rudimentary fetus. Histocompatibility studies and gene markers do not support parthenogenesis as a likely etiology.

In the continuum theory of monozygous twin, there is a progression from normal twins to conjoined symmetrical twins to asymmetrical twins (acardiac twins), and then to parasitic twins, and then teratoma is hypothesized. As mentioned under Prevalence, the incidence is about equally divided between sexes (with a slight male predominance in this review), which is an argument against the continuum theory and the highly differentiated sacrococcygeal teratoma theory because conjoint twins and sacrococcygeal teratomas are more common in females.

Willis considered that the fetus-in-fetu did not represent a monoamniotic twin but rather included a monozygotic di-amniotic parasitic twin within the host twin: "It is, I believe, a mistake to suppose that a gentle series of gradations exists between double monsters and malformed twins on one hand and teratomas on the other—a mistake widely promulgated because of the prevalent view that teratomas are included monsters or malformed twins. The sooner this misconception is abandoned, the better."[417] His postulate explains why in all extracranial locations the fetus-in-fetu is embedded in a gestational sac. If the fetus-in-fetu was a conjoined twin, it would have to be monoamniotic and thus would not have its own gestational sac. This theory has been widely accepted.

Pathogenesis

The currently accepted mechanism is the embedding of a twin due to vitelline circulation anastomoses. (Fig. 24–47).

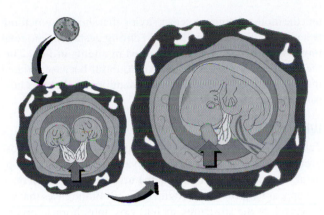

Figure 24–47. Anastomoses between vitelline vessels are believed to cause the common form of fetus-in-fetu.

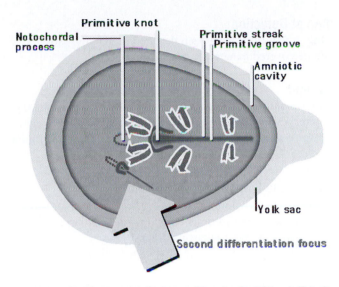

Figure 24–48. The cause of intracranial and spinal fetus-in-fetu is probably due to the presence of a second differentiation focus in the bilaminar embryo.

Vascular anastomoses between twins have variable repercussions, depending on the vessels anastomosed and the location of the anastomoses. The most benign anastomoses are superficial connections of similar vessels on the surface of the placenta. These connections between artery and artery or between vein and vein are common and of limited significance when they occur after the first few weeks of gestation. When they occur early and one fetus has a slight developmental delay, they result in the TRAP syndrome. Anastomoses that are between dissimilar vessels and occur in the placenta are responsible for the twin-to-twin transfusion syndrome.

Anastomoses between vitelline vessels, which are only possible when the twins are monochorionic, are assumed to cause fetus-in-fetu by a mechanism similar to that which produces acardiac twins. The cardiac development of the affected twin is impaired by the reversal of the flow in its heart. This stunts the growth of the affected fetus, and as the host grows it progressively embeds the smaller twin around the third week.

A few intracranial cases have been described. The location in the skull results from a different embryologic mechanism. To be imbedded in the ventricle, a fetus-in-fetu has to separate at a much later date than those that are imbedded in the retroperitoneum. At 15 days, when the embryo is at the bilaminar disk level, the primitive streak develops. At the cephalic end of the streak, a depression, the primitive knot or Hensen's node, forms and extends cranially. The invagination of the cells into the depression is at the origin of the mesoderm and forms the notochordal process (or blastopore). The blastopore extends to become the notochord, which elongates toward the cranial end. If a second differentiation focus occurs in the bilaminar embryo and grows at the same rate as the primary focus, it will form a craniopagus conjoint twin. If the second differentiation focus grows more slowly than the primary focus, it will be engulfed in the invagination of cells and may arrest in what will ultimately become the ventricles. A fetus-in-fetu thus may also settle along the central canal of the spinal cord. In intracranial fetus-in-fetu, one does not expect to find a gestational sac (amnion or chorion equivalent),

and indeed none of the intracranial cases have described any surrounding membranes (Fig. 24–48).

Localization

Most cases of fetus-in-fetu are retroperitoneal, but some have been found in the mesentery, adrenal cranial cavity, lateral ventricles, pelvis, coccyx, inguinal region, testicles, and scrotum. Thus, most of the resting places are retroperitoneal or on the path that the germ cells follow on their way back from the yolk sac to the retroperitoneum and into the gonads. When located on ectopic testes, they may be intraperitoneal. The affected testicle is usually ectopic or undescended, probably because the added bulk impairs the migration of the cells.

Vascularization

As expected from the etiologies, most cases of fetus-in-fetu are connected to the host by vessels originating from or around the superior mesenteric artery, a derivative of the right vitelline artery in mammals. The artery of the fetus-in-fetu derives from the vitelline artery and thus is the equivalent of a superior mesenteric artery. In the host, if the superior mesenteric artery is not directly involved, the connection is usually with direct branches from the aorta and the small retroperitoneal or diaphragmatic vessels. In a testicular location, spermatic vessels or even renal and adrenal vessels may be involved. In only a few cases, a definite vascular connection can be recognized between the fetus-in-fetu and the host. In other cases, a capillary system exists between the two circulations. Because the fetus-in-fetu does not have a cardiac system, the severe hypoxia is responsible for the lack of evolution.

Age at Detection

Only a few cases have been detected prenatally. Most cases are discovered in newborns or small children.

Weight

The weight varies from a few grams to 2000 or even 4000 g. There is some inexactitude in the reporting of the weights because some reports mention the weight of the whole tumor and others report the weight of the fetus-in-fetu alone.

Presenting Symptoms in Children

Aside from a few fortuitous discoveries, the disorder usually becomes apparent from its compression of adjacent organs, principally the gastrointestinal tract.

Number

Usually one fetus is found, but several instances of two, three, five, or even more have been described. When several fetuses are present, they usually share the same sac, but some may have their own sacs.

Zygosity

Studies of gonads,[418] blood types, chromosomes, and red cell antigens (ABO, Rh, M, N, S, P_1, K, Fy, and Jk) have shown the fetus-in-fetu to be monozygotic to the host. It is not surprising, however, that the fetus-in-fetu has the same blood type as the host because it is perfused by the host. There have been no recorded cases of dizygosity. However, as in acardiac twins, the combination of a normal twin with a twin that has lost a gonosomic chromosome and thus appears as a 45,X0 could potentially be found.

Macroscopic Appearance

At surgery, the fetus-in-fetu appears as a well-circumscribed mass bound by a fibrous membrane. Inside the mass the fetus-in-fetu is suspended in straw-colored fluid by a pedicle. Two vessels (an artery and a vein) travel along the pedicle. The fluid is generally not abundant and has been described as containing sebaceous material. The origin of this fluid is uncertain. Several investigators have pointed out that the membranes of a normal embryo are not responsible for the production of amniotic fluid. They would more likely act as a semipermeable membrane. In fetuses past 12 weeks, the urinary system produces the fluid and the gastrointestinal system reabsorbs it. Because no fetus-in-fetu has ever been described to contain a urinary system and the segments of gastrointestinal tract that are found are too incomplete to have any reabsorptive capabilities, the fluid is probably in communication with the extracellular fluid of the fetus-in-fetu and is maintained in the amniotic cavity solely by osmotic and oncotic pressure.

The presence of chorionic villi has only been reported in one case. Except for one quotation of a 15-year-old saying "Mother, do come to me, I have something alive in my body" and the mother being quoted as saying that she felt something resembling "the motion of a child during gestation," no fetal movements have ever been recorded in a fetus-in-fetu. This record of movement is somewhat doubtful because striated muscles have rarely been found around joints. Yet this host is one of the older hosts described.

What Is Included

Fetus-in-fetu resemble poorly formed acardiac twins. Almost every organ has been recognized in various stages of development. The notable exception is the urinary tract, which does not appear to have been recognized in any of the cases that we reviewed. Some structures such as ribs, intrathoracic organs (lung, heart, and thymus), and retroperitoneal organs (liver, spleen, kidneys, adrenal glands, pancreas, and gonads) are rarely described. An incomplete heart has been found. In one instance, a rudimentary two-chamber heart was found, with the atrium in the caudal position and the ventricle in the cranial position. This is the stage normally reached in a 22-day embryo.[419] Facial and cranial structures also are seldom seen, yet eyes, ears, mouth and poorly organized brain and cerebellum have been observed.

The cord that connects the fetus to the membrane has different characteristics than a normal cord: it contains vasa vasorum and nerve fibers.

The evolution of the fetus-in-fetu is usually arrested at the first trimester, and further evolution is by mass accretion more than by development. Overall structures derived from the ectoderm are better represented than structures derived from the other two layers. The mesoderm contributes the musculoskeletal system, which is usually well represented, but the other derivatives (the vascular and urogenital system, the spleen, and adrenal glands) are seldom found. The most commonly represented derivative from the endodermal layer is the gastrointestinal tract, but the liver and pancreas are also often recognized.

Ultrasound Appearance

The few cases detected prenatally all presented as a complex mass. The general appearance is a well-delineated capsule, with an echogenic mass suspended in fluid or partly surrounded by fluid. Occasionally the diagnosis can be suggested by the recognition of a rudimentary spine (Fig. 24–49).

Differential Diagnosis

When discovered in a newborn child during physical examination, the differential diagnosis includes all the common masses such as Wilms' tumor, hydronephrosis, and neuroblastomas. Prenatally, the main differential diagnosis is with teratoma. Teratomas are disorganized congregations of pluripotential cells from all three primitive tissue layers. By differentiation and induction, they can achieve striking organization, with examples of several organs being well formed. However, teratomas do not have vertebral segmentation,

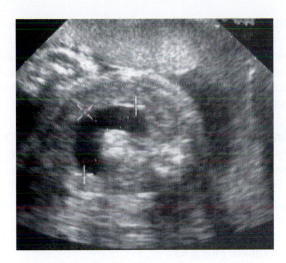

Figure 24–49. A fetus-in-fetu, with a rudimentary spinal organization. *(Courtesy K. Caldwell and P. Dix.)*

craniocaudal and lateral differentiation, body coelom, or systemic organogenesis. Thus, the presence of a mass with a spinal organization and surrounded by fluid suggests the correct diagnosis. When spinal structures are not present, most investigators have considered that the diagnosis of fetus-in-fetu can still be made when the alternate criteria described under Definition are found. These criteria are sufficiently restrictive that even well-organized teratomas cannot fulfill all of them. Teratomas have a definite malignant potential, a feature that has not been reported in fetus-in-fetu. Teratomas occur predominantly in the lower abdomen, not in the upper retroperitoneum. Nonetheless, the coexistence of a fetus-in-fetu and a teratoma and the occurrence of a teratoma 14 years after removal of a twin fetus-in-fetu have been reported, thus supporting the older hypothesis of a continuum between twin and teratoma. Cases of sacrococcygeal fetus-in-fetu should probably be regarded and treated as teratoma because of the high incidence of teratoma in this region.[420]

Ectopic testicles have a higher incidence of germ cell tumors,[421] and the differentiation between fetus-in-fetu and teratoma is particularly important. Although the characteristics of intracranial teratoma differ from those of intracranial fetus-in-fetu, Wakai et al. found, in a large review of 245 intracranial teratomas, that there are some transitions between certain teratomas and fetus-in-fetu.[422]

In the older literature, several descriptions of fetus-in-fetu were too vague to be acceptable by current criteria. For example, the case reported by Phillips[368] does not unequivocally suggest the criteria described above and therefore should probably be considered a teratoma. Some have argued that fetus-in-fetu should be considered teratomas because they do not evolve into lithopedion-like fetuses of abdominocyesis. That argument is probably not valid because in abdominocyesis the antigen complements of the host and fetus are different, which contrasts with fetuses-in-fetu.

Associated Anomalies

Every organ of the fetus-in-fetu has undergone hypoxic growth and is deformed. Most cases are anencephalic. Usually the body is closed, but ventral wall defects such as omphalocele are common, and a case that suggests a limb–body wall complex has also been described. The host rarely presents any anomalies, except those related to the presence of a space-occupying lesion. Those manifestations have rarely been severe, even in the case of intracranial fetus-in-fetu, although in rare cases severe hydrocephalus was responsible for the death of the host. One case of Meckel diverticulum and another of skin hemangioma have been described. A malignant degeneration has never been reported, even in the cases that have been allowed to evolve for several years.

Evolution

If conservative management is chosen, the fetus-in-fetu does not seem to be harmful to the host. However, in every case in which the fetal mass was not removed at the time of discovery, a slow growth has been described.

Prognosis

In the literature of the 19th century, fetus-in-fetu was fatal to the host because of the compression on adjacent organs. In the more recent literature, the outcome for the host twin is usually favorable. Only a few cases of spontaneous or postsurgical deaths have been recorded.

Recurrence Risk

There is no report of recurrence.

Management

Aside from a few attempts, in the first half of the 20th century, to marsupialize the fetus-in-fetu, surgical removal is the treatment of choice. The membranous capsule can usually be enucleated from the host with minimal problems. In only a few cases, removal is difficult because of adhesions, and this difficulty may precipitate the end of the operation or even be the reason of the postoperative death of the host. Leaving the capsule, or part of it, has not led to complications except in very rare cases in which fluid reaccumulated in it.

HETEROTOPIC GESTATION

Definition

A heterotopic pregnancy is the occurrence of a multiple pregnancy in which one or more gestational sacs are implanted outside the uterine cavity (ectopic pregnancy) and is associated with a single or multiple intrauterine pregnancy (eutopic pregnancy)[423–427] (Fig. 24–50). It occurs in 1 to 2.9% of pregnancies after *in vitro* fertilization and embryo transfer.[428–432]

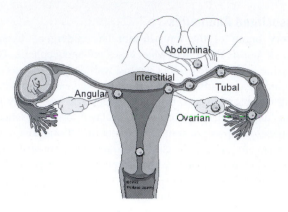

Figure 24–50. A heterotopic pregnancy is the combination of an ectopic pregnancy and an intrauterine pregnancy.

Sonographic Features

Visualization of one or more intrauterine gestational sacs is associated with one or more ectopic pregnancies, which are classified depending on the site of implantation: tubal,[433,434] cervical,[435] cornual,[436–439] abdominal,[440,441] and ovarian.[442–444]

The diagnosis can be made by transvaginal ultrasound during the first trimester. This diagnosis should particularly be considered in cases with abdominal pain (vaginal bleeding may be absent[445]) and in those with a failed pregnancy with rising human chorionic gonadotropin (β-hCG).

Differential Diagnosis

The presence of a small pelvic mass associated with an early intrauterine pregnancy is also suggestive of heterotopic pregnancy. The differential diagnosis can be made by the identification of the heartbeat. Patients with diagnosis of ectopic pregnancy, in particular the ones who have undergone infertility treatment, must have the uterine cavity investigated to exclude heterotopic pregnancy. The presence of an intrauterine gestation sac in a patient without symptoms should not exclude the diagnosis of a concomitant extrauterine pregnancy until the pelvis is carefully visualized.[446,447] Heterotopic pregnancies can occur even in patients without risk factors.

Associated Syndromes

This condition is particularly associated with infertility cases that have undergone assisted reproductive techniques.[448–455]

MOLAR GESTATION WITH A CONCURRENT PREGNANCY

The recognition of twin pregnancies that include a complete hydatidiform mole and coexisting fetus have a greater malignant potential and thus should be differentiated from simple partial hydatidiform moles.[456–459]

VANISHING TWIN

The three common forms of spontaneous fetal loss in multiple gestation are 1) the vanishing twin syndrome, which occurs in the first trimester; 2) the fetus papyraceous in the second trimester; and 3) stillbirth in the third trimester.

Definition

The vanishing twin is the first-trimester loss of a member of a twin gestation.[460,461] The incidence of twinning has been reported to be 3.29%, and of these 21.2% have demonstrated the vanishing twin phenomenon.[462] The vanishing twin is simply reabsorbed.

Sonographic Features

The gestational sac is small, and the development of one fetus lags behind that of the other fetus; there is no detectable fetal heart activity. The spectrum varies, from a crescent-shaped sac adjacent, to a normal early gestation (between 10 and 14 weeks), to a well-formed but dead fetus (fetus papyraceous in the second trimester). Early vanishing twins should be distinguished from implantation bleeds that are not surrounded by a trophoblastic ring.[463] Sonographic evaluation of early gestational bleeds frequently leads to the diagnosis of a vanishing twin, and this is apparently the single complication associated with the disappearance of a twin at this stage.[464,465] A vanishing twin does not adversely affect the development of a coexisting singleton pregnancy; therefore, the exact distinction between implantation bleed and vanishing twin may be academic (Figs. 24–51 to 24–53).

Differential Diagnosis

The differential diagnosis includes implantation bleeds in the early pregnancy, artifactual error (rectus muscle artifact), incomplete scanning technique, poor-quality ultrasound equipment, and placental cysts after the second trimester (Fig. 24–54). Tomko and Baltarowich showed that a synechia may also resemble a vanishing twin.[466]

Associated Syndromes

Fetus papyraceus is a macerated fetus delivered with a normal co-twin and is usually embedded in the placental membranes.[467–469]

MULTIFETAL PREGNANCY REDUCTION

Multifetal pregnancy reduction is the elective termination of a variable number of fetuses, preferably done between the 10th and the 13th weeks of gestation, to improve the perinatal outcome of the remaining fetuses.[470–481] It is well known that high-order multiple gestations have increased risks for both maternal and fetal complications, and the most common are loss of the entire pregnancy, maternal high blood pressure,

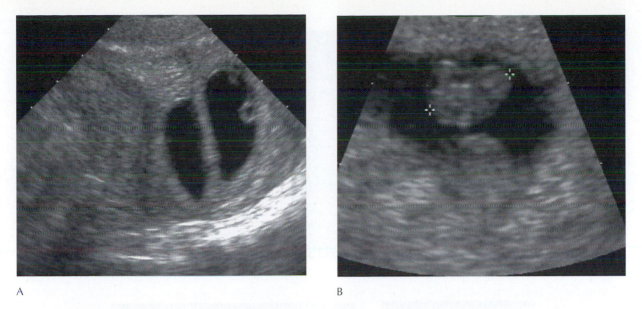

Figure 24–51. At 5 to 6 weeks two gestational sacs are seen **(A).** Two weeks later, **(B)** a single fetus is visible and the sac of the other is already partly resorbed at the lower aspect of the image.

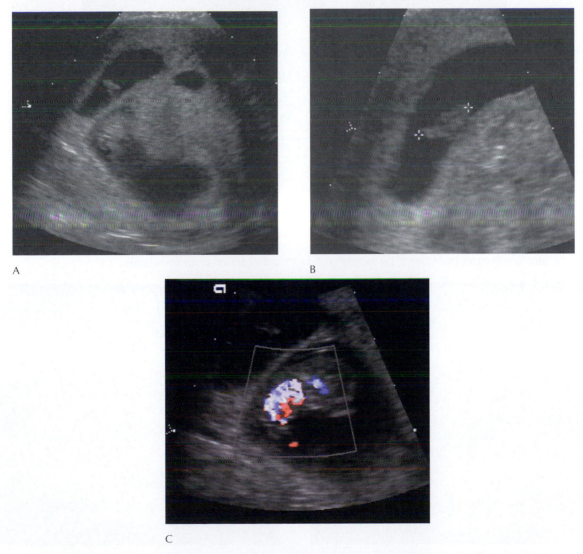

Figure 24–52. In this sequence of images, **(A)** demonstrates the two main gestational sacs. The upper fetus is visible but with a questionable slow heartbeat. The lower fetus appears normal. A repeat scan 10 days later **(B)** demonstrates some growth of the first fetus but cessation of cardiac activity. The other fetus **(C)** has grown appropriately.

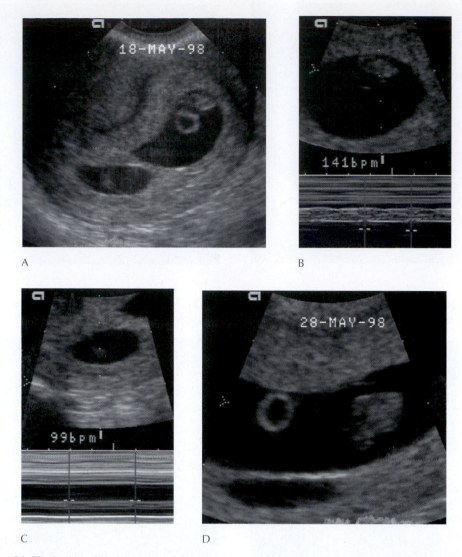

A

B

C

D

Figure 24–53. In these four images, a vanishing twin was suspected in the early examination (image 1, **A**). Both embryos had heartbeats but of different rhythms (99 and 141 bpm, **B, C**). A repeat examination 10 days later demonstrates resorption of the vanishing twin with normal growth of the co-twin **(D)**.

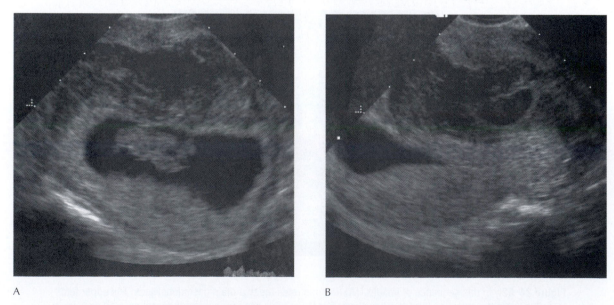

A

B

Figure 24–54. Although a implantation bleed can occasionally resemble a vanishing twin **(A)**, the lack of a trophoblastic ring demonstrates the distinction **(B)**.

666

IUGR, premature rupture of membranes, and preterm delivery. The occurrence of any of these events increases the risk of perinatal death and that of sequelae, such as interventricular hemorrhage, cerebral palsy, retinopathy, and respiratory diseases.[482,483] The procedure may improve maternal and fetal conditions, thereby reducing the risk of prematurity and its associated complications.[484–488] Although it confers unequivocal benefits to the pregnancy when successful, fetal reduction itself carries risks. The risk of losing the entire pregnancy is the major concern and occurs in approximately 12% of cases.

Basically the procedure consists of a transabdominal needle injection of potassium chloride into the fetal thorax.[489,490] If reduction of both fetuses of a monochorionic pair is desired, the procedure may be successfully accomplished with a single injection in one of the pair.[491] Special attention should be given to the appropriate use of the terminology *selective termination* and *elective fetal reduction*. Although both are procedures applied only in multiple gestations, there are some differences between them.

Selective termination is a procedure in which an anomalous fetus in a multifetal pregnancy is terminated to improve the prognosis of the normal co-twin.[492–498] It is usually a second-trimester procedure that follows the same routine as a first-trimester reduction.

Elective fetal reduction describes the reduction of triplets or higher-order fetuses to a smaller set (in general, to twins) for medical, psychological, and socioeconomic reasons, thus improving the outcome of the remaining fetuses and reducing the maternal risks. Some controversy still persists regarding the impact of fetal reduction from triplets to twins. Some investigators have stated that triplet-to-twin fetal reduction significantly reduces the risk for prematurity and low birth weight and may be even associated with a reduction of the overall pregnancy loss rate, suggesting that it is a medically justifiable procedure and should be offered in these cases.[499–502] Others who recommend the maintenance of the entire pregnancy, have stated that bed rest starting at the 20th week of gestation, with special diet and close prenatal care, reduces the prematurity rate and optimizes fetal growth, thereby improving the outcome to the levels of a twin pregnancy.

Selective termination can be performed any time during pregnancy, with good outcome in approximately 90% of cases and a total pregnancy loss rate of 11.7%.[503,504]

AMNIOCENTESES IN TWINS

Diagnostic Amniocentesis

Although amniocentesis is a well-known, safe technique that has been employed in prenatal diagnosis for many years, the risks and benefits should be considered when a multiple gestation is involved. The risk of pregnancy loss when amniocentesis is performed in twins is higher than in singletons. Some investigators have attributed this increased loss rate to the natural tendency of miscarriage observed in multiple gestations.[505–507]

In the past, the most common technique employed the injection of dye into one of the amniotic cavities to differentiate one sac from the other (Fig. 24–55). Since 1990, the avoidance of methylene dye in prenatal diagnosis has been recommended because of its fetotoxicity and a weak association with intestinal atresia.[508–510] More recently, Jeanty et al. successfully used a single needle puncture with no need of dye injection, with the advantages of being less invasive and less painful[511] (Fig. 24–56). Their results have been reproduced by others.[512–514]

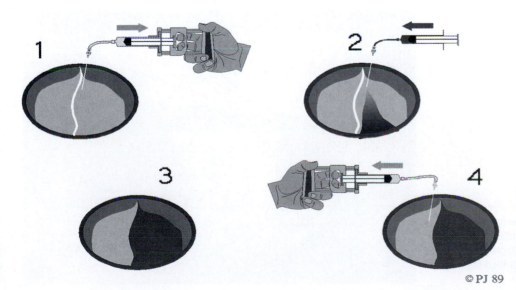

Figure 24–55. In the double stick technique, a needle is inserted into one sac, the fluid is sampled *(1)*, and blue dye is injected *(2)*. The fluid equilibrates for a few minutes *(3)*. The second sample is then obtained *(4)*, hopefully clear of the dye.

© PJ 89

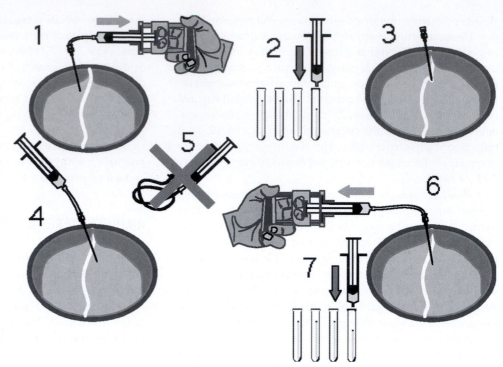

Figure 24–56. In the single insertion technique, the needle is inserted near the membrane attachment at a location where both sacs are visible *(1)*. The fluid is then obtained and transferred to the appropriate containers *(2)*. The plastic tubing is disconnected and the stylet of the needle is reinserted. The needle is then advanced through the membrane *(3)* under ultrasound guidance. A few cubic centimeter of fluid from the second sac are aspirated *(4)* and then the whole assembly (syringe) and tubing are discarded *(5)* to prevent contamination of the second sample by cells from the first sample. The proper sample is then obtained *(6)* and transferred to the containers.

Therapeutic Amniocentesis

Amniocentesis may also have therapeutic applications, in particular in acute polyhydramnios, a common complication in twin pregnancies, with elevated perinatal mortality if not treated. The overdistention of the uterus provokes maternal discomfort, premature labor, and premature rupture of membranes. The treatment consists of serial amniocenteses to normalize the intrauterine pressure, prevent premature labor, and relieve maternal symptoms (see Twin-to-Twin Transfusion Syndrome, above).

CERVICAL CERCLAGE

Cervical cerclage in multiple gestations remains a controversial matter in prenatal care. Some investigators have demonstrated a satisfactory fetal survival rate with minimal incidence of maternal complications postcerclage and thus recommend the routine use of the procedure in multiple pregnancies.[515] Other groups have shown a higher risk for premature rupture of membranes, with no evident benefit for the pregnancy outcome.[516–520] We believe the twin pregnancy

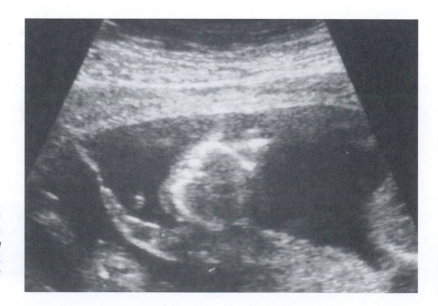

Figure 24–57. This triplet's placenta is inserted at the membrane with the left-sided twin. Although part of this placenta is in contact with the myometrium *(bottom right)*, this was insufficient for adequate growth of this fetus, which was several weeks smaller then the other two.

by itself does not justify the procedure. In multiple pregnancies with sets of triplets or more, the cerclage should be discussed with the patient, considering risks and benefits on each case. If there is a history of cervical incompetence, the procedure must be offered independently of the number of fetuses.

MEMBRANOUS INSERTION OF PLACENTA

Membranous insertion of placenta is a complication that mainly affects higher-order gestations (triplets or higher). In such pregnancies, a centrally located fetus may have a trophoblast developing predominantly on the uterine tissue between the gestational sacs of the other embryos (Fig. 24–57). As the sac grows, that trophoblast will transform into a placenta that is predominantly over the membranes of the other embryos. Even with trophotropism (the tendency of the placenta to preferentially develop where maternal exchanges are best), this embryo is at great risk of growth restriction. Should a fetal reduction be considered, this embryo would be a prime candidate.

REFERENCES

1. Sebire NJ, Nicolaides KH. Screening for fetal abnormalities in multiple pregnancies. *Baillieres Clin Obstet Gynaecol.* 1998; 12:19–36.
2. Benson CB, Doubilet PM. Sonography of multiple gestations. *Radiol Clin North Am.* 1990;28:149–161.
3. Moore KL, Persaud TVN. The placental and fetal membranes. In: *The Developing Human—Clinical Oriented Embryology,* 5th ed. Philadelphia: WB Saunders; 1993.
4. Sebire NJ, Snijders RJM, Hughes K, et al. The hidden mortality of monochorionic twin pregnancies. *Br J Obstet Gynaecol.* 1997;104:1203–1207.
5. Van Heteren CF, Nijhuis JG, Semmekrot BA, et al. Discordant fetal growth in multiple pregnancy: Intervention should be based on chorionicity. *Ned Tijdschr Geneeskd.* 1999;143: 1017–1121.
6. Nicolaides KH, Sebire NJ, Snijders RJM. *The 11–14 Week Scan: The Diagnosis of Fetal Abnormalities.* London: Parthenon Publishing; 1999.
7. Cameron AH. The Birmingham twin survey. *Proc R Soc Med.* 1968;61:229–234.
8. Benirschke K. The biology of the twinning process: How placentation influences outcome. *Semin Perinatol.* 1995;19: 342–350.
9. Husby H, Holm NV, Gernow A, et al. Zygosity, placental membranes and Weinberg's rule in a Danish consecutive twin series. *Acta Genet Med Gemellol.* 1991;40:147–152.
10. Denbow ML, Fisk NM. The consequences of monochorionic placentation. *Baillieres Clin Obstet Gynaecol.* 1998;12: 37–51.
11. Thigpen J. Discordant twins: A case report. *Neonatal Netw.* 1996;15:35–39.
12. McCulloch K. Neonatal problems in twins. *Clin Perinatol.* 1988;15:141–158.
13. Minakami H, Honma Y, Matsubara S, et al. Effects of placental chorionicity on outcome in twin pregnancies. A cohort study. *J Reprod Med.* 1999;44:595–600.
14. Malinowski W. Very early and simple determination of chorionic and amniotic type in twin gestations by high-frequency transvaginal ultrasonography. *Acta Genet Med Gemellol.* 1997;46:167–173.
15. Monteagudo A, Timor-Tritsch IE, Sharma S. Early and simple determination of chorionic and amniotic type in multifetal gestations in the first fourteen weeks by high-frequency transvaginal ultrasonography. *Am J Obstet Gynecol.* 1994;170: 824–829.
16. Finberg HJ. The "twin peak" sign: Reliable evidence of dichorionic twinning. *J Ultrasound Med.* 1992;11:571–577.
17. Rode ME, Jackson M. Sonographic considerations with multiple gestation. *Semin Roentgenol.* 1999;34:29–34.
18. Sepulveda W, Sebire NJ, Hughes K, et al. The lambda sign at 10–14 weeks of gestation as a predictor of chorionicity in twin pregnancies. *Ultrasound Obstet Gynecol.* 1996;7:421–423.
19. Kurtz AB, Wapner RJ, Mata J, et al. Twin pregnancies: Accuracy of first trimester abdominal US in predicting chorionicity and amnionicity. *Radiology.* 1992;185:759–762.
20. Hertzberg BS, Kurtz AB, Choi HY, et al. Significance of membrane thickness in the sonographic evaluation of twin gestations. *AJR.* 1987;148:151–153.
21. Ayala Mendez JA, Jimenez Solis G, Fernandez Martinez LR, et al. Determination by ultrasound of chorionicity in twin pregnancy. *Ginecol Obstet Mex.* 1997;65:111–113.
22. Vayssiere CF, Heim N, Camus EP, et al. Determination of chorionicity in twin gestations by high-frequency abdominal ultrasonography: Counting the layers of the dividing membrane. *Am J Obstet Gynecol.* 1996;75:1529–1533.
23. D'Alton ME, Dudley DK. The ultrasonographic prediction of chorionicity in twin gestation. *Am J Obstet Gynecol.* 1989; 160:557–561.
24. Townsend RR, Simpson GF, Filly RA. Membrane thickness in ultrasound prediction of chorionicity of twin gestations. *J Ultrasound Med.* 1988;7:327–332.
25. Cheung A, Wan M, Collins RJ. Differentiation of monochorionic and dichorionic twin placentas by antenatal ultrasonic evaluation. *Aust NZ J Obstet Gynaecol.* 1990;30:134–136.
26. Uccello N, Daniele F, Sannino F, et al. Ultrasonic criteria for the evaluation of placentation in twin pregnancies. *Minerva Ginecol.* 1989;41:75–77.
27. Winn HN, Gabrielli S, Reece EA, et al. Ultrasonographic criteria for the prenatal diagnosis of placental chorionicity in twin gestations. *Am J Obstet Gynecol.* 1989;161:1540–1542.
28. Bajoria R, Kingdom J. The case for routine determination of chorionicity and zygosity in multiple pregnancy. *Prenat Diagn.* 1997;17:1207–1225.
29. Zondervan HA, Stoutenbeek P, Arabin B, et al. Third circulation: Twin transfusion syndrome. *Ned Tijdschr Geneeskd.* 1999;143:1022–1027.
30. Van Heteren CF, Nijhuts JG, Semmekrot BA, et al. Risk for surviving twin after fetal death of co-twin in twin–twin transfusion syndrome. *Obstet Gynecol.* 1998;92:215–219.
31. Brackley KJ, Kilby MD. Twin–twin transfusion syndrome. *Hosp Med.* 1999;60:419–424.

32. Brown DL, Benson CB, Driscoll SG, et al. Twin–twin transfusion syndrome: Sonographic findings. *Radiology.* 1989;170: 61–63.

33. Mari G, Detti L, Levi-D'Ancona R, et al. "Pseudo" twin-to-twin transfusion syndrome and fetal outcome. *J Perinatol.* 1998;18:399–403.

34. Weston PJ, Ives EJ, Honore RL, et al. Monochorionic diamniotic minimally conjoined twins: A case report. *Am J Med Genet.* 1990;37:558–561.

35. Law KS, Chang SD, Chen FP, et al. Acardiac acephalus: A case report and implications on expectant management. *Chang Keng I Hsueh Tsa Chih.* 1999;22:334–338.

36. Benirschke K. Intrauterine death of a twin: Mechanisms, implications for surviving twin, and placental pathology. *Semin Diagn Pathol.* 1993;10:222–231.

37. Ries M, Beinder E, Gruner C, et al. Rapid development of hydrops fetalis in the donor twin following death of the recipient twin in twin–twin transfusion syndrome. *J Perinat Med.* 1999;27:68–73.

38. Lin IJ, Chen CH, Wang TM, et al. Infants of twin pregnancies with one twin demise in the uterus: A retrospective study. *Chung Hua Min Kuo Hsiao Erh Ko I Hsueh Hui Tsa Chih.* 1999;40:92–96.

39. Krayenbuhl M, Huch A, Zimmermann R. Single intrauterine fetal death in twin pregnancy. *Z Geburtshilfe Neonatol.* 1998;202:60–63.

40. Kilby MD, Govind A, O'Brien PM. Outcome of twin pregnancies complicated by a single intrauterine death: A comparison with viable twin pregnancies. *Obstet Gynecol.* 1994;84: 107–109.

41. Chen CD, Ko TM, Hsieh FJ, et al. Intrauterine death of co-twin in the third trimester: A case report of twin-to-twin transfusion syndrome and cord accident. *J Formos Med Assoc.* 1993;92:665–667.

42. Gold F, Saliba E, Grangeponte MC, et al. Cerebral lesions observed in a twin after the in utero death of the other twin. Fetal anoxia-ischemia can be the possible mechanism (3 cases). *Arch Fr Pediatr.* 1992;49:529–533.

43. Choulot JJ, Fescharek R, Saint Martin J, et al. In utero death of one twin and cerebral complications in the surviving twin. *Presse Med.* 1985;14:1077–1080.

44. Fusi L, MacParland P, Fisk N, et al. Acute twin–twin transfusion: A possible mechanism for brain damaged survivors after intrauterine death of a monozygotic twin. *Obstet Gynecol.* 1991;78:517–522.

45. Jou HJ, Ng KY, Teng RJ, et al. Doppler sonographic detection of reverse twin–twin trans fusion after intrauterine death of the donor. *J Ultrasound Med.* 1993;12:307–309.

46. Pharoah PO, Cooke RW. A hypothesis for the aetiology of spastic cerebral palsy—The vanishing twin. *Dev Med Child Neurol.* 1997;39:292–296.

47. Perlman JM, Burns DK, Twickler DM, et al. Fetal hypokinesia syndrome in the monochorionic pair of a triplet pregnancy secondary to severe disruptive cerebral injury. *Pediatrics.* 1995;96:521–523.

48. Fleischer AC, Romero R, Manning F, et al, eds. *Principles and Practice of Ultrasonography in Obstetrics and Gynecology,* 4th ed. Norwalk, Conn: Appleton & Lange; 1991.

49. Baldwin, VJ. *Pathology of Multiple Pregnancies.* New York: Springer-Verlag; 1994.

50. Rumack CM, Wilson SR, Charboneau JW, eds. *Diagnostic Ultrasound.* St Louis; Mosby-Year Book; 1991:745–758.

51. Overton TG, Denbow ML, Duncan KR, Fisk NM. First-trimester cord entanglement in monoamniotic twins. *Ultrasound Obstet Gynecol.* 1999;13:140–142.

52. Lumme R, Saarikoski S. Monoamniotic twin pregnancy. *Acta Genet Med Gemellol.* 1986;35:99–105.

53. Filly RA, Goldstein RB, Callen PW. Monochorionic twinning: Sonographic assessment. *AJR.* 1990;154:459–469.

54. Aisenbrey GA, et al. Monoamniotic and pseudomonoamniotic twins: Sonographic diagnosis, detection of cord entanglement, and obstetric management. *Obstet Gynecol.* 1995;86:218–222.

55. Tannirandorn Y, Phaosavasdi S. Accuracy of ultrasonographic criteria for the prenatal diagnosis of placental amnionicity and chorionicity in twin gestations. *J Med Assoc Thai.* 1993; 76:190–195.

56. Levi CS, et al. Yolk sac number, size and morphologic features in monochorionic monoamniotic twin pregnancy. *Can Assoc Radiol J.* 1996;47:98–100.

57. Carlan SJ, Angel JL, Sawai SK, et al. Late diagnosis of nonconjoined monoamniotic twins using computed tomographic imaging: A case report. *Obstet Gynecol.* 1990;76:504–506.

58. Strohbehn K, Dattel BJ. Pitfalls in the diagnosis of nonconjoined monoamniotic twins. *J Perinatol.* 1995;15:484–493.

59. Blane CE, DiPietro MA, Johnson MZ, et al. Sonographic detection of monoamniotic twins. *J Clin Ultrasound.* 1987;15: 394–396.

60. Bajoria R. Abundant vascular anastomoses in monoamniotic versus diamniotic monochorionic placentas. *Am J Obstet Gynecol.* 1998;179:788–793.

61. Ritossa M, et al. Monoamniotic twin pregnancy and cord entanglement: A clinical dilemma. *Aust NZ J Obstet Gynaecol.* 1996;36:309–312.

62. D'Alton ME, et al. Syndromes in twins. *Semin Perinatol.* 1995; 19:375–386.

63. Arabin B, Laurini RN, van Eyck J. Early prenatal diagnosis of cord entanglement in monoamniotic multiple pregnancies. *Ultrasound Obstet Gynecol.* 1999;13:181–186.

64. Sherer DM, Anyaegbunam A. Prenatal ultrasonographic morphologic assessment of the umbilical cord: A review. Part I. *Obstet Gynecol Surv.* 1997;52:506–514.

65. Sherer DM, Anyaegbunam A. Prenatal ultrasonographic morphologic assessment of the umbilical cord: A review. Part II. *Obstet Gynecol Surv.* 1997;52:515–523.

66. Peek MJ, et al. Medical amnioreduction with sulindac to reduce cord complications in monoamniotic twins. *Am J Obstet Gynecol.* 1997;176:334–336.

67. Westover T, Guzman ER, Shen-Schwartz S. Prenatal diagnosis of an unusual nuchal cord complication in monoamniotic twins. *Obstet Gynecol.* 1994;84:689–691.

68. Krussel JS, von Eckardstein S, Schwenzer T. Double umbilical cord knot in mono-amniotic twin pregnancy as the cause of intrauterine fetal death of both twins. *Zentralbl Gynakol.* 1994;116:497–499.

69. Hod M, Merlob P, Friedman S, et al. Single intrauterine fetal death in monoamniotic twins due to cord entanglement. *Clin Exp Obstet Gynecol.* 1988;15:63–65.

70. Beck R. Monoamniotic twin pregnancy with knotted umbilical cords. *Zentralbl Gynakol.* 1985;107:688–692.

71. McLeod FN, McCoy DR. Monoamniotic twins with an

unusual cord complication. Case report. *Br J Obstet Gynaecol.* 1981;88:774–775.

72. Foglmann R. Monoamniotic twins. *Acta Genet Med Gemellol.* 1976;25:62–65.

73. Hansen LM, Donnenfeld AE. Concordant anencephaly in monoamniotic twins and an analysis of maternal serum markers. *Prenat Diagn.* 1997;17:471–473.

74. McCoy MC, Chescheir NC, Kuller JA, et al. A fetus with sirenomelia, omphalocele, and meningomyelocele, but normal kidneys. *Teratology.* 1994;50:168–171.

75. Cilento BG Jr, Benacerraf BR, Mandell J. Prenatal and postnatal findings in monochorionic monoamniotic twins discordant for bilateral renal agenesis-dysgenesis (perinatal lethal renal disease). *J Urol.* 1994;151:1034–1035.

76. Langer JC, Brennan B, Lappalainen RE, et al. Cloacal exstrophy: Prenatal diagnosis before rupture of the cloacal membrane. *J Pediatr Surg.* 1992;27:1352–1355.

77. Neal GS, Hankins GD. Left microtia in one monozygotic twin. A case report. *J Reprod Med.* 1992;37:375–377.

78. Berry SA, Johnson DE, Thompson TR. Agenesis of the penis, scrotal raphe, and anus in one of monoamniotic twins. *Teratology.* 1984;29:173–176.

79. Vaughn TC, Powell LC. The obstetrical management of conjoined twins. *Obstet Gynecol.* 1979;53:67S–72S.

80. James WH. The sex ratio of monoamniotic twin pairs. *Ann Hum Biol.* 1977;4:143–153.

81. Myrianthopoulos NC. Congenital malformations in twins: Epidemiologic survey. *Birth Defects Orig Art Ser.* 1975;11:1–39.

82. Entazami M, Ragosch V, Hopp H, et al. Notch in the umbilical artery Doppler profile in umbilical cord compression in a twin. *Ultraschall Med.* 1997;18:277–279.

83. Carr SR, Aronson MP, Couston DR. Survival rates of monoamniotic twins do not decrease after 30 weeks gestation. *Am J Obstet Gynecol.* 1990;163:719–722.

84. Townsend RR, Filly RA. Sonography of nonconjoined monoamniotic twin pregnancies. *J Ultrasound Med.* 1988;7:665–670.

85. Rosemond RL, Hinds NE. Persistent abdominal umbilical cord Doppler velocimetry in a monoamniotic twin with cord entanglement. *J Ultrasound Med.* 1998;17:337–338.

86. Tessen JA, Zlatnik FJ. Monoamniotic twins: A retrospective study controlled study. *Obstet Gynecol.* 1991;77:832–834.

87. Dorum A, Nesheim BL. Monochorionic monoamniotic twins—The most precarious of twin pregnancies. *Acta Obstet Gynecol Scand.* 1991;70:381–383.

88. Fraser RB, Liston RM, Thompson DL, et al. Monoamniotic twins delivered liveborn with a forked umbilical cord. *Pediatr Pathol Lab Med.* 1997;17:639–644.

89. Multiple gestation. *ACOG Tech Bull,* 1989;131.

90. Benirschke K, Kim CK. Multiple pregnancy. *N Engl J Med.* 1973;228:1276–1284.

91. Reece EA, Yarkoni S, Abdalla M, et al. A prospective longitudinal study of growth in twin gestations compared with growth in singleton pregnancies. I. The fetal head. *J Ultrasound Med.* 1991;10:439–443.

92. Reece EA, Yarkoni S, Abdalla M, et al. A prospective longitudinal study of growth in twin gestations compared with growth in singleton pregnancies. II. The fetal limbs. *J Ultrasound Med.* 1991;10:445–450.

93. Rode ME, Jackson M. Sonographic considerations with multiple gestation. *Semin Roentgenol.* 1999;34:29–34.

94. Sherer DM, Divon MY. Fetal growth in multifetal gestation. *Clin Obstet Gynecol.* 1997;40:764–770.

95. Caravello JW, Chauhan SP, Morrison JC, et al. Sonographic examination does not predict twin growth discrepancy accurately. *Obstet Gynecol.* 1997;89:529–533.

96. Talbot GT, Goldstein RF, Nesbitt T, et al. Is size discordancy an indication for delivery of preterm twins? *Am J Obstet Gynecol.* 1997;177:1050–1054.

97. Bajoria R. Vascular anatomy of monochorionic placenta in relation to discordant growth and amniotic fluid volume. *Hum Reprod.* 1998;13:2933–2940.

98. Sonntag J, Waltz S, Schollmeyer T, et al. Morbidity and mortality of discordant twins up to 34 weeks of gestational age. *Eur J Pediatr.* 1996;155:224–229.

99. Rizzo G, Arduini D, Romanini C. Cardiac and extracardiac flows in discordant twins. *Am J Obstet Gynecol.* 1994;70:1321–1327.

100. Eberle AM, Levesque D, Vintzileos AM, et al. Placental pathology in discordant twins. *Am J Obstet Gynecol.* 1993;169:931–935.

101. Yalcin HR, Zorlu CG, Lembet A, et al. The significance of birth weight difference in discordant twins: A level to standardize? *Acta Obstet Gynecol Scand.* 1998;77:28–31.

102. Tadmor O, Nitzan M, Rabinowitz R, et al. Prediction of second trimester intrauterine growth retardation and fetal death in a discordant twin by first trimester measurements. Case report and review of the literature. *Fetal Diagn Ther.* 1995;10:17–21.

103. Weissman A, Achiron R, Lipitz S, et al. The first trimester growth discordant twin: An ominous prenatal finding. *Obstet Gynecol.* 1994;84:110–114.

104. Chitkara U, Berkowitz GS, Levine R, et al. Twin pregnancy: Routine use of ultrasound examinations in the perinatal diagnosis of intrauterine growth retardation and discordant growth. *Am J Perinatol.* 1985;2:49–54.

105. Divon MY, Weiner Z. Ultrasound in twin pregnancy. *Semin Perinatol.* 1995;19:404–412.

106. Blickstein I, Goldman RD, Smith-Levitin M, et al. The relation between intertwin birth weight discrepancy and total twin birth weight. *Obstet Gynecol.* 1999;93:113–116.

107. Lemery DR, Santolaya-Forgas J, Serre AF, et al. Fetal serum erythropoietin in twin pregnancies with discordant growth. A clue for prenatal diagnosis of monochorionic twins with vascular communications. *Fetal Diagn Ther.* 1995;10:86–91.

108. Hsieh TT, Chang TC, Chiu TH, et al. Growth discordancy, birth weight, and neonatal adverse events in third trimester twin gestations. *Gynecol Obstet Invest.* 1994;38:36–40.

109. Chauhan SP, Washburne JF, Martin JN Jr, et al. Intrapartum assessment by house staff of birth weight among twins. *Obstet Gynecol.* 1993;82:523–526.

110. Sayegh SK, Warsof SL. Ultrasonic prediction of discordant growth in twin pregnancies. *Fetal Diagn Ther.* 1993;8:241–246.

111. Mordel N, Benshushan A, Zajicek G, et al. Discordancy in triplets. *Am J Perinatol.* 1993;10:224–225.

112. Jakobovits AA. The significance of birth weight discrepancy in twins. *Acta Med Hung.* 1992–1993;49:195–200.

113. Chamberlain P, Murphy M, Comerford FR. How accurate

is antenatal sonographic identification of discordant birth weight in twins? *Eur J Obstet Gynecol Reprod Biol.* 1991;40: 91–96.

114. Blickstein I, Shoham-Schwartz Z, Lancet M. Growth discordancy in appropiate for gestational age, term twins. *Obstet Gynecol.* 1988;72:582–584.

115. Blickstein I, Shoham-Schwartz Z, Lancet M, et al. Characterization of the growth-discordant twin. *Obstet Gynecol.* 1987; 70:11–15.

116. Philip AG. Term twins with discordant birth weights: Observations at birth and one year. *Acta Genet Med Gemellol.* 1981;30:203–212.

117. Devoe LD, Ware DJ. Antenatal assessment of twin gestation. *Semin Perinatol.* 1995;19:413–423.

118. Fraser D, Picard R, Picard E, et al. Birth weight discordance, intrauterine growth retardation and perinatal outcomes in twins. *J Reprod Med.* 1994;39:504–508.

119. Storlazzi E, Vintzileos AM, Campbell WA, et al. Ultrasonic diagnosis of discordant fetal growth in twin gestations. *Obstet Gynecol.* 1987;69:363–367.

120. Blickstein I, Manor M, Levi R, et al. The intrauterine ponderal index in relation to birth weight discrepancy in twin gestations. *Int J Gynaecol Obstet.* 1995;50:253–255.

121. Cheung VY, Bocking AD, Dasilva OP. Preterm discordant twins: What birth weight difference is significant? *Am J Obstet Gynecol.* 1995;172:955–959.

122. Blickstein I. The definition, diagnosis, and management of growth-discordant twins: An international census survey. *Acta Genet Med Gemellol.* 1991;40:345–351.

123. Blickstein I, Manor M, Levi R, et al. Is intertwin birth weight discrepancy predictable? *Gynecol Obstet Invest.* 1996;42:105–108.

124. Divon MY, Girz BA, Sklar A, et al. Discordant twins—A prospective study of the diagnostic value of real-time ultrasonography combined with umbilical artery velocimetry. *Am J Obstet Gynecol.* 1989;161:757–760.

125. Blickstein I, Friedman A, Caspi B, et al. Ultrasonic prediction of growth discordancy by intertwin difference in abdominal circumference. *Int J Gynaecol Obstet.* 1989;29:121–124.

126. Brown CE, Guzick DS, Leveno KJ, et al. Prediction of discordant twins using ultrasound measurement of biparietal diameter and abdominal perimeter. *Obstet Gynecol.* 1987;70: 677–681.

127. Crane JP, Tomich PG, Kopta M. Ultrasonic growth patterns in normal and discordant twins. *Obstet Gynecol.* 1980;55:678–683.

128. Chittacharoen A, Leelapattana P, Phuapradit W. Umbilical Doppler velocimetry prediction of discordant twins. *J Obstet Gynaecol Res.* 1999;25:95–98.

129. Grab D, Hutter W, Haller T, et al. Discordant growth in twin pregnancy—Value of Doppler ultrasound. *Geburtshilfe Frauenheilkd.* 1993;53:42–48.

130. Giles WB. Doppler ultrasound in multiple pregnancies. *Baillieres Clin Obstet Gynaecol.* 1998;12:77–89.

131. Clode N, Casal E, Graca LM. Umbilical flowmetry in twin pregnancy. A method for identifying discordant fetal growth? *Acta Med Port.* 1992;5:483–484.

132. Behrens O, Wedeking-Schohl H, Mesrogli M, et al. Doppler ultrasound in monitoring twin pregnancies with early discordant growth. *Z Geburtshilfe Perinatol.* 1992;196:209–212.

133. Gerson AG, Wallace DM, Bridgens NK, et al. Duplex Doppler ultrasound in the evaluation of growth in twin pregnancies. *Obstet Gynecol.* 1987;70:419–423.

134. Giles WB, Trudinger BJ, Cook CM. Fetal umbilical artery flow velocity-time waveforms in twin pregnancies. *Br J Obstet Gynaecol.* 1985;92:490–497.

135. Oberg KC, Pestaner JP, Bielamowicz L, et al. Renal tubular disgenesis in twin–twin transfusion syndrome. *Pediatr Dev Pathol.* 1999;2:25–32.

136. Lazda EJ. Endocardial fibroelastosis in growth-discordant monozygotic twins. *Pediatr Dev Pathol.* 1998;1:522–527.

137. Weiner CP, Ludomirski A. Diagnosis, pathophysiology, and treatment of chronic twin-to-twin transfusion syndrome. *Fetal Diagn Ther.* 1994;9:283–290.

138. Salvolini E, Lucarini G, Cester N, et al. Growth retardation and discordant twin pregnancy. An immunomorphological and biochemical characterisation of the human umbilical cord. *Biochem Mol Biol Int.* 1998;46:795–805.

139. D'Alton ME, Mercer BM. Antepartum management of twin gestation: Ultrasound. *Clin Obstet Gynecol.* 1990;33:42–51.

140. Bruner JP, Anderson TL, Rosemond RL. Placental pathophysiology of the twin oligohydramnios–polyhydramnios sequence and the twin–twin transfusion syndrome. *Placenta.* 1998;19:81–86.

141. Blickstein I, Weissman A. Birth weight discordancy in male-first and female-first pairs of unlike-sexed twins. *Am J Obstet Gynecol.* 1990;162:661–663.

142. Vetter K. Considerations on growth discordant twins. *J Perinat Med.* 1993;21:267–272.

143. Blickstein I, Lancet M. The growth discordant twin. *Obstet Gynecol Surv.* 1998;43:509–515.

144. Fakeye O. Twin birth weight discordancy in Nigeria. *Int J Gynaecol Obstet.* 1986;24:235–238.

145. Bernasko J, Lynch L, Lapinsky R, et al. Twin pregnancies conceived by assisted reproductive techniques: Maternal and neonatal outcomes. *Obstet Gynecol.* 1997;89:368–372.

146. Johnson JM, Harman CR, Evans JA, et al. Maternal serum alpha-fetoprotein in twin pregnancy. *Am J Obstet Gynecol.* 1990;162:1020–1025.

147. Samuels, P. Ultrasound in the management of the twin gestation. *Clin Obstet Gynecol.* 1988;31:110–122.

148. Gaziano EP, Knox GE, Bendel RP, et al. Is pulsed Doppler velocimetry useful in the management of multiple-gestations pregnancies? *Am J Obstet Gynecol.* 1991;164:1425–1431.

149. Chittacharoen A, Leelapattana P, Phuapradit W. Umbilical Doppler velocimetry prediction of discordant twins. *J Obstet Gynaecol Res.* 1999;25:95–98.

150. Schwarzler P, Ville Y, Moscoso G, et al. Diagnosis of twin reversed arterial perfusion sequence in the first trimester by transvaginal color Doppler ultrasound. *Ultrasound Obstet Gynecol.* 1999;13:143–146.

151. Donner C, Noel JC, Rypens F, et al. Twin–twin transfusion syndrome—Possible roles for Doppler ultrasound and amniocentesis. *Prenat Diagn.* 1995;15:60–63.

152. Sohl S, David M. Doppler ultrasound study of a twin pregnancy with feto-fetal transfusion syndrome. *Geburtshilfe Frauenheilkd.* 1994;54:475–477.

153. Ohno Y, Ando H, Tanamura A, et al. The value of Doppler ultrasound in the diagnosis and management of twin-to-twin transfusion syndrome. *Arch Gynecol Obstet.* 1994;255:37–42.

154. Overton TG, Denbow ML, Duncan KR, et al. First-trimester cord entanglement in monoamniotic twins. *Ultrasound Obstet Gynecol.* 1999;13:140–142.

155. Rodis JF, Egan JFX, Craffey A, et al. Calculated risk of chromosomal abnormalities in twin gestations. *Obstet Gynecol.* 1990;76:1037–1041.

156. Appelman Z, Vinkler C, Caspi B. Chorionic villus sampling in multiple pregnancies. *Eur J Obstet Gynecol Reprod Biol.* 1999;85:97–99.

157. Wapner RJ, Johnson A, Davis G, et al. Prenatal diagnosis in twin gestations: A comparison between second-trimester amniocentesis and first-trimester chorionic villus sampling. *Obstet Gynecol.* 1993;82:49–56.

158. Mielke G, Kiesel L, Backsch C, et al. Fetal sex determination by high resolution ultrasound in early pregnancy. *Eur J Ultrasound.* 1998;7:109–114.

159. Costa T, Lambert M, Teshima I, et al. Monozygotic twins with 45,X/46,XY mosaicism discordant for phenotypic sex. *Am J Med Genet.* 1998;75:40–44.

160. Kurosawa K, Kuromaru R, Imaizumi K, et al. Monozygotic twins with discordant sex. *Acta Genet Med Gemellol.* 1992;41:301–310.

161. Fujimoto A, Boelter WD, Sparkes RS, et al. Monozygotic twins of discordant sex both with 45,X/46,X,idic(Y) mosaicism. *Am J Med Genet.* 1991;41:239–245.

162. Gonsoulin W, Copeland KL, Carpenter RJ Jr, et al. Fetal blood sampling demonstrating chimerism in monozygotic twins discordant for sex and tissue karyotype (46,XY and 45,X). *Prenat Diagn.* 1990;10:25–28.

163. Reindollar RH, Byrd JR, Hahn DH, et al. A cytogenetic and endocrinologic study of a set of monozygotic isokaryotic 45,X/46,XY twins discordant for phenotypic sex: Mosaicism versus chimerism. *Fertil Steril.* 1987;47(4):626–633.

164. Schmidt R, Sobel EH, Nitowsky HM, et al. Monozygotic twins discordant for sex. *J Med Genet.* 1976;13:64–68.

165. Schinzel A. Karyotype–phenotype correlations in autosomal chromosomal aberrations. *Prog Clin Biol Res.* 1993;384:19–31.

166. Nieuwint A, Van Zalen-Sprock R, Hummel P, et al. 'Identical' twins with discordant karyotypes. *Prenat Diagn.* 1999;19:72–76.

167. Carta G, Iovenitti P, D'Alfonso A, et al. Fetal malformations and chromosome abnormalities diagnosed at the Center of Prenatal Diagnosis of the University of Aquila in the 1995–1998 triennium. *Minerva Ginecol.* 1999;51:393–398.

168. Loevy HT, Miller M, Rosenthal IM. Discordant monozygotic twins with trisomy 13. *Acta Genet Med Gemellol.* 1985;34:185–188.

169. Mielke G, Enders H, Goelz R, et al. Prenatal detection of double aneuploidy trisomy 10/monosomy X in a liveborn twin with exclusively monosomy X in blood. *Clin Genet.* 1997;51:275–277.

170. Pedersen IK, Philip J, Sele V, et al. Monozygotic twins with dissimilar phenotypes and chromosome complements. *Acta Obstet Gynecol Scand.* 1980;59:459–462.

171. Cussen LJ, MacMahon RA. Germ cells and ova in dysgenetic gonads of a 46-XY female dizygotic twin. *Am J Dis Child.* 1979;133:373–375.

172. Qureshi F, Jacques SM, Yaron Y, et al. Prenatal diagnosis of cloacal dysgenesis sequence: Differential diagnosis from other forms of fetal obstructive uropathy. *Fetal Diagn Ther.* 1998;13:69–74.

173. Peng Y, Shieh JL, Jung SM, et al. Cyclopia in one of discordant twins: A case report. *Chang Keng I Hsueh.* 1997;20:232–236.

174. Shih TY, Liu YJ, Lin YZ, et al. Amniotic band disruption complex: Report of one case in twins. *Chung Hua Min Kuo Hsiao Erh Ko I Hsueh Hui Tsa Chih.* 1991;32:115–121.

175. Nguyen Tan Lung R, Lalau P. Echographic diagnosis of cystic hygroma. Apropos of a case. *J Gynecol Obstet Biol Reprod.* 1987;16:893–900.

176. Weill J, Boudailliez B, Piussan C, et al. Cerebral and ocular abnormalities with anterior pituitary insufficiency of familial nature. *J Hum Genet.* 1985;33:31–35.

177. Fried K, Micle S, Goldberg MD. Genetic microcephaly in a pair of monozygous twins. *Teratology.* 1984;29:177–180.

178. Sagot P, David A, Talmant C, et al. Russell–Silver syndrome: An explanation for discordant growth in monozygotic twins. *Fetal Diagn Ther.* 1996;11:72–78.

179. Bailey W, Popovich B, Jones KL. Monozygotic twins discordant for the Russell–Silver syndrome. *Am J Med Genet.* 1995;58:101–105.

180. Mahony BS, Filly RA, Callen PW. Amnionicity and chorionicity in twin pregnancies: Prediction using ultrasound. *Radiology.* 1985;155:205–209.

181. Mari G, Detti L, Levi-D'Ancona R, et al. "Pseudo" twin-to-twin transfusion syndrome and fetal outcome. *J Perinatol.* 1998;18:399–403.

182. Nores J, Athanassiou A, Elkadry E, et al. Gender differences in twin–twin transfusion syndrome. *Obstet Gynecol.* 1997;90:580–582.

183. Patten RM, Mack LA, Harvey D, et al. Disparity of amniotic fluid volume and fetal size: Problem of the stuck twin–US studies. *Radiology.* 1989;172:153–157.

184. Brown DL, Benson CB, Driscoll SG, et al. Twin–twin transfusion syndrome: Sonographic findings. *Radiology.* 1989;170:61–63.

185. Weiner CP, Ludomirsky A. Diagnosis, pathophisiology and treatment of chronic twin-to-twin transfusion syndrome. *Fetal Diagn Ther.* 1994;9:283–290.

186. Farmakides G, Schulman H, Saldona LR, et al. Surveillance of twin pregnancy with umbilical artery velocimetry. *Am J Obstet Gynecol.* 1985;153:789–792.

187. Giles WB. Doppler ultrasound in multiple pregnancies. *Baillieres Clin Obstet Gynaecol.* 1998;12:77–89.

188. Hecher K, Ville Y, Nicolaides KH. Color Doppler ultrasonography in the identification of communicating vessels in twin–twin transfusion syndrome and acardiac twins. *J Ultrasound Med.* 1995;14:37–40.

189. Hecher K, Ville Y, Nicolaides KH. Fetal arterial Doppler studies in twin–twin transfusion syndrome. *J Ultrasound Med.* 1995;14:101–108.

190. Hecher K, Ville Y, Snidjers R, et al. Doppler studies of the fetal circulation in twin–twin transfusion syndrome. *Ultrasound Obstet Gynecol.* 1995;5:318–324.

191. Sohl S, David M. Doppler ultrasound study of a twin pregnancy with feto–fetal transfusion syndrome. *Geburtshilfe Frauenheilkd.* 1994;54:475–477.

192. Donner C, Noel JC, Rypens F, et al. Twin–twin transfusion syndrome–Possible roles for Doppler ultrasound and amniocentesis. *Prenat Diagn.* 1995;15:60–63.

193. Weiner CP, Ludomirski A. Diagnosis, pathophysiology, and treatment of chronic twin-to-twin transfusion syndrome. *Fetal Diagn Ther.* 1994;9:283–290.

194. Wittman BK, Baldwin VJ, Nichol B. Antenatal diagnosis of twin transfusion syndrome by ultrasound. *Obstet Gynecol.* 1981;58:123–126.

195. Brennan JN, Diwan RV, Roscn MG, et al. Fetofetal transfusion syndrome: Prenatal ultrasonographic diagnosis. *Radiology.* 1982;143:535–536.

196. Ville Y. Management of twin–twin transfusion syndrome: An open multicentre randomized trial to evaluate serial amniodrainage versus endoscopic placental laser surgery with amniodrainage. *Front Fetal Health.* 1999;1:2–5.

197. Berry SM, Puder KS, Bottoms SF, et al. Comparison of intrauterine hematologic and biochemical values between twin pairs with and without stuck twin syndrome. *Am J Obstet Gynecol.* 1995;172:1403–1410.

198. Arts H, van Eyck J, Arabin B. Fetal death of one twin in a monochorionic pregnancy with twin–twin transfusion syndrome. *J Reprod Med.* 1996;4:775–778.

199. Braat DD, Exalto N, Bernardus RE, et al. Twin pregnancy: Case reports illustrating variations in transfusion syndrome. *Eur J Obstet Gynecol Reprod Biol.* 1985;19:383–390.

200. Rumack CM, Wilson SR, Charboneau JW, eds. *Diagnostic Ultrasound.* St. Louis: Mosby-Year Book; 1991:745–758.

201. Dickinson JE. Severe twin–twin transfusion syndrome: Current management concepts. *Aust NZ Obstet Gynaecol.* 1995;35:16–21.

202. Van Gemert MJ, Sterenborg HJ. Haemodynamic model of twin–twin transfusion syndrome in monochorionic twin pregnancies. *Placenta.* 1998;19:195–208.

203. Wax JR, Blakemore KJ, Blohm P, et al. Stuck twin with cotwin noninmune hydrops: Successful treatment by amniocentesis. *Fetal Diagn Ther.* 1991;6:126–131.

204. Bajoria R. Abundant vascular anastomoses in monoamniotic versus diamniotic monochorionic placentas. *Am J Obstet Gynecol.* 1998;179:788–793.

205. Hecher K, Ville Y, Nicolaides KH. Color Doppler ultrasonography in the identification of communicating vessels in twin–twin transfusion syndrome and acardiac twins. *J Ultrasound Med.* 1995;14:37–40.

206. Mielke G, Gonser M. Prenatal diagnosis and therapy of fetofetal transfusion syndrome. *Z Geburtshilfe Neonatol.* 1998;202:141–148.

207. Urig MA, Clewell WH, Elliot JP. Twin–twin transfusion syndrome. *Am J Obstet Gynecol.* 1990;163:1522–1526.

208. Ries M, Beinder E, Gruner C, et al. Rapid development of hydrops fetalis in the donor twin following death of the recipient twin in twin–twin transfusion syndrome. *J Perinat Med.* 1999;27:68–73.

209. Mahony BS, Petty CN, Nyberg DA, et al. The "stuck twin" phenomenon: Ultrasonographic findings, pregnancy outcome, and management with serial amniocenteses. *Am J Obstet Gynecol.* 1990;163:1513–1522.

210. Bajoria R, Wigglesworth J, Fisk NM. Angioarchitecture of monochorionic placentas in relation to the twin–twin transfusion syndrome. *Am J Obstet Gynecol.* 1995;172:856–863.

211. Brackley KJ, Kilby MD. Twin–twin transfusion syndrome. *Hosp Med.* 1999;60:419–424.

212. Filkins KA, Beverly SE. Twin–twin transfusion syndrome: The challenge of etiology-based management decisions. *Curr Opin Obstet Gynecol.* 1998;10:441–446.

213. Kilby MD, Howe DT, McHugo JM, et al. Bladder visualization as a prognostic sign in oligohydramnious-polyhydramnios sequence in twin pregnancies treated using therapeutic amniocentesis. *Br J Obstet Gynaecol.* 1997;104:939–942.

214. Elliot JP, Urig MA, Clewell WH. Aggressive therapeutic amniocentesis for treatment of twin–twin transfusion syndrome. *Obstet Gynecol.* 1991;77:537–540.

215. Golaszewski T, Plockinger B, Golaszewski S, et al. Prenatal management of fetofetal transfusion syndrome. *Geburtshilfe Frauenheilkd.* 1995;55:218–222.

216. Pinette MG, Pan Y, Pinette SG, et al. Treatment of twin–twin transfusion syndrome. *Obstet Gynecol.* 1993;82:841–846.

217. Dennis LG, et al. Twin-to-twin transfusion syndrome: Aggressive therapeutic amniocentesis. *Am J Obstet Gynecol.* 1997;177:342–347.

218. Trespidi L, Boschetto C, Caravelli E, et al. Serial amniocenteses in the management of twin–twin transfusion syndrome: When is it valuable? *Fetal Diagn Ther.* 1997;12:15–20.

219. Garry D, Lysikiewicz A, Mays J, et al. Intra-amniotic pressure reduction in twin–twin transfusion syndrome. *J Perinatol.* 1998;18:284–286.

220. Bajoria R. Chorionic plate vascular anatomy determines the efficacy of amnioreduction therapy for twin–twin transfusion syndrome. *Hum Reprod.* 1998;13:1709–1713.

221. Larroche JC, Droulle P, Delezoide AL, et al. Brain damage in monozygous twins. *Biol Neonate.* 1990;57:261–278.

222. Saunders NJ, Snijders RJM, Nicolaides KH. Therapeutic amniocentesis in twin–twin transfusion syndrome appearing in the second trimester of pregnancy. *Am J Obstet Gynecol.* 1992;166:820–824.

223. Pinette MG, Pan Y, Pinette SG, et al. Treatment of twin–twin transfusion syndrome. *Obstet Gynecol.* 1993;82:841–846.

224. Trespidi L, Boschetto C, Caravelli E, et al. Serial amniocentesis in the management of twin–twin transfusion syndrome: When is it valuable? *Fetal Diagn Ther.* 1997;12:15–20.

225. Mahony BS, Petty CN, Nyberg DA, et al. The stuck twin phenomenon: Ultrasonographic findings, pregnancy outcome and management with serial amniocentesis. *Am J Obstet Gynecol.* 1990;163:1513–1522.

226. Urig MA, Clewell WH, Elliott JP. Twin–twin transfusion syndrome. *Am J Obstet Gynecol.* 1990;163:1522–1526.

227. Elliott JP, Urig MA, Clewell WH. Aggressive therapeutic amniocentesis for treatment of twin–twin transfusion syndrome. *Obstet Gynecol.* 1991;77:537–540.

228. Reisner DP, Mahony BS, Petty CN, et al. Stuck twin syndrome: Outcome in thirty-seven consecutive cases. *Am J Obstet Gynecol.* 1993;169:991–995.

229. Bruner JP, Rosemond RL. Twin-to-twin transfusion syndrome. A subset of the twin oligohydramnios–polyhydramnios sequence. *Am J Obstet Gynecol.* 1993;169:925–930.

230. Dickinson JE. Severe twin–twin transfusion syndrome: Current management concepts. *Aust NZ J Obstet Gynecol.* 1995;35:16–21.

231. Bernirschke K, Kim CK. Multiple pregnancy. *N Engl J Med.* 1973;288:1276–1284.

232. Fusi L, Gordon H. Twin pregnancy complicated by single intrauterine death. Problems and outcome with conservative management. *Br J Obstet Gynaecol.* 1990;97:511–516.

233. Liu S, Bernirschke K, Scioscia AL, et al. Intrauterine death in multiple gestation. *Acta Genet Med Gemellol.* 1992;41: 5–26.

234. Bejar R, Vigliocco G, Gramajo H, et al. Antenatal origin of neurologic damage in newborn infants II. Multiple gestations. *Am J Obstet Gynecol.* 1990;162:1230–1236.

235. Evrard VA, et al. Underwater Nd:YAG laser coagulation of blood vessels in a rat model. *Fetal Diagn Ther.* 1996;11: 422–426.

236. Evrard VA, Deprest JA, Van Ballaer P, et al. Treatment of the twin–twin transfusion syndrome: Initial experience using laser-induced interstitial thermotherapy. *Fetal Diagn Ther.* 1996;11:390–397.

237. Ville Y, et al. Endoscopic laser coagulation in the management of severe twin-to-twin transfusion syndrome. *Br J Obstet Gynaecol.* 1998;105:446–453.

238. Deprest J, et al. Laser-induced thermotherapy for severe twin–twin transfusion syndrome. *Fetal Diagn Ther.* 1997;12: 193–194.

239. Hecher K, et al. Umbilical cord coagulation by operative microendoscopy at 16 weeks' gestation in an acardiac twin. *Ultrasound Obstet Gynecol.* 1997;10:130–132.

240. Lundvall L, Skibsted L, Graem N. Limb necrosis associated with twin-twin transfusion syndrome treated with YAG-laser coagulation. *Acta Obstet Gynecol Scand.* 1999;78:349–350.

241. Quintero RA, Morales WJ, Mendoza G, et al. Selective photocoagulation of placental vessels in twin–twin transfusion syndrome: Evolution of a surgical technique. *Obstet Gynecol Surv.* 1998;53(12, suppl):S97–S103.

242. Rodeck C, Deans A, Jauniaux E. Thermocoagulation for the early treatment of pregnancy with an acardiac twin. *N Engl J Med.* 1998;339:1293–1295.

243. Arabin B, Laurini RN, van Eyck J, et al. Treatment of twin–twin transfusion syndrome by laser and digoxin. Biophysical and angiographic evaluation. *Fetal Diagn Ther.* 1998;13:141–146.

244. Stone CA, Quinn MW, Saxby PJ. Congenital skin loss following Nd:YAG placental photocoagulation. *Burns.* 1998;24: 275–277.

245. Deprest JA, Van Schoubroeck D, Van Ballaer PP, et al. Alternative technique for Nd:YAG laser coagulation in twin-to-twin transfusion syndrome with anterior placenta. *Ultrasound Obstet Gynecol.* 1998;11:347–352.

246. Sohn C, Wallwiener D, Kurek R, et al. Treatment of the twin–twin transfusion syndrome: Initial experience using laser-induced interstitial thermotherapy. *Fetal Diagn Ther.* 1996;11:390–397.

247. Ville Y, Hyett J, Hecher K, et al. Preliminary experience with endoscopic laser surgery for severe twin–twin transfusion syndrome. *N Engl J Med.* 1995;332:224–227.

248. De Lia JE, Kuhlmann RS, Lopez KP. Treating previable twin–twin transfusion syndrome with fetoscopic laser surgery: Outcomes following the learning curve. *J Perinat Med.* 1999; 27:61–67.

249. De Lia JE, Kuhlmann RS, Harstad TW, et al. Fetoscopic laser ablation of placental vessels in severe previable twin–twin transfusion syndrome. *Am J Obstet Gynecol.* 1995;172:1202–1208.

250. Hecher K, Plath H, Bregenzer T, et al. Endoscopic laser surgery versus serial amniocenteses in the treatment of severe twin–twin transfusion syndrome. *Am J Obstet Gynecol.* 1999; 180(3, Pt 1):717–724.

251. van Gemert MJ, Major AL, Scherjon SA. Placental anatomy, fetal demise and therapeutic intervention in monochorionic twins and the transfusion syndrome: New hypotheses. *Eur J Obstet Gynecol Reprod Biol.* 1998;78:53–62.

252. Saade GR, Belfort MA, Berry DL, et al. Amniotic septostomy for the treatment of twin oligohydramnios–polyhydramnios sequence. *Fetal Diagn Ther.* 1998;13:86–93.

253. Suzuki S, Ishikawa G, Sawa R, et al. Iatrogenic monoamniotic twin gestation with progressive twin–twin transfusion syndrome. *Fetal Diagn Ther.* 1999;14:98–101.

254. Quintero RA. Twin-to-twin transfusion syndrome. http://www.fetalmd.com.

255. Lenery DJ, Vanlieferinghen P, Gasq M, et al. Fetal umbilical cord ligation under ultrasound guidance. *Ultrasound Obstet Gynecol.* 1994;330:469–471.

256. Jones JM, Sbarra AJ, Dilillo L, et al. Indomethacin in severe twin-to-twin transfusion syndrome. *J Perinat.* 1993;10:24–26.

257. DeLia JE, Emery MG, Sheafor SA, et al. Twin–twin transfusion syndrome: Successful in-utero treatment with digoxin. *Int J Gynecol Obstet.* 1985;23:197–201.

258. Bromley B, Benacerraf BR. Acute reversal of oligohydramnios–polyhydramnios sequence in monochorionic twins. *Int J Gynaecol Obstet.* 1996;55:281–283.

259. Bruner JP, Rosemond RL. Twin-to-twin transfusion syndrome: A subset of the twin oligohydramnios–polyhydramnios sequence. *Am J Obstet Gynecol.* 1993;169:925–930.

260. Shih JC, Shyu MK, Hsieh MH, et al. Agenesis of the ductus venosus in a case of monochorionic twins which mimics twin–twin transfusion syndrome. *Prenat Diagn.* 1996;16: 243–246.

261. Machin GA. Re. Agenesis of the ductus venosus in a case of monochorionic twins which mimics twin–twin transfusion syndrome. *Prenat Diagn.* 1996;16:971–972.

262. Kuller JA, Coulson CC, McCoy MC, et al. Prenatal diagnosis of renal agenesis in a twin gestation. *Prenat Diagn.* 1994; 14:1090–1092.

263. Wada H, Nunogami K, Wada T, et al. Diffuse brain damage caused by acute twin–twin transfusion during late pregnancy. *Acta Paediatr Jpn.* 1998;40:370–373.

264. Zosmer N, Bajoria R, Weiner E, et al. Clinical and echographic features of in utero cardiac dysfunction in the recipient twin in twin–twin transfusion syndrome. *Br Heart J.* 1994;72:74–79.

265. Fesslova V, Villa L, Nava S, et al. Fetal and neonatal echocardiographic findings in twin–twin transfusion syndrome. *Am J Obstet Gynecol.* 1998;179:1056–1062.

266. Simpson LL, Marx GR, Elkadry EA, et al. Cardiac dysfunction in twin–twin transfusion syndrome: A prospective, longitudinal study. *Obstet Gynecol.* 1998;92:557–562.

267. Watson WJ, Munson DP, Ohrt DW, et al. Polyhydramnios-oligohydramnios in a twin pregnancy complicated by fetal glomerulocystic kidney disease. *Am J Perinatol.* 1995;12: 379–381.

268. Oberg KC, Pestaner JP, Bielamowicz L, et al. Renal tubular dysgenesis in twin–twin transfusion syndrome. *Pediatr Dev Pathol.* 1999;2:25–32.

269. Murphy KW. Intrauterine death in a twin: Implications for the survivor. In: Ward RH, Whittle M, eds. *Multiple Pregnancy.* London: RCOG Press; 1995:218–230.

270. Saier F, Burden L, Cavanagh D. Fetus papyraceus: An unusual case with congenital anomaly of the surviving fetus. *Obstet Gynecol.* 1975;45:217–220.

271. Wagner DS, Klein RL, Robinson HB, et al. Placental emboli from a fetus papyraceous. *J Pediatr Surg.* 1990;25:538–542.

272. Boente M del C, Frontini M del V, Acosta MI, et al. Extensive symmetric truncal aplasia cutis congenita without fetus papyraceous or macroscopic evidence of placental abnormalities. *Pediatr Dermatol.* 1995;12:228–230.

273. Visva-Lingam S, Jana A, Murray H, et al. Preterm premature rupture of membranes associated with aplasia cutis congenita and fetus papyraceous. *Aust NZ J Obstet Gynaecol.* 1996;36:90–91.

274. Patten RM, Mack LA, Nyberg DA, et al. Twin embolization syndrome: Prenatal sonographic detection and significance. *Radiology.* 1989;173:685–689.

275. Dallay D, Soumireu-Mourat J. Problems posed by the death of one fetus in a twin pregnancy. *Rev Fr Gynecol Obstet.* 1985; 80:877–879.

276. Schinzel AA, Smith DW, Miller JR. Monozygotic twinning and structural defects. *J Pediatr.* 1979;95:921–930.

277. Caballero P, Del Campo L, Ocon E. Cystic encephalomalacia in twin embolization syndrome. *Radiology.* 1991;178: 892–893.

278. Fuentes A, Porter KB, Torres BA, et al. A twin gestation complicated by gastroschisis in both twins. *J Clin Ultrasound.* 1996;24:48–50.

279. Yancey MK, Brady K, Read JA. Sonographic evidence of fetal hydrothorax after in-utero death of monozygotic twin. *J Clin Ultrasound.* 1991;19:162–166.

280. Harrison SD, Cyr DR, Patten RM, et al. Twin growth problems: Causes and sonographic analysis. *Semin Ultrasound CT MR.* 1993;14:56–67.

281. Elchalal U, Tanos V, Bar-Oz B, et al. Early second trimester twin embolization syndrome. *J Ultrasound Med.* 1997;16: 509–512.

282. Sogaard K, Skibsted L, Brocks V. Acardiac twins: Pathophisiology, diagnosis, outcome and treatment. Six cases and review of the literature. *Fetal Diagn Ther.* 1999;14:53–59.

283. Zhioua F, Rezigua H, Khouja H, et al. Acardiac malformation: Ultrasonographic diagnosis. A case report. *Rev Fr Gynecol Obstet.* 1993;88:267–272.

284. Landy HJ, Larsen JW Jr, Schoen M, et al. Acardiac fetus in a triplet pregnancy. *Teratology.* 1988;37:1–6.

285. Gibson JY, D'Cruz CA, Patel RB, et al. Acardiac anomaly: Review of the subject with case report and emphasis on practical sonography. *J Clin Ultrasound.* 1986;14:541–545.

286. Cardwell MS. The acardiac twin. A case report. *J Reprod Med.* 1988;33:320–322.

287. Hecher K, Ville Y, Nicolaides KH. Color Doppler ultrasonography in the identification of communicating vessels in twin–twin transfusion syndrome and acardiac twins. *J Ultrasound Med.* 1995;14:37–40.

288. Schwarzler P, Ville Y, Moscoso G, et al. Diagnosis of twin reversed arterial perfusion sequence in the first trimester by transvaginal color Doppler ultrasound. *Ultrasound Obstet Gynecol.* 1999;13:143–146.

289. Papa T, Dao A, Bruner JP. Pathognomonic sign of twin reversed arterial perfusion using color Doppler sonography. *J Ultrasound Med.* 1997;16:501–503.

290. Benson CB, Bieber FR, Genest DR, et al. Doppler demonstration of reversed umbilical blood flow in an acardiac twin. *J Clin Ultrasound.* 1989;17:291–295.

291. Sepulveda WH, Quiroz VH, Giuliano A, et al. Prenatal ultrasonographic diagnosis of acardiac twin. *J Perinat Med.* 1993; 21:241–246.

292. Shalev E, Zalel Y, Ben-Ami M, et al. First trimester ultrasonic diagnosis of twin reversed arterial perfusion sequence. *Prenat Diagn.* 1992;12:219–222.

293. Hanafy A, Peterson CM. Twin-reversed arterial perfusion (TRAP) sequence: Case reports and review of literature. *Aust NZ J Obstet Gynaecol.* 1997;37:187–191.

294. Benirschke K, des Roches Harper V. The acardiac anomaly. *Teratology.* 1977;15:311–316.

295. Kaplan C, Benirschke K. The acardiac anomaly new case reports and current status. *Acta Genet Med Gemellol.* 1979;28: 51–59.

296. Moore CA, Buehler BA, McManus BM, et al. Acephalusacardia in twins with aneuploidy. *Am J Med Genet.* 1987; 3(Suppl):139–143.

297. Chaliha C, Schwarzler P, Booker M, et al. Trisomy 2 in an acardiac twin in a triplet in vitro fertilization pregnancy. *Hum Reprod.* 1999;14:1378–1380.

298. Faguer C, Bonan J, Mulliez N, et al. Acardiac fetus. *Presse Med.* 1996;25:1191–1194.

299. Blaicher W, Repa C, Schaller A. Acardiac twin pregnancy: Associated with trisomy 2: Case report. *Hum Reprod.* 2000; 5:474–475.

300. Pavlova M, Fouron JC, Proulx F, et al. Importance of intrauterine diagnosis of rudimentary autonomic circulation in an acardiac twin. *Arch Mal Coeur Vaiss.* 1996;89:629–632.

301. Imai A, Hirose R, Kawabata I, et al. Acardiac acephalic monster extremely larger than its co twin. A case report. *Gynecol Obstet Invest.* 1991;32:62–64.

302. Pezzati M, Cianciulli D, Danesi G. Acardiac twins. Two case reports. *J Perinat Med.* 1997;25:119–124.

303. Sanjaghsaz H, Bayram MO, Qureshi F. Twin reversed arterial perfusion sequence in conjoined, acardiac, acephalic twins associated with a normal triplet. A case report. *J Reprod Med.* 1998;43:1046–1050.

304. Cox M, Murphy K, Ryan G, et al. Spontaneous cesation of umbilical blood flow in the acardius fetus of a twin pregnancy. *Prenat Diagn.* 1992;12:689–693.

305. Chang DY, Chang RY, Chen RJ, et al. Triplet pregnancy complicated by intrauterine fetal death of conjoined twins from an umbilical cord accident of an acardius. A case report. *J Reprod Med.* 1996;41:459–462.

306. Willcourt RJ, Naughton MJ, Knutzen VK, et al. Laparoscopic ligation of the umbilical cord of an acardiac fetus. *J Am Assoc Gynecol Laparosc.* 1995;2:319–321.

307. Quintero R, Munoz H, Hasbun J, et al. Fetal endoscopic surgery in a case of twin pregnancy complicated by reversed arterial perfusion sequence. *Rev Chil Obstet Ginecol.* 1995; 60:112–116.

308. Sepulveda W, Bower S, Hassan J, et al. Ablation of acardiac twin by alcohol injection into the intraabdominal umbilical artery. *Obstet Gynecol.* 1995;86:680–681.

309. Hecher K, Reinhold U, Gbur K, et al. Interruption of umbilical blood flow in an acardiac twin by endoscopic laser coagulation. *Geburtshilfe Frauenheilkd.* 1996;56:97–100.

310. Hecher K, Hackeloer BJ, Ville Y. Umbilical cord coagulation by operative microendoscopy at 16 weeks' gestation in an acardiac twin. *Ultrasound Obstet Gynecol*. 1997;10:130–132.

311. Sanchioni L, Presti C, Morotti R, et al. Twin pregnancy with acephalic acardiac fetus. Anatomo-clinical description cases. *Ann Ostet Ginecol Med Perinat*. 1990;111:174–180.

312. Ko TM, Tzeng SJ, Hsieh FJ, et al. Acardius anceps: Report of 3 cases. *Asia Oceania J Obstet Gynaecol*. 1991;17:49–56.

313. Natho W, Kirsch M, Abet L, et al. Perinatal imaging diagnosis in twin pregnancies with humanus amorphus. *Zentralbl Gynakol*. 1990;112:679–688.

314. Wigglesworth JS, Singer DB, eds. *Textbook of Fetal and Perinatal Pathology*. Cambridge, MA: Blackwell Scientific Publications, 1991:221–262.

315. Chan DP. Thoracomphalopagus diagnosed before delivery. *Med J Aust*. 1976;1:480–483.

316. Monteagudo A, Timor-Tritsch IE. *Ultrasound and Multifetal Pregnancy*, 1st ed. Parthenon Publishing Group; New York. 1998:87–112.

317. Hernandez-Valencia M, Baruch Pavon Rojas A, Ferrer Ponce LA, et al. Janiceps cephalo-thoraco-abdominopagus pregnancy. *Ginecol Obstet Mex*. 1998;66:499–502.

318. Quiroz VH, Sepulveda WH, Mercado M, et al. Prenatal ultrasonographic diagnosis of thoracopagus conjoined twins. *J Perinat Med*. 1989;17:297–303.

319. Grutter F, Marguerat P, Maillard-Brignon C, et al. Thoracopagus fetus. Ultrasonic diagnosis at 16 weeks. *J Gynecol Obstet Biol Reprod*. 1989;18:355–359.

320. Spencer R. Conjoined twins: Theoretical embryologic basis. *Teratology*. 1992;45:591–602.

321. Divon MY, Weiner Z. Ultrasound in twin pregnancy. *Semin Perinatol*. 1995;19:404–412.

322. Koontz WL, Herbert WN, Seeds JW, et al. Ultrasonography in the antepartum diagnosis of conjoined twins. A report of two cases. *J Reprod Med*. 1983;28:627–630.

323. Weston PJ, Ives EJ, Honore RLH, et al. Monochorionic diamniotic minimally conjoined twins: A case report. *Am J Med Genet*. 1990;37:558–561.

324. Boulot P, Deschamps F, Hedon B, et al. Conjoined twins associated with a normal singleton: Very early diagnosis and successful selective termination. *J Perinat Med*. 1992;20:135–137.

325. Demidov VN, Stygar AM, Voevodin SM, et al. Ultrasonic diagnosis of malformations during the 1st trimester of pregnancy. *Sov Med*. 1991;12:25–28.

326. Lam YH, Sin SY, Lam C, et al. Prenatal sonographic diagnosis of conjoined twins in the first trimester: Two case reports. *Ultrasound Obstet Gynecol*. 1998;11:289–291.

327. Bonilla-Musoles F, Raga F, Bonilla F Jr, et al. Early diagnosis of conjoined twins using two-dimensional color Doppler and three-dimensional ultrasound. *J Natl Med Assoc*. 1998;90:552–556.

328. Maymon R, Halperin R, Weinraub Z, et al. Three-dimensional transvaginal sonography of conjoined twins at 10 weeks: A case report. *Ultrasound Obstet Gynecol*. 1998;11:292–294.

329. Hubinont C, Kollman P, Malvaux V, et al. First-trimester diagnosis of conjoined twins. *Fetal Diagn Ther*. 1997;12:185–187.

330. Cazeneuve C, Nihoul-Fekete C, Adafer M, et al. Conjoined omphalopagus twins separated at fifteen days of age. *Arch Pediatr*. 1995;2:452–455.

331. Yang CC, Wu RC, Kuo PL, et al. Prenatal diagnosis of dicephalic conjoined twins: Report of a case. *J Formos Med Assoc*. 1994;93:626–628.

332. Barth RA, Filly RA, Goldberg JD, et al. Conjoined twins: Prenatal diagnosis and assessment of associated malformations. *Radiology*. 1990;177:201–207.

333. Monni G, Useli C, Ibba RM, et al. Early antenatal sonographic diagnosis of conjoined syncephalus-craniothoracoomphalopagus twins. Case report. *J Perinat Med*. 1991;19:489–492.

334. Conjoined twins—An epidemiological study based on 312 cases. The International Clearinghouse for Birth Defects Monitoring Systems. *Acta Genet Med Gemellol*. 1991;40:325–335.

335. Abossolo T, Dancoisne P, Tuaillin J, et al. Early prenatal diagnosis of asymmetric cephalothoracopagus twins. *J Gynecol Obstet Biol Reprod*. 1994;23:79–84.

336. Furuya A, Okawa I, Matsukawa T, et al. Anesthetic management of cesarean section for conjoined twins. *Masul*. 1999;48:195–197.

337. Van der Brand SF, Nijhuis JG, van Dongen PW. Prenatal ultrasound diagnosis of conjoined twins. *Obstet Gynecol Surv*. 1994;49:656–662.

338. Hilfiker ML, Hart M, Holmes R, et al. Expansion and division of conjoined twins. *J Pediatr Surg*. 1998;33:768–770.

339. Karsdorp VH, van der Linden JC, Sobotka-Plojhar MA, et al. Ultrasonographic prenatal diagnosis of conjoined thoracopagus twins: A case report. *Eur J Obstet Gynecol Reprod Biol*. 1991;39:157–161.

340. Vaughn TC, Powell LC. The obstetrical management of conjoined twins. *Obstet Gynecol*. 1979;53(3 suppl):67S–72S.

341. Stoll-Simona U, Ingold W, Tanner H. A rare increase in the incidence of Siamese twin deliveries. *Geburtshilfe Frauenheilkd*. 1979;39:147–151.

342. Al Muti Zaitoun A, Chang J, Booker M. Diprosopus (partially duplicated head) associated with anencephaly: A case report. *Pathol Res Pract*. 1999;195:45–50.

343. Amr SS, Hammouri MF. Craniofacial duplication (diprosopus): Report of a case with a review of the literature. *Eur J Obstet Gynecol Reprod Biol*. 1995;58:77–80.

344. La Torre R, Fusaro P, Anceschi MM, et al. Unusual case of caudal duplication (dipygus). *J Clin Ultrasound*. 1998;26:163–165.

345. Mir E, Sencan A, Karaca I, et al. Truncal duplication: A case report. *Pediatr Surg Int*. 1998;14:227–228.

346. Spencer R, Robichaux WH. Prosopo-thoracopagus conjoined twins and other cephalopagus–thoracopagus intermediates: Case report and review of literature. *Pediatr Dev Pathol*. 1998;1:164–171.

347. Chen CP, Lee CC, Liu FF, et al. Prenatal diagnosis of cephalothoracopagus janiceps monosymmetros. *Prenat Diagn*. 1997;17:384–388.

348. Ramadani HM, Johnsrud N, al Nasser M, et al. The antenatal diagnosis of cephalothoracopagus Janiceps conjoined twins. *Aust NZ J Obstet Gynaecol*. 1994;34:113–115.

349. Koltuksuz U, Eskicioglu S, Mehmetoglu F. Minimally conjoined omphalopagus twinning: A case report. *Eur J Pediatr Surg*. 1998;8:368–370.

350. Jain PK, Budhwani KS, Gambhir A, et al. Omphalopagus parasite: A rare congenital anomaly. *J Pediatr Surg*. 1998;33:946–947.

351. Sathekge MM, Venkannagari RR, Clauss RP. Scintigraphic evaluation of craniopagus twins. *Br J Radiol.* 1998;71:1096–1099.

352. Nicolini U, Dell'Agnola CA, Ferrazzi E, et al. Ultrasonic prenatal diagnosis of fetus in fetu. *J Clin Ultrasound.* 1983;11:321–322.

353. Bomsel F, Stroh-Marcy A, Thabaut S, et al. Fœtus in fœtu: Un cas dépisté par échographie anténatale. *JEMU.* 1985;6:163–8.

354. Heifetz SA, Alrabeeah A, Brown BS, et al. Fetus in fetu: A fetiform teratoma. *Pediatr Pathol.* 1988;8:215–226.

355. Chitrit Y, Zorn B, Scart G, et al. Fœtus in fœtu surrenalien: Un cas evoque par l'echographie prenatale. Revue de la litterature. *J Gynecol Obstet Biol Reprod (Paris).* 1990;19:1019–1022.

356. Martinez Urrutia MJ, Lopez Pereira P, et al. Abdominal mass: "Fetus in fetu." *Acta Pædiatr Scand.* 1990;79:121–122.

357. Sada I, Shiratori H, Nakamura Y. Antenatal diagnosis of fetus in fetu. *Asia Oceania J Obstet Gynaecol.* 1986;12:353–356.

358. Grant P, Pearn JH. Fœtus in fœtu. *Med J Aust.* 1969;1:1016–1019.

359. Krafka J. Teratoma: An explanation of its cause based on the organizer theory of embryology. *Arch Pathol.* 1936;21:756.

360. Carles D, Alberti EM, Serville F, et al. Fœtus in fetu et monstre acardiaque: Un mécanisme morphogénique commun explique-t-il les similitudes de ces deux malformations? *Arch Anat Cytol Pathol.* 1991;39:77–82.

361. Chateil JF, Diard F, Bondonny JM, et al. Foetus in foetu testiculaire intraperitoneal. *Pediatrie.* 1990;45:255–257.

362. Alpers CE, Harrison MR. Fetus in fetu associated with an undescended testis. *Pediatr Pathol.* 1985;4(1–2):37–46.

363. Corona Reyes D, Navarro Cruz RA, Toxtle Tlamani R, et al. Fetus in fetu originado en un testiculo criptorquidico. *Bol Med Hosp Infant Mex.* 1982;39:680–684.

364. Potter EL. *Pathology of the Fetus and Newborn,* 2nd ed. Chicago: Year Book Medical Publishing; 1962:183–187.

365. Willis RA. The structure of teratoma. *J Pathol Bacteriol.* 1935;40:1–36.

366. Young GW. Case of a fœtus found in the abdomen of a boy. *Med Chir Trans.* 1809;1:234.

367. Highmore N. Case of a fœtus found in the abdomen of a young man, at Sherborne, in Dorsetshire. *R Coll Surg.* 1815.

368. Phillips E. Account of a case in which parts of a fœtus were found in a tumour situated in the abdomen of a girl two and a half year old. *Medico-Chirug Trans.* 1815;6:124–127.

369. Taylor S. Case of included ovum. *Trans Pathol Soc Lond.* 1887;38:440–444.

370. McNutt WF. Case report. *Pacific Med J.* 1894;37:118.

371. von Haberer H. Operativ entferater Fötus in Föto. *Zentralbl Chir.* 1939;66:840.

372. Eng HL, Chuang JH, Lee TY, et al. Fetus in fetu: A case report and review of the literature. *J Pediatr Surg.* 1989;24:296–299.

373. Kimmel DL, Moyer EK, Peale AR, et al. A cerebral tumor containing five human fetuses. A case of fetus in fetu. *Anat Rec.* 1950;106:141–165.

374. Povysilova V. Encranius s mnohotnymi rudimentarnimi fetus in fetu u nedonoseneho chlapce [Encranius with multiple rudimentary fetus in fetu in a premature boy]. *Cesk Patol.* 1983;19:49–54.

375. Brines R.I. A large teratoma containing rudimentary arm bones and a hand. *JAMA.* 1934;103:338.

376. Gale CW, Willis RA. A retroperitoneal digit-containing teratoma. *J Pathol Bacteriol.* 1944;56:403–409.

377. Wollin E, Ozonoff MB. Serial development of teeth in an ovarian teratoma. *N Engl J Med.* 1961;265:897–898.

378. Oberman B. Intracranial teratoma replacing brain: Report of a case. *Arch Neurol.* 1964;11:423–426.

379. Afshar F, King TT, Berry CL. Intraventricular fetus in fetu. Case report. *J Neurosurg.* 1982;56:845–849.

380. Bernal Sprekelsen JC, Bernal Cascales M. Fetus in Fetu: Ein Fallbericht einer extrem seltenen Ursache von Bauchtumoren beim Sling. *Z Kinderchir.* 1990;45:317–318.

381. Bomsel F, Stroh-Marcy A, Thabaut S, et al. Fœtus in fœtu: Un cas dépisté par échographie anténatale. *JEMU.* 1985;6:163–168.

382. Boyce MJ, Lockyer JW, Wood CBS. Fœtus in fœtu: Serological assessment of monozygotic origin by automated analysis. *J Clin Pathol.* 1972;25:793–798.

383. Broghammer BJ, Wolf RS, Geppert CH. The included twin or fetus in fetu—A case report. *Radiology.* 1963;80:849–846.

384. Burtner CD, Conn AG. Fetus in fetu: Case report. *WV Med J.* 1988;84:123–125.

385. Chi JG, Yoon SL, Park YS, et al. Fetus in fetu: Report of a case. *Am J Clin Pathol.* 1984;82:115–119.

386. Du Plessis JPG, Winship WS, Kirstein JDL. Fetus in fetu and teratoma: A case report and review. *S Afr Med J.* 1974;48:2119–2212.

387. Farris JM, Bishop RC. Surgical aspects of included twins. *Surgery.* 1950;28:443–448.

388. Fujikura T, Hunter WC. Retroperitoneal fetus in fetu. *Obstet Gynecol.* 1959;13:547–554.

389. Galatius-Jensen F, Rah DH, Uhm IK, et al. Fetus in fetu. *Br J Radiol.* 1965;38:305–308.

390. George V, Khanna M, Dutta T. Fetus in fetu. *J Pediatr Surg.* 1983;18:288–289.

391. Griscom T. The roentgenology of abdominal masses. *AJR.* 1965;93:447–463.

392. Grosfeld JL, Stepita DS, Nance WE, et al. Fetus in fetu: An unusual cause for abdominal mass in infancy. *Ann Surg.* 1974;180:80–84.

393. Gross RE, Clatworthy HW. Twin fetuses in fetu. *J Pediatr.* 1951;38:502–508.

394. Gürses N, Gürses N, Bernay F. Twin fetuses in fetu and a review of the literature. *Z Kinderchir.* 1990;45:319–322.

395. Janovski NA. Fetus in fetu. *J Pediatr.* 1962;61:100–104.

396. Kakizoe T, Tahara M. Fetus in fetu located in the scrotal sac of a newborn infant: A case report. *J Urol.* 1972;107:506–508.

397. Karasimbarao KL, Mitra SK, Pathak IC. Sacrococcygeal fetus in fetu. *Indian Pediatr.* 1984;21:820–822.

398. Knox AJS, Webb AJ. The clinical features and treatment of a fetus in fetu: Two cases reports and a review of the literature. *J Pediatr Surg.* 1972;7:434.

399. Lal M. A fœtus in the abdomen of a young boy. *Med J Malaya.* 1971;25:307–310.

400. Lamabadusarya SP, Atukrale AW, Soysa PE, et al. A case of fetus in fetu. *Arch Dis Child.* 1972;47:305–307.

401. Lee EYC. Fœtus in fœtu. *Arch Dis Child.* 1965;40:689–693.

402. Lewis PH. Fœtus in fœtu and the retroperitoneal teratoma. *Arch Dis Child.* 1961;36:220–226.

403. Lord JM. Intra-abdominal fœtus in fœtu. *J Pathol Bacteriol.* 1956;72:627–641.

404. Maxwell RW. Endocyme fœtus in a Fiji infant. *Br Med J.* 1947;732–733.

405. Montupet P, Sinico M, Soulier YA, et al. Fœtus in fœtu: Rapport de 2 cas et analyse de la littérature. *Chir Pediatr.* 1984; 25:37–42.

406. Nadimpalli VR, Reyes II, Manaligold JR. Retroperitoneal teratoma with fetuses. *Teratology.* 1989;39:233–236.

407. Nocera RM, Davis M, Hayden CK Jr, et al. Fetus-in-fetu. *AJR.* 1982;138:762–764.

408. Numanoglu I, Yavuz Gödemir A, et al. Fetus in fetu. *J Pediatr Surg.* 1970;5:472–473.

409. Ouimet A, Russo P. Fetus in fetu or not? *J Pediatr Surg.* 1989; 24:926–927.

410. Prasad KR, Rai VK, Chowdhary DK. Fetus in fetu. *J Indian Med Assoc.* 1981;77:134–136.

411. Rastogi V, Singhal PK, Taneja SB. Fetus in fetu. *Indian Pediatr.* 1988;25:584–586.

412. Sangvichien S, Sutthiwan P. Fetus in fetu and teratoma: Their genesis and the formation of vertebral column. *J Med Assoc Thai.* 1982;65:505–510.

413. Sutthiwan P, Sutthiwan I, Tree-trakan T. Fetus in fetu. *J Pediatr Surg.* 1983;18:290–292.

414. Wiel MA, Tortollo G, Butti A, et al. Teratoma fetiforme breve nota su di un caso. *Chir Pat Sper.* 1970;3:178–181.

415. Yasuda Y, Mitomori T, Matsuura A, et al. Fetus-in-fetu: Report of a case. *Teratology.* 1985;31:337–344.

416. Hing A, Corteville J, Foglia RP, et al. Fetus in fetu: Molecular analysis of a feti-form mass. *Am J Med Genet.* 1993;47: 333–341.

417. Willis RA. *Pathology of Tumors.* St. Louis: CV Mosby; 1948: 941.

418. Brunkow CW. *Pediatric Gynecology.* Chicago: Schouffler; 1942:220–226.

419. Sadler TW. *Langman's Medical Embryology,* 5th ed. Baltimore: Williams & Wilkins; 1985:171.

420. Hawkins EP. Fetus in fetu or not. *J Pediatr Surg.* 1990;25: 583–584.

421. Nochomovitz LE, Rosai J. Current concepts on the histogenesis, pathology and immunochemistry of germ cells tumors of the testis. *Pathol Ann.* 1978;13:327–362.

422. Wakai S. On the origin of intracranial teratomas. *No To Shinkei.* 1989;41:947–953.

423. Wang PH, Chao HT, Taeng JY, et al. Laparoscopic surgery for heterotopic pregnancies: A case report and a brief review. *Eur J Obstet Gynecol Reprod Biol.* 1998;80:267–271.

424. Giacomello F, Larciprete G, Valensise H, et al. Spontaneous heterotopic pregnancy with live embryos: An insidious echographic problem in the first trimester. Therapeutic problems. A clinical case and review of the literature. *Minerva Ginecol.* 1998;50:151–155.

425. Kably Ambe A, Werner von der Meden Alarcon J, et al. Early diagnosis of heterotopic pregnancy with viability of the intrauterine fetus. Report of two cases and review of the literature. *Ginecol Obstet Mex.* 1995;63:346–348.

426. Bassil S, Pouly JL, Canis M, et al. Advanced heterotopic pregnancy after in vitro fertilization and embryo transfer, with survival of both the babies and the mother. *Hum Reprod.* 1991;6:1008–1010.

427. Jerrard D, Tso E, Salik R, et al. Unsuspected heterotopic pregnancy in a woman without risk factors. *Am J Emerg Med.* 1992;10:58–60.

428. Tummon IS, Whitmore NA, Daniel SA, et al. Transferring more embryos increases risk of heterotopic pregnancy. *Fertil Steril.* 1994;61:1065–1067.

429. Svare JA, Norup PA, Thomsen SG, et al. Heterotopic pregnancy after in vitro fertilization. *Ugeskr Laeger.* 1994;156: 2230–2233.

430. Barron Vallejo J, Ortega Diaz R, Kably Ambe A. Heterotopic pregnancy with intrauterine dizygotic twins following embryo transfer in the blastocyst phase. *Ginecol Obstet Mex.* 1999;67:169–172.

431. Pistofidis GA, Mastrominas MJ, Dimitropoulos K. Laparoscopic management of heterotopic pregnancies. *J Am Assoc Gynecol Laparosc.* 1995;2:42–43.

432. Loret de Mola JR, Austin CM, Judge NE, et al. Cornual heterotopic pregnancy and cornual resection after in vitro fertilization/embryo transfer. A report of two cases. *J Reprod Med.* 1995;40:606–610.

433. Hanf V, Dietl J, Gagsteiger F, et al. Bilateral tubal pregnancy with intra-uterine gestation after IVF-ET: Therapy by bilateral laparoscopic salpingectomy; a case report. *Eur J Obstet Gynecol Reprod Biol.* 1990;37:87–90.

434. Rondeau JA, Hibbert ML, Nelson KM. Combined tubal and cornual pregnancy in a patient without risk factors. A case report. *J Reprod Med.* 1997;42:675–677.

435. Ginsburg ES, Frates MC, Rein MS, et al. Early diagnosis and treatment of cervical pregnancy in an in vitro fertilization program. *Fertil Steril.* 1994;61:966–969.

436. Andersen BB. Succesful intrauterine term pregnancy after resection of corneal pregnancy. *Eur J Obstet Gynecol Reprod Biol.* 1999;84:99–100.

437. Beck P, Silverman M, Oehninger S, et al. Survival of the cornual pregnancy in a heterotopic gestation after in vitro fertilization and embryo transfer. *Fertil Steril.* 1990;53: 732–734.

438. Chen SU, Yang YS, Ho HN, et al. Combined cornual pregnancy and intrauterine twin pregnancy after in vitro fertilization and embryo transfer: Report of a case. *J Formos Med Assoc.* 1992;91:1002–1005.

439. Leach RE, Ney JA, Ory SJ. Selective embryo reduction of an interstitial heterotopic gestation. *Fetal Diagn Ther.* 1992;7: 41–45.

440. Scheiber MD, Cedars MI. Successful non-surgical management of a heterotopic abdominal pregnancy following embryo transfer with cryopreserved-thawed embryos. *Hum Reprod.* 1999;14:1375–1377.

441. Pisarska MD, Casson PR, Moise KJ Jr, et al. Heterotopic abdominal pregnancy treated at laparoscopy. *Fertil Steril.* 1998;70:159–160.

442. Fernandez H, De Ziegler D, Imbert MC, et al. Advanced combined intra-uterine and ovarian gestations: Case report. *Eur J Obstet Gynecol Reprod Biol.* 1990;37:293–296.

443. Ogunniyi SO, Faleyimu BL, Odesanmi WO, et al. Ovarian pregnancy causing obstructed labor at term in a heterotopic gestation. *Int J Gynaecol Obstet.* 1990;31:283–285.

444. De Muylder X, De Loecker P, Campo R. Heterotopic ovarian pregnancy after clomiphene ovulation induction. *Eur J Obstet Gynecol Reprod Biol.* 1994;53:65–66.

445. Svare J, Norup P, Grove Thomsen S, et al. Heterotopic pregnancies after in-vitro fertilization and embryo transfer—A Danish survey. *Hum Reprod*. 1993;8:116–118.

446. Rizk B, Tan SL, Morcos S, et al. Heterotopic pregnancies after in vitro fertilization and embryo transfer. *Am J Obstet Gynecol*. 1991;164:161–164.

447. Wu MY, Chen HF, Chen SU, et al. Heterotopic pregnancies after controlled ovarian hyperstimulation and assisted reproductive techniques. *J Formos Med Assoc*. 1995;94:600–604.

448. Botta G, Fortunato N, Merlino G. Heterotopic pregnancy following administration of human menopausal gonadotropin and following in vitro fertilization and embryo transfer: Two case reports and review of the literature. *Eur J Obstet Gynecol Reprod Biol*. 1995;59:211–215.

449. Li HP, Balmaceda JP, Zouves C, et al. Heterotopic pregnancy associated with gamete intra-fallopian transfer. *Hum Reprod*. 1992;7:131–135.

450. Goldman JA, Dicker D, Dekel A, et al. Successful management and outcome of heterotopic triplet in vitro fertilization (IVF) gestation: Twin tubal and surviving instrauterine pregnancy. *J In Vitro Fert Embryo Transf*. 1991;8:300–302.

451. Prapas Y, Prapas N, Chatziparasidou A, et al. Ovarian hyperstimulation syndrome and heterotopic pregnancy after IVF. *Acta Eur Fertil*. 1994;25:331–333.

452. Mascarenhas L, Elliot B. Severe ovarian hyperstimulation syndrome, embryo reduction and heteropic pregnancy. *Hum Reprod*. 1993;8:1329–1331.

453. Su WH, Wang PH, Chang SP. Unusual presentation of heterotopic pregnancy: A case report. *Chung Hua I Hsueh Tsa Chih*. 1998;61:608–612.

454. Johnson N, McComb P, Gudex G. Heterotopic pregnancy complicating in vitro fertilization. *Aust NZ J Obstet Gynaecol*. 1998;38:151–155.

455. Mantzavinos T, Kanakas N, Zourlas PA. Heterotopic pregnancies in an in-vitro fertilization program. *Clin Exp Obstet Gynecol*. 1996;23:205–208.

456. Fishman DA, Padilla LA, Keh P, et al. Management of twin pregnancies consisting of a complete hydatidiform mole and normal fetus. *Obstet Gynecol*. 1998;91:546–550.

457. Choi-Hong SR, Genest DR, Crum CP, et al. Twin pregnancies with complete hydatidiform mole and coexisting fetus: Use of fluorescent in situ hybridization to evaluate placental X- and Y chromosomal content. *Hum Pathol*. 1995;26:1175–1180.

458. Steller MA, Genest DR, Bernstein MR, et al. Natural history of twin pregnancy with complete hydatidiform mole and coexisting fetus. *Obstet Gynecol*. 1994;83:35–42.

459. Miller D, Jackson R, Ehlen T, et al. Complete hydatidiform mole coexistent with a twin live fetus: Clinical course of four cases with complete cytogenetic analysis. *Gynecol Oncol*. 1993;50:119–123.

460. Jeanty P, Rodesch F, Struyven J. The vanishing twin. *Ultrasonics*. 1981;2:25–31.

461. Landy HJ, Keith L, Keith D. The vanishing twin. *Acta Genet Med Gemellol*. 1982;31:179–194.

462. Landy HJ, Weiner S, Corson SL, et al. The "vanishing twin": Ultrasonographic assessment of fetal disappearance in the first trimester. *Am J Obstet Gynecol*. 1986;155:14–19.

463. Sulak LE, Dodson MG. The vanishing twin: Pathologic confirmation of an ultrasonographic phenomenon. *Obstet Gynecol*. 1986;68:811–815.

464. Saidi MH. First trimester bleeding and the vanishing twin. A report of three cases. *J Reprod Med*. 1988;33:831–834.

465. Jauniaux E, Elkazen N, Leroy F, et al. Clinical and morphologic aspects of the vanishing twin phenomenon. *Obstet Gynecol*. 1988;72:577–581.

466. Tomko J, Baltarowich O. Synechial band (or amniotic fold) as a differential diagnosis for vanishing twin. www.TheFetus.net.

467. Benirschke K. Intrauterine death of a twin: Mechanisms, implications for surviving twin, and placental pathology. *Semin Diagn Pathol*. 1993;10:222–231.

468. Wagner DS, Klein RL, Robinson HB, et al. Placental emboli from a fetus papyraceous. *J Pediatr Surg*. 1990;25:538–542.

469. Csecsei K, Toth Z, Szeifert GT, et al. Pathological consequences of the vanishing twin. *Acta Chir Hung*. 1988;29:173–182.

470. Bergh C, Moller A, Nilsson L, et al. Obstetric outcome and psychological follow-up of pregnancies after embryo reduction. *Hum Reprod*. 1999;14:2170–2175.

471. De Catte L, Camus M, Bonduelle M, et al. Prenatal diagnosis by chorionic villus sampling in multiple pregnancies prior to fetal reduction. *Am J Perinatol*. 1998;15:339–343.

472. Fasouliotis SJ, Schenker JG. Multifetal pregnancy reduction: A review of the world results for the period 1993–1996. *Eur J Obstet Gynecol Reprod Biol*. 1997;75:183–190.

473. Evans MI, Dommergues M, Wapner RJ, et al. International, collaborative experience of 1789 patients having multifetal pregnancy reduction: A plateauing of risks and outcomes. *J Soc Gynecol Invest*. 1996;3:23–26.

474. Ormont MA, Shapiro PA. Multifetal pregnancy reduction. A review of an evolving technology and its psychosocial implications. *Psychosomatics*. 1995;36:522–530.

475. Stone J, Berkowitz RL. Multifetal pregnancy reduction and selective termination. *Semin Perinatol*. 1995;19:363–374.

476. Fang Q, Zhuang G, Zhou C. Clinical use of selective reduction in multifetal pregnancies. *Chung Hua I Hsueh Tsa Chih*. 1995;75:459–462.

477. Brambati B, Tului L. First trimester fetal reduction: Its role in the management of twin and higher order multiple pregnancies. *Hum Reprod Update*. 1995;1:397–408.

478. Brambati B, Tului L, Baldi M, et al. Genetic analysis prior to selective fetal reduction in multiple pregnancy: Technical aspects and clinical outcome. *Hum Reprod*. 1995;10:818–825.

479. Stone J, Lynch L. Multifetal pregnancy: Risks and methods of reduction. *Mt Sinai J Med* 1994;61:404–408.

480. Chen SC, Lee FK, Chang SP, et al. Selective embryo reduction in multiple pregnancies resulting from assisted conception. *Chung Hua I Hsueh Tsa Chih (Taipei)*. 1994;53:37–41.

481. Check JH, Nowroozi K, Vetter B, et al. The effects of multiple gestation and selective reduction on fetal outcome. *Perinat Med*. 1993;21:299–302.

482. Sebire NJ, D'Ercole C, Sepulveda W, et al. Effects of embryo reduction from trichorionic triplets to twins. *Br J Obstet Gynaecol*. 1997;104:1201–1203.

483. Maymon R, Herman A, Shulman A, et al. First trimester embryo reduction: A medical solution to an iatrogenic problem. *Hum Reprod*. 1995;10:668–673.

484. Papiernik E, Grange G, Zeitlin J. Should multifetal pregnancy reduction be used prevention of preterm deliveries in triplet or higher order multiple pregnancies? *J Perinat Med*. 1998;26:365–370.

485. Evans MI, Littman L, Richter R, et al. Selective reduction for multifetal pregnancy. Early opinions revisited. *J Reprod Med.* 1997;42:771–777.

486. Haning RV Jr, Seifer DB, Wheeler CA, et al. Effects of fetal number and multifetal reduction on length of in vitro fertilization pregnancies. *Obstet Gynecol.* 1996;87:964–968.

487. Berkowitz RL, Lynch L, Stone J, et al. The current status of multifetal pregnancy reduction. *Am J Obstet Gynecol.* 1996; 174:1265–1272.

488. Dommergues M, Aknin J, Boulot P, et al. Embryo reduction in multiple pregnancies. A French multicenter study. *J Gynecol Obstet Biol Reprod (Paris).* 1994;23:415–418.

489. Evans MI, Hume RF Jr, Yaron Y, et al. Multifetal pregnancy reduction. *Baillieres Clin Obstet Gynaecol.* 1998;12: 147–159.

490. Chitkara U, Berkowitz RL, Wilkins IA, et al. Selective second-trimester termination of the anomalous fetus in twin pregnancies. *Obstet Gynecol.* 1989;73(5, Pt 1):690–694.

491. Benson CB, Doubilet PM, Acker D, et al. Multifetal pregnancy reduction of both fetuses of a monochorionic pair by intrathoracic potassium chloride injection of one fetus. *J Ultrasound Med.* 1998;17:447–449.

492. Yaron Y, Johnson KD, Bryant-Greenwood PK, et al. Selective termination and elective reduction in twin pregnancies: 10 Years experience at a single centre. *Hum Reprod.* 1998; 13:2301–2304.

493. Berkowitz RL. Ethical issues involving multifetal pregnancies. *Mt Sinai J Med.* 1998;65:185–190; discussion 215–223.

494. Berkowitz RL, Stone JL, Eddleman KA. One hundred consecutive cases of selective termination of an abnormal fetus in a multifetal gestation. *Obstet Gynecol.* 1997;90(4, Pt 1): 606–610.

495. Lipitz S, Peltz R, Achiron R, et al. Selective second-trimester termination of an abnormal fetus in twin pregnancies. *J Perinatol.* 1997;17:301–304.

496. Stewart KS, Johnson MP, Quintero RA, et al. Congenital abnormalities in twins: Selective termination. *Curr Opin Obstet Gynecol.* 1997;9:136–139.

497. Sebire NJ, Sepulveda W, Hughes KS, et al. Management of twin pregnancies discordant for anencephaly. *Br J Obstet Gynaecol.* 1997;104:216–219.

498. Lipitz S, Shalev E, Meizner I, et al. Late selective termination of fetal abnormalities in twin pregnancies: A multicentre report. *Br J Obstet Gynaecol.* 1996;103:1212–1216.

499. Yaron Y, Bryant-Greenwood PK, Dave N, et al. Multifetal pregnancy reductions of triplets to twins: Comparison with nonreduced triplets and twins. *Am J Obstet Gynecol.* 1999; 180:1268–1271.

500. Smith-Levitin M, Kowalik A, Birnholz J, et al. Selective reduction of multifetal pregnancies to twins improves outcome over nonreduced triplet gestations. *Am J Obstet Gynecol.* 1996; 175(4, Pt 1):878–882.

501. Bollen N, Camus M, Tournaye H, et al. Embryo reduction in triplet pregnancies after assisted procreation: A comparative study. *Fertil Steril.* 1993;60:504–509.

502. Vauthier-Brouzes D, Lefebvre G. Selective reduction in multifetal pregnancies: Technical and psychological aspects. *Fertil Steril.* 1992;57:1012–1016.

503. Evans MI, Goldberg JD, Horenstein J, et al. Selective termination for structural, chromosomal, and mendelian anomalies: International experience. *Am J Obstet Gynecol.* 1999;181: 893–897.

504. Coffler MS, Kol S, Drugan A, et al. Early transvaginal embryo aspiration: A safer method for selective reduction in high order multiple gestations. *Hum Reprod.* 1999;14:1875–1878.

505. Wapner RJ. Genetic diagnosis in multiple pregnancies. *Semin Perinatol.* 1995;19:351–362.

506. Anderson RL, Goldberg JD, Golbus MS. Prenatal diagnosis in multiple gestations: 20 Years' experience with amniocentesis. *Prenat Diagn.* 1991;11:263–270.

507. Ghidini A, Lynch L, Hicks C, et al. The risk of second-trimester amniocentesis in twin gestations: A case-control study. *Am J Obstet Gynecol.* 1993;169:1013–1016.

508. Kidd SA, Lancaster PA, Anderson JC, et al. Fetal death after exposure to methylene blue dye during mid-trimester amniocentesis in twin pregnancy. *Prenat Diagn.* 1996;16:39–47.

509. Gluer S. Intestinal atresia following intraamniotic use of dyes. *Eur J Pediatr Surg.* 1995;5:240–242.

510. Van der Pol JG, Wolf H, Boer K, et al. Jejunal atresia related to the use of methylene blue in genetic amniocentesis in twins. *Br J Obstet Gynaecol.* 1992;99:141–143.

511. Jeanty P, Shah D, Roussis P. Single-needle insertion in twin amniocentesis. *J Ultrasound Med.* 1990;9:511–517.

512. Buscaglia M, Ghisoni L, Bellotti M, et al. Genetic amniocentesis in biamniotic twin pregnancies by a single transabdominal insertion of the needle. *Prenat Diagn.* 1995;15:17–19.

513. Van Vugt JM, Nieuwint A, van Geijn HP. Single-needle insertion: An alternative technique for early second-trimester genetic twin amniocentesis. *Fetal Diagn Ther.* 1995;10: 178–181.

514. Sebire NJ, Noble PL, Odibo A, et al. Single uterine entry for genetic amniocentesis in twin pregnancies. *Ultrasound Obstet Gynecol.* 1996;7:26–31.

515. Benifla JL, Goffinet F, Dorai E, et al. Emergency cervical cerclage after 20 weeks' gestation: A retrospective study of 6 years' practice in 34 cases. *Fetal Diagn Ther.* 1997;12:274–278.

516. Lewis R, Mercer BM. Selected issues in premature rupture of the membranes: Herpes, cerclage, twins, tocolysis and hospitalization. *Semin Perinatol.* 1996;20:451–461.

517. Maly Z, Deutinger J. Decrease in cerclage incidence in multiple pregnancies by vaginal ultrasound monitoring. *Z Geburtshilfe Perinatol.* 1993;197:162–164.

518. Michaels WH, Schreiber FR, Padgett RJ, et al. Ultrasound surveillance of the cervix in twin gestations: Management of cervical incompetency. *Obstet Gynecol.* 1991;78:739–744.

519. Jones JM, Sbaua AJ, Cetrulo CL. Antepartum management of twin gestation. *Clin Obstet Gynecol.* 1990;33:32–41.

520. Newton ER. Antepartum care in multiple gestation. *Semin Perinatol.* 1986;10:19–29.

Ultrasound in the Management of the Alloimmunized Pregnancy

Chris Harman

Ultrasound-facilitated management of the patient with alloimmune disease is an ideal model for assessment of the practice of perinatal medicine. It demonstrates the mature integration of an understanding of the disease process, the etiology, pathologic change, approaches to investigation, mechanisms for treatment, and, perhaps most importantly, the means of prevention. High-resolution fetal imaging has led to highly specific, detailed physical examination. Invasive testing guided by real-time ultrasound yields direct biochemical, hematologic, and respiratory measurements that quantify fetal disease. Ultrasound-guided transfusion procedures allow treatment of even the most severely ill, with the expectation of excellent results at virtually all levels of alloimmune disease over a broad range of gestational ages. The roles of Doppler velocimetry in preinvasive monitoring and intraprocedure evaluation continue to be clarified. No better model exists to illustrate the fundamental role of ultrasonic fetal evaluation in the new obstetrics.

Anti-D sensitization (Rh disease) remains the cause of 80 to 90% of clinical hemolytic diseases of the fetus and newborn (HDFN), although "atypical" blood group antigens are assuming a larger role in the etiology of alloimmune disease, more so in the case of hydropic disease (Fig. 25–1).[1–5] The mortality of serious HDFN has continued to decrease with ongoing improvements in neonatal care. An equally impor-

tant factor in overall decline of this disease entity is a lower incidence (Table 25–1). Better management of those who are sick combined with fewer sick babies means perinatal death due to alloimmunization is seldom encountered in the general population (5 to 8 per 10,000 live births). Thus, Rh disease has become an unusual category of fetal disease, but it remains a correctable cause of perinatal mortality and neonatal morbidity, which deserves careful attention. With the application of the principles described in this chapter for detection, monitoring, and treatment, survival can approach 100%.

BASIC PATHOPHYSIOLOGY

In any pregnancy where the mother and fetus have differing blood types (and, therefore, in virtually all pregnancies where the mother and *father* have different blood types), maternal sensitization can occur.[6] To effect a mature antibody response, the mother must have been sensitized at some prior point, perhaps even as remote as the mother's time as a fetus (Fig. 25–2).[7] With a first immune exposure to a given antigen, a primary immune response follows, in the form of immunoglobulin M (IgM), which does not cross the placenta. The second exposure to that antigen results in the mature immune response. A "sensitized" woman is one with a

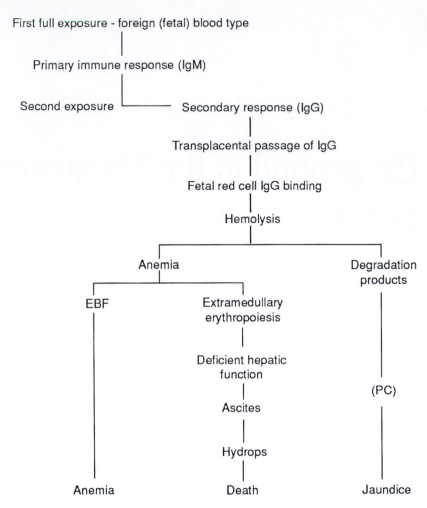

Figure 25–1. Development and impact of maternal sensitization. IgM, immunoglobulin M; IgG, immunoglobulin G; EBF, erythroblastosis fetalis; PC, placental clearance.

detectable antibody. When this antibody is immunoglobulin G (IgG), it readily crosses the placenta, as early as 10 weeks, and can cause fetal disease.

The pathophysiology is well understood (see Fig. 25–2). The fetus expresses Rh antigens on the red blood cells (RBCs), virtually as early in gestation as these are present. Once exposed, the mother mounts a competent antibody response against the fetal RBC antigens. As the antibody binds fetal

RBCs in circulation, it triggers fetal reticuloendothelial system digestion. Deformed cells are removed from circulation, mainly in the spleen, and disposed of ultimately by hemolysis and phagocytosis. Kell alloimmunization is an exception to this model: the secondary immune response produces IgG which is complement fixing. It attacks Kell-positive RBC and progenitor cells and produces direct injury within the bone marrow, essentially suppressing erythropoiesis without generating the detectable products of hemolysis.[8]

With worsening anemia, the fetus compensates by maximizing RBC production in the liver, spleen, intestinal wall, and other sites to a minor extent, mediated by fetal erythropoietin. In the liver, the erythropoietic islands of cells enlarge and, when subjected to further demands, coalesce and occupy the majority of hepatic structure, causing displacement of hepatic cellular function, occlusion of transport pathways, and disruption of enzyme systems on a cellular basis.[8,9] The ultimate result of this "hepatotoxic" hematopoiesis is liver failure. Hemolysis continues, so the anemia remains uncorrected and worsens. Physically, this amounts to the ultimate form of fetal disease, hydrops fetalis: hepatosplenomegaly, hypoproteinemia, hypoalbuminemia, ascites, complete

TABLE 25–1. FACTORS IN THE DECLINING FREQUENCY OF HEMOLYTIC DISEASE OF THE FETUS AND NEWBORN

Reduced exposure to Rh+ blood
  Later first pregnancy
  Lower parity
  Detailed cross-matching
Reduced sensitization with transplacental hemorrhage
  Postpartum prophylaxis (90%)
  Antepartum prophylaxis (8%)
  Prophylaxis for specific events
  Therapeutic immunoglobulin G for massive exposure

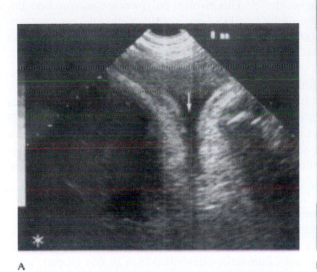
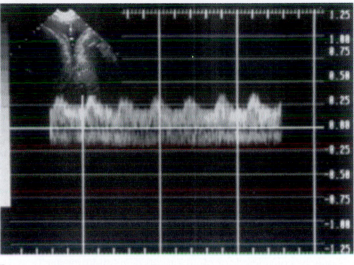

A   B

Figure 25–2. Doppler ultrasound in amniocentesis. **(A)** An apparently clear pocket of fluid *(arrow)*. **(B)** It contains arterial and venous waveforms. A different site was chosen.

anasarca, pericardial effusions, pleural effusions, cardiac failure, impaired placental circulation and function, and ultimately intrauterine death.

Hydrops fetalis presents many neonatal management problems, including difficulties in ventilation, enormous tissue edema, metabolic acidosis, cardiac instability, pulmonary immaturity, and abnormal chest wall compliance. Even the nonhydropic infant is at substantial risk of bilirubin toxicity, which in its most serious form (kernicterus) can cause death or severe cerebral damage.

The ultimate goals of management of alloimmunization are to reduce even further the sensitization of women at risk, to facilitate timely diagnosis and investigation of fetuses affected with disease, and to provide treatment when disease is severe enough to pose a threat to intrauterine survival. The essential role of ultrasound in all three processes will become clear to the reader.

PREVENTION OF ALLOIMMUNIZATION

In almost all instances, Rhesus sensitization is a result of exposure to fetal blood. This may happen spontaneously, as a result of transplacental hemorrhage (TPH) or several other factors (Table 25–2). At least 75% of TPHs occur at delivery, but up to 10% happen by 28 weeks of gestation.

Obstetric interference adds substantially to the risk of TPH before term. Procedures such as genetic amniocentesis, chorionic villus sampling (CVS), percutaneous umbilical blood sampling, and external version are all associated with increased risk of TPH and, therefore, of maternal sensitization. Detailed application of Rh immune globulin (Winrho,

intravenously or intramuscularly [IM]; RhoGAM, only IM) will prevent sensitization in many such cases.[10,11] A primary approach in controlling sensitization, however, is to reduce the frequency of TPH.

Ultrasound-guided procedures are less likely to generate TPH. For example, genetic amniocenteses with ultrasound direction produce only one-tenth the TPH of those done without ultrasound guidance.[12] Current studies show that patients do not become sensitized when ultrasound and immune prophylaxis are combined for genetic amniocentesis ($n > 3000$). Adequate ultrasound guidance for any procedure includes identification of the origin of the cord at the placenta, the entire course of the free umbilical cord, and accurate placental localization. Placental abnormalities, including succenturiate lobes, vasa previa, and so forth, are within the

TABLE 25–2. MATERNAL EXPOSURE TO Rh+ BLOOD

Spontaneous transplacental hemorrhage (TPH)
    At delivery
    Abruptio placentae
    Antepartum
    Miscarriage
    Fetal death
Traumatic TPH
    Chorionic villus sampling
    Amniocentesis
    Cordocentesis
    Therapeutic abortion
    Dilation and curettage
    Intrauterine fetal transfusion
    External version
    Obstetric manipulation

definition of *placental localization*. Emphasis on choosing a route that does not traverse the placenta has undoubtedly reduced the frequency of TPH. At the same time, diligent application of Rh immune prophylaxis with the procedure and Kleihauer testing to detect any fetal-to-maternal hemorrhage after transplacental procedures can produce the ideal result: no woman is sensitized as a result of the intervention.

In the pregnant woman already sensitized, however, a different level of concern is present. The pregnant woman who is already sensitized cannot be protected by any amount of Rh immune globulin or by carefully selecting a "thin" area of the placenta to traverse; the placenta should be avoided completely. We defer genetic amniocentesis, for example, when the pregnant woman is seriously sensitized, and the placenta is completely anterior. We do not recommend CVS in sensitized women.[13,14] Fetal blood sampling by cordocentesis may be considered for rapid karyotype in midtrimester, but it is important to remember that cordocentesis in the sensitized woman is associated with a very high frequency of TPH and subsequent increase in sensitization.[15]

INVESTIGATION OF THE ALLOIMMUNIZED PREGNANCY

"Critical levels" of maternal antibody that mandate testing are defined on an institutional basis. Once the mother demonstrates significant sensitization, however, further calibration of her antibody level may not accurately reflect the likelihood of fetal disease. A mother with a titer of 1:128 in albumin is just as likely to have severe disease if the titer remains stable as another patient whose antibody titer rises from 1:64 to 1:256 at the same gestational age. In women so sensitized, information must be obtained directly from the fetus.

Fetal Blood Typing

If the father is heterozygous for the antigen, then the fetus has a 50% chance of being negative and unaffected; thus, determining fetal blood type is important. A number of invasive procedures, all guided by real-time ultrasound, have been used to identify the antigen-positive (e.g., Rh-positive) fetus at risk. These procedures include use of fetal blood obtained at CVS, at amniocentesis when a bloody tap occurs, or by deliberate fetal blood sampling by cordocentesis. Any of these procedures, but especially CVS and cordocentesis, carries a definite risk of major acceleration of fetal disease: We do not recommend CVS in this situation and employ cordocentesis in very few cases (e.g., Kell alloimmunization, where the father is known heterozygous, because it would be more informative than amniocentesis in the case of a positive fetus, and the same information if the fetus were negative).

Although these blood typing methods may be employed occasionally, routine determination of fetal blood type genes using DNA technology (polymerase chain reaction) on ordinary amniocytes from routine amniocentesis is now

practicable.[16,17] This involves polymerase chain reaction amplification of fetal DNA and identification of the *gene*, not typing of RBCs from the antigen. Expert ultrasound guidance, to avoid the placenta and cord, is critical in such amniocenteses.

Amniocentesis for Amniotic Fluid Bilirubin

Bilirubin is the endproduct of fetal disposal of the waste products of hemolysis. Amniotic fluid spectrophotometry (ΔOD 450, a measure of the fluid's "yellowness") correlates with the amount of bilirubin present and, therefore, the amount of hemolysis. Indications for amniocentesis are summarized in Table 25–3.

Amniocentesis provides ongoing reassurance that more invasive fetal testing is not yet necessary but rarely may provide false reassurance,[18] and serial values are more reliable than single ones, especially in early gestation.[19] Detailed physical examination, described later in this chapter, must be added to amniocentesis to determine the extent of fetal disease.[20] If there is evidence of accelerated fetal disease, the amniocentesis may be properly deferred in favor of fetal blood sampling. Clearly, amniocentesis in the face of obvious hydropic fetal disease is superfluous. Having been scanned to determine the extent and severity of hydropic fetal disease, such a patient should be referred promptly to a center capable of fetal intravascular transfusion (IVT).

Amniocentesis is done under continuous ultrasound direction. When the placenta is posterior or when a clear path (at least 1 cm by 1 cm) is visible lateral to an anterior placenta, the needle is inserted in the sterile area, while the transducer is angled from a distance, to allow visualization. When access is limited and the transducer must be placed adjacent to the needle, a sterile plastic bag and sterile mineral oil allow the transducer to be positioned without contaminating the field. Transplacental amniocentesis with a 25-gauge needle rather than the 22-gauge spinal needle normally used is increasingly infrequent; fetal blood sampling is the superior choice. Some investigators believe that amniocentesis should play an extremely minor role in the management of such patients.[18,21] The argument on this issue has not been resolved.[22–25] In our team's experience, amniocentesis remains a valuable component of our ability to investigate fetal disease at an early stage of pregnancy.

Careful note is taken of the location of the cord and, if at all possible, the target pocket of amniotic fluid should contain

---

TABLE 25–3. INDICATIONS FOR AMNIOCENTESIS FOR ΔOD 450

Previous intrauterine death related to Rh disease

Neonatal disease requiring exchange transfusion

Significant antibody titer rise[a]

"Suggestive" ultrasound findings but no hydrops, when serial data are not available, cordocentesis not available

[a]Specific to the lab concerned. In the University of Manitoba program, 1:16 albumin titer, or absolute level of $>1.0~\mu g/L$.

no loops of cord, at any depth. If there is any doubt about the quality of image, Doppler ultrasound can be valuable in certifying a cord-free pocket (see Fig. 25–2).[26] To achieve these criteria, the ultrasonographer must have an open mind as to the angle of approach, and continuous real-time ultrasound imaging of the needle as it advances should be used to avoid maternal structures. A 10-mL aliquot is obtained and rapidly decanted into a light-proof container. Unless the fluid is grossly contaminated with particulate matter such as blood or vermix or deeply stained with heme pigment (green) or denatured blood (brown or red), the fluid should be analyzed directly and not centrifuged. Analysis of other metabolites in amniotic fluid remains experimental.[27]

After removal of the amniocentesis needle, careful observation is made to detect any intraamniotic bleeding. Bleeding of *maternal* origin may persist for some time, tends to be "gentle" in its appearance ("falling leaves"), and does not produce a "plume" or a "jet" within the amniotic fluid.[28] Very small amounts of *fetal* blood under pressure can produce these ultrasound appearances (Fig. 25–3). In all cases, a maternal blood sample for Kleihauer investigation is drawn 2 to 5 mins after the procedure. Fetal cells present in the maternal circulation may be cleared extremely rapidly and not be detected if the Kleihauer is drawn more than 10 mins after the procedure in a sensitized woman. If blood is accidentally obtained at the time of amniocentesis, it can be sent for Kleihauer examination and blood typing, if proven fetal.

Kleihauer testing demonstrating significant amounts of fetal blood in maternal circulation, whether after an invasive procedure or occurring spontaneously, calls for more frequent testing. Maternal antibody titer measurements are also impor-

tant in advancing the date of any investigation. In either case, maternal antibody production may have been provoked and fetal disease accelerate, making the assumption of a steady state of disease unreliable.

EXAMINATION OF THE ALLOIMMUNIZED FETUS

The reasons for detailed fetal examination in the alloimmunized pregnancy are basically the same as the reasons for testing (either amniocentesis or fetal blood sampling). The sonographer should be made aware of the mode of sensitization, antibody quantification and qualification, and a firm gestational age on which to base appraisal of the fetus. For subsequent amniocentesis, the sonographer must be aware that the fetus is positive and likely to be affected. Evaluation of subtle signs of incipient disease can be accomplished within the context of a normal obstetric scan, but a formatted examination ("data sheet") is helpful in ensuring consistency.

There are two primary components: physical examination to detect signs of hydropic disease and Doppler velocimetry to detect hemodynamic signs of fetal anemia. These components have not been compared in randomized fashion, and there is no apparent reason to perform either one in isolation. In the course of the examination, if either component is abnormal, biophysical profile scoring should also be completed.

Objective data are necessary because the physical examination has limited sensitivity in the nonhydropic fetus,[29] but laboratory data in isolation are not sufficient in formulating prognosis and management plans.

Fetal Examination

Physical examination is quite subjective, is highly variable from fetus to fetus, and may change rapidly in a given individual.[30,31] The examination, however, is an important part of the investigative process of the alloimmunized pregnancy and part of the effort to define the extremes of compromise to which the fetus has gone in trying to alleviate the anemia. Comprehensive examination includes the fetus, cord, placenta, and amniotic fluid.[32]

Anemia does not appear to bear any pathognomonic fetal physical signs, and a serious degree of fetal anemia may be present without frank hydrops.[33,34] First, especially before 24 weeks of gestation, many fetuses tolerate low hemoglobin concentrations without major hepatic compromise due to overwhelming hematopoiesis; this may well be dependent on tissue oxygenation remaining normal despite very low hematocrit levels. In other situations, hemolysis may be so rapid, in the form of a fetal hemolytic crisis, that fetal physical changes do not have time to evolve to the full-blown picture that "ought to" accompany profound fetal anemia.[34] There is much additional variability even when hydrops develops, with hemoglobulin values ranging from seriously low

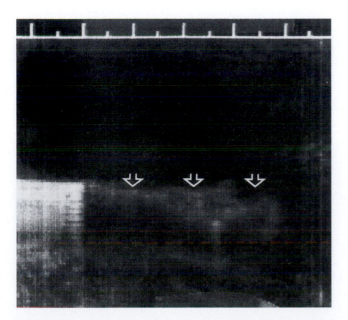

Figure 25–3. Waterbath image of infusion of only 0.025 mL of blood through a 25-gauge needle (bright linear echoes at left), producing turbulence *(arrows)*.

to profoundly low among fetuses with very similar physical appearances.

Fetal examination when the fetus is not yet hydropic is relatively straightforward.[26,34] Routine biometry establishes gestational age, using the mean of multiple gestational age parameters (head circumference, biparietal diameter, femur length, abdominal circumference, and foot length).[35] This aids in interpreting ΔOD 450 values, establishes where on the gestationally dependent slope the mean hemoglobin should lie, and helps predict lung maturity in terms of intrauterine versus extrauterine management. A careful screen of possible anomalies is performed, and detailed examination of fetal anatomy is performed. The example of a fetus with trisomy 21 with thickened occipital region, moderate ascites, and elevated ΔOD 450 (secondary to gastrointestinal obstruction, not hemolysis) reinforces the need to consider a differential ultrasound diagnosis even when the laboratory data seem obvious.

Subtle signs of impending ascites include double outlining of hollow organs, such as the stomach, gallbladder, and urinary bladder (Fig. 25–4), and later in gestation, fluid separating loops of small bowel.[36] Male fetuses may show expanding hydroceles (Fig. 25–5), and identification of maleness in itself may be a significant indicator of increased risk of severe disease.[37]

The few milliliters of fluid normally present in the abdomen may be detected by high-resolution ultrasound instruments. Further, *pseudoascites,* may be noted in fetal cross-section at the level of the dome of the diaphragm descend-

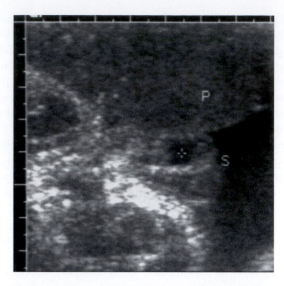

Figure 25–5. Male fetus with serious anti-D hemolysis, 30 weeks of gestation. First sign of progression to hydropic disease was a small hydrocele *(caliper).* S, scrotum; P, placenta, which is bulging.

ing to the anterior abdominal wall, where the abdominal wall musculature and the diaphragm may lie in apposition.[38] Because both of these skeletal muscle structures are echo poor, an apparent fluid rim may be visualized at this level (Fig. 25–6). True ascites does not usually accumulate at this level. If it is not continuous with the same fluid rim at the dome of the diaphragm or situated in the fetal pelvis, it is probably pseudoascites. A fluid rim also should be clearly visible in both longitudinal and transverse planes.

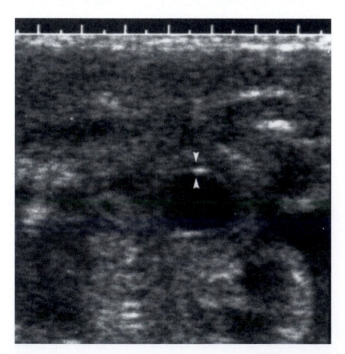

Figure 25–4. Impending ascites. The fetal bladder wall outlined *(arrowheads)* on both sides, by urine inside and a small amount of ascites on the peritoneal surface.

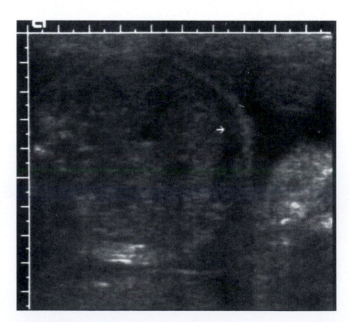

Figure 25–6. Pseudoascites. The apparent "fluid rim" *(arrow)* was not seen in the fetal pelvis or at the top of the liver and disappeared when the fetus changed position.

In the absence of overt ascites, other generalized signs of fetal edema or anasarca are seldom present. In our experience, it is of little value to perform systematic serial measurement of abdominal wall thickness, scalp thickness, or assessment of other areas of the integument. Without ascites, significant peripheral edema is usually a combination of artifact and wishful thinking, or it may be associated with other abnormalities of the fetus independent of the alloimmune process. Similar comments can be made for pleural effusions, which are seldom present in the absence of ascites and are statistically more common in nonimmune hydrops than in alloimmunization even when ascites is present.

The same may not be true of pericardial effusions. DeVore and others rely on the presence of pericardial effusions detected by M-mode ultrasound examination to initiate invasive therapy.[39,40] Such monitoring in sensitized patients may detect minor pericardial effusions as small as 2 to 3 mm. In our laboratory, high-resolution ultrasound instruments are sometimes able to demonstrate small amounts of pericardial fluid in the healthiest, nonaffected fetuses. No randomized study of such fetuses has been published, and we do not rely on this subtle finding to initiate investigation. It is our experience that large pericardial effusions (larger than 4 mm) are usually associated with other obvious signs of fetal disease. Large effusions, such as those shown in Fig. 25–13, are prognostically significant and may alter some aspects of management (e.g., the total volume of blood administered as a single IVT, being aware of the possibility of cardiac tamponade with hypervolemia).

Small pericardial effusions may appear as an early manifestation of the hyperkinetic fetal circulation of mild to moderate anemia. Fetal cardiac output is increased proportionately to the degree of anemia, corrected for gestational age, and may reach 150 to 175% of normal.[41] If this is analogous to cardiac function in the anemic preterm infant, red cell mass (i.e., hematocrit) and not oxygen-carrying capacity (hemoglobin concentration) is a critical determinant.[42] The increased cardiac output may be affected by a combination of mechanical factors (e.g., cardiac dilatation[43]), humoral factors (noradrenaline among them[44]), structural cardiac changes (such as the classic ventricular hypertrophy), and the relative ease of pumping blood with lower viscosity. An apparent increase in fetal coronary artery blood flow seen in severe anemia may be an important factor allowing this dramatically increased cardiac work.[45] Effusions larger than 4 mm, biventricular outer diameter in millimeters greater than 1.1 times the number of weeks (e.g., larger than 36.3 mm at 33 weeks), and subjective indications of a hyperdynamic cardiac examination would all be included in a general picture favoring invasive testing and would be enhanced by the Doppler examinations, discussed later.

Change in serial abdominal circumference may be a valuable ultrasound sign of impending disease in the nonhydropic fetus, especially if Doppler velocities are rising concurrently. Special care must be taken in performing this measurement in sensitized pregnancies to observe the landmarks (bifurcation of the portal vein within the liver and a smooth oval cross-section). Measurement should be taken from skin to skin, using an elliptical caliper when possible (Fig. 25–24). Sudden increases in percentile ranking of the fetal abdominal circumference suggest significant hepatomegaly secondary to advancing hepatopoiesis (Fig. 25–7).[46,47] Changes in fetal position may produce artifactual rises in percentile ranking, as demonstrated in Fig. 25–7B, but one should not ignore significant changes in established percentile ranking. If a sharp rise in abdominal circumference growth is shown in association with a serious antibody titer, serial amniocenteses or fetal blood sampling should be initiated. In the fetus already being followed by amniocentesis, a sudden rise in abdominal circumference calls for confirmation of the "benign" amniotic fluid results by fetal blood sampling. It is worth emphasizing that a "stable") ΔOD 450 does *not* guarantee a stable fetal hemoglobin.

Subjective signs of hepatosplenomegaly, such as the bottom edge of the liver lying as low as the fetal right iliac crest or splenomegaly with the spleen extended more than 2 cm below the left costal margin, may suggest accelerating disease. Measuring the spleen directly has been effective in prediction of fetal anemia for some investigators,[48] but our experience has included fetuses in whom the measurement was technically unsatisfactory and others with marked variability depending on fetal position. The general principles of strengths in serial assessments and cordocentesis when in doubt are emphasized.

Hydrops Fetalis

The original description of hydrops fetalis refers to the appearance of stillborn infants who had suffered the ultimate consequence of intrauterine alloimmune disease. In most centers, the neonatologist is not often confronted by this awful appearance, but the intrauterine ultrasound correlates of this appearance may still present antenatally (Figs. 25–8 through 25–13). The classic findings of the most severe form of disease, preceding fetal death by only days, are illustrated in these figures.

Ascites. The threshold for ascites being visualized is not certain, but based on serial observations of intraperitoneal transfusion, estimates can be made. At 30 mL, the double outlining (see Fig. 25–4) and an increased contrast of the abdominal contents first appear. At 50 mL, a distinct fluid rim (such as in Fig. 25–8) begins to be visible. At 100 mL, a classic picture of ascites is clear[28] (see Fig. 25–9).

At the other end of the scale, changes in large volumes of ascites may be difficult to monitor, because abdominal wall tension and intraabdominal organs will cause the fluid to appear in fairly consistent fashion over a wide range of volumes. In our experience, serial measurement of fetal ascites is a poor way of documenting response to therapy.

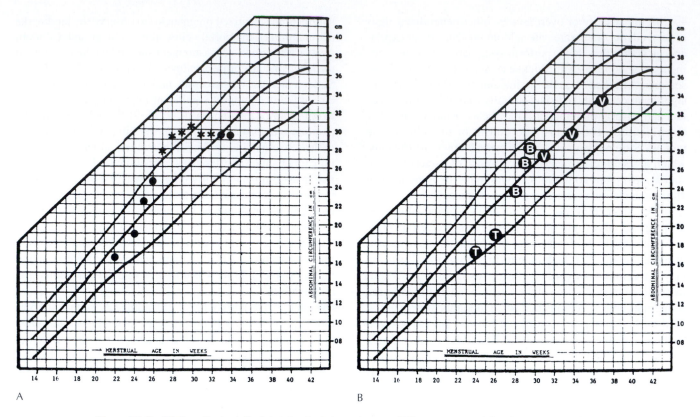

A   B

Figure 25–7. **(A)** Growth chart. Serial abdominal circumference (AC) measurements in a fetus who developed severe anti-D alloimmune disease. Starting at 22 weeks, four measurements show acceleration in AC (accompanied by rising amniotic fluid bilirubin). At 26 weeks, intravascular fetal transfusions were begun, three procedures over 6½ weeks, with weekly AC measurements (∗). Measurements taken at 33 and 34 weeks of gestation, after the transfusions were complete, showed fetal AC at the previously established level (40th percentile) with a corresponding decrease in liver size. **(B)** Serial AC in a fetus who switched from transverse lie (T), to breech (B), to vertex (V). Mother had stable 1:8 titer anti-Kell, but the rise in AC was troubling. A single amniocentesis at 30 weeks demonstrated a low zone I fluid.

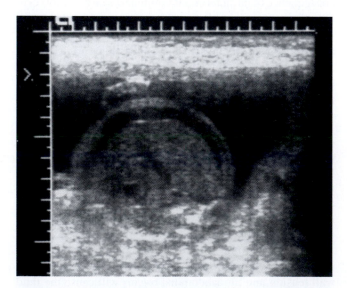

Figure 25–8. "Early" ascites. Small rim of intraperitoneal fluid not associated with significant fetal edema or other effusions. Fetal hemoglobin 66 g/L at 26 weeks of gestation.

Before onset of any therapy, the ascites is bright yellow and crystal clear. If intraperitoneal transfusions (IPTs) are used in managing such fetuses, the blood introduced into the peritoneal cavity produces changes notable by ultrasound. Turbidity of intraperitoneal fluid, when the fetus moves and in more or less static views, can be observed but is not a reliable indicator of the amount of the blood absorption. It may well be that the same examiner following the patient will produce the best evidence of improvement after IPT.

Fetal Edema. Figure 25–10 shows the most severe form of fetal facial edema, the so-called Buddha face. Forehead and cheeks are so waterlogged with edema that the eye sockets are lost in contour; head and body size can be overestimated due to intense tissue swelling (see Fig. 25–11). In some cases, abdominal wall edema can be seen first, but serial measurements of abdominal wall thickness are not helpful in predicting severity or rate of deterioration. Expression of abdominal wall edema differs greatly with gestational age and fetal position and may be reduced as further deterioration leads to tense

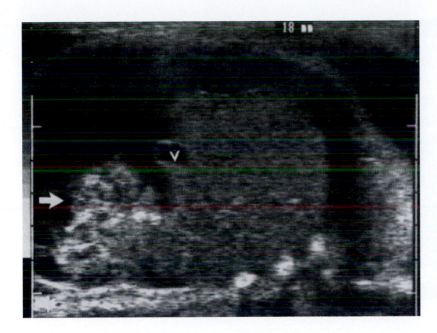

Figure 25–9. Massive fetal ascites. Longitudinal view of the abdomen of a hydropic fetus at 24 weeks. The chest is to the right, with lower three ribs seen at lower right. Ascites outlines the liver, with umbilical vein entering at V. The more echogenic small bowel *(arrow)* hangs freely in the fluid. The abdominal circumference was >97.5 percentile; the abdominal wall was not thicker than normal.

ascites. Especially in the occipital region, normal scalp thickness may be exaggerated simply by fetal posture, creating an impression of scalp edema. It is most helpful, therefore, to obtain serial examinations by the same observer, using each available area to monitor edema. A careful review of the following structures will illustrate fetal edema if present: face, including eyelids, nostrils, lips, and ears; scalp, frontal and occipital; abdominal wall thickness; and hands and feet.

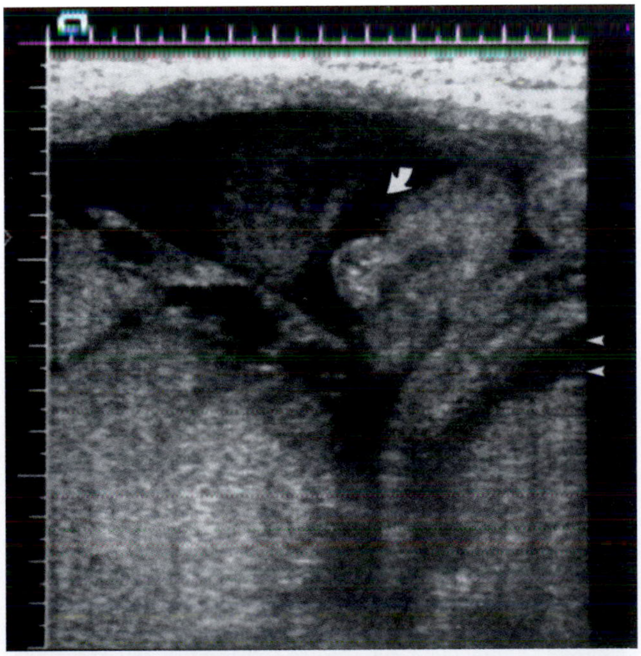

Figure 25–10. "The Buddha face." The forehead is at upper center, with the swollen face angled down to the right. The left eye *(arrow)* is closed by edema. The chin rests on the chest, which shows a pleural effusion *(double arrowhead)*.

Particularly helpful in the evaluation of hands and feet and in some areas of the face is to observe the fetus while it moves. The edematous hand cannot close properly, and although movements may be seen, these are stiff and limited in range (see Fig. 25–12).

Pericardial and Pleural Effusions. When present in the severely hydropic fetus, these effusions are very obvious. Pericardial effusions may reach large dimensions (see Fig. 25–13) and interfere with myocardial contractility. Such observations are important in the occasional fetus in whom cardiac output is impaired and call for reduced volumes at the initial IVTs.[34] Pleural effusions are seen with less frequency and should be regarded with some suspicion when the fetus is responding to therapy, especially if they persist longer than pericardial effusions and ascites. Invasive testing will provide adequate fetal samples of either amniotic fluid or blood for genetic studies to exclude the unusual but definite possibility of maternal alloimmunization that exists in conjunction with serious fetal anomalies that lead to effusions, ascites, or both. Pleural effusions usually resolve quite rapidly with therapy, although pericardial effusions in a number of infants treated in our center were the last to resolve while the fetus was improving. It is not uncommon for pericardial effusion to last 3 weeks after fetal hemoglobin has been restored to a normal level or even longer after *intracardiac* transfusion.

Fetal Behavior. Fetal well-being is assessed with the biophysical profile score (BPS)[20,49] Behavioral indices monitored by ultrasound, including fetal body and limb movement, fetal tone, fetal breathing movements, and amniotic fluid volume, are assessed in the same fashion as for other high-risk pregnancies. Cardiotocography is frequently used in completing the antenatal assessment of such fetuses,

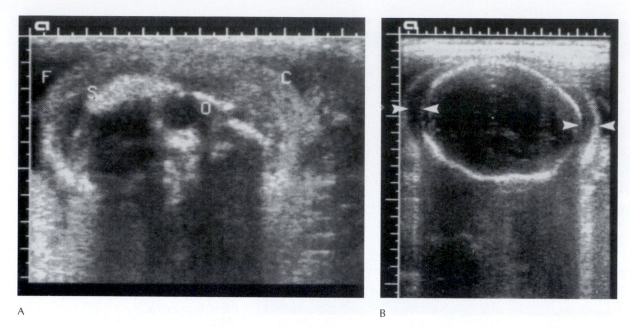

A   B

Figure 25–11. Scalp edema. **(A)** The fetus is surrounded by a 2-cm thick mass of edema. The face, identified by O (left orbit) and S (top of skull), is dwarfed by edema, shown by C (surface of left cheek) and F (forehead). This fetus survived intact, after seven intravascular transfusions. **(B)** In axial plane, the "halo" of edema is best seen anteriorly and posteriorly *(between arrowheads)*.

especially in observations immediately before and after intrauterine procedures. The BPS is usually normal (8–10/10) through a wide range of fetal disease. This is functional evidence that the fetus is able to maintain homeostasis despite severe impairment of hematologic function. A BPS of 4/10 or less (the moribund fetus) is almost exclusively found in fetuses with the most severe structural evidence of hydrops fetalis and is a severe prognostic sign.[20,30,50,51] The complete

absence of fetal behavior in a fetus illustrating typical signs of hydrops fetalis constitutes a fetal emergency for which the only means of rescue is direct vascular access, either intrauterine or after emergency cesarean section. Such fetuses do not respond to series of intraperitoneal fetal transfusion, perhaps on the basis of absent fetal breathing movements.[52] If treatment by IVT is successful, it is usually the result of multiple small transfusions, with interval BPS monitoring to ensure fetal stability between procedures.[34]

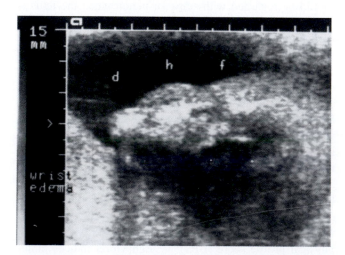

Figure 25–12. Skin edema. Scan shows the fetal arm in longitudinal view. Distorted by edema, the forearm (f), hand and wrist (h), and digits (d) remained in a fixed position for several days after hemoglobin and pH were restored to normal by a series of intravascular transfusions. The fetus regained normal movement before normal anatomy, resulting in limbs that moved "like paddles."

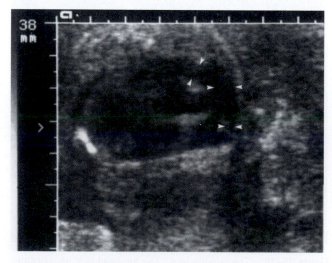

Figure 25–13. Pericardial effusions. This fetus at 23 weeks had striking ascites, placental edema, and severe facial and scalp edema. The large pericardial effusion *(arrowheads)* was the last sign to resolve, 3 weeks after restoration of normal hemoglobin levels.

Intravascular fetal data available suggest that these fetuses are indeed acidotic and hypoxic and have serious perfusion problems. The sickest of these may have a pH as low as 6.90 and be beyond resuscitation, but we have been successful in resuscitating moribund fetuses with a pH as low as 7.11. Among alloimmunized fetuses in general, there is good correlation between formal BPS and fetal umbilical venous pH,[53] and at least part of the success with such previously lethal disease is attributable to serial BPS.

In such situations, the return of normal fetal behavior, shown by rapid increase in fetal movements with normal tone and soon after that the return of regular, cyclic, fetal breathing movements, demonstrates the value of BPS in the posttransfusion phase. In several instances, restoration of hemoglobin to a normal range, associated with a rise in PO_2 and correction of acidotic pH, along with resumption of normal behavior, has been demonstrated within 30 mins of transfusion.[30,50] The survival of the majority of fetuses in this condition demonstrates the maxim that no fetus with a heartbeat is beyond treatment (see Fig. 25–14). [51]

Amniotic Fluid Volume

Fetuses with early stages of disease tend to have increased amniotic fluid. This may not always exceed the ultrasound threshold for hydramnios (greater than 8.0 cm in maximum vertical amniotic fluid pocket depth), but it certainly meets subjective impressions of increased fluid. Although some have found this to be a reliable first indicator of the onset of fetal disease,[54] it may not be a reliable enough sign on which to base management.[29] Reduced amniotic fluid volume is an ominous sign. A maximum pocket depth of less

than 2 cm (amniotic fluid index < 10) signifies reduced production of amniotic fluid, as can be seen in end-stage disease or when intrauterine growth retardation is associated with alloimmunization. Fetal vascular access should be sought urgently when such a finding is associated with hydropic fetal disease, including assessment of karyotype, viral infection markers, and potential hereditary disorders in the blood samples submitted.

Quantitative examination of the amniotic fluid includes documentation of backbleeding after vascular access, approximation of volume of blood lost at the end of the transfusion, and noting the presence of any intraamniotic clot (Fig. 25–15). In the case illustrated, fetal thrombocytopenia was so severe that backbleeding of greater volume than had been given at the first transfusion occurred rapidly after withdrawal of the needle.[55] The intraamniotic clot formed quickly after the backbleeding and rapidly contracted around the cord and fetal limbs adherent to the fetal abdomen. An increase in the amount of free-floating particles after transfusion correlates with a small amount of backbleeding and normal hemostasis. Masses of such particles (evident as a snowstorm) when the fetus moves a limb vigorously are of little significance when detailed fetal hematology is known. Such particles may persist for several weeks after the last fetal transfusion, noting that the fetus active enough to stir up the particles has *not* been exsanguinated!

Umbilical Cord

Detailed identification of the umbilical cord at its two ends is an integral part of preparation for a fetal IVT. The placental end of the cord is the target of first choice in IVT and is

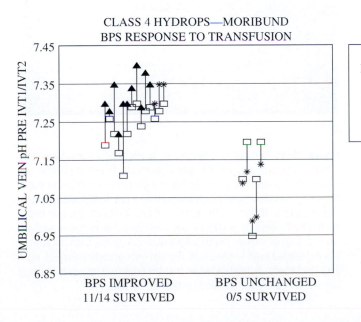

CLASS 4 HYDROPS—MORIBUND
BPS RESPONSE TO TRANSFUSION

BPS IMPROVED
11/14 SURVIVED

BPS UNCHANGED
0/5 SURVIVED

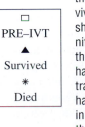

PRE–IVT

▲ Survived

✳ Died

Figure 25–14. Biophysical profile score (BPS) and response to intravascular transfusion. In 19 moribund fetuses (class 4 hydrops, BPS ≤ 4/10, flat or decelerative cardiotocogram, and gross physical hydrops), the BPS was used to monitor the fetus between transfusions. In those fetuses with improved BPS after the first or second transfusion *(n = 14, left),* 11 survived, with their pH at the time of the next procedure shown by the *solid triangles.* In 8 cases *(asterisk,* signifying pH at the time of the subsequent procedure), the fetus died. In 3 fetuses, in the left-hand group, BPS had improved, and pH was somewhat improved, but traumatic complications led to fetal demise. In the right-hand group, with no improvement in BPS, mean pH fell in this group between the first and second procedures; there was no resumption of normal fetal behavior, and all fetuses died. Fetuses in the right-hand group had more severe disease; lower pre-intravascular transfusion (IVT) pH and lower pre-IVT hemoglobin level. The BPS reflected the success or failure of IVT to return pH toward normal. This study demonstrates the sensitivity of BPS behaviors to pH, not only in worsening acidosis but in improving fetal acidemia. This suggests that the success of efforts at intrauterine resuscitation for fetal asphyxia can be monitored successfully by BPS.

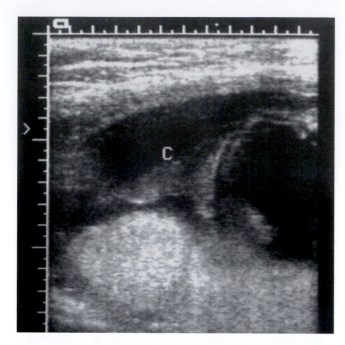

Figure 25–15. Large intraamniotic clot after thrombocytopenic hemorrhage after intravascular fetal transfusion. This image was obtained approximately 30 mins after the needle was removed from posterior cord insertion, as the clot (C) gradually contracted up against the abdominal wall. Retransfusion was necessary due to extensive back-bleeding.

identified in maximum detail. With the anterior placenta or with the posterior placenta and generous amniotic fluid, this identification is not difficult (Fig. 25–20). In the more mature fetus with a posterior cord insertion, the area of the placenta where the cord is anchored may be completely obscured. Similarly, the anterior cord insertion may not be ideally visualized when the fetus is large, the fluid is reduced, and the cord wrapped around a fetal limb, neck, or torso. From performing more than 2000 cord procedures, the lesson we learned has been to take as much time as necessary, to use maternal repositioning or fetal manipulation, or simply to defer the procedure to another time to obtain optimal visualization.

Serial fetal umbilical vein diameter does not correlate with onset or extent of fetal disease.[56–58] In addition to its lack of correlation, this measurement itself differs significantly with fetal position, tension on the cord, nuchal or other loops, and with advancing gestational age. Variations in cord anatomy, discussed later, may also change with position and age.

Placenta

This may be the earliest site of manifestations of accelerated fetal alloimmune hemolysis. As disease progresses, placental architecture is lost, with gradual assumption of the "ground glass" appearance (Fig. 25–16). The placenta becomes more erect and stiffer, and the presence of maternal "lakes," as seen

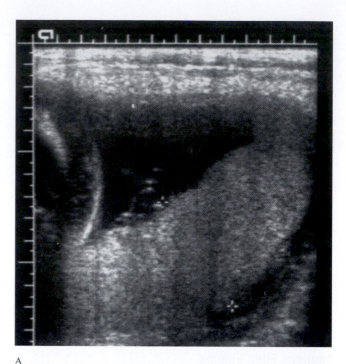

A

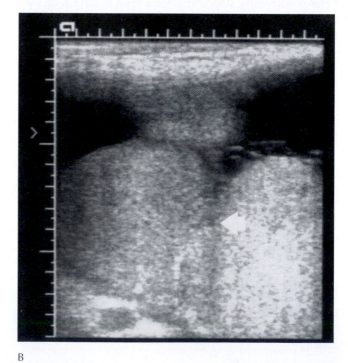

B

Figure 25–16. Placental changes in accelerated alloimmune fetal disease. **(A)** Typical "ground glass" placenta found in serious alloimmune disease. The placenta has lost much of its architecture and shows a generally uniform appearance with ablation of maternal intervillous spaces. Maximum thickness >6 cm *(calipers)*, grossly thickened for 22 weeks of gestation. Cord insertion lies to the immediate left of the upper caliper. **(B)** Hydropic placenta. In this case the edema has proceeded even further, with the placenta grossly enlarged, rigid very thickened, and distended so that the true cord insertion *(arrow)* lies >2 cm below the buckled surface of the placenta.

in the more relaxed placenta, is progressively lost. Eventually, the placenta assumes a rigid, spherical appearance with a puckered chorionic surface. In the most severe forms of placental edema, the placenta may reach thicknesses of 8 to 10 cm and weigh as much as 2.0 kg at the time of delivery. One such example is shown in Fig. 25–16B, which demonstrates the cord insertion puckered as much as 3 cm below the interface between the amniotic fluid and the membrane. The most severe form of placental distortion may not resolve even over a successful course of intrauterine fetal therapy and may be a causal factor in the generation of maternal "mirror syndrome," premature labor, or both.

PHYSICAL CLASSIFICATION OF DISEASE STATE

Based on the rather straightforward findings described, the physical extent of fetal disease can be classified as shown in Table 25–4.[20] *The reader should be careful not to infer that fetal disease proceeds in a regular, step-by-step fashion, or that disease neatly segregates into these classifications.* Nicolaides et al.[29] demonstrated in convincing fashion that morphometrics, whatever the object measured, are probably not of much use in quantifying fetal anemia. The purpose of the classification described in this section is not to refute that argument but simply to illustrate the levels of physical compromise that are associated with different depths of fetal anemia. The classification assists in standardization of results for comparison and helps formulate prognosis. Brief description of the classes follows.

Class 0 fetuses underwent cordocentesis due to suspected alloimmune disease, based on historical data, marginal or suspicious ΔOD 450 values, or suspicious ultrasound findings. A pure fetal blood sample was obtained, but no transfusion was performed. All fetuses ($n = 68$) were delivered with normal hemoglobin levels at mature gestation without transfusion. Most fetuses were proven not to have the antigen in question, whereas nine were antigen positive but did

not require transfusion. None had any of the serious findings of accelerated alloimmune disease on serial examination.

Class 1 fetuses all had elevated ΔOD 450 amniocentesis and were antigen-positive, Coombs' complete in less than 1 min, had elevated serum bilirubin, and demonstrated progressive, accelerated loss of fetal hemoglobin on serial fetal blood sampling. In 11 of these fetuses, initial cordocentesis values showed normal hemoglobin concentration, with subsequent cordocenteses at intervals of 7 to 14 days, demonstrating the need for initiation of therapy. None demonstrated fetal signs of accelerated disease, but almost all demonstrated increased amniotic fluid (greater than 8.0 cm in maximum vertical amniotic fluid pocket depth) and loss of detailed placental architecture. Fetal hemoglobin in these fetuses ranged from 120 g/L, the threshold for initiating transfusion, to as low as 52 g/L in a fetus at $31^{6/7}$ weeks. In that particular patient, the placenta was grossly edematous, but the fetus demonstrated no other signs of accelerated disease. For this class, the mean hemoglobin at first sampling was 81.4 g/L. In cases where serial abdominal circumference measurements were available, two-thirds showed a rise in percentile rank of 20 or more. Subjective evidence of hepatomegaly was cited in one-half.

Class 2 fetuses have been described as "mild hydrops." The findings include hydramnios and loss of placental architecture, with a trend toward an increased placental thickness, a homogeneous placental appearance, and a uterine shape that is spherical as opposed to oval in cross-section, signifying an increase in uterine tone. The fetus demonstrates ascites of varying extent, the minimum threshold for diagnosis of ascites being 5 mm of transverse fluid rim width. Fetuses in this group do not have generalized body edema, with maximum occipital scalp thickness of less than 7 mm. Fetal behavior is normal, with a BPS of 8/8 or 10/10. Fetal hemoglobin in these fetuses range from 32 to 66 g/L at first sample. In all cases of class 2 disease, the ascites reversed promptly (mean 11 days) and fetal appearance did not deteriorate into class 3 or 4 once IVT was initiated. As seen in Fig. 25–17, there is significant overlap of class 2 disease with classes 3 and 4 disease (as discussed below). Peripheral smears of blood from these fetuses contain few if any erythroblasts.

Class 3 fetuses have very severe-appearing fetal disease, including massive fetal ascites, scalp edema, skin edema, digital and facial edema, of the extent illustrated in Figures 25–8 through 25–13. Despite this accelerated disease and very low hemoglobin levels ranging from 13 g/L at 22 weeks to 56 g/L at 29 weeks, these fetuses maintain normal P_{O_2} and normal pH, as demonstrated by normal BPSs. In cases where serial IVT was performed, normal BPS was maintained and intact survival was achieved. Exsanguination during IVT accounted for three of the four deaths in this class. Class 3 disease tends to occur at earlier gestation and, therefore, requires an increased number of procedures compared with class 2 disease. Cardiac overload and the risk of hemorrhage differentiate class 3 from class 2 fetuses.

TABLE 25–4. ULTRASOUND CLASSIFICATION OF ALLOIMMUNE DISEASE

Class	Elevated MCA Doppler	Ultrasound Appearance			Abnormal BPS <4/10
		Placenta	Effusion	Anasarca	
0	—	—	—	—	—
1	+	+	—	—	—
2	+	+	+	—	—
3	+	+	+	+	—
4	a	+	+	+	+

BPS, biophysical profile score; MCA, middle cerebral artery peak systolic velocity.
[a] In severe hydrops with cardiac compromise, MCA velocity may be reduced, with absent or reversed end-diastolic velocity.

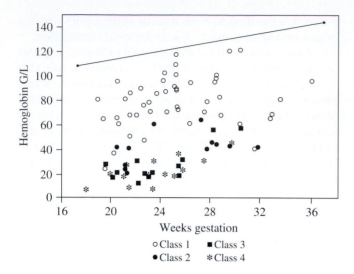

Figure 25–17. Distribution plot of fetal hemoglobin concentration at time of first fetal blood sampling. Note the wide range covered by class 1 (nonhydropic) fetal disease. There is also significant overlap among classes 2, 3, and 4. Mean normal hemoglobin concentration is shown by the regression line at the top.

Class 4 is clearly differentiated from the other classes by the absence of fetal behavior. The fetus hangs completely limp, although posture may be stiffened to some extent by the extreme nature of peripheral edema. These fetuses constitute a fetal emergency. Delay of even a few hours may result in an irretrievable level of acidosis and hypoxemia. Fetal death among most of these class 4 infants was related to absent fetal cardiac output. Despite pH as low as 7.11 and fetal hemoglobin levels as low as 6 g/L (0.6 g%), many of these fetuses can be salvaged.

These classifications illustrate that certain appearances may correlate reasonably well with the more "objective" data from fetal blood sampling (Fig. 25–17). There is significant overlap among fetuses with similar classifications of disease; one could not by any means predict fetal hematocrit on the basis of ultrasound appearance alone. It is a clinical reality, however, that more severe physical disease correlates with poorer prognosis. Taken from another point of view, fetal hemoglobin measurement may not necessarily indicate completely the depth of disease to which the fetus has dropped.

DOPPLER ULTRASOUND

The roles of Doppler evaluation of fetal circulation in the immunized pregnancy have not yet been completely defined; many applications have been developed, but their limits and advantages are not yet clear. The principal application, the use of blood flow velocity in the systemic fetal circulation to determine which fetuses do or do not require invasive fetal testing, is gaining acceptance and is the focus of this dis-

cussion. The second application, to cardiac physiology and the understanding of treatment requirements and responses, continues to evolve.

The circulation of the anemic fetus is hyperdynamic.[59] As discussed above, increased cardiac output is likely multifactorial but includes a marked increase in peak systolic velocity of the thinner fetal blood, documented in almost every fetal vessel detectable by Doppler. Originally described in *umbilical arteries*,[60] the correlation between severity of anemia and degree of Doppler abnormality in the *descending aorta* (possibly reflecting peripheral vasodilation in response to anemia),[59,61] *middle cerebral artery* (relating decreased viscosity to higher velocity,[62–64] and *precordial veins* (reflecting cardiac compensation or compromise in most severely affected)[59,65,66] has been clinically significant.

Initial research described the changes before and after transfusion, when acute, known changes in hematocrit could be related to the major changes in flow velocity.[67,68] Doppler indices showed very little change, although the absolute velocities dropped dramatically. Subsequently, major effort has been focused on the *prediction* of fetal anemia. Prospective studies have used the descending aorta[69] plus the umbilical vein,[70] umbilical vein plus ultrasound and maternal serology,[71] and the middle cerebral artery.[72,73] The following is a summary of current investigations.

Umbilical Artery

Positive correlations exist, but there is wide variation, with no relation to acid–base status,[74] and it is only overtly abnormal in hydrops. Because it is not reliable after the first transfusion, this Doppler modality is not presently used to defer invasive testing (Fig. 25–18).

Descending Aorta

The correlations are reasonable and improve when other data (e.g., venous Dopplers and ultrasound visualization) are added, reaching a positive predictive value of 89% and a negative predictive value of 100%.[70] Studies suggest this parameter is not reliable enough by itself to defer testing; it is being used in combination with other parameters in a number of research protocols.

Precordial Veins and Cardiac Evaluation

These vessels illustrate cardiac effects and volume status; thus, they may be valuable in hydrops or individual fetuses with inadequate response, but correlations to nonhydropic anemia are poor, so the utility of these vessels in the prediction of anemia is not clinically important.

Regional Arterial Beds

Splenic artery Doppler may reflect an erythropoietic effect in that organ and serve as a marker for accelerated production.[75] Alternatively, the splenic artery may directly reflect the

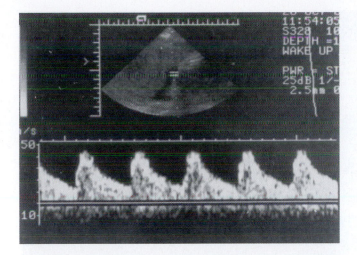

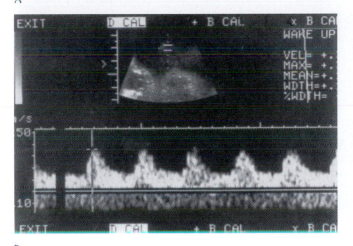

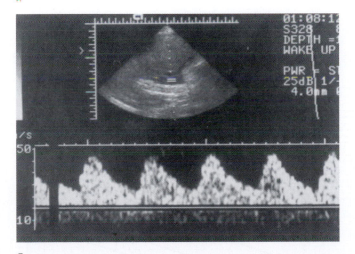

Figure 25–18. Umbilical vein velocity waveforms from a 30-week fetus at the time of the fourth intravascular transfusion. **(A)** Pretransfusion. Hemoglobin 96 g/L. **(B)** At the 90-mL mark of the transfusion. **(C)** Eighteen hours posttransfusion. Hemoglobin 190 g/L. There are significant changes in **B**, probably related to the large volume expansion given over only 20 mins. Despite doubling of the hematocrit, the pretransfusion and posttransfusion waveforms are virtually identical.

velocity changes associated with anemia. In any case, sensitivity for severe anemia has reached 100%, with elimination of many procedures which would have been scheduled by that group.[75] As illustrated by several studies evaluating multiple vessels,[45,59,63,67,68,70] however, the advantages of the middle cerebral artery and descending aorta in ease, reproducibility, and standard interpretation mean that splenic, renal, adrenal, coronary, portal, and other vessels, will remain of primarily research interest.

Middle Cerebral Artery (MCA)

The MCA is short and straight, the Doppler angle can be standardized easily, and the measurement has low observer-dependent variation.[64] Gestational age variations are smooth and predictable, and the increases in velocity with anemia have been demonstrated by many groups. In anemic fetuses, transfusion produces measurable Doppler changes that parallel the known changes in fetal hematocrit[76] (Fig. 25–19). Prospective evaluation in a multicenter trial has shown high sensitivity (100%, 95% confidence interval = 86 to 100%) for the detection of moderate to severe anemia.[74] The arbitrary categorization of anemia in this study may mean that prospective application achieves less than perfect results; all fetuses in this trial had cordocentesis and standard treatment regardless of the MCA values. In our experience, MCA has less reliability in predicting hematocrit levels after the initial transfusion, another aspect of this technique that requires further structured evaluation. Regardless of these hesitations, MCA peak velocity should be evaluated serially in all fetuses at risk of anemia by using curves normalized for gestational age (Fig. 25–20).

The considerable overlap between classes of disease, groups of hemoglobin measurements, or depictions of fetal blood smear evaluation emphasizes the importance of gathering all available data before assigning prognosis, determining management plans, or electing delivery over intrauterine management. The degree of anemia that may be present with normal ultrasound appearance emphasizes the need for a comprehensive plan of investigation: Do not defer planned tests because the "fetus looks fine"; continue with the plan!

INVASIVE FETAL PROCEDURES

Indications

Mandatory indications for gaining fetal vascular access include confirmation of a therapeutic range ΔOD 450 (either a single high zone III fluid or an inevitable progression of serial measurements greater than 80% of zone II) or any hydropic class of fetal disease. Relative indications can be summarized to reflect any situation in which 1) there may be a large discrepancy between ΔOD 450 and fetal hemoglobin or 2) cordocentesis may be safer than amniocentesis. Situation 1 includes any mother with historically demonstrated virulent antibody or when there is a recent dramatic rise in

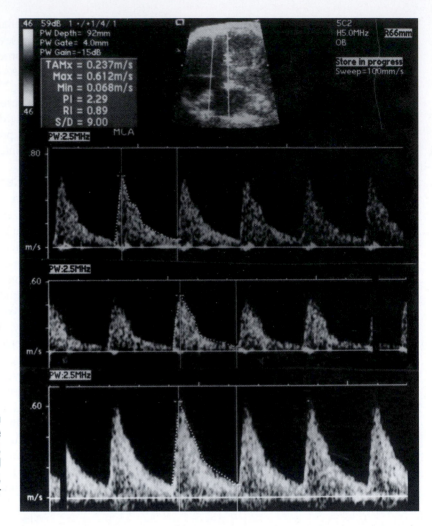

Figure 25–19. Middle cerebral artery waveforms in an anemic fetus requiring serial transfusions for severe Rh (D) disease. The peak systolic velocities of 62, 50, and 61 cm per second *(top to bottom)* corresponded to fetal hematocrits of 19%, 44%, and 32%, before, at the time of, and a week after the first intravascular transfusion, respectively.

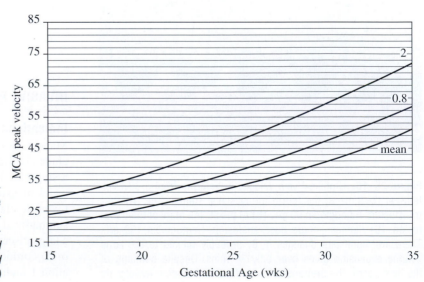

Figure 25–20. Middle cerebral artery peak systolic velocity plotted as a function of gestational age. Above the upper line (1.5 multiples of the median), invasive testing and treatment are indicated. Below that line, individual monitoring regimes are established. *(Reproduced with permission from Mari G, Adrignolo A, Abuhamad AZ, et al. Ultrasound Obstet Gynecol. 1995;5:400–405.)*

titer, suggesting the possibility of fetal hemolytic crisis.[77] If a placenta-free route for the amniocentesis is not available, cordocentesis (also known as *percutaneous umbilical blood sampling*) should be considered for any stage of gestation (situation 2). This will frequently be the ultrasonographer's decision.

Cordocentesis

Cordocentesis is always diagnostic in nature, but in many cases the need for immediate transfusion will be quite evident. All cases of hydropic disease, for example, should be transfused at the same time the initial fetal blood sample is obtained. Thus, a team approach is essential in organizing these procedures. If it is certain that the fetus will require transfusion immediately (all hydropic disease, hemoglobin falling rapidly on previous cordocentesis), then fetal blood sampling is done in continuity with fetal transfusion. With nonhydropic disease, cordocentesis is generally done as a solitary procedure, with transfusion to follow later as indicated. In intermediate situations (suggestive ΔOD 450, very aggressive history, suspicious ultrasound, and so on), the "cordo-IVT" is used. In this procedure, all preparations are made for IVT, cordocentesis is done, and the needle is kept in place until the hemoglobin level is measured at the bedside.

For cordocentesis as a solitary procedure, light maternal sedation is used only if the placenta is posterior, and prophy-lactic antibiotics are not routinely employed. The cord insertion is identified meticulously, as shown in Figures 25–21 and 25–22, making full use of the "zoom" feature on the high-resolution ultrasound instrument. It would appear from a close review of the literature that no particular scan head offers distinct advantages over another. Pulsed Doppler is useful in distinguishing the maternal venous "lake" that frequently overlies the cord insertion from the fetal vessels at the placental surface. Color Doppler flow mapping is efficient in illustrating the sometimes complicated anatomy of the cord insertion (Fig. 25–22). Finding the ideal route to the cord insertion may include manipulation of the mother or fetus to obtain better views.

Cord insertion variants may also complicate the approach. Careful review may reveal a safe route (e.g., Fig. 25–22B), but in some cases (Fig. 25–23) the placental insertion is not acceptable. Alternate targets include the umbilical vein as it runs through the fetal liver[78] or a free loop of cord pinned against the posterior wall (Fig. 25–24). Selection of the target will also change with fetal activity, the presence of tension on the cord by nuchal or body loops, and the urgency of the situation. Secure access may be found up to 3 to 5 cm from the origin (there may actually be less backbleeding here, because the needle will traverse Wharton's jelly en route). Beyond this point, the cord is mobile and will move away from the needle. An absolutely vertical approach, with the cord pinned against the (usually) underlying placenta, is

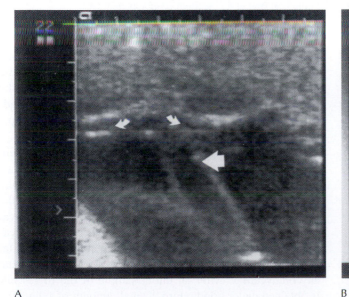

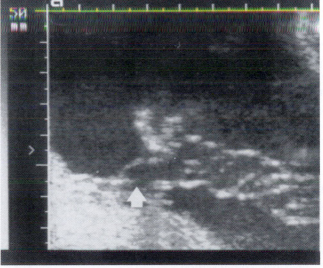

A

B

Figure 25–21. Visualization of cord insertion into the placenta. **(A)** Large umbilical vein *(large arrow)* inserting into an anterior placenta. In this case, needle penetration into the vessel is extraamnionic, and there is potential for contamination with maternal intervillous blood. There would usually be no backbleeding after transfusion in this case. The arteries *(small arrows)* run along the surface of the placenta. **(B)** Posterior cord insertion, vein at *arrow*. In this case, vessel entry would be through the amniotic fluid; therefore, maternal blood would be an unlikely contaminant, although the sample may be diluted with amniotic fluid present in the needle. Following removal of the needle after a transfusion, backbleeding could be documented easily.

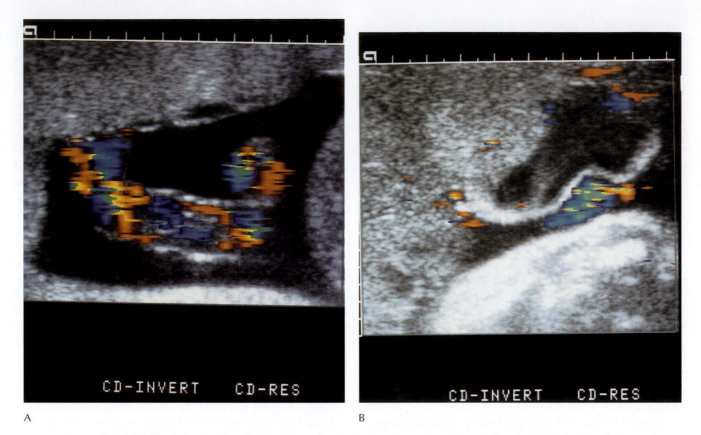

A   B

Figure 25–22. (A) Color Doppler depiction of orthodox cord insertion into anterior placenta, with small maternal venous spaces (no flow depicted) to right of insertion. Blue venous velocities. **(B)** Large maternal vascular space directly overlying cord insertion with broad separation of arteries *(red)*. In this fetus, all of the four serial intravascular transfusions were done using the umbilical vein at its insertion *(blue)*, in each case traversing this maternal "lake."

necessary for successful needling of such free loops. Earlier fears of cord laceration from free loop puncture have not been substantiated, but needle dislodgement and the risk of intrafunic hematoma due to fetal movement have occurred, so we advocate fetal paralysis with intravenous pancuronium in virtually all free loop procedures.[34] Confirmation of *pure* fetal blood is critical in this case, considering the possibility of amniotic fluid contaminating hematocrit measurement.

Identifying the target is the most important part of cordocentesis or IVT. Take as much time as necessary and proceed only when a clear approach to an umambiguous target is achieved. It is notable at this point in the discussion that *deferring the procedure* is also a useful way of ensuring safety. Sending the mother for a walk is often an effective answer to an "invisible" cord insertion.

The technique described is used for both cordocenteses and intrauterine transfusion procedures. There are many variations.[34,79] This routine has been applied to more than 1500 intrauterine procedures over the past 14 years. Two operators perform the procedure, one manipulating the ultrasound instrument and the other the needle. The ultrasound instrument is enclosed in a sterile plastic bag, with ordinary ultrasound gel within the bag. A Bridine prep is used, and

acoustic coupling is ensured with sterile oil on the maternal abdomen. The needle (a 22-gauge, 9-cm-long spinal needle in most situations) is introduced into the maternal skin at the target site. Under continuous visualization, the needle is gradually advanced to the cord insertion and, with a firm "pop," is inserted into the lumen of the vessel.

There are several reasons for selecting the umbilical vein for sampling. It is a larger vessel with thinner walls and thus is easier to cannulate. Turbulence down the vessel (toward the fetus) from the point of entry is easier to visualize within the umbilical cord, compared with small tributaries of umbilical arteries running along the surface of the placenta. Identification of the vessel entered is necessary to confirm pure fetal sampling, interpret blood gases and pH properly, and evaluate any bradycardia. After an initial sample of 0.6 to 1.0 mL is obtained under good return, a small amount of saline, 0.5 to 0.8 mL, is injected to identify the vessel. The remainder of the sample is then obtained. If only hematologic data are sought, a total of 1.6 mL suffices. The needle is then removed under direct visualization, and the vessel is observed for backbleeding (Fig. 25–25).

Teamwork is essential. The individual manipulating the needle should receive unequivocal instructions from the

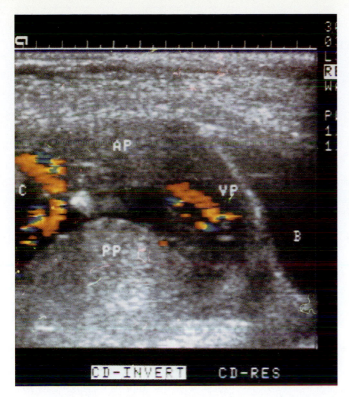

Figure 25–23. Vasa previa (VP), with cord insertion into membranes overlying the cervix (B, maternal bladder), separating anterior and posterior halves of the placenta (AP, PP, respectively). This highly mobile insertion close to the cervix, inserting in the membranes, is not an acceptable target for fetal vascular access.

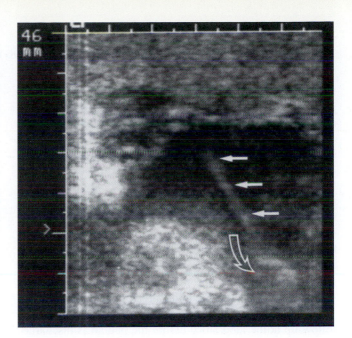

Figure 25–25. Backbleeding at 30 weeks of gestation. The pronounced jet of blood *(arrows)* ricochets off the fetal limb *(curved arrow)*. This fetus has a normal platelet count of 140,000, and backbleeding stopped after 50 s.

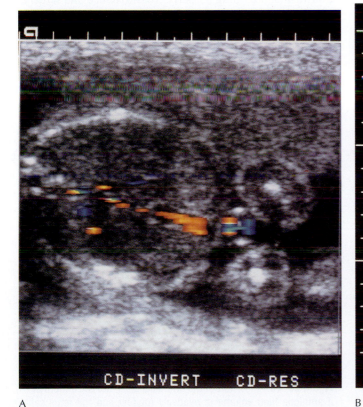

A

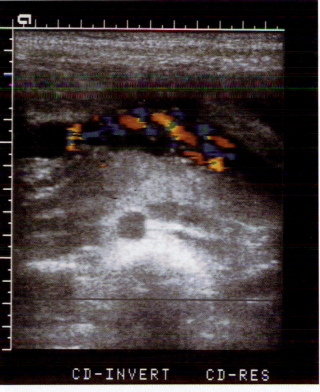

B

Figure 25–24. Alternate targets for cordocentesis or intravascular transfusion (IVT). **(A)** Abdominal umbilical cord insertion or intrahepatic portion of the umbilical vein *(red)*. **(B)** Ideal situation for use of free loop of cord for cordocentesis or IVT. There is a short, directly vertical approach to clearly seen individual vessels (umbilical vein, *red* here, is preferred), with the posterior placenta directly below providing a surface to pin the cord against.

701

ultrasonographer, noting that the rectangular vertical plane presented on the screen may not correspond to the tangential angled vantage point of the scan head from which the image is obtained. In addition, although the procedure is started with a lubricated needle with a stylet in place, the stylet is removed once the vessel is thought to be entered. If proper vessel entry is not achieved, *under no circumstances* should the stylet be reinserted. This would introduce microbubbles of air into the substance of the placenta, which are not dangerous but immediately obscure the target and cause acoustic shadowing below it. This is particularly true of the anterior placenta, but it may also complicate proper sampling in the posterior placenta. Pull the needle back from the target, reinsert the stylet, then advance again to the target.

Detailed testing is performed at the bedside and in follow-up at the laboratory before the patient is discharged after the procedure to confirm that the samples on which management is based are absolutely pure fetal blood.

Intravascular Fetal Transfusion[34,80,81]

Intravascular transfusion owes its existence to high-resolution ultrasonography. This procedure has proved lifesaving for fetuses previously out of the reach of intrauterine therapy. The procedure is indicated at any point in gestation when fetal anemia poses a danger to the fetus, and when extrauterine life is associated with significant risk of mortality or serious morbidity. The reasoning behind these indications has been alluded to previously and can be summarized as follows: gestation at or before 34 weeks, class 2 disease or greater or class 1 disease with a hemoglobin level below 120 g/L, and significant evidence of hemolysis. (Normally fetal hemoglobin increases linearly, from a mean of 110 g/L at 20 weeks to a mean of 150 g/L at 40 weeks; therefore, the value of 120 g/L may be quite normal at earlier gestations. It is intended merely as a general guideline. See Fig. 25–17 for the regression line of normal hemoglobin versus gestational age.)

If the placenta is anterior, the fetus will interfere very little with correct placement of the needle for sampling; thus, only light maternal sedation is given. If the cord insertion is posterior and the fetus is very vigorous or if the amniotic fluid not very generous, it is anticipated that the fetus will interfere with correct needle placement or dislodge it partway through the procedure. In that case, fairly heavy maternal sedation (morphine 5 mg IM with promethazine 25 mg IM) 1 hour before the onset of the procedure is given. Prophylactic antibiotics have not been studied in randomized fashion, but no fetus has died from chorioamnionitis in more than 1600 intrauterine transfusion procedures using our protocol.

The detailed fetal evaluation previously described is undertaken before sedation; the moribund hydropic fetus needs no sedation to remain motionless.

The cord site is carefully identified: an ideal target should be visualized before commencing. One might accept a less-than-ideal site if the needle needs to remain in the vessel

for only the few seconds needed for fetal blood sampling. In cases of IVT, however, an ideal target is needed, that is, one without significant threat of dislodgement by fetal movement, the excursion due to maternal respiratory movements, or the change in the uterine shape with uterine contractions.

If an excellent target site for IVT cannot be identified, there are several alternatives. Maternal repositioning may work, but often simply waiting 24 h and having the mother rest mainly in one lateral position will suffice. In the mature fetus with posterior cord, IPT (see following discussion) may be considered.

If indications to proceed are urgent (e.g., in hydropic disease), the fetal end of the cord should be considered (Fig. 25–26). All of the alternate sites considered for cordocentesis are also eligible for IVT *provided* a stable, clearly visualized portion of the umbilical vein is accessible. However, choosing an unsatisfactory target is *not* justified by severe fetal disease. The circulation of the hydropic fetus may tolerate only one attempt before vascular collapse. It is better to take "hours" to find a safe site than to exsanguinate the fetus to "give it a try." On rare occasions, the fetal heart may represent the only suitable target for use when urgent need is clear.

The IVT procedure used by our team is similar to that described for cordocentesis.[34] Preparation must be made for transfusion, providing properly cross-matched and screened, densely packed, maternally compatible, irradiated donor

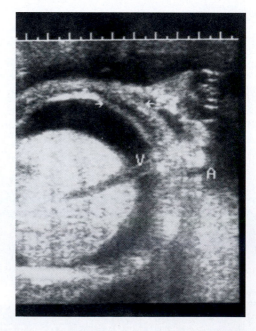

Figure 25–26. Insertion of the umbilical cord into the abdomen (A). If amniotic fluid volume is relatively modest and the fetus can be pinned against the lateral wall of the uterus, this may represent a stable target. This fetus has significant ascites and a thickened abdominal wall *(arrows)*. Intrahepatic portion of umbilical vein (V) has been the primary target in some techniques.

blood close to room temperature and ready for infusion at the bedside. Infusion is done through Y-tubing with a stopcock to allow filling and refilling of the 10-mL glass syringe. Because of the high density of the blood (280 g/L or greater) and the narrow lumen of the needle, significant pressure is necessary to infuse the blood. At early gestations, a 22-gauge needle is used, and at later gestations a 20-gauge spinal needle is used, depth permitting.

The ultrasonographer's role in this procedure is crucial. Not only must the needle be guided successfully to the target and a good vessel entry ensured, but every second of the infusion must be monitored by observation of continuous turbulence in the vessel being infused, as shown in Figure 25–27. In some cases, return may seem excellent but is of mixed maternal and fetal origin when the needle is not properly placed in the anterior placenta. In some hydropic fetuses, the blood is so thin, it looks exactly like blood-tinged amniotic fluid, so the ultrasonographer needs to be very careful in this situation before allowing either saline injection (to prove vessel cannulation) or needle movement (possibly out of the vessel). In other cases, needle placement in the vessel may be somewhat tenuous so that the downward pressure exerted each time the infusion is resumed causes the needle to penetrate the posterior vessel wall. The ultrasonographer must be particularly alert in identifying any interruptions in turbulence, noting that turbulence ceases immediately when infusion ceases. On occasion, turbulence may persist simply due to the presence of the needle in the lumen, even when the vessel is totally transfixed and infusion is out the other side of the cord into the amniotic fluid! The

point deserves emphasis: Only by observing continuous turbulence can the ultrasonographer permit continued infusion of blood.

The ultrasonographer must also monitor fetal heart rate, because bradycardia is frequently the first sign of complication in the procedure. This may signify the development of an intramural or extravascular hematoma within the cord substance, a potentially lethal complication if the hematoma is enlarged by continued infusion. Other cases of bradycardia seem to occur spontaneously, although they may be related to infusion of microbubbles, cold blood, rapid dilation of the right atrium, or irritation and spasm of the adjacent artery. Relative bradycardia may occur as a natural consequence of expansion of blood volume and is particularly notable in the mature fetus; establishing a normal baseline pre-procedure has obvious benefit.

One should be aware of the possibility of laceration of small placental vessels when the needle traverses the placenta. Transplacental needle passage occurs with an anterior placenta, with a target made anterior by maternal repositioning, or in the fundal placenta, where the needle must actually go through the placenta and then traverse the amniotic fluid to reach the fundal posterior cord. In such situations, the bleeding may not be dramatic, but it may occur simply as "streamers" or spaghetti-like strings of blood gradually settling downward in the fluid (Fig. 25–28). Only when there is significant pressure will blood form a jet, as seen with typical backbleeding after large volume transfusion. Rarely, fetal venous hypertension is so severe as to allow backbleeding with the needle still in place.

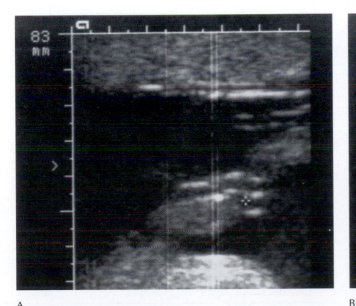
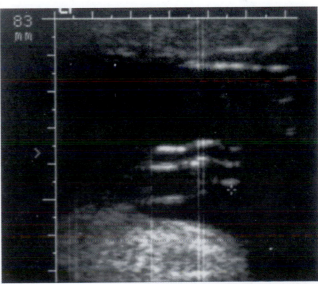

A   B

Figure 25–27. Intravenous turbulence must be observed continuously throughout the transfusion process. **(A)** Turbulence of the high-pressure injection of dense donor blood "lights up" the cord. **(B)** Equally important is the complete absence of turbulence when infusion is stopped while the syringe is refilled.

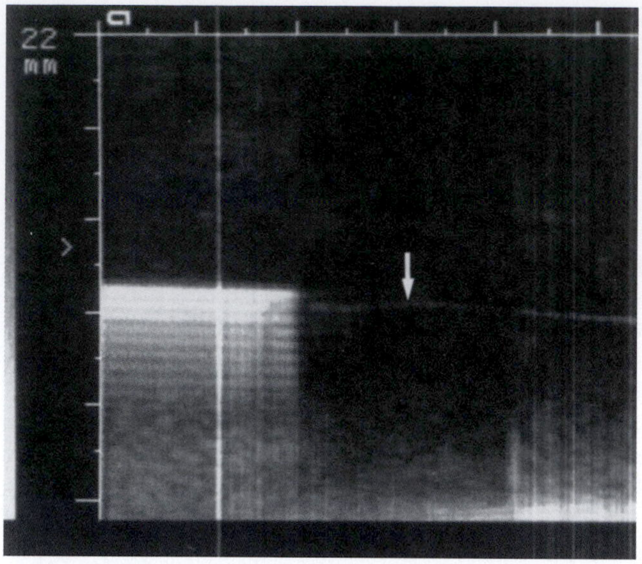

Figure 25–28. Waterbath experiment in which no pressure was exerted on the syringe, but the weight of the blood, elevated 5 cm above the 25-gauge needle, caused the minute leakage of blood, evident as a tiny stream *(arrow).* This simulates the bleeding observed from small placental vessels that have been damaged during transplacental procedures.

Hemorrhagic complications and a variety of miscellaneous problems have accounted for deaths in fetuses in classes 1 through 3, whereas the severity of fetal disease and maternal interference resulted in falure of class 4 fetuses to be resuscitated in the initial course of therapy (Table 25–5).

Overall, the results speak for themselves (Table 25–6). Comparable figures for IPT are displayed in Table 25–7.[82] At this point, it is no exaggeration to say that high-resolution ultrasonography provided the impetus for the development of fetal IVT, which has raised the possibility of a high frequency of intact survival in severe alloimmune disease from the theoretical to the practical realm. Longterm survival figures confirm the lifesaving nature of this advance: More than 90% of long-term hydropic survivors have normal neurologic outcome.[83–85]

TABLE 25–5. CAUSES OF DEATH WITH INTRAVASCULAR TRANSFUSIONS

Class	Deaths	GA (weeks)
1	Delayed F-M hemorrhage	29
	Nursery accident (non-IVT)	37
2	Abruptio (non-IVT)	36
	IVT hemorrhage	21
3	Delayed F-M hemorrhage	21
	IVT hemorrhage (2)	19, 22
	NND premature labor	25
4	No cardiac output (4)	20–25
	Maternal IV cocaine	20, 21
	NND premature labor	25

F-M, fetal–maternal; GA, gestational age; IV, intravenous; IVT, intravascular transfusion; NND, neonatal death.

TABLE 25–6. RESULTS WITH INTRAVASCUALR TRANSFUSION (IVT) 1986–1999

Fetuses treated	166
Transfusions	679
Overall survival	149 (90%)
Survivors/class 1[a]	96/98 (98%)
Survivors/classes 2–3	33/40 (83%)
Survivors/class 4	20/28 (71%)
Procedures total	717
Attempts/IVT	2.1
Failed procedures[b]	38

[a]Class assigned at first vascular access.
[b]Cordocentesis, not satisfactory for infusion = 28, no vascular access = 10. Twenty-seven fetuses were concerned.

Intraperitoneal Fetal Transfusion[34]

The use of IPT has shown a corresponding decline as IVT has expanded in application. The substantial improvement in performance of IPT due to enhanced ultrasonic visualization has ultimately given way to the advantages of IVT in many situations.[58] For example, in the past 14 years, we have used IPT only 8 times versus 657 IVT and 14 intracardiac transfusions. However, there are situations in which IPT may be advantageous or even essential.[86,87]

With careful application, IPT can deliver large volumes of donor blood with reasonable efficiency, safety, and potential for very good results (see Table 25–7). In general, the

TABLE 25–7. INTRAPERITONEAL TRANSFUSIONS AT THE UNIVERSITY OF MANITOBA, 1980–1986

Fetuses treated	75
Total procedures	202
Overall survival	57 (76%)
Survivors/class 1[a]	41/46 (89%)
Survivors/class 2–3	16/21 (76%)
Survivors/class 4	0/8 (0%)
Procedures total	216
Successful	202
Attempts/IPT	2.4
Failed procedures	14
Deaths	18
Trauma: Fetal	4
Neonatal	3
Moribund hydropic disease	8
Newborn complications[b]	3

Does not include 8 fetuses who had a single intraperitoneal transfusion (IPT) in the course of management with intravascular transfusion.
[a]Class assigned at first IPT.
[b]Hyaline membrane disease due to prematurity (2) and iatrogenic complications of exchange transfusion (1).

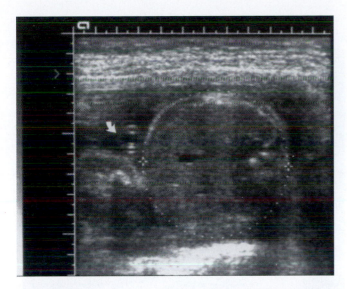

Figure 25–29. Ideal fetal position for intraperitoneal transfusion. Spine is lateral *(right caliper)*, the placenta is posterior *(bottom of image)*, and the cord *(arrow)* and limbs are in front of the fetus *(left caliper)*.

indications are the same as those for IVT, with additional provisos of posterior placenta, *nonhydropic disease,* and premature gestation. It follows that, because nonhydropic disease does not represent a fetal emergency, fetal position should be ideal (Fig. 25–29) or the procedure is deferred. *Transplacental* IPT is never indicated. In this circumstance, IVT should be performed.

With the fetus in a stable position lying on its side, a vertical approach is selected. The cord must be visualized in detail and avoided absolutely (if the abdominal insertion is prominent and available, an intravascular approach is suggested). Maternal sedation is given to reduce fetal movement. The fetus will almost always move vigorously as the needle enters the abdominal wall, so the approach must not be tangential to any degree. The ultrasonographer works in close tandem with the operator by guiding the needle to the fetal surface and attempting placement in the midanterior to lateral lower quadrant.

Traditional IPT calls for placement of a modified epidural catheter, inserted through a 16-gauge Tuohy needle.[46] This large needle undeniably causes significant pain and trauma, factors that encourage use of smaller bore needles without catheter placement.[88] In either case, after the firm thrust necessary to completely enter the fetal peritoneal cavity, the most important aspect of IPT ultrasound guidance takes place: Free intraperitoneal placement must be verified. To establish that the needle tip is free after the needle movement has stopped: 1) the catheter can be seen coiling within the fetal peritoneal cavity in large loops; 2) no aspirate can be removed (nonhydrops only; clear fluid under pressure equals fetal urine); 3) a small bubble of air (0.5 to 1.0 mL) injected alone or with 1 to 2 mL of agitated saline will rise freely to the top of the cavity; and 4) further agitated saline injected can be seen tracking freely within the cavity.

In the past, instillation of dye and x-ray confirmation was mandated. The criteria for ultrasonic confirmation are met unequivocally in 60 to 75% of cases. When they are not, a single flatplate abdominal film, demonstrating classic intraperitoneal contrast (outlining of the diaphragm and "semilunes" of dye between adjacent bowel loops are dependent on pooling of the dye), is required.[89]

Correct placement is confirmed as the transfusion mass is administered. Total volume of less than 50 mL may produce only suggestive changes, such as increased contrast of abdomen contents and double outlining without an overt fluid rim. Above this volume, progressive increase in width of fluid rim and development of a diaphragm blood-to-liver interface will become visible. In the larger fetus, this may not be evident until the end of the procedure (with more than 100 mL) or afterward, with distribution cephalad within the fetus. During the procedure, the fetal heart is visualized, and a rate is obtained with each 10-mL aliquot of densely packed donor blood. Tachycardia (stretch or pain response) is frequent; bradycardia (intrahepatic umbilical vein compression) calls for a pause in the infusion. If bradycardia is persistent, the procedure is terminated.[63]

The precise role of IPT in overall management of severe Rh disease has not been completely defined.[82,90] Some teams have converted to a combination of IPT and IVT,[87] whereas others have abandoned IPT altogether.[91] Our use is limited, but we do continue to use IPT with confidence, especially as the final procedure (at 33 to 35 weeks of gestation) when the large fetus covers a posterior cord insertion.

Intracardiac Fetal Transfusion[34]

As illustrated by the losses presented in Table 25–5, fetal exsanguination is a significant cause of mortality complicating severe, early disease treated with IVT. In such a critical situation, only seconds exist in which resuscitation by reinserting the needle in a fetal vessel is possible. Afterward, vascular collapse makes this route impossible, and fetal demise is likely. Intracardiac transfusion (ICT) in these circumstances is a desperate, sometimes lifesaving, maneuver. Under other even rarer circumstances, ICT may be the only available approach in very early hydropic disease before 18 weeks of gestation or very severe disease after IVT has failed due to severe placental edema and fetal position.

We have used ICT in 13 fetuses on 14 occasions, all but 4 of these in exsanguination following IVT. The majority had class 4 disease at less than 22 weeks (11 of 13 fetuses). On 10 of 14 occasions, the fetus survived the acute event due to successful intracardiac resuscitation. Westgren et al.[92] also had limited success with this approach, mainly in similar circumstances. At present, there are no large series reporting use in nonextreme situations.

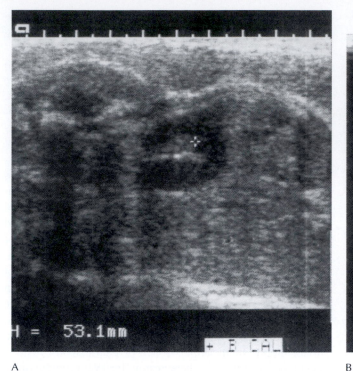

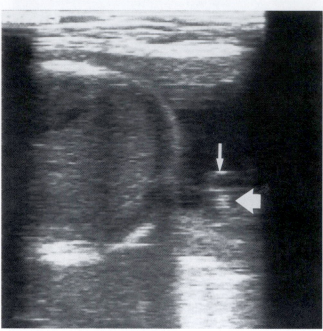

A

B

Figure 25–30. Intracardiac fetal transfusion (ICT). **(A)** Infusion of blood in right ventricle produces typical turbulence *(caliper)* during ICT. **(B)** Turbulence may also be documented in umbilical arteries *(large arrow)*, proving that the transfused blood has entered the fetal circulation, and illustrating fetal cardiac output. Note there is no turbulence in the umbilical vein *(small arrow)* above the arteries in this loop of cord.

Technically ICT is straightforward. A 20-gauge needle is used, because the increased rigidity allows steering of the needle while it is within the fetal chest. The needle is aimed for the right side of the anterior chest, if possible. Although the right ventricle is favored, one accepts any direct access available in such dire circumstances. Turbulence during infusion is as critical in ICT as it is in IVT, and it is visible in the chamber cavity and in distal arteries (Fig. 25–30). The intent is resuscitation, not comprehensive therapy, so that a much smaller volume is given. The moribund condition of the exsanguinated fetus, the damage incurred during profound hypotension, the large pericardial effusions that may already be present, and hemopericardium during the procedure may all prove lethal in these situations.

Because all class 3 or 4 fetuses are at risk for thrombocytopenia, vessel wall edema, or both, they may be at risk for exsanguinating hemorrhage at IVT.[34,55] Therefore, in the preparation for IVT, the ultrasonographer should also identify the route to the fetal heart in case ICT becomes necessary.

Posttransfusion Monitoring

Ultrasound monitoring of fetal structural and functional indices is imperative in the posttransfusion period, and the ultrasonographer is key. Recovery from paralytic agents may confound fetal assessment,[93] another reason not to "paralyze" the moribund hydrops, because recovery of biophysi-

cal variables is a fundamental indicator of the success of the treatment.[51] Recovery of normal fetal behavior (BPS of 8/8 or 10/10) after transfusion is almost always an indicator of normal, stable fetal respiratory status.

With IPT, serial observations will show resolution of the intraperitoneal fluid mass, usually 4 to 8 days after the procedure. Failure of diminution by 5 days suggests impaired absorption, possibly with onset of hydrops. Fetal vascular access should then be sought. In either case, therapeutic effect is not guaranteed by an apparently satisfactory procedure. Backbleeding, hemolysis of donor blood, mistaken placement, or very accelerated fetal disease may supervene.

With hydropic disease, because IVT is now the only recommended approach, there is no longer a question of worsening hydrops versus nonabsortion. Ascites reverses relative to the stage of disease. In class 2, the ascites may disappear within 7 to 10 days; in class 3 or 4, it may be 5 weeks or more before every vestige of ascites and pericardial effusion has resolved. In this situation, BPS provides essential reassurance. If it is not proceeding promptly and fetal vascular access is not available, delivery may be indicated.

After ICT, in addition to the functional demonstration of fetal recovery by BPS, fetal cardiac function is evaluated. A significant post-ICT pericardial effusion is not uncommon and may take 8 to 10 days to resolve in the otherwise healthy fetus. Ultrasound confirmation of fetal well-being is the most important aspect of monitoring between the frequent serial procedures required by such fetuses. When done by the same ultrasound observer and using the range of parameters described, serial examinations can provide an accurate evaluation of therapeutic response. The exact timing of the next procedure depends on the class of disease, gestational age, and the hemoglobin level achieved with the transfusion. That timetable being set, deterioration, failure of ongoing improvements, or an abnormal BPS (less than or equal to 6/10) would call for advancement. Thus, the fetus is monitored both for immediate welfare (BPS) and structural changes indicating onset or persistence of severe disease. Biophysical profile scoring is performed 24 h postprocedure and then at a frequency appropriate to the severity of fetal disease (once per week to as often as once per day) until the next procedure. Interval cordocentesis, without transfusion, is required occasionally, if ultrasound findings are equivocal.

SUMMARY

Detailed ultrasound visualization and Doppler velocimetry of the fetus affected with alloimmune disease form the basis of intrauterine investigation and delivery of therapy. Ultrasound has provided key ingredients in the development and enhancement of invasive fetal testing and innovative fetal treatment. With the high-resolution instruments now available, a systematic approach to the sensitized pregnant patient offers the promise of early and complete detection and evaluation and of intact fetal survival even when disease is worst. Intravascular monitoring and transfusion have demonstrated clear benefits over the relatively short time they have been used, and more precise application may now be possible through the use of ultrasound and Doppler in predicting anemia. The continuing role of preventive measures, many of them associated with ultrasound-facilitated care, deserves further emphasis.

REFERENCES

1. Bowman JM. Maternal blood group immunization. In: Creasy RK, Resnik R, eds. *Maternal–Fetal Medicine: Principles and Practice*, 2nd ed. Philadelphia: Saunders; 1989:613–649.
2. Bowman JM, Pollock JM, Manning FA, et al. Maternal Kell blood group alloimmunization. *Obstet Gynecol.* 1992;79:239–244.
3. Bowman PJ, Brown SE, Inskip MJ. The significance of anti-C alloimmunization in pregnancy. *Br J Obstet Gynaecol.* 198;693:1044–1048.
4. Bowman JM, Pollock JM, Manning FA, et al. Severe anti-C hemolytic disease of the newborn. *Am J Obstet Gynecol.* 1992;166:1239–1243.
5. Bowman JM, Harman CR, Manning FA, et al. Severe erythroblastosis fetalis produced by anti-cellano. *Box Sang.* 1989;56:187–189.
6. Harman CR, Manning FA. Alloimmune disease. In: Pauerstein CJ, ed. *Clinical Obstetrics.* New York: Wiley; 1987:441–469.
7. Paoloni-Giacobino A, Dutoit MH, Morris MA, Dahoun SP. A proven case of materno-foetal transfusion determined by cytogenetic and DNA analysis. *Clin Genet.* 1999;55:256–258.
8. Vaughan JI, Manning M, Warwick RM, et al. Inhibition of erythroid progenitor cells by anti-Kell antibodies in fetal alloimmune anemia. *N Engl J Med.* 1998;338:798–803.
9. Bowman JM. Blood group immunization in obstetric practice. *Curr Probl Obstet Gynecol.* 1983;7:1.
10. Urbaniak SJ. The scientific basis of antenatal prophylaxis. *Br J Obstet Gynaecol.* 1998;105 (suppl 18):11–18.
11. Hartwell EA. Use of Rh immune globulin: ASCP practice parameter. *Am J Clin Pathol.* 1998;110:281–292.
12. Bowman JM, Pollock JM. Transplacental fetal hemorrhage after amniocentesis. *Obstet Gynecol.* 1985;66:749–754.
13. Blakemore KJ, Baumgarten A, Schoenfeld-Dimaio M, et al. Rise in maternal serum α-fetoprotein concentration after chorionic villus sampling and the possibility of isoimmunization. *Am J Obstet Gynecol.* 1986;155:988–993.
14. Jansen MW, Brandenburg H, Wilschut HI, et al. The effect of chorionic villus sampling on the number of fetal cells isolated from maternal blood and on maternal serum alpha-fetoprotein levels. *Prenat Diagn.* 1997;10:953–959.
15. Bowman JM, Pollock JM, Peterson LE, et al. Fetomaternal hemorrhage following funipuncture: Increase in severity of maternal red cell alloimmunization. *Obstet Gynecol.* 1994;84:839–843.
16. Bennett PR, Le Van KC, Colin Y, et al. Prenatal determination of fetal RhD type by DNA amplication. *N Engl J Med.* 1993;329:607–610.
17. Lee S, Bennett PR, Overton T, Warwick R, et al. Prenatal diagnosis of Kell blood group genotypes: KEL1 and KEL2. *Am J Obstet Gynecol.* 1996;175:455–459.
18. Nicolaides KH, Rodeck CH, Mibashan RS, et al. Have Liley charts outlived their usefulness? *Am J Obstet Gynecol.* 1986;155:90.
19. Rahman F, Detti L, Ozcan T, et al. Can a single measurement of amniotic fluid delta optical density be safely used in the clinical management of Rhesus-alloimmunized pregnancies before 27 weeks' gestation? *Acta Obstet Gynecol Scand.* 1998;77:804–807.
20. Harman CR, Bowman JM, Menticoglou SM, et al. Ultrasound classification of fetal alloimmune disease. Correlation with fetal hematology (abstract 19). Proceeding of the Society for Perinatal Obstetrics, New Orleans, February 1989.
21. Reece EA, Copel JA, Scioscia AL, et al. Diagnostic fetal umbilical blood sampling in the management of isoimmunization. *Am J Obstet Gynecol.* 1988;159:1059–1062.
22. Spinnato JA. Hemolytic disease of the fetus: A plea for restraint. *Obstet Gynecol.* 1992;80:873–877.
23. Weiner CP. Hemolytic disease of the fetus (letter). *Am J Obstet Gynecol.* 1992;166:1590.
24. Bowman JM, Pollock J, Menticoglou S, et al. Hemolytic disease of the fetus: A plea for restraint. *Obstet Gynecol.* 1993;81:478.
25. Spinnato JA, Clark AL, Ralston KK, et al. Hemolytic disease of the fetus: A comparison of the Queenan and extended Liley methods. *Obstet Gynecol.* 1998;92:441–445.
26. Harman CR. Comprehensive examination of the fetus. *Fetal Med Rev.* 1989;1:125–176.
27. Egberts J, van den Bosch N, Soederhuizen P. Amniotic fluid

nitric oxide metabolites, cyclic guanosine 3′,5′ monophosphate and dimethylarginine in alloimmunized pregnancies. *Eur J Obstet Gynecol Reprod Biol.* 1999;85:209–214.

28. Harman CR. Specialized applications of obstetric ultrasound: Management of the alloimmunized pregnancy. *Semin Perinatol.* 1985;9:184.

29. Nicolaides KH, Fontanarosa M, Gabbe SG, et al. Failure of ultrasonographic parameters to predict the severity of fetal anemia in rhesus isoimmunization. *Am J Obstet Gynecol.* 1988; 158:920.

30. Harman CR, Bowman JM, Manning FA, et al. Moribund alloimmune hydrops: Intravascular fetal transfusion is the only hope. Proceedings of the Society for Obstetrics and Gynecology, Vancouver, BC, June 1988.

31. Bakos O, Ewald U, Lindgren PG. Fetal cardiocentesis in care of severe Kell immunisation. *Fetal Diagn Ther.* 1998;13: 372–374.

32. Harman CR. Fetal monitoring in the alloimmunized pregnancy. In: Smith MK, ed. *Clinics in Perinatology.* Philadelphia: Saunders; 1989.

33. Nicolaides KH, Warenski JC, Rodeck CH. The relationship of fetal plasma protein concentration and hemoglobin level to the development of hydrops in rhesus isoimmunization. *Am J Obstet Gynecol.* 1985;152:341–344.

34. Harman CR. Invasive techniques in management of alloimmune anemia. In: Harman CR, ed. *Invasive Fetal Testing and Treatment.* Cambridge: Blackwell Scientific Publications; 1995:107–191.

35. Hadlock FP, Deter RL, Harrist RB, et al. Estimating fetal age: Computer-assisted analysis of multiple fetal growth parameters. *Radiology.* 1984;152:497–501.

36. Benacerraf BR, Frigoletto FD. Sonographic sign for the detection of early fetal ascites in the management of severe isoimmune disease without intrauterine transfusion. *Am J Obstet Gynecol.* 1985;152:1039–1041.

37. Ulm B, Svolba G, Ulm MR, et al. Male fetuses are particularly affected by maternal alloimmunization to D antigen. *Transfusion.* 1999;39:169–173.

38. Hashimoto BE, Filly RA, Callen PW. Fetal pseudoascites: Further anatomic observations. *J Ultrasound Med.* 1986;5:151.

39. DeVore GR. The prenatal diagnosis of congenital heart disease: A practical approach for the fetal sonographer. *J Clin Ultrasound.* 1985;13:229–245.

40. DeVore GR, Donnerstein RI, Kleinman CS, et al. Fetal echocardiography. II: The diagnosis and significance of a pericardial effusion in the fetus using real-time directed M-mode ultrasound. *Am J Obstet Gynecol.* 1982;144:693–701.

41. Copel JA, Grannum PA, Green JJ, et al. Fetal cardiac output in the isoimmunized pregnancy: A plused Doppler-echocardiographic study of patients undergoing intravascular intrauterine transfusion. *Am J Obstet Gynecol.* 1989;161: 361–365.

42. Hudson I, Cooke A, Holland B, Houston A, Jones JG, Turner T, Wardrop CA. Red cell volume and cardiac output in anaemic preterm infants. *Arch Dis Child.* 1990;65:672–675.

43. Ouzounian JG, Monteiro HA, Alsulyman OM, Songster GS. Ultrasonographic fetal cardiac measurement in isoimmunized pregnancies. *J Reprod Med.* 1998;105:567.

44. Oberhoffer R, Grab D, Keckstein J, et al. Cardiac changes in fetuses secondary to immune hemolytic anemia and their rela-

tion to hemoglobin and catecholamine concentrations in fetal blood. *Ultrasound Obstet Gynecol.* 1999;13:396–400.

45. Baschat AA, Harman CR, Alger LS, Weiner CP. Fetal coronary and cerebral blood flow in acute fetomaternal hemorrhage. *Ultrasound Obstet Gynecol.* 1998;12:128–131.

46. Harman CR, Bowman JM. Intraperitoneal fetal transfusion. In: Chervenak F, Issacson G, Campbell S, eds. *Textbook of Ultrasound in Obstetrics and Gynecology.* Boston: Little, Brown;1993.

47. Vintzileos AM, Cambell WA, Storlazzi E, et al. Fetal liver ultrasound measurements in isoimmunized pregnancies. *Obstet Gynecol.* 1986;68:162–167.

48. Bahado-Singh R, Oz U, Mari G, et al. Fetal splenic size in anemia due to Rh-alloimmunization. *Obstet Gynecol.* 1998;92: 828–832.

49. Manning FA, Menticoglou S, Harman CR, et al. Antepartum fetal risk assessment: The role of the fetal biophysical profile score. *Bailliere Clin Obstet Gynecol.* 1987;1:55–72.

50. Harman CR, Manning FA, Bowman JM, et al. Use of intravascular transfusion to treat hydrops fetalis in a moribund fetus. *Can Med Assoc J.* 1988;138:827–830.

51. Harman CR, Menticoglou SM, Manning FA. Fetal biophysical variables and fetal status. In: Maulik D, ed. *Asphyxia and Brain Damage.* New York: Wiley-Liss, 1998:279–320.

52. Menticoglou SM, Harman Cr, Manning FA, et al. Intraperitoneal fetal transfusion: Paralysis inhibits red cell absorption. *Fetal Ther.* 1987;2:154–159.

53. Manning FA, Snijders R, Harman CR, et al. Fetal biophysical profile score. VI: Correlation with antepartum umbilical venous fetal pH. *Am J Obstet Gynecol.* 1993;169:755–763.

54. Chitkara U, Wilkins I, Lynch L, et al. The role of sonography in assessing severity of fetal anemia in Rh- and Kell-isoimmunized pregnancies. *Obstet Gynecol.* 1988;71:393–398.

55. Harman CR, Bowman JM, Menticoglou SM, et al. Profound fetal thrombocytopenia in rhesus disease: Serious hazard at intravascular transfusion. *Lancet.* 1988;2:741–742.

56. DeVore GR, Mayden K, Tortora M, et al. Dilatation of the fetal umbilical vein in rhesus hemolytic anemia: A predictor of severe disease. *Am J Obstet Gynecol.* 1981;141:464.

57. Witter FR, Graham D. The utility of ultrasonically measured umbilical vein diameter in isoimmunized pregnancies. *Am J Obstet Gynecol.* 1983;146:225.

58. Reece EA, Gabrielli S, Abdalla M, et al. Reassessment of the utility of fetal umbilical vein diameter in the management of isoimmunization. *Am J Obstet Gynecol.* 1988;159:937–938.

59. Hecher K, Snijders R, Campbell S, Nicolaides K. Fetal venous, arterial, and intracardiac blood flows in red blood cell isoimmunization. *Obstet Gynecol.* 1995;85:122–128.

60. Rightmire DA, Nicolaides KH, Rodeck CH, et al. Fetal blood velocities in Rh isoimmunization: Relationship to gestational age and to fetal hematocrit. *Obstet Gynecol.* 1986;68:233–236.

61. Steiner H, Schaffer H, Spitzer D, et al. The relationship between peak velocity in the fetal descending aorta and hematocrit in rhesus isoimmunization. *Obstet Gynecol.* 1995;85(5, Pt 1):659–662.

62. Vyas S, Nicolaides KH, Campbell S. Doppler examination of the middle cerebral artery in anemic fetuses. *Am J Obstet Gynecol.* 1990;162:1066–1068.

63. Mari G, Moise KJ Jr, Deter RL, Carpenter RJ Jr. Flow velocity waveforms of the umbilical and cerebral arteries before

and after intravascular transfusion. *Obstet Gynecol.* 1990;75: 584–589.

64. Mari G, Adrignolo A, Abuhamad AZ, et al. Diagnosis of fetal anemia with Doppler ultrasound in the pregnancy complicated by maternal blood group immunization. *Ultrasound Obstet Gynecol.* 1995;5:400–405.

65. Oepkes D, Vandenbussche FP, Van Bel F, Kanhai HH. Fetal ductus venosus blood flow velocities before and after transfusion in red-cell alloimmunized pregnancies. *Obstet Gynecol.* 1993;82:237–241.

66. D'Ancona RL, Rahman F, Ozcan T, et al. The effect of intravascular blood transfusion on the flow velocity waveform of the portal venous system of the anemic fetus. *Ultrasound Obstet Gynecol.* 1997;10:333–337.

67. Mari G, Moise KJ Jr, Deter RL, et al. Flow velocity waveforms of the vascular system in the anemic fetus before and after intravascular transfusion for severe red blood cell alloimmunization. *Am J Obstet Gynecol.* 1990;162:1060–1064.

68. Copel JA, Grannum PA, Belanger K, et al. Pulsed Doppler flow-velocity waveforms before and after intrauterine intravascular transfusion for severe erythroblastosis fetalis. *Am J Obstet Gynecol.* 1988;158:768–774.

69. Nicolaides KH, Bilardo CM, Campbell S. Prediction of fetal anemia by measurement of the mean blood velocity in the fetal aorta. *Am J Obstet Gynecol.* 1990;162:209–212.

70. Oepkes D, Brand R, Vandenbussche FP, et al. The use of ultrasonography and Doppler in the prediction of fetal haemolytic anaemia: A multivariate analysis. *Br J Obstet Gynaecol.* 1994; 101:680–684.

71. Iskaros J, Kingdom J, Morrison JJ, Rodeck C. Prospective non-invasive monitoring of pregnancies complicated by red cell alloimmunization. *Ultrasound Obstet Gynecol.* 1998;11: 432–437.

72. Mari G, Deter RL, Carpenter RL, et al. Noninvasive diagnosis by Doppler ultrasonography of fetal anemia due to maternal red-cell alloimmunization. *N Engl J Med.* 2000;342:9–14.

73. Saade GR. Noninvasive testing for fetal anemia. *N Engl J Med.* 2000;342:52–53.

74. Legarth J, Lingman G, Stangenberg M, Rahman F. Umbilical artery Doppler flow-velocity waveforms and fetal acid–base balance in Rhesus-isoimmunized pregnancies. *J Clin Ultrasound.* 1994;22:37–41.

75. Onderoglu L. A new splenic artery Doppler velocimetric index for prediction of severe fetal anemia associated with Rh alloimmunization. *Am J Obstet Gynecol.* 1999;180(1, Pt 1): 49–54.

76. Mari G, Rahman F, Olofsson P, et al. Increase of fetal hematocrit decreases the middle cerebral artery peak systolic velocity in pregnancies complicated by rhesus alloimmunization. *J Matern Fetal Med.* 1997;6:206–208.

77. Pollock JM, Bowman JM, Manning FA, et al. Fetal blood sampling in Rh hemolytic disease. *Vox Sang.* 1987;53:139–142.

78. Nicolini U, Santolaya J, Ojo OE, et al. The fetal intrahepatic umbilical vein as an alternative to cord needling for prenatal diagnosis and therapy. *Prenat Diagn.* 1988;8:665–671.

79. Harman CR. Fetal blood sampling. In: Creasy R, Resnick R, eds. *Fetal–Maternal Medicine.* Philadelphia: WB Saunders; 1998.

80. DeCrespigny LCH, Robinson HP, Quinn M, et al. Ultrasound-guided fetal blood transfusion for severe rhesus isoimmunization. *Obstet Gynecol.* 1985;66:529.

81. Nicolaides KH, Soothill PW, Clewell W, et al. Rh disease: Intravascular fetal blood transfusion by cordocentesis. *Fetal Ther.* 1986;1:185.

82. Harman CR, Bowman JM, Manning FA, et al. Intrauterine transfusion—Intraperitoneal versus intravascular approach: A case-control comparison. *Am J Obstet Gynecol.* 1990;1672: 1053–1059.

83. Janssens HM, de Haan MJ, van Kamp IL, et al. Outcome for children treated with fetal intravascular transfusions because of severe blood group antagonism. *J Pediatr.* 1997;131:373–380.

84. Hudon L, Moise KJ Jr, Hegemier SE, et al. Long-term neurodevelopmental outcome after intrauterine transfusion for the treatment of fetal hemolytic disease. *Am J Obstet Gynecol.* 1998;179:858–863.

85. Grab D, Paulus WE, Bommer A, et al. Treatment of fetal erythroblastosis by intravascular transfusions: Outcome at 6 years. *Obstet Gynecol.* 1999;93:165–168.

86. Watts DH, Lathy DA, Benedetti TJ, et al. Intraperitoneal fetal transfusion under direct ultrasound guidance. *Obstet Gynecol.* 1988;71:84.

87. Moise KH, Carpenter RJ Jr, Kirshon B, et al. Comparison of four types of intrauterine transfusion technique for the treatment of red cell alloimmunization (abstract 187). Proceedings of the Society for Perinatal Obstetrics, New Orleans, February 1989.

88. Barss VA, Benacerraf BR, Greene MF, et al. Use of a small-gauge needle for intrauterine fetal transfusions. *Am J Obstet Gynecol.* 1986;155:1057–1058.

89. Harman CR, Menticoglou SM, Bowman JM, et al. Current technique of intraperitoneal transfusion: Do not throw away the Renografin. *Fetal Ther.* 1989;4:78–82.

90. Harman CR, Manning FA, Bowman JM, et al. Severe Rh disease—Poor outcome is not inevitable. *Am J Obstet Gynecol.* 1983;145:823–829.

91. Poissonnier M-H, Brossard Y, Demedeiros N, et al. Two hundred intrauterine exchange transfusions in severe blood incompatibilities. *Am J Obstet Gynecol.* 1989;161:709–713.

92. Westgren M, Selbing A, Stangenberg M. Fetal intracardiac transfusions in patients with severe rhesus isoimmunization. *Br Med J.* 1988;296:885–886.

93. Mouw RJ, Klumper F, Hermans J, et al. Effect of atracurium or pancuronium on the anemic fetus during and directly after intravascular intrauterine transfusion. A double blind randomized study. *Acta Obstet Gynecol Scand.* 1999;78: 763–767.

26

Fetal Biophysical Profile Score:

Theoretical Consideration and Practical Application

Frank A. Manning

The development of objective clinical methods for the detection of the fetus at risk for death or damage *in utero* began in earnest only in the past few decades. The initial forays were in the measurement of endocrine products released by the placenta into the maternal circulation. A wide range of compounds, including placental enzymes (alkaline phosphatase, leucine amino-peptidase), placental specific hormones (placental lactogen), and placental conversion products (estriols, estetrol), were studied. For most there was a relation to fetal outcome, but none of these measures had the necessary accuracy to become a useful adjunct to clinical management. In the early 1960s two clinical investigative teams, one headed by Hon in Yale, the other by Caldero-Barcia in Uruguay, reported methods for continuous recording of the fetal heart rate.[1,2] This innovation ushered in the contemporary era of fetal evaluation based on dynamic biophysical monitoring. Although designed for the intrapartum period, the application of heart rate monitoring in the antepartum period was quickly realized, and a generation of tests based on heart rate responses to contractions (the contraction stress test), fetal movements (the nonstress test [NST]), or both came into vogue[3] and quickly supplanted the biochemical tests. In the late 1960s two groups, those of Dawes in Oxford and Tchobroutsky in Paris, reported fetal breathing

movements as a normal characteristic of intrauterine life.[3,4] Dawes and colleagues in a series of elegant experiments in the chronic fetal lamb preparation were able to demonstrate an exquisite sensitivity of the fetal respiratory center to experimental hypoxemia,[5] thereby creating interest in the potential of this measurement in predicting human fetal compromise. The clinical application of these observations was thwarted by the inability to record human fetal breathing accurately.

In the mid-1970s a revolutionary clinical tool, dynamic real-time B-mode ultrasound, became available. Through this method observation of a broad range of dynamic fetal biophysical activities became clinically facile. From the outset of clinical testing it was evident that observation of the presence or absence of breathing movements in the human fetus was as predictive as the NST[6] was useful in the differentiation of true-positive and false-positive contraction stress test results[7] and, when combined with heart rate test, yielded a better prediction than any single test.[8] Further, it became evident that objective recording of gross body movements was predictive of fetal health and disease[9] and that, when combined with other biophysical variables, predictive accuracy was improved. The preliminary observations provided a first insight into a fundamental tenet of antepartum risk assessment: *the predictive accuracy of fetal testing methods improves as more fetal variables are considered.* Even from what would be crude ultrasound images by today's standards, it was patently evident that the wealth of fetal information that could be assessed was vast and included a wide spectrum of acutely dynamic biophysical activities, ranging from gross body movements to fine finger control, an objective means of determining the presence (or lack of) and distribution of amniotic fluid, a detailed measurement of fetal structures (morphometrics), and an evaluation of the organ system's structural and functional integrity (morphology). From these observations arose the now entrenched concept of composite fetal assessment. The fetal biophysical profile scoring method emerged from this rich clinical milieu as a means of integration of dynamic biophysical activities into a workable clinical format.[10] As from the inception it remains *critical today to interpret the results of the biophysical profile score (BPS) within the context of all the information concurrently rendered accessible by dynamic ultrasound fetal imaging.*

It is the intent of this chapter to review the clinical role of the fetal BPS in the prediction and prevention of perinatal mortality, perinatal morbidity as reflected by antenatal acidosis, immediate neonatal compromise, and longterm sequelae and to review application of the testing method to discrete at-risk pregnancy categories.

FETAL ADAPTIVE RESPONSES TO ACUTE AND CHRONIC HYPOXEMIA OR ACIDEMIA

Whereas in the majority of high-risk pregnancies there are either no or minimal noxious fetal consequences, in a small percentage, estimated to be in the range of 2 to 3% based on our large clinical trials of more than 82,000 referrals, the fetus will be exposed to potentially damaging or even lethal interruptions in placental respiratory function. Unable to extricate itself from this hostile environment the mammalian fetus has evolved remarkable protective compensatory mechanisms. It is these adaptations to hypoxemia and acidemia (asphyxia) that result in the deviation from normal of the components of the BPS. In response to acute hypoxemia, for example, as may occur with fulminant preeclampsia or abruption, the fetus ceases all acute biophysical activities nonessential to immediate survival: the fetus will stop moving and breathing and will lose flexor tone. In the fetal lamb, abolition of all skeletal muscle activity, as induced by pharmacologic footplate blockade (e.g., gallamine), produces an immediate reduction in oxygen consumption by up to 17% and yields a rise in fetal PO_2.[11] In the human fetus, we have observed a similar effect: In alloimmune anemic fetuses undergoing intravascular transfusion, the measured PO_2 in venous blood increases after pancuronium blockade.[12] This adaptive response is mediated by acute tissue hypoxia in central nervous system neurons that initiate the discrete biophysical activities (Fig. 26–1). Evidence of this adaptive response in high-risk human fetuses is demonstrated by

antenatal venous cord blood analysis. For each of the individual acute biophysical variables, the mean pH was always significantly higher when the activity was observed than when the activity was absent (Fig. 26–2).[13] Further, there appears to be a differential sensitivity between these acute variables: The NST and fetal breathing movements were absent with the least decline in pH, whereas larger falls were observed before fetal body movement and tone became abnormal. The animal fetus with mild to moderate sustained stable nonacidemic hypoxemia may exhibit the return of acute biophysical activities, albeit at a lower frequency.[14] The physiologic basis for this partial recovery is complex and involves such factors as increased oxygen-carrying capacity, improved oxygen extraction, resetting of receptor thresholds, and increased cerebral blood flow. Thus, the BPS is a coreflection of tissue hypoxemia but may not predict circulating PO_2. The statistically significant but clinically poor correlation between the fetal BPS and antenatal venous PO_2 confirms this explanation.[14] It is of clinical importance to note that progressive hypoxemia, acidemic hypoxemia (asphyxia), or both have not been associated with reemergence of acute biophysical variables in either animal or human fetuses.

The fetus has a second adaptive response to hypoxemia, which is the aortic arch chemoreceptor reflex redistribution of cardiac output. This reflex, which probably requires either more severe hypoxemia or acidemia to be triggered, results in preferential shunting of blood flow away from all nonessential organs to essential organs (the heart, brain, placenta, and adrenals).[15] The measurable clinical effect manifest over days is oliguric oligohydramnios and over weeks is intrauterine growth restriction (IUGR). This reflex accounts for an important principle of fetal assessment by the BPS, which is that *in the presence of intact membranes and a functional genitourinary tract oligohydramnios is near certain presumptive evidence of fetal compromise.* Although exceptions to this clinical dictum may occur, they must be exceedingly rare because our group has yet to identify one in more than 160,000 tests.

The time differential between the immediate adaptive response to hypoxemia, acidemia (loss of acute biophysical variables), or both and the delayed reflex response (oliguric oligohydramnios) permits an assessment of the chronicity of the insult. The differential sensitivity of the regulatory centers provides some insight into the severity of the insult. These two components are critical to the testing frequency and interpretation in specific risk categories. Thus, for example, in clinical circumstances in which fetal compromise is apt to be sudden (e.g., insulin-dependent diabetes), testing is frequent (twice weekly) with an emphasis on acute biophysical variables. In other conditions where fetal compromise is rapidly progressive, as, for example, with severe alloimmune anemia, testing may occur very frequently (daily or twice daily), with emphasis on the acute variables, and continue until treatment (intravascular transfusion) restores normal oxygen-carrying

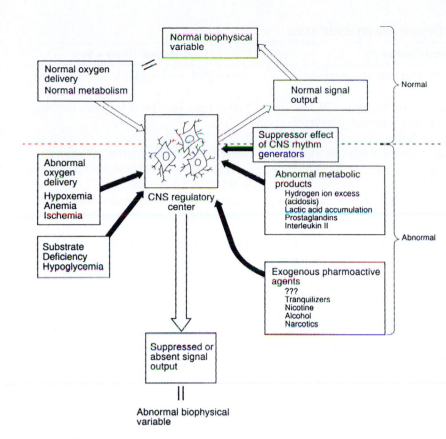

Figure 26–1. A schematic of the factors, both normal and pathologic and both intrinsic and extrinsic, that modulate dynamic fetal biophysical activities. The observation of a normal given biophysical activity is strong presumptive evidence that the central nervous system (CNS) regulatory neurons are not hypoxic. In contrast, the failure to observe a variable necessitates a differential diagnosis. *(Reproduced with permission from Manning FA, ed. Fetal Medicine: Principles and Practice. Norwalk, CT: Appleton & Lange; 1995.)*

capacity. With indolent progressive placental failure, as may occur in the postdate pregnancy, the focus of biophysical scoring is to detect evidence of chronic adaptation (oligohydramnios), the superimposition of acute on chronic hypoxemia (loss of some or all acute variables), or both. Because the rate of deterioration in these circumstances may be rapid, the testing interval is shortened to at least twice weekly. It is likely that, as our understanding of the pathophysiology of other abnormal fetal conditions improves, the frequency and emphasis of fetal biophysical profile scoring will be altered.

FETAL BIOPHYSICAL PROFILE SCORE: METHOD AND MODIFICATION

The original method of fetal biophysical profile scoring was based on a composite assessment of five variables: fetal breathing, gross body movements, tone, heart rate acceleration with fetal movement (NST), and semiquantitative amniotic fluid volume as measured by the ventricle diameter of the largest pocket. Each of these variables, with the exception of fetal tone, had been evaluated in separate studies, and the norms and predictive accuracies determined.[6,16,17] Based on cumulative experience we introduced modification of the original criteria; the definition of oligohydramnios was increased from a pocket of 1 cm to a pocket of 2 cm,[18] and the definition of fetal tone was advanced to

include the dynamics of opening and closing of the fetal hand and the nondynamics of sustained closure in the absence of active movement.[19] The contemporary criteria for interpretation of the BPS variable are given in Table 26–1. In a subsequent modification, based on a prospective study, we excluded the result of the NST in those fetuses in whom the other dynamic ultrasound-monitored variables were normal.[20] This modification yielded a new score category of 8/8.

Additional modifications have been proposed by other investigators. Phelan and coworkers modified the determination of amniotic fluid volume by summing the vertical diameters of the largest pocket in each uterine quadrant (amniotic fluid index [AFI]).[21] Because this method appears equivalent in predictive accuracy to the single pocket method,[22] the substantiation of the AFI for the single pocket measurement seems reasonable. To date, however, there are no prospective clinical trials of sufficient size to establish the validity of this substantiation. Vintzileos and associates modified the original method by introducing graduated scoring of each of the original five variables and by inclusion of a sixth variable, placental grade.[23] This modification has not been shown to confer any clinical advantage. The value of including static placental morphology to an acute assessment method is not clear, particularly because the clinical value of placental grade is controversial.[24,25] Eden and colleagues described a "modified BPS" method by which only two variables, the NST and amniotic fluid, were considered.[25] The advantages of this

TABLE 26–1. BIOPHYSICAL PROFILE SCORING: TECHNIQUE AND INTERPRETATION

Biophysical Variable	Normal (Score = 2)	Abnormal (Score = 0)
FBM	At least one episode of FBM of at least 30 s duration in 30 min observation	Absent FBM or no episode of >30 s in 30 min
Gross body movement	At least three discrete body/limb movements in 30 min (episodes of active continuous movement considered movements as single movement)	Two or fewer episodes of body/limb in 30 min
Fetal tone	At least one episode of active extension with return to flexion of fetal limb(s) or trunk; opening and closing of hand considered normal tone	Either slow extension with return to partial flexion or movement of limb in full extension; absent fetal movement
Reactive FHR	At least two episodes of FHR acceleration of >15 beats/min and of at least 15 s duration associated with fetal movement in 30 min	Less than two episodes of acceleration of FHR or acceleration of <15 beats/min in 30 min
Qualitative AFV	At least one pocket of AF that measures at least 2 cm in two perpendicular planes	Either no AF pockets or a pocket <2 cm in two perpendicular planes

FBM, fetal breathing movement; FHR, fetal heart rate; AFV, amniotic fluid volume; AF, amniotic fluid.

modification seem unclear because it requires collection of some ultrasound data (amniotic fluid volume) yet ignores other information (fetal breathing movements, fetal body movements, and fetal tone); further, because the method is in conflict with the principle that the more information collected the better, so is the evaluation. Nonetheless, despite these concerns, this modification has proven to be clinically useful by some groups. The definitive answer to the value of the modified BPS awaits larger trials that include comparison with the original method. Other modifications, such as including acoustic stimulation[26] and umbilical artery flow velocity waveform assessments, although intriguing, have not been sufficiently evaluated.

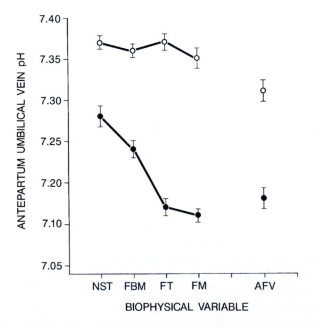

Figure 26–2. The mean pH ± 2 SD observed in antenatal cord blood (cordocentesis) for each of the components of the biophysical profile score when normal *(open circles)* or abnormal *(closed circles)*. A differential effect is observed with the nonstress test (NST), requiring the least perturbation in pH to become abnormal and fetal movement requiring the greatest. FBM, fetal breathing movement; FT, fetal tone; FM, fetal movement; AFV, amniotic fluid volume. *(Reproduced with permission from Manning FA, Snijders RL, Harman CR, et al. Am J Obstet Gynecol. 1993;165:755.)*

FETAL BIOPHYSICAL PROFILE SCORING: CLINICAL APPLICATION, PREDICTIVE ACCURACY, AND IMPACT ON OUTCOME

Clinical Application

Fetal biophysical profile scoring is used to predict the presence or absence of fetal asphyxia. Both the gestational age at which testing is begun and the testing frequency will differ by both the maternal and fetal risk factors. In general, testing is not begun at a gestational age before which intervention for fetal reasons is contemplated. This age will differ across centers; in our facility, testing is not started before 26 weeks except in clinical circumstances where fetal therapy is possible (e.g., alloimmune anemia). In most cases, testing is not instituted until there is demonstrable clinical evidence of maternal (e.g., preeclampsia) or fetal (e.g., IUGR) disease. The exception is the diabetic pregnancy: Testing is begun at 28 weeks in class 1 diabetics and at 32 weeks in gestational diabetics, even if there is no other evidence of pregnancy complications.

The distribution of BPS test results across all high-risk pregnancies studied ($n = 155,000$ tests) is quite remarkable in that most test results are normal (~98%), equivocal results (BPS 6/10) are uncommon (~1.5%), most (66%) revert to normal on repeat testing, and abnormal tests (BPS ≤ 4/10) are decidedly rare (0.5%).[27] This distribution of test results mirrors the incidence of perinatal compromise in the

TABLE 26–2. INTERPRETATION OF FETAL BIOPHYSICAL PROFILE SCORE RESULTS AND RECOMMENDED CLINICAL MANAGEMENT

Test Score Result	Interpretation	PNM[1] Within 1 wk Without Intervention	Management
10 of 10 8 of 10 (normal fluid), 8 of 8 (NST not done)	Risk of fetal asphyxia extremely rare	1 per 1000	Intervention only for obstetric and maternal factors; no indication for intervention for fetal disease
8 of 10 (abnormal fluid)	Probable chronic fetal compromise	89 per 1000[1]	Determine that there is functioning renal tissue and intact membranes; if so, deliver for fetal indications
6 of 10 (normal fluid)	Equivocal test, possible fetal asphyxia	Variable	If the fetus is mature, deliver; in the immature fetus, repeat test within 24 h; if <6/10, deliver
6 of 10 (abnormal fluid)	Probable fetal asphyxia	89 per 1000[11]	Deliver for fetal indications
4 of 10	High probability of fetal asphyxia	91 per 1000[1]	Deliver for fetal indications
2 of 10	Fetal asphyxia almost certain	125 per 1000[1]	Deliver for fetal indications
0 of 10	Fetal asphyxia certain	600 per 1000[1]	Deliver for fetal indications

[1]PNM, perinatal mortality; NST, nonstress test.

untested population, implying that the test is selecting those fetuses at risk. Given the high probability of a normal test result even in the pregnancy considered at risk, the false-negative rate (defined as stillbirth within a week of a normal test result) is of critical importance. In an initial study we observed a false-negative rate of 0.645 per 1000 among 19,221 referred high-risk pregnancies,[27] and this rate has remained at or below this value over the past 10 years ($n = 82,000$ patients).

Management has been based on the BPS result as interpreted within the overall clinical context including gestational age, maternal condition, and obstetric factors. The management criteria based on BPS results are given in Table 26–2. The gestational age at which intervention will occur varies by BPS result (Fig. 26–3).

Perinatal Outcome: Mortality and Morbidity

The relation between the last BPS result and perinatal mortality has been confirmed in several large studies involving 3000 or more high-risk patients.[27–31] All of these studies have demonstrated a significant increase in gross and corrected perinatal death among fetuses with an abnormal (low) score. In our studies a highly significant inverse exponential correlation between the last test score and perinatal mortality was observed.[32] There have been no randomized control trials contrasting perinatal mortality between patients managed by BPS results and patients who were not subjected to any antepartum testing; however, comparison of observed perinatal mortality between tested patients and concurrent untested (historical) controls has yielded encouraging results. Chamberlain reported a corrected perinatal mortality of 4.16 among 3202 tested high-risk pregnancies as compared with a rate of 10.7 among 5814 untested historical controls (net decrease 61%).[30] Our group observed a corrected perinatal mortality of 1.86 per 1000 among tested and managed

55,661 high-risk pregnancies as compared with a rate of 7.69 per 1000 in 104,337 untested historical controls (net decrease 76%): these differences were highly significant.[31]

The relation between last BPS result and perinatal morbidity has been studied extensively by our group and

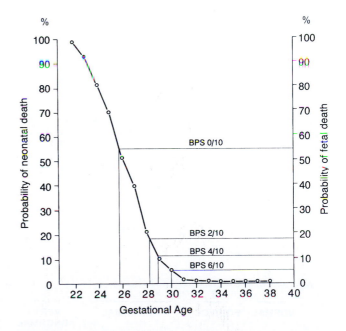

Figure 26–3. A schematic of the interaction of gestational age, the predictor of neonatal death, and the biophysical profile score (BPS), the predictor of fetal death, in the management of the high-risk fetus. Timing of intervention depends on these relative risks. The fetal mortality prediction by BPS should be uniform and accurate across centers, but the neonatal survival curves may differ by center. *(Reproduced with permission from Manning FA, Harman CR, Morrison I, et al.* Am J Obstet Gynecol. *1990;162:703.)*

others.[28,29,32] Unlike perinatal mortality the incidence of immediate perinatal morbidity, as reflected by fetal distress in labor (with or without lower-segment cesarean section), low Apgar score (≤ 7 at 5 mins), cord vein acidosis (≤ 7.20), and admission to an intensive care unit for reasons other than immaturity alone, showed a direct inverse relation to the last BPS. These differences are predicted because mortality must reflect a failure of compensation (hence, the exponential curve), whereas immediate morbidity (a linear curve) is a reflection of either compensation per se (e.g., low Apgar) or failure of compensation with added stress (fetal distress in labor). A highly significant inverse linear correlation between cumulative (any) immediate morbidity and the last BPS is observed (Fig. 26–4). It is of interest to note that no correlation between meconium staining of amniotic fluid and the last BPS result is observed.

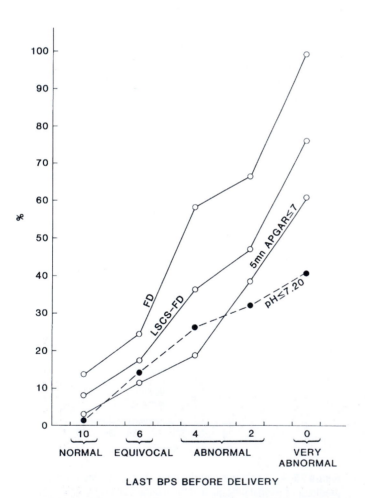

Figure 26–4. The relation between the incidence (percentage of occurrence) of indices of perinatal morbidity and the last fetal biophysical profile score (BPS). Note the inverse linear correlation. FD, fetal distress; LSCS, lower-segment cesarean section. *(Reproduced with permission from Manning FA, ed. Fetal Medicine: Principles and Practice. Norwalk, CT: Appleton & Lange; 1995.)*

BIOPHYSICAL PROFILE SCORE AND FETAL CORD BLOOD ACID–BASE AND PH VALUES

The relation between the BPS result and fetal blood gas and pH has been studied in several clinical settings. A highly significant direct linear correlation between the BPS result and cord blood obtained at delivery has been reported.[32] Vintzileos and associates compared cord blood gas and pH values with the BPS result in samples collected at cesarean section before the onset of labor in 124 cases and reported a highly significant direct linear correlation with both arterial and venous pH.[33] The mean pH in 102 fetuses with a last normal score (Vintzileos method) was 7.28 and two (1.9%) were mildly acidotic; in 13 fetuses with an equivocal BPS, the mean pH was 7.19 and nine (69%) were acidotic, and in nine fetuses with an abnormal score, the mean pH was 6.99 and all (100%) were acidotic.[33] Our group studied 557 fetuses delivered by elective cesarean section and noted a similar relation.[27] Extrapolation of cord blood obtained at elective cesarean section to antenatal values has been shown to be inexact, tending to significantly underestimate antenatal values.[34] The advent of ultrasound-guided cordocentesis now permits direct comparison of immediate BPS results and antenatal venous pH. At the time of this writing there are at least four reported studies of this comparison. Ribbert and coworkers compared BPS and venous blood gas and pH values in 14 severely nonanomalous IUGR fetuses[15]: A highly significant direct correlation between BPS and venous pH (standard deviation [SD] below normal) was reported, but no relation between BPS and PO_2, PCO_2, oxygen saturation, or content was identified. Manning and colleagues reported comparative results in 493 structurally normal fetuses, of which 104 were severely growth retarded and 393 had alloimmune anemia.[13] A highly significant linear correlation between BPS and mean pH was observed (Fig. 26–5). The mean pH with a normal score was 7.37 ± 0.06 (± 2 SD), and the lowest observed pH was 7.26. In contrast, with a very abnormal score (BPS = 0), the mean pH was 7.07 ± 0.15 and ranged from 7.17 to 6.86. The distribution of abnormal results defined as a pH below an arbitrary threshold differed by the selected threshold and assumed a curvilinear distribution at a pH cutoff of 7.20. Serial sampling in some patients confirmed that the BPS result mirrored the change in fetal venous pH. Salversen and coworkers compared the BPS and antenatal cord pH in 41 diabetic pregnancies.[35] A significant correlation between BPS and pH was reported. In this study one fetus had a normal score and a venous pH of 7.228. Because, by comparison with established normal pH distribution for gestational age, the mean pH among these diabetics was significantly reduced, interpretation of the relation of BPS to pH in these diabetics is difficult. A fourth study by Okamura and colleagues of 150 fetuses, including 79 anomalous fetuses, failed to demonstrate any correlation between the BPS (Vintzileos method) and antenatal venous pH.[36] Because values for structurally

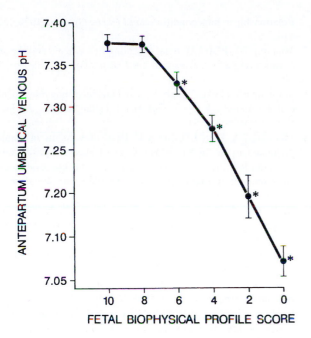

Figure 26–5. The relation between mean umbilical vein pH (± 2 SD) and the fetal biophysical profile score. The correlation is direct, linear, and highly significant (R^2 0.912; $p < 0.01$). The asterisks denote a pH value significantly less than the immediate. *(Reproduced with permission from Manning FA, Snijders RL, Harman CR, et al. Am J Obstet Gynecol. 1993;165:755.)*

normal fetuses are not given in this study, direct comparison with studies having conflicting results is difficult.

FETAL BIOPHYSICAL PROFILE SCORING: OUTCOME IN SELECTED HIGH-RISK SUBGROUPS

As the experience with the fetal biophysical profile scoring method has accumulated, it has become possible to assess its impact, if any, on perinatal outcome in relatively large numbers of patients in specific high-risk subgroups.

The adjunctive value of BPS in the management of the postdate pregnancy has been studied by several groups. It is important to stress that in these studies BPS testing is reserved for those patients in whom the cervix is unfavorable for induction or unresponsive to attempts at cervical ripening by local prostaglandin. In an initial study, Johnson and associates used BPS to guide management in 243 postdate patients with an unfavorable cervix.[37] These patients were tested twice weekly, and intervention was delayed until either the cervix became favorable or the score became equivocal or abnormal (13.2% of cases). There were no perinatal deaths in this series. The incidence of cesarean section was 17.7%, of which 5.3% were performed for fetal distress. In contrast, in a control group of 50 patients induced electively at 42 weeks regardless of cervical findings, although there were no fetal deaths, the overall cesarean section rate was 42%, of which

14% were for fetal distress. There were no significant differences in perinatal morbidity between the conservative (BPS) and actively managed patients; however, in patients with an abnormal BPS (32 of 243 fetuses) perinatal morbidity was significantly increased. Our experience with selected postdates pregnancies managed conservatively by BPS exceeds 1400 cases, yielding a perinatal mortality of 0.7 per 1000.

Outcome among diabetic pregnancies managed by serial BPS testing has been reported by our group and others. Johnson and coworkers studied 235 diabetics (50 class 1) and reported an intervention rate of 3.3% for an abnormal BPS and no perinatal deaths.[38] Dicker and associates studied 98 insulin-dependent diabetics, with no perinatal deaths: the intervention rate for an abnormal BPS result was 2.9%.[39] Manning and colleagues reported outcomes in 1153 diabetics (252 class 1) and observed an intervention rate for abnormal BPS of 3.1% and corrected perinatal mortality rate of 1.73 per 1000.[28] In our extended experience, we have used BPS in the management of 4973 diabetics (1087 class 1). The intervention rate for an abnormal BPS was 3.2%, the corrected stillbirth rate was 1.2 per 1000, and the corrected perinatal mortality was 2.01 per 1000.[27]

The use of BPS in the management of the IUGR fetus has reduced perinatal mortality, but the relative rate remains high.[27] In our experience of 2218 IUGR fetuses (below the third percentile for age and sex) we have observed a gross perinatal mortality of 31 per 1000 (versus 6.69 per 1000 in 53,443 appropriate-for-gestational age [AGA] tested controls) and a corrected perinatal mortality of 7.42 per 1000 versus 1.86 per 1000 in AGA tested controls. Although high, the perinatal mortality results observed in test IUGR fetuses compares favorably with 1765 untested historical IUGR controls in whom the gross perinatal mortality was 56 per 1000 and the corrected perinatal mortality was 37 per 1000.[27] Recently, we reported outcomes in 731 structurally normal IUGR fetuses delivered at or beyond 34 weeks; there were no perinatal deaths among these mature IUGR fetuses.[40]

Biophysical profile scoring plays a valuable clinical role in the management of the alloimmune anemic fetus. In these fetuses, the assessment of fetal condition by BPS is used as a secondary adjunct to determine the timing and urgency of fetal transfusion both initial and subsequent. There is a highly significant relation between disease severity, as assessed by ultrasound pathomorphology or by fetal blood indices, and the BPS result.[41] Specific determination of the positive contribution of BPS for such patients is difficult to ascertain because fetal treatment by transfusion yields such excellent results.[42] The observation of a deteriorating BPS despite fetal intravascular transfusion has been lifesaving in some cases, prompting repeat invasive testing (cordocentesis) and repeat transfusion for unrecognized bleeding from the puncture site.

The role of BPS testing in other high-risk subgroups, such as the hypertensive patient, the patient reporting decreased fetal movement, and the anomalous fetus, has yet to be systematically analyzed; however, given the low corrected perinatal mortality rate in the high-risk group at large (1.86 per 1000), such analysis holds promise.

BIOPHYSICAL PROFILE SCORE: RELATION TO NEUROLOGIC CONDITIONS OF CHILDHOOD

The association of the fetal BPS to childhood diseases known or suspected to be a consequence of perinatal asphyxia or infection has been area of active research. Because the BPS is an accurate proxy for the presence and extent of fetal acidemia and because intervention for fetal indication is based on the BPS results, it follows that some relation between the fetal condition, as reflected by the BPS, and postnatal outcome may exist. Recently, we examined these relations for four childhood diseases, namely cerebral palsy, attention deficit disorders, cortical blindness, and mental retardation.[43] Among 19,660 high-risk patients subjected to serial testing by BPS and managed according to the last BPS result, there was a highly significant inverse exponential relation between last test score and incidence of each of these conditions. In contrasting the prevalence of these disorders between the 19,660 tested high-risk fetuses and 63,540 contemporaneous nontested control patients, we noted a highly significant lowering of disease prevalence for each endpoint in the tested population. Interestingly, for conditions not suspected to be associated with fetal asphyxia (e.g., emotional disorders of childhood, brachial plexus injury), we noted no relation between prevalence and last BPS result, and the incidence of these disorders did not differ significantly between tested and nontested populations. These data imply that intervention for the abnormal BPS result not only can reduce perinatal mortality and immediate neonatal morbidity but also may prevent some of the devastating asphyxia-related diseases of childhood.

REFERENCES

1. Hon EH. The electronic evaluation of the fetal heart rate. *Am J Obstet Gynecol*. 1980;75:1215.
2. Caldero-Barcia R, Poseiro JJ, Pantle G, et al. Effects of uterine contraction on the heart rate of the human fetus. *Proceedings of the Fourth International Conference on Medical Electronics*. New York, 1961.
3. Dawes GS, Fox HE, Leduc BM, et al. Respiratory movements and paradoxical sleep in foetal lambs. *J Physiol (Lond)*. 1970;210:77.
4. Merlet C, Hoertner J, Devilleneuve C, et al. Mise en evidence de movements respiratoires chez la foetus d'argeau in utero au cours du dernier mois de la gestation. *Can R Acad Sci*. 1970;270:2462.
5. Boddy K, Dawes GS, Fisher R, et al. Foetal respiratory movements, electrocortical and cardiovascular responses to hypoxemia and hypercapnia in sheep. *J Physiol (Lond)*. 1974;243:599.
6. Platt LD, Manning FA, LeMay M. Human fetal breathing: Relationship to fetal condition. *Am J Obstet Gynecol*. 1978;132: 514.
7. Manning FA, Platt LD. Fetal breathing movements and the abnormal contraction stress test. *Am J Obstet Gynecol*. 1979;133: 590.
8. Manning FA, Platt LD, Sipos L, et al. Fetal breathing movements and the non-stress test in high risk pregnancies. *Am J Obstet Gynecol*. 1979;135:511.
9. Manning FA, Platt LD, Sipos L. Fetal movements in human pregnancy in the third trimester. *Obstet Gynecol*. 1979;54:699.
10. Manning FA, Platt LD, Sipos L. Antepartum fetal evaluation: Development of a fetal biophysical profile score. *Am J Obstet Gynecol*. 1980;136:787.
11. Rurak DW, Gruber NC. Effect of neuromuscular blockade on oxygen consumption and blood gases. *Am J Obstet Gynecol*. 1983;145:258.
12. Harman CR, Manning FA. Unpublished observations, 1994.
13. Manning FA, Snijders RL, Harman CR, et al. Fetal biophysical profile score. VI: Correlation with antepartum umbilical venous pH. *Am J Obstet Gynecol*. 1993;165:755.
14. Bocking AD, Gagnon R, Milne KM, et al. Behavioural activity during prolonged hypoxemia in fetal sheep. *J Appl Physiol*. 1988;65:2420.
15. Ribbert LSM, Snijders RJM, Nicolaides KH, et al. Relationship of fetal biophysical profile score and blood gas values at cordocentesis in severely growth-retarded fetuses. *Am J Obstet Gynecol*. 1990;163:569.
16. Cohn HE, Sacks GT, Heyman M, et al. Cardiovascular responses to hypoxemia and acidemia in fetal lambs. *Am J Obstet Gynecol*. 1974;120:817.
17. Manning FA, Hill LM, Platt LD. Qualitative amniotic fluid volume determination by ultrasound: Antepartum detection of intrauterine growth retardation. *Am J Obstet Gynecol*. 1981;139:254.
18. Chamberlain PF, Manning FA, Morrison I, et al. Ultrasound evaluation of amniotic fluid volume. I: Relationship of marginal and decreased amniotic fluid to perinatal outcome. *Am J Obstet Gynecol*. 1984;150:245.
19. Manning FA, Baskett TF, Morrison I, et al. Fetal biophysical profile scoring: A prospective study in 1184 high risk patients. *Am J Obstet Gynecol*. 1981;140:289.
20. Manning FA, Morrison I, Lange IR, et al. Fetal biophysical profile scoring: Selective use of the non-stress test. *Am J Obstet Gynecol*. 1987;156:709.
21. Phelan JP, Ahn MO, Smith CV, et al. Amniotic fluid index measurements during pregnancy. *J Reprod Med*. 1987;32:601.
22. Moore TR. Superiority of the four quadrant sum over the single-deepest-pocket technique in ultrasound identification of abnormal amniotic fluid volume. *Am J Obstet Gynecol*. 1990;163: 762.
23. Vintzileos AM, Campbell WA, Ingardia CT, et al. The fetal biophysical profile score and its predictive value. *Obstet Gynecol*. 1983;62:271.
24. Manning FA, Hohler C. Intrauterine growth retardation: Diagnosis, prognostication, and management based on ultrasound methods. In: Fleischer AC, Romero R, Manning FA, et al, eds. *The Principles and Practice of Ultrasonography in Obstetrics and Gynecology*, 4th ed. Norwalk, CT: Appleton & Lange, 1991: 331–347.
25. Eden RD, Gargely RZ, Schifrin BS, et al. Comparison of

antepartum testing methods for the management of the post-date pregnancy. *Am J Obstet Gynecol.* 1982;144:683.

26. Clark SL, Sabey P, Jolley K. Non-stress testing with acoustic stimulation and amniotic fluid volume assessment: 5973 tests without unexpected fetal death. *Am J Obstet Gynecol.* 1989; 160:694.

27. Manning FA. Fetal biophysical profile scoring. In: Manning FA, ed. *Fetal Medicine: Principles and Practice.* Norwalk, CT: Appleton & Lange; 1995.

28. Manning FA, Morrison I, Harman CR, et al. Fetal assessment based on fetal biophysical profile scoring: Experience in 19,221 referred high risk pregnancies. II: An analysis of false negative fetal death. *Am J Obstet Gynecol.* 1987;157:880.

29. Baskett TF, Allen AC, Gray JH, et al. Fetal biophysical profile and perinatal death. *Obstet Gynecol.* 1987;70:357.

30. Chamberlain PF. Late fetal death—Has ultrasound a role to play in its prevention? *Irish J Med Sci.* 1991;160:251.

31. Manning FA, Harman CR, Morrison I, et al. Fetal assessment based on fetal biophysical profile scoring. IV: Positive predictive accuracy of the abnormal test. *Am J Obstet Gynecol.* 1990;162:703.

32. Vintzileos AM, Fleming AD, Sconza WE, et al. Relationship between fetal biophysical activities and cord blood gas values. *Am J Obstet Gynecol.* 1991;165:707.

33. Vintzileos AM, Campbell WA, Rodis JF, et al. The relationship between fetal biophysical profile score and cord pH in patients undergoing elective cesarean section before the onset of labour. *Obstet Gynecol.* 1987;70:196.

34. Khoury AD, Morehi ML, Barton JR, et al. Fetal blood sampling in patients undergoing elective cesarean section: A correlation with cord blood gases obtained at delivery. *Am J Obstet Gynecol.* 1991;165:1026.

35. Salversen DR, Freeman J, Brudenell JM, et al. Prediction of foetal acidaemia in pregnancies complicated by maternal diabetes mellitus by biophysical profile scoring and fetal heart rate monitoring. *Br J Obstet Gynecol.* 1993;100:227.

36. Okamura K, Watanabe T, Endo H, et al. Biophysical profile and its relationship to fetal blood gases obtained by cordocentesis. *Acta Obstet Gynaecol Jpn.* 1991;43:1573.

37. Johnson JM, Harman CR, Lange IR, et al. Biophysical profile scoring in the management of the postdates pregnancy: An analysis of 307 patients. *Am J Obstet Gynecol.* 1986;154:269.

38. Johnson JM, Lange IR, Harman CR, et al. Biophysical profile scoring in the management of the diabetic pregnancy. *Obstet Gynecol.* 1988;72:841.

39. Dicker D, Feldberg D, Yeshaya A, et al. Fetal surveillance in insulin dependent diabetics: Predictive value of the fetal biophysical profile score. *Am J Obstet Gynecol.* 1988;159:800.

40. Morrison I, Manning FA, Harman CR, et al. Unpublished observations, 1995.

41. Harman CR. Ultrasound in the management of the alloimmunized pregnancy. In: Fleischer AC, Romero R, Manning FA, et al, eds. *The Principles and Practice of Ultrasonography in Obstetrics and Gynecology,* 4th ed. Norwalk, CT: Appleton & Lange; 1991:393–416.

42. Harman CR, Bowman JM, Manning FA, et al. Intrauterine transfusion: Intraperitoneal versus intravascular approach: A case-control comparison. *Am J Obstet Gynecol.* 1990;162:1053.

43. Manning FA. Fetal assessment: 1999 Update. *Clin Obstet Gynecol.* 2000;26:557.

27

Chorionic Villus Sampling

Ronald J. Wapner

Sonographically guided chorionic villus sampling (CVS) has been available in the United States since the early 1980s and has offered couples at genetic risk an early and rapid prenatal diagnosis. The procedure, which can be performed as early as 10 weeks of menstrual age, provides preliminary cytogenetic results within 48 h and final culture results within 7 days. In contrast, genetic amniocentesis is not routinely performed until approximately 16 weeks of menstrual age with an additional 7 to 10 days required to culture the amniotic fluid cells. Thus, pregnancy is nearly half completed before a definitive diagnosis can be established. If a significant fetal abnormality is identified, the prospective parents must make a difficult choice of whether to continue or terminate the pregnancy. Postponing this decision until the midtrimester is extremely difficult because fetal movement has been perceived and significant bonding between the parent and fetus has occurred. In addition, the pregnancy is public knowledge, thereby precluding an element of privacy in decision making. If termination is chosen, maternal risks are greater than in the first trimester, with maternal mortality being up to five times higher.[1]

Despite the advantages of CVS, the procedure has struggled to become universally accepted. This has been due predominately to a perception that the sampling and laboratory procedures are more complex than amniocentesis. In addition, there have been concerns that the procedure may induce fetal limb defects. Recently, however, enthusiasm for CVS has been renewed. First, contemporaneous studies have demonstrated the accuracy of the laboratory results, the reliability of the sampling, and the safety of the procedure if performed after 10 weeks of gestation by experienced operators. Second, recent concerns have been raised about the safety of the alternative approach of first-trimester amniocentesis,[2,3] Third, the recent success of first-trimester screening for fetal chromosomal abnormalities requires a first-trimester diagnostic procedure.[4]

CONCEPTS AND INDICATIONS FOR CHORIONIC VILLUS SAMPLING

For years, prenatal diagnosis has relied on the analysis of amniotic fluid fibroblasts as an indirect reflection of the fetal genetic makeup. Similarly, chorionic villi are fetal in origin and as such are also an appropriate and useful source of tissue for the evaluation of fetal genetic disease. Their cytogenetic, molecular, and biochemical properties reflect those of the fetus. In addition, the villi are partly composed of cytotrophoblast cells, which are an actively dividing source of spontaneous mitoses that can be used to obtain a rapid chromosomal analysis. Finally, villi can be easily obtained without requiring puncture of the chorion or amnion membrane.

With the exception of α-fetoprotein analysis, the indications for CVS are essentially the same as those for amniocentesis. The major indications are listed in Table 27–1.

TABLE 27–1. MAJOR INDICATIONS FOR CHORIONIC VILLUS SAMPLING

Maternal age: 35 years or older at delivery
Previous child with nondisjunctional chromosome abnormality
Parent is carrier of balanced translocation or other chromosome disorder
Both parents are carriers of autosomal recessive disease
Women who are carriers of a sex-linked disease
Positive first-trimester screen for trisomy 21 or 18

Advanced maternal age (older than 35 years) is the most common, accounting for 90% of procedures.[5] In addition, parents who have previously had a child with a chromosomal abnormality that may recur are likely to request early invasive testing, as are couples who are carriers of chromosome translocations or autosomal recessive biochemical or molecular diseases. First-trimester prenatal diagnosis is often requested by women who carry sex-linked diseases because of the 50% recurrence risk in male offspring. Recently, screening for trisomics 21 and 18 in the first trimester has become possible by using a combination of biochemical analysis [PAPP-A (pregnancy-associated plasma protein A) and HCG (human chorionic gonadotropin)] and measurement of the fetal nuchal translucency.[4] If the preliminary work demonstrating almost 90% sensitivity is substantiated, a positive screen could become a major indication for CVS.

HISTORY OF CHORIONIC VILLUS SAMPLING

First-trimester prenatal diagnosis is not a new concept. The ability to sample and analyze villus tissue was demonstrated more than 25 years ago by the Chinese who, in an attempt to develop a technique for fetal sex determination inserted a thin catheter into the uterus guided only by tactile sensation.[6] When resistance from the gestational sac was felt, suction was applied and small pieces of villi aspirated. Although this approach seems relatively crude by today's standards of ultrasonically guided invasive procedures, the diagnostic accuracy and low miscarriage rate demonstrated the feasibility of first-trimester sampling.

In 1968, Hahnemann and Mohr attempted blind transcervical (TC) trophoblast biopsy in 12 patients using a 6-mm-diameter instrument.[7] Although successful tissue culture was possible, half of these subjects subsequently aborted. In 1973, Kullander and Sandahl used a 5-mm-diameter fiberoptic endocervoscope with biopsy forceps to perform TC CVS in patients requesting pregnancy termination.[8] Although tissue culture was successful in approximately half of the cases, two of the subjects subsequently became septic.

In 1974, Hahnemann described further experience with first-trimester prenatal diagnosis using a 2.5-mm hysteroscope and cylindrical biopsy knife.[9] Once again, significant complications, including inadvertent rupture of the amniotic sac, were encountered. By this time, the safety of midtrimester genetic amniocentesis had become well established, and further attempts at first-trimester prenatal diagnosis were temporarily abandoned in the Western hemisphere.

Two technological advances occurred in the early 1980s to allow reintroduction of CVS. The first of these was the development of real-time sonography, making continuous guidance possible. At the same time, sampling instruments were miniaturized and refined. In 1982, Kazy et al. reported the first TC CVS performed with real-time sonographic guidance.[10] That same year, Old reported the first-trimester diagnosis of beta-thalassemia major using DNA from chorionic villi obtained by sonographically guided TC aspiration with a 1.5-mm-diameter polyethylene catheter.[11] Using a similar sampling technique, Brambati and Simoni diagnosed trisomy 21 at 11 weeks of gestation.[12]

After these preliminary reports, several CVS programs were established in both Europe and the United States, with the outcomes informally reported to a World Health Organization (WHO)–sponsored registry maintained at Jefferson Medical College. This registry and single-center reports were used to estimate the safety of CVS until 1989, when two prospective multicentered studies, one from Canada[13] and one from the United States,[14] were published and confirmed the safety of the procedure.

CHORIONIC VILLUS SAMPLING: THE PROCEDURE

Procedure-Related Anatomy (Fig. 27–1)

Between 9 and 12 weeks after the last menstrual period, the developing gestation does not yet fill the uterine cavity. The sac is surrounded by the thick leathery chorionic membranes within which is both the amniotic cavity and the extraembryonic coeloem. The amniotic cavity contains the embryo and is enclosed by the thin, whispy, freely mobile amniotic membrane. The extraembryonic coeloem is located between the amniotic and chorionic membranes, contains a tenacious mucoid-like substance, and disappears as the amniotic sac grows toward the chorion and the two membranes becomes juxtaposed.

Before 9 weeks, chorionic villi cover the entire outer surface of the gestational sac. As growth continues, the developing sac begins to fill the uterine cavity, and most villi regress except at the implantation site, where they are associated with the decidua basalis (see Fig. 27–1). Villi in this area rapidly proliferate to form the chorion frondosum, or fetal component of the placenta. Between 9 and 12 weeks of gestation, the villi float freely within the blood of the intervillus space and are only loosely anchored to the underlying decidua basalis.

Sampling Techniques

Sampling by CVS is performed between 70 and 91 days after the last menstrual period. This window is chosen to minimize

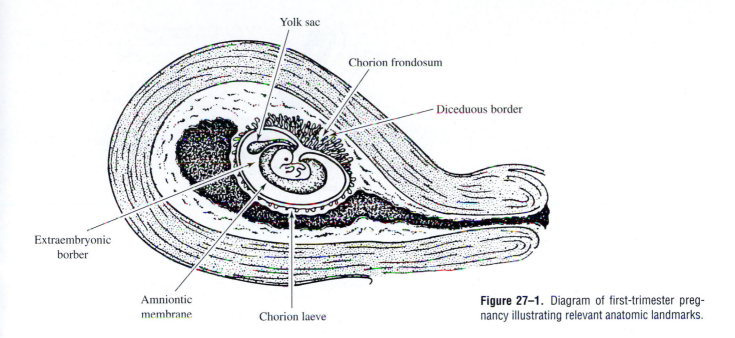

Yolk sac

Chorion frondosum

Diceduous border

Extraembryonic borber

Amniontic membrane

Chorion laeve

Figure 27–1. Diagram of first-trimester pregnancy illustrating relevant anatomic landmarks.

the background spontaneous miscarriage rate that is higher in early pregnancy, yet still allows sufficient time for results to be available within the first trimester. The chorion frondosum is easily localized by ultrasound as a hyperechoic homogeneous area by this gestational age (Fig. 27–2). In addition, fusion of the amnion and chorion has not yet occurred, thereby decreasing the risk of amnion rupture during the procedure. Sampling significantly earlier in gestation may be associated with an increased risk of fetal abnormalities and should not routinely be done.[15] Transcervical sampling may be more difficult after 12 weeks of menstrual age due to the increasing distance between the cervix and placental site as uterine growth continues.

Chorionic villus sampling can be performed by either the TC or the transabdominal (TA) approach (Fig. 27–3). The techniques are equally safe and efficacious and the majority of patients can be sampled by either technique.[16] In most cases, physician or patient preference will dictate which approach is used; however, in approximately 3 to 5% of patients, clinical circumstances will support one approach over the other (Table 27–2) requiring operators to be proficient in both.[16,17] Transcervical CVS is preferred when the placenta is located on the posterior uterine wall, whereas TA sampling is particularly useful when the placenta is implanted in a fundal or high anterior location. Transcervical sampling has the advantage of minimal patient discomfort but is somewhat more difficult to learn.[18] Both approaches are best performed by using a two-person technique, with one individual performing the sampling and the other guiding the ultrasound. Communication between the sonographer and sampler is imperative, and the best results have come from centers in which a limited numbers of samplers and sonographers perform CVS.

Transcervical Sampling

Transcervical CVS is performed by using a polyethylene catheter through which a stainless-steel malleable stylet has been inserted. The stylet fits snugly through the catheter and provides sufficient rigidity for adequate passage through the cervix and into the frondosum. The stylet has a rounded, blunt end that protrudes slightly beyond the end of the catheter to prevent sharp edges that may potentially perforate the membranes. The catheter has a luerlock end to accommodate

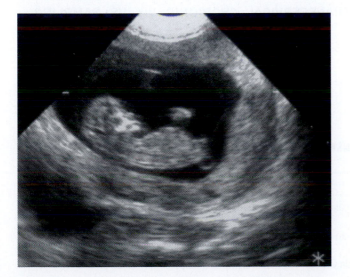

Figure 27–2. Sonogram at 10.8 weeks of gestation. The chorion frondosum (placenta) is located posteriorly and appears as a homogeneous hyperechoic area.

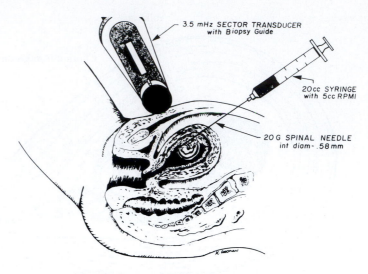

TRANSABDOMINAL CHORIONIC VILLUS SAMPLING

A

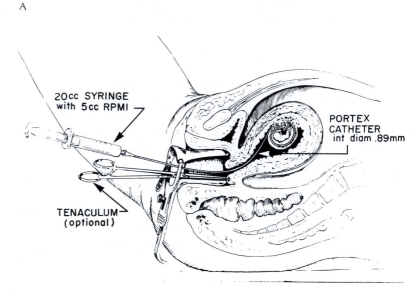

TRANSCERVICAL CHORIONIC VILLUS SAMPLING

B

Figure 27–3. Diagram illustrating the technique of sonographically guided chorionic villus sampling: **(A)** transcervical sampling, **(B)** transabdominal sampling.

TABLE 27–2. COMPARISON OF TRANSCERVICAL AND TRANSABDOMINAL CHORIONIC VILLUS SAMPLING PROCEDURES

	Transcervical	Transabdominal
Relative contraindications	Cervical polyps, active cervical or vaginal herpes	Interceding bowel
Ease of learning	Somewhat more complex than transabdominal approach	Adaptation of amniocentesis technique but learning curve still required
Sample size	Large sample; includes whole villi	Smaller sample; includes many small pieces
Patient discomfort	Minimal to absent	Moderate
Placental location	Better for posterior placenta	Better for fundal placenta

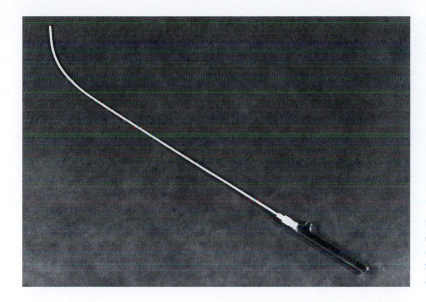

Figure 27–4. Cook catheter used for transcervical chorionic villus sampling. Note the general curvature of the distal end, which is aligned with the notch on the handle. This allows the operator to be aware of the direction of the curve.

a syringe. The Trophcan catheter (Portex Company, Concord, MA, USA) had been the one most frequently used in the United States. However, this catheter has recently been removed from the market by the manufacturer, leaving the catheter manufactured by the Cook Company (Spencer, IN) as the only commercially available TC sampling device (Fig. 27–4).

Before performing the CVS procedure, ultrasound scanning confirms fetal viability and establishes the area of the chorion frondosum. An approach is mentally mapped that allows catheter placement parallel to the chorionic membrane. Uterine contractions may be present and obstruct or alter the sampling path (Fig. 27–5). They may also alter the appearance and location of the placenta by pulling it into unusual locations. When contractions significantly interfere with a proposed sampling path, delaying the procedure for 15 to 30 minutes until they abate is suggested. The presence of large placental lakes should also be noted so they can be avoided because sampling through these lakes has been associated with increased postprocedure bleeding.[19]

The maternal bladder should be sufficiently full to provide an acoustic window through which the vagina, cervix, and uterus can be visualized. Overfilling makes retrieval more difficult by increasing patient discomfort and displacing the uterus out of the pelvis, which extends and fixes the sampling path.

The procedure is performed in the lithotomy position on a standard examination table with foot stirrups. A speculum is inserted, and the vagina and cervix are cleansed with antiseptic solution. The catheter is prepared by slightly curving its distal 3- to 5-cm part with the guidewire in place to allow easy insertion through the cervix. In most cases, only a minimal amount of curvature is required. The cervical canal is then reimaged by ultrasound, and the catheter is introduced through the cervix until loss of resistance at the internal os is

felt. Once the sonographer clearly identifies the catheter tip, it is guided by real-time sector scanning to the placental site (Fig. 27–6A). The catheter is directed by gently maneuvering the curved periphery of the gestational sac. A greater amount of upward or downward movement of the tip can be accomplished by manipulating the speculum to redirect the angle of approach. Severe bending of the stylet is rarely, if ever, required but, occasionally, use of a single-tooth tenaculum on the cervix is needed to alter uterine position.

Insertion of the catheter in the correct tissue plane between the inner uterine wall and gestational sac is critical to safe sampling. Although sonographic guidance is crucial, tactile sensation is equally important. The catheter can be easily advanced if it is in the proper tissue plane, whereas resistance is encountered if it is against the chorionic membrane or uterine wall. A gritty sensation is felt if the catheter is inserted too deeply into the decidua. Slight readjustment of the angle of direction corrects the problem. To ensure an adequate sample, the catheter should be advanced through the full length of the placenta. The guide wire is then removed, and a 20-cc syringe containing approximately 5 cc of a collection medium is attached. The sample is collected by aspiration using negative pressure as the catheter is slowly withdrawn. Slight distortion of the placental surface may be noted sonographically during this process, and larger villus fragments may be visualized as they pass through the catheter lumen.

Transabdominal Chorionic Villus Sampling

Two techniques for TA sampling are presently used. In the single-needle approach a 20-gauge spinal needle is used.[20] Alternatively, some operators perform a double-needle technique that uses an outer guide needle (18-gauge thin wall or a 16- to 17-gauge standard spinal needle) and a smaller sampling needle (20 gauge).[21] In general, a 3.5-in.-long needle

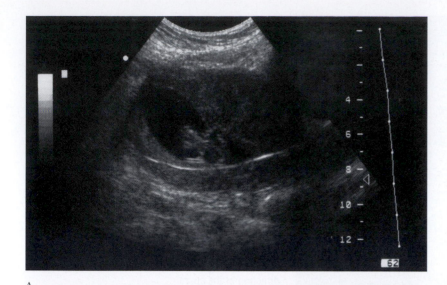

A

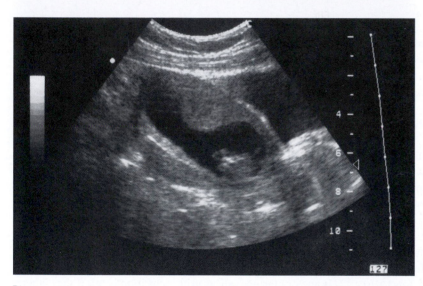

B

Figure 27–5. Sonogram illustrating sonographically guided transcervical chorionic villus sampling at 11.5 weeks of menstrual age. **(A)** The tip of the catheter is visible at the internal os before farther advancement. **(B)** The catheter is correctly placed within the corion frondosum parallel to the chorionic membrane.

Figure 27–6. Sonogram illustrating transabdominal chorionic villus sampling. The needle is parallel to the chorionic plate.

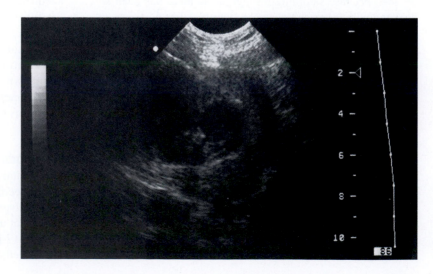

is sufficient for most patients, but a 5- or 6-in.-long needle should be available for very obese women.

With the single-needle technique, a sampling path is chosen so that the tip of the needle passes within the chorion frondosum parallel to the chorionic membrane. Intervening bowel and bladder must be avoided. The needle tip is first inserted into the myometrium and then redirected parallel to the membrane. As with cervical sampling, the needle should be passed through as much villus tissue as possible and remain parallel to the chorionic membrane to avoid inadvertent puncture (Fig. 27–6B). Once appropriately placed within the placenta, the stylet is removed, and a syringe containing 5 cc of media attached. Under continuous suction, 4 or 5 to-and-fro passes within the frondosum are made. The needle is then removed from the abdomen while suction is continued. This "vacuuming" technique is required to assure retrieval of sufficient villus tissue because the diameter of the 20-gauge needle is slightly smaller than that of a TC catheter.

The two-needle technique uses a slightly larger gauge spinal needle as a trocar, which is inserted into the myometrium. A thinner (19 to 20 gauge) and longer sampling needle is passed through the trocar into the chorion frondosum. The stylet of the sampling needle is then replaced with a syringe, and sampling is performed as with a single needle.

Both TA sampling approaches appear to be equally safe. The two-needle technique is theoretically less traumatic because the outer trocar remains still during sampling. It also has the advantage of allowing the operator to obtain additional villi by reinserting the sampling needle without requiring a second skin puncture. The single-needle approach is quicker, less uncomfortable, able to retrieve adequate tissue with minimal insertions, and appears to be the technique that has gained widest acceptance.

Confirmation of Adequate Tissue Retrieval

The presence of adequate villus tissue can usually be confirmed by visual inspection of the syringe contents, but occasionally the sample may need to be evaluated under a dissecting microscope. Samples typically contain a mixture of predominately villi with a small amount of maternally derived decidua. The chorionic villi appear as free-floating, white, structures with fluffy, filiforme branches (Fig. 27–7A). Contaminating decidua tissue has a more amorphous appearance and lacks distinct branches. Although these two tissues can usually be grossly distinguished by virtue of their respective morphology, confirmation under a dissecting microscope is required if there is uncertainty that adequate villi have been retrieved. Microsopically, the villi have a distinctive branched appearance. Their surface is punctuated by small buds consisting of an outer syncytiotrophoblast covering and a core of mitotically, active cytotrophoblast cells (Fig. 27–7B). Within the center of each villus is the mesenchymal core, through which capillaries carrying fetal blood cells course.

A minimum of 5 mg of villus tissue is required for most genetic analyses. If insufficient villi are present with the ini-

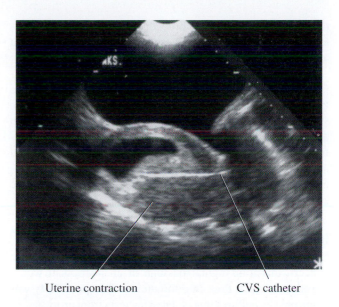

Uterine contraction   CVS catheter

Figure 27–7. Transcervical chorionic villus sampling catheter forced anteriorally by posterior uterine contraction.

tial attempt, a second aspiration may be performed without additional risk.[5] Pregnancy loss rates increase significantly when more than two insertions are required, and may be as high as 10% if three attempts are made.[14,22] Therefore, a third pass should only be attempted if successful retrieval seems certain. Before a third attempt, the anatomic relationships should be reevaluated, interfering contractions should have abated, and consideration should be given to sampling by the alternative route. In most experienced centers, more than 99% of patients can be successfully sampled with two or fewer insertions. In our center, we have not had a failed procedure in our last 15,000 patients.

Patients may resume normal physical activity after CVS, although strenuous exercise should be avoided for 24 h. Sexual abstinence is recommended for a short period of time to minimize any risk of ascending infection. Patients may have some mild vaginal bleeding after CVS; therefore, they should be counseled about this possibility before sampling.

RISKS ASSOCIATED WITH CHORIONIC VILLUS SAMPLING

Bleeding

Vaginal bleeding is uncommon after TA CVS but is seen in 7 to 10% of patients sampled transcervically. Minimal spotting is a common occurrence and may occur in almost one-third of women sampled by the TC route.[14] In most cases, the bleeding is self-limited and the pregnancy outcome is excellent. However, a subchorionic hematoma may be visualized immediately after sampling in up to 4% of TC samples.[23] The hematoma usually disappears before the 16th week of pregnancy and is only rarely associated with adverse outcome. Of the more than 15,000 CVS procedures performed in our center, we have never needed to terminate a pregnancy or admit a patient for excessive postprocedural bleeding.

Cases of heavy bleeding and resulting hematoma formation occur from accidental placement of the TC catheter into the vascular decidua basalis underlying the chorion frondosum. In extreme cases, the development of the hematoma can actually be seen on ultrasound. In most of these cases, a gritty feeling indicates penetration into the decidual layer. Careful attention to the feel of the catheter and avoidance of unnecessary manipulation can prevent most of these hemorrhagic episodes and minimize this complication.

Infection

Since the initial development of TC CVS, there has been concern that transvaginal passage of an instrument would introduce vaginal flora into the uterus. This possibility was confirmed by cultures that isolated bacteria from up to 30% of catheters used for CVS.[24,25,26] However, in clinical practice, the incidence of post-CVS chorioamnionitis is low.[13,14,27,28] In a recently published U.S. study of more than 2000 cases of TC CVS, infection was suspected as a possible etiology of pregnancy loss in only 0.3% of cases.[14] Infection after TA CVS also occurs and has been demonstrated, at least in some cases, to be secondary to bowel flora introduced by inadvertent puncture by the sampling needle.

In our own series of more than 15,000 procedures, in which prophylactic antibodies are not used, we have not observed any cases of chorioamnionitis requiring uterine evacuation. Our incidence of periabortion chorioamnionitis was 0.08% for both TC and TA sampling; this rate is about the same as that seen in series of spontaneous abortions that have not been sampled.[29,30] At present, because of the clinically low incidence of post-CVS chorioamnionitis, routine pre-CVS vaginal or cervical cultures for any organism other than gonococcus is not indicated.

Early in the development of TC CVS, two life-threatening pelvic infections were reported.[31,32] Each initially presented with a mild prodrome of maternal myalgias and low-grade fever without localized adnexal or uterine tenderness and subsequently led to maternal sepsis. Both occurred early in the respective center's experience, and in both the same catheter was used for repeat insertions. Since these reports, a practice of using a new sterile catheter for each insertion has been universally adopted, with only exceedingly rare reports of serious infectious complications.

Ruptured Membranes

Acute rupture of the membranes, documented by either obvious gross fluid leakage or a decrease in measurable amnionic fluid on ultrasound evaluation, is a very rare complication of CVS.[14,33] In our own experience, acute rupture of the membranes has not occurred. Experimental attempts to rupture membranes intentionally with a TC catheter have confirmed

that the chorion can withstand significant punishment without perforation.

Gross rupture of the membranes days to weeks after the procedure is acknowledged as a possible post-CVS complication. Delayed rupture can result from either mechanical injury to the chorion at the time of sampling with rupture from exposure of the amnion or chronic irritation or inflammation from a hematoma on low-grade infection, allowing exposure of the amnion to subsequent damage or infection. One group reported a 0.3% incidence of delayed rupture of the membranes after CVS,[28] a rate confirmed by Bramabati et al.[23]

Unexplained midtrimester oligohydramnios has been suggested as a rare complication of TC CVS and may occur from delayed chorioamnion rupture with slow leakage of amniotic fluid.[33] These cases are frequently associated with postprocedure bleeding and an elevated maternal serum α-fetoprotein (MSAFP). Operator experience will markedly reduce the risk of this complication, probably by decreasing hematoma formation with its potential to serve as either a nidus for a smoldering infection or a chemical irritant of the membranes.

Elevated MSAFP

An acute rise in MSAFP after CVS has been consistently reported, implying a detectable degree of fetal maternal bleeding.[34-36] The elevation is transient, occurs more frequently after TA CVS, and appears to be dependent on the quantity of tissue aspirated.[36] Some studies have also demonstrated a correlation between the degree of elevation and the incidence of pregnancy loss.[37] Levels will drop to normal ranges by 16 to 18 weeks, which allows neural tube defect (NTD) serum screening to proceed according to usual prenatal protocols.

Rh Isoimmunization

In Rh-negative women, the otherwise negligible fetal maternal bleeding that follows CVS accrues special importance because Rh-positive cells in volumes as low as 0.1 mL have been shown to cause Rh sensitization.[38] Because all women with even a single pass of a catheter or needle show detectable rises in MSAFP, it seems prudent that all Rh-negative nonsensitized women undergoing CVS receive Rho (D) immunoglobulin subsequent to the procedure.

The potential for a CVS-induced maternal-to-fetal transfusion to worsen already existing Rh immunization has been described, suggesting that sampling sensitized patients represents a contraindication to the procedure.[39]

Pregnancy Loss

Multiple reports from individual centers have demonstrated the safety and low pregnancy loss rates after CVS.[5,40-47] In experienced centers, the rate of miscarriage from the time of CVS until 28 weeks of gestation is approximately 2 to

3%.[16] However, to determine the incidence of procedure-induced pregnancy loss, adjustments for the relatively high background loss at this gestational age must be made.

First-trimester spontaneous abortion in women not undergoing CVS is a common event, occurring in one in every six clinically recognized pregnancies.[48] However, miscarriage rates after ultrasound confirmation of a viable gestation are expected to be less. Simpson et al. reported that, when ultrasound confirmation of fetal viability was noted at 8 weeks, 3.2% of 220 women with a mean age of 30 years aborted.[49] Christiaens and Stoutenbeek noted a 3.3% fetal loss rate in 274 women with proven fetal viability at 10 weeks.[50] Because the majority of woman undergoing CVS are older than 35 years and the spontaneous miscarriage rate increases with advancing maternal age, this variable must also be considered. Wilson et al. found a total fetal loss rate after proven viability by first-trimester ultrasonography of 1.4% in women younger than 30 years, 2.6% in those between 30 and 34 years old, and 4.3% in women older than 35 years.[51] It appears that the best estimate of the background spontaneous miscarriage rate in a population of woman similar to those undergoing CVS is approximately 2 to 3%. Although this rate is similar to the postprocedure loss rate in other centers, a randomized clinical trial is necessary to quantify the procedure-induced risk precisely. Unfortunately, no randomized comparison of sampled with unsampled patients is likely; however, comparisons to amniocentesis have been performed.

Because the background loss rate is higher in the first trimester than in the second, any comparison of CVS to second-trimester amniocentesis must enroll all patients before the gestational age at which CVS is performed. The total loss rates can then be compared. All losses must be included, whether from a spontaneous miscarriage or an induced termination for abnormal results. This approach eliminates any bias that may occur when comparing procedures performed at significantly different gestational ages and also takes into account cytogenetically abnormal embryos that miscarry before an amniocentesis, which would be electively terminated after CVS.

The largest demonstrations of data evaluating the relative safety of CVS and amniocentesis come from three recent collaborative reports. In 1989, the Canadian Collaborative CVS-Amniocentesis Clinical Trial Group reported its experience with a prospective, randomized trial comparing TC CVS with second-trimester amniocentesis.[13] During the study period, patients across Canada were only able to undergo CVS in conjunction with the randomized protocol. There were 7.6% fetal losses (spontaneous abortions, induced abortions, and late losses) in the CVS group and 7.0% in the amniocentesis group. Thus, in desired pregnancies, an excess loss rate of 0.6% for CVS over amniocentesis was obtained; this difference was not statistically significant.

Two months after the publication of the Canadian experience, the first American collaborative report appeared.[14] This study was a prospective, although nonrandomized, trial of more than 2200 women who chose either TC CVS or second-trimester amniocentesis. Patients in both groups were recruited in the first trimester of pregnancy. As in the Canadian study, advanced maternal age was the primary indication for prenatal testing. When the loss rates were adjusted for slight group differences in maternal and gestational ages at enrollment, an excess pregnancy loss rate of 0.8% referable to CVS over amniocentesis was calculated, which was not statistically significant.

Whereas both North American trials showed no statistical difference in pregnancy loss when CVS was compared with amniocentesis, a prospective, randomized collaborative comparison of more than 3200 pregnancies sponsored by the European MRC Working Party on the Evaluation of CVS demonstrated a 4.6% greater pregnancy loss rate after CVS (95% confidence interval [CI], 1.6 to 7.5%).[32] This difference reflected more spontaneous deaths before 28 weeks of gestation (2.9%), more terminations of pregnancy for chromosomal anomalies (1.0%), and more neonatal deaths (0.3%) in the CVS group.

The factors responsible for the discrepant results between the European and North American studies remain uncertain, but it is probable that inadequate operator experience with CVS accounted for a large part of this difference. Whereas the United States trial consisted of 7 centers and the Canadian trial 11 centers, the European trial included 31 sampling sites. There were, on average, 325 cases per center in the United States study, 106 in the Canadian study, and only 52 in the European trial. Although no significant change in pregnancy loss rate was demonstrated during the course of the European trial, it appears that the learning curve for both TC and TA CVS may exceed 400 or more cases.[52,53] Operators having performed fewer than 100 cases may have two or three times the postprocedure loss rate of operators who have performed more than 1000 procedures.

There have been similar comparisons between CVS and *early amniocentesis,* defined as amniocentesis performed before 14 weeks of gestation. In these comparisons of two first-trimester procedures, consideration of gestational age differences is not necessary. Nicolaides et al. compared TA CVS with amniocentesis performed between 10 and 13 weeks and gestation.[54] In this prospective comparison, the spontaneous loss rate was significantly higher after early amniocentesis (5.3%) than after CVS (2.3%). Also, a significant increase in the incidence of talipes equinovarus was seen after early amniocentesis. In another recent comparison, Sundberg randomized patients to either amniocentesis between 11 and 13 weeks or TA CVS between 10 and 12 weeks.[2] Although the initial endpoint of this trial was intended to be pregnancy loss, the trial was stopped early because of an increased risk of talipes equinovarus in the early amniocentesis group. Although the power of the trial to compare fetal loss rates was limited by the incomplete sample, no significant difference was demonstrated. The amniocentesis loss rate, however, was 0.6% higher. Leakage of amniotic fluid after sampling occurred significantly more frequently after amniocentesis. Overall, the higher loss rates and increased risk of fluid leakage and subsequent club-foot deformity with early amniocentesis suggest that CVS is the preferred technique for first-trimester sampling.

Pregnancy Loss: Transcervical Versus Transabdominal Chorionic Villus Sampling

Randomized trials have compared the TC and TA approaches.[16,53,55–57] The United States collaborative CVS project performed a randomized, prospective study and found no difference in the postprocedure pregnancy loss rates between the two approaches (TC, 2.5%; TA, 2.3%).[16] Equally important was that the overall post-CVS loss rate in the study (2.5%) was 0.8% lower than that in the initial United States study, which compared CVS with second-trimester amniocentesis. Because 0.8% was the quantitative difference in loss rates between amniocentesis and CVS in the original study, this finding suggests that, when centers become equivalently experienced, amniocentesis and CVS may have the same risk of pregnancy loss.

Smidt-Jensen et al., pioneers of TA CVS, added additional information to the comparative safety of the procedures.[57] In a prospective, randomized study, they found no difference in pregnancy loss between TA CVS and second-trimester amniocentesis but did demonstrate an increased risk for TC CVS, the procedure for which their center was least experienced. Chueh et al. in a retrospective review of more than 9000 CVS procedures showed that in their center TC CVS had a slightly greater risk of pregnancy loss than TA sampling.[58] It appears safe to speculate that fetal loss rates between TC and TA sampling will be similar in most centers once equivalent expertise is gained with either approach. Integration of both methods into the program of any single center will offer the most complete, practical, and safe approach to first-trimester diagnosis.

Risk of Fetal Abnormalities After Chorionic Villus Sampling

It has recently been suggested that CVS may be associated with the occurrence of specific fetal malformations. The first suggestion of this was reported by Firth et al.[59] In a series of 539 CVS-exposed pregnancies, they identified five infants with severe limb abnormalities, all of which came from a cohort of 289 pregnancies sampled at 66 days of gestation or less. Four of these infants had the unusual and rare oromandibular-limb hypogenesis syndrome, and the fifth had a terminal transverse limb reduction defect. Oromandibular-limb hypogenesis syndrome occurs with a birth prevalence of 1 per 175,000 live births,[60] and limb reduction defects occur in 1 per 1690 births.[61] Therefore, the occurrence of these abnormalities in more than 1% of CVS-sampled cases raised strong suspicion of an association. In this initial report, all of the limb abnormalities followed TA sampling performed between 55 and 66 days of gestation.

Subsequent to this initial report, others added supporting cases to this list. Using the Italian multicenter birth defects registry, Mastroiacovo et al. reported, in a case control study, an odds ratio of 11.3 (CI 5.6 to 2.13) for transverse limb abnormalities after first-trimester CVS.[62] When stratified by gestational age at sampling, pregnancies sampled before 70 days had a 19.7% increased risk of transverse limb reduction defects, whereas patients sampled later did not demonstrate a significantly increased risk. Other single-center and case control studies, however, have been inconclusive about an association of CVS with limb reduction defects, with the majority demonstrating no increased risk (Table 27–3).

There is support of the notion that CVS may increase the risk of limb defects when sampling is performed before 63 days of gestation. Most notably, Brambati et al., an extremely experienced group who have reported no increased risk of limb defects in patients sampled after 9 weeks, have reported a 1.6% incidence of severe limb reduction defects when patients were sampled at 6 and 7 weeks.[63] This rate decreased to 0.1% for sampling at 8 to 9 weeks. Hsieh et al., in a report of the Taiwan CVS experience, reported 29 cases of limb reduction defects after CVS from September 1990 until June 1992; four case had oromandibular-limb hypogenesis syndrome.[64] There were two remarkable aspects of this report. First, although the gestational age at sampling was not known with certainty in all cases, the majority were performed at less than 63 days after the last menstrual period. Second, very inexperienced community-based operators performed the cases with limb reduction defects, whereas no defects were seen from the major centers. This experience suggests that very early sampling with excessive placental trauma may be etiologic in some reports of post-CVS limb reduction defects.

The question continues to be debated of whether CVS sampling after 70 days has the potential of causing more subtle defects, such as shortening of the distal phalanx or nail hypoplasia.[65] At present, there are few data to substantiate this concern. On the contrary, most experienced centers performing CVS after 10 weeks have not seen an increase in limb defects of any type. A recent review of more than 200,000 CVS procedures reported to the WHO registry was reported and demonstrated no increase in the overall incidence of limb reduction defects after CVS or in any specific type or pattern of defect.[66] In a similar review of more than 65,000 procedures performed in 10 of the most experienced centers in the world, no increase in limb reduction defects was identified.[67]

Mechanisms by which early CVS could potentially lead to fetal malformations continue to be disputed. Placental thrombosis with subsequent fetal embolization has been raised as a potential etiology but is unlikely, because fetal clotting factors appear to be insufficient at this early gestational age. Inadvertent entry into the extraembryonic coelom with resulting amnionic bands, has also been raised as a potential mechanism but appears unlikely as well, because actual bands have not been observed in the majority of the

TABLE 27–3. STUDIES EVALUATING THE ASSOCIATION OF CHORIONIC VILLUS SAMPLING (CVS) AND LIMB REDUCTION DEFECT (LRD): PROCEDURES PERFORMED AFTER 63 DAYS

	No Association			Association	
Reference	***n* Post-CVS Liveborns**	***n* LRDs**	**Reference**	***n* Post-CVS Liveborns**	***n* LRDs**
Jahoda et al.[120]	3973	3	Burton et al.[131]	394	4
Halliday et al.[121]	2071	3*	Mastroiacovo et al.[132]	2759	3
Canadian group[13]	905	0	Bissonnette et al.[129]‡	507	5
Schloo et al.[122]	3120	2			
Monni et al.[123]	2752	2			
Blakemore et al.[124]	3709	3			
Silver et al.[125]	1048	1*			
Mahoney et al.[126]	4588	8**			
Jackson et al.[127]	12,863	5			
Smidt-Jensen et al.[128]	2624	0			
Bissonnette et al.[129]‡	269	0			
Case Control Studies	**OR**	**CI**		**OR**	**CI**
Dolk et al.[130]	1.8	0.7–5	Mastroiacovo and Botto[133]§	19	9–37
Williams et al.[73]			Williams et al.[73]		
Overall LRD	1.7	0.4–6	Terminal Digital LRD	6.4	1.1–38
Transverse LRD	4.7	0.8–28			

*Uncertain association: There was no statistical increase in LRDs, but absolute incidence was higher than general risk.
†Includes known syndromal defects.
‡Single report comparing two sampling sites.
§Less than 76 days.
CI, confidence interval; OR, odds ratio.

cases. In addition, many of the cases of oromandibular-limb hypogenesis syndrome had internal central nervous system anomalies that cannot be accounted for by fetal entanglement or compression.

Uterine vascular disruption appears to be the most plausible mechanism at present.[60] In this hypothesis, CVS causes placental injury or vasospasm that subsequently results in underperfusion of the fetal peripheral circulation. After the initial insult, there may be subsequent rupture of the thin-walled vessels of the damaged distal embryonic circulation, leading to further hypoxia, necrosis, and eventual resorption of preexisting limb structures. A similar mechanism leading to limb defects has been demonstrated in animal models after uterine vascular clamping, maternal cocaine exposure, or even simple uterine palpitation.[67,68]

In a recent report, Quintero et al. added additional information about a possible etiology.[69,70] Using TA embryoscopic visualization of the first-trimester embryo, they demonstrated the occurrence of fetal facial, head, and thoracic ecchymotic lesions after traumatically induced detachment of the placenta with subchorionic hematoma formation. No changes in fetal heart rate were seen. Although these lesions consistently appeared after major physical trauma to the placental site, they were not able to be produced by the passage of a standard CVS catheter.

Any theory of CVS-induced limb defects must consider that there are different stages of fetal sensitivity and should demonstrate a correlation between the severity of the defects and the gestational age at sampling. Firth et al. recently presented evidence that appears to illustrate that sampling before 9 weeks of gestation induces the most severe and proximally located fetal limb defects.[71] These severe defects are not seen after later CVS. Alternatively, Jackson and Froster reviewed the severity of the post-CVS limb defects reported to the WHO registry and found no such correlation.[66]

At the present time, patients planning to have CVS can be counseled that there is no increased risk of severe limb defects if CVS is performed after 70 days of gestation. They should be made aware of the present controversy concerning more subtle defects and reassured that this has not been seen in most experienced centers. If such a risk does exist, the magnitude based on case control studies can be estimated to be no higher than 1 in 3000.[72] Ideally, centers performing CVS should have aggressive follow-up systems in place and be capable of giving patients information about the rate of congenital abnormalities in their center. Sampling before 10 weeks of gestation should be limited to very exceptional cases, and these patients must be informed of a 1% or higher risk of limb reduction defects.

Perinatal Risks and Impact on Long-Term Development of the Infant

No increases in preterm labor, premature rupture of the membranes, small-for-gestational-age infants, maternal morbidity, or other obstetric complications have occurred in sampled patients.[73] Although the Canadian collaborative study showed an increased perinatal mortality in CVS sampled patients, with the greatest imbalance being beyond 28 weeks, no obvious recurrent event was identified.[13] To date, no other studies have seen a similar increase in perinatal loss.

Long-term infant follow-up has been performed by Chinese investigators who evaluated 53 children from their initial placental biopsy experience of the 1970s. All were reported in good health, with normal development and school performance.[74]

Laboratory Aspects of Chorionic Villus Sampling

CVS is now considered a reliable method of prenatal diagnosis, but early in its development incorrect results were reported.[75-77] The major sources of these errors included maternal cell contamination and misinterpretation of mosaicism confined to the placenta. Today, genetic evaluation of chorionic villi provides a high degree of success and accuracy, in particular with regard to the diagnosis of common trisomies.[78,79] In 1990, the United States collaborative study reported a 99.7% rate of successful cytogenetic diagnosis, with 1.1% of the patients requiring a second diagnostic test, such as amniocentesis or fetal blood analysis to further interpret the results.[78] In most cases, the additional testing was required to delineate the clinical significance of mosaic or other ambiguous results (76%), and laboratory failure (21%) and maternal cell contamination (3%) also required follow-up

testing. Continued experience has almost eliminated maternal cell contamination as a source of clinical errors. In addition, we now have a better understanding of the biology of the placenta so that confined placental mosaicism no longer leads to incorrect diagnosis but provides us with information predictive of pregnancy outcome and can serve as a clue to the presence of uniparental disomy. Therefore, an understanding of villus morphology and CVS laboratory techniques is required to provide correct clinical interpretation.

Chorionic villi have three major components: 1) an outer layer of hormonally active and invasive syncytiotrophoblast, 2) a middle layer of cytotrophoblast from which syncytiotrophoblast is derived, and 3) an inner mesodermal core containing blood, capillaries for oxygen, and nutrient exchange (Fig. 27–8). After collection, the villi are cleaned of any adherent decidua and then exposed to trypsin to digest and separate the cytotrophoblast from the underlying mesodermal core. The cytotrophoblast has a high mitotic index, with many spontaneous mitoses available for immediate chromosomal analysis. The liquid suspension containing the cytotrophblast is either dropped immediately onto a slide for analysis or may undergo a short incubation.[80-82] This "direct" chromosomal preparation can provide preliminary results within 2 to 3 h. However, most laboratories now use overnight incubation to improve karyotype quality and thus report results within 2 to 4 days (Fig. 27–9). The remaining villus core is placed in tissue culture and is typically ready for harvest and chromosome analysis within 1 week.[83] The

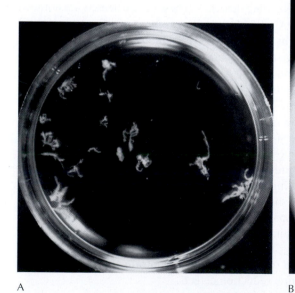

A

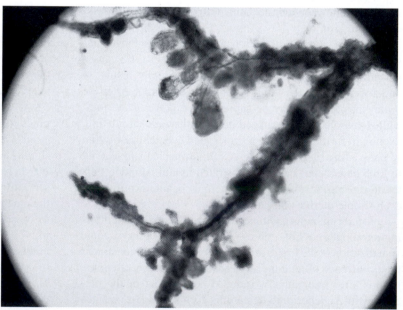

B

Figure 27–8. (A) Photograph of chorionic villus fragments in a Petri dish after collection by chorionic villus sampling. **(B)** Magnified image of chorionic villus. Note the cytotrophoblastic bud. Within the center of the villus is the mesymchal core and fetal blood vessels.

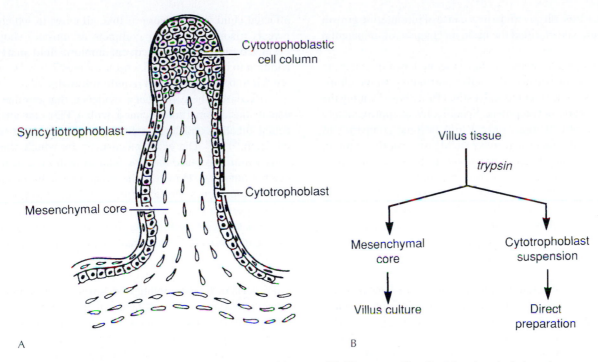

Figure 27–9. (A) Diagram of normal villus architecture. **(B)** Diagram outling the laboratory technique for chorionic villus sampling direct chromosomal preparation and villus culture.

direct method has the advantage of providing a rapid result and minimizing the decidual contamination, whereas tissue culture is better for interpreting discrepancies between the cytotrophoblast and the actual fetal state. Ideally, both the direct and culture methods should be used because they each evaluate slightly different tissue sources. Abnormalities in either may have clinical implications. However, the direct preparation is labor intensive, adds additional cost, and is not routinely available in some laboratories.

Maternal Cell Contamination

Chorionic villus samples typically contain a mixture of placental villi and maternally derived decidua. Although specimens are thoroughly washed and inspected under a microscope after collection, some maternal cells may remain and grow in the culture. As a result, two cell lines, one fetal and the other maternal, may be identified. In other cases, the maternal cell line may completely overgrow the culture, thereby leading to diagnostic errors including incorrect sex determination[5,84,85,86] and potentially to false-negative diagnoses, although there are no published reports of the latter. Direct preparations of chorionic villi are generally thought to prevent maternal cell contamination,[82,85] whereas long-term culture has a rate ranging from 1.8 to 4%.[86] Because, in contrast to cytotrophoblast, maternal decidua has a low mitotic index, it is highly desirable for laboratories to offer a direct chromosomal preparation and a long-term culture on all samples of chorionic villus. Even in culture, the contam-

inating cells are easily identified as maternal and should not lead to clinical errors. Interestingly, for reasons still uncertain, maternal cell contamination occurs more frequently in specimens retrieved by the TC route.[86]

Contamination of samples with significant amounts of maternal decidual tissue is almost always due to small sample size, making selection of appropriate tissue difficult. In experienced centers in which adequate quantities of villi are available, this problem has disappeared. Choosing only whole, clearly typical villus material and discarding any atypical fragments, small pieces, or fragments with adherent decidua will avoid confusion.[87] Therefore, if the initial aspiration is small, a second pass should be performed rather than risk inaccurate results. When proper care is taken and good cooperation and communication exists between the sampler and the laboratory, even small amounts of contaminating maternal tissue can be absent.

Confined Placental Mosaicism

The second major source of potential diagnostic error associated with CVS is mosaicism confined to the placenta. Although the fetus and placenta have a common ancestry, chorionic villus tissue will not always reflect fetal genotype.[78,88] Although there was concern that this might invalidate CVS as a prenatal diagnostic tool, subsequent investigations have led to a clearer understanding of villus biology so that accurate clinical interpretation is now possible. This understanding has also revealed new information about the etiology of pregnancy loss, discovered a new cause of intrauterine growth retardation, and clarified the basic mechanism of uniparental disomy.

Discrepancies between the cytogenetics of the placenta and fetus occur because the cells contributing to the chorionic villi become separate and distinct from those forming the embryo in early development. Specifically, at approximately the 32- to 64-cell stage, only 3 to 4 become compartmentalized into the inner cell mass (ICM) to form the embryo, and the remainder become precursors of the extraembryonic tissues.[89] Mosaicism can then occur through two possible mechanisms.[90] An initial meiotic error in one of the gametes can lead to a trisomic conceptus that normally would spontaneously abort. However, if one of the early aneuploid precursor cells loses one of the chromosomes contributing to the trisomic set during subsequent mitotic divisions, the embryo can be "rescued" by reduction of a portion of its cells to disomy. This will result in a mosaic morula, with the percentage of normal cells dependent on the cell division at which rescue occurred. More abnormal cells will be present when correction is delayed to the second or a subsequent cell division. Because the majority of cells in the morula proceed to the trophoblast cell lineage (processed by the direct preparation), it is highly probable that that lineage will continue to contain a significant number of trisomic cells. Alternatively, because only a small number of cells are incorporated into the ICM, involvement of the fetus will depend on the chance distribution of the aneuploid progenitor cells. Involvement of the mesenchymal core of the villus, which also evolves from the ICM, is similarly dependent on this random cell distribution. Noninvolvement of the fetal cell lineage will produce *confined placental mosaicism* (CPM) in which the trophoblast and perhaps the extra-embryonic mesoderm will have aneuploid cells, but the fetus will be euploid.

Alternatively, mitotic postzygotic errors can produce mosaicism, with the distribution and percentage of aneuploid cells in the morula or blastocyst dependent on the timing of nondisjunction. If mitotic errors occur early in the development of the morula, they may segregate to the ICM and have the same potential to produce an affected fetus as do meiotic errors. Mitotic errors occurring after primary cell differentiation and compartmentalization has been completed, leading to cytogenetic abnormalities in only one lineage.

Meiotic rescue can lead to uniparental disomy (UPD). This occurs because the original trisomic cell contained two chromosomes from one parent and one from the other. After rescue, there is a theoretical 1 in 3 chance that the resulting pair of chromosomes came from the same parent, which is called *uniparental disomy*. UPD may have clinical consequences if the chromosomes involved carry imprinted genes in which expression is based on the parent of origin. For example, Prader–Willi syndrome may result from uniparental maternal disomy for chromosome 15. Therefore, a CVS diagnosis of confined placental mosaicism for trisomy 15 may be the initial clue that UPD could be present and lead to an affected child.[91,92] Because of this, all cases in which CVS reveals trisomy 15 (either complete or mosaic) should be evaluated for UPD by subsequent amniotic fluid analysis. In addition to chromosome 15, chromosomes 7, 11, 14, and 22 are felt to be imprinted and require follow-up.[93]

Recently, there has been evidence that confined placental mosaicism (unassociated with UPD) can alter placental function and lead to fetal growth failure or perinatal death.[90,94–99] The exact mechanism by which abnormal cells within the placenta alter fetal growth or lead to fetal death is unknown. However, the effect may be limited to specific chromosomes. For example, CPM for chromosome 16 leads to severe intrauterine growth restriction, prematurity, or perinatal death, with fewer than 30% of pregnancies resulting in normal full-term infants appropriate for gestational age.[100–107]

CVS mosaic results require diligent follow-up by amniocentesis or fetal sampling to determine their clinical significance because, in most cases, if the mosaic results are confined to the placenta, fetal development will be normal. However, if the mosaic cell line also involves the fetus, there may be significant phenotypic consequences. Mosaicism occurs in about 1% of all CVS samples[79,86,103,104] but is confirmed in the fetus in only 10 to 40% of these cases. The probability of fetal involvement appears to be related to the tissue source in which the aneuploid cells were detected and the specific chromosome involved.[93] Mesenchymal core culture results are more likely than direct preparation to reflect a true fetal mosaicism.

In a recent review, Phillips et al. demonstrated that autosomal mosaicism involving common trisomies (i.e., 21, 18, and 13) was confirmed in the fetus in 19% of cases, whereas uncommon trisomies involved the fetus in only 3%.[105] When sex chromosome mosaicism was found in the placenta, the abnormal cell line was confirmed in the fetus in 16% of cases. When a nonfamilial marker chromosome was involved, it was confirmed in the fetus in more than one-fourth of cases, whereas mosaic polyploidy was confirmed in only 1 of 28 cases. Chromosomal structural abnormalities were confirmed in 8.6% of cases.

When placental mosaicism is discovered, amniocentesis is frequently performed to elucidate the extent of fetal involvement. When mosaicism is limited to the direct preparation only, amniocentesis appears to correlate perfectly with fetal genotype.[105] However, when a mosaicism is observed in tissue culture, both false-positive and false-negative amniocentesis results occur. In these cases, amniocentesis will predict the true fetal karyotype in approximately 94% of cases.[105] Most importantly, these discrepancies may involve the common autosomal trisomies. There have been three cases reported of mosaic trisomy 21 on villus culture, a normal amniotic fluid analysis, followed by a fetus or newborn with mosaic aneuploidy.[78]

At present, the following clinical recommendations may be used to assist in the evaluation of CVS mosaicism. Analysis of CVS samples should, if possible, include both direct preparation and tissue culture. Although the direct preparation is less likely to be representative of the fetus, its use will minimize the likelihood of maternal cell contamination; and if culture fails, a nonmosaic normal direct preparation result can be considered conclusive, although rare cases of false-negative results for trisomies 21 and 18 have been reported.[106–110] If mosaicism is found on either culture or direct preparation, follow-up amniocentesis should be offered. Under no circumstances should a decision to terminate a pregnancy be based entirely on a CVS mosaic result. For CVS mosaicism involving sex chromosome abnormalities, polyploidy, marker chromosomes, structural rearrangements, and uncommon trisomies, the patient can be reassured if amniocentesis results are euploid and detailed ultrasonographic examination is normal. However, no guarantees should be made and, as described above, in certain cases testing for UPD will be indicated. If common trisomies 21, 18, and 13 are involved, amniocentesis should be offered, but the patient must be advised of the possibilities of a false-negative result. Follow-up may include detailed ultrasonography, fetal blood sampling, or fetal skin biopsy. At present, the predictive accuracy of these additional tests is uncertain.

Biochemical and DNA Procedures

Most biochemical and molecular diagnosis that can be made from amnionic fluid or cultured amniocytes can also be made from chorionic villi. In many cases, the results will be available more rapidly and more efficiently by using villi, because sufficient enzyme or DNA is present in villus samples to allow direct analysis rather than wait for tissue culture. For example, the analysis of Tay-Sachs disease can be performed in less than 30 mins using fresh villi.[111]

A discussion of individual biochemical or molecular diagnoses is beyond the scope of this chapter and is impractical because techniques are changing so rapidly. A registry of diagnoses performed by CVS is kept and updated through the WHO by Dr. Hans Galjaard in Rotterdam, The Netherlands, and a published summary of the early worldwide experience is available.[112]

It cannot be assumed that biochemical or molecular results from villus tissue will always be a true reflection of the fetal state. Recently, misdiagnosis of the peroxisomal disorder, X-linked adrenoleukodystrophy, from cultured villus cells has been reported.[113] In addition, tests requiring determination of DNA methylation status, such as that for fragile X,[114] are also not always reliable in villus tissue. This does not, however, preclude CVS from making these prenatal diagnoses because other molecular approaches can be used. It does emphasize that all tests on villus tissue must be validated by testing sufficient numbers of affected and unaffected pregnancies before being used clinically. Because of the rarity and unique aspects of most biochemical and molecular disorders, specific diagnoses are usually performed by only a few laboratories. Before performing a CVS, the clinician should contact the center analyzing the tissue so that the details of testing can be discussed.

Chorionic Villus Sampling in Multiple Gestations

Chorionic villus sampling is a safe and effective approach to examining twins. Not only does it provide results early in pregnancy, but, if discordancy is discovered, the medical and psychological difficulties encountered with selective termination can be minimized. However, it can be technically more demanding because it requires an experienced operator and sonographer. The ideal time to perform a twin CVS is similar to that for singletons. Ultrasound initially identifies placental locations, determines chorionicity, and confirms fetal sizes and viability. Sampling of each sac is independently performed by either a TC or TA approach, with separate passes of a new sampling instrument for each attempt. Because no unique marker is available to ensure that the samples have been retrieved from distinct placentas, it is imperative that insertion of the instrument into each frondosum is certain. Longitudinal and transverse scanning planes should be used to ensure proper location. If any doubt exists, a repeat procedure is required, but with increased experience, the need for repeat procedure is rare.[115]

Contamination of one sample with villi from the other sac is possible and occurs most commonly when retrieval is performed near the dividing membrane or if a needle or catheter is dragged through one frondosum while sampling another. When the chorions appear fused, sampling near the cord insertion sites, with avoidance of the area of confluence of the two placentas, should prevent contamination and ensure sampling of each fetus. A combination of TC and TA sampling can minimize co-twin contamination by ensuring unique sampling paths. For example, if both chorion frondosa are situated along the anterior uterine wall, the lower one can be sampled transcervically and the upper transabdominally without contaminating either sample. Despite meticulous sampling techniques, co-twin contamination occurs in up to 4% of cases[116] but is rarely of clinical concern. If the cytogenetic laboratory is aware of the presence of a multiple gestation, the presence of both normal and aneuploid cells in the sample will be correctly interpreted. The possibility of contamination is of greater consequence if sampling is being performed for biochemical analysis, where a small amount of contaminating tissue could lead to an incorrect diagnosis. For this reason, instead of pooling a sample, we recommend analyzing individual villi when biochemical studies are to be performed. An experienced sampler and an aware and knowledgeable laboratory are extremely important in such cases.

The need to map the placental location clearly and accurately is mandatory, because the risk of discordant results is higher early in the pregnancy and selective termination may be required. The relative positions of the placentas will remain stable over the time frame that results are obtained, so that identification of the affected fetus can usually be

TABLE 27–4. SAFETY OF CHORIONIC VILLUS SAMPLING (CVS) WITH TWINS COMPARED WITH AMNIOCENTESIS

	n	Success Rate	Pregnancy Loss Rate to 28 Weeks
CVS			
Wapner et al.[115]*	440[†]	100%	2.8%
Pergament et al.[116]	128	99.2%	2.4%
Brambati et al.[119]	66	100%	1.6%
Amniocentesis			
Wapner et al.[115]*	73	100	2.9%

*Contemporaneously collected comparison of CVS with amniocentesis in a single center.

[†]Additional cases added since original publication.

determined even 2 or 3 weeks after the procedure. However, if there is uncertainty, a repeat CVS with direct villus analysis can confirm the position immediately before the termination.

Procedure-related loss rates after CVS sampling of twins are well studied. In experienced centers, no increased procedure related loss risks are seen compared with second-trimester amniocentesis.[115,116] Table 27–4 presents overall pregnancy loss rates to 28 weeks of 1.6 to 2.8% in sampled twins. When compared with a contemporaneously sampled group of patients choosing either CVS or second-trimester amniocentesis, we found no difference in the overall risk of pregnancy loss (2.9% amniocentesis vs. 3.2% CVS). There was, however, a slightly increased risk of losing one fetus in the group sampled by amniocentesis.[115]

The choice of the appropriate technique for sampling twins depends on a number of factors including locally available skill and expertise. In centers in which amniocentesis and CVS are both available, CVS may be the preferred approach because it provides results 1 month sooner, thus providing earlier reassurance. When discordant results are encountered, complications and loss rates are decreased when selective termination is performed before 16 weeks of gestation.[117]

Chorionic Villus Sampling and Multifetal Pregnancy Reduction

Multifetal pregnancy reduction (MFPR) to improve perinatal outcome is an unfortunate but accepted part of reproductive medicine. As with selective termination, MFPR is most safely performed in the first trimester.[118] Therefore, in high order gestations at increased risk for a genetic abnormality, CVS before a reduction can avoid the potential need for a later selective termination. The CVS can be performed between 10 and 11.5 weeks of gestation, and a rapid karyotype can be available within 24 to 48 hours, after which the MFPR is performed. Villus mesenchymal core tissue culture is also performed, but results are usually not available for 7 to 10 days. Because of the small increased risk of confined placental mosaicism with the direct preparation, awaiting culture results when time allows is suggested. The positions of the sampled fetuses will be the same when the patient returns for the MFPR. In most cases, only the two fetuses most likely to remain after the MFPR are sampled. If an abnormality is identified, an additional fetus can be sampled at the time of the MFPR and the patient can return if this is also abnormal. Of 745 MFPR reductions performed at our center, 254 had an initial CVS. Abnormal chromosomal results were present in approximately 2.5% of pregnancies, and the abnormal fetus was terminated as part of the reduction procedure. The pregnancy loss rate to 24 weeks of gestation of those having a preceding CVS was 5.5% versus 5.6% in those having only MFPR. This encouraging outcome is similar to that described by Brambati et al.[119] in which the cohort of patients undergoing CVS before MFPR demonstrated no increased risk of pregnancy loss, prematurity, or small-for-gestational-age infants.

SUMMARY

Chorionic villus sampling is a safe technique for first-trimester prenatal diagnosis of genetic disorders. Real-time sonography and technologic advances of sampling instruments have been critical in establishing a safe technique for retrieving villus tissue for genetic analysis. Clinical trials suggest that CVS carries a low risk of pregnancy loss, which is comparable to that of second-trimester amniocentesis. An understanding of the laboratory techniques and human embryology is essential in avoiding diagnostic errors related to confined placental mosaicism.

To maximize outcome, CVS should be performed by an experienced team of physicians, ultrasonographers, and genetic laboratory technicians. Before initiating a CVS program, operators should have considerable experience in the placement of the catheter, which can be achieved either in a formal training program with observation of 50 procedures followed by close hands-on supervision of another 100 cases[5] or by supervised practice on pregnancies undergoing subsequent abortion. In addition, it is advisable to limit the number of ultrasonographers assigned to assist in this procedure because sampling success is equally dependent on skillful ultrasound guidance. Similar to the physician retrieving the villi, the guiding sonographer should be knowledgable in the didactics of CVS sampling and should obtain adequate hands-on training before beginning work in this area. This can be achieved in a formal training program or by visiting centers performing this procedure.[5] In this setting, CVS will continue to be an important, reliable, and safe contributor to prenatal genetic diagnosis.

REFERENCES

1. Grimes DA, Schultz KF. Morbity and mortality from second trimester abortion. *J Repro Med.* 1985;30:505–514.

2. Sundberg K, Bang J, Smidt-Jensen S, et al. Randomized study of risk of fetal loss related to early amniocentesis versus chorionic villus sampling. *Lancet*. 1997;350:697–703.

3. CEMAT Group. Randomized trial to assess safety and fetal outcomes of early and midtrimester amniocentesis. *Lancet*. 1998; 351:1435.

4. Spencer K, Souter V, Tul N, et al. A screening program for trisomy 21 at 10–14 weeks using fetal nuchal translucency, maternal serum free B-human chorionic gonadotrophin and pregnancy-assoicarted plasma protein A. *Ultrasound Obstet Gynecol*. 1991;13:231–231.

5. Boehm FH, Salyer SL, Dev VG, et al. Chorionic villus sampling: Quality control-m-A continuous improvement model. *Am J Obstet Gynecol*. 1993;168:1766–1777.

6. Department of Obstetrics and Gynecology. Tietung Hospital of Anshan Iron and Steel Co. Anshan, China. Fetal sex prediction by sex chromatin of chorionic villi cells during early pregnancy. *Chinese Med J*. 1975;1:117.

7. Hahnemann N, Mohr J. Genetic diagnosis in the embryo by means of biopsy from extraembryonic membranes. *Bull Eur Soc Hum Genet*. 1968;2:23–29.

8. Kullander S, Sandahl B. Fetal chromosome analysis after transcervical placental biopsies during early pregnancy. *Acta Obstet Gynecol Scand*. 1973;52:355–359.

9. Hahnemann N. Early prenatal diagnosis: A study of biopsy techniques and cell culturing from extraembryonic membranes. *Clin Genet*. 1974;6:294–306.

10. Kazy Z, Rozovsky I, Bakhaey V. Chorion biopsy in early pregnancy: A method of early prenatal diagnosis for inherited disorders. *Prenat Diagn*. 1982;2:39–45.

11. Old J. First trimester fetal diagnosis for haemoglobinopathies: Three cases. *Lancet*. 1982;2:1413–1416.

12. Brambati B, Simoni G. Diagnosis of fetal trisomy 21 in first trimester. *Lancet*. 1983;1:586.

13. Canadian Collaborative CVS Amniocentesis Clinical Trial Group. Multicentre randomized clinical trial of chorion villus sampling and amniocentesis. *Lancet*. 1989;i:1.

14. Rhoads GG, Jackson IG, Schlesselman SE, et al. The safety and efficacy of chorionic villus sampling for early prenatal diagnosis of cytogenetic abnormalities. *N Engl J Med*. 1989;320:609–619.

15. Committee on Genetics. *ACOG Committee Opin*. 1995;160.

16. Jackson LG, Zachary JM, Fowler SE, et al. Randomized comparison of transcervical and transabdominal chorionic villus sampling. *N Engl J Med*. 1992;327:594–598.

17. Silver RK, MacGregor SN, Sholl JS, et al. Initiating a chorionic villus sampling program. Relying on placental location as the primary determinant of the sampling route. *J Reprod Med*. 1990;35:964–968.

18. Brambati B, Oldrini A, Lanzani A. Transabdominal and trans-cervical chorionic villus sampling: Efficiency and risk evaluation of 2,411 cases. *Am J Med Genet*. 1990;35: 160–164.

19. Liu DT, Agbaje R, Preston C, Savage J. Intraplacental sonolucent spaces: Incidences and relevance to chorionic villus sampling. *Prenat Diagn*. 1991;11:805.

20. Brambati B, Oldrini A, Lanzani A. Transabdominal chorionic villus sampling: A freehand ultrasound-guided technique. *Am J Obstet Gynecol*. 1987;157:134.

21. Smidt-Jensen S, Hahnemann N. Transabdominal chorionic villus sampling for fetal genetic diagnosis. Technical and obstetric evaluation of 100 cases. *Prenat Diagn*. 1988;8:7.

22. Jackson LG, Wapner RJ. Risks of chorionic villus sampling. *Clin Obstet Gynecol*. 1987;1:513.

23. Brambati B, Oldrini A, Ferrazzi E, et al. Chorionic villus sampling: An analysis of the obstetric experience of 1000 cases. *Prenat Diagn*. 1987;7:157–169.

24. Brambati B, Matarrelli M, Varotto F. Septic complications after chorionic villus sampling. *Lancet*. 1987;i(8543):1212a.

25. Wass D, Bennett MJ. Infection and chorionic villus sampling. *Lancet*. 1985;ii:338.

26. Scialli AR, Neugebauer DL, Fabro SE. Microbiology of the endcervix in patients undergoing chorionic villus sampling. In: Fracearo M, Simoni G, Brambati B, eds. *First Trimester Fetal Diagnosis*. Berlin: Springer-Verlag; 1985;69–73.

27. Brambati B, Varotti F. Infection and chorionic villus sampling. *Lancet*. 1985;ii:609.

28. Hogge WA, Schonberg SA, Golbus MS. Chorionic villus sampling: Experience of the first 1000 cases. *Am J Obstet Gynecol*. 1986;154:1249.

29. Gilmore DH, McNay MB. Spontaneous fetal loss rate in early pregnancy. *Lancet*. 1985;i:107.

30. Wilson RD, Kendrick V, Witmann BK. Risks of spontaneous abortion in ultrasonographically normal pregnancies. *Lancet*. 1984;ii:920.

31. Barela A, Kleinman GE, Golditch IM, et al. Septic shock with renal failure after chorionic villus sampling. *Am J Obstet Gynecol*. 1986;154:1120.

32. Blakemore KJ, Mahoney MJ, Hobbins JC. Infection and chorionic villus sampling. *Lancet*. 1985;2:339.

33. Cheng EY, Luth DA, Hickok D, et al. Transcervical chorionic villus sampling and midtrimester oligohydramnios. *Am J Obstet Gynecol*. 1991;165:1063.

34. Blakemore KJ, Baumgarten A, Schoenfeld-Dimaio M, et al. Rise in maternal serum alpha fetoprotein concentration after chorionic villus sampling. *Lancet*. 1985;ii:339.

35. Bramabati B, Guercilena S, Bonacchi I, et al. Fetomaternal transfusion after chorionic villus sampling: Clinical implications. *Hum Reprod*. 1986;37.

36. Shulman LP, Meyers CM, Simpson JL, et al. Fetomaternal transfusion depends on amount of chorionic villi aspirated but not on method of chorionic villus sampling. *Am J Obstet Gynecol*. 1990;162:1185.

37. Smidt-Jensen S, Philip J, Zachary J, et al. Implications of maternal serum alpha-fetoprotein elevation caused by transabdominal and transcervical CVS. *Prenat Diagn*. 1994; 14:35–46.

38. Zipursky A, Israels LG. The pathogenesis and prevention of Rh immunization. *Can Med Assoc J*. 1967;97:1245–1257.

39. Moise KJ, Carpenter RJ: Increased severity of fetal hemolytic disease with known Rhesus alloimmunization after first trimester transcervical chorionic villus biopsy. *Fetal Diagn Ther*. 1990;5:76.

40. Clark BA, Bissonnette J, Olson SB, et al. Pregnancy loss in a small chorionic villus sampling series. *Am J Obstet Gynecol*. 1989;161:301.

41. Green JE, Dorfman A, Jones SL, et al. Chorionic villus sampling: Experience with an initial 940 cases. *Obstet Gynecol*. 1988;71:208.

42. Gustavii B, Claesson V, Kristoffersson U, et al. Risk of

miscarriage after chorionic biopsy is probably not higher than after amniocentesis. *Lakartidningen*. 1989;86:4221.

43. Jahoda MGJ, Pijpers L, Reuss A, et al. Evaluation of transcervical chorionic villus sampling with a completed follow-up of 1550 consecutive pregnancies. *Prenat Diagn*. 1989;9:621.

44. Young SR, Shipley CF, Wade RV, et al. Single-center comparison of results of 1000 prenatal diagnoses with chorionic villus sampling and 1000 diagnoses with amniocentesis. *Am J Obstet Gynecol*. 1991;165:255.

45. Hogge WA, Schonberg SA, Golbus MS. Chorionic villus sampling: Experience of the first 1000 cases. *Am J Obstet Gynecol*. 1986;154:1249–1252.

46. Jackson LG. *CVS Newslett*. 1988;25–27.

47. Wade RV, Young SR. Analysis of fetal loss after transcervical chorionic villus sampling: A review of 719 patients. *Am J Obstet Gynecol*. 1989;161:513–519.

48. Warburton D, Fraser FC. Spontaneous abortion risks in man: Data from reproductive histories collected in a medical genetics unit. *Hum Genet*. 1964;16:1–25.

49. Simpson JL, Mills ML, Holmes LB, et al. Low fetal loss rates after ultrasound-proved viability in early pregnancy. *JAMA*. 1987;258:2555–2557.

50. Christiaens GC, Stoutenbeck MC. Spontaneous abortion in proven intact pregnancies. *Lancet*. 1984;2:571–572.

51. Wilson RD, Kendrick V, Wirtman BP, et al. Spontaneous abortion and pregnancy outcome after normal first-trimester ultrasound examination. *Obstet Gynecol*. 1986;67:352–355.

52. Saura R, Gauthier B, Taine L, et al. Operator experiences and fetal loss rate in transabdominal CVS. *Prenat Diagn*. 1994;14:70.

53. Wapner RJ, Barr MA, Heeger S, et al. Chorionic villus sampling: A 10-year, over 13,000 consecutive case experience (abstract). Presented at the First Annual Meeting of the American College of Medical Genetics, Orlando, Florida, March 1994.

54. Nicolaides K, Brizot M de L, Patel F, Snijders R. Comparison of chorionic villus sampling and amniocentesis for fetal karyotyping at 10–13 weeks' gestation. *Lancet*. 1994; 344(8920):435.

55. Brambati B, Lanzani A, Tului L. Transabdominal and transcervical chorionic villus sampling: Efficacy and risk evaluation of 2411 cases. *Am J Hum Genet*. 1990;35:160.

56. Brambati B, Terzian E, Tognoni G. Randomized clinical trial of transabdominal versus transcervical chorionic villus sampling methods. *Prenat Diagn*. 1991;11:285.

57. Smidt-Jensen S, Permin M, Philip J. Sampling success and risk by transabdominal chorionic villus sampling, transcervical chorionic villus sampling and amniocentesis: A randomized study. *Ultrasound Obstet Gynecol*. 1991;1:86.

58. Chuch JT, Goldberg JD, Wohlfered MM, Golbus MS. Comparison of transcervical and transabdominal chorionic villus sampling loss rates in nine thousand cases from a single center. *Am J Obstet Gynecol*. 1995;173:1277.

59. Firth HV, Boyd P, Chamberlain P, et al. Severe limb abnormalities after chorion villus sampling at 56–66 days gestation. *Lancet*. 1991;337:726.

60. Hoyme F, Jones KL, Van Allen MI, et al. Vascular pathogenesis of transverse limb reduction defects. *J Pediatr*. 1982;101:839.

61. Foster-Iskenius U, Baird P. Limb reduction defects in over 1,000,000 consecutive live births. *Teratology*. 1989;39:127.

62. Mastroiacovo P, Botto LD, Cavalcanti DP. Limb anomalies following chorionic villus sampling: A registry based case control study. *Am J Med Genet*. 1992;44:856–863.

63. Brambati B, Simoni G, Traui M. Genetic diagnosis by chorionic villus sampling before 8 gestational weeks: Efficiency, reliability, and risks on 317 completed pregnancies. *Prenat Diagn*. 1992;12:784–799.

64. Hsieh FJ, Shyu MK, Sheu BC, et al. Limb defects after chorionic villus sampling. *Obstet Gynecol*. 1995;85:84.

65. Burton BK, Schultz CJ, Burd LI. Spectrum of limb disruption defects associated with chorionic villus sampling. *Pediatrics*. 1993;91:989–993.

66. Froster UG, Jackson L. Limb defects and chorionic villus sampling: Results from an international registry. 1992–1994. *Lancet*. 1996;347(9000):489.

67. Brent RL. Relationship between uterine vascular clamping, vascular disruption syndrome and cocaine teratology. *Teratology*. 1990;41:757.

68. Webster W, Brown-Woodman T. Cocaine as a cause of congenital malformations of vascular origin: Experimental evidence in the rat. *Teratology*. 1990;41:689.

69. Quintero R, Romero R, Mahoney M, et al. Fetal haemorrhagic lesions after chorionic villus sampling. *Lancet*. 1992;339:193.

70. Quintero RA, Romero R, Mahoney MJ, et al. Embryoscopic demonstration of hemoagic lesions on the human embryo after placental tauma. *Am J Obstet Gynecol*. 1993;168:756–759.

71. Firth HV, Boyd PA, Chamberlain PF, et al. Analysis of limb reduction defects in babies exposed to chorionic villus sampling. *Lancet*. 1994;343(8905):1069.

72. Olney RS, Khoury MJ, Alo CJ, et al. Increased risk for transverse digital deficiency after chorionic villus sampling: Results of the United States Multistate Case-Control Study. 1988–1992. *Teratology*. 1995;5(1):20–29.

73. Williams J, Medearis AL, Bear MD, et al. Chorionic villus sampling is associated with normal fetal growth. *Am J Obstet Gynecol*. 1987;157:708.

74. Angue H, Bingru Z, Hong W. Long-term follow-up results after aspiration of chorionic villi during early pregnancy. In: Fraccaro M, Simoni G, Brambati B, eds. *First Trimester Fetal Diagnosis*. New York: Springer; 1995:1.

75. Martin AO, Simpson JL, Rosinksy BJ, et al. Chorionic villus sampling in continuing pregnancies II: Cytogenetic reliability. *Am J Obstet Gynecol*. 1986;154:1653–1662.

76. Simoni G, Gimelli G, Cuoco C, et al. Discordance between prenatal cytogenetic diagnosis after chorionic villi sampling and chromosomal constitution of the fetus. In: Fraccaro M, Simoni G, Brambati B, eds. *First Trimester Fetal Diagnosis*. Heidelberg: Springer-Verlag; 1985:137–143.

77. Cheung SW, Crane JP, Beaver HA, et al. Chromosome mosaicism and maternal cell contamination in chorionic villi. *Prenat Diagn*. 1987;7:535–542.

78. Ledbetter DH, Martin AO, Verlinsky Y, et al. Cytogenetic results of chorionic villus sampling: High success rate and diagnostic accuracy in the United States collaborative study. *Am J Obstet Gynecol*. 1990;162:495.

79. Mikkelsen M, Ayme S. Chromosomal findings in chorionic villi. In: Vogel F, Sperling K, eds. *Human Genetics*. Heidelberg: Springer-Verlag; 1987:597.

80. Simoni G, Brambati B, Danesino C, et al. Efficient direct chromosome analyses and enzyme determinations from chorionic

villi samples in the first trimester of pregnancy. *Hum Genet.* 1983;63:349.

81. Ford JH, Jahnke AB. Handling of chorionic villus for direct chromosome studies. *Lancet.* 1983;2:1491.

82. Gregson NM, Seabright N. Handling of chorionic villi for direct chromosome studies. *Lancet.* 1983;2:1491.

83. Chang HC, Jones OW, Masui H. Human amniotic fluid cells grown in a hormone-supplemented medium: Suitability for prenatal diagnosis. *Proc Natl Acad Sci U S A.* 1982;79:4795.

84. Hogge WA, Schonberg SA, Golbus MS. Prenatal diagnosis by chorionic villus sampling: Lessons of the first 600 cases. *Prenat Diagn.* 1985;5:393.

85. Williams J, Madearis AL, Chun WH, et al. Maternal cell contamination in cultured chorionic villi: Comparison of chromosome Q-polymorphisms derived from villi, fetal skin, and maternal lymphocytes. *Prenal Diagn.* 1987;7:315.

86. Ledbetter DH, Zachary JL, Simpson MS, et al. Cytogenetic results from the U.S. collaborative study on CVS. *Prenat Diagn.* 1992;12:317.

87. Elles RG, Williamson R, Niazi D, et al. Absence of maternal contamination of chorionic villi used for fetal gene analysis. *N Engl J Med.* 1983;308:1433.

88. Karkut I, Zakrzewski S, Sperling K. Mixed karyotypes obtained by chorionic villi analysis: Mosaicism and maternal contamination. In: Fraccaro M, Simoni G, Brambati B, eds. *First Trimester Fetal Diagnosis.* Heidelberg: Springer-Verlag; 1985:144–146.

89. Markert C, Petters R. Manufactured hexaparenteral mice show that adults are derived from three embryonic cells. *Science.* 1978;202:56.

90. Wolstenholine J. Confined placental mosaicism for trisomies 2, 3, 7, 8, 9, 16, and 22: Their incidence, likely origins, and mechanisms for cell lineage compartmentalization. *Prenat Diag.* 1996;16:511.

91. Cassidy SB, Lai LW, Erickson RP, et al. Trisomy 15 with loss of the paternal 15 as a cause of Prader–Willi syndrome due to maternal disomy. *Am J Hum Genet.* 1992;51:701.

92. Purvis-Smith SG, Sayille T, Manass S, et al. Uniparental disomy 15 resulting from "correction" of an initial trisomy 15. *Am J Hum Genet.* 1992;50:1348.

93. Ledbetter DH, Engel E. Uniparental disomy in humans: Development of an imprinting map and its implications for prenatal diagnosis. *Hum Mol Genet.* 1995;4:1757–1764.

94. Kalousek DK, Dill FJ, Pantzar T, et al. Confined chorionic mosaicism in prenatal diagnosis. *Hum Genet.* 1987;77:163.

95. Johnson A, Wapner RJ, Davis GH, et al. Mosaicism in chorionic villus sampling: An association with poor perinatal outcome. *Obstet Gynecol.* 1990;75:573.

96. Wapner RJ, Simpson MS, Golbus MS, et al. Chorionic mosaicism: Association with fetal loss but not with adverse perinatal outcome. *Prenat Diagn.* 1992;12:347.

97. Goldberg JD, Proter AE, Golbus MS. Current assessment of fetal losses as a direct consequence of chorionic villus sampling. *Am J Med Genet.* 1990;35:174.

98. Kalousek DK, Howard-Pebbles PN, Olson SB, et al. Confirmation of CVS mosaicism in term placentae and high frequency of intrauterine growth retardation association with confined placental mosaicism. *Prenat Diagn.* 1991;11:743.

99. Worton RG, Stern R. A. Canadian collaborative study of mosaicism in amniotic fluid cell cultures. *Prenat Diagn.* 1984;4:131.

100. Kalousek DK, Langlois S, Barrett I, et al. Uniparental disomy for chromosome 16 in humans. *Am J Hum Genet.* 1993;52:8.

101. Post JG, Nijhuis JG. Trisomy 16 confined to the placenta. *Prenat Diagn.* 1992;12:1001.

102. Benn P. Trisomy 16 and trisomy 16 mosaicism: A review. *Am J Med Genet.* 1998;79:121–133.

103. Vejerslev LO, Mikkelsen M. The European collaborative study on mosaicism in chorionic villus sampling: Data from 1986–1987. *Prenal Diagn.* 1989;9:575.

104. Breed ASPM, Mantingh A, Vosters R, et al. Follow-up and pregnancy outcome after a diagnosis of mosaicism in CVS. *Prenat Diagn.* 1991;11:577.

105. Phillips OP, Tharapel AT, Lerner JL, et al. Risk of fetal mosaicism when placental mosaicism is diagnosed by chorionic villus sampling. *Am J Obstet Gynecol.* 1996;174:850.

106. Bartels I, Hansmann I, Holland U, et al. Down syndrome at birth not detected by first trimester chorionic villus sampling. *Am J Med Genet.* 1989;34:606.

107. Lilford RJ, Caine A, Linton G, et al. Short-term culture and false-negative results for Down's syndrome on chorionic villus sampling. *Lancet.* 1991;337:861.

108. Miny P, Basaran S, Holzgreve W, et al. False-negative cytogenetic result in direct preparations after CVS. *Prenat Diagn.* 1988;8:633.

109. Simoni G, Fraccaro M, Gimelli G, et al. False-positive and false-negative findings on chorionic villus sampling. *Prenat Diagn.* 1987;7:671.

110. Martin AO, Elias S, Rosinsky B, et al. False-negative findings on chorion villus sampling. *Lancet.* 1986;2:391.

111. Grebner EE, Jackson LG. Prenatal diagnosis for Tay–Sachs disease using chorionic villus sampling. *Prenat Diagn.* 1985;5:313.

112. Galjaard H. Biochemical analyses of chorionic villi: A worldwide survey of first trimester fetal diagnosis of inborn errors of metabolism. In: Fraccaro M, Simoni G, Brambati B, eds. *First Trimester Fetal Diagnostic.* Berlin: Springer-Verlag: 1985:205.

113. Gray RG, Green A, Cole T, et al. A misdiagnosis of X-linked adrenoleukodystrophy in cultured chorionic villus cells by the measurement of very long chain fatty acids. *Prenat Diagn.* 1995;15:486.

114. Castellvi-Bel S, Mila M, Solor A, et al. Prenatal diagnosis of fragile X syndrome: Expansion and methylation of chorionic villus samples. *Prenat Diagn.* 1995;15:801.

115. Wapner RJ, Johnson A, Davis G, et al. Prenatal diagnosis in twin gestations: A comparison between second trimester amniocentesis and first trimester chorionic villus sampling. *Obstet Gynecol.* 1993;82:49–56.

116. Pergament E, Schulman J, Copeland K, et al. The risk of and efficacy of chorionic villus sampling in multiple gestations. *Prenatal Diagn.* 1992;12:377–384.

117. Evans MI, Goldberg J, Horenstein J, et al. Selective termination for structural chromosomal and mendelian anomalies: International experience. *Obstet Gynecol.* 1999;180:S31.

118. Evans MI, Wapner RJ, Carpenter R, et al. International collaboration on multifetal pregnancy reduction: Dramatically improved outcomes with increased experience. *Obstet Gynecol.* 1999;180:S28.

119. Brambati B, Tului L, Lanzana A, et al. First trimester gentic diagnosis in multiple pregnancies: Principles and potential pitfalls. *Prenat Diagn.* 1991;11:767–774.

120. Jahoda MGJ, Brandenberg H, Cohen-Overbeek TE, et al. Terminal transverse limb defects and early chorionic villus sampling: Evaluation of 4,300 cases with completed follow-up. *Am J Med Genet.* 1993;46:483.

121. Halliday J, Lumley J, Sheffield LJ, et al. Limb deficiencies, chorion villus sampling, and advanced maternal age. *Am J Med Genet.* 1993;47:1096.

122. Schloo R, Miney P, Holzgreve W, et al. Distal limb deficiency following chorionic villus sampling? *Am J Med Genet.* 1992;42:404.

123. Monni G, Ibba RM, Lai R, et al. Limb-reduction defects and chorion villus sampling. *Lancet.* 1991;337:1091.

124. Blakemore K, Filkins K, Luthy DA, et al. Cook Obstetrics and Gynecology Catheter Multicenter Chorionic Villus Sampling Trial: Comparison of birth defects with expected rates. *Am J Obstet Gynecol.* 1993;169:1022.

125. Silver RK, Macgregor SN, Muhlbach LH, et al. Congenital malformations subsequent to chorionic villus sampling: Outcome analysis of 1048 consecutive procedures. *Prenat Diagn.* 1994;14:421.

126. Mahoney MJ for the USNICHD Collaborative CVS Study Group. Limb abnormalities and chorionic villus sampling. *Lancet.* 1991;37:1422.

127. Jackson LG, Wapner RJ, Brambati B. Limb abnormalities and chorionic villus sampling. *Lancet.* 1991;337:1423.

128. Smidt-Jensen S, Permin M, Philip J, et al. Randomized comparison of amniocentesis and transabdominal and transcervical chorionic villus sampling. *Lancet.* 1992;340:1237.

129. Bissonnette JM, Busch WL, Buckmaster JG, et al. Factors associated with limb anomalies after chorionic villus sampling (letter). *Prenat Diagn.* 1993;13:1163–1165.

130. Dolk H, Bertrend F, Lechat MF. Chorionic villus sampling and limb abnormalities. The EUROCAT Working Group. *Lancet.* 1992;339:876.

131. Burton BK, Schulz CH, Burd LI. Limb anomalies associated with chorionic villus sampling. *Obstet Gynecol.* 1992;79:726.

132. Mastroiacovo P, Tozzi AE, Agosti S, et al. Transverse limb reduction defects after chorion villus sampling: A retrospective cohort study. *Prenat Diagn.* 1993;13:1051.

133. Mastroiacovo P, Botto LD. Chorionic villus sampling and transverse limb deficiencies: Maternal age is not a confounder. *Am J Med Genet.* 1994;53:182.

28

Amniocentesis

*Eli Maymon • Roberto Romero • Luís Gonçalves •
Maria-Teresa Gervasi • Mark Redman • Fabio Ghezzi*

Amniocentesis is the oldest invasive procedure for prenatal diagnosis. It has been in use for more than 100 years. First employed for the treatment of polyhydramnios in the 19th century,[1–3] it has been used subsequently for amniography[4] and elective termination of pregnancy.[5,6] As a diagnostic procedure, amniocentesis gained popularity in the management of pregnancies complicated by isoimmunization,[7] and genetic amniocentesis has been in use for almost three decades. In 1956, Fuchs and Riis[8] reported prenatal gender determination by analysis of the sex chromatin of cells obtained by amniocentesis. Human cytogenetics emerged as a field in 1966 when Steele and Breg reported the successful determination of a human karyotype from cultured amniotic fluid cells.[9] A year later, the first prenatal diagnosis of a chromosomal abnormality was reported, a balanced translocation.[10] Trisomy 21 was initially diagnosed in 1968 by Valenti et al.,[11] and the first congenital metabolic disorder diagnosed by amniotic fluid analysis was adrenogenital syndrome in 1965.[12]

INDICATIONS

Table 28–1 presents the most frequent indications for amniocentesis. The most common indication is prenatal diagnosis. Evaluation of fetal lung maturity has been the leading indication for the procedure in the third trimester. The role of amniotic fluid analysis in the diagnosis of intrauterine infection has increased over the past few years and will be discussed in detail later in this chapter.

TECHNICAL ASPECTS OF THE PROCEDURE

An ultrasound is performed before amniocentesis to establish fetal viability, gestational age, number of fetuses, placental location, adequacy of amniotic fluid volume, and the presence of any abnormality that might impact on the performance of the procedure (i.e., uterine leiomyoma, fetal anomaly, etc.).

Gestational Age

Genetic amniocentesis is usually performed after 15 weeks (most commonly between 16 and 18 weeks of gestation). Before the introduction of ultrasonographic guidance, early studies of amniocentesis indicated a lower success rate in retrieving amniotic fluid when the procedure was performed at gestational ages equal to or less than 15 weeks.[13,14] The maternal risks associated with late second-trimester termination of pregnancy and the psychologic trauma of terminating a pregnancy that is both visible and felt led to the search for alternative procedures for earlier prenatal diagnosis, namely chorionic villus sampling (CVS) and early

TABLE 28–1. INDICATIONS FOR AMNIOCENTESIS

Purpose	Indication
Late first- and second-trimester diagnosis	Cytogenetic diagnosis, diagnosis of neural tube defects, diagnosis of metabolic disorders
Late second- and third-trimester diagnosis	Evaluation of the severity of isoimmunization, evaluation of fetal lung maturity, diagnosis of intra-amniotic infection, confirmation of ruptured membranes
Therapeutic	Drainage of polyhydramnios, medical treatment of fetal disorders

amniocentesis.[15–47] Early amniocentesis is discussed in detail in the next section. For a discussion of CVS, please refer to Chapter 27.

Needle Selection

Amniocentesis is performed with a regular spinal needle. It has been recommended that the needle bore should be between 20 and 22 gauge. Larger bore needles have been associated with an increased incidence of fetal loss.[13,26] Smaller bore needles prolong the period of time required to obtain amniotic fluid and are more difficult to guide if intraoperative manipulations are required. The standard length of a spinal needle is 8.89 cm, excluding the hub. Longer needles are required for procedures in obese patients. Recently, needles that optimize sonographic visualization have been made commercially available (Cooke Catheter, Bloomington, IN, USA). Acoustic visualization is improved by roughening the needle, and Teflon coating is added to decrease needle friction.[48–51] Needles with side orifices are also commercially available. This design allows fluid to flow not only through the needle tip but also through the side orifices. This may have some advantages in cases of severe oligohydramnios. Although *in vitro* studies have shown that the flow rate during aspiration doubles with 22-gauge needles with side holes when compared with standard spinal needles of the same caliber, the use of these new needle types is strictly dependent on personal preference until an adequate clinical trial is performed.[52]

Ultrasound

Ultrasound has become an integral part of the amniocentesis procedure. The term *sonographically guided technique* refers to the use of ultrasound for selecting the site of needle insertion before amniocentesis; then, the needle is inserted blindly into the amniotic cavity. In contrast, the term *sonographically monitored technique* describes the continuous use of ultrasound throughout the procedure so that the movement of the needle and the fetus are under constant surveillance.[53]

The sonographically monitored technique has been shown to reduce the frequency of bloody and dry taps (and multiple needle insertions) in comparison with the sonographically guided technique.[53] The monitored technique also adds to the ease and expedience of the procedure, improves the patient's understanding of amniocentesis, and allows the operator to correct for potential difficulties during the procedure, such as tenting of the membranes or uterine contractions.

Operative Technique

After the ultrasound examination, asepsis of the skin is performed with wide boundaries, and then the field is draped. Needle insertion is performed under sonographic visualization. Several techniques have been described for this purpose. We have described a technique that continues to be employed in our institution.[53,54] A sterile coupling agent is applied to the skin (Fig. 28–1), and a nonsterile coupling agent is applied to the surface of a linear array real-time transducer, which is placed into a sterile glove or a sterile plastic bag (Fig. 28–2). A site for needle insertion is selected, while trying to avoid the placenta, a localized contraction, a uterine leiomyoma, or the umbilicus. An anterior placenta does not contraindicate the procedure, but if a transplacental puncture is necessary, preference is given to the thinnest portion of the organ.

Investigators have assessed the potential role of transplacental needle passage in procedure-related pregnancy loss in early amniocentesis and in second-trimester amniocentesis. A study of 380 cases of amniocentesis before 14.9 weeks at the University of Tennessee, Memphis, found 147 cases of transplacental needle passage (38.7%).[55] The frequency of bloody fluid was higher in cases of transplacental (6) versus

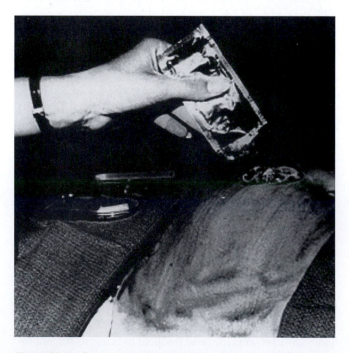

Figure 28–1. Preparation of a sterile field using antiseptic and sterile drapes and application of sterile gel.

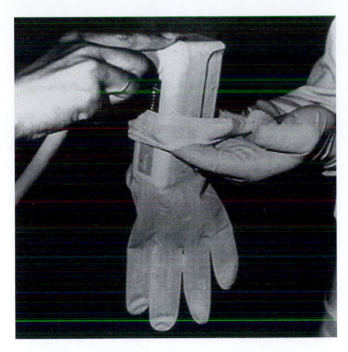

Figure 28–2. Insertion of the transducer into a sterile glove.

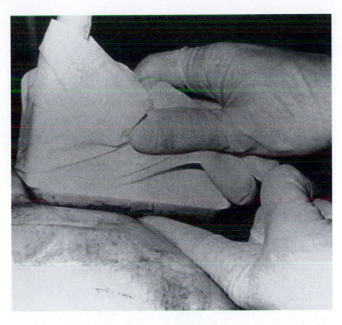

Figure 28–3. Placing the gloved finger at the puncture site, underneath the linear transducer, produces a shadow in the ultrasound image that allows identification of the needle path.

nontransplacental (1) needle passage ($p < 0.05$). The rate of pregnancy loss, however, did not differ between cases of transplacental (3.6%) and nontransplacental (3.6%) needle passage ($p > 0.4$). These results were similar to those obtained in second-trimester amniocentesis. An investigation of 1000 consecutive patients referred for genetic amniocentesis showed a nonsignificant difference in pregnancy loss between 306 cases with transplacental needle passage (1.96%) and 694 cases without transplacental needle passage (1%, $p = 0.23$).[56] Similarly, a retrospective review of 2083 second-trimester amniocenteses showed no increased risk of pregnancy loss for 476 patients exposed to transplacental needle passage.[57] None of the studies had adequate power to rule out a difference between groups, and the investigators reported that, when transplacental needle passage was unavoidable, the thinnest accessible portion of placenta was traversed.

Once the insertion site has been selected, a finger is placed under the transducer (Fig. 28–3). Decoupling of the transducer from the skin's surface produces a shadow that allows the identification of the needle path. Under direct sonographic visualization, the needle is inserted along the side of the transducer, and the tip, which appears as a bright echo, is continuously monitored throughout the procedure. The stylet is removed, and an extension tube is attached to the hub of the needle and connected to the syringe (Fig. 28–4). The purpose of the plastic tube is to allow the needle to float freely in the amniotic cavity, thereby decreasing the likelihood of fetal injury. This method also prevents operator movements (i.e., sneezing) from being transmitted to the needle. The first

0.5 cc of amniotic fluid is discarded to decrease the likelihood of contamination of the fluid with maternal cells. After obtaining the fluid, the stylet is replaced, and the needle is removed. Fetal cardiac activity is documented with ultrasound after the procedure. An alternative method to performing a sonographically monitored procedure is to use a convex or

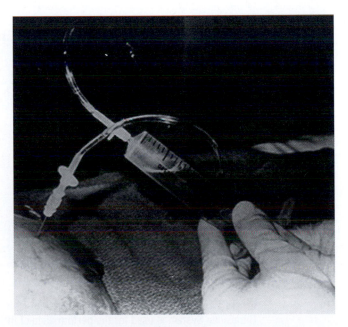

Figure 28–4. Withdrawal of amniotic fluid using a 22-gauge needle, extension tubing, and a 20-cc syringe.

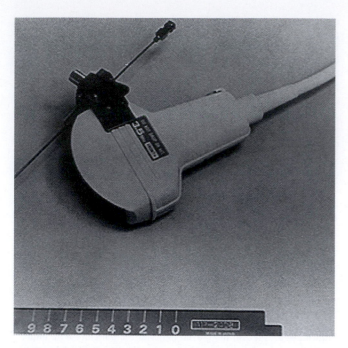

Figure 28–5. Transducer with an attached needle guide device. *(Reproduced with permission from Corometrics Medical Systems, Inc.)*

a sector scanner to visualize the path of the needle. The advantage of this approach is that the needle can be visualized in its entirety, and the transducer can be located away from the sterile field. This technique requires expertise with the needle-to-transducer spatial orientation. Needle-guiding devices have been introduced as another technical modifi-

cation for use in invasive prenatal diagnosis. Some investigators have reported a reduced risk of amniocentesis with devices that affix to the ultrasound transducer and mechanically guide the needle[58] (Fig. 28–5). Because this modification can limit the operator's ability to maneuver the needle, the technique has been further modified to incorporate an articulated needle guide to combine the advantages of the needle guide procedure and the free-hand technique.[59] Still further evolution of the needle guide technique has produced a system that provides needle guidance via graphic display. The UltraGuide 1000 system (Fig. 28–6A and B), for example, displays continuously on the ultrasound image the projected trajectory of the needle, regardless of whether the needle is in the image or in plane with the image.[60] This technical modification allows the operator to manipulate the needle as in a free-hand technique while following a continuous image on the ultrasound display of the projected needle path before and during insertion and advancement of the needle (Fig. 28–7).

The technique for early amniocentesis is basically the same as for midtrimester amniocentesis, with minor modifications. Most investigators have recommended the use of a smaller bore (22-gauge) spinal needle.[15–40] The fluid should be aspirated slowly to prevent collapse of the amniotic sac.[33] Because the amniotic membrane may not be completely fused with the chorion at this state in pregnancy, membrane tenting (separation of the chorioamniotic membrane from the anterior uterine wall during needle insertion) is a more frequent complication than with midtrimester amniocentesis. This difficulty may be overcome by a more vigorous thrust, twisting, or redirecting the needle during perforation of the amniotic membrane. If these maneuvers fail, the needle may

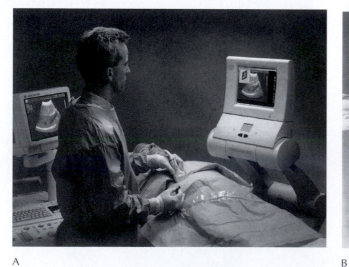

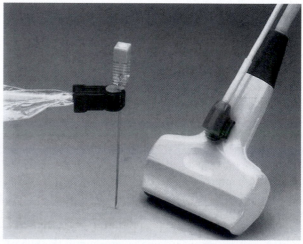

A

B

Figure 28–6. (A) The UltraGuide 1000 System is connected to the ultrasound system. The monitor of the UltraGuide System is used for the performance of the procedure as it displays the ultrasound image as well as information about the needle pathway. **(B)** Two sensors are used by the system: A needle sensor *(on the left)* and a transducer sensor *(on the right)* is placed on the side of the device.

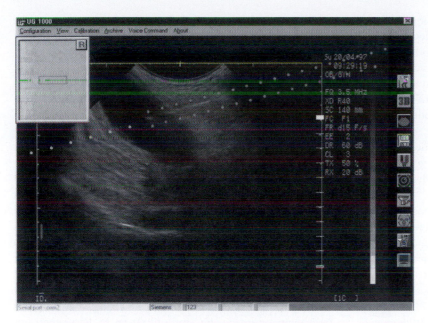

Figure 28–7. The UltraGuide 1000 System calculates the needle projection on the ultrasound screen and computes its predicted future path. The system determines the future trajectory of the needle even before its insertion into the abdominal wall.

be advanced into the posterior uterine wall, physically displacing the obstructing membrane down the shaft and away from the tip.[29,39,61–64]

At the conclusion of the procedure, either the syringe or the tubes in which the amniotic fluid will be transported to the laboratory are labeled with the name of the patient. The patient is asked to verify the identification of her own sample. An amniocentesis report should include the ultrasound findings, number of needle insertions, color and volume of the amniotic fluid retrieved, whether or not the placenta was penetrated, and any other unusual finding or event occurring during the procedure. The patient is instructed to report any signs of infection or vaginal leakage of fluid. There is no evidence to support restriction of normal activity after an uneventful procedure. If the patient is Rh-negative and not sensitized, Rh immunoglobulin is administered.

Local anesthesia is not routinely employed at our institution. The administration of local anesthesia requires an additional needle puncture and will only provide subcutaneous and dermal anesthesia. Some patients, however, may benefit from its use. If used, administration of the anesthetic should be limited to the skin and subcutaneous tissue.

All patients undergoing genetic amniocentesis should have been fully informed about the objectives, procedure, and potential complications of amniocentesis. An informed consent is signed before the procedure.

Transvaginal aspiration of amniotic fluid has been proposed as an alternative to the transabdominal approach for early amniocentesis. Potential advantages include the high resolution of the transvaginal probe and easy access to the amniotic sac. Jorgensen et al.[38] attempted the procedure in 36 women between 7 and 12 weeks of gestation. Although amniotic fluid was obtained in all cases and the patients tolerated the procedure well, culture was unsuccessful in six cases

(16.7%) because of bacterial or fungal overgrowth. In contrast, culture success was reported in all 96 control samples obtained by the transabdominal route. Shalev et al.[65] compared the clinical and laboratory results of first-trimester transvaginal amniocentesis with those of transcervical CVS and midtrimester amniocentesis. Transvaginal amniocentesis was performed in 355 women between 10 and 12 weeks of gestation using a 20-cm-long 22-gauge needle. The volume of amniotic fluid retrieved was 1 mL per week of gestation. Three hundred fifty-six consecutive transcervical CVS and 356 consecutive midtrimester transabdominal amniocenteses were matched for maternal age and indication for the procedure and selected as controls. Amniotic fluid was successfully retrieved in 99.7% (355 of 356) of the first-trimester amniocenteses and 100% (356 of 356) of the midtrimester amniocenteses. In comparison, CVS was successful in only 97.8% (346 of 356) of the cases ($p < 0.05$ vs. first-trimester and midtrimester amniocenteses, respectively). No significant differences in culture success rates were observed between patients undergoing early transvaginal amniocentesis [97.9% (344 of 355)], midtrimester transabdominal amniocentesis [97.2% (348 of 356)], and CVS [96.5% (335 of 346)]. The spontaneous pregnancy loss, however, was significantly higher in patients undergoing early transvaginal amniocentesis than in patients who had midtrimester transabdominal amniocentesis [3.2% (11 of 345) vs. 0.9% (3 of 350), $p < 0.05$]. There were no differences in total pregnancy loss between either group and the patients who had CVS [2.9% (10 of 344)].

Volume of Amniotic Fluid

The volume of amniotic fluid drawn at the time of genetic amniocentesis has differed from 8 to 45 cc. Most centers retrieve between 20 and 25 cc. This represents approximately 10% of the mean volume of amniotic fluid for 16 weeks of gestation. The effect of amniotic fluid volume on pregnancy loss has been the subject of contradictory reports. Whereas the American Collaborative Study concluded that the volume removed was unrelated to fetal loss,[26] the Canadian report suggested an increased prevalence of neonatal complications with volumes greater than 16 cc.[13] The volume of amniotic fluid retrieved in early amniocentesis programs (before 15 weeks) has ranged between 8 and 25 cc. The recommended amount of fluid to be withdrawn is 1 mL per week of gestation.[28] The first 0.5 to 1 mL of fluid aspirated should be discarded to decrease the risk of maternal cell contamination.[16] The time required to replace the volume of fluid aspirated has not been established. Although a 3-hour period has been cited as an average replacement time for midtrimester amniocentesis (16 to 18 weeks), there are no adequate data to support this view.[66–68]

Amniotic fluid cell filtration (amniofiltration) has been proposed to retrieve amniotic fluid cells in early amniocentesis without removing a relatively large amount of amniotic fluid.[15,36,69,70] The basic principle is to interpose a filter membrane with appropriate pore size between the syringe and the needle, recirculate the amniotic fluid back to the amniotic cavity, and retrieve the amniotic fluid cells directly from the filter membrane (Fig. 28–8). A three-way tap is interposed between the syringe and the filter membrane and a second one between the filter membrane and the needle. Both three-way taps are connected through a bypassing T tube. Fluid is aspirated through the bypassing tube until air is drawn into the syringe. The three-way taps are then directed to allow aspiration of fluid through the filter membrane. Once the desired amount of fluid is aspirated, the three-way taps are redirected to permit the amniotic fluid to bypass the membrane through the T tube back into the amniotic cavity. The process may be repeated as many times as necessary. Amniotic fluid cells are retrieved for culture by reverse flushing.[36] A 0.9-μm cellulose acetate membrane has been compared to a 1.2-μm cellulose acetate membrane and a 1.2-μm polyamide

membrane by Byrne et al.[36] The 0.8-μm cellulose acetate membrane proved to be the most efficient filter because it not only trapped all amniotic fluid cells but also allowed easy release of the trapped cells once the membrane was reverse flushed. Kennerknecht et al.[15] compared the prolongation in culture time for amniocytes obtained by amniofiltration using four different sets of filters: 1) 5.0-μm polyvinylidene difluoride filter (70% porosity), 2) 0.45-μm polyvinylidene difluoride filter (75% porosity), 3) 5.0-μm mixed cellulose ester filter (84% porosity), and 4) 0.45-μm mixed cellulose ester filter (79% porosity). The control group consisted of fluid obtained without a filter. The mixed cellulose ester and the polyvinylidene difluoride filters with 5.0-μm pore size had the shortest mean prolongation in culture time for filtered amniocytes when compared with amniocytes without filtration from the amniotic fluid (2.4 and 3.0 days, respectively, vs. 6.5 and 6.3 days for the 0.45-μm mixed cellulose ester and polyvinylidene difluoride filters).

Byrne and Nicolaides[70] studied changes in amniotic fluid temperature during amniofiltration in 10 women undergoing surgical termination of the pregnancy between 9 and 12 weeks of gestation. They observed a gradual decrease in temperature from a mean of 36.8°C before amniofiltration to 36.5°C after one fluid circuit (8 mL), 36.3°C after two fluid circuits (16 mL), and 36.2°C after three fluid circuits (24 mL). They speculated that, although fetal cooling (unlike hyperthermia) has not been implicated in teratogenesis, measures to avoid a decrease in amniotic fluid temperature (such as isolated syringes and tubing), should probably be considered when performing amniofiltration.

INTRAOPERATIVE COMPLICATIONS

Membrane Tenting

The term *membrane tenting* refers to the separation of the chorioamniotic membrane from the anterior uterine wall

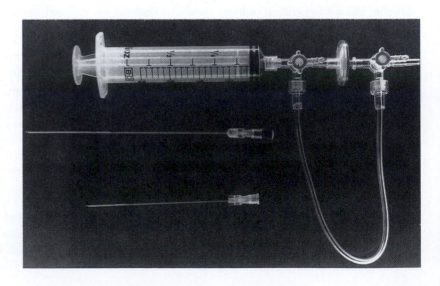

Figure 28–8. Amniotic cell filtration apparatus.

during needle insertion. It is a frequent cause of amniocentesis failure and multiple needle insertions. The diagnosis is made when the tip of the needle is visualized within a clearly defined pocket and no fluid is obtained. The membranes can sometimes be visualized in contact with the tip of the needle. Tenting of the membranes can be overcome by twisting or redirecting the needle. If these maneuvers fail, another approach is to advance the needle into the posterior uterine wall, physically displacing the obstructing membrane down the shaft and away from the tip.[29,39,61–64] On occasion, patients will be referred to a different center when amniocentesis has failed and significant chorioamniotic separation has occurred. Amniocentesis can be deferred until reattachment is documented (1 or 2 weeks) or a transplacental needle insertion can be attempted, because membrane tenting is unlikely to occur at this site. Chorioamniotic membranes are more adherent on the surface of the chorionic plate. Dombrowski et al. reported a modified stylet technique to overcome failed aspiration of amniotic fluid in cases complicated by tenting of amniotic membranes.[71] The technique of advancing a stylet from a 12.7-cm spinal needle through the original 8.9-cm 22-gauge spinal needle yielded successful aspiration of fluid in 21 of 22 cases of tenting of amniotic membranes. This technique can be used to avoid multiple needle insertions or postponement of the procedure when tenting of membranes persists despite rotating or advancing the needle.

Multiple Needle Insertions

The American Collaborative Study of midtrimester amniocentesis reported an increased frequency of spontaneous abortion and stillbirth after multiple needle insertions (more than two).[72] Similarly, the Canadian Trial found an association between multiple needle insertions (more than two) and total fetal losses.[13] Other studies examining this relationship, however, have not confirmed these findings. Since the introduction of sonographic monitoring of amniocentesis, the frequency of dry taps and multiple needle insertions has decreased significantly.[53,73,74] For example, only 1.9% of all patients in the trial by Tabor et al. required more than one needle insertion, and no patient required more than two needle insertions.[69] These investigators could not demonstrate an association between the number of taps and fetal loss.

Bloody Taps

Bloody amniotic fluid can result from contamination with maternal blood, fetal blood, or both. The prevalence of this complication has also decreased with the use of the sonographically monitored technique.[36,73–77] The American Collaborative Study did not demonstrate an increased risk of fetal loss with bloody taps,[72] whereas most other studies did not comment on this issue (i.e., the Canadian and British Collaborative Studies).[13,78] Ron et al.[79] specifically addressed the clinical significance of blood contaminated amniotic fluid. They studied 706 women undergoing midtrimester amnio-

centesis. The first 2 mL of amniotic fluid was examined for the presence of blood from maternal or fetal origin. The prevalence of bloody taps was 25.5% (180 of 706). Maternal contamination occurred most frequently 84.4% (152 of 180), and fetal contamination occurred in 15.5% (28 of 180). A mixture of fetal and maternal blood was present in eight cases. The incidence of spontaneous abortion was significantly greater in patients with bloody taps than in patients with clear taps (maternal blood contamination = 6.6%, fetal blood contamination = 14.3%, and clear taps = 1.7%). The incidence of pregnancy loss when fetal blood contamination occurred was twice as that observed when maternal blood contamination was documented. This difference, however, did not reach statistical significance. The investigators did not provide separate risk figures for microscopic versus gross bloody taps.

Fetomaternal Transfusion

Fetomaternal transfusion (FMT) can be detected by performing a Kleihauer–Betke test after the procedure or by determinations of maternal serum AFP before and after the procedure.[80,81] The frequency of FMT depends on the test employed to diagnose this complication. The AFP method is more sensitive than the Kleihauer–Betke test. For example, Lele et al. reported that the frequency of FMT was 1.8 and 7.02%, as detected with the Kleihauer–Betke test and the AFP method, respectively.[82] It has been suggested, however, that in some cases the rise of AFP concentration in maternal serum after the procedure is due to contamination with amniotic fluid and not FMT. Fetomaternal transfusion is important because it can lead to isoimmunization (see section on Isoimmunization) and an increased frequency of pregnancy loss. Mennutti et al.[81] reported that spontaneous abortion occurred more frequently in patients with an elevation of maternal serum AFP after amniocentesis than in patients with no elevation (14.2 vs. 0.98%). Fetomateranl transfusion is more common with anterior placentae.

Discolored Amniotic Fluid

Brown- and green-stained amniotic fluids are occasionally obtained in midtrimester amniocenteses.[83–94] Whereas brown amniotic fluid is considered an indicator of an intra-amniotic hemorrhage, green fluid had been attributed to meconium staining or an old hemorrhage. Hankins et al.[91] presented compelling evidence to suggest that both green and brown amniotic fluids probably represent the occurrence of previous intra-amniotic bleeding. Indeed, both green- and brown-stained amniotic fluids are positive for free hemoglobin. Furthermore, they have a similar specrophotometric pattern that is consistent with the presence of oxyhemoglobin and free hemoglobin. It has been suggested that the color of the fluid correlates with the amount of hemoglobin present. *In vitro* experiments, in which amniotic fluid is contaminated with blood, have indicated a sequential color change. Green-colored fluid was seen after 3 days and brown-colored fluid after 7 days of incubation. This interpretation is consistent with the clinical observation that women with green or brown amniotic fluid have a positive history of vaginal bleeding, but little is known about the etiology of the bleeding episode. Cassell et al.[95] reported the recovery of *Mycoplasma hominis* and *Ureaplasma urealyticum* in 4 of 33 samples with discolored, second-trimester amniotic fluid. Similarly, Gray et al.[96] found the amniotic fluid to be discolored in 4 of 8 amniotic fluid samples positive for *U. urealyticum.* It is possible that an intrauterine infection may lead to bleeding or that bleeding and clot formations provide an adequate nidus for microbial growth. The possibility that some green-stained amniotic fluid could be due to meconium passage cannot be ruled out entirely. The human fetus produces and can pass meconium before the 20th week of gestation.[97] Although the evidence is not consistent, most studies examining the prognostic significance of dark-stained amniotic fluid have suggested an increased risk of pregnancy loss. The relative risk for spontaneous abortion after retrieval of discolored amniotic fluid has been reported to be 9.9 by Tabor et al.[73] King et al. suggested that the prognosis is worse if discolored fluid is associated with an elevated maternal serum AFP determined before the amniocentesis. These findings are at variance with those of Hankins et al.[91] who did not find an increased frequency of poor pregnancy outcome after examining data from 83 patients with dark or green fluid (77 green and 6 brown) from 1227 women undergoing midtrimester amniocenteses.

AMNIOCENTESIS RISKS

Maternal Risks

Maternal complications are extremely rare. They include perforation of intraabdominal viscera with subsequent intraabdominal infection, bleeding, and blood group sensitization. One case of amniotic fluid embolism has been reported after a third-trimester amniocentesis.[98] The patient presented at 32 weeks of gestation with polyhydramnios. After draining 200 cc, the patient developed respiratory distress and disseminated intravascular coagulation. The mother was treated with exchange transfusions and survived. The fetus died *in utero*. Severe hemorrhage due to laceration of the inferior epigastric vessels has also been reported after a third-trimester amniocentesis.[99]

Fetal Risks

Fetal complications can be grouped into fetal loss and needle injuries. Fetal loss can be idiopathic or due to direct fetal injury resulting in exsanguination or infection. The term *idiopathic* refers to unexplained fetal death that occurs during the procedure, and in which postmortem examination yields no demonstrable reason for the demise. In these cases, fetal heart activity is detected before but not after the amniocentesis. A neurogenic mechanism has been postulated, but there is no evidence to support this mechanism.

Amniocentesis may lead to intra-amniotic infection by introducing microorganisms into the amniotic cavity (i.e., contaminated instruments, passage of the needle through contaminated skin or intraabdominal viscera). Alternatively, if amniocentesis results in the rupture of membranes, ascending infection may occur. The midtrimester period seems to be particularly vulnerable to microbial invasion, as the antibacterial activity of amniotic fluid is at its nadir.[100] Antibiotic prophylaxis is not a routine practice. Blood cultures obtained around the time of the procedure have been negative in a small study.[101]

The prevalence of intra-amniotic infection after midtrimester amniocentesis is unknown. However, there is evidence implicating infection/inflammation as an etiologic factor for pregnancy loss after midtrimester amniocentesis. There have been case reports in which there was a temporal association between the procedure and clinical chorioamnionitis. Positive microbial cultures of amniotic fluid obtained at the time of midtrimester amniocentesis in asymptomatic patients suggest that, in some cases, intraamniotic infection may precede the procedure rather than follow it.[95,96] In a series of 2641 second-trimester genetic amniocenteses reported by Gray et al.,[96] all of which were cultured for mycoplasmas (*M. hominis and U. urealyticum*), 9 patients had a positive culture for *U. urealyticum.* One patient was excluded from the analysis because of a subsequent therapeutic abortion. The perinatal outcome of the other 8 patients was compared with 86 patients with complete follow-up having genetic amniocenteses during the same study period and negative cultures for mycoplasmas. Among the 8 patients who cultured positive for *U. urealyticum,* 75% (6 of 8) had a spontaneous abortion within 4 weeks of the procedure as compared with only 1.2% (1 of 86) of the patients with negative cultures. The other 2 patients in the positive culture group delivered prematurely at 24 and 30 weeks, and only 1 of the infants survived. All 8 placentas had evidence of chorioamnionitis on histologic examination. Fifty percent (4 of 8) of the samples obtained from *Ureaplasma*-positive patients were discolored while only 2.3% (2 of 86) of the fluid obtained from *Ureaplasma*-negative patients had this characteristic. Discolored amniotic fluid was significantly associated with the presence of *Ureaplasma urealyticum* in amniotic fluid ($p < 0.001$) and an adverse perinatal outcome.

Ager and Oliver[100] analyzed the results of 28 different reports of midtrimester amniocenteses published between 1977 and 1985. The total fetal loss rate [(total spontaneous abortions + stillbirths + neonatal deaths)/effective total number of pregnancies] differed considerably across the studies (range = 2.4–5.2%). [Note: The effective total number of pregnancies = total number of pregnancies − (deaths prior to amniocentesis + total elective abortions + pregnancies lost to follow-up)]. Ager and Oliver concluded, however, that these estimations of risk are questionable because of differences in amniocentesis procedures, patient populations, methods of risk estimation, and problems in the design and analysis of the different studies. Most studies do not have a control group, or the control group was the result of matching. Non-randomized studies are susceptible to bias. Furthermore, most studies do not have the adequate sample size to detect a significant difference in the risk associated with the procedure.

Tabor et al.[73] reported a randomized controlled trial of genetic amniocentesis in 4606 low-risk women. This study provides the best risk estimation available in the literature. Patients were invited to participate in a study in which they were randomized to have an amniocentesis or an ultrasound in the midtrimester. The patient population consisted of low-risk women. Patients at increased risk for chromosomal anomalies, neural tube defects, metabolic disorders, or spontaneous abortions were excluded. Amniocenteses were performed under sonographic guidance with a 20-gauge needle by a group of five physicians.[73] The rate of spontaneous abortion was higher in the study group than in the control group (1.7 vs. 0.7%, $p < 0.01$). The excess spontaneous abortion rate of 1% (95% CI 0.3 to 1.5) corresponds to a relative risk of 2.3 (95% CI 1.3 to 4.0). There was a different distribution of the time elapsed between procedure and spontaneous abortion in the study and control groups. The median time interval was 21.5 days (range 5 to 67) in the study group versus 46.5 days (range 8 to 70) in the control group. An elevated maternal serum AFP (greater than 2 multiples of the median for gestational age), perforation of the placenta, and discolored amniotic fluid were identified as risk factors for spontaneous abortion. The relative risks for fetal loss were 8.3 (95% CI 2.4 to 19.8), 2.6 (1.3 to 5.4), and 9.9 (4.3 to 22.6), respectively. The researchers pointed out that the 1% increased risk of spontaneous abortion after midtrimester amniocentesis may be an underestimation of the real risk. Termination of pregnancies with fetuses affected with chromosomal abnormalities (identified in the study group and not in the control group) may have artificially reduced the rate of spontaneous abortion of the study group. Contrary to what has been reported in previous studies, no correlation was found between the rate of spontaneous abortion and number of needle insertions, placental site, or experience of the operator.

Whereas amniotic fluid leakage occurred more commonly in the study group than in the control group (1.7 vs. 0.4%, $p < 0.001$), vaginal bleeding occurred with similar frequency in both groups (2.4 vs. 2.6%). Other obstetric complications, such as preterm delivery, spontaneous rupture of membranes, and abruption placentae, had similar prevalence in both groups.

The frequency of orthopedic congenital anomalies was not different in the amniocentesis and control groups. These results are compatible with the findings of a case control study in which amniocentesis had not been performed more often in mothers of newborns with orthopedic abnormalities than in a control group.[102] In contrast, the British[78] and American[72] Collaborative Studies reported an increased incidence of orthopedic abnormalities (talipes equinovarus, congenital dis-

location of the hip, and metatarsus abductus) in the newborns of mothers who underwent amniocentesis.

The prevalence of respiratory distress syndrome was higher in neonates born to mothers in the study group than in those born to mothers in the control group (1.1 vs. 0.5%, $p < 0.05$). A similar finding was reported for neonatal pneumonia (0.7 vs. 9.3%, $p < 0.05$). These observations are of considerable interest because they are consistent with those of the British Collaborative Study[78] in which there was an increased incidence of respiratory distress (defined as respiratory difficulties requiring oxygen and lasting more than 24 hours) in neonates born to mothers who had undergone amniocentesis in comparison with those in the control group [1.27% (30 of 2370) vs. 0.38% (9 of 2402)].[73] In addition, the mean crying vital capacity, a measure of lung volume, was found to be lower in 10 neonates of mothers undergoing midtrimester amniocentesis in comparison with those in a control group.[103] Studies in monkeys (*Macaca fascicularis*), specifically designed to study the effect of amniocentesis on lung development, have indicated that a reduction in the number of alveoli and in lung volume can occur after amniocentesis at a period equivalent to 14 to 17 weeks of gestation in humans.[104,105]

Thompson et al.[106] evaluated the prevalence of respiratory distress and lung growth by measuring the functional residual capacity (FRC) in 74 newborns of mothers who had an amniocentesis at 10 to 13 weeks and 86 newborns of mothers who had a CVS during the same gestational age interval. Six infants in the CVS group, but none in the amniocentesis group, required admission to the intensive care unit because of respiratory distress ($p < 0.005$). The FRC was not different between the two groups. The overall incidence of FRC values below the 2.5th percentile was higher than expected (9%), indicating however, that both amniocentesis and CVS performed in the first trimester of pregnancy may impair antenatal lung growth.

Although other clinical studies have not demonstrated an increased incidence of pulmonary complications after amniocentesis, their design and sample size are not as adequate as those reported by Tabor et al.[73]

Leakage of Amniotic Fluid

Transient vaginal leakage of small volumes of amniotic fluid after genetic amniocentesis occurs in approximately 1 to 2% of all cases and resolves spontaneously within 48 h.[107] Chronic leakage of amniotic fluid is rare. Of the 8 cases reviewed by Crane and Rohland,[107] preterm delivery (before 32 weeks) occurred in 3, and clubfoot deformity in 2 cases with chronic leakage. One death occurred in an infant delivered at 31 weeks of gestation with clubfoot deformity and Potter's facies. Although there is not enough data at present to support definitive conclusions, expectant management was employed successfully in 6 of 7 patients who experienced amniotic fluid leakage within 24 h of a genetic amniocentesis in a series of 603 patients reported by Gold et al.[108] All patients were placed on bed rest, had digital cervical examination prohibited, frequent white blood cell counts with differential analysis, and close maternal surveillance for clinical evidence of chorioamnionitis. Six patients delivered healthy neonates at term, and one patient had an intrauterine fetal demise at 25 weeks. In this case, an unsuccessful amniocentesis was attempted 6 weeks before delivery.

Fetal Injuries Associated With Amniocentesis

Table 28–2 presents the fetal injuries that have been attributed to amniocentesis and whether or not ultrasound was employed during the procedure. The spectrum of lesions ranges from mild skin dimples to fetal death due to exsanguination.[109–140] Although fetal injuries are generally associated with bloody taps, they have also been reported after clear taps. If a fragment of tissue is retrieved with amniotic fluid, histologic examination is recommended to establish its origin. Fetal injuries have occurred even with the use of a sonographically monitored technique.

Several ocular injuries have been attributed to amniocentesis.[112,116,127,135,138,140] Typically, these are unilateral lesions detected shortly after birth. In one case, the newborn had a small and cloudy eye, a coloboma of the upper lid, and a hazy and edematous cornea. The combination of lesions in the eyelid and cornea suggests that the injury occurred before separation of the eyelids. The mother had an amniocentesis at 19 weeks; the first 2 cc of fluid were bloody, but the subsequent 30 cc were clear.[127] In two cases, a red and photophobic eye in the newborn period was subsequently associated with the development of an enlarging cystic mass in the anterior chamber of the eye. The cystic lesions evolved over a period of several months and were lined by a stratified squamous epithelium.[112,116] Similar findings have been reported for two children with unilateral and progressively large epithelial iris cysts occupying nearly half of the pupil. The lesions were diagnosed at 8 months and 5 years of age, respectively, and both mothers had an amniocentesis performed at 18 and 43 weeks. The children had no history of postnatal ocular trauma.[140] Five other children were reported with lesions attributed to ocular perforation during amniocentesis: the first child had an amniocentesis at 16 weeks and was found at birth to have a cystic lesion communicating with the right lateral ventricle, left homonymous hemianopia, and possible damage to the right optic tract; the second child had an amniocentesis at 30 weeks and presented in the neonatal period with a distorted pupil toward the 3 o'clock position and a small tag or iris drawn up toward the full-thickness corneal scar; the third child had an amniocentesis performed at 16 weeks and presented at birth with left exotrophia, limitation of abduction, and microphthalmia; the fourth child had an amniocentesis performed at 15 weeks and was noted at $3^{1}/_{2}$ years to have a small adherent leukoma near the limbus at the 7 o'clock position; the last child in this series had an amniocentesis performed during the second trimester and was found at 5 years of age to have a small chalazion on its

right upper lid with a small full-thickness scar near the limbus at the 9 o'clock position.[138]

A porencephalic cyst in a newborn with two subcutaneous nodules in the right and left occipital region (suggesting a needle tract) has been reported.[128] An amniocentesis had been performed at 18 weeks. *In utero* injection of contrast in the ventricular system during the course of amniograms has been reported.[110,111]

Thoracic lesions associated with amniocentesis include hemothorax,[113,132] pneumothoraces,[110,113] and fetal cardiac tamponade.[111] In the abdomen, injuries have ranged from laceration of the liver, kidney, and spleen to ileocutaneous fistula with ileal atresia.[114,120,121,126,129] In one case, a fragment of tissue retrieved during amniocentesis grew small bowel mucosa in culture, confirming intraoperative bowel injury.[129]

Limb lesions have included disruption of the patellar tendon,[125] gangrene of one arm (perforation of the subclavian artery),[117] and an arteriovenous fistula between the popliteal artery and vein.[139] Amniocentesis has been implicated by some investigators in the etiology of amniotic band syndrome;[123,124,130,133] however, there is no agreement regarding a cause-and-effect relationship between this syndrome and amniocentesis.

Two cases of hematomas of the umbilical cord have been reported.[112,134] Fetal exsanguination due to vascular puncture has also been reported.[109,122]

The most frequent lesion associated with amniocentesis is skin puncture. Although a cause-and-effect relationship is difficult to establish, needle injuries should be suspected if the shape of the lesion resembles a needle tract or a depressed punctiform scar.[118,119,125]

Long-Term Outcome

Midtrimester amniocentesis has been used as a diagnostic procedure for more than 20 years. A Canadian trial[141] compared the long-term outcome (7 to 18 years) of 1297 children whose mothers had midtrimester amniocentesis for advanced maternal age with a group of 3704 controls matched for maternal age, sex, date, and place of birth. With the exception of a higher risk of ABO isoimmunization [9.46% (6 of 1297) vs. 0.027% (1 of 3704); relative risk 3.32, 95% CI 2.44 to 4.51], the offspring of women who had midtrimester amniocenteses did not have more disabilities than those who did not (including cerebral palsy, delayed speech, intellectual impairment, hearing deficits, epilepsy, asthma, and limb anomalies).

Fluorescence In Situ Hybridization Analysis

The time required to obtain results of genetic amniocentesis can be 10 to 16 days. In recent years, fluorescence *in situ* hybridization (FISH) has been proposed as an adjunctive tool for a rapid diagnosis of the most frequent chromosomal aberration. FISH on uncultured amniocytes with use of chromosome-specific probes has been utilized for the diagnosis of numeric abnormalities affecting chromosomes 13, 18, 21, X, and Y.[142] Morris et al. reported the results of

TABLE 28–2. FETAL INJURY DUE TO AMNIOCENTESIS AND MONITORING TECHNIQUE USED

Reference	Year	Lesion	Outcome	Bloody Tap	US	GA	Indication for Amnio
Misenhimer[109]	1966	Fetomaternal transfusion > 100 mL	Neonatal death: 1 hour	Y	N	35	Preeclampsia, PROM
		Fetomaternal transfusion > 100 mL	Preterm labor: Neonatal death		N	30	Placental localization
Creasman et al.[110]	1968	Hematoma on thorax, skin dimple on arm	No limitation	N	N	30	Placental localization
		Pneumothorax 40%	Thoracentesis	N	N	Term	
		Subdural hemorrhage	Stillborn	N	N	28	Placental localization
Berner et al.[111]	1972	Fetal cardiac tamponade	Stillborn	N	N	31	Rh negative
Cross and Maumenee[112]	1973	Coloboma, epthelial cyst, intermittent glaucoma, chronic irritation	Stillborn	N	N	31	Rh negagive
Grove et al.[113]	1973	Pneumothorax	Thoracentesis; Neonatal death	Y	N	42	Fetal assessment
		Cord Hematoma	Healthy newborn	N	N	Postterm	Gestational age
Egley[114]	1973	Fetal spleen laceration	C/S fetal distress	Y	N	44	Gestational age
Cook et al.[115]	1974	Pneumothorax	Thoracostomy	Y	N	32	Fetal assessment
Fortin and Lemire[116]	1975	Corneal perforation	Enucleation	Y	N	39	Fetal lung maturity
Lamb[117]	1975	Supraclavicular puncture; fetal arm gangrene	Elective abortion		Y	15	Anencephaly
Broome et al.[118]	1976	Scar on arm	Normal newborn	N		17	Genetic indication
		Scars on arm and chest	Normal newborn	N		16	Genetic indication
		Scars on chest and thigh	Normal newborn	Y		16	Genetic indication
		Scars on neck	Normal newborn	N	Y	17	Genetic indication
		Scars on inferior limb and genital area	Normal newborn	N	Y	15	Genetic indication
Karp and Hayden[119]	1976	Punctate lesion on right arm	Normal newborn	N		14.5	Genetic indication
		Punctate lesion on abdomen	Normal newborn	N		14.5	Genetic indication
		Punctate lesion on back	Normal newborn	N		16	Genetic indication
		Punctate lesion on chest	Normal newborn	N		16	Genetic indication
Rickwood[120]	1977	Fistula, ileal atresia	Bowel resection	N	N	18	Genetic indication
Cromie et al.[121]	1978	Renal trauma	Normal	Y	N	35	Fetal assessment
Young et al.[122]	1977	Fetal exsanguination	Stillbirth	Y	Y[a]	22.5	Genetic indication
Rehder[123]	1978	Amniotic band syndrome	Spontaneous abortion	N		14	Genetic indication
Rehder and Weitzel[124]	1978	Amniotic band syndrome	Malformation; preterm delivery, neonatal death	Y	Y	16	Genetic indication
Epley et al.[125]	1979	Patellar tendon disruption	Surgical repair	N	N	14–16	Genetic indication
Swift et al.[126]	1979	Small bowel obstruction	Bowel resection	N	Y	16	Genetic indication
Merin and Beyth[127]	1980	Coloboma, corneal perforation	Unilateral undeveloped eye, blindness		Y[a]	19	Genetic indication
Youroukos et al.[128]	1980	Porencephalic cyst	Opsoclonus; unilateral hemiparesis	Y	Y	18	Genetic indication
Therkelsen and Rehder[129]	1981	Ileal atresia	Abortion	N	Y	16	Genetic indication
Moessinger et al.[130]	1981	Amniotic band syndrome	Elective abortion	N	Y[a]	17	Genetic indication
Isenberg and Heckenlively[131]	1985	Scleral perforation, exposed uvea		N	Y[a]	20	Genetic indication
Achiron and Zakut[132]	1986	Right hemothorax	Neonatal death	Y	Y	32	Fetal lung maturity
Kohn[133]	1987	Amniotic band syndrome	Shortened fingers; nail aplasia/hypoplasia	N	N	16	Genetic indication
Morin et al.[134]	1987	Cord hematoma		N	N	17	Genetic indication
Admoni and Ben Ezra[135]	1988	Leukocoria, globe perforation, retinal traction and detachment	Spontaneous resolution	Y	Y	17	Genetic indication

[a] Ultrasound guidance only, not ultrasound monitoring.
C/S, cesarean section; GA, gestational age; N, no; PROM, premature rupture of the membranes; US, Ultrasonography; Y, yes.

a prospective study using FISH on uncultured amniocytes. Of 1504 amniotic fluid samples tested, 1467 were correctly identified as having two copies of chromosomes 21, and 35 samples were correctly scored as having three copies of chromosome 21. Only 2 samples failed to produce results. On average, results were reported 48 hours after sampling (range 1 to 7 days).[143] These findings are consistent with those of Eiben et al. who reported a correct identification of a normal karyotype in 98% (727 of 741) of cases and of an abnormal karyotype in 95.8% (68 of 71) of cases.[144] Fluorescence *in situ* hybridization has the advantage over routine cytogenetic analysis that it requires a small amount of amniotic fluid and it provides rapid and accurate diagnosis of the most frequent chromosomal abnormalities within 24 hours from the procedure.[145] This makes this method of particular value when an early amniocentesis is performed. There is, however, the disadvantage that FISH can be used to detect only abberrations for which it has been designed; therefore, most structural and some numerical chromosomal abnormalities cannot be diagnosed with this method. In addition, the procedure requires considerable laboratory expertise.[146]

The American College of Medical Genetics still recommends that FISH on uncultured amniocytes be considered investigational, and clinical actions should not be based on the results of FISH alone.[147] However, some investigators have suggested that, in the presence of an abnormal ultrasonographic finding in the second trimester, an informative FISH result can be used to make management decisions even before the final cytogenetic result is available.[145]

Isoimmunization

Fetal red blood cells contain the D antigen on their surface and are capable of immunizing the Rh-negative mother after an FMT in the midtrimester. This event can occur spontaneously during pregnancy or after an amniocentesis. The World Health Organization (WHO) and the American College of Obstetrics and Gynecology (ACOG) have recommended the administration of the anti-D immunoglobulin G (IgG) to women after midtrimester amniocentesis. There is no agreement on the dose; the WHO recommends 50 μg, whereas the ACOG recommends 300 μg.[148]

The basis for this recommendation is that midtrimester amniocentesis has been associated with an increased incidence of transplacental hemorrhage, a risk factor for isoimmunization. The precise risk of isoimmunization after midtrimester amniocentesis has not been well defined, however. The incidence of Rh isoimmunization in the randomized controlled clinical trial reported by Tabor et al.[73] was 0.3% (7 of 370) in the study group and 0.1% (3 of 347) in the control group (anti-D IgG was not administered to Rh-negative patients undergoing amniocentesis). Although this difference is not significant, the number of patients required to detect a difference of 1% between the amniocentesis and the control group would be 2896 in each group.[73] The analysis of the previous reports suggests that midtrimester amniocentesis is

associated with an increased risk of isoimmunization. The magnitude of the increased risk seems to be approximately 1%.[100]

Murray et al.[149] provided a comprehensive analysis of the advantages and disadvantages of anti-D IgG administration. The objections that have been raised against the routine use of anti-D IgG are unproven efficacy (isolated case reports have indicated that sensitization can occur after anti-D IgG administration[150,151]) and unproven long-term safety. Anti-D IgG crosses the placenta and coats Rh-positive fetal red cells. It is unclear if this could have adverse effects. The theoretic risk of augmentation has been suggested. This phenomenon consists of an enhancement of the immune response in the context of small amounts of antibody. Furthermore, the long-term effects of exposing the immunologically "naïve" fetal immune system to human immunoglobulins are unknown.[152]

Although there is no incontrovertible evidence to support the routine administration of anti-D IgG after midtrimester amniocentesis, it has become the standard practice in the United States.

Early Amniocentesis

Traditionally, genetic amniocentesis has been carried out after the 16th week of gestation. To obtain results earlier, several centers have introduced the performance of "early amniocentesis" at a gestational age lower than 15 weeks. Early amniocentesis is an attractive approach because it provides early cytogenetic diagnosis and amniotic fluid for alpha-fetoprotein (AFP) determinations for the assessment of neural tube defects.[28,29,38] Wald and Cukle[153] demonstrated that amniotic fluid AFP obtained between 13 and 15 weeks had a 100% sensitivity for the diagnosis of anencephaly and a 96% sensitivity for the diagnosis of spina bifida when using cutoff levels greater than 2.0 and 2.5 multiples of the normal median, respectively.

Although early amniocentesis has been performed as early as the 7th week of gestation,[38] it is usually performed between 11 and 15 weeks of gestation. Early amniocentesis has been compared with both mid-trimester amniocentesis and CVS. The major concern with early amniocentesis is the increased risk of spontaneous fetal loss in comparison with either CVS or conventional amniocentesis. The Canadian Early and Mid-Trimester Amniocentesis Trial (CEMAT) Group conducted a randomized trial in 4374 patients to assess safety and efficacy of early and midtrimester amniocentesis. The group reported a post-procedure spontaneous loss rate (excluding intrauterine and neonatal death) of 2.6% and 0.8% for early amniocentesis and midtrimester amniocentesis, respectively.[154] Early amniocentesis was associated with a higher rate of multiple needle insertions (5.4 vs. 2.1%, $p < 0.0001$) and amniotic fluid leakage before 22 weeks of gestation (3.5 vs. 1.7%, $p = 0.0007$) than in midtrimester amniocentesis. The incidence of talipes equinovarus was higher in the early amniocentesis group than in the midtrimester group (1.3 vs. 0.1%, $p = 0.0001$). A possible explanation for talipes

TABLE 28–3. SAMPLING SUCCESS AND PREGNANCY LOSS IN EARLY AMNIOCENTESIS

Reference	Year	No. of Cases	% Sampling Failure	Needle Size (gauge)	% Leakage	% Unintended Pregnancy Loss
Hanson et al.[21]	1987	541	0	20		4.7
Godmillow et al.[24]	1987	600	1.6			3.1
Elejalde et al.[28]	1990	323	0.2	20	1.6	2.5
Hanson et al.[156]	1990	527	0.2	20	1.5	2.3
Nevin et al.[32]	1990	222	0	20		1.9
Penso and Frigoletto[29]	1990	407		22	2.6	3.8
Stripparo et al.[33]	1990	505	0.3	22	1.2	3.4
Thayer et al.[157]	1990	348	2.7		2.1	3.4
Hackett et al.[37]	1991	106	2.8	20	1.0	3.2
Assel et al.[158]	1992	301	1.7			2.1
Hanson et al.[43]	1992	936	0.1	22	1.1	3.4
Henry and Miller[39]	1992	428	1.0	22	1.7	1.6
Yang et al.[159]	1993	311	0.6			1.0
Crandall et al.[160]	1994	693	<1	22,25	1.2	1.5
Shulman et al.[161]	1994	250	0.8	22	1.2	3.6
Nicolaides et al.[162]	1994	731	2.5	20		5.3
Rousseau et al.[163]	1995	242	1.2	19		1.6
Sundberg et al.[164]	1995	249	0.8	20	4.8	2
Brumfield et al.[165]	1996	315		22	2.9	2.2
Johnson et al.[166]	1996	344	0.6	22	2.1	2.4
Diaz Vega et al.[167]	1996	181	1.6	22	1.6	1.6
Eiben et al.[168]	1997	2976	0.25	22	0.9	1.9
Wilson et al.[169]	1997	349	3.3	22	3.9	2.3
Sundberg et al.[170]	1997	548	0.2	20	4.4	2.6
Daniel et al.[171]	1998	279	4.3	22		2.2
Collins et al.[172]	1998	1207				2.2
CEMAT[154]	1998	2183	1.7	22	4.6	2.6
Jörgensen et al.[173]	1998	1624	1.9	22		1.5
Roper et al.[174]	1999	417		20,22		1.0
Total		18,179	1.1%		2.2%	2.5%

is the removal of a relatively large amount of amniotic fluid (11 mL, about 20% of the total amount of amniotic fluid) during early amniocentesis in the CEMAT study. Cytogenetic results from the CEMAT study—including culture success, detection of chromosome abnormalities, frequency of mosaicism, and maternal cell contamination—showed no difference between early and midtrimester amniocentesis. A repeat amniocentesis was required more frequently after early amniocentesis than after midtrimester amniocentesis.[155]

Table 28–3 displays the overall spontaneous pregnancy loss of early amniocentesis reported in published studies including at least 100 cases.[21,28,29,32,33,37,39,43,47,154–174] The fetal loss rate is related to the gestational age at which the procedure is performed. Table 28–4 shows data of four different studies in which the fetal loss rate by gestational age at amniocentesis was reported. The overall fetal loss rate was significantly higher when the amniocentesis was performed before 12 weeks of gestation than after this gestational age [8.1%

TABLE 28–4. EARLY AMNIOCENTESIS: FETAL LOSS BEFORE 28 WEEKS OF GESTATION

Reference	9 Weeks		10 Weeks		11 Weeks		12 Weeks		13 Weeks		14 Weeks		Total	Loss
	n	Loss	n	Loss	n	Loss	n	Loss	n	Loss	n	Loss		
Hanson et al.[21,43]	1	0	3	0	4	0	12	0	215	4	255	5	490	9
Henry and Miller[39]					14	0	193	1	426	3	1172	7	1805	11
Stripparo et al.[33]					13	3	41	5	154	6	176	1	384	15
Elejalde et al.[28]	3	0	6	0	18	2	77	3	98	2	121	1	323	8
Total	4	0	9	0	49	5	323	9	893	15	1724	14	3002	43
% Loss	0.00		0.00		10.20		2.79		1.68		0.81		1.43	

TABLE 28–5. FETAL LOSS WITHIN 2 WEEKS OF PROCEDURE

Reference	9 Weeks		10 Weeks		11 Weeks		12 Weeks		13 Weeks		14 Weeks		Total	Loss
	n	Loss	*n*	Loss	*n*	Loss	*n*	Loss	*n*	Loss	*n*	Loss		
Elias and Simpson[47]	1	0	3	0	4	0	12	0	47	0			67	0
Hanson et al.[21,43]									215	2	255	2	470	4
Henry and Miller[39]					14	0	193	1	426	3	1172	7	1805	11
Stripparo et al.[33]					13	3	41	3	154	3	110	1	318	10
Elejalde et al.[28]	3	0	6	0	18	2	77	2	98	0	121	14	323	18
Nevin et al.[32]	1	0	2	0	2	0	25	0	56	0	121	0	207	0
Hackett et al.[37]					5	0	24	1	42	0	35	0	106	1
Total	5	0	11	0	56	5	372	7	1038	8	1814	24	3296	44
% Loss	0.00		0.00		8.93		1.88		0.77		1.32		1.33	

(5 of 62) vs. 1.29% (38 of 2950), $p < 0.001$.[21,28,33,39,43] The combined experience of 7 centers which data are available (Table 28–5) shows an overall loss rate of 1.33% (44 of 3296) within 14 days of the procedure, with a significant increase when amniocentesis is performed before 12 weeks [6.94% (5 of 72) vs. 1.21% (39 of 3224), $p < 0.001$].[21,28,32,33,37,39,43,47]

In assessing the ability to culture amniocytes, Nelson and Emery[176] demonstrated that the largest percentage of viable cells were present between 13 and 16 weeks of gestation. Several studies have reported a higher culture failure rate and a longer time to reach a final diagnosis after early amniocentesis than after midtrimester amniocentesis.[28,159,176–178] This has been attributed to a lower cell concentration in the amniotic fluid.[28] Moreover, confined mosaicism may be more likely in fluid retrieved after an early amniocentesis. Up to 70% of cells in amniotic fluid during the first trimester are derived from the membranes and trophoblast rather than from the fetus.[179]

With the use of a new filter technique some problems of early amniocentesis have been, in part, overcome. In 1996, Sundberg et al. reported the pregnancy outcome for 249 patients subjected to an early amniocentesis with a filtration technique.[60] Sampling failure occurred in 8 cases (3.2%). Spontaneous losses before 28 weeks occurred in 5 cases (2.0%). A subsequent report by Sundberg et al. described the use of early amniocentesis with filtration in 44 pregnancies with a previous finding of mosaicism.[177] Amniocenteses were performed at a mean gestational age of 12.5 weeks (range of 11 to 14 weeks) after CVS had demonstrated mosaicism. In all 44 cases, culture of the filtered fluid was successful, and cultures were harvested after a mean time of 8.8 days. Mosaicism was confirmed in 7 cases, and non-mosaic karyotypes were found in 36.

The question of whether early amniocentesis is a reasonable alternative to CVS has been addressed by randomized clinical trials. In one trial, 488 patients were randomized to either early amniocentesis ($n = 238$) or CVS ($n = 250$) at 10 to 13 weeks. An additional group of 813 patients had either an early amniocentesis ($n = 493$) or CVS ($n = 321$) by choice.[162] Patients who were randomized to

CVS had a lower spontaneous fetal loss rate (intrauterine or neonatal deaths) than patients randomized to early amniocentesis {1.2% [3 of 250; 95% confidence interval (CI) 0.3–3.5] vs. 5.9% [14 of 238; 95% CI 3.3–9.7], $p < 0.01$}. Cultures obtained by CVS demonstrated more mosaicism than cultures obtained by early amniocentesis [1.2% (7 of 556) vs. 0.1% (1 of 731), $p < 0.05$], although a larger number of culture failures occurred in the early amniocentesis group [2.32% (17 of 731) vs. 0.53% (3 of 566), $p < 0.05$]. In another randomized trial, early amniocentesis was compared to transabdominal CVS;[181] 115 patients were randomized to either early amniocentesis ($n = 55$) or transabdominal CVS ($n = 60$). Seventy patients who refused randomization chose early amniocentesis, and 25 chose transabdominal CVS. Several patients did not have the procedure to which they had been assigned. Thus, 130 had early amniocentesis and 74 received transabdominal CVS. Spontaneous fetal loss occurred with 8 patients who had early amniocentesis (6.2%) and with none of the patients who had transabdominal CVS. Talipes equinovarus complicated 4 pregnancies who underwent early amniocentesis (3.1%) and none of the pregnancies exposed to transabdominal CVS. Early amniocentesis performed with a filter technique has also been compared with CVS. A 1999 report compared 555 cell cultures and karyotypes obtained by CVS with 548 obtained by early amniocentesis with a filter technique.[181] No significant difference in culture success, pseudomosaicism, preparation problems, or maternal cell contamination were found between the groups.

In addition to filtration, other technical modifications have been proposed to improve the results of early amniocentesis. For example, Eiben et al.[168] reported an incidence of talipes equinovarus of only 0.43% when removing 3.5 mL of amniotic fluid during early amniocentesis.

AMNIOCENTESIS IN MULTIPLE GESTATION

The prevalence of chromosomal abnormalities is estimated to be higher in twins than in singleton pregnancies (for advanced maternal age indication).[182] Similarly, the incidence of neural tube defects in a patient with a previous history of a child with a neural tube defect is higher in a twin gestation (as much as doubled) than in a singleton gestation.[129,182]

Before amniocentesis is performed in a multiple gestation, the possible outcome, risks, and management alternatives need to be discussed with the patient. The major issue is the possibility of discrepant results regarding cytogenetic diagnosis. If only one fetus is affected, the options available to the patient include abortion of both fetuses, continuation of the pregnancy, or selective feticide of the affected fetus. Feticide is associated with potential complications, such as infection, disseminated intravascular coagulation, and spontaneous abortion.[183] Under these circumstances, pregnancy termination implies the abortion of an unaffected fetus.

The technique for amniocentesis in multiple gestations is different from that in singleton gestations. The number of fetuses, location within the uterine cavity, presence of an interamniotic membrane, placentation, sex, fetal biometry, and anatomy need to be documented. An important step is the topographic location of the fetus. This becomes critical in cases where discrepant results are reported and selective feticide is considered. Identification of the fetuses should be based on the relation to the maternal hemipelvis (left vs. right, anterior vs. posterior, and superior vs. inferior). We recommend that a diagram of the procedure be drawn and kept in the medical record for reference.

Several techniques have been proposed to ensure that fluid is retrieved from each amniotic cavity.[184–188] After amniotic fluid is obtained from the first sac, before removing the needle, an indicator dye is injected into the cavity. Indigo carmine is presently the dye of choice.[183,189–194] Other alternatives are Congo red[146,196] and Evan's blue.[197] The use of a solution of maternal hemoglobin as a dye has also been reported.[198] The use of methylene blue is discouraged because of the risk of fetal hemolytic anemia due to methamobloginemia[199–200] and a possible association with gastrointestinal obstruction.[201,202] The association between the use of methylene blue and multiple ileal occlusions was first reported by Nicolini and Monni[201] in seven babies born to mothers who had a midtrimester amniocentesis and the injection of 10 to 30 mg of methylene blue into one of the amniotic sacs. Pruggmayer et al.[202] compared the incidence of gastrointestinal obstruction among 474 twin pregnancies who had either indigo carmine ($n = 351$) or methylene blue ($n = 123$) injected as a dye during midtrimester amniocentesis. Seventeen percent (21 of 123) of the fetuses who had the sacs injected with methylene blue required a postnatal operation to correct jejunal atresia as opposed to 0.3% (1 of 351) of fetuses who had the sacs injected with indigo carmine and who presented with duodenal atresia in the neonatal period ($p < 0.0001$). It is expected that clear amniotic fluid will be obtained when the second sac is punctured. The same procedure is applicable to amniocentesis for a multiple gestation with more than two fetuses. The technique consists of sequential injections of dye into different sacs before removal of the needle. The number of clear amniotic fluid aspirations should equal the number of fetuses.

A technique for single needle insertion in twin amniocentesis was described by Jeanty et al.[187] Briefly, a puncture site clear of placental tissue demonstrating both gestational sacs and the interamniotic membrane is selected with real-time ultrasound. The most proximal sac is tapped first; the stylet is then replaced into the needle and advanced under ultrasound guidance through the interamniotic membrane into the second sac; finally, fluid is aspirated from the second sac. Amniotic fluid was successfully retrieved from both sacs in 17 of the 18 patients included in their study, and no adverse perinatal outcomes were reported. Alternatively, two needle insertions may be performed simultaneously by two operators into two separate sacs under direct ultrasonographic guidance.[188] The procedure has been reported in a series of 7 patients, with successful retrieval of fluid in all cases and no perinatal complications.[188] A shortcoming of this technique is that it may not be used by a single operator. The overall success rate in obtaining fluid from both sacs is greater than 90%. A challenging situation occurs when one sac is behind the other. In this case, the second is sampled by advancing the needle to penetrate the inter-amniotic membrane under direct visualization, as described earlier. The first 2 cc of amniotic fluid retrieved from the second sac is discarded to decrease the likelihood of contamination.

Another difficult situation arises when an inter-amniotic membrane cannot be identified. This can occur in the setting of polyhydramnios and in monoamniotic twins. A practical approach consists of sampling two sites in close proximity to each fetus but distant from each other. We have found it helpful to place a linear or convex array transducer along the transverse axis of the uterus and to monitor the turbulence created by the injection of the indicator dye. Before injection, the dye is diluted with 10 cc of amniotic fluid. The mixture is then injected into the amniotic cavity, producing a typical particulate image that identifies the boundaries of that sac. The operator must be ready to proceed with the second puncture because the image is short-lived. Tabsh described another interesting approach.[186] After aspirating the amniotic fluid sample from the first sac, 0.1 mL of air and 0.5 mL of dye are drawn through a 15-μm filter into a 6-mL syringe. The syringe is then reattached to the needle hub, and 5 mL of amniotic fluid is aspirated into the syringe. The mixture of dye, air, and amniotic fluid is then reinjected into the amniotic sac with gentle pressure, but enough to create microbubbles that will serve as an ultrasonographic contrast within the amniotic sac. If the microbubbles are seen around both fetuses, the diagnosis of monoamniotic twinning is made.

The risk of pregnancy loss in multiple gestations has been addressed in several reports[190,191,193–196,198,202–209]

TABLE 28–6. PERINATAL OUTCOME IN MULTIPLE PREGNANCIES UNDERGOING MIDTRIMESTER AMNIOCENTESIS

Reference	Period	Timing of Amniocentesis	n	Loss of Both Twins <20 wk		Loss of Both Twins <28 wk		Loss of Both Twins >28 wk		Loss of Only One Twin	
				n	%	n	%	n	%	n	%
Elias et al.[185]	1979–	>17 week	20	0	0	0	0	0	0	2	10
Bovicelli et al.[186]	1979–1982	Midtrimester	13	0	0	1	7.69	0	0		
Palle et al.[187]	1973–1979	16–17 week	29	3	10.35	6	20.69	0	0	0	0
Goldstein and Stills[190]	1978–1982	Midtrimester	22	0	0	1	4.55	1	4.55	0	0
Filkins et al.[193]	1976–1982	17–18 week	31	2	6.45	1	3.23	0	0	0	0
Librach et al.[191]	1972–1983	16–17 week	70	3	4.29	4	5.71	4	5.71	0	0
Tabsh et al.[194]	1972–1983	Midtrimester	48	0	0	1	2.08	0	0	5	10.42
Kappel et al.[205]	1980–1983	Midtrimester	48			6	12.5	0	0	0	0
Pjipers et al.[203]	1980–1995	16–20 week	83	1	1.20	4	4.82	0	0	3	3.61
Anderson et al.[209]	1969–1990	Midtrimester	336			12	3.57	6	1.79	1	0.30
Beekhuis et al.[198]		16 week	63	1	1.59	2	3.17	0	0	1	1.59
Pruggmayer et al.[202]	1985–1991	14–19 week	529	12	2.27	20	3.78	11	2.08	31	5.86
Wapner et al.[204]	1984–1990	16–18 week	70	1	1.43	2	2.86	1	1.43	7	10.00
Ko et al.[211]	1986–1997	18–19 week	128	0	0	5	3.9	0	0	0	0
Total			1490	23/949	2.42	65/1490	4.36	23/1362	1.69	50/1349	3.71

(Table 28–6). Anderson et al.[209] compared the risk of spontaneous abortion after midtrimester amniocentesis in 353 twin pregnancies with 687 singleton pregnancies matched for gestational age and indication for prenatal diagnosis (one preceding and one following each twin). Fourteen cases were excluded because of congenital anomalies, growth retardation, twin-to-twin transfusion, or death of one twin at the time of the procedure, leaving 339 patients for subsequent analysis. The groups were not different with regard to maternal age or experience of the physician performing the procedure. Three pregnancies were terminated after the diagnosis of aneuploidy in one of the fetuses. After terminations for chromosomal abnormalities were excluded, the spontaneous fetal loss rate before 28 weeks was significantly higher for multiple pregnancies than for singleton pregnancies [3.57% (12 of 336) vs. 0.60% (4 of 671), $p < 0.001$]. The perinatal mortality rate, however, was not different between the two groups [12.6 of 1000 (8 of 633) vs. 12.1 of 1000 (8 of 659), not significant]. In another large series assessing the perinatal outcome of 529 twin pregnancies undergoing genetic amniocentesis, the combined fetal loss rate before 28 weeks was 3.78% (20 of 529)[202] and comparable to the 3.57% rate reported by Anderson et al.[209] Both studies concluded that, although there is an increased risk of spontaneous pregnancy loss for twin pregnancies undergoing amniocentesis, it is unlikely that this increased risk exceeds the normal biologic loss rate in twins. This conclusion is also supported by the analysis of the risks of midtrimester amniocentesis in twin gestations conducted by Ager and Oliver,[130] even with a different outcome measure: total fetal loss rate. Total fetal loss rate is defined as follows: total spontaneous abortions + stillbirths + neonatal deaths. According to their analysis, the to-

tal fetal loss rate is 10.8% (range 3.6 to 22.2%), which is not different from the natural fetal loss rate for twin gestations after 17 weeks as estimated from 12,392 twin pregnancies collected in Japan.[210]

AMNIOCENTESIS FOR THE DIAGNOSIS OF MICROBIAL INVASION OF THE AMNIOTIC CAVITY

Definition

The amniotic cavity is normally sterile; therefore, isolation of any microorganisms from the amniotic fluid constitutes evidence of microbial invasion. Microorganisms may gain access to the amniotic cavity and fetus using any of the following pathways: 1) ascending from the vagina and the cervix, 2) hematogenous dissemination through the placenta (transplacental infection), 3) retrograde seeding from the peritoneal cavity through the fallopian tubes, and 4) accidental introduction at the time of invasive procedures, such as amniocentesis, percutaneous fetal blood sampling, CVS, or shunting. The most common pathway of intrauterine infection is the ascending route.[212–217]

We have proposed a four-stage process leading to intrauterine infection (Fig. 28–9)[218] The first stage consists of an overgrowth of facultative organisms or the presence of the pathologic organisms (i.e., *Neisseria gonorrhoeae*) in the vagina, cervix, or both. Bacterial vaginosis may be an early manifestation of stage I. Once microorganisms gain access to the intrauterine cavity, they reside in the decidua (stage II). A localized inflammatory reaction leads to deciduitis and further extension to chorionitis. The infection may invade the

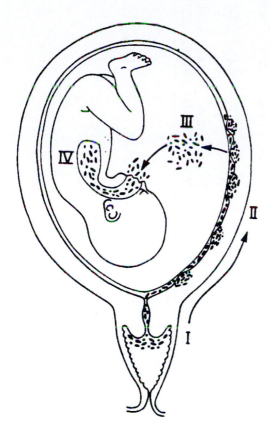

Figure 28–9. Pathways and stages of intrauterine infection.

fetal vessels (choriovasculitis) or proceed through the amnion (amnionitis) into the amniotic cavity, leading to microbial invasion of the amniotic cavity (stage III). Rupture of the membranes is not a prerequisite for this condition, as microorganisms are capable of crossing intact membranes.[219] Once in the amniotic cavity, the bacteria may gain access to the fetus (stage IV) by different ports of entry. Aspiration of infected fluid by the fetus may lead to congenital pneumonia. Otitis, conjunctivitis, and omphalitis are localized infections that occur by direct spread of microorganisms from infected amniotic fluid. Seeding from any of these sites to the fetal circulation may lead to bacteremia and sepsis.

Frequency

The frequency of microbial invasion of the amniotic cavity differs according to the presence of labor, cervical dilation, and the state of the fetal membranes, and it ranges from 0.4% in patients in the midtrimester of pregnancy to 51.5% in patients with cervical incompetence (Table 28–7).[212,220–232] The most common microbial isolates from the amniotic cavity from women with preterm labor and intact membranes and women with preterm rupture of the membranes are *U. urealyticum, Fusobacterium* species, and *M. hominis* (Table 28–8).[212,218,220–232,232–237]

TABLE 28–7. PREVALENCE OF MICROBIAL INVASION OF THE AMNIOTIC CAVITY ACCORDING TO PREGNANCY STATUS

Pregnancy Status	Prevalence of Infection (%)
Gestational age < 37 years	
Midtrimester[227]	9/2461 (0.4)
PROM, no labor[225]	41/160 (25.6)
PROM, labor[225]	24/61 (39)
Labor, intact membranes[228]	214/1675 (12.8)
Cervical incompetence[229]	17/33 (51.5)
Labor, twin gestation[230]	5/46 (10.8)
Gestational age ≥ 37 years	
Intact membranes, no labor[231]	2/143 (1.4)
Intact membranes, labor[231]	17/90 (18.8)
PROM[232]	11/32 (34.3)

PROM, premature rupture of membranes.

Importance of the Diagnosis

Accumulating evidence supports an association between microbial invasion of the amniotic cavity and preterm labor and delivery.[228] Microbial invasion of the amniotic cavity has been reported in 21.6% of women with preterm labor and intact membranes who subsequently delivered a preterm neonate.[212] This condition is often subclinical in nature and requires microbiologic studies of amniotic fluid for diagnosis. The early identification of microbial invasion of the amniotic cavity is a desirable clinical goal because neonates born to mothers with intra-amniotic infection are at higher risk for both infectious and noninfectious complications (Table 28–9).[212,220–222,224,237,239–243] Moreover, patients with microbial invasion of the amniotic cavity are at risk for the development of clinical chorioamnionitis, failure to respond to tocolysis, subsequent rupture of membranes, and puerperal endometritis (Table 28–9).[228] Despite the importance of microbial invasion of the amniotic cavity, an early diagnosis is difficult to accomplish. Clinical signs of infection (fever, uterine tenderness, foul-smelling vaginal discharge, fetal tachycardia, and maternal leukocytosis) occur late and

TABLE 28–8. MICROORGANISMS ISOLATED FROM AMNIOTIC FLUID IN PATIENTS WITH PRETERM LABOR AND INTACT MEMBRANES AND IN WOMEN WITH PRETERM PREMATURE RUPTURE OF THE MEMBRANES

	Preterm Labor, Intact Membranes[212]	Preterm Premature Rupture of Membranes[225]
Prevalence of MIAC	9.1% (24/264)	27% (65/241)
Ureaplasma urealyticum	6	4
Mycoplasma hominis	4	6
Fusobacterium species	5	5
Other	14	20
No. of cases with CFU > 10⁵	83.3% (20/24)	30.8% (20/65)

MIAC, microbial invasion of the amniotic cavity; CFU, colony forming unit.

TABLE 28–9. MATERNAL AND NEONATAL COMPLICATIONS IN PATIENTS WITH PRETERM LABOR AND INTACT MEMBRANES AND IN PATIENTS WITH PREMATURE RUPTURE OF THE MEMBRANES WITH AND WITHOUT MICROBIAL INVASION OF THE AMNIOTIC CAVITY

Reference	Year	Condition	n	Positive Culture					Negative Culture				
				Chorioamnionitis	Endometritis	Neonatal Sepsis	RDS	Other	Chorioamnionitis	Endometritis	Neonatal Sepsis	RDS	Other
Garite et al.[239]	1979	PROM	30	66.6%	33.3%	11.1%			4.7%	4.7%	0		
Bobitt et al.[240]	1981	PTL	31	50%	0	50%	37.5%		21.7%	0	21.7%	8.7%	
Garite and Freeman[220]	1982	PROM	86	55%	25%	25%	25%		7.5%	1.5%	4.5%	6.1%	
Cotton et al.[221]	1984	PROM	47	100%		16.6%			2.5%		0		
Broekhuizen et al.[222]	1985	PROM	53	20%	33.3%	16.6%			0	2.6%	2.6%		
Feinstein et al.[224]	1986	PROM	15	16.6%		16.6%			5.2%		2.6%		
Skoll et al.[237]	1989	PTL	127	14.3%		14.3%			3.3%		0		
Romero et al.[212]	1989	PTL	111	12.5%	8.3%	4.1%	54.2%	41.7%	1.1%	4.6%	1.1%	23%	10.3%
Romero et al.[243]	1990	PTL	168	13%		4.3%			0.6%		0		
Romero et al.[241]	1993	PTL	120	18.2%		27.3%	54.5%	54.5%	0		1%	12.6%	10.7%
Romero et al.[242]	1993	PROM	110	11.9%		4.8%			4.4%		3%		
Total				26% (46/177)	19.7% (15/16)	12.4% (22/177)	42.9% (27/63)	45.7% (16/35)	3% (23/755)	3% (7/235)	1.9% (14/749)	14% (39/279)	10.5% (20/190)

PROM, premature rupture of the membranes; PTL, preterm labor; RDS, respiratory distress syndrome.

are found only in 12% of these patients.[212] However, amniotic fluid cultures, considered the gold standard for diagnosis, are not immediately available for clinical management, and their results may take several days. Consequently, there has been considerable interest in the development of rapid tests for the diagnosis of this condition by analysis of amniotic fluid.

Amniotic Fluid Collection

The method of amniotic fluid collection for microbiologic studies is critical. The two techniques that have been used are transabdominal amniocentesis and transcervical retrieval either by needle puncturing of the membranes or by aspiration through an intrauterine catheter. Transcervical amniotic fluid collection is associated with an unacceptable risk of contamination with vaginal flora and is contraindicated in both preterm labor and nonlaboring patients with premature rupture of the membranes (PROM). Successful retrieval of amniotic fluid by ultrasonographically monitored amniocentesis is possible in virtually all patients with preterm labor with intact membranes and in more than 90% of patients with PROM, making it the method of choice to obtain amniotic fluid from these patients.

Tests for Diagnosis of Microbial Invasion of the Amniotic Cavity

In the following sections, we review the clinical value of amniotic fluid Gram stain, acridine orange tests, limulus ame-bocyte lysate assays, white blood cell count, glucose concentration, and interleukin-6 in the identification of microbial invasion of the amniotic cavity.

__Amniotic Fluid Gram Stain.__ The Gram stain is the most frequently used rapid diagnostic test for detecting intra-amniotic infection and has been used extensively for making clinical decisions in patients at risk for intra-amniotic infection.

Some technical aspects should be taken into account to obtain optimal results using this test. The slide should be prepared with fluid obtained directly from the syringe because swabs absorb both fluid and cells, decreasing the likelihood of observing organisms in a smear or culture. Although centrifugation of amniotic fluid at low speed does not improve the detection of bacteria with the Gram stain,[244] the use of a cytocentrifuge increases the concentration of bacteria in the sediment and probably allows an easier identification of the microorganisms.

Table 28–10 shows the diagnostic accuracy of the Gram stain as a diagnostic tool in the detection of microbial invasion of the amniotic cavity in different studies.[212,220–222,224–226,236,237–243,245–250] The overall indices are: sensitivity 49.5% (196 of 396), specificity 97.5% (1388 of 1423), positive predictive value 79.4% (196 of 247), and negative predictive value 87.4% (1387 of 1587). The sensitivity increases significantly with a higher inoculum ($>10^5$ colony forming units per milliliter).[244] It is important to note

TABLE 28–10. SENSITIVITY, SPECIFICITY, AND POSITIVE AND NEGATIVE PREDICTIVE VALUES OF THE GRAM STAIN IN DETECTING MICROBIAL INVASION OF THE AMNIOTIC CAVITY IN PATIENTS WITH PRETERM LABOR AND INTACT MEMBRANES AND IN PATIENTS WITH PREMATURE RUPTURE OF THE MEMBRANES

| Reference | Year | Condition | n | % Sensitivity | % Specificity | Predictive Value | |
						% Positive	% Negative
Garite et al.[239]	1979	PROM	30	55.6	100	55.6	84
Miller et al.[245]	1980	PROM	37	84.6	87.5	78.6	91.3
Bobitt et al.[240]	1981	PTL	31	75	100	75	92
Garite and Freeman[220]	1982	PROM	86	70	97	63.6	91.4
Cotton et al.[221]	1984	PROM	41	85.7	100	85.7	100
Zlatnik et al.[246]	1984	PROM	29	25	95.2	75	76.9
Hameed et al.[247]	1984	PTL	37	50	100	50	94.2
Broekhuizen et al.[222]	1985	PROM	53	60	89.2	78.9	70.6
Feinstein et al.[224]	1986	PROM	50	75	92.1	75	92.1
Gravett et al.[248]	1986	PTL	54	50	100	100	93.2
Duff and Kopelman[236]	1987	PTL	18	0	100	0	94.4
Romero et al.[225]	1988	PROM	114	44.8	97.7	86.7	83.8
Skoll et al.[237]	1989	PTL	127	28.6	95.8	28.6	95.8
Romero et al.[212]	1989	PTL	264	79.2	99.6	95	97.5
Romero et al.[243]	1990	PTL	168	65.2	99.3	93.7	94.7
Gauthier et al.[250]	1991	PROM/PTL	204	29.9	97.8	87.0	74.0
Coultrip and Grossman[249]	1992	PROM/PTL	136	62.5	93.8	68.2	92.1
Gauthier and Meyer[226]	1992	PROM	117	39	96.7	91.7	63
Romero et al.[241]	1993	PTL	120	63.6	99.1	87.5	96.4
Romero et al.[242]	1993	PROM	110	23.8	98.5	90.9	67.7
Total				49.5	97.5	79.4	87.4

PROM, premature rupture of membranes; PTL, preterm labor.

TABLE 28–11. DIAGNOSTIC INDICES OF GRAM AND ACRIDINE ORANGE STAINS

			Predictive Value	
	% Sensitivity	% Specificity	% Positive	% Negative
Gram stain	46.8 (15/32)	98.1 (104/106)	88.2 (15/17)	86 (104/121)
Acridine orange	43.8 (14/32)	96.2 (102/106)	82.4 (14/17)	85.1 (103/121)
Both tests	53.1 (17/32)	95.3 (101/106)	77.3 (17/22)	95.3 (101/106)

Reproduced with permission from Romero R, Emamian M, Quintero R, et al. Am J Perinatol. 1989;6:41.

that *Mycoplasma* species, which are frequently isolated in the amniotic fluid of patients in preterm labor with intact membranes or PROM, are not visible on Gram stain examination.

Acridine Orange Stain.

Acridine orange (AO) stain is a fluorochrome dye that, when buffered at low pH, binds to the nucleic acid of bacteria and stains them an orange color. The nucleus of human epithelial and inflammatory cells shows a green to yellow fluorescence, with no orange or green fluorescence in the cytoplasm. Therefore, bacteria should be readily identified as bright orange structures against a dark background.

Several investigators have claimed that AO stain is more sensitive than the Gram stain in the detection of bacteria in biologic fluids.[251–254] Data generated by our group, however, indicate that AO cannot replace the Gram stain as a method to diagnose microbial invasion of the amniotic fluid, because the sensitivity, specificity, and predictive values of the test are not superior to those obtained when using Gram stain (Table 28–11).[255] The potential use of AO stain would be to identify *Mycoplasma,* but this potential advantage needs to be weighed against the risk of increasing the false-positive diagnosis.

Limulus Amebocyte Lysate Assay.

Limulus amebocyte lysate (LAL) assay is a rapid, inexpensive, and sensitive bioassay for the detection of bacterial lipopolysaccharide. It is based on the gelation of the lysate of blood cells (amebocyte) of the horseshoe crab, *Limulus polyphemus,* in the presence of endotoxin.[256–258] Gram-negative organisms are frequently found in microbial invasion of the amniotic cavity. Their cell walls contain lipopolysaccaride, which can be detected either free after cell lysis or as part of the intact bacteria.

Gram stain and LAL have comparable diagnostic performances for the diagnosis of microbial invasion of the amniotic cavity (sensitivity of 69%, specificity of 95%), but when used in combination, there is a remarkable improvement of the sensitivity (from 69 to 96%) with a small decrease in the specificity (from 95 to 86).[257] Although the LAL assay test would be expected to detect only gram-negative microorganisms, it also identifies 33% of pure gram-positive infections and cases of intra-amniotic infection produced by *Mycoplasma* or *Candida.* Two explanations have been proposed for these findings. The infection could have included gram-negative organisms that were not grown in culture because of their fastidious nature or because they were not visible. In the latter case, free lipopolysaccharide released at the time of cell death could lead to a positive LAL result, although the organism may not grow in culture. An alternative explanation is that cross-reacting microbial products could induce gelation of the limulus lysate.[257] For example, peptidoglycans, a component of gram-positive bacteria, and mannan, a carbohydrate molecule isolated from *Candida* species, have been reported to produce a positive LAL test result.[258,259]

Amniotic Fluid White Blood Cell Count.

Neutrophils are infrequently found in the amniotic fluid of women who are not in labor. Their presence in the amniotic fluid indicates the existence of an inflammatory reaction, usually caused by microbial invasion of the amniotic cavity. Table 28–12 summarizes the results of three different studies examining the performance of amniotic fluid white blood cell count in the identification of microbial invasion of the amniotic cavity

TABLE 28–12. DIAGNOSTIC INDICES OF AMNIOTIC FLUID WBC IN DETECTING MICROBIAL INVASION OF THE AMNIOTIC CAVITY IN PATIENTS WITH PRETERM LABOR AND INTACT MEMBRANES AND IN PATIENTS WITH PROM

Reference	Year	Condition	n	WBC Cutoff Value (cell/mm³)	% Sensitivity	% Specificity	Predictive Value	
							% Positive	% Negative
Romero et al.[260]	1991	PTL	195	100	68	92.9	58.6	95.2
Romero et al.[260]	1991	PTL	195	50	80	87.6	48.8	96.7
Romero et al.[241]	1993	PTL	120	50	63.6	94.5	53.8	96.3
Romero et al.[242]	1993	PROM	110	50	57.1	77.9	61.5	74.7

PROM, premature rupture of membranes; PTL, preterm labor; WBC, white blood cell count.

in patients with preterm labor and intact membranes and in women with PROM.[242,260,261] In a study of 195 patients in preterm labor with intact membranes who underwent amniocentesis for the assessment of the microbiologic status of the amniotic cavity, a white blood cell count greater than or equal to 50 cells/mm[3] had a sensitivity of 80% (20 of 25) and a specificity of 87.6% (149 of 170) in the detection of a positive amniotic fluid culture.[260] Although the sensitivity was higher than the Gram stain (80 vs. 48%, $p < 0.05$), the specificity was lower (87.6 vs. 98.8%, $p < 0.05$); thus, the false-positive rate was high (12.45%). Patients with an amniotic fluid white blood cell count greater than or equal to 50 cells/mm[3] but a negative amniotic fluid culture are at risk for preterm delivery.[260] Therefore, independently of the culture results, an elevated amniotic fluid white blood cell count identifies a subset of patients at risk for failure to respond to tocolysis and impending preterm delivery. These patients may have microbiologic invasion of the amniotic cavity that escapes detection with standard microbiologic techniques, or a noninfectious process may have driven neutrophil recruitment into the amniotic cavity. We have proposed a different cutoff value for the diagnosis of microbial invasion of the amniotic cavity in patients with PROM (30 cells/mm[3]) (Fig. 28–10).[242]

Glucose Concentration in the Amniotic Fluid. Glucose determination has been used extensively to diagnose infection in other body fluids (i.e., cerbrospinal fluid, pleural fluid,

and synovial fluid).[261–263] It does not require sophisticated interpretation by trained personnel. Amniotic fluid glucose concentration is significantly lower in patients with microbial invasion of the amniotic cavity (identified by a positive amniotic fluid culture or clinical signs of infection) and in patients with PROM who develop clinical infection.[241–243,249,250,264] The mechanism responsible for the lower amniotic fluid glucose concentration in the setting of infection has not been established but probably relates to glucose metabolism by both microorganisms and polymorphonuclear leukocytes.[249]

The diagnostic indices of amniotic fluid glucose concentration in the diagnosis of microbial invasion of the amniotic cavity according to various published reports are displayed in Table 28–13. Collectively, these data indicate that the sensitivity and specificity of amniotic fluid glucose concentrations for the diagnosis of intra-amniotic infection range from 57 to 87% and from 51 to 100%, respectively, when using different cutoff values.

As in the case of white blood cell count, the false-positive rates of amniotic fluid glucose concentration are high (8 to 48%) (Tables 28–12 and 28–13). The seriousness of a false-positive result is dependent on the action taken after an abnormal test result. If the course of action is to perform additional tests for the identification of intra-amniotic infection, then a false-positive result is not clinically problematic; however, if the course of action is to deliver a preterm neonate believed to be infected, then there is the potential for serious consequences.[243]

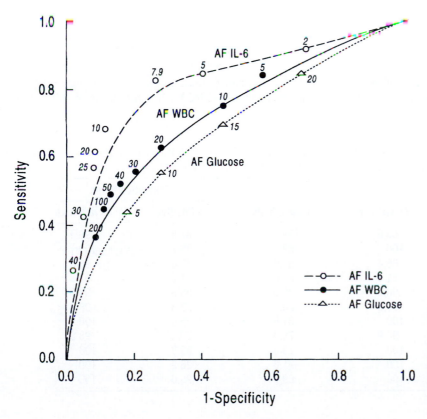

Figure 28–10. Receiver-operator characteristic curves for amniotic fluid white blood cell count (AF WBC), glucose, and interleukin-6 (IL-6) in the detection of microbial invasion of the amniotic cavity in patients with preterm premature rupture of the membranes, indicating that IL-6 performs better than other amniotic fluid tests.

TABLE 28–13. SENSITIVITY, SPECIFICITY, AND POSITIVE AND NEGATIVE PREDICTIVE VALUES OF AMNIOTIC FLUID GLUCOSE FOR POSITIVE AMNIOTIC FLUID CULTURE IN PATIENTS WITH PRETERM LABOR

Reference	Condition	n	Cutoff (mb/dL)	% Sensitivity	% Specificity	Predictive Value % Positive	% Negative
Romero et al.[243]	PTL	168	14	86.9	91.7	62.5	97.8
Gauthier et al.[250]	PROM/PTL	204	16	79.1	94.2	86.9	90.2
Kirsnon et al.[264]	PROM/PTL	39	10	75.0	100	100	90.0
Coutrip and Grossman[249]	PROM/PTL	107	10	91.7	89.5	52.4	97.7
Coutrip and Grossman[249]	PROM/PTL	107	15	91.7	74.7	31.4	98.6
Coutrip and Grossman[249]	PROM/PTL	29	15	25.0	64.7	33.3	55.0
Coutrip and Grossman[249]	PROM/PTL	29	15	33.3	58.8	44.4	55.6
Romero et al.[241]	PTL	120	14	81.8	81.6	53.8	96.3
Romero et al.[242]	PROM	110	14	71.4	51.5	47.6	74.5
Romero et al.[242]	PROM	110	10	57.1	73.5	57.1	73.5

PROM, premature rupture of membranes; PTL, preterm labor.

Amniotic Fluid Interleukin-6 Concentrations. Interleukin-6 (IL-6) has been implicated as a major mediator of the host response to infection and tissue damage. A growing body of evidence indicates that preterm parturition in the setting of infection is associated with dramatic alterations in the amniotic fluid concentration of several cytokines, including IL-6.[265–272] This cytokine is a glycoprotein that is produced in a wide variety of cells, such as fibroblasts, monocyte/macrophages, endothelial cells, keratinocytes, and endometrial stromal cells. Interleukin-6 expression is induced by several inflammation-associated cytokines, including IL-1, tumor necrosis factor and interferons, bacterial products, RNA- and DNA-containing viruses, and second messenger agonists (diacylglycerol, cAMP, and Ca^{2+}) that activate any of the three major signal transduction pathways. Interleukin-6 elicits major changes in the biochemical, physiologic, and immunologic status of the host, including the acute phase plasma protein response, activation of T and natural killer cells, and stimulation and proliferation of Ig production by B cells. It induces the production of C-reactive protein (CRP). This may be important in the context of intra-amniotic infection, because clinical studies have indicated that an increase in maternal serum CRP often precedes the development of clinical chorioamnionitis and the onset of preterm labor in women with PROM.[273–278] In addition, it has been demonstrated that IL-6 stimulates prostaglandin production by human amnion and decidual cells in primary cultures.[279]

Interleukin-6 has been studied as a rapid test for the detection of microbial invasion of the amniotic cavity.[241,242,250] Patients with a positive amniotic fluid culture have significantly higher amniotic fluid IL-6 concentrations than patients with a negative culture. In patients with preterm labor and intact membranes, a cutoff level of 11.3 ng/mL has a sensitivity of 100% and a specificity of 82.6% in the detection of microbial invasion of the amniotic cavity (Table 28–14).[270] Among patients with PROM, a cutoff level of 7.9 ng/mL

TABLE 28–14. DIAGNOSTIC INDICES AND PREDICTIVE VALUES OF AMNIOTIC FLUID TESTS FOR DETECTION OF POSITIVE AMNIOTIC FLUID CULTURE IN PATIENTS WITH PRETERM LABOR AND INTACT MEMBRANES

	% Sensitivity	% Specificity	Predictive Value % Positive	% Negative
Gram stain	63.6	99.1	87.5	96.4
IL-6 $\geq$ 11.3 ng/mL	100	82.6	36.7	100
WBC $\geq$ 50/mm^3	63.4	94.5	53.8	96.3
Glucose < 14 mg/dL	81.8	81.6	31.0	97.8
Gram stain + WBC	90.9	93.6	58.8	99.0
Gram stain + glucose	90.9	80.7	32.3	98.9
Gram stain + IL-6	100	81.6	35.5	100
Gram stain + glucose + WBC	90.9	78.0	29.4	98.8
Gram stain + WBC + IL-6	100	79.8	33.3	100
Gram stain + glucose + IL-6	100	71.6	26.2	100
Gram stain + WBC + glucose + IL-6	100	69.7	25.0	100

IL-6, interleukin-6; WBC, white blood cell count.

results in a sensitivity of 80.9% and a specificity of 75% (Table 28–14).[242] Moreover, an elevated amniotic fluid IL-6 is an independent predictor of the likelihood of preterm delivery and a risk factor for neonatal complications.[241,242]

Another important clinical role for IL-6 determination has been proposed by our group in patients undergoing midtrimester amniocentesis. Amniotic fluid IL-6 concentrations were higher in patients with a pregnancy loss than in patients with normal pregnancy outcome. An amniotic fluid IL-6 concentration greater than or equal to 2.8 ng/mL has been associated with an odds ratio of 8.1 (95% CI 1.9 to 36.3) for pregnancy loss.[280] We propose that a preexisting but subclinical inflammatory process is an important risk factor for pregnancy loss after midtrimester amniocentesis. This finding may have relevant clinical and legal implications.

Comparison Between Frequently Used Amniotic Fluid Tests

The diagnostic performance of amniotic fluid IL-6 determination, glucose concentration, white blood cell count, and Gram stain in patients with preterm labor and intact membranes[241] and patients with PROM[242] has been studied. Figure 28–11 shows the receiver-operator characteristic (ROC) curves for the performance of amniotic fluid IL-6, white blood cell count, and glucose in the detection of a positive amniotic fluid culture in patients with preterm labor and intact membranes. Diagnostic indices and prognostic values for each

test and their potential combinations are displayed in Table 28–15. Interleukin-6 was the most sensitive test for the detection of microbial invasion of the amniotic cavity (100%), followed by glucose concentration (81.8%), white blood cell count (63.6%), and Gram stain (63.6%). The most specific test was Gram stain (99.1%), followed by white blood cell count (94.5%), IL-6 (82.6%), and glucose (81.6%).

Figure 28–10 shows the ROC curves for amniotic fluid IL-6, white blood cell count, and glucose concentration in the detection of a positive amniotic fluid culture in patients with PROM. Interleukin-6 was the most sensitive test in the detection of microbial invasion of the amniotic cavity (80.9%), followed by white blood cell count (57.1%), glucose concentration (57.1%), and Gram stain (23.8%). The most specific test for the detection of microbial invasion of the amniotic cavity was the Gram stain (98.5%), followed by the white blood cell count (77.9%), IL-6 (75%), and glucose concentration (73.5%) (Table 28–15).[242] IL-6 was the only proven test to have an independent relationship with the amniocentesis to delivery interval and likelihood of neonatal complications.

Significant progress has been made in the development of rapid tests for the diagnosis of microbial invasion of the amniotic cavity. Although the determination of IL-6 in amniotic fluid seems to be better than any other current method for the detection of microbial invasion of the amniotic cavity, the use of Gram stain, white blood cell count, and glucose determination remain valuable tools for clinical decision making.

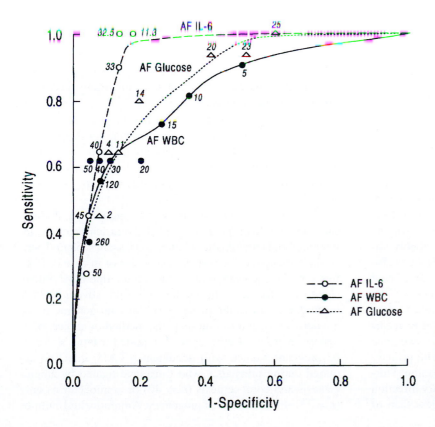

Figure 28–11. Receiver-operator characteristic curves for amniotic fluid white blood cell count (AF WBC), glucose, and interleukin-6 (IL-6) in the detection of microbial invasion of the amniotic cavity in patients with preterm labor and intact membranes, demonstrating the superior performance of IL-6.

TABLE 28–15. DIAGNOSTIC INDICES AND PREDICTIVE VALUES OF AMNIOTIC FLUID TESTS FOR DETECTION OF POSITIVE AMNIOTIC FLUID CULTURE IN PATIENTS WITH PRETERM PREMATURE RUPTURE OF THE MEMBRANES

	% Sensitivity	% Specificity	Predictive Value	
			% Positive	% Negative
Gram stain	23.8	98.5	90.9	67.7
IL-6 ≥ 7.9 ng/mL	80.9	75.0	66.7	86.4
WBC ≥ 30/mm³	57.1	77.9	61.5	74.6
WBC ≥ 50/mm³	52.4	83.8	66.7	74.0
Glucose < 10 mg/dL	57.1	73.5	57.1	73.5
Glucose < 14 mg/dL	71.4	51.5	47.6	74.5
Gram stain + WBC	61.9	77.9	63.4	76.8
Gram stain + glucose	66.7	73.5	60.9	78.1
Gram stain + IL-6	80.9	75.0	66.7	86.4
Gram stain + glucose + WBC	76.2	60.3	54.2	80.4
Gram stain + WBC + IL-6	85.7	61.8	58.1	87.5
Gram stain + glucose + IL-6	85.7	52.9	52.9	85.7
Gram stain + WBC + glucose + IL-6	92.9	47.1	52.0	91.4

IL-6, interleukin-6; WBC, white blood cell count.

CONGENITAL VIRAL AND PARASITIC INFECTIONS

Traditionally, viral congenital infections have been diagnosed by the use of fetal blood sampling. With the introduction of the polymerase chain reaction (PCR), the identification of genome fragments of parasites, viruses, and bacteria is now possible by the use of amniocentesis in most of the congenital infections. In one series, PCR analysis of amniotic fluid obtained in second-trimester amniocenteses for genetic indications showed evidence of a single virus in 14 of 122 specimens (11.5%).[281] The viruses identified were adenovirus, parvovirus, cytomegalovirus, Epstein–Barr virus, herpes simplex virus, enterovirus, and influenza A virus.

Cytomegalovirus

Cytomegalovirus (CMV) is the most common perinatal viral infection, with a prevalence ranging between 0.4 and 2.3 per 100 live-births. Forty percent of infants delivered to mothers with primary CMV will have congenital infection, accounting for approximately 33,110 infected newborns annually in the United States.[282] Of these, 5 to 10% are symptomatic at birth. Mortality may be as high as 20 to 30%, with 90% of survivors suffering long-term sequelae. Among asymptomatic infants, 5 to 15% develop some abnormalities in the first 2 years of life.[283,284] Although CMV can also be transmitted to the fetus during a reactivation of a latent infection, long-term sequelae are less likely to occur.[285,286] Symptoms at birth are present in 18% of infants following primary infection, but it is extremely rare after recurrent infection.[287] After a mean follow-up of 4.7 years, one or more sequelae were seen in 25% of infants with primary infection and in 8% of infants with recurrent-infection. Thirteen percent of infants whose mothers had primary infection during pregnancy had mental impairment (IQ less than or equal to 70) as opposed to none of those whose mothers had recurrent CMV infections. Sensorineural hearing loss was found in 15% of infants with primary infection and in only 5% of those with recurrent infection. Bilateral hearing loss was identified only among children in the primary infection group (8%).

The route of infection is mainly transplacental, although the fetus can acquire the infection by exposure to CMV from the cervix.[288] Transmission from the mother to the fetus can occur any time during gestation and with equal frequency throughout the three trimesters. However, the most serious sequelae are observed when the fetus is infected in the first half of pregnancy.[285,286] Pregnant women at greatest risk of CMV infection are those working in day care centers, hospital nurseries, dialysis units, and areas providing services to immunosupressed hosts.[288]

Universal screening for evidence of prior infection is not considered cost effective. The rationale for this is based on the fact that, with 1% prevalence of CMV primary infection during pregnancy, the incidence of infants with CMV-related problems in a low-risk population is approximately 0.9%.[289]

In the presence of suspicious ultrasound findings (non-immune hydrops, microcephaly, ventriculomegaly, intracranial and intrahepatic calcifications, ascites, pleural pericardial effusion, or hepatosplenomegaly) or in case of positive serology, an evaluation of the intrauterine environment should be offered to the mother. With the advent of PCR technique to assess the presence of the viral genome in the amniotic fluid, amniocentesis is the method of choice to diagnose infection. Lipitz et al.[290] reported a large series of 63 pregnant women with documented CMV infection acquired during pregnancy who were investigated by amniocentesis and cordocentesis (n = 40) or amniocentesis only (n = 23) after 21 weeks of pregnancy. Amniotic fluid cultures or PCR analysis and fetal blood CMV IgM determinations were performed. Twenty-two (35%) pregnancies showed evidence of vertical transmission: 13 of them underwent cordocentesis, but only 77% of the 13 showed positive IgM results in fetal blood. There were no cases of positive fetal serum IgM with negative amniotic fluid culture or PCR. In 41 (65%) pregnancies, no evidence of vertical transmission was found, and 37 continued to term. Only one newborn from this subgroup subsequently showed mild motor disability during a median 23 months of follow-up. Other investigators have confirmed the accuracy of PCR analysis to identify CMV in amniotic fluid.[291–294] However, false-negative results with the use of PCR analysis have also been reported. They have been attributed to performance of the tests too soon after primary maternal infection.[104,295–298] Donner et al. reported a study in which PCR analysis for the detection of CMV genome in amniotic fluid was performed in 35 women between 14 and 20 weeks (mean of 17 weeks) of gestation and, if negative, repeated at a gestational age greater than 21 weeks. Over a total of 11 positive cases, 6 were negative at first sampling.[296] Considering that 1) CMV is a slow-growing virus and viremia is not detected before 2 or 3 weeks after primary infection; 2) 2 to 3 weeks can elapse before a significant amount of virus passes into the fetal compartment; and 3) another 2 to 3 weeks could be necessary for CMV excretion by the fetal kidney; therefore, at least 6 to 9 weeks should pass from maternal infection for the virus to be present in amniotic fluid.[299,300]

Once the diagnosis of vertical transmission to the fetus is established, only ultrasound examination can provide information as to the presence of fetal damage. Moreover, in the absence of ultrasonographic findings, we are unable to predict which fetuses will be clinically affected.

Toxoplasmosis

Toxoplasmosis is caused by infection with *Toxoplasma gondii,* an obligate intracellular parasite. In the United States, between 400 and 4000 cases of acute infection are recognized each year.[301] Human infection with *Toxoplasma gondii* is frequently asymptomatic and is acquired by ingestion of either oocysts of tissue cysts or congenital transmission. Acute toxoplasmosis is diagnosed by demonstrating seroconversion from a negative to a positive test, (IgM antibodies), or a four-fold increase in specific IgG titer over a 3-week interval in the absence of treatment. Congenital transmission of *T. gondii* only occurs during pregnancy or reactivated infection in immunocompromised persons.[302–304] Of infants who have acquired toxoplasmosis during fetal life, 15% become infected in the first trimester, 25% in the second trimester, and 60% in the third trimester.[305–306] The incidence of fetal or congenital toxoplasmosis is 0.65 when the mother acquires the infection in the periconceptional period, 3.7% from 6 to 16 weeks, and 20% from 16 to 25 weeks.[306] The delay between maternal and fetal infection differs, from less than 4 to more than 16 weeks.[307] The clinical manifestations

associated with transplacental infection differ, depending on the gestational age at which infection occurs. Although more than 90% of fetal infections acquired in the third trimester are asymptomatic, those occurring in the first trimester often result in fetal death, abortion, or overt clinical disease. The lesions observed in infants born to mothers who acquired *T. gondii* infection in pregnancy include chorioretinitis, microcephaly, hydrocephalus, cerebral calcifications, and mental retardation. The sonographic finding of ventriculomegaly, intracranial calcifications, hepatomegaly, ascites, and thickened placenta are suggestive of congenital toxoplasmosis. The sensitivity of ultrasonography alone in detecting fetal infection is as low as 20%.[308]

Amniocentesis and detection of the *T. gondii* DNA in amniotic fluid using PCR analysis has been described by several investigators as a highly sensitive and specific method.[309–312] Hohlfeld et al. reported a study in which congenital infection was demonstrated in 34 of 339 fetuses at risk by conventional methods, and the PCR test was positive in all 34. In three other fetuses, only the PCR test gave positive results, and follow-up testing confirmed the presence of congenital toxoplasmosis. The major advantage of PCR analysis is that it is a rapid method and results can be obtained in less than 24 hours, compared with the gold standard of mouse inoculation that takes 3 to 6 weeks. In addition, after the start of antibiotic treatment PCR analysis seems more sensitive.[309] Considering that false-negative results have been reported, a close ultrasonographic and clinical surveillance should be considered in all *T. gondii*–infected patients. To reduce the occurrence of false-negative results, prenatal diagnosis should be timed to approximately 4 weeks after acute infection in the mother.

Varicella Zoster

Varicella is one of the most common communicable diseases in the United States, where the annual incidence is 3.7 million.[313–314] More than 90% of adults living in temperate areas are immune. The incidence of varicella in pregnancy is approximately 0.7 per 1000 patients.[315] The incubation period is 15 ± 5 days, and it is contagious between 2 days before and 5 days after the outbreak of the rash. After maternal chickenpox, the rate of intrauterine transmission of the infection has been estimated to be 24%,[316,317] and it is highest during the last 4 weeks before delivery, reaching almost 50%. Fetal infection during early pregnancy has been associated with a variety of congenital anomalies termed *congenital varicella syndrome.*[318–326] Anomalies associated with this syndrome include cutaneous scars, limb hypoplasia, malformed digits, microcephaly, hydrocephalus, muscle atrophy, neurologic abnormalities (paralysis, seizures), micropthalmia, cataracts, and chorioretinitis. In a study of 1373 women who had varicella during pregnancy the highest risk (2.0%) of the varicella syndrome was observed between 13 and 20 weeks of gestation, with 7 affected infants identified among 351 pregnancies. Only 0.4% ($n = 2$)

cases of congenital varicella syndrome were identified among 472 pregnancies in which maternal varicella occurred before 13 weeks. No cases occurred after 20 weeks of gestation (0 of 477).[327]

Although the varicella virus can be isolated from the amniotic cavity and identified by PCR techniques, the role of amniocentesis for the diagnosis of fetal varicella infection is limited. The reason for this is that the detection of the virus in the fetal compartment is most informative about the severity of fetal infection.[321,328] Varicella infection may be suspected if targeted ultrasound detects associated fetal anomalies. Pretorius et al. reported on 37 cases of mothers who had varicella virus infection during early pregnancy and subsequently underwent fetal sonography between 13 and 37 weeks of gestation.[322] Of the 5 infants subsequently shown to have congenital varicella infection after birth, all showed ultrasonographic abnormalities suggesting infection, and all died by 4 months of age. All sonographic abnormalities were observed in the first half of pregnancy. None of the 32 unaffected infants demonstrated *in utero* ultrasonographic abnormalities.

Rubella

It has been estimated that the risk of congenital rubella in infants born to seronegative pregnant patients is 0.5 per 1000. The rate of transplacental infections changes with the gestational age at which the infection occurs. In the first 12 weeks of pregnancy, it is 80%; between 13 and 14 weeks, it is 54%; and during the late second trimester, it is 25%.[329–331] Enders et al. reported that no evidence of intrauterine infection was found in 38 pregnancies in which the mother's rash appeared before or within 11 days after the last menstrual period.[331] The risk of fetal damage in cases of fetal infection decreases from almost 100% in the first trimester to 35% in the early second trimester.[329,331–333] Although rubella infections during the 17th to 24th weeks of pregnancy result in transmission to the fetus in about one-fifth of the cases, sequelae seem to be a rare event.[332,334]

Prenatal diagnosis of infection by using PCR technique to assess the viral DNA in amniotic fluid seems promising. Revello et al. reported that reverse transcription-nested PCR had a 100% (8 of 8) sensitivity and 100% (8 of 8) specificity for the identification of the virus. Others have also reported high accuracy of PCR analysis in the detection of intraamniotic rubella infection.[335,336]

REFERENCES

1. Prochnownick L. Bietrage zur lehre vom frachtawasser und entstehung. *Arch Gynaekol.* 1877;11:304.
2. Lambl D. Ein seltener fall van hydramnios. *Zentralbl Gynaekol.* 1881;5:329.
3. Von Schatz F. Eine besondere art von einseitiger polyhydramnic mit anderseitiger oligohydramnie bie eineiigen zwillingen. *Arch Gynaekol.* 1882;19:329.
4. Menees TO, Miller JD, Holly LE. Amniography: Preliminary report. *AJR.* 1930:24:363.
5. Boero E. Intra-amniotiques. Semana Medica Buenos-Aires, August 15, 1935.
6. Aburel ME. Le declanchement du travail par injections intraamniotiques du serum sale hypertonique. *Gynecol Obstet.* 1937;36:393.
7. Bevis DCA. Composition of liquor amnii in haemolytic disease of newborn. *Lancet.* 1950;2:443.
8. Fuchs F, Riis P. Antenatal sex determination. *Nature.* 1956;177:330.
9. Steele MW, Breg WR Jr. Chromosome analysis of human amniotic fluid cells. *Lancet.* 1966;1:383.
10. Jacobson CB, Barter RH. Intrauterine diagnosis and management of genetic defects. *Am J Obstet Gynecol.* 1967;99:796.
11. Valenti C, Schutta EJ, Kehaty T. Prenatal diagnosis of Down's syndrome (letter). *Lancet.* 1968;2:220.
12. Jeffcoate TNA, Fliegner JRH, Russell SH, et al. Diagnosis of the adrenogenital syndrome before birth. *Lancet.* 1965;2:553.
13. Simpson NE, Dallaire L, Miller JR, et al. Prenatal diagnosis of genetic disease in Canada: Report of a collaborative study. *Can Med Assoc J.* 1976;115:739.
14. Golbus MS, Loughman WD, Epstein CH, et al. Prenatal genetic diagnosis in 3000 amniocentesis. *N Engl J Med.* 1979;300:157.
15. Kennerknecht I, Kramer S, Grab D, et al. Evaluation of amniotic fluid cell filtration: An experimental approach to early amniocentesis. *Prenat Diagn.* 1993;13:247.
16. Johnson A, Godmilow L. Genetic amniocentesis at 14 weeks or less. *Clin Obstet Gynecol.* 1988;31:345.
17. Kerber S, Held KR. Early cytogenetic amniocentesis—4 years experience. *Prenat Diagn.* 1993;13:21.
18. Henry G, Peakman DC, Winkler W, et al. Amniocentesis before 155 weeks instead of CVS for earlier prenatal cytogenetic diagnosis (abstract 650). *Am J Hum Genet.* 985;37(S).
19. Luthardt FW, Luthy DA, Karp LE, et al. Prospective evaluation of early amniocentesis for prenatal diagnosis (abstract 659). *Am J Hum Genet.* 1985;37(S).
20. Luthy DA, Hickok DE, Luthardt FW, et al. A prospective evaluation of early amniocentesis: An alternative to chorionic villus sampling for prenatal diagnosis (abstract 268). Presented at the *6th Annual Meeting of the Society of Perinatal Obstetricians,* San Antonio, TX, January 30–February 1, 1986.
21. Hanson FW, Zorn EM, Tennant FR, et al. Amniocentesis before 15 weeks' gestation: Outcome, risks and technical problems. *Am J Obstet Gynecol.* 1987;156:1524.
22. Miller WA, Davies RM, Thayer BA, et al. Success, safety and accuracy of early amniocentesis (EA) (abstract 835). *Am J Hum Genet.* 1987;42(S).
23. Weiner CP. Genetic amniocentesis at, or before, 14.0 weeks gestation (abstract 63). Presented at the *7th Annual Meeting of the Society of Perinatal Obstetricians,* Lake Buena Vista, FL, February 5–7, 1987.
24. Godmilow L, Weiner S, Dunn LK. Genetic amniocentesis performed between 12 and 14 weeks gestation (abstract 818). *Am J Hum Genet.* 1987;41(S).
25. Benacerraf BR, Greene MF, Saltzman DH, et al. Early amniocentesis for prenatal cytogenetic evaluation. *Radiology.* 1988;169:708.
26. Lowe BY, Alexander D, Bryla D, et al. *The NICHD Amniocentesis Registry. The Safety and Accuracy of Midtrimester*

Amniocentesis. DHEW Publication No. (NIH) 78-190. Washington, DC: U.S. Department of Health, Education, and Welfare; 1978.

27. Evans MI, Drugan A, Koppitch FC, et al. Genetic diagnosis in the first trimester: The norm for the 1990s. *Am J Obstet Gynecol.* 1989;160:1332.

28. Elejalde BR, de Elejalde MM, Acuna JM, et al. Prospective study of amniocentesis performed between weeks 9 and 16 of gestation: Its feasibility, risks, complications and use in early genetic prenatal diagnosis. *Am J Med Genet.* 1990;35:188–196.

29. Penso CA, Frigoletto FD Jr. Early amniocentesis. *Semin Perinatol.* 1990;14:465.

30. Penso CA, Dandstrom MM, Garber MF, et al. Early amniocentesis: Report of 407 cases with neonatal follow-up. *Obstet Gynecol.* 1990;76:1032.

31. Hanson FW, Happ RL, Rennant FR, et al. Ultrasonography-guided early amniocentesis in singleton pregnancies. *Am J Obstet Gynecol.* 1990;162:1376–1383.

32. Nevin J, Nevin NC, Dornan JC, et al. Early amniocentesis: Experience of 222 consecutive patients. 1987–1988. *Prenat Diagn.* 1990;10:79.

33. Stripparo L, Buscaglia M, Longatti L, et al. Genetic amniocentesis: 505 cases performed before the sixteenth week of gestation. *Prenat Diagn.* 1990;10:350.

34. Klapp J, Nicolaides KH, Hager HD, et al. Early amniocentesis. *Geburtshilfe Frauenheilkd.* 1990;50:443.

35. Lindner C, Huneke B, Masson D, et al. Early amniocentesis for cytogenetic diagnosis. *Geburtshilfe Frauenheilkd.* 1990;50:954.

36. Byrne DL, Marks K, Braude PR, et al. Amnifiltration in the first trimester: Feasibility, technical aspects and cytological outcome. *Ultrasound Obstet Gynecol.* 1991;1:320.

37. Hackett GA, Smith JH, Rebello MT, et al. Early amniocentesis at 11–14 weeks' gestation for the prenatal diagnosis of fetal chromosomal abnormality: A clinical evaluation. *Prenat Diagn.* 1991;11:311–315.

38. Jorgensen FS, Bang J, Lind A, et al. Genetic amniocentesis at 7–14 weeks of gestation. *Prenat Diagn.* 1992;12:277.

39. Henry GP, Miller WA. Early amniocentesis. *J Reprod Med.* 1992;37:396.

40. Djalali M, Barbi G, Kennerknecht I, et al. Introduction of early amniocentesis to routine prenatal diagnosis. *Prenat Diagn.* 1992;12:661.

41. Assel BG, Lewis SM, Dickerman LH, et al. Single-operator comparison of early and mid-second trimester amniocentesis. *Obstet Gynecol.* 1992;79:940.

42. Bombard T, Rigson T. Prospective pilot evaluation of early (11–14 weeks' gestation) amniocentesis in 75 patients. *Military Med.* 1992;157:339.

43. Hanson FW, Tennant F, Hune S, et al. Early amniocentesis: Outcome, risks, and technical problems at ≤12.8 weeks. *Am J Obstet Gynecol.* 1992;166:1707.

44. Frydman R, Pons JC, Borghi E, et al. Periurethral transvestical first-trimester amniocentesis. *Eur J Obstet Gynecol Reprod Biol.* 1993;48:99.

45. Eiben B, Goebel R, Rutt G, et al. Early amniocentesis between the 12th–14th week of pregnancy. Clinical experiences with 1,100 cases. *Geburtshilfe Fraunheilkd.* 1993;53:554.

46. Gabriel R, Harika G, Carre-Pigeon F, et al. Amniocentesis to study the fetal karyotype before 16 weeks of amenorrhea.

Prospective study comparing it with conventional amniocentesis. *J Gynecol Obstet Biol Reprod.* 1993;22:169.

47. Elias S, Simpson JL. Amniocentesis. In: Simpson JL, Elias S. eds. *Essentials of Prenatal Diagnosis.* New York: Churchill Livingston; 1993:27–44.

48. McGahan JP. Aspiration and drainage procedures in the intensive care unit: Percutaneous sonographic guidance. *Radiology.* 1985;154:531.

49. McGahan JP, Walter JP. Diagnostic percutaneous aspiration of the gallbladder. *Radiology.* 1985;155:619.

50. McGahan JP. Laboratory assessment of ultrasonic needle and catheter visualization. *J Ultrasound Med.* 1986;5:373.

51. McGahan JP, Tennant F, Hanson FW, et al. Ultrasound needle guidance for amniocentesis in pregnancies with low amniotic fluid. *J Reprod Med.* 1987;32:513.

52. Hurwitz SR, Nagotte MP. Amniocentesis needle with improved sonographic visualization. *Radiology.* 1989;171:576.

53. Romero R, Jeanty P, Reece EA, et al. Sonographically monitored amniocentesis to decrease intraoperative complications. *Obstet Gynecol.* 1985;65:426.

54. Jeanty P, Rodesch F, Romero R, et al. How to improve your amniocentesis technique. *Am J Obstet Gynecol.* 1983;146:593.

55. Bravo RR, Shulman LS, Phillips OP, et al. Transplacental needle passage in early amniocentesis and pregnancy loss. *Obstet Gynecol.* 1995;86:437–440.

56. Bombard AT, Powers JF, Carter S, et al. Procedure-related fetal losses in transplacental versus nontransplacental genetic amniocentesis. *Am J Obstet Gynecol.* 1995;172:868–872.

57. Marthin T, Liedgren S, Hammar M. Transplacental needle passage and other risk factors associated with second trimester amniocentesis. *Acta Obstet Gynecol Scand.* 1997;76:728–732.

58. Williamson RA, Varner MW, Grant SS. Reduction in amniocentesis risks using a real-time needle guide procedure. *Obstet Gynecol.* 1985;83:751–755.

59. Sonek J, Nicolaides K, Sadowsky G, et al. Articulated needle guide: Report on the first 30 cases. *Obstet Gynecol.* 1989;74:821–823.

60. UltraGuide. *UltraGuide 1000 Instruction Manual.* 1998.

61. Bowerman RA, Barclay ML. A new technique to overcome failed second trimester amniocentesis due to membrane tenting. *Obstet Gynecol.* 1987;70:806.

62. Platt LD, Manning FA, Lemay M. Real-time B-scan—Directed amniocentesis. *Am J Obstet Gynecol.* 1978;130:700.

63. Benacerraf BR, Frigoletto FD. Amniocentesis under continuous ultrasound guidance: A series of 232 cases. *Obstet Gynecol.* 1983;62:760.

64. McArdle CR, Cohen W, Nickerson C, et al. The use of ultrasound in evaluating problems and complications of genetic amniocentesis. *J Clin Ultrasound.* 1983;11:427.

65. Shalev E, Weiner E, Yanai N, et al. Comparison of first-trimester transvaginal amniocentesis with chorionic villus sampling and mid-trimester amniocentesis. *Prenat Diagn.* 1994;14:279.

66. Fuchs F. Volume of amniotic fluid at various stages of pregnancy. *Clin Obstet Gynecol.* 1966;9:449.

67. Abramovich DR. The volume of amniotic fluid in early pregnancy. *J Obstet Gynaecol Br Commonw.* 1968;75:728.

68. Finegal JK. Amniotic fluid and midtrimester amniocentesis: A review. *Br J Obstet Gynaecol.* 1984;91:745.

69. Sundberg K, Smidt-Jenson S, Philip J. Amniocentesis with

increased cell yield, obtained by filtration and reinjection of the amniotic fluid. *Ultrasound Obstet Gynecol.* 1991;1:91–94.

70. Byrne DL, Nicolaides KH. Amniotic fluid temperature change during first trimester amnifiltration. *Br J Obstet Gynaecol.* 1994;101:304.

71. Dombrowski MP, Isada NB, Johnson MP, Berry SM. Modified stylet technique for tenting of amniotic membranes. *Obstet Gynecol.* 1996;87:455–456.

72. NICHD National Registry for Amniocentesis Study Group. Midtrimester amniocentesis for prenatal diagnosis, safety and accuracy. *JAMA.* 1976;236:1471.

73. Tabor A, Mmadsen M, Obel EB, et al. Randomized controlled trial of genetic amniocentesis in 4606 low-risk women. *Lancet.* 1986;1:1287.

74. Williamson RA, Varner MW, Grant SS. Reduction in amniocentesis risks using a real-time needle guide procedure. *Obstet Gynecol.* 1985;65:751.

75. Dacus JV, Wilroy RS, Summitt RL, et al. Genetic amniocentesis: A twelve years' experience. *Am J Med Genet.* 1985;20:443.

76. Katayama KP, Roesler MR. Five hundred cases of amniocentesis without bloody tap. *Obstet Gynecol.* 1986;68:70.

77. Crandon AJ, Peel KR. Amniocentesis with and without ultrasound guidance. *Br J Obstet Gynaecol.* 1979;86:1.

78. Chayen S, ed. An assessment of the hazards of amniocentesis. Report to the Medical Research Council by their Working Party on Amniocentesis. *Br J Obstet Gynaecol.* 1978;85(suppl 2):1.

79. Ron M, Cohen T, Taffe H, et al. The clinical significance of blood-contaminated midtrimester amniocentesis. *Acta Obstet Gynecol Scand.* 1982;61:43.

80. Harwood LM. Detection of fetal cells in maternal circulation. *J Med Lab Technol.* 1961;19:19.

81. Mennuti MT, Brummond W, Crombleholme WR, et al. Fetal–maternal bleeding associated with genetic amniocentesis. *Obstet Gynecol.* 1980;55:48.

82. Lele AS, Carmody PJ, Hurd ME, et al. Feto–maternal bleeding following diagnostic amniocentesis. *Obstet Gynecol.* 1982;60:60.

83. Robinson A, Bowes W, Droegememueller W, et al. Intrauterine diagnosis: Potential complications. *Am J Obstet Gynecol.* 1973;116:937.

84. Karp LE, Schiller HS. Meconium staining of amniotic fluid at midtrimester amniocentesis. *Obstet Gynecol.* 1977;50(S):47.

85. Seller M. Dark-brown amniotic fluid. *Lancet.* 1977;2:983.

86. King CR, Prescott G, Pernoll M. Significance of meconium in midtrimester diagnostic amniocentesis. *Am J Obstet Gynecol.* 1978;132:667.

87. Bartsch FK, Lundberg J, Wahlstrom J. One thousand consecutive midtrimester amniocenteses. *Obstet Gynecol.* 1980;55:305.

88. Crandall BF, Howard J, Lebherz TB, et al. Follow-up of 2000 second-trimester amniocenteses. *Obstet Gynecol.* 1980;56:625.

89. Svbigos JM, Stewart-Rattray SF, Pridmore BR. Meconium-stained liquor at second trimester amniocentesis: Is it significant? *Aust NZ J Obstet Gynaecol.* 1981;21:5.

90. Cruikshank DP, Varner MW, Cruikshank JE, et al. Midtrimester amniocentesis. *Am J Obstet Gynecol.* 1983;146:204.

91. Hankins GDV, Rowe J, Quirk JG, et al. Significance of brown and/or green amniotic fluid at the time of second trimester genetic amniocentesis. *Obstet Gynecol.* 1984;64:353.

92. Allen R. The significance of meconium in midtrimester genetic amniocentesis. *Am J Obstet Gynecol.* 1985;152:413.

93. Hess LW, Anderson RL, Golbus MS. Significance of opaque discolored amniotic fluid at second-trimester amniocentesis. *Obstet Gynecol.* 1986;67:44.

94. Zorn EM, Hanson FW, Greve LC, et al. Analysis of the significance of discolored amniotic fluid detected at midtrimester amniocentesis. *Am J Obstet Gynecol.* 1986;154:1234.

95. Cassell GH, Davis RO, Waites KB, et al. isolation of *Mycoplasma hominis* and *Ureaplasma urealyticum* from amniotic fluid at 16–20 weeks of gestation: Potential effect on outcome of pregnancy. *Sex Transm Dis.* 1983;10:294.

96. Gray DJ, Robinson H, Malone J, et al. Adverse outcome in pregnancy following amniotic fluid isolation of *Ureaplasma urealyticum. Prenat Diagn.* 1992;12:111–117.

97. Abramovich DR, Gray ES. Physiologic fetal defecation in midpregnancy. *Obstet Gynecol.* 1982;60:294.

98. Dodgson J, Martin J, Boswell J, et al. Probable amniotic fluid embolism precipated by amniocentesis and treated by exchange transfusion. *Br Med J.* 1987;294:1322.

99. Galle PC, Meis PJ. Complications of amniocentesis. *J Reprod Med.* 1982;27:149.

100. Ager RP, Oliver RWA. *The Risks of Midtrimester Amniocenteses.* Lancashire, UK: University of Salford; 1986.

101. Klein SA, Gobbo PN, Ristuccia PA, et al. Diagnostic amniocentesis and bacteremia. *J Hosp Infect.* 1987;9:81.

102. Wald NJ, Terzian E, Vickers PA. Congenital talipes and hip malformation in relation to amniocentesis: A case-control study. *Lancet.* 1983;2:246.

103. Vyas H, Milner AD, Hopkin IE. Amniocentesis and fetal lung development. *Arch Dis Child.* 1982;57:627.

104. Hislop A, Fairweather DVI. Amniocentesis and lung growth: An animal experiment with clinical implications. *Lancet.* 1982;2:1271.

105. Hislop A, Fairweather FVI, Blackwell RJ, et al. The effect of amniocentesis and drainage of amniotic fluid on lung development in *Maccaca fascicularis. Br J Obstet Gynaecol.* 1984;91:835.

106. Thompson PJ, Greenough A, Nicolaides KH. Lung volume measured by functional residual capacity in infants following first trimester amniocentesis or chorion villus sampling. *Br J Obstet Gynaecol.* 1992;99:479.

107. Crane JP, Rohland BM. Clinical significance of persistent amniotic fluid leakage after genetic amniocentesis. *Prenat Diagn.* 19867;6:25.

108. Gold RB, Goyert GL, Schwartz DB, et al. Conservative management of second trimester post-amniocentesis fluid leakage. *Obstet Gynecol.* 1989;74:745.

109. Misenhimer HR. Fetal hemorrhage associated with amniocentesis. *Am J Obstet Gynecol.* 1966;94:1133.

110. Creasman WT, Lawrence RA, Thiede HA. Fetal complications of amniocentesis. *JAMA.* 1968;204:91.

111. Berner HW, Seisler EP, Barlow J. Fetal cardiac tamponade: A complication of amniocentesis. *Obstet Gynecol.* 1972;40:599.

112. Cross HE, Maumenee AE. Ocular trauma during amniocentesis. *N Engl J Med.* 1972;287:993.

113. Grove CS, Trombetta GC, Amstey MS. Fetal complications of amniocentesis. *Am J Obstet Gynecol.* 1973;115:1154.

114. Egley CC. Laceration of fetal spleen during amniocentesis. *Am J Obstet Gynecol.* 1973;116:482.

115. Cook LN, Shott RJ, Andrews BF. Fetal complications of diagnostic amniocentesis: A review and report of a case with pneumothorax. *Pediatrics.* 1974;53:421.

116. Fortin JG, Lemire J. Une complication oculaire de l'amniocenteses. *Can J Opthalmol.* 1975;10:551.

117. Lamb MP. Gangrene of a fetal limb due to amniocentesis. *Br J Obstet Gynaecol.* 1975;82:829.

118. Broome DL, Wilson MG, Weiss B, et al. Needle puncture of fetus: A complication of second-trimester amniocentesis. *Am J Obstet Gynecol.* 1976;126:247.

119. Karp LE, Hayden PW. Fetal puncture during midtrimester amniocentesis. *Obstet Gynecol.* 1977;49:115.

120. Rickwood AMK. A case of ileal atresia and ileo-cutaneous fistula caused by amniocentesis. *J Pediatr.* 1977;91:312.

121. Cromie WJ, Bates RD, Duckett JW Jr. Penetrating renal trauma in the neonate. *J Urol.* 1978;119:259.

122. Young PE, Matson MR, Jones OW. Fetal exsanguination and other vascular injuries from midtrimester genetic amniocentesis. *Am J Obstet Gynecol.* 1977;129:21.

123. Rehder H. Fetal limb deformities due to amniotic constrictions (a possible consequence of preceding amniocentesis). *Pathol Res Pract.* 1978;162:316.

124. Rehder H, Weitzel H. Intrauterine amputations after amniocentesis. *Lancet.* 1978;1:382.

125. Epley SL, Hanson JW, Cruikshank DP. Fetal injury with midtrimester diagnostic amniocentesis. *Obstet Gynecol.* 1979;53:77.

126. Swift PGF, Driscoll IB, Vowles KDJ. Neonatal small-bowel obstruction associated with amniocentesis. *Br Med J.* 1979;1:720.

127. Merin S, Beyth Y. Uniocular congenital blindness as a complication of midtrimester amniocentesis. *Arch Dis Child.* 1980;55:814.

128. Youroukos S, Papedelis F, Matsaniotis N. Porencephalic cysts after amniocentesis. *Arch Dis Child.* 1980;55:814.

129. Therkelsen AJ, Rehder H. Intestinal atresia caused by second trimester amniocentesis. *Br J Obstet Gynaecol.* 1981;88:559.

130. Moessinger AC, Blanc WA, Byrne J, et al. Amniotic band syndrome associated with amniocentesis. *Am J Obstet Gynecol.* 1981;141:588.

131. Isenberg SJ, Heckenlively Jr. Traumatized eye with retinal damage from amniocentesis. *J Pediatr Ophthalmol Strabismus.* 1985;22:65.

132. Achiron R, Zakut H. Fetal hemothorax complicating amniocentesis—Antenatal sonographic diagnosis. *Acta Obstet Gynecol Scand.* 1986;65:869.

133. Kohn G. The amniotic band syndrome: A possible complication of amniocentesis. *Prenat Diagn.* 1987;7:303.

134. Morin LRM, Bonan J, Vendrolini G, et al. Sonography of umbilical cord hematoma following genetic amniocentesis. *Acta Obstet Gynecol Scand.* 1987;66:669.

135. Admoni M, Ben Exra D. Ocular trauma following amniocentesis as the cause of leukocoria. *J Pediatr Ophthalmol Strabismus.* 1988;25:196–197.

136. Wiener JJ, Farrow A, Farrow SC. Audit of amniocentesis from a district general hospital: Is it worth it? *Br Med J.* 1998;300:1243.

137. Chong SKF, Levitt GA, Lawson J, et al. Subarachnoid cyst with hydrocephalus—A complication of mid-trimester amniocentesis. *Prenat Diagn.* 1989;9:677.

138. Naylor G, Roper JP, Wilshaw HE. Ophthalmic complications of amniocentesis. *Eye.* 1990;4:845.

139. Ledbetter DJ, Hall DG. Traumatic arteriovenous fistula: A complication of amniocentesis. *J Pediatr Surg.* 1992;27:720.

140. Rummelt V, Rummelt C, Naumann GOH. Congenital nonpigmental epithelial iris cyst after amniocentesis: Clinicopathologic report on two children. *Ophthalmology.* 1993;100:776.

141. Baird PA, Yee IML, Sadovnick AD. Population-based study of long-term outcomes after amniocentesis. *Lancet.* 1994;344:1134–1136.

142. D'Alton ME, Malone FD, Chelmow D, et al. Defining the role of fluorescence in situ hybridization on uncultured amniocytes for prenatal diagnosis of aneuploidies (and discussion). *Am J Obstet Gynecol.* 1997;176:769–774, 774–776.

143. Morris A, Boyd E, Dhanjal S, et al. Two years' prospective experience using fluorescence in situ hybridization on uncultured amniotic fluid cells for rapid prenatal diagnosis of common chromosomal aneuploidies. *Prenat Diagn.* 1999;19:546–551.

144. Eiben B, Trawicki W, Hammans W, et al. A prospective comparative study on fluorescence in situ hybridization (FISH) of uncultured amniocytes and standard karyotype analysis. *Prenat Diagn.* 1998;18:901–906.

145. Aviram-Goldring A, Daniely M, Chaki R, et al. Advanced FISH with directly labeled X, Y and 18 DNA probes as a tool for rapid prenatal diagnosis. *J Reprod Med.* 1999;44:497–503.

146. Velagelati GV, Shulman LP, Phillips OP, et al. Primed in situ labeling for rapid prenatal diagnosis. *Am J Obstet Gynecol.* 1998;178:1313–1320.

147. American College of Medical Genetics. Prenatal interphase fluorescence in situ hybridization (FISH) policy statement. *Am J Hum Genet.* 1993;53:526–527.

148. American College of Obstetricians and Gynecologists. Prevention of RhD alloimmunization. *ACOG Practice Bulletin, 4,* Washington DC: ACOG; 1999.

149. Murray JC, Karp LE, Williamson RA, et al. Rh isoimmunization related to amniocentesis. *Am J Med Genet.* 1983;16:527.

150. Henry G, Wexler P, Robinson A. Rh-immune globulin after amniocentesis for genetic diagnosis. *Obstet Gynecol.* 1976;48:557.

151. Golbus MS, Stephens JD, Cann HM, et al. Rh isoimmunization following genetic amniocentesis. *Prenat Diagn.* 1982;2:149.

152. Frigoletto FD, Jewett JF, Konugres AA, eds. *Rh Hemolytic Disease: New Strategy for Eradication.* Boston: GK Hall Medical Publishers; 1982.

153. Wald NJ, Cuckle HS. Amniotic fluid alpha-fetoprotein measurement in antenatal diagnosis of anencephaly and open spina bifida in early pregnancy. *Lancet.* 1979;2:651.

154. The Canadian Early and Mid-Trimester Amniocentesis Trial (CEMAT) Group. Randomized trial to assess safety and fetal outcome of early and midtrimester amniocentesis. *Lancet.* 1998;351:242.

155. Winsor EJT, Tomkins DJ, Kalousek D, et al. Cytogenetic aspects of the Canadian early and mid-trimester amniotic fluid trial (CEMAT). *Prenat Diagn.* 1999;19:620–627.

156. Hanson FW, Happ RL, Tennant FR et al. Ultrasonography-guided early amniocentesis in singleton pregnancies. *Am J Obstet Gynecol.* 1990;162:1376.

157. Thayer B, Braddock B, Spitzer K, Miller W. Clinical and laboratory experience with early amniocentesis. *Birth Defects Original Article Series.* 1990;26:58.

158. Assel BG, Lewis SM, Dickerman LH, et al. Single-operator comparison of early and mid-second-trimester amniocentesis. *Obstet Gynecol.* 1992;79:940.

159. Yang CH, Chu Ho ES, Liu CC, et al. Prenatal cytogenetic diagnosis by amniocentesis before 15 weeks' gestation. *Chung Hua I Hsueh Tsa Chih (Taipei).* 1993;52:81.

160. Crandall BF, Kulch P, Tabsh K. Risk assessment of amniocentesis between 11 and 15 weeks: Comparison to later amniocentesis controls. *Prenat Diagn.* 1994;14:913–919.

161. Shulman LP, Elias S, Phillips OP, et al. Amniocentesis performed at 14 weeks' gestation or earlier: Comparison with first-trimester transabdominal chorionic villus sampling. *Obstet Gynecol.* 1994;83:543.

162. Nicolaides K, Brizot M de L, Patel F, Snijders R. Comparison of chorionic villus sampling and amniocentesis for fetal karyotyping at 10–13 weeks' gestation. *Lancet.* 1994;344:435.

163. Rousseau O, Boulot P, Lefort G, et al. Amniocentesis before 15 weeks' gestation: Technical aspects and obstetric risks. *Eur J Obstet Gynecol Reprod Biol.* 1995;58:127.

164. Sundberg K, Bang J, Brocks V, et al. Early sonographically guided amniocentesis with filtration technique: Follow-up on 249 procedures. *J Ultrasound Med.* 1995;14:585.

165. Brumfield CG, Lin S, Conner W, et al. Pregnancy outcome following genetic amniocentesis at 11–14 versus 16–19 weeks' gestation. *Obstet Gynecol.* 1996;88:114–118.

166. Johnson JAM, Douglas Wilson R, Winsor EJT, et al. The early amniocentesis study: A randomized clinical trial of early amniocentesis versus midtrimester amniocentesis. *Fetal Diagn Ther.* 1996;11:85.

167. Diaz Vega M, De La Cueva P, Leal C, Aisa P. Early amniocentesis at 10–12 weeks' gestation. *Prenat Diagn.* 1996;16:307.

168. Eiben B, Hammans W, Hansen S, et al. On the complication risk of early amniocentesis versus standard amniocentesis. *Fetal Diagn Ther.* 1997;12:140.

169. Wilson RD, Johnson J, Windrim R, et al. The early amniocentesis study: A randomized clinical trial of early amniocentesis and midtrimester amniocentesis. *Fetal Diagn Ther.* 1997; 12:97.

170. Sundberg K, Bang J, Smidt-Jensen S, et al. Randomized study of risk of fetal loss related to early amniocentesis versus chorionic villus sampling. *Lancet.* 1997;350:697.

171. Daniel A, Ng A, Kuah KB, et al. A study of early amniocentesis for prenatal cytogenetic diagnosis. *Prenat Diagn.* 1998;18: 21.

172. Collins VR, Webley C, Sheffield LJ, Halliday JL. Fetal outcome and maternal morbidity after early amniocentesis. *Prenat Diagn.* 1998;18:767.

173. Jörgensen C, Andolf E. Amniocentesis before the 15th gestational week in single and twin gestations—Complications and quality of genetic analysis. *Acta Obstet Gynecol Scand.* 1998;77:151.

174. Roper EC, Konje JC, DeChazal RC, et al. Genetic amniocentesis: Gestation-specific pregnancy outcome and comparison of outcome following early and traditional amniocentesis. *Prenat Diagn.* 1999;19:803–807.

175. Nelson MM, Emery AEH. Amniotic fluid cells: Prenatal sex prediction and culture. *Br Med J.* 1970;1:523.

176. Sundberg K, Lundsteen C, Philip J. Early amniocentesis for further investigation of mosaicism diagnosed by chorionic villus sampling. *Prenat Diagn.* 1996;16:1121.

177. Byrne D, Marks K, Azar G, Nicolaides K. Randomized study of early amniocentesis versus chorionic villus sampling: A technical and cytogenetic comparison of 650 patients. *Ultrasound Obstet Gynecol.* 1991;1:235.

178. Rooney DE, MacLachlan N, Smith J, et al. Early amniocentesis: A cytogenetic evaluation. *Br Med J.* 1989;299:25.

179. Wilson RD. Early amniocentesis: A clinical review. *Prenat Diagn.* 1995;15:1259.

180. Nagel HTC, Vandenbussche FPHA, Keirse MJNC, et al. Amniocentesis before 14 completed weeks as an alternative to transabdominal chorionic villus sampling: A controlled trial with infant follow-up. *Prenat Diagn.* 1998;18:465–475.

181. Sundberg K, Lundsteen C, Philip J. Comparison of cell cultures, chromosome quality and karyotypes obtained after chorionic villus sampling and early amniocentesis with filter technique. *Prenat Diagn.* 1999;19:12–16.

182. Hunter AGW, Cox DM. Counseling problems when twins are discovered at genetic amniocentesis. *Clin Genet.* 1979;16:34.

183. Rodeck CH, Mibashan RS, Campbell S. Selective feticide of the affected twin by fetoscopic air embolism. *Prenat Diagn.* 1982;2:189.

184. Elias S, Gerbie AB, Simpson JL, et al. Genetic amniocentesis in twin gestations. *Am J Obstet Gynecol.* 1980;138:169.

185. Bang J, Nielsen H, Philip J. Prenatal karyotyping of twins by ultrasonically guided amniocentesis. *Am J Obstet Gynecol.* 1975;123:695.

186. Tabsh K. Genetic amniocentesis in multiple gestation: A new technique to diagnose monoamniotic twins. *Obstet Gynecol.* 75:296;1990.

187. Jeanty P, Shah D, Roussis P. Single-needle insertion in twin amniocentesis. *J Ultrasound Med.* 1990;9:511.

188. Bahado-Singh R, Schmitt R, Hobbins JC. New technique for genetic amniocentesis in twins. *Obstet Gynecol.* 1992;79:304.

189. Fribourg S. Safety of intra-amniotic injection of indigo carmine. *Am J Obstet Gynecol.* 1981;140:350.

190. Goldstein AI, Stills SM. Midtrimester amniocentesis in twin pregnancies. *Obstet Gynecol.* 1983;62:659.

191. Librach CL, Doran TA, Benzie RJ, et al. Genetic amniocentesis in seventy twin pregnancies. *Am J Obstet Gynecol.* 1984;148:585.

192. Di-lin L, Zhi-long Z. Double sacs amniocentesis in twin pregnancy. *Chin Med J.* 1984;97:465.

193. Fillkins K, Russo J, Brown T, et al. Genetic amniocentesis in multiple gestations. *Prenat Diagn.* 1984;4:223.

194. Tabsh KMA, Crandall B, Lebherz TB, et al. Genetic amniocentesis in twin pregnancy. *Obstet Gynecol.* 1985;65:843.

195. Bovicelli L, Michelacci L, Rizzo N, et al. Genetic amniocentesis in twin pregnancy. *Prenat Diagn.* 1983;3:101.

196. Palle C, Andersen JW, Tabor A, et al. Increased risk of abortion after genetic amniocentesis in twin pregnancies. *Prenat Diagn.* 1983;3:83.

197. Wolf DA, Scheible FW, Young PE, et al. Genetic amniocentesis in multiple pregnancy. *J Clin Ultrasound.* 1979;7:208.

198. Beekhuis JR, DeBruijn HWA, Van Ligh JMM, et al. Second trimester amniocentesis in twin pregnancies: Maternal hemoglobin as a dye marker to differentiate diamniotic twins. *Br J Obstet Gynaecol.* 1992;99:126.

199. Cowett RM, Kakanson DO, Kocon RW, et al. Untoward neonatal effect of intraamniotic administration of methylene blue. *Obstet Gynecol.* 1976;48:74s.

200. Plunkett GD. Neonatal complications. *Obstet Gynecol.* 1973; 41:476.

201. Nicolini U, Monni G. Intestinal obstruction in babies exposed to in utero methylene blue. *Lancet.* 1990;336:1258.

202. Pruggmayer MRK, Jahoda MGJ, Van der Pol JG, et al. Genetic amniocentesis in twin pregnancies: Results of a multicenter trial in 529 pregnancies. *Ultrasound Obstet Gynecol.* 1992;2:6.

203. Pjipers L, Jahoda MGJ, Vosters RPL, et al. Genetic amniocentesis in twin pregnancies. *Br J Obstet Gynaecol.* 1988;95:323.

204. Wapner RJ, Johnson A, David G, et al. Prenatal diagnosis in twin gestations: A comparison between second-trimester amniocentesis and first-trimester chorionic villus sampling. *Obstet Gynecol.* 1993;82:49.

205. Kappel B, Nielsen J, Hansen KB, et al. Spontaneous abortion following mid-trimester amniocentesis. Clinical significance of placental perforation and blood-stained amniotic fluid. *Br J Obstet Gynaecol.* 1987;94:50.

206. Grau P, Tabsh K, Crandall B. Genetic amniocentesis in twin gestation. *Am J Hum Genet.* 1989;45:A259.

207. Pruggmayer M, Bartels I, Rauskolb R, et al. Abortrisiko nach genetischer Amniozentese im II. Trimenon be Zwillingsschwangerschaften. *Geburtshilfe Frauenheilkd.* 1990;50:810.

208. Pruggmayer M, Baumann P, Schuttel H, et al. Incidence of abortion after genetic amniocentesis in twin pregnancies. *Prenat Diagn.* 1991;11:637.

209. Anderson RL, Goldberg JD, Golbus MS. Prenatal diagnosis in multiple gestation: 20 years' experience with amniocentesis. *Prenat Diagn.* 1991;11:263.

210. Imaizumi Y, Asaka A, Inouye E. Analysis of multiple birth rates in Japan. VII: Rates of spontaneous and induced terminations of pregnancy in twins. *Jpn J Hum Genet.* 1982; 27:235.

211. Ko TM, Tseng LH, Hwa HL. Second-trimester genetic amniocentesis in twin pregnancy. *Int J Obstet Gynecol.* 1998;61; 285.

212. Romero R, Sirtori M, Oyarzun E, et al. Infection and labor: V. Prevalence, microbiology, and clinical significance of intraamniotic infection in women with preterm labor and intact membranes. *Am J Obstet Gynecol.* 1989;161:817–824.

213. Blanc WA. Infection amniotique et neonatal. *Gynaecologia.* 1953;136:101.

214. Blanc WA. Pathways of fetal and early neonatal infection: Viral placentitis, bacterial and fungal chorioamnionitis. *J Pediatr.* 1964;473:59.

215. Benirschke K, Clifford SH. Intrauterine bacterial infection of the newborn infant. *J Pediatr.* 1959;54:11.

216. Driscoll SG. Pathology and the developing fetus. *Pediatr Clin North Am.* 1965;12:493.

217. Benirschke K. Routes and types of infection in the fetus and newborn. *Am J Dis Child.* 1965;28:714.

218. Romero R, Mazor M. Infection and preterm labor. *Clin Obstet Gynecol.* 1988;31:553.

219. Galask RP, Varner MW, Petzold CR, et al. Bacterial attachment to the chorioamniotic membranes. *Am J Obstet Gynecol.* 1984;148:915.

220. Garite TJ, Freeman RK. Chorioamnionitis in the pre-term gestation. *Obstet Gynecol.* 1984;73:38.

221. Cotton DB, Hill LM, Strassner HT, et al. Use of amniocentesis in preterm gestation with ruptured membranes. *Obstet Gynecol.* 1984;63:38.

222. Broekhuizen FF, Gilman M, Hamilton PR. Amniocentesis for Gram stain and culture in preterm premature rupture of the membranes. *Obstet Gynecol.* 1985;66:316.

223. Vintzileos AM, Campbell WA, Nochimson DJ, et al. Qualitative amniotic fluid volume versus amniocentesis in predicting infection in preterm rupture of the membranes. *Obstet Gynecol.* 1986;67:579.

224. Feinstein ST, Vintzileos AM, Lodeiro JG, et al. Amniocentesis with premature rupture of membranes. *Obstet Gynecol.* 1986;68:147.

225. Romero R, Quintero R, Oyarzun E, et al. Intraamniotic infection and the onset of labor in preterm premature rupture of membranes. *Am J Obstet Gynecol.* 1988;159;661.

226. Gauthier DW, Meyer W. Comparison of Gram stain, leukocyte esterase activity and amniotic fluid glucose concentration in predicting amniotic fluid culture results in preterm premature rupture of membranes. *Am J Obstet Gynecol.* 1992;167:1092.

227. Gray DJ, Robinson HB, Malone J, et al. Adverse outcome in pregnancy following amniotic isolation of *Ureaplasma urealyticum. Prenat Diagn.* 1992;12:111.

228. Romero R, Munoz H, Gomez R, et al. Does the infection cause preterm labor and delivery? *Semin Reprod Endocrinol.* 1994;12:227.

229. Romero R, Gonzales R, Sepulveda W, et al. Infection and labor: VII. Microbial invasion of the amniotic cavity in patients with suspected cervical incompetence: Prevalence and clinical significance. *AJOB.* 1992;167:1086.

230. Romero R, Shamma F, Avila C, et al. Infection and labor: VI. Prevalence, microbiology, and clinical significance of intraamniotic infection in twin gestations with preterm labor. *Am J Obstet Gynecol.* 1992;166:129.

231. Romero R, Nores J, Mazor M, et al. Microbial invasion of the amniotic cavity during term labor. Prevalence and clinical significance. *J Reprod Med.* 1993;38:543.

232. Romero R, Mazor M, Morrotti R, et al. Infection and labor: VII. Microbial invasion of the amniotic cavity in spontaneous rupture of membrane at term. *Am J Obstet Gynecol.* 1992;166: 129.

233. Leigh J, Garite TJ. Amniocentesis and the management of premature labor. *Obstet Gynecol.* 1986;67:513.

234. Altshuler G, Hyde S. Clinicopathologic consideration of fusobacteria chorioamnionitis. *Acta Obstet Gynecol Scand.* 1988; 67:513.

235. Hillier SL, Martius J, Krohn M, et al. A case-control study of chorioamnionic infection and histologic chorioamnionitis in prematurity. *N Engl J Med.* 1988;319:972.

236. Duff P, Kopelman JN. Subclinical intraamniotic infection in asymptomatic patients with refractory preterm labor. *Obstet Gynecol.* 1987;69:756.

237. Skoll MA, Moretti ML, Sibai BM. The incidence of positive amniotic fluid cultures in patients in preterm labor with intact membranes. *Am J Obstet Gynecol.* 1989;161:813.

238. Gibbs RS, Blanco JD, St. Clair PJ, et al. Quantitative bacteriology of amniotic fluid from women with clinical intraamniotic infection at term. *J Infect Dis.* 1982;145:1.

239. Garite TJ, Freeman RK, Linzey EM, et al. The use of amniocentesis in patients with premature rupture of membranes. *Obstet Gynecol.* 1979;54:226.

240. Bobitt JR, Hayslip CC, Damato JD. Amniotic fluid infection as determined by transabdominal amniocentesis in patients with

intact membranes in premature labor. *Am J Obstet Gynecol.* 1981;140:947.

241. Romero R, Yoon BH, Mazor M, et al. The diagnostic and prognostic value of amniotic fluid white blood cell count, glucose, interleukin-6 Gram stain in patients with preterm labor and intact membranes. *Am J Obstet Gynecol.* 1993;169:805.

242. Romero R, Yoon BH, Mazor M, et al. A comparative study of the diagnostic performance of amniotic fluid glucose, white blood cell count, interleukin-6, and Gram stain in the detection of microbial invasion in patients with preterm premature rupture of membranes. *Am J Obstet Gynecol.* 1993;169:839.

243. Romero R, Jimenez C, Kohda AK, et al. Amniotic fluid glucose concentration: A rapid and simple method for the detection of intraamniotic infection in preterm labor. *Am J Obstet Gynecol.* 1909;163:968.

244. Romero R, Emamian M, Quintero R, et al. The value and limitations of the Gram stain examination in the diagnosis of intraamniotic infection. *Am J Obstet Gynecol.* 1988;159:114.

245. Miller JM Jr, Hill GB, Welt SL, et al. Bacterial colonization of amniotic fluid in the presence of ruptured membranes. *Am J Obstet Gynecol.* 1980;137:151.

246. Zlatnik FJ, Cruikshank DP, Petzold CR, et al. Amniocentesis in the identification of inapparent infection in preterm patients with premature rupture of the membranes. *J Reprod Med.* 1984;29:656.

247. Hameed C, Tejani N, Verma UL, et al. Silent chorioamnionitis as a cause of preterm labor refractory to tocolytic therapy. *Am J Obstet Gynecol.* 1984;149:726.

248. Gravett MG, Hummel D, Eschenbach DA, et al. Preterm labor associated with subclinical amniotic fluid infection with bacterial vaginosis. *Obstet Gynecol.* 1986;67:229.

249. Coultrip LL, Grossman JH. Evaluation of rapid diagnostic tests in the detection of microbial invasion of the amniotic cavity. *Am J Obstet Gynecol.* 1992;167:1231.

250. Gauthier DW, Meyer WJ, Bieniarz A. Correlation of amniotic fluid glucose concentration and intraamniotic infection in patients with preterm labor or premature rupture of membranes. *Am J Obstet Gynecol.* 1991;165:1105.

251. Kronvall G, Myhre E. Differential staining of bacteria in clinical specimens using acridine orange buffered at low pH. *Acta Pathol Microbiol Scand.* 1977;85:249.

252. Kleimann MB, Reynolds KJ, Screiner RL, et al. Rapid diagnosis of neonatal bacteremia with acridine orange stain buffy coat smears. *J Pediatr.* 1984;105:149.

253. Kleimann MB, Reynolds JK, Watts NJ, et al. Superiority of acridine orange stain versus Gram stain in partially treated bacterial meningitis. *J Pediatr.* 1984;104:401.

254. Lauer BA, Reller LB, Mirret S, et al. Comparison of acridine orange and Gram stains for detection of microorganisms in cerebrospinal fluid and other clinical specimens. *J Clin Microbiol.* 1989;6:41.

255. Romero R, Emamian M, Quintero R, et al. Diagnosis of intrauterine infection: The acridine orange stain. *Am J Perinatol.* 1989;6:41.

256. Ellin RJ, Hosseini J. Clinical utility of limulus amebocyte lysate test. Bacterial endotoxin, structure, biomedical significance and detection with the limulus amebocyte lysate test. In: Ten Cate JW, Buller HR, Sturke A, et al., eds. *Progress in Clinical and Biological Research.* New York: Liss; 1985:307.

257. Romero R, Kadar N, Hobbins JC, et al. Infection and labor: The detection of endotoxin in amniotic fluid. *Am J Obstet Gynecol.* 1987;157:815.

258. Wildfauber A, Heymer B, Schleiffer KH, et al. Investigation on the specificity of the limulus test for the detection of endotoxin. *Appl Microbiol.* 1974;28:269.

259. Ray TL, Hanson A, Ray LF, et al. Purification of mannan from *Candida albicans* which activates serum complement. *J Invest Dermatol.* 1979;73:269.

260. Romero R, Quintero R, Nores J, et al. Amniotic fluid white blood cell count: A rapid and simple test to diagnose microbial invasion of the amniotic cavity and preddict preterm delivery. *Am J Obstet Gynecol.* 1991;165:821.

261. Overtufr GD. Infections of the central nervous system. In: Hoeproch PD, Jordan MC, eds. *Infectious Diseases,* 4th ed. Philadelphia: Lippincott; 1989:1114.

262. Brody JS. Diseases of the pleura, mediastinum, diaphragm and chest wall. In: Wyngaarden JB, Smith LH Jr, eds. *Cecil Textbook of Medicine,* 17th ed. Philadelphia: Saunders; 185:447.

263. Parker RH. Skeletal infections. In: Hoeproch PD, Jordan MC, eds. *Infectious Diseases,* 4th ed. Philadelphia: Lippincott; 1989:1376.

264. Kirshon B, Rosenfeld B, Mari G, et al. Amniotic fluid glucose and intraamniotic infection. *Am J Obstet Gynecol.* 1991;164:818.

265. Romero R, Brody DT, Oyarzun E, et al. Infection and labor: III. Interleukin-1: A signal for the onset of parturition. *Am J Obstet Gynecol.* 160:1117.

266. Romero R, Mazor M, Brandt F, et al. Interleukin-1 alpha and interleukin-1 beta in human preterm and term parturition. *Am J Reprod Immunol.* 1992;27:117.

267. Romero R, Manogue KR, Mitchell MD, et al. Infection and labor: IV. Cachectin tumor necrosis factor in the amniotic fluid of women with intraamniotic infection and preterm and term labor. *Am J Obstet Gynecol.* 1989;161:336.

268. Romero R, Mazor M, Sepulveda W, et al. Tumor necrosis factor in preterm and term labor. *Am J Obstet Gynecol.* 1992;166:1576.

269. Romero R, Avila C, Santhanam U, et al. Amniotic fluid interleukin-6 in preterm labor. Association with infection. *J Clin Invest.* 1990;85:1392.

270. Romero R, Yoon BH, Kenney JS, et al. Amniotic fluid IL-6 determinations are of diagnostic and prognostic value in preterm labor. *Am J Reprod Immunol.* 1993;30:167.

271. Romero R, Ceska M, Avila C, et al. Neutrophil attractant/activating peptide-1/interleukin-8 in term and preterm parturition. *Am J Obstet Gynecol.* 1991;165:813.

272. Cherouny P, Pankuch G, Botti J, et al. The presence of amniotic fluid leukoattractants accurately identifies histologic chorioamnionitis and predicts tocolytic efficacy in patients with idiopathic preterm labor. *Am J Obstet Gynecol.* 1992;167:683.

273. Evans MI, Hajj SN, Devoe LD, et al. C-reactive protein with premature rupture of membranes and preterm labor. *Obstet Gynecol.* 1983;62:49.

274. Farb HF, Arnesen M, Geistler P, et al. C-reactive protein with premature rupture of membranes and preterm labor. *Obstet Gynecol.* 1983;62:49.

275. Gawrylyshyn P, Bernstein P, Milligan JE, et al. Premature rupture of membranes. The role of C-reactive protein in the

prediction of chorioamnionitis. *Am J Obstet Gynecol.* 1983; 147:240.

276. Romem Y, Artal R. C-reactive protein as a predictor for chorioamnionitis in cases of premature rupture of the membranes. *Am J Obstet Gynecol.* 1984;150:546.

277. Hadwerker SM, Tejani NA, Verma UL, et al. Correlation of maternal serum C-reactive protein with outcome of tocolysis. *Obstet Gynecol.* 1984;63:220.

278. Potkul RK, Moawad AH, Ponto KL. The association of subclinical infection with preterm labor: The role of C-reactive protein. *Am J Obstet Gynecol.* 1985;153:642.

279. Mitchell MD, Dudley DJ, Edwin SS, et al. Interleukin-6 stimulates prostaglandin production by human amnion and decidual cells. *Eur J Pharmacol.* 1991;192:189.

280. Romero R, Munoz H, Gomez R, et al. Two thirds of spontaneous abortion/fetal deaths after genetic midtrimester amniocentesis are the result of a pre-existing subclinical inflammatory process of the amniotic cavity (abstract). *Am J Obstet Gynecol.* 1995;172:257.

281. Wenstrom KD, Andrews WW, Bowles NE, et al. Intrauterine viral infection at the time of second trimester genetic amniocentesis. *Obstet Gynecol.* 1998;92:420.

282. Griffiths PD, Campbell-Benzie A, Heath RB. A prospective study of primary cytomegalovirus infection in pregnant women. *Br J Obstet Gynaecol.* 1980;87:308.

283. Stagno S, Whitley RJ. Herpesvirus infections of pregnancy. Part I: Cytomegalovirus and Epstein-Barr virus infections. *N Engl J Med.* 1985;313:1270.

284. Demmler GJ. Infectious Diseases Society of America and Centers for Disease Control. Summary of a workshop on surveillance for congenital cytomegalovirus disease. *Rev Infect Dis.* 1991;13:315.

285. Griffiths PD, Baboonian C. A prospective study of primary cytomegalovirus infection during pregnancy: Final report. *Br J Obstet Gynaecol.* 1984;91:307.

286. Rudd P, Peckham C. Infection of the fetus and the newborn: Prevention, treatment and related handicap. *Bailliere Clin Obstet Gynaecol.* 1988;2:55.

287. Fowler KB, Stagno S, Pass RF, et al. The outcome of congenital cytomegalovirus infection in relation to maternal antibody status. *N Eng J Med.* 1992;326:663.

288. Brown HL, Abernathy MP. Cytomegalovirus infection. *Semin Perinatol.* 1998;22:260.

289. Stagno S, Pass RF, Sworsky ME, et al. Maternal cytomegalovirus infection and perinatal transmission. *Clin Obstet Gynecol.* 1982;25:563.

290. Lipitz S, Yagel S, Shalev E, Achiron R, Mashiach S, Schiff E. Prenatal diagnosis of fetal primary cytomegalovirus infection. *Obstet Gynecol.* 1997;89(5, Pt 1):763.

291. Labouret N, Cecille A, Wendling MJ, et al. Prenatal diagnosis of viral infections. A two year study in Strasbourg. *Pathol Biol (Paris).* 1999;47:526.

292. Revello MG, Sarasini A, Zavattoni M, et al. Improved prenatal diagnosis of congenital human cytomegalovirus infection by a modified nested polymerase chain reaction. *J Med Virol.* 1998;56:99.

293. Van den Veyver IB, Ni J, Bowles N, et al. Detection of intrauterine viral infection using the polymerase chain reaction. *Mol Genet Metab.* 1998;63:85.

294. Lazzarotto T, Guerra B, Spezzacatena P, et al. Prenatal diagno-sis of congenital cytomegalovirus infection. *J Clin Microbiol.* 1998;36:3540.

295. Donner C, Liesnard C, Content J, et al. Prenatal diagnosis of 52 pregnancies at risk for congenital cytomegalovirus infection. *Obstet Gynecol.* 1993;82(4, Pt 1):481.

296. Donner C, Liesnard C, Brancart F, Rodesch F. Accuracy of amniotic fluid testing before 21 weeks' gestation in prenatal diagnosis of congenital cytomegalovirus infection. *Prenat Diagn.* 1994;14:1055.

297. Revello MG, Baldanti F, Furione M, et al. Polymerase chain reaction for prenatal diagnosis of congenital human cytomegalovirus infection. *J Med Virol.* 1995;47:462.

298. Ruellan-Eugene G, Barjot P, Campet M, et al. Evaluation of virological procedures to detect fetal human cytomegalovirus infection: Avidity of IgG antibodies, virus detection in amniotic fluid and maternal serum. *J Med Virol.* 1996;50: 9–15.

299. Apperley JF, Goldman JM. Cytomegalovirus: Biology, clinical features and methods for diagnosis. *Bone Marrow Transplant.* 1988;3:253–264.

300. Dummer JS. Cytomegalovirus infection after liver transplantation: Clinical manifestations and strategies for prevention. *Rev Infect Dis.* 1990;12(suppl 7):S767–S775.

301. Boyer KM. Diagnosis and treatment of congenital toxoplasmosis. *Adv Pediatr Infect Dis.* 1996;11:449–467.

302. Desmonts G, Couvreur J, Thulliez P. Toxoplasmose congenitale: Cinq cas de transmission a l'enfant d'une infection maternelle anterieure a la grossesse. *Presse Med.* 1990;19:1445.

303. Remington JS, Desmonts G. Toxoplasmosis. In: Remington JS, Klein JO, eds. *Infectious Diseases of the Fetus and Newborn Infant.* Philadelphia: Saunders; 1976:171.

304. Ades AE. Evaluating the sensitivity and predictive value of tests of recent infection: Toxoplasmosis in pregnancy. *Epidemiol Infect.* 1991;107:527–535.

305. Beazley DM, Egerman RS. Toxoplasmosis. *Semin Perinatol.* 1998;22:332–338.

306. Sever JL, Larsen JW, Grossman III JH. *Handbook of Perinatal Infections.* Boston: Little Brown; 1979.

307. Daffos F, Forester F, Capella-Pavlovsky M, et al. Prenatal management of 746 pregnancies at risk for congenital toxoplasmosis. *N Engl J Med.* 1988;318:271–275.

308. Virkola K, Lappalainen M, Valanne L, Koskiniemi M. Radiological signs in newborns exposed to primary *Toxoplasma* infection in utero. *Pediatr Radiol.* 1997;27:133–138.

309. Jenum PA, Holberg-Peterson M, Melby KK, Stray-Pederson B. Diagnosis of congenital *Toxoplasma gondii* infection by polymerase chain reaction (PCR) on amniotic fluid samples. The Norwegian experience. *APMIS.* 1998;106:680–686.

310. Hohlfeld P, Daffos F, Costa JM, et al. Prenatal diagnosis of congenital toxoplasmosis with a polymerase-chain-reaction test on amniotic fluid. *N Engl J Med.* 1994;331:695–699.

311. Johnson JD, Butcher PD, Sarra D, Holliman RE. Application of the polymerase chain reaction to the diagnosis of human toxoplasmosis. *J Infect.* 1993;26:147–158.

312. Dupouy-Camet J, Bougnoux ME, Lavareda de Sooza S, et al. Comparative value of polymerase chain reaction and conventional biological tests for the prenatal diagnosis of congenital toxoplasmosis. *Ann Biol Clin (Paris).* 1992;50:315.

313. Chapman SJ. Varicella in pregnancy. *Semin Perinatol.* 1998; 22:339.

314. Centers for Disease Control and Prevention. Recommend-dations of the Immunization Practices Advisory Committee: Varicella-zoster immune globulin for the prevention of chickenpox. *MMWR.* 1984;33:84.

315. Balducci J, Rodis JF, Rosengren S, et al. Pregnancy outcome following first-trimester varicella infection. *Obstet Gynecol.* 1992;79:5.

316. Paryani SG, Arvin AM. Intrauterine infection with varicella-zoster virus after maternal varicella. *N Engl J Med.* 1986;314: 1542.

317. Liesnard C, Donner C, Brancart F, Rodesch F. Varicella in pregnancy. *Lancet.* 1994;344(8927):950.

318. Higa K, Dan K, Manabe H. Varicella-zoster virus infections during pregnancy: Hypothesis concerning the mechanisms of congenital malformations. *Obstet Gynecol.* 1987;69:214.

319. Cuthbertson G, Weiner CP, Giller RH, et al. Prenatal diagnosis of second-trimester congenital varicella syndrome by virus-specific immunoglobulin M. *J Pediatr.* 1987;111:592–595.

320. Harding B, Baumer JA. Congenital varicella-zoster. A sero-logically proven case with necrotizing encephalitis and mal-formation. *Acta Neuropathol (Berl).* 1988;76:311–315.

321. Scharf A, Scherr O, Enders G, et al. Virus detection in the fetal tissue of a premature delivery with a congenital varicella syndrome. A case report. *J Perinat Med.* 1990;18:317–322.

322. Pretorius DH, Hayward I, Jones KL, Stamm E. Sonographic evaluation of pregnancies with maternal varicella infection. *J Ultrasound Med.* 1992;11:459–463.

323. Salzman MB, Sharrar RG, Steinbera S, et al. Transmission of varicella-vaccine virus from a healthy 12-month-old child to his pregnant mother. *J Pediatr.* 1997;131:151–154.

324. Salzman MB, Sood SK. Congenital anomalies resulting from maternal varicella at $25^1/2$ weeks of gestation. *Pediatr Infect Dis J.* 1992;11:504–505.

325. Magliocco AM, Demetrick DJ, Sarnat HB, et al. Varicella em-bryopathy. *Arch Pathol Lab Med.* 1992;116:181–186.

326. Hartung J, Enders G, Chaoui R, et al. Prenatal diagnosis of con-genital varicella syndrome and detection of varicella-zoster virus in the fetus: A case report. *Prenat Diagn.* 1999;19: 163–166.

327. Enders G, Miller E, Cradock-Watson J, et al. Consequences of varicella and herpes zoster in pregnancy: Prospective study of 1739 cases. *Lancet.* 1994;343:1548–1551.

328. Isada NB, Paar DP, Johnson MP, et al. In utero diagnosis of congenital varicella zoster virus infection by chorionic villus sampling and polymerase chain reaction. *Am J Obstet Gynecol.* 1991;165:1727–1730.

329. Miller E, Cradock-Watson JE, Pollock TM. Consequences of confirmed maternal rubella at successive stages of pregnancy. *Lancet.* 1982;2:781–784.

330. Freij BJ, South MA, Sever JL. Maternal rubella and the con-genital rubella syndrome. *Clin Perinatol.* 1988;15:247–257.

331. Enders G, Nickerel-Pacher U, Miller E, et al. Outcome of confirmed periconceptional maternal rubella. *Lancet.* 1988;1:1445–1447.

332. Grillner L, Forsgren M, Barr B, Bottiger M, et al. Outcome of rubella during pregnancy with special reference to the 17th–24th weeks of gestation. *Scand J Infect Dis.* 1983;15: 321–325.

333. Munro ND, Sheppard S, Smithells RW, et al. Temporal rela-tions between maternal rubella and congenital defects. *Lancet.* 1987;2:201–204.

334. Ghidini A, Lynch L. Prenatal diagnosis and significance of fetal infections. *West J Med.* 1993;159:366–373.

335. Tanemura M, Suzumori K, Yagani U, et al. Diagnosis of fetal rubella infection with reverse transcription and nested poly-merase chain reaction: A study of 34 cases diagnosed in fe-tuses. *Am J Obstet Gynecol.* 1996;174:578–582.

336. Segondy M, Boulot P. RT-PCR in the prenatal diagnosis of rubella. Report of 2 cases. *J Gynecol Obstet Biol Reprod (Paris).* 1998;27:708–713.

Fetal Blood Sampling

Fabio Ghezzi • Roberto Romero • Eli Maymon • Mark Redman •
Sean Blackwell • Stanley M. Berry

Fetal blood sampling was performed for the first time almost 30 years ago under fetoscopic visualization.[1–3] In the early 1980s, advances in ultrasound technology allowed the introduction of the technique of cordocentesis under ultrasound guidance.[4] This new method opened a new era in fetal assessment and therapy.[5] During the following years, several studies were conducted to investigate the fetal chromosomal, immunologic, hematologic, and metabolic status.[4–9] Between 1987 and 1991, Ludomirsky et al.[10,11] established a multicentric registry of cordocentesis performed in 11 centers in the United States and Canada to document the indications for cordocentesis. At the conclusion of this registry, the most frequent indication for cordocentesis was the need of rapid karyotyping (40%), followed by fetal red cell isoimmunization (8%) and nonimmune hydrops fetalis (7%). In the past few years, the advent of new and widely available methods for molecular biology and genetic analysis have changed the role of fetal blood testing in clinical practice. Polymerase chain reaction (PCR) allows DNA analysis for the diagnosis of most hereditary genetic disorders on chorionic villous or amniotic fluid samples; the Rh status of the fetus can be easily established by PCR analysis of amniotic fluid or chorionic villi; rapid evaluation of the fetal chromosomal status for the most common aneuploidies can be achieved within a few hours with fluorescence *in situ* hybridization.[12–17]

Today, new and more challenging conditions may require direct access to the fetal circulation. With the increasing knowledge of fetal pathophysiology, the evaluation of the fetal metabolism plays a crucial role in the diagnosis and management of intrauterine infection and endocrinological diseases. Moreover, the intravenous administration of therapeutic agents to the fetus has been used recently.

The purpose of this chapter is to briefly review the techniques and indications of cordocentesis and to discuss the actual role of this procedure in clinical practice.

TECHNIQUES OF FETAL BLOOD SAMPLING

Cordocentesis

Before fetal viability, percutaneous umbilical blood sampling (PUBS) can be performed in an outpatient facility. After viability, the procedure should be performed in proximity to an operating room because cesarean section may be required if fetal distress develops during or after the procedure.[18]

An ultrasound examination is performed before the procedure to determine fetal viability, position, biometry, location of the placenta, and the presence of associated anomalies. Clear identification of the insertion site of the umbilical cord in the placenta or a fixed segment of cord is a critical step, because this will be the target of the procedure; at times, a loop of cord adjacent to the placental mass can be confused with the actual insertion site. Color Doppler can be helpful in difficult cases by showing the branching of the cord vessels within the placenta. Cordocentesis is easiest when the placenta is anterior because access to the target portion of the cord with a posterior placenta may be hampered by the fetus. Under these circumstances, access to the sampling site can be achieved by external manipulation on the maternal abdomen to move the fetus. If indicated, a path is chosen for the needle that allows amniocentesis and cordocentesis to be accomplished with one insertion.

The abdomen is cleaned with an antiseptic solution and draped. The use of local anesthesia for diagnostic procedures is a matter of choice, and it can ease the patient's discomfort in cases of prolonged procedures. Maternal sedation (diazepam) can be used for prolonged therapeutic procedures. Diazepam is preferred to meperidine because the latter can induce nausea and vomiting. Prophylactic administration of antibiotics is routinely given in many centers because the risk of chorioamnionitis far outweighs the risks of adverse reactions to the antibiotics; in some reports chorioamnionitis was responsible for up to 40% of the fetal losses.[19] A sample of maternal blood should be drawn before the procedure for the cell size analyzer so that quality control of the fetal samples can be performed later.

Several different approaches can be used for cordocentesis. All require that the needle be inserted under sonographic monitoring and the tip of the needle be maintained under visualization. Three major considerations are the type of transducer, whether the operator employs a needle guiding device or a "free-hand technique," and whether the ultrasound guidance is performed by the operator or an assistant. The type of ultrasound transducer used is a matter of personal preference. Most of the experienced operators use a free-hand technique because of its flexibility in the adjustment of the needle path. An alternative approach is to employ a needle guiding device attached to the transducer.[20] Modern real-time machines are equipped with an on-screen template of the needle tract that is used to target the sampling site. It has been suggested that needle guidance may decrease the risk of cord laceration or needle displacement when the tip is properly placed.[21] The needle guiding device restricts the lateral motion of the needle, however, which may hamper the procedure if the needle needs repositioning. This problem can be solved by removing the guiding device during the procedure, if it becomes necessary.

A new computerized system (UltraGuide 1000) that enhances the image of the needle and provides guidance information has recently been introduced in clinical practice (Fig. 29–1A and B). The system provides continuous graphic display of the needle trajectory on the ultrasound image, regardless of whether or not the needle is in the image plane or is actually visible in the ultrasound image. These images are shown before the actual insertion and throughout the entire procedure. Thus, the system enables physicians using it to independently position both the needle and the transducer for the safest target access and best imaging before the insertion. Then the operator can monitor the needle's progress, thereby avoiding accidental contact with the fetus. The needle spatial

position, orientation, and its predicted future path are transformed into two-dimensional display and are overlaid over the ultrasound B-scan. The display is color coded, facilitating differentiation between the actual and future needle path (Fig. 29–2).

A regular 20- to 25-gauge spinal needle is used for cordocentesis. Most centers use a 20- to 22-gauge needle. Larger bore needles are not necessary for either diagnostic or therapeutic procedures. Smaller bore needles prolong the period of time required to obtain fetal blood and are more difficult to guide if intraoperative manipulations are required. An alternative technique first uses a biopsy guide 20-gauge needle to reach the amniotic cavity close to the umbilical cord and then a 25-gauge needle, which is threaded into the 20-gauge needle and advanced into the umbilical vein.[22] The incidence of procedure-related complications using this needle-within-needle technique is claimed to be lower than that reported using a single needle technique (bleeding from puncture site, 23.1%; fetal bradycardia, 0%; and pregnancy loss rate, 0.9%).

The standard length of the spinal needle is 8.89 cm, excluding the hub. The length of the needle should take into account the thickness of maternal panniculus and the location of the target segment of cord within the uterus. A few additional centimeters should be considered to avoid underestimation due to intervening events, such as uterine contractions. Priming of the needle with sodium citrate solution immediately before the procedure has been proposed to prevent clot formation.[6] Needles designed to optimize sonographic visualization (Cooke Catheter, Bloomington, IN, USA) are also available, but a clear benefit of these new designs has not been adequately documented.

If amniocentesis is to be performed, it should be done before cordocentesis to avoid contamination of the specimen. The needle is inserted into the amniotic cavity, and amniotic fluid is aspirated. It is then either advanced into the cord or, in cases of anterior placenta, it can be withdrawn within the placental mass, reoriented, and advanced into the cord. Within the umbilical cord, it is easier and safer to sample the vein rather than an artery. Puncture of the artery has been associated with a greater incidence of bradycardia and longer postprocedural bleeding.[21] The vessels can be distinguished by their relative size and by determination of the flow waveform using Doppler ultrasound. Distinction of the origin of the sample (arterial vs. venous) is crucial for interpretation of the acid–base and oxygentation status of the fetus.

Upon entering the umbilical cord, the stylet is removed, and fetal blood is withdrawn into a syringe attached to the hub of the needle. The syringe may be primed with a small amount of anticoagulant, such as heparin or citrate. After flow is documented, an initial sample should be submitted for blood cell size determination with an electronic cell analyzer (Coulter Electronics, Hialeah, FL, USA) to distinguish fetal from maternal cells (Fig. 29–3).[23,24] The proper positioning of the needle can be confirmed by injection of saline solution into the cord and observation of turbulence along the vessel.

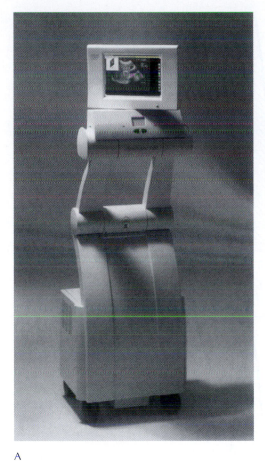

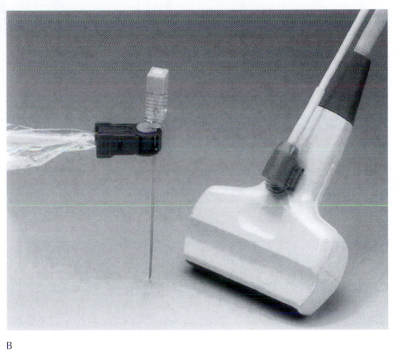

A   B

Figure 29–1. (A) The UltraGuide 1000 System is connected to the ultrasound system. The monitor of the UltraGuide System is used to view the performance of the procedure as it displays the ultrasound image and information about the needle pathway. **(B)** Two sensors are used by the system: A needle sensor *(left)* and a transducer sensor *(right)* is placed on the side of the device.

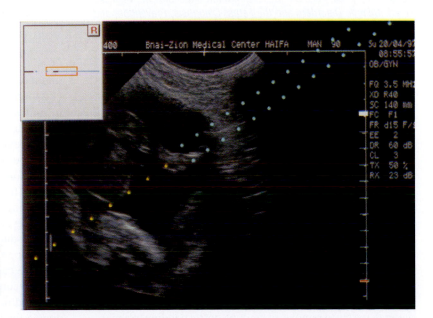

Figure 29–2. The UltraGuide 1000 System calculates the needle projection on the ultrasound screen and computes its predicted future path. The system determines the future trajectory of the needle even before its insertion into the abdominal wall.

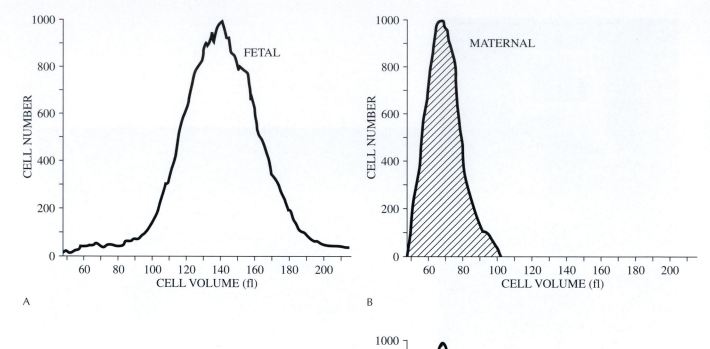

Figure 29–3. Cell-size distribution of maternal and fetal blood. **(A)** One hundred percent fetal blood. **(B)** One hundred percent maternal blood. **(C)** Mixture of maternal and fetal blood (30%). (*A and C reprinted with permission from Devore GR, Venus I, Hobbins JC, et al. Fetoscopy: General clinical approach. In: Rocker I, Laurence KM, eds. Fetoscopy. Amsterdam: Elsevier/North Holland Biomedical Press; 1981;60. B reprinted with permission from Romero R, Hobbins JC, Mahoney MJ. Fetal blood sampling and fetoscopy. In: Milunsky A, ed. Genetic Disorders and the Fetus: Diagnosis, Prevention, and Treatment. New York: Plenum; 1986;579.*)

The use of paralytic agents to decrease fetal movement is left to the discretion of the operator. When indicated, atracuronium (0.4 mg/kg fetal weight intravenously) or pancuronium (0.1 mg/kg fetal weight) can be used. Once the needle is in place, the sample(s) required for diagnostic purposes is (are) taken using different syringes. Transfer to the appropriate tubes should occur immediately after collection. Tubes containing citrate are for coagulation studies; tubes with ethylene-diaminetetraacetic acid are for complete blood cell count and platelets; blood group typing requires serum; karyotype and molecular biologic analysis require anticoagulation with sodium heparin.[25] Blood gas analysis can be performed directly on a sample in a heparin-primed syringe. The volume of blood removed differs with the number of tests required and should take into account the gestational age. In general, we try to remove an amount corresponding to a maximum of 6 to 7% of the fetoplacental blood volume for that gestational age. The fetoplacental blood volume, as expressed in milliliters per kilogram of fetal weight, decreases with advancing gestational age.[26] Several studies have evaluated fetoplacental blood volume using different techniques. The average estimate of fetoplacental blood volume is 125 mL/kg of ultrasonographically estimated fetal weight. Monitoring of the fetal heart rate during fetal transfusions can be performed by placing a Doppler gate on an umbilical artery near the sampling area. This approach makes it unnecessary to move the transducer from the sampling site to the fetal chest. After an appropriate volume of blood is removed, 2 to 3 mL of saline can be injected as volume replacement and to confirm the correct position of the needle tip. If turbulence is not observed in the umbilical cord vessel, it may be prudent to draw a final sample to confirm the fetal origin of the blood.

The needle is withdrawn, and the puncture site is monitored for bleeding. If the patient has a viable fetus, the fetal heart rate is monitored for 1 to 2 h after the procedure.

Intrahepatic Fetal Blood Sampling

This technique consists of the introduction of a 20-gauge needle into the fetal abdomen aiming for the intrahepatic portion of the umbilical vein or the left portal vein. Although this technique has some advantages over sampling of the umbilical cord (such as avoidance of the umbilical arteries, certainty of the venous origin of the sample, and lack of need for immediate laboratory support to confirm the fetal origin of the sample), it is considered to be the second choice after cordocentesis because it has a higher rate of fetal losses (6.2% in low-risk patients).[27,28] Fetal liver necrosis after blood sampling from the intrahepatic vein has also been reported.[29] This technique is, therefore, reserved for cases in which cordocentesis fails or cannot be performed due to fetal position and lack of change. No significant changes in the concentrations of liver enzymes have been noted after the procedure in fetuses undergoing sampling at the intrahepatic vein as opposed to the umbilical cord, suggesting absent or minimal fetal liver injury.[28] Similarly, acid–base and blood gas status in appropriate-for-gestational-age (AGA) fetuses is not affected by the site of sampling; therefore, values obtained at the intrahepatic vein may be interpreted by using reference ranges derived from sampling at the placental cord insertion.[30]

Cardiocentesis

This method for fetal blood sampling has limited indications because of the high rate of fetal loss. In a large series of 158 cardiocenteses during the second trimester for the prenatal diagnosis of hemoglobinopathies, the procedure-related fetal loss rate was 5.6%.[31] No cases of fetal cardiac trauma or hemopericardium were encountered among living infants. Cardiocentesis should be reserved for cases in which PUBS is technically impossible; for example, after repeated failed attempts, and when there is a substantial risk that the fetus is affected with a serious disorder. Ideally, the needle should enter the fetal heart, preferably the right ventricle, through the anterior thoracic wall.[32] To prevent fetal movements from interfering with the procedure, the needle should be introduced swiftly into the fetal thorax.

Quality Control of the Specimen

A crucial step is the assessment of the quality of the blood sample. Contamination with maternal blood and amniotic fluid can alter the diagnostic value of the specimen. For example, contamination with amniotic fluid of as little as 1% leads to a significant increase in factor V and VIII activity; therefore, it interferes with the diagnostic accuracy of some congenital hemostatic disorders.[25] To assess the purity of the fetal blood sample, the profile of the mean corpuscular volume of red blood cells (RBCs) has been the method commonly used, because fetal RBCs are larger than maternal RBCs. This difference decreases, however, with advancing gestational age. Furthermore, the profile can be misinterpreted in the presence of some maternal hematologic disorders, such as macrocytic anemia. Other hematologic indices can be used to differentiate maternal from fetal blood. For instance, lymphocytes are the predominant white blood cells (WBC) in the fetus, whereas neutrophils are in the mother. Tables 29–1 and 29–2 present normal hematologic and biochemical values in fetal blood. The Kleihauer–Betke test may be used

TABLE 29–1. HEMATOLOGIC VALUES IN FETAL, NEONATAL, AND ADULT BLOOD

Component	Adult	Fetus Weeks 16–19	Fetus Weeks 20–27	Neonate
Platelet count ($\times 10^9$/L)	268 ± 54	185 ± 31[a]	218 ± 21	306 ± 46
Erythrocyte count ($\times 10^{12}$/L)	4.7 ± 0.5	2.5 ± 0.1[a]	2.9 ± 0.2[a]	4.6 ± 0.4
Hemoglobin (g/L)	147 ± 18	110 ± 7[a]	121 ± 8[a]	163 ± 17[a]
Hematocrit (L)	0.43 ± 0.05	0.33 ± 0.02[a]	0.36 ± 0.02[a]	0.49 ± 0.05
MCV (fL)	92 ± 2	134 ± 11[a]	121 ± 8[a]	105 ± 3[a]
Mean corpuscular hemoglobin (pg)	31 ± 1	45 ± 3[a]	39 ± 5[a]	35 ± 2[a]
MCHC (g/L)	330 ± 10	330 ± 50	330 ± 10	330 ± 10
Nucleated cells ($\times 10^9$/L)	6.0 ± 1.4	4.7 ± 0.8[a]	4.3 ± 0.9[a]	14.1 ± 3.0[a]
Differential count ($\times 10^9$/L)				
Neutrophils	3.2 ± 0.8	0.2 ± 0.1[a]	0.2 ± 0.1[a]	6.5 ± 1.7[a]
Basophils	0.03 ± 0.03	0.01 ± 0.02	0.02 ± 0.02	0.1 ± 0.1
Eosinophils	0.09 ± 0.06	0.02 ± 0.02[a]	0.08 ± 0.1	0.4 ± 0.3[a]
Lymphocytes	2.1 ± 0.7	1.9 ± 0.7	2.6 ± 0.7	5.6 ± 1.0[a]
Monocytes	0.5 ± 0.2	0.1 ± 0.1[a]	0.2 ± 0.1[a]	0.9 ± 0.4[a]
Erythroblasts	<0.01	2.5 ± 1.3[a]	0.9 ± 0.4[a]	0.5 ± 0.5[a]

Note: The results are expressed as mean value ± one standard deviation. MCV, Mean corpuscular volume; MCHC, mean corpuscular hemoglobin concentration.
[a]Statistically different ($p < 0.05$) from adult values (Student's t-test).
Reproduced with permission from De Waele, Foulon W, Renmans W, et al. Am J Clin Pathol. 1988;89:742.

TABLE 29–2. COMPARATIVE FETAL (WEEKS 20–26) AND MATERNAL BIOCHEMISTRY (MEAN AND SD)

	Fetuses (n = 63)	Mothers (n = 63)
Glucose	2.8 ± 0.2 mmol/L (51 ± 3.8 mg/dL)	4.4 ± 0.1 mmol/L (79 ± 1.8 mg/dL)
Triglycerides	0.89 ± 0.03 mmol/L (78 ± 2 mg/dL)	1.4 ± 0.07 mmol/L (122 ± 6 mg/dL)
Cholesterol	1.5 ± 0.05 mmol/L (58 ± 2 mg/dL)	6.6 ± 0.2 mmol/L (255 ± 7 mg/dL)
Total protein	30.4 ± 0.6 g/L (3.04 ± 0.06 g/dL)	69.6 ± 0.9 g/L (6.96 ± 0.09 g/dL)
Albumin	21.4 ± 0.4 g/L (2.14 ± 0.04 g/dL)	34.9 ± 0.5 g/L (3.49 ± 0.05 g/dL)
Calcium	2.25 ± 0.2 mmol/L (9.02 ± 0.8 mg/dL)	2.27 ± 0.1 mmol/L (9.1 ± 0.4 mg/dL)
Phosphorus	2.65 ± 0.1 mmol/L (8.31 ± 0.29 mg/dL)	1.45 ± 0.1 mmol/L (4.55 ± 0.18 mg/dL)
Urea	2.6 ± 0.16 mmol/L (16 ± 0.1 mg/dL)	4.3 ± 0.2 mmol/L (26 ± 0.1 mg/dL)
Creatinine	64 ± 2 mol/L (0.726 ± 0.021 mg/dL)	67 ± 1.5 mol/L (0.765 ± 0.016 mg/dL)
Uric acid	167 ± 10 mol/L (2.80 ± 0.17 mg/dL)	215 ± 9.5 mol/L (3.62 ± 0.16 mg/dL)
Total bilirubin	26.8 ± 1 mol/L (1.57 ± 0.06 mg/dL)	8.6 ± 0.4 mol/L (0.504 ± 0.025 mg/dL)
Direct bilirubin	16.1 ± 0.6 mol/L (0.943 ± 0.035 mg/dL)	0.9 ± 0.4 mol/L (0.05 ± 0.021 mg/dL)

Reproduced with permission from Forestier F, Daffos F, Rainaut M, et al. Pediatr Res. 1987;21:579.

for second-trimester samples, at which time it can accurately detect a maternal contamination.[26] The utility of the test is limited during the late third trimester of pregnancy because fetal erythrocytes contain increasing amounts of hemoglobin A. Blood typing can confirm the fetal origin of a sample because antigen I is present only in adult RBCs. Monoclonal antibodies for antigen I can detect as little as a 5% maternal blood contamination.[26] Human chorionic gonadotropin (hCG) determination is the best marker for detection of maternal blood contamination in the specimen.[26] Maternal blood contains high concentrations of this hormone, whereas fetal blood is practically devoid of it. The ratio of fetal to amniotic fluid to maternal blood of hCG is 1:100:400. Determination of this hormone by an enzyme-linked assay using monoclonal antibodies against the beta-subunit of hCG can detect as little as 0.2% contamination with maternal blood.[26]

The hCG concentration can also be used to rule out contamination of the blood sample with as little as 1% of amniotic fluid.[26] Alternatively, dilution with amniotic fluid can be inferred by a proportional decrease in the number of RBCs, WBCs, and platelets in the specimen or by the presence of ferning or multiple desquamated epithelial cells on a smear.[33,34] The most accurate test for amniotic fluid contamination is the increased activity of factors V and VIII. Factors II and IX are not activated by amniotic fluid and can be used as internal controls.[26]

Duration of the Procedure

The duration of the procedure is related to placental location, fetal interference, quality of ultrasound image, and operator expertise. In a series of 606 cordocenteses, 70% of the first 100 procedures were performed in less than 10 mins, whereas the percentage rose to 90% in the last 100 cases.[6] A second needle insertion was required in 2.9% of the cases. Oligohydramnios can interfere with visualization of the insertion site of the cord. In these cases, amnioinfusion or needling of a fixed loop of cord may overcome the difficulty. In cases of polyhydramnios with posterior placenta, it may be necessary to perform therapeutic amniocentesis to gain access to the cord insertion.

Training

Fetal blood sampling is a surgical procedure. In the United States, it is performed by specialists in maternal–fetal medicine. Training is difficult to obtain because of the limited number of cases available at any given institution, and because of the risks associated with the procedure. Ideally, the operator should have a strong background in obstetric ultrasonography and experience with other invasive procedures of prenatal diagnosis. Training can be first provided with *in vitro* models.[35] Once proficiency is acquired with *in vitro* models, the procedure can be performed in patients having elective midtrimester termination of pregnancy.[36]

Normal Values for Fetal Blood

Tables 29–3 and 29–4 display the distribution of the most common hematologic and acid–base parameters in fetal blood in relation to the gestational age.[37] Drug levels in the fetal blood have also been determined, including those of spyramicin, folic acid, fluorides, and vitamin K.[38–40]

COMPLICATIONS

The maternal risks of PUBS are minimal but should not be minimized. Chorioamnionitis is a rare (1%) complication, but it is responsible for up to 40% of pregnancy losses after PUBS.[19,41,42] An isolated case of maternal respiratory distress syndrome in association with *Corynebacterium amnionitis* after cordocentesis has also been reported.[43] For these reasons, a policy of antibiotic prophylaxis has been advocated and implemented in many centers, despite the absence of any trials documenting its benefit.

Fetal Losses

The risk of procedure-related pregnancy loss is difficult to assess because many centers do not have long-term follow-up on all cases. Losses are usually considered to be procedure related if they occur within a short time interval from the cordocentesis. A review of the published series of low-risk cases reported an overall risk of fetal loss before 28 weeks of 1.4% and an additional 1.4% risk of perinatal death after 28 weeks.[44] This loss rate is greater than that related to amniocentesis and about six times greater than that of a general population obtaining prenatal care. The most important risk factors implicated in the occurrence of complications are:

1. Indication for the procedure. In the presence of fetal pathology, the risks are substantially higher. A review of the risks of PUBS in relation to the indication showed that the total loss rate of desired ongoing pregnancies within 2 weeks of the procedure was 1.3% when the indication was prenatal diagnosis of genetic disorders of karyotyping, 6.6% in the presence of structural fetal anomalies, 13.8% among small-for-gestational-age (SGA) fetuses, and 25% in fetuses with nonimmune hydrops.[41]

2. Operator experience. The published reports show that the smaller the series size, the higher the incidence of fetal losses.[19] This is relevant because more centers now offer and perform PUBS, leading to a dispersion of the case load.

3. Technique. Both puncture of the intrahepatic portion of the umbilical vein and cardiocentesis carry an increased risk of fetal death (6.2% and 5.4%, respectively, among low-risk cases).[28,31]

4. Gestational age at procedure. Even though PUBS before 20 weeks is a more challenging procedure, it does not seem to have a significantly higher risk of fetal loss.[45] Smaller bore needles (25 gauge), however, ought to be used at 12 to 15 weeks than at later gestational ages (20 to 22 gauge after 16 weeks).

Hemorrhage

Bleeding from the puncture site is the most common, although usually benign, complication of cordocentesis. It occurs in 41 to 53% of cases, with a mean duration of 35 s.[6,19,46] At gestational age of less than 21 weeks, postprocedural bleeding has been associated with nearly a threefold increase in the fetal loss rate.[45] Bleeding seems to be dependent on the technique used. Use of a 25-gauge rather than a 21-gauge needle is associated with a lower bleeding rate (23%).[22] Similarly, the use of a fixed needle guide has a lower bleeding rate from the puncture site (29%).[47] This has been attributed to decreased lateral motion of the needle in comparison to a free-hand technique, thus, decreasing the risk of laceration of the cord. Puncture of the umbilical artery is associated with a

GA	5th	Mean	95th
TABLE 29–3. FETAL HEMATOLOGIC INDICES DURING GESTATION			
	Erythroblast Count (10⁹/L)		
20	0.34	1.19	4.15
22	0.23	0.79	2.77
24	0.16	0.55	1.92
26	0.11	0.40	1.38
28	0.08	0.29	1.03
30	0.06	0.23	0.79
32	0.05	0.18	0.63
34	0.04	0.15	0.53
36	0.04	0.13	0.45
38	0.03	0.11	0.41
40	0.03	0.10	0.38

TABLE 29–3. FETAL HEMATOLOGIC INDICES DURING GESTATION — Erythroblast Count (10^9/L)

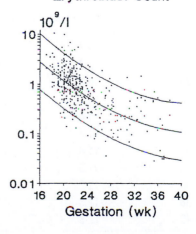

Erythroblast Count

TABLE 29–3. *(Continued)*

Mean Corpuscular Volume (fL)			
20	119	129	140
22	114	124	134
24	110	119	130
26	107	116	126
28	104	113	123
30	103	112	122
32	102	111	121
34	102	110	120
36	102	110	120
38	102	110	120
40	102	110	120

Mean Corpuscular Volume

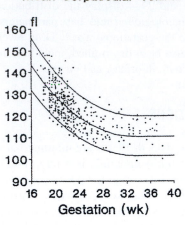

Platelet Count (10⁹/L)			
20	145	219	293
22	148	222	297
24	151	225	300
26	154	229	303
28	157	232	306
30	160	235	310
32	163	238	313
34	166	241	316
36	169	244	319
38	172	247	323
40	175	250	326

Platelet count

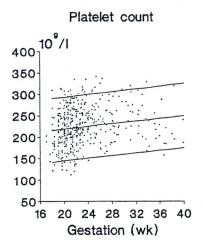

Hemoglobin (g/dL)			
20	9.7	11.3	12.8
22	10.0	11.6	13.1
24	10.3	11.9	13.4
26	10.7	12.2	13.8
28	11.0	12.5	14.1
30	11.3	12.8	14.4
32	11.6	13.1	14.7
34	11.9	13.5	15.0
36	12.2	13.8	15.3
38	12.5	14.1	15.6
40	12.8	14.4	16.0

Hemoglobin

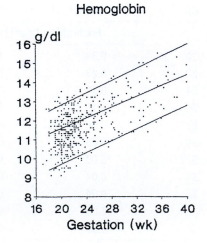

TABLE 29–3. *(Continued)*

Total Leucocyte Count

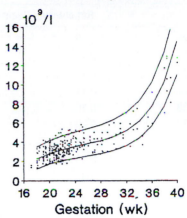

	Total Leukocyte Count (10⁹/L)		
20	1.73	2.82	4.16
22	2.07	3.23	4.67
24	2.33	3.56	5.07
26	2.56	3.84	5.42
28	2.81	4.16	5.81
30	3.15	4.58	6.34
32	3.65	5.21	7.12
34	4.45	6.19	8.34
36	5.71	7.75	10.26
38	7.73	10.26	13.39
40	10.98	14.45	18.77

Neutrophil Count

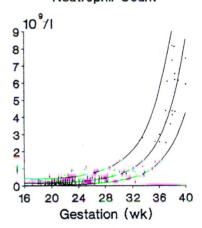

	Neutrophil Count (10⁹/L)		
20	0.03	0.16	0.42
22	0.04	0.19	0.47
24	0.07	0.23	0.55
26	0.10	0.31	0.70
28	0.17	0.43	0.94
30	0.27	0.63	1.33
32	0.44	0.96	1.98
34	0.74	1.55	3.12
36	1.28	2.60	5.19
38	2.28	4.59	9.14
40	4.23	8.53	17.09

Lymphocyte Count

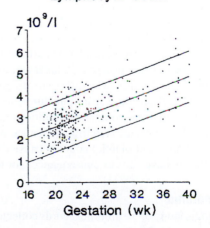

	Lymphocyte Count (10⁹/L)		
20	1.40	2.56	3.72
22	1.63	2.79	3.94
24	1.86	3.02	4.17
26	2.09	3.24	4.40
28	2.31	3.47	4.63
30	2.54	3.70	4.86
32	2.77	3.93	5.09
34	3.00	4.16	5.33
36	3.22	4.39	5.56
38	3.45	4.62	5.79
40	3.67	4.85	6.02

TABLE 29–3. *(Continued)*

Reticulocyte Count (10^{12}/L)		
20	0.15	0.33	0.73
22	0.13	0.30	0.66
24	0.12	0.27	0.60
26	0.11	0.25	0.55
28	0.10	0.22	0.50
30	0.09	0.20	0.46
32	0.08	0.19	0.41
34	0.08	0.17	0.38
36	0.07	0.15	0.35
38	0.06	0.14	0.32
40	0.06	0.13	0.29

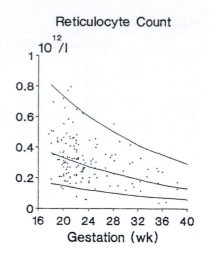

Reticulocyte Count

Erythrocyte Count (10^{12}/L)		
20	2.26	2.70	3.14
22	2.41	2.85	3.29
24	2.56	3.00	3.43
26	2.71	3.14	3.58
28	2.85	3.29	3.73
30	3.00	3.44	3.88
32	3.15	3.59	4.03
34	3.30	3.74	4.18
36	3.44	3.88	4.33
38	3.59	4.03	4.48
40	3.74	4.18	4.62

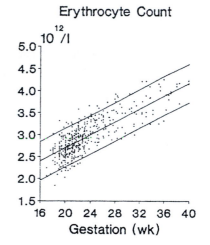

Erythrocyte Count

Reproduced with permission from Davies NP, Buggins AGS, Snijders RJM, et al. Arch Dis Child. 1992;67:399–403; Nicolaides KH, Snijders RJM, Thorpe-Beeston G, et al. Fetal Diagn Ther. 1989;4:1–13; Nicolaides KH, Thilaganathan B, Mibashan RS. Am J Obstet Gynecol. 1989;161:1197–1200; Van den Hof MC, Nicolaides KH. Am J Obstet Gynecol. 1990;162:735–739.
GA, Gestational age.

significantly longer duration of bleeding than venipuncture.[47] The fetal platelet count does not seem to determine the severity of bleeding from the puncture site. In a series inclusive of 20 fetuses with platelet counts below 50×10^9/L and 8 fetuses with a platelet count below 10×10^9/L, there was no correlation between fetal platelet count and either the incidence or duration of bleeding.[47] However, fetuses affected by defects in platelet number or function (e.g., Glanzmann's thrombasthenia or alloimmune thrombocytopenia), are at significant risk for potentially fatal bleeding from puncture site.[48,49] When PUBS is performed to rule out these conditions, it is prudent to slowly transfuse concentrated irradiated maternal platelets while awaiting the fetal platelet count because dislodgment of the needle can have serious consequences for the fetus.

Cord Hematoma

In a pathologic study of 50 umbilical cords collected between 1 and 20 h after PUBS, hematomas were noted in as many as 17% of cases.[50] No relationship could be documented between transient fetal bradycardia or bleeding from the cord puncture site and the size of the hematoma. A hematoma is generally asymptomatic, but it can be associated with prolonged bradycardia and rapid fetal deterioration.[46,50,51] On occasion, cord hematomas can be visualized by ultrasound as an echogenic area near the puncture site.[52,53] In the absence of signs of fetal distress, expectant management is recommended.

Bradycardia

A transient fetal bradycardia is a complication reported in 3 to 12% of cases.[6,9,19,47] It is usually a self-limited phenomenon. In most cases, bradycardias are thought to be manifestations of a vasovagal response caused by local vasospasm; this hypothesis is supported by a higher incidence of bradycardia in cases of puncture of an umbilical artery.[47] The occurrence of bradycardia does not seem to be related to the sampling

TABLE 29–4. FETAL BLOOD GAS VALUES DURING GESTATION

Gestation (wks)	Umbilical Vein pH			Umbilical Artery pH		
	5th	Mean	95th	5th	Mean	95th
18	7.385	7.423	7.461	7.360	7.398	7.435
20	7.382	7.420	7.458	7.357	7.394	7.431
22	7.379	7.417	7.454	7.353	7.390	7.427
24	7.376	7.414	7.451	7.350	7.386	7.423
26	7.373	7.410	7.448	7.346	7.383	7.419
28	7.370	7.407	7.445	7.342	7.379	7.416
30	7.366	7.404	7.442	7.338	7.375	7.412
32	7.363	7.401	7.439	7.334	7.371	7.409
34	7.360	7.398	7.436	7.330	7.368	7.406
36	7.357	7.395	7.433	7.325	7.364	7.403
38	7.353	7.392	7.430	7.321	7.360	7.399
40	7.350	7.388	7.427	7.317	7.357	7.396

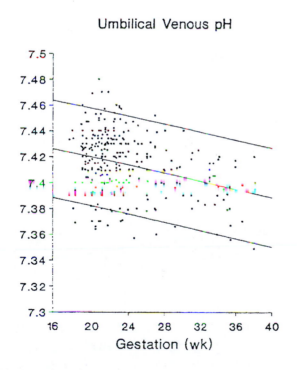

Umbilical Venous pH

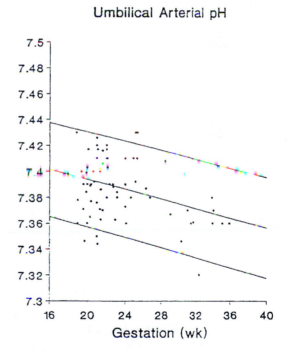

Umbilical Arterial pH

site (placental insertion or free-floating loop of the cord) or to the number of puncture attempts.[54] Ulm et al.[54] reported a series of 339 cordocentesis in which perinatal mortality was significantly higher among cases with bradycardia (61.5%) than among those without bradycardia (3.1%). A significantly higher incidence of bradycardia has also been noted among SGA fetuses than among AGA fetuses (17.2 vs. 4.1%, respectively; $p = 0.001$) and among fetuses with absent diastolic flow by Doppler analysis of the umbilical artery compared with present end diastolic velocities (21.4 vs. 5.3%).[47]

Fetomaternal Hemorrhage

Cordocentesis performed for therapeutic purposes is often associated with fetomaternal transfusion (FMT). In a study of consecutive diagnostic cordocentesis, FMT (defined as a $\geq 50\%$ postprocedural increase in maternal serum α-fetoprotein concentration) occurred in about 40% of cases, and it was more common when the procedure was performed with an anterior rather than a posterior placenta (65.6 vs. 16.6%, $p < 0.001$).[55] These findings have been confirmed by independent investigators.[56,57] The mean estimated volume of hemorrhage was 2.4 mL (3.1% of the total fetoplacental

TABLE 29–4. *(Continued)*

Gestation (wks)	Umbilical Vein Po$_2$ (mm Hg)			Umbilical Artery Po$_2$ (mm Hg)		
	5th	Mean	95th	5th	Mean	95th
18	40.6	51.4	62.2	23.9	29.7	35.5
20	38.7	49.5	60.3	23.2	29.0	34.8
22	36.8	47.6	58.4	22.6	28.3	34.1
24	35.0	45.8	56.5	21.9	27.7	33.4
26	33.1	43.9	54.7	21.2	27.0	32.8
28	31.2	42.0	52.8	20.5	26.3	32.1
30	29.3	40.1	50.9	19.8	25.6	31.5
32	27.4	38.2	49.0	19.1	25.0	30.9
34	25.4	36.3	47.2	18.3	24.3	30.3
36	23.5	34.4	45.3	17.6	23.6	29.7
38	21.6	32.5	43.5	16.8	23.0	29.1
40	19.7	30.6	41.6	16.0	22.3	28.5

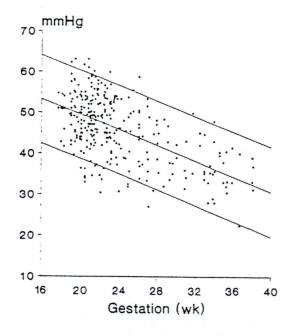

Umbilical Venous pO2

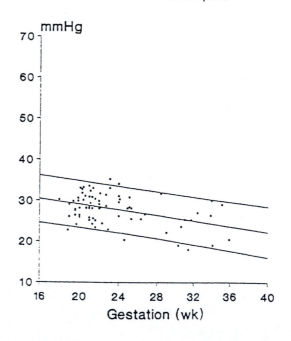

Umbilical Arterial pO2

blood volume). Fetomaternal transfusions have been noted to occur more frequently with a procedure duration of 3 minutes or more and with two or more needle insertions.[58] No relationship has been noted between the degree of fetomaternal hemorrhage, gestational age, or type of procedure (diagnostic vs. therapeutic cordocentesis).[47]

Abruptio Placentae

Despite the use of a transplacental approach, the incidence of this complication is negligible, and only one documented case has been reported thus far.[59]

Preterm Delivery

In 7% of cases, cordocentesis is associated with an irregular pattern of uterine contractions.[42] The preterm delivery rate in a low-risk population was 5.0 to 5.7%.[6,45] Therefore, the procedure does not seem to increase the incidence of prematurity.

Fetal Resuscitation

The risk of life-threatening fetal complications during or immediately after cordocentesis is small. After viability, the option of emergent abdominal delivery and *ex utero* resuscitation

TABLE 29–4. *(Continued)*

Gestation	Umbilical Vein Pco$_2$ (mm Hg)			Umbilical Artery Pco$_2$ (mm Hg)		
(wks)	5th	Mean	95th	5th	Mean	95th
18	27.9	32.7	37.5	31.9	37.2	42.6
20	28.3	33.1	37.9	32.5	37.9	43.3
22	28.8	33.6	38.3	33.2	38.6	43.9
24	29.2	34.0	38.8	33.9	39.2	44.6
26	29.7	34.4	39.2	34.5	39.5	45.2
28	30.1	34.9	39.7	35.2	40.2	45.9
30	30.5	35.3	40.1	35.8	40.9	46.6
32	30.9	35.8	40.6	36.4	41.8	47.3
34	31.4	36.2	41.0	37.0	42.5	48.0
36	31.8	36.6	41.5	37.5	43.2	48.8
38	32.2	37.1	41.9	38.1	43.8	49.5
40	32.6	37.5	42.4	38.7	44.5	50.3

Reproduced with permission from Nicolaides KH, Economides KH, Soothill PW. Am J Obstet Gynecol. 1989;161:996–1001.

Umbilical Venous pCO2

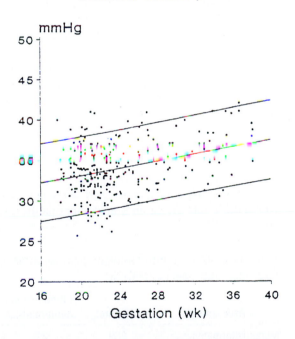

Umbilical Arterial pCO2

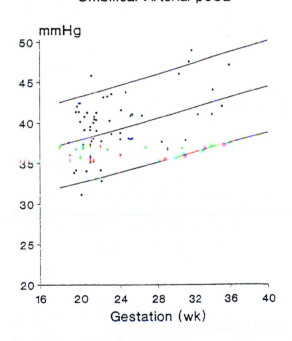

is available. If fetal lung maturity is not documented or is suspected not to be present, it may be prudent to administer a brief course of oral steroids to the patient during the days before the procedure to enhance fetal lung maturity. The risk-to-benefit ratio of this recommendation has not been evaluated.

Before viability or at an extremely premature gestational age, when emergent cesarean delivery is not desirable, fetal resuscitation can be attempted *in utero*. In the presence of unremitting fetal bradycardia, the common maneuvers to improve uterine perfusion and enhance fetal oxygenation should be implemented immediately. These include adopting the left lateral decubitus, intravenous hydration, and administer-

ing oxygen by mask.[60] If the bradycardia is associated with uterine contractions, subcutaneous or intravenous tocolytics can be administered to the mother.[61] If the bradycardia persists or worsens, a more aggressive approach is necessary because little or no flow is present in the fetal circulation to provide peripheral oxygenation and feto-maternal gas and drug exchange. Only anecdotal case reports of *in utero* resuscitation have been published, and a selection bias in favor of successful procedures is likely to exist.[19,62–64] External maneuvers on the mother's abdomen in an attempt to perform an indirect fetal cardiac massage, as proposed by a case report, are anecdotal.[62] If the needle is still in the

TABLE 29–5. MEDICATIONS FOR FETAL RESUSCITATION

Medication	Preparation	Dosage/Route	Total Dose EFW	Total Dose mL
Epinephrine	1:10,000 (1mL)	0.1–0.3 mL/kg[a]	500 g 1000 g	0.05–0.15 0.1–0.3
Volume expanders	Whole blood or normal saline	14 mL/kg[b]	500 g 1000 g	7 14

EFW, Estimated fetal weight.
[a]Can be repeated every 3 to 5 mins if required.
[b]The dosage takes into consideration the fetoplacental blood volume.

umbilical vessel, immediate administration of epinephrine or volume expanders may be attempted. Table 29–5 displays a protocol for potentially useful treatments that have been derived from recommendations of the American Academy of Pediatrics and the American Heart Association for neonatal resuscitation.[65] The dosages have been adjusted for the estimated fetal weight and the fetoplacental blood volume. There is no evidence in the neonatal literature to suggest that atropine is useful in the acute phase of resuscitation.[65] If the bradycardia is secondary to documented or suspected prolonged bleeding from the puncture site, hypovolemic shock is likely to be present and volume restoration would be the treatment of choice. The operator should be aware that no medication will be delivered to the fetal heart if there is no venous flow.[65] In this condition, or if a new needle insertion is required, cardiocentesis may be considered. This has been accomplished successfully in a 20-week fetus affected with von Willebrand disease. Cordocentesis was followed by a severe 5-min bradycardia secondary to a large fetomaternal transfusion. An intracardiac puncture and transfusion with 30 mL of maternal blood was used to resuscitate the fetus.[64] An emergency resuscitation kit should be available and ready for use. The establishment of a centralized registry of cases of attempted *in utero* resuscitation would be ideal to determine which procedures and medications are effective.

INDICATIONS

Cytogenetic Diagnosis

During the past few years, the use of cordocentesis in clinical practice has been replaced by late chorionic villus sampling (CVS) in most situations. The success rate of CVS in the second and third trimesters of pregnancy has been reported to be more than 99%, with a risk of spontaneous loss within 4 to 6 weeks from the procedure lower than 0.3%.[66,67] In addition, Cameron et al.[68] reported a series of 551 late CVSs in which a fetal karyotype was obtained within a mean interval of 4.4 days (with a standard deviation of 0.86 days) in 96.3% of cases.

Fetal karyotype from cultured human lymphocytes obtained from fetal blood has a limited role in clinical practice for cytogenetic diagnosis and is considered useful in the following circumstances: 1) when karyotype results are necessary within a short time interval (2 to 3 days); 2) when mosaicism or pseudomosaicism is detected at amniocentesis or CVS; and 3) when karyotype by CVS in the second and third trimesters of pregnancy has failed.

The workup of a fetus with a structural anomaly at a gestational age near the time limit for legal termination is one of the most common indications for diagnostic cordocentesis. The objective of the procedure is to exclude the presence of chromosomal anomalies and congenital infection. In a comprehensive study of 936 fetuses with structural anomalies identified by ultrasound, the overall prevalence of chromosomal aberrations was 12.1% in cases of an isolated anomaly and 29.2% in cases of multiple anomalies.[69] Table 29–6 presents the prevalence of chromosomal anomalies per structural defect. Trisomies 21, 18, and 13 and monosomy X accounted for 80% of all anomalies. Triploidy (4.9%) and balanced (4.9%) and unbalanced (9.8%) non-Robertsonian translocations were also frequently found. These observations are consistent with those of smaller reports.[70–73] Unexplained polyhydramnios (amniotic fluid index $\geq$ 25 cm) in the absence of sonographically detected anomalies is associated with a 3.2% rate of chromosomal abnormalities, including

TABLE 29–6. FETAL BLOOD CHROMOSOMAL ABNORMALITIES AND "ISOLATED" MALFORMATIONS

Assessment	Number	Chromosomal Abnormalities	%
Monomalformations	239	29	12.1
Central nervous system	51	4	7.8
Cardiovascular	21	3	14.3
Gastrointestinal	20	3	15.0
Genitourinary	55	1	1.8
Facial	4	0	—
Extremities	7	0	—
Ventral wall defects	42	3	7.1
Hygromas	20	14	70.0
Fetal effusions	15	1	6.7
Placenta	2	0	—
Other	2	0	—
Polymalformations	65	19	29.2

From Eydoux P, Choiset A, Le Porrier N, et al. Prenat Diagn. 1989;9:235.

trisomies 21 and 18.[74] Similarly, severe oligohydramnios or anhydramnios in the second and third trimesters is associated with a rate of aneuploidy of at least 4.4%.[75]

Another cytogenetic indication for cordocentesis is the presence of mosaicism at amniocentesis or CVS. Mosaicism has been reported in 2 to 3% of amniotic fluid cultures,[76–78] but has been confirmed by amniocentesis or PUBS in only 0.2 to 0.4% of cases.[77,79–83] Possible explanations for this discrepancy include *in vitro* changes in cultured amniotic fluid cells (pseudomosaicism), a postzygotic error that is restricted to the extraembryonic membranes (amnion or trophoblast), an unrecognized dizygotic twin pregnancy with early death of an abnormal twin, or contamination with maternal tissue. If mosaicism is not confirmed in fetal blood, patients should be informed that it is not possible to exclude that the mosaicism cell line may be present in fetal tissues other than blood cells (i.e., liver, brain, etc.).

A supernumerary chromosome (marker chromosome) represents a heterogeneous group of disorders characterized by the presence of fragments of chromosomes that can be inherited from one of the parents or that may arise *de novo*. Percutaneous umbilical blood sampling can be offered to the couple to rule out mosaicism for the marker chromosome in cases of *de novo* occurrences. Regrettably, this extrachromosomal material is easily lost from the leukocytes. Identification of mosaicism for the marker chromosome in fetal blood is diagnostic, but a negative result is not helpful.[79,80]

The role of PUBS in the prenatal diagnosis of fragile X syndrome is very limited, because the PCR technique complemented by direct genomic Southern blot analysis has been found to have close to 100% diagnostic accuracy.[84]

Congenital Infections

In the past, fetal blood sampling has been used in the prenatal diagnosis of several congenital infections including toxoplasmosis, rubella, cytomegalovirus, varicella, and parvovirus.[8,85–95] The general approach consists of obtaining material to isolate the infectious agent or documenting a specific fetal immune response. This response is variable, and it is influenced by the maturity of the fetal immune system so that a consistent response may not be detected before 20 to 22 weeks. The response can also be transient and, therefore, affected by the time interval between infection and blood sampling. Moreover, fetal immune response may be weak or undetectable, and the formation of antigen–antibody complexes under conditions of excess antigen may interfere with the immunologic assay used. For these reasons, documentation of a specific fetal immunoglobulin M (IgM) response is diagnostic of recent infection, but absence of specific IgM response is not helpful. Actually, with the availability of fast and reliable PCR techniques to amplify microbial genomes present in the amniotic fluid, fetal blood sampling has a limited role in the prenatal diagnosis of several congenital infections. In addition, PUBS performed in cases of documented maternal infection to exclude fetal involvement has the po-

tential to increase transplacental passage of the infectious agent.

Toxoplasmosis. Identification of the parasite in the fetal blood requires up to 45 days to achieve optimum results. Amplification by PCR of the *Toxoplasma gondii* genome is the fastest and most sensitive diagnostic test;[95–100] it can be performed on either fetal blood or amniotic fluid, and it seems particularly helpful in cases in which the parasite burden is small. Fetal blood sampling has considerable value for the detection of infected fetuses but also carries some risks and is currently being abandoned in favor of amniocentesis alone with gene amplification.[99,101]

Rubella. Prenatal diagnosis of fetal infection can be made by cordocentesis measuring fetal levels of specific IgM antibodies that are persistently found only after the 22nd week.[87] The overall sensitivity of prenatal diagnosis with this method in the largest series available ($n = 119$ cases) has been 98% (59 of 60) with a specificity of 100% (59 of 59).[87] The only incorrect diagnosis was thought to be due to sampling too early during pregnancy (20 weeks). Fetal rubella infection can also be diagnosed by amniocentesis by using a reverse transcription–PCR method. Revello et al. reported that this method has 100% sensitivity and specificity and has the advantage of producing results in 24 to 48 h after sampling.[102]

Cytomegalovirus. The role of PUBS in the diagnosis of cytomegalovirus (CMV) infection is quite limited. Lipitz et al.[103] compared the accuracy of amniocentesis (cultures and/or PCR analysis) combined with PUBS for specific IgM determination and amniocentesis alone. Of the two procedures, the less-invasive amniocentesis identified all infected fetuses. Therefore, PUBS did not add diagnostic information and had a sensitivity of only 77% in identifying affected fetuses. Once the diagnosis of vertical transmission is established, ultrasound examination can provide information as to the presence of fetal damage. Ultrasound findings of fetal CMV infection include ascites, generalized hydrops, ventriculomegaly, intracranial calcifications, increased bowel echodensity, and growth retardation.[89,104]

Varicella Zoster Virus. Fetal blood sampling has limited application because viremia is present for a limited time, and specific IgM antibodies are absent in more than half of infected newborns. Recently, it has been documented that PCR analysis of the viral genome in the amniotic fluid is far more sensitive than detection of specific IgM antibodies in the fetal blood for the diagnosis of fetal infection.[105]

Parvovirus. Human parvovirus B19 is the etiologic agent of erythema infectiosum in children, and it manifests with flu-like symptoms and arthralgias in adults. However, parvovirus can be entirely asymptomatic in about 20% of adults. The primary sites for parvovirus replication are the erythroid progenitor cells in the bone marrow.[106] The infection is lytic in nature, leading to erythrocytes failing to mature. The aplastic event lasts 7 to 10 days, after which time reticulocytes appear; the bone marrow fully recovers within approximately 3 weeks. Adults with normal hematopoiesis tolerate this transient red cell aplasia with a minimal decrease in hemoglobin; however, anemia may develop in cases of infection when there is rapid erythrocyte turnover (i.e., fetuses). The transplacental transmission rate of parvovirus is about 33%.[107] It has been estimated that the risk of fetal death due to parvovirus is 9%.[107] Data from a prospective cohort study of 200 women with serologic evidence of acute parvovirus infection have indicated that there is a 2 to 3% increase in fetal death among infected women compared with control subjects.[108] Parvovirus infection can affect the fetus at any gestational age. Severe anemia and hydrops, probably due to high output cardiac failure, precede fetal death in most cases.[109] When present, hydrops generally occurs 3 to 5 weeks after symptomatic infection in the mother, but it has been reported up to 12 weeks later.[107,109] Therefore, once maternal infection has been documented, serial sonographic examinations every 1 to 2 weeks are indicated to detect early signs of hydrops. Some fetuses can become hydropic without evidence of anemia. Because viral particles have been recovered from the myocardium, hydrops could be due to viral cardiomyopathy.[110–112] Although most fetuses with hydrops die *in utero* if not transfused, cases of transient hydrops and survival have been reported.[113–116] A finding at PUBS of an elevated reticulocyte count suggests resolution of the anemia and may indicate that fetal transfusion is not required. Infants who survive fetal anemia with or without transfusion appear to develop normally, but cases of chronic anemia resistant to immunoglobulin treatment have been reported.[117] It has been postulated that in these cases an anti-idiotypic response to parvovirus might be directed against erythroid precursors. There is no conclusive evidence that parvovirus infection is associated with structural abnormalities. A prenatal diagnosis of parvovirus fetal infection can be made in the presence of hydrops using amniocentesis. Viral infection can be detected with a high accuracy using PCR amplification of the viral genome in the amniotic fluid[110,118–120] or by using monoclonal antibodies directed against the two viral capsid antigens.[121] Despite this, PUBS remains the method of choice to assess the degree of fetal anemia. The clinical situation in which the performance of PUBS is warranted is in cases of overt fetal hydrops in a patient with suspicion of acute infection (IgG and IgM positive) at a gestational age in which fetal viability is not guaranteed. Recently, Schild et al.[122] reported a series of 35 cases of fetal hydrops in the presence of a maternal parvovirus B19 infection in which PUBS was performed to assess the presence of viral genome and the degree of fetal anemia. Whereas IgM titers were negative or equivocal in 67.6% of cases, the PCR technique for the presence of parvovirus B19 yielded positive results in 93.7% of cases. During PUBS, fetal hemoglobin was measured within 1 minute and, in case of fetal anemia, a transfusion of packed red cells was performed while the

needle was left in the umbilical vein. The majority of pregnancies (31 of 35) had a successful outcome with a live birth. Although assessing the reticulocyte count may help in deciding if the fetus would not need transfusion, this procedure takes too long to have clinical management value.

Preterm Labor and Preterm Premature Rupture of Membranes

Prematurity is the leading cause of perinatal morbidity and mortality worldwide, affecting 5 to 10% of births.[123–126] Microbial invasion of the amniotic cavity is present in 10% of patients with preterm labor and intact membranes and in 30% of patients with preterm premature rupture of membranes (PROM).[127–134] Recent evidence indicates that the human fetus plays a central role in determining the onset of preterm labor.[135–137] A condition termed *fetal inflammatory response syndrome* (FIRS), defined as an elevated fetal plasma interleukin-6 (IL-6) value greater than 11 pg/mL at PUBS, has been found in 39% of patients with preterm PROM and in 48% of patients with preterm labor and intact membranes.[135,136] An elevation of fetal plasma IL-6 is a marker for the acute phase response to infection and is considered to have survival value. Fetuses who subsequently develop neonatal morbidity have higher concentrations of plasma IL-6 than those who do not have complications during the neonatal period. A plot of the predicted probability that neonatal morbidity will develop according to gestational age at delivery for fetuses with and without a systemic inflammatory response is displayed in Fig. 29–4. Yoon et al. recently reported that an elevation in fetal plasma cortisol at PUBS is followed by the onset of spontaneous preterm labor in patients with preterm PROM.[136] These findings suggest that a population of fetuses presenting with preterm labor or preterm

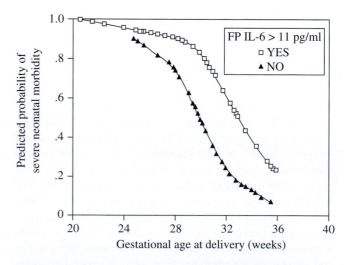

Figure 29–4. Plot of predicted probability of severe neonatal morbidity as a function of gestational age at delivery and presence or absence of fetal plasma IL-6 > 11 pg/mL. *(Reprinted with permission from Gomez R, Romero R, Ghezzi F, et al. Am J Obstet Gynecol. 1998;179:194.)*

PROM are ill and that PUBS may be useful in identifying them. Indeed, a proportion of fetuses with infection or an inflammatory response are not detected by maternal monitoring (maternal temperature, heart rate, leukocyte count, C-reactive protein)[138] or by amniotic fluid analysis.[135,136] Moreover, fetuses with FIRS have an impending onset of preterm labor and delivery, regardless of the inflammatory state of the amniotic cavity. A crucial question is whether or not PUBS should be used routinely in patients with preterm labor or preterm PROM. Although some investigators have advocated its use routinely in patients with preterm labor and preterm PROM and it has been demonstrated that the procedure-related mortality associated with PUBS appears to be comparable with midtrimester amniocentesis, further studies are required to assess the clinical value of PUBS.

Congenital Immunodeficiency

Four components of the immune system play a role in the host defense against infection: phagocytosis, antibody-mediated immunity (B cells), cell-mediated immunity (T cells), and complement. Congenital disorders of any of these components can impair the ability of the host to deal with infection, and, in some cases, they may result in early death due to opportunistic infections.

Prenatal diagnosis can be done using 1) determination of gene products in chorionic villi or amniocytes (e.g., adenosine deaminase and purine nucleoside phosphorylase deficiencies); 2) determination of immunologic markers on fetal blood lymphocytes (specific lymphocyte subpopulations can be counted, and functional assays, such as stimulation with phytohemagglutinin, can be used adjunctively); 3) in informative families, linkage analysis using flanking DNA markers, such as restriction fragment length polymorphisms

(RFLPs), dinucleotide repeats, or short tandem sequences; and 4) ultrasonographic visualization of associated structural fetal abnormalities (e.g., short limb dwarfism associated with immunodeficiency). The advantage of PUBS is that it is useful to diagnosis immunodeficiencies of unknown etiology. Table 29–7 displays the normal values of T cells and B cells at different gestational ages. Because immune elements are present in the peripheral circulation in significant numbers only after 18 to 20 weeks, PUBS should be postponed to this gestational age. Quantitative disorders of T cells can be diagnosed using monoclonal antibodies to cell surface markers present only in T cells. In the normal fetus, T cells are detectable at approximately 16 weeks and increase during the remainder of pregnancy.[139–141] Similarly, enumeration of B cells in fetal blood has permitted the diagnosis (or its exclusion) of immunoglobulin associated deficiencies.[142] Prenatal diagnosis by PUBS of qualitative defects of host defense cells has also been reported.[143–148] A detailed discussion of congenital immunodeficiencies is beyond the scope of this chapter. Advances in the cloning of the responsible genes and definition of specific molecular defects are allowing earlier and more precise diagnosis of some congenital immunodeficiencies on chorionic villi or amniotic fluid cells. Therefore, before attempting prenatal diagnosis of any of these conditions, updated genetic services should be contacted to determine the optimal technique recommended for prenatal diagnosis.

Coagulopathies

The majority of inherited hematologic disorders can now be diagnosed by molecular genetic testing on amniocytes or chorionic villi. Fetal blood sampling still has a role, although minor, in the prenatal diagnosis of some congenital hemostatic disorders. Because excessive bleeding after sampling

TABLE 29–7. LYMPHOCYTE SUBSETS IN FETAL BLOOD[a]

Component	Fetus 16th–20th Week	Fetus 20th–27th Week	Neonate	Adult
Lymphocyte count ($\times 10^9$/L)	1.9 ± 0.7	2.6 ± 0.7	5.6 ± 1.0[†]	2.1 ± 0.7
Reactivity with (%)				
OKT6 CD1[b]	3.9 ± 4.3	0.2 ± 0.3	1.2 ± 1.3	0.8 ± 1.1
OKT3 CD3[c]	68.2 ± 10.3[g]	71.1 ± 8.7	73.2 ± 6.4	76.9 ± 5.6
OKT4 CD4[c]	47.7 ± 6.0	50.2 ± 7.2	51.3 ± 4.8[g]	46.1 ± 4.2
OKT8 CD8[c]	18.2 ± 6.9[†g]	23.1 ± 7.6	24.3 ± 4.5	27.8 ± 4.8
Leu-12 CD19[d]	15.6 ± 8.7	22 ± 8.1[g]	16.3 ± 7.9	9.4 ± 5.5
OKT10 CD38[b,c,e]	83.9 ± 8.5[†g]	87.2 ± 9.4[g]	85.3 ± 8.1[g]	23.2 ± 6.5
OKIa[c,d]	24.1 ± 11.1[†g]	26.3 ± 9.6[g]	22.5 ± 9.0[g]	16.2 ± 5.6
Leu-7 CD57[f]	0.3 ± 0.6[†g]	1.4 ± 2.2[g]	0.6 ± 0.7[g]	6.4 ± 4.2
OKT4/OKT8 ratio	2.95 ± 1.14[†g]	2.41 ± 0.99[g]	2.17 ± 0.50[g]	1.65 ± 0.35

[a]Results expressed as mean value ± one standard deviation.
[b]Thymocyte surface antigen.
[c]T-cell surface antigen.
[d]B-cell surface antigen.
[e]Plasma cells surface antigen.
[f]Natural killer cells surface antigen.
[g]Statistically different ($p < 0.05$) in comparison with adult values (Student's t-test).
Modified with permission from De Waele M, Foulon W, Renmans W, et al. Am J Clin Pathol. 1988;89:242.

in fetuses with coagulopathies, such as severe von Willebrand disease and hemophilia, has been reported,[64,149] concentrated products and/or platelets for transfusion should be available at the time of PUBS in these cases.

Hemophilia A. Factor VIII is a protein formed by two different components: a small molecule, coded by the X chromosome, that is involved in the coagulation pathway, and a large, multimeric molecule (von Willebrand factor), coded by a gene located on chromosome 12, that functions as a carrier protein for factor VIII moieties. The recommended nomenclature for factor VIII and von Willebrand factor uses the following abbreviations:

- Factor VIII: Protein lacking or aberrant in hemophilia A.
- Factor VIIIC: Functional attribute of factor VIII responsible for coagulant activity and measured using coagulation techniques.
- Factor VIIIAg: Antigenic expression of factor VIII as measured by immunoassays.
- vWF: Von Willebrand factor, a protein required for normal platelet adhesion; also acts as carrier of factor VIII.
- vWFAg: Antigenic expression of vWF as measured by immunoassays.

In hemophilia A there is deficiency of factor VIIIC that, in 90 to 95% of cases, is associated with a deficiency in factor VIIIAg; in the remaining 5 to 10%, a variant of factor VIII is present that interacts with autologous antibodies (factor VIIIAg present) but has no functional activity. In von Willebrand disease, there is an abnormal or deficient vWF. This is manifested by both abnormality in platelet function and a factor VIII deficiency.

Diagnosis of factor VIII disorders must consider the properties tested by the assay employed. Factor VIIIC is measured by its ability to shorten the clotting time of hemophilic plasma. This assay was the method used for many years to assess factor VIII levels in the postnatal period. Shortcomings of this assay were that it required a relatively large amount of blood, that it was affected by coagulation of the sample (factor VIII is not present in serum because it is consumed during normal clotting), and that it is affected by contamination with amniotic fluid. An advance was the development of an immunoassay for the antigenic portion of factor VIII. Antibodies against factor VIII develop in some hemophilic patients after transfusions. These antibodies can be used to detect an antigenic determinant of factor VIII. This antigen is present in both serum and plasma. In addition, this assay is not significantly affected by contamination with amniotic fluid. In normal individuals, factors VIIIC and VIIIAg are highly correlated and inferences can be drawn from either assay. In some hemophilic patients, however, there is a discrepancy between factors VIIIC and VIIIAg, with an excess of the latter. The substance responsible for this difference

is a cross-reactive material (CRM), an antigenically recognizable protein without functional activity. A false-negative diagnosis of hemophilia A can occur if the clinician relies solely on the immunologic assay of factor VIII. Therefore, for prenatal diagnostic purposes, it was important to know if the index case in the family has CRM. If the affected individual was CRM-positive, diagnosis would have required a functional clotting assay. About 95% of families with severe hemophilia A (VIIIC below 1%) are CRM-negative.

Prenatal Diagnosis. Hemophilia A is inherited in an X-linked recessive pattern. Its estimated incidence is 1 in 10,000 with male births. Its severity is related to the degree of reduction of factor VIIIC. The first and crucial step involved in the prenatal diagnosis of hemophilia A is an assessment of the carrier risk. Overall, 80% of mothers of isolated hemophiliacs are expected to be carriers.[150] This assessment can be accomplished by family history, laboratory techniques, and the demonstration of linkage between hemophilia A and other genetic markers.[151,152] Carrier status cannot be established unambiguously by coagulation tests due to considerable overlap between the levels of factor VIIIC in carriers and normal women.

The size and complexity of the gene and the wide range of mutations responsible for hemophilia A (mainly point mutations) have made direct detection of hemophilic mutation quite challenging.[153] As a consequence, carrier detection and prenatal diagnosis are still made by linkage analysis.[152] Several intragenic and extragenic polymorphic markers can now be identified with the use of PCR and Southern blotting.[151] The rate of informativeness for these polymorphisms depends on the ethnic background. Among those of European descent, more that 95% of females are informative for intragenic markers,[151,154] but among other ethnic groups, informativeness can be as low as 63%.[155,156] If genetic markers are informative, prenatal diagnosis has a greater than 96% accuracy rate,[151] which can be close to 100% if intragenic probes are informative, because no intragenic recombination events for hemophilia A have been reported thus far.

The most reliable method for prenatal diagnosis of hemophilia A and B is direct identification of the mutation. This is possible once the mutation and family tree have been characterized. This allows identification of carriers and prenatal diagnosis even if no living hemophiliac remains in the family without the need for blood samples from other family members. However, in 50% of cases, hemophilia A is due to inversion of the X chromosome.

Chorionic villus sampling is the method most widely used today for hemophilia A diagnosis. In a male fetus, further DNA analysis has to be performed to make the diagnosis. This can be accomplished by sequencing a known mutation by RFLP or PCR.[157]

In cases where early genetic diagnosis has, for some reason, not been possible or was inconclusive, PUBS can be used for diagnosis.[158] Several laboratories have established normal values for factors VIIIC and VIIIAg from midtrimester fetuses that are disease free.[159–161] It is prudent, however, that centers involved in the prenatal diagnosis of coagulopathies derive their own control data before undertaking diagnostic efforts in patients at risk. Mibashan and Rodeck[162] reported their results in the prenatal diagnosis of 153 consecutive male fetuses at risk for hemophilia A. Of these fetuses, 47 were found to be affected. There were no false-positive or false-negative diagnoses in the abortuses or infants delivered at the time of the report. The incidence of CRM-positive families in their first 100 cases was 8%. In all cases, the correct diagnosis could be made by using a functional clotting assay for factor VIIIC.

Hemophilia B. Hemophilia B (factor IX deficiency) is an X-linked recessive disorder due to a deficiency in factor IX activity. Clinical presentation is quite similar to that of the hemophilia A. The diagnosis is made by demonstrating reduced factor IX coagulant (IXC) activity in a functional assay. An immunoassay is also available for the detection of factor IX antigen (IXAg), but unlike hemophilia A, there is a high prevalence of CRM-positive families with hemophilia B.[163] The considerations already stated for carrier detection and prenatal diagnosis of hemophilia A using linkage analysis also hold true for hemophilia B. The only difference is a higher rate (about 10% among those of European descent) of hemophilia B families with uninformative intragenic polymorphisms compared with hemophilia A.[151,164,165] These families require diagnostic studies with linked extragenic markers that carry a possibility of genetic recombination between the polymorphic site and the hemophilic mutation and, hence, a lower accuracy of prenatal genetic diagnosis.

If fetal blood sampling is performed, it is important that a functional assay for factor IXC be performed, unless the proband has been clearly demonstrated to be CRM-negative.[166] All necessary tubes should be prepared before cordocentesis. Determination of factor IXC studies (for both activity and antigen) requires tubes with citrate as the anticoagulant. Both factors VIII and IX should be measured in all cases to verify the validity of the samples, as well as factors V and X, as indicators of possible consumption or activation of the coagulation cascade. Mibashan and Rodeck[162] examined 19 male fetuses at risk for hemophilia B. Of these, 16 were normal and 3 were affected. All diagnoses were confirmed in blood specimens from the abortuses or from infants after birth. Similar results have been reported by other groups.[48] Prenatal diagnosis of hemophilia B has been achieved by PCR analysis at CVS.[167]

von Willebrand Disease. von Willebrand disease is the most common inherited bleeding disorder and is characterized by a prolonged bleeding time associated with qualitative or quantitative abnormalities of vWF. More than 70% of von Willebrand cases are inherited as an autosomal dominant trait. The precise prevalence of this disorder is difficult to establish because it has only 60% penetrance and a mild case may go unnoticed. The disease can be classified as homozygous or heterozygous. Only in homozygous cases of von Willebrand disease (i.e., in the offspring of two heterozygote cases of von Willebrand disease) are hemorrhagic manifestations severe enough to warrant prenatal diagnosis. The disorder is characterized by low vWFAg and reduced VIIIC and VIIIAg; however, there is a significant overlap between the levels of vWFAg in von Willebrand disease and the normal range. The vWF is critical for normal platelet adhesion, and this explains the abnormalities in bleeding time.

Mibashan and Rodeck[162] examined three couples at risk for an infant with homozygous disease. The diagnosis was excluded in two fetuses and made in one. The affected fetus had extremely low levels of all components of the factor VIII complex. The diagnosis has been made in a second case[64] and excluded in three other cases.[48,168]

Other Congenital Hemostatic Disorders. Several congenital hemostatic disorders are associated with a risk of intrauterine or early postnatal hemorrhage. Table 29–8 displays the normal values for the activity of coagulation factors. Antenatal diagnoses of deficient factors V, VII, and XIII have been reported.[48]

Platelet Disorders

Fetal blood sampling can be useful in the prenatal diagnosis and management of congenital quantitative (thrombocytopenias) and qualitative (thrombocytopathies) platelet disorders.

Exsanguination after cordocenteses has been reported in fetuses affected with alloimmune thrombocytopenia and

---

TABLE 29–8. THE EVOLUTION OF COAGULATION FACTOR OF 103 NORMAL FETUSES DURING PREGNANCY AND THEIR RELATIVE MOTHERS (MEAN ± SD)

Weeks of Gestation	VIII (%)	vWFAg (%)	IXC (%)	VC (%)	IIC (%)
Fetuses					
19–21 ($n = 51$)	40 ± 12	59 ± 12.5	9 ± 2.5	39 ± 11	13 ± 4
22–24 ($n = 44$)	39 ± 13.5	64 ± 13	9 ± 3	40.5 ± 5	14 ± 2
25–27 ($n = 44$)	42.5 ± 12	63 ± 13	12 ± 4	39 ± 9	14 ± 3.5
Mothers	160 ± 80	190 ± 110	90 ± 20	85 ± 10	95 ± 15

Reproduced with permission from Forestier F, Daffos F, Galactéros F, et al. Pediatr Res. 1986;20:342–346.

Glanzmann's thrombasthenia.[48,49] To avoid it, it is important to have concentrated platelets available for transfusion before needle withdrawal. In thrombocytopenias, the transfusion volume can be calculated according to the formula:

$$V + EFBV(C_{desired} = C_{observed}/C_{transfused})$$

where EFBV is the estimated fetal blood volume, $C_{desired}$ is the platelet concentration desired at the end of transfusion, $C_{observed}$ is the platelet concentration before transfusion, and $C_{transfused}$ is the platelet concentration in the product to be transfused.

Thrombocytopenias. These include immunologic thrombocytopenias and genetic syndromes in which thrombocytopenia is one of the features.

In immune thrombocytopenic purpura (ITP), there is a small but definite risk of intracranial hemorrhage that is related to the severity of fetal thrombocytopenia.[169] Fetal blood sampling by cordocentesis was recommended at term to evaluate fetal platelet count before labor.[170,171] Because the risk of intracranial hemorrhage before the onset of labor is negligible,[172] the performance of a fetal scalp platelet count during labor as soon as the cervical dilation permits has been proposed.[170,173,174] However, it has been demonstrated that results obtained using this technique can differ by more than 35% in estimating neonatal counts in almost half the cases and that in some cases this could affect obstetric management. In addition, a moderate correlation has been noted between fetal and neonatal platelet count in fetuses with ITP.[175] Performance of serial postnatal platelet counts is crucial because the count reaches a nadir at about 3 to 4 days of life.[169,173]

Alloimmune thrombocytopenia (ATP) occurs in about 1 per 5000 births, and in the majority (more than 75%) of cases, it involves the platelet-specific antigen 1 (PLA 1). The disease can be considered as the counterpart of Rh immunization in the platelet system, with the important difference that the first born is commonly affected (more than 50%) and maternal antibody titers are not predictive of the severity of fetal thrombocytopenia. Most commonly, a PLA1-negative mother is immunized by fetal PLA1-positive platelets. An antiplatelet IgG antibody crosses the placenta and produces thrombocytopenia in the PLA1-positive fetus. Severe intracranial hemorrhage *in utero* or during the perinatal period is a major cause of death and of neurologic impairment.[176,177] In families with an affected infant, the rate of recurrence is in excess of 90%,[178] and the thrombocytopenia in the second infant is always at least as severe as the previous infant.[179] Intracranial hemorrhage occurs in 10 to 30% of cases, and in 25 to 50% of cases it occurs *in utero*.[179,180] For the management of the pregnancy, it is important to know whether the father is homozygous or heterozygous for the offending antigen.[181] In the latter case, it may be useful to perform genotyping of the fetus on amniocytes or chorionic villi by PCR. Genotyping for all important human platelet alloantigens is feasible.

Cordocentesis is the only tool available to assess the severity of this condition because the monitoring of anti-human platelet antibodies does not accurately predict the severity of fetal thrombocytopenia.[178] However, PUBS carries significant risks: 14 cases of fetal death caused by hemorrhage at the puncture site have been reported after the procedure for this disorder.[182] Currently, fetal blood sampling is recommended at 18 to 20 weeks of gestation, which is the earliest gestational age that an intracranial hemorrhage has been documented.[180,183] If the fetus is affected, different management protocols have been proposed. The most aggressive entails serial cordocentesis every 2 to 3 weeks with platelet transfusions if the platelet count is below 100×10^9/L (the life span of transfused platelets is only 5 to 7 days).[184] Delivery is accomplished by cesarean section as soon as fetal lung maturity is documented.[184] The major problem with this protocol lies in its invasiveness. Serial cordocenteses increase the risks inherent in the procedure. Serial maternal thrombocytophereses are debilitating for the mother. Platelet transfusions with pooled donor platelets carry a risk of transfusion-related infections; and cases of adverse fetal outcome due to platelet transfusion itself have been reported.[185] A second protocol recommends careful home rest until 37 weeks, when cordocentesis is repeated. If necessary, platelets are transfused to a count above 50×10^9/L, and vaginal delivery is induced within 36 h of the cordocentesis.[178] Another approach consists of parenteral administration of high doses (1 g/kg of maternal weight once a week) of immunoglobulin to the mother in the presence of a PLA1-positive fetus with a platelet count below 100×10^9/L.[178,179,186] Fetal blood sampling would still be required, although at wider intervals (every 4 to 6 weeks), to monitor the response to treatment and to document the presence and severity of thrombocytopenia before labor. Washed maternal platelets are transfused only to prevent fetal exsanguination from the cord puncture site (i.e., if the fetal platelet count is below 50×10^9/L). This protocol results in a significant increase in platelet count (mean $\times 10^9$/L between pretreatment fetal platelet count and the one at birth) and improved pregnancy outcome of the index pregnancies when compared with the previously affected pregnancies.[178,179,186] A randomized prospective study has been conducted on 54 cases of ATP with a platelet count at first PUBS below 100×10^9/L to evaluate the efficacy of immunoglobulin alone or in combination with steroids (prednisone).[186] There were no differences in the success rate (as documented by the increase in platelet count) between the two therapies. There were no cases of intracranial hemorrhage. It was noted, however, that there was a lower response rate in fetuses with an initial platelet count below 20×10^9/L. It would seem that the optimal treatment and frequency of PUBS should be tailored to the risk of a severe form of ATP.

Thrombocytopenia with absent radius (TAR) syndrome is an autosomal recessive condition characterized by the absence or hypoplasia of the radius and hematologic abnormalities. Fetal blood sampling is indicated in the presence of prenatal sonographic evidence of radial abnormalities.[187] Differential diagnosis includes mainly Fanconi's

TABLE 29–9. CONGENITAL DISORDERS OF PLATELET FUNCTION

Disorders of adhesion
  Von Willebrand disease[48,163,169,189]
  Bernard–Soulier syndrome[188]
Disorders of aggregation
  Glanzmann's thrombasthenia[48]
  Congenital afibrinogenemia
Disorders of secretion
  Storage pool deficiency[48]
  Miscellaneous congenital disorders
    May–Hegglin anomaly[48]
    Hermansky–Pudlak syndrome[190,191]
    TAR syndrome[48,187]
    Wiskott–Aldrich syndrome[192]
    Chédiak–Higashi syndrome[143]

pancytopenia syndrome, which is diagnosed by a characteristic high frequency of diepoxybutane-induced chromosomal breakage on karyotype.

Thrombocytopathies. Table 29–9 displays the most common congenital qualitative platelet disorders and cases of prenatal diagnosis reported.

Hemoglobinopathies

Hemoglobin is a tetrameric molecule composed of four polypeptide chains in a stoichiometric fashion. Adult hemoglobin, or hemoglobin A, contains two α-globin chains and two β-globin chains. The major component of fetal hemoglobin, hemoglobin F, has two gamma chains instead of beta chains. The fetal red blood cells are capable of synthesizing fetal and adult hemoglobin from early gestation. The hemoglobinopathies can be divided into two major groups: those secondary to a quantitative defect in the rate of synthesis of the globin chains (e.g., thalassemias) and those resulting from inherited structural alterations in the globin chains, such as sickle cell anemia, which is characterized by an amino acid substitution in the beta chains.

Alpha-thalassemia is a condition with different presentations, depending on the number of the four α-globin genes involved. The lack of one or two α-globin genes is generally asymptomatic. If three α-globin genes are missing (hemoglobin H disease, characterized by β-44 tetramers), moderate or marked anemia is present at birth, although the condition is not lethal. If all four α-globin genes are deleted or inactive, fetal erythrocytes contain γ-globin tetramers (hemoglobin Bart). The condition presents with nonimmune hydrops usually leading to fetal demise at 28 to 37 weeks.[194] Prenatal diagnosis is indicated only in couples at risk for hemoglobin Bart's hydrops fetalis (i.e., those in which both parents can contribute a haplotype devoid of active α-globin genes). Carrier screening is indicated in the presence of hemoglobin H on electrophoresis or unexplained low mean RBC volumes. Mean cell volume determination alone cannot be used to distinguish patients with two or three deleted genes

because of a significant overlap in values. Restriction enzyme testing can determine the deletion haplotype present and, hence, determine the need for prenatal diagnosis.[194] Originally, prenatal diagnosis of hemoglobinopathies was accomplished on fetal blood by assessment of the rate of synthesis of different globin chains.[195] Blood cells were incubated with radio-labeled leucine for 2 h to label the nascent hemoglobin. Red cells were then lysed and the globin precipitated and separated into carboxyl-methylcellulose columns. The presence of only hemoglobin S identifies a fetus with sickle cell anemia. Quantitation of the amount of beta chains in relation to the amount of gamma chains synthesized was necessary for the diagnosis of beta-thalassemia. No beta chain would be synthesized in beta-thalassemia (ratio of beta to gamma below 0.02), and only a very small amount, if any, in beta-positive thalassemia. Fetuses with beta-thalassemia trait will have intermediate beta-to-gamma ratios.[195]

Currently, fetal diagnosis is done with the use of DNA techniques (restriction enzyme analysis and PCR) in amniotic fluid cells or chorionic villi.[196] The accuracy of the testing is greater than 99% because only three common deletions in southeast Asia and eight common deletions throughout the world account for nearly all alpha-thalassemia mutations.[194]

The diagnosis of sickle cell disease can be made reliably with the use of restriction endonucleases in cultured chorionic villi or amniotic cells.[197] Because the gene defect is known and arises from a single mutation, molecular techniques with direct mutation detection (e.g., allele-specific oligonucleotide probe analysis) are nearly 100% accurate and rapid.[198] Beta-thalassemias can be caused by more than 60 different mutations. Four to six mutations account for more than 90% of beta-thalassemia cases worldwide, however, so that most mutations can be detected by direct methods, such as PCR coupled with allele-specific oligonucleotide hybridization, restriction endonuclease digestion of amplified product, or both.[199,200] The accuracy of these tests is close to 100%. Direct sequence analysis of the hot regions of the gene is necessary only when screening of the couple for the mutations known to occur in that ethnic group fails to show the most common mutation.

Small-for-Gestational Age Fetus

In the presence of a severely SGA fetus of early onset, diagnostic cordocentesis can be used to identify possible causes, such as aneuploidy or fetal infection, and to assess fetal hematologic and acid–base status. Table 29–10 displays the prevalence and type of aneuploidy and congenital infections found in the largest published series.[69,201–215] The risk of aneuploidy seems to increase with the severity of SGA. The prevalence of aneuploidy increases if SGA is associated with polyhydramnios (27%), with structural anomalies (31%), or with both (50%).[69]

In the absence of aneuploidy or congenital infection, SGA is thought to be due to placental insufficiency. Indeed, the levels of most essential amino acids and glucose are

TABLE 29–10. FINDINGS AT PERCUTANEOUS UMBILICAL BLOOD SAMPLING IN SMALL-FOR-GESTATIONAL AGE FETUSES

Reference	Number of Cases	Definition of IUGR	Aneuploidy	Infections
Bilardo et al.[202]	239	NA	17% (40/239) of which triploidy 19/40	NA
Weiner et al.[203]	21	BPD < 10th percentile; AC < 2nd percentile	24% (5/21)	9.5% (2/21)
Eydoux et al.[69]	180	AC < 10th percentile	4% (7/180) Trisomy 13, 18, and 21	NA
Economides et al.[204]	38	AC < 2 SD	8% (3/38) Triploidy and trisomy 21	0/38
Nicolini et al.[205]	58	AC < 5th percentile	7% (4/58) Trisomy 18 and 21 triploidy	0/31
Pardi et al.[206]	56	HC and AC < 5th percentile	0% (0/56)	NA

IUGR, Intrauterine growth retardation; NA, not available; AC, abdominal circumference; BPD, biparietal diameter; HC, head circumference.

lower in SGA than in AGA fetuses of similar gestational ages.[204,207–209] Severe SGA fetuses have signs of chronic hypoxia, as manifested by significantly increased levels of hemoglobin and erythropoietin,[210,211] increased erythroblast count, and elevated gamma-glutamyl-transferase and lactate dehydrogenase levels.[210] In growth-restricted fetuses, the triglyceride levels are increased due to enhanced lipolysis and impaired utilization.[212] Hypertriglyceridemia is most pronounced in cases of fetal hypoxia.[213] In SGA fetuses the cortisol concentration is increased and the adrenocorticotropin level is decreased.[213] The increased plasma cortisol level is probably a response to hypoglycemia. In growth-restricted fetuses, growth hormone and prolactin levels are higher and insulin-like growth factor I is lower than in normal fetuses.[214]

Fetuses who are SGA also have an elevated thyroid-stimulating hormone level and low thyroid hormone[215] and reduced platelet counts[216] than do AGA fetuses of similar gestational age; the pathogenesis of these findings is unknown. Because SGA fetuses have a higher prevalence of hypoxia and acidemia than AGA fetuses,[217] assessment of fetal oxygenation and acid–base balance in SGA fetuses has been proposed to optimize the timing of delivery. Such an approach has several limitations, however. The acid–base status has been shown to correlate with noninvasive tests, such as Doppler velocimetry studies, nonstress test, and biophysical profile.[202,203,206,218–222] Falsely reassuring noninvasive testing (i.e., normal fetal heart rate tracings in the presence of severe acidosis before labor) are exceedingly rare.[223,224] The management of cases with nonreassuring, noninvasive testing and normal fetal acid–base status by cordocentesis is undetermined. Cases with absent end diastolic flow and acidemia/hypoxemia may persist for weeks before fetal delivery is required.[225] Fetal blood sampling is an invasive procedure that is difficult to perform for longitudinal assessment of fetal well-being. A negative result does not guarantee that fetal distress will not develop in the future, within hours or days.[226,227] Finally, acid–base determination has not been shown to predict perinatal mortality in karyotypically normal SGA fetuses without end-diastolic flow on Doppler velocimetry studies.[205]

One study has found that children who had been SGA fetuses with acidemia (blood pH below 2 standard deviations

for gestational age) had a significantly lower developmental score at 29 months of age than SGA fetuses with normal pH.[228] A strong correlation ($r = 0.41$, $p = 0.012$) was also found between severity of antenatal acidemia and developmental score. Acidemic fetuses were significantly more premature and had lower birth weights than nonacidemic fetuses, however; and no information was provided as to the results of fetal surveillance tests (e.g., nonstress test, biophysical profile, Doppler velocimetry studies) to determine whether or not fetal blood sampling can provide additional information in the prediction of long-term postnatal outcome.

FETAL BLOOD SAMPLING IN MULTIPLE GESTATIONS

Two indications for PUBS are specific to multiple gestations, namely twin-to-twin transfusion syndrome and selective termination. Obviously, all the indications for singletons can also apply to multiple gestations.

Twin-to-Twin Transfusion Syndrome

The conditions which should be entertained in the differential diagnoses of discordant growth in twins, include uteroplacental insufficiency, congenital infection, and aneuploidy. Fetal blood sampling is a rapid and informative method of assessing the etiology of the discrepancy.[229] Twin-to-twin transfusion is a complication of monozygotic twin pregnancies and is found in 3.3% of monozygotic twins. Communications between the twins' placental circulations, as documented by dye infusion, are present in 98% (55 of 56) of monochorionic twin placentas and in only 1.5% (1 of 68) of dichorionic twin placentas.[230] The diagnosis of the twin transfusion syndrome in neonates is suspected in the presence of 1) monochorionic twins, 2) clinical evidence of weight discrepancy above 20%, 3) oligohydramnios in the smaller twin, 4) plethora in the larger twin and pallor in the smaller one, and 5) a difference at birth of more than 5 g/dL in hemoglobin between the twins.[231–233] The clinical suspicion should be confirmed by pathologic evidence of communication within the placenta between the twin circulations. Acute events occurring at the time of delivery may reverse the flow, however, leading to a plethoric donor twin with a higher hemoglobin level than the recipient twin. Unfortunately, there is not a gold standard for the diagnosis.[233–235] The *in utero* diagnosis of twin-to-twin transfusion syndrome is suspected when ultrasound reveals discordant growth between members of a twin pair with the same sex and a single placenta in the setting of coexisting oligohydramnios and polyhydramnios. Color flow mapping has allowed visualization of the communicating vessel in several cases in which the vessel was laser coagulated under fetoscopic guidance.[236] It is unknown at present how sensitive this technique can be in the diagnosis of twin-to-twin transfusion syndrome.

Sonographic criteria, however, appear insufficient for establishing the diagnosis of twin-to-twin transfusion syndrome. One series describes the findings in seven patients who had cordocentesis and serial amniocentesis for treatment of twin-to-twin transfusion syndrome diagnosed by sonographic criteria.[235] Only four of the seven cases were confirmed to have twin-to-twin transfusion syndrome by the recovery of adult cells injected into the suspected donor twin in the circulation of the suspected recipient twin. Of these four, only one twin pair exhibited a hemoglobin difference greater than 5g/dL. Additional criteria involving data obtained from cordocentesis have been recommended when considering the diagnosis of twin-to-twin transfusion syndrome. For example, a difference in hemoglobin concentration above 2.4 g/dL had a sensitivity of 50% (4 of 8) and a specificity of 100% for the diagnosis of twin-to-twin syndrome in a series of 38 cases.[237] Recovery of adult cells in the circulation of the suspected recipient twin after injection into the suspected donor twin during cordocentesis had a sensitivity of 83% (10 of 12) in the diagnosis of twin-to-twin transfusion syndrome in a combination of three published series.[235,238,239] Fetal erythropoietin levels were consistently elevated in the recipient twin in three cases of twin-to-twin transfusion syndrome but not in four cases of twin pairs with discordant growth without other features of twin-to-twin transfusion syndrome.[239]

Investigations using cordocentesis for the diagnosis of twin-to-twin transfusion syndrome have continued to evaluate the proposed additional criteria for twin-to-twin transfusion syndrome described above. A small series of patients in London were found to have a mean hemoglobin difference of only 1.7 g/dL in twin pairs with other findings strongly suggestive of twin-to-twin transfusion syndrome.[241] The investigators reporting this finding hypothesized that acute shifts in blood volume between donor and recipient twins with twin-to-twin transfusion syndrome may represent only part of a more complex etiology to the syndrome. They proposed that uteroplacental insufficiency, affecting predominantly one twin, may cause both oligohydramnios in the smaller twin and shunting of blood to the larger twin. However, a recent study of 11 cases of twin-to-twin transfusion syndrome described a significant difference in hemoglobin values obtained during cordocentesis between discordant twins (mean of 4.8 g/dL) and not between nondiscordant twins.[242]

Selective Termination

Selective termination is a procedure used in multiple gestations in which one of the fetuses is abnormal. The most common indications include chromosomal abnormalities (52%), structural abnormalities (42%), and Mendelian disorders (5%).[243] The presence of monochorionicity is a contraindication for the procedure because, in this form of placentation, vascular communications between the twins are almost universally present. Selective termination in a monochorionic twin would carry high risks of exsanguination of the live fetus into the dead one, embolic phenomena in the surviving co-twin, and passage of potassium chloride into the surviving twin circulation. Techniques employed include: 1) intracardiac of intravascular injection of potassium chloride (5 to 15 mEq) to cause cardiac arrest, 2) cardiac puncture to achieve exsanguination, 3) intravascular or intracardiac air embolism (10 to 20 mL of air), and 4) intracardiac injection of calcium gluconate.[244–248] The first method appears to be the safest. In the largest series to date ($n = 183$ cases), the procedure was successful in 100% of cases.[243] No maternal morbidity was reported. The most common complication was PROM (7%). No cases of intraamniotic infection, preterm labor, and clinical or laboratory evidence of disseminated intravascular coagulation were reported. Anecdotal evidence suggests that the risk of the last complication is higher in triplet pregnancies in which two fetuses are selectively terminated. The optimal management in the presence of decreasing fibrinogen levels or prolonged aPTT is undetermined.

The crucial step in the procedure consists of correctly identifying the affected fetus. This is easy in the presence of a gross structural anomaly or discordant gender. In the absence of an anatomical marker, fetal blood sampling for rapid karyotyping may be required before termination. After selective termination, a sample of blood should be obtained to confirm that the procedure was performed on the correct fetus.

FETAL THERAPY

Access to the fetal circulation offers the possibility of infusing biologic (e.g., transfusions) or pharmacologic agents for therapeutic purposes. Several clinical conditions may require treatment with transfusion via cordocentesis. Anemia due to isoimmunization is the most common indication for intravascular transfusion, and anemia due to other causes may require transfusion.[249–252] A recent report has described the use of cordocentesis for transfusion in three cases of Smith–Lemli–Opitz syndrome (SLOS).[253] A defect in cholesterol biosynthesis affects patients with SLOS and is associated with severe growth and developmental retardation. Cholesterol is an important component of myelin and other cell membranes and has recently been implicated in the activation of the important signaling protein sonic hedgehog. Irons et al. initiated prenatal therapy by providing the fetus with cholesterol contained in frozen plasma to arrest some of the adverse consequences of cholesterol deficiency.[253] In their case, they performed three sequential *in utero* transfusions in a patient with SLOS and were able to show that these transfusions resulted in increased fetal plasma cholesterol, as measured by cordocentesis. Cordocentesis has been undertaken for *in utero* exchange transfusion in a case of homozygous alpha-thalassemia.[254] Intrauterine platelet transfusion in cases of alloimmune thrombocytopenia has already been discussed. Weinblatt et al. also reported use of intrauterine platelet transfusion in the antenatal management of TAR syndrome.[256]

Antenatal intravascular pharmacologic therapy may be advantageous when the transplacental passage of an indicated drug is poor (e.g., digoxin in hydropic fetuses with supraventricular tachycardia) or when the drug must be administered as a bolus (e.g., adenosine in persistent supraventricular tachycardia resistant to digoxin). Cordocentesis may also be used to guide fetal therapy administered through the amniotic fluid, as in the treatment of fetal hypothyroidism. Noia et al. reported the use of cordocentesis to diagnose hypothyroidism in a fetus with a goiter, which persisted despite maternal treatment, and resolution of the goiter after intraamniotic administration of levothyroxine.[256] Subsequent case reports have described further experience with the use of cordocentesis to guide intrauterine therapy for fetal hypothyroidism.[257–259]

Another exciting application of access to the fetal circulation is therapy *in utero,* particularly of inherited disorders amenable to treatment with bone marrow transplantation. Whereas extensive animal data are available to suggest that stem cells transplanted earlier in gestation are associated with a lower risk of rejection, human data are limited.[260–262]

REFERENCES

1. Valenti C. Endoamnioscopy and fetal biopsy; a new technique. *Am J Obstet Gynecol.* 1972;114:561.
2. Hobbins JC, Mahoney MJ. In utero diagnosis of hemoglobinopathies: Techniques for obtaining fetal blood. *N Engl J Med.* 1974;290:1065.
3. Rodeck CH, Campbell S. Umbilical cord insertion as a source of pure fetal blood for prenatal diagnosis. *Lancet.* 1979;1:1244.
4. Daffos F, Capella-Pavlovsky M, Forestier F. A new procedure for fetal blood sampling in utero: Preliminary results of fifty-three cases. *Am J Obstet Gynecol.* 1983;152:47.
5. Hobbins JC, Grannum PA, Romero R, et al. Percutaneous umbilical cord blood sampling. *Am J Obstet Gynecol.* 1985;152:47.
6. Daffos F, Capella-Pavlovsky M, Forestier F. Fetal blood sampling during pregnancy with use of a needle guided by ultrasound: A study of 606 consecutive cases. *Am J Obstet Gynecol.* 1985;153:655.
7. Forestier F, Daffos F, Galacteros F. Hematological values of 163 normal fetuses between 18 and 30 weeks of gestation. *Pediatr Res.* 1986;20:342.
8. Daffos F, Forestier F, Capella-Pavlovsky M, et al. Prenatal management of 746 pregnancies at risk for congenital toxoplasmosis. *N Engl J Med.* 1988;318:271.
9. Weiner CP. Cordocentesis for diagnostic indications: Two years' experience. *Obstet Gynecol.* 1987;70:664.
10. Ludomirsky A. Intrauterine fetal blood sampling—A multicenter registry: Evaluation of 7462 procedures between 1987–1991 (abstract 69). *Am J Obstet Gynecol.* 1993;168:318.
11. Megerian G, Ludomirsky A. Role of cordocentesis in perinatal medicine. *Curr Opin Obstet Gynecol.* 1994;6:30.
12. Bodeus M, Hubinont C, Bernard P, et al. Prenatal diagnosis of human cytomegalovirus by culture and polymerase chain reaction: 98 pregnancies leading to congenital infection. *Prenat Diagn.* 1999;19:314.
13. Mouly F, Mirlesse V, Meritet JF, et al. Prenatal diagnosis of fetal varicella-zoster virus infection with polymerase chain reaction of amniotic fluid in 107 cases. *Am J Obstet Gynecol.* 1997;177:894.
14. Crombach G, Picard F, Beckmann M, et al. Fetal rhesus D genotyping on amniocytes in alloimmunised pregnancies using fluorescence duplex polymerase chain reaction. *Br J Obstet Gynaecol.* 1997;104:15.
15. Van Den Veyver IB, Subramanian SB, Hudson KM, et al. Prenatal diagnosis of the RhD fetal blood type on amniotic fluid by polymerase chain reaction. *Obstet Gynecol.* 1996;87:419.
16. D'Alton ME, Malone FD, Chelmow D, et al. Defining the role of fluorescence in situ hybridization on uncultured amniocytes for prenatal diagnosis of aneuploidies. *Am J Obstet Gynecol.* 1997;176:769.
17. Morris A, Boyd E, Dhanjal S, et al. Two years' prospective experience using fluorescence in situ hybridization on uncultured amniotic fluid cells for rapid prenatal diagnosis of common chromosomal aneuploidies. *Prenat Diagn.* 1999;19:546.
18. Benecerraf BR, Barss VA, Saltzman DH, et al. Acute fetal distress associated with percutaneous umbilical blood sampling. *Am J Obstet Gynecol.* 1987;145:1218.
19. Boulot P, Deschamps F, Lefort G, et al. Pure fetal blood samples obtained by cordocentesis: Technical aspects of 322 cases. *Prenat Diagn.* 1990;10:93.
20. Sonek J, Nicolaides K, Sadowsky G, et al. Articulated needle guide: Report on the first 30 cases. *Obstet Gynecol.* 1989;74:821.
21. Weiner CP, Wenstrom KD, Sipes SL, et al. Risk factors for cordocentesis and fetal intravascular transfusion. *Am J Obstet Gynecol.* 1991;165:1020.
22. Bovicelli L, Orsini LF, Grannum PAT, et al. A new funipuncture technique: Two needle ultrasound and needle biopsy-guided procedure. *Obstet Gynecol.* 1989;73:428.
23. Devore GR, Venus I, Hobbins JC, et al. Fetoscopy: General clinical approach. In: Rocker I, Laurence KM, eds. *Fetoscopy.* Amsterdam: Elsevier/North Holland Biomedical Press; 1981:60.
24. Romero R, Hobbins JC, Mahoney MJ. Fetal blood sampling and fetoscopy. In: Milunsky A, ed. *Genetic Disorders and the Fetus: Diagnosis, Prevention, and Treatment.* New York: Plenum; 1986:579.
25. Forestier F, Cox WL, Daffos F, et al. The assessment of fetal blood sample. *Am J Obstet Gynecol.* 1988;158:1184.
26. Nicolaides KH, Clewell WH, Rodeck CH. Measurement of human fetoplacental blood volume in erythroblastosis fetalis. *Am J Obstet Gynecol.* 1987;157:50.
27. Nicolini U, Santolaya J, Ojo OE, et al. The fetal intrahepatic

umbilical vein as an alternative to cord needling for prenatal diagnosis and therapy. *Prenat Diagn.* 1988;8:665.

28. Nicolini U, Nicolaides P, Fisk NM, et al. Fetal blood sampling from the intrahepatic vein: Analysis of safety and clinical experience with 214 procedures. *Obstet Gynecol.* 1990;76:47.

29. Sturgiss SN, Wright C, Davison JM, et al. Fetal hepatic necrosis following blood sampling from the intrahepatic vein. *Prenat Diagn.* 1966;16:866.

30. Zosmer N, Vaughan J, Fisk NM. Fetal blood sampling from intrahepatic vein versus cord insertion: Effect on pH and blood gases. *Obstet Gynecol.* 1993;82:504.

31. Antsaklis AI, Papantoniou NE, Mesogitis SA, et al. Cardiocentesis: An alternative method of fetal blood sampling for the prenatal diagnosis of hemoglobinopathies. *Obstet Gynecol.* 1992;79:630.

32. Westgreen M, Selbing A, Staugenbert M. Fetal intracardiac transfusions in patients with severe rhesus isoimmunization. *Br Med J.* 1988;295:885.

33. Lazebnik N, Hendrix PV, Ashmead GG, et al. Detection of fetal blood contamination by amniotic fluid obtained during cordocentesis. *Am J Obstet Gynecol.* 1990;163:78.

34. Chao A, Herd JP, Tabsh KMA. The ferning test for detection of amniotic fluid contamination in umbilical blood samples. *Am J Obstet Gynecol.* 1990;172:1207.

35. Timor-Tritsch IE, Yeh MN. In vitro training model for diagnostic and therapeutic fetal intravascular needle puncture. *Am J Obstet Gynecol.* 1987;157:858.

36. Angel JL, O'Brien WF, Michelson JA, et al. Instructional model for percutaneous fetal umbilical blood sampling. *Obstet Gynecol.* 1989;73:669.

37. Soothill PW, Nicolaides KH, Rodeck CH, et al. Blood gases and acid–base status of the human second-trimester fetus. *Obstet Gynecol.* 1986;68:173.

38. Mandelbrot L, Guillaumont M, Leclercq M, et al. Placental transfer of vitamin K and its implications in fetal hemostasis. *Thromb Haem.* 1988;60:39.

39. Daffos F, Forestier F. Pharmacologic antenatale. In: Daffos F, Forestier F, eds. *Medicine et Biologie due Foetus Humain.* Paris: Maloine; 1988:431.

40. Daffos F. Fetal blood sampling. *Annu Rev Med.* 1989;40:319.

41. Maxwell DJ, Johnson P, Hurley P, et al. Fetal blood sampling and pregnancy loss in relation to indication. *Br J Obstet Gynecol.* 1991;98:892.

42. Ludomirsky A, Weiner S, Ashmead GG, et al. Percutaneous fetal umbilical blood sampling: Procedure safety and normal fetal hematologic indices. *Am J Perinatol.* 1988;5:264.

43. Wilkins I, Mezrow G, Lynch L, et al. Amnionitis and life-threatening respiratory distress after percutaneous umbilical blood sampling. *Am J Obstet Gynecol.* 1989;160:427.

44. Ghidini A, Sepulveda W, Lockwood CJ, et al. Complications of fetal blood sampling. *Am J Obstet Gynecol.* 1993;179:1339.

45. Orlandi F, Damiani G, Jakil C, et al. The risks of early cordocentesis (12–21 weeks): Analysis of 500 procedures. *Prenat Diagn.* 1990;10:425.

46. Hogge WA, Ghiagarajah S, Brenbridge AN, et al. Fetal evaluation by the percutaneous blood sampling. *Am J Obstet Gynecol.* 1988;158:132.

47. Weiner CP, Wenstrom KD, Sipes SL, et al. Risk factors for cordocentesis and fetal intravascular transfusion. *Am J Obstet Gynecol.* 1991;165:1020.

48. Daffos F, Forestier F, Kaplan C, et al. Prenatal diagnosis and management of bleeding disorders with fetal blood sampling. *Am J Obstet Gynecol.* 1988;158:939.

49. Rightmire DA, Ertmoed EE. Fetal exsanguination following umbilical cord blood sampling (abstract). *Am J Obstet Gynecol.* 1991;175:339.

50. Jauniaux E, Donner C, Simon P, et al. Pathologic aspects of the umbilical cord after percutaneous umbilical blood sampling. *Obstet Gynecol.* 1989;73:215.

51. Chenard E, Bastide A, Fraser WD. Umbilical cord hematoma following diagnostic funipuncture. *Obstet Gynecol.* 1990;76:994.

52. Moise KJ Jr, Carpenter RK Jr, Huhta JC, et al. Umbilical cord hematoma secondary to *in utero* intravascular transfusion for Rh isoimmunization. *Fetal Ther.* 1987;2:65.

53. Keckstein G, Tschurtz S, Schneider V, et al. Umbilical cord haematoma as a complication of intrauterine intravascular blood transfusion. *Prenat Diagn.* 1990;10:59.

54. Ulm MR, Bettelheim D, Ulm B, et al. Fetal bradycardia following cordocentesis. *Prenat Diagn.* 1997;17:919.

55. Nicolini U, Kochenour NK, Greco P, et al. Consequences of feto-maternal hemorrhage following intrauterine transfusion. *Br Med J.* 1988;297:1379.

56. Bowell PJ, Selinger M, Ferguson J, et al. Antenatal fetal blood sampling for the management of alloimmunized pregnancies: Effect upon maternal anti-D potency levels. *Br J Obstet Gynaecol.* 1988;95:759.

57. Weiner C, Grant S, Hudson J, et al. Effect of diagnostic and therapeutic cordocentesis on maternal serum α-fetoprotein concentration. *Am J Obstet Gynecol.* 1989;161:706.

58. Feinkind L, Nanda D, Delke I, et al. Abruptio placentae after percutaneous umbilical cord sampling: A case report. *Am J Obstet Gynecol.* 1990;162:1203.

59. Chitrit Y, Caubel P, Lusina D, et al. Detection and measurement of fetomaternal hemorrhage following diagnostic cordocentesis. *Fetal Diagn Ther.* 1998;13:253.

60. Campbell WA, Vintzileos AM, Nochimson DJ. Intrauterine versus extrauterine management. Resuscitation of the fetus/neonate. *Clin Obstet Gynecol.* 1986;29:33.

61. Patriarco MS, Viechnicki VM, Hutchinson TA, et al. A study on intrauterine fetal resuscitation with terbutaline. *Am J Obstet Gynecol.* 1987;157:384.

62. Nicolaides KH, Rodeck CH. In utero resuscitation after cardiac arrest in fetus. *Br Med J.* 1984;288:900.

63. Shalev E, Peleg D. Fetal cardiac resuscitation. *Lancet.* 1993;341:305.

64. Ash KM, Mibashan RS, Nicolaides KH. Diagnosis and treatment of feto-maternal hemorrhage in a fetus with homozygous von Willebrand's disease. *Fetal Ther.* 1988;3:189.

65. Benitz WE, Frankel LR, Stevenson DK. The pharmacology of neonatal resuscitation and cardiopulmonary intensive care. Part I: Extended intensive care. *West J Med.* 1986;145:47.

66. Podobnik M, Ciglar S, Singer Z, et al. Transabdominal chorionic villus sampling in the second and third trimesters of high-risk pregnancies. *Prenat Diagn.* 1997;17:125.

67. Smidt-Jensen S, Lundsteen C, Lind AM, et al. Transabdominal chorionic villus sampling in the second and third trimesters of pregnancy: Chromosome quality, reporting time, and feto-maternal bleeding. *Prenat Diagn.* 1993;13:957.

68. Cameron AD, Murphy KW, McNay MB, et al. Midtrimester chorionic villus sampling: An alternative approach? *Am J Obstet Gynecol.* 1994;171:1035.

69. Eydoux P, Choiset A, Le Porrier N, et al. Chromosomal prenatal diagnosis: Study of 936 cases of intrauterine abnormalities after ultrasound assessment. *Prenat Diagn*. 1989;9:235.

70. Nicolaides KH, Rodeck CH, Gosden CM. Rapid karyotyping in non-lethal fetal malformations. *Lancet*. 1986;1:283.

71. Williamson RA, Weiner CP, Patil S, et al. Abnormal pregnancy sonograph: Selective indication for fetal karyotype. *Obstet Gynecol*. 1987;69:15.

72. Rizzo N, Pittalis MC, Pilu G. Prenatal karyotyping in malformed fetuses. *Prenat Diagn*. 1990;10:17.

73. Shah DM, Roussis P, Ulm J, et al. Cordocentesis for rapid karyotyping. *Am J Obstet Gynecol*. 1990;162:1548.

74. Brady K, Polzin WJ, Kopelman JN, et al. Risk of chromosomal abnormalities in patients with idiopathic polyhydramnios. *Obstet Gynecol*. 1992;79:234.

75. Shipp TD, Bromley B, Pauker S, et al. Outcome of singleton pregnancies with severe oligohydramnios in the second and third trimesters. *Ultrasound Obstet Gynecol*. 1996;7:108.

76. Peakman DC, Moreton MF, Corn BJ, et al. Chromosomal mosaicism in amniotic fluid cell cultures. *Pediatr Res*. 1978;12:455.

77. Hsu LYF, Perlis TE. United States survey on chromosome mosaicism and pseudomosaicism in prenatal diagnosis. *Prenat Diagn*. 1985;4:97.

78. Benn PA, Hsu LYF, Perlis TE, et al. Prenatal diagnosis of chromosome mosaicism. *Prenat Diagn*. 1984;4:1.

79. Gosden C, Nicolaides KH, Rodeck CH. Fetal blood sampling in investigation of chromosome mosaicism in amniotic fluid cell culture. *Lancet*. 1988;1:613.

80. Kaffe S, Benn PA, Hsu LYF. Fetal blood sampling in investigation of chromosome mosaicism in amniotic fluid cell culture. *Lancet*. 1988;2:284.

81. Bui TH, Iselius L, Lindstein J. European collaborative study on prenatal diagnosis: Mosaicism, pseudo-mosaicism and single abnormal cells in amniotic fluid cell cultures. *Prenat Diagn*. 1984;4:145.

82. Worton RG, Stern RA. Canadian collaborative study of mosaicism in amniotic fluid cell cultures. *Prenat Diagn*. 1984;4:131.

83. Watson MS, Breg WR, Hobbins JC, et al. Cytogenetic diagnosis using midtrimester fetal blood samples: Application to suspected mosaicism and other diagnostic problems. *Am J Med Genet*. 1984;19:805.

84. Brown WT, Houck G, et al. Rapid fragile X carrier screening and prenatal diagnosis using a nonradioactive PCR test. *JAMA*. 1993;270:1569.

85. Thilaganathan B, Carroll SG, Plachouras N, et al. Fetal immunological and haematological changes in intrauterine infection. *Br J Obstet Gynaecol*. 1994;102:418.

86. Hohlfeld P, Vial Y, Maillard-Brignon C, et al. Cytomegalovirus fetal infection: Prenatal diagnosis. *Obstet Gynecol*. 1991;78:615.

87. Daffos F, Forestier F, Lynch L, et al. Fetal infectious diseases. In: Harman CR, ed. *Invasive Fetal Testing and Treatment*. Cambridge, MA. Blackwell Publications; 1994:79.

88. Skvorc-Ranko R, Lavoie H, St Denis P, et al. Intrauterine diagnosis of cytomegalovirus and rubella infections by amniocentesis. *Can Med Assoc J*. 1991;145:649.

89. Lynch L, Daffos F, Emanuel D, et al. Prenatal diagnosis of fetal cytomegalovirus infection. *Am J Obstet Gynecol*. 1991;165:714.

90. Hogge WA, Buffonte GJ, Hogge JS. Prenatal diagnosis of cytomegalovirus (CMV) infection: A preliminary report. *Prenat Diagn*. 1993;13:131.

91. Donner C, Liesard C, Content J, et al. Prenatal diagnosis of 52 pregnancies at risk for congenital cytomegalovirus infection. *Obstet Gynecol*. 1993;82:481.

92. Catanzarite V, Dankner WM. Prenatal diagnosis of congenital cytomegalovirus infection: False-negative amniocentesis at 20 weeks' gestation. *Prenat Diagn*. 1993;13:1021.

93. Donner C, Liesnard C, Brancart F, et al. Accuracy of amniotic fluid testing before 21 weeks' gestation in prenatal diagnosis of congenital cytomegalovirus infection. *Prenat Diagn*. 1994;14:1055.

94. Lamy ME, Mulongo KN, Gadisseux J-F, et al. Prenatal diagnosis of fetal cytomegalovirus infection. *Am J Obstet Gynecol*. 1992;166:91.

95. Cuthbertson G, Weiner CP, Gilles RH, et al. Prenatal diagnosis of second trimester congenital varicella syndrome by virus-specific immunoglobulin M. *J Pediatr*. 1987;111:592.

96. Hohlfeld P, Daffos F, Costa JM, et al. Prenatal diagnosis of congenital toxoplasmosis with a polymerase-chain reaction test on amniotic fluid. *N Engl J Med*. 1994;331:695.

97. Cazenave J, Forestier F, Bessieres MH, et al. Contribution of a new PCR assay to the prenatal diagnosis of congenital toxoplasmosis. *Prenat Diagn*. 1992;12:119.

98. Grover CM, Thulliez P, Remington JS, et al. Rapid prenatal diagnosis of congenital toxoplasma infection by using polymerase chain reaction and amniotic fluid. *J Clin Microbiol*. 1990;28:2297.

99. Jenum PA, Holberg-Petersen M, Melby KK, et al. Diagnosis of congenital *Toxoplasma gondii* infection by polymerase chain reaction (PCR) on amniotic fluid samples. The Norwegian experience. *APMIS*. 1998;106:680.

100. Johnson JD, Butcher PD, Savva D, et al. Application of the polymerase chain reaction to the diagnosis of human toxoplasmosis. *J Infect*. 1993;26:147.

101. Hezard N, Marx-Chemla C, Foudrinier F, et al. Prenatal diagnosis of congenital toxoplasmosis in 261 pregnancies. *Prenat Diagn*. 1997;17:1047.

102. Revello MG, Baldanti F, Sarasini A, et al. Prenatal diagnosis of rubella virus infection by direct detection and semiquantitation of viral RNA in clinical samples by reverse transcription–PCR. *J Clin Microbiol*. 1997;35:708.

103. Lipitz S, Yagel S, Shalev E, et al. Prenatal diagnosis of fetal primary cytomegalovirus infection. *Obstet Gynecol*. 1997;89:763.

104. Pletcher BA, Williams MK, Mulivor RA, et al. Intrauterine cytomegalovirus infection presenting as fetal meconium peritonitis. *Obstet Gynecol*. 1991;78:903.

105. Mouly F, Mirlesse V, Meritet JF, et al. Prenatal diagnosis of fetal varicella-zoster virus infection with polymerase chain reaction of amniotic fluid in 107 cases. *Am J Obstet Gynecol*. 1997;177:894.

106. Knisely AS, O'Shea PA, McMillan P, et al. Electron microscopic identification of parvovirus virions in erythroid-line cells in fatal hydrops fetalis. *Pediatr Pathol*. 1988;8:163.

107. Public Health Laboratory Service Working Party on Fifth

Disease. Prospective study of human parvovirus (B19) infection in pregnancy. *Br Med J*. 1990;300:1166.

108. Torok TJ. Human parvovirus B19 infection in pregnancy. *Pediatr Infect Dis J*. 1990;9:772.

109. Schwarz TF, Nerlich A, Hottentrager B, et al. Parvovirus B19 infection of the fetus: Histology and in situ hybridization. *Am J Clin Pathol*. 1991;96:121.

110. Torok TJ, Wang QY, Gary GW, et al. Prenatal diagnosis of intrauterine infection with parvovirus B19 by the polymerase reaction technique. *Clin Infect Dis*. 1992;14:149.

111. Porter HJ, Khong TY, Evans MF, et al. Parvovirus as a cause of hydrops fetalis: Detection by in situ DNA hybridization. *J Clin Pathol*. 1988;41:381.

112. Naides SJ, Weiner CP. Antenatal diagnosis and palliative treatment of non-immune hydrops fetalis secondary to fetal parvovirus B-19 infection. *Prenat Diagn*. 1989;9:105.

113. Humphrey W, Magoon M, O'Shaughnessy R. Severe nonimmune hydrops secondary to parvovirus B-19 infection: Spontaneous reversal in utero and survival of a term infant. *Obstet Gynecol*. 1991;78:900.

114. Morey AL, Nicolini U, Welch CR, et al. Parvovirus B19 infection and transient fetal hydrops. *Lancet*. 1991;337:496.

115. Pryde PG, Nugent CE, Prodjian G, et al. Spontaneous resolution of nonimmune hydrops fetalis secondary to human parvovirus B19 infection. *Obstet Gynecol*. 1992;79:859.

116. Sheikh AU, Ernest JM, O'Shea M. Long-term outcome in fetal hydrops from parvovirus B19 infection. *Am J Obstet Gynecol*. 1992;167:337.

117. Brown KE, Green SW, de Mayolo JA, et al. Congenital anemia after transplacental B19 parvovirus infection. *Lancet*. 1994;343:895.

118. Salimans MMM, van de Rijke FM, Raap AK, et al. Detection of parvovirus DNA in fetal tissues by in situ hybridization and polymerase chain reaction. *J Clin Pathol*. 1989;42:525.

119. Sahakian V, Weiner CP, Naides SJ, et al. Intrauterine transfusion treatment of nonimmune hydrops fetalis secondary to human parvovirus B10 infection. *Am J Obstet Gynecol*. 1991;164:1090.

120. Kovacs BW, Carlson DE, Shahbahrami B, et al. Prenatal diagnosis of human parvovirus B19 in nonimmune hydrops fetalis by polymerase chain reaction. *Am J Obstet Gynecol*. 1992;167:461.

121. Gentilomi G, Zerbini M, Gallinella G, et al. B19 parvovirus induced fetal hydrops: Rapid and simple diagnosis by detection of B19 antigens in amniotic fluids. *Prenat Diagn*.1998;18:363.

122. Schild RL, Bald R, Plath H, et al. Intrauterine management of fetal parvovirus B19 infection. *Ultrasound Obstet Gynecol*. 1999;13:161.

123. Van den Berg B, Oeshsli FW. Prematurity. In: Bracken MB, ed. *Perinatal Epidemiology*. London: Oxford University Press; 1984:69.

124. Kessel SS, Villar J, Berendes HW, et al. The changing pattern of low birth weight in the United States (1970 to 1980). *JAMA*. 1984;251:1978.

125. Main DM, Main EK. Management of preterm labor and delivery. In: Gabbe SG, Niebyl J, Simpson JL, eds. *Obstetrics: Normal and Problem Pregnancies*. New York: Churchill Livingston; 1986:689.

126. Rush RW, Keirse MJNC, Howat P, et al. Contribution of preterm delivery to perinatal mortality. *Br Med J*. 1976;2:965.

127. Gomez R, Ghezzi F, Romero R, et al. Premature labor and intra-amniotic infection: Clinical aspects and role of the cytokines in diagnosis and pathophysiology. *Clin Perinatol*. 1995;22:281.

128. Arias F, Rodriquez L, Rayne S, et al. Maternal placental vasculopathy and infection: Two distinct subgroups among patients with preterm labor and preterm ruptured membranes. *Am J Obstet Gynecol*. 1993;168:585.

129. Duff P, Kopelman J. Subclinical intra-amniotic infection in asymptomatic patients with refractory preterm labor. *Obstet Gynecol*. 1987;69:756.

130. Romero R, Sirtori M, Oyarzun E, et al. Infection and labor. Prevalence, microbiology, and clinical significance of intraamniotic infection in women with preterm labor and intact membranes. *Am J Obstet Gynecol*. 1989;161:817.

131. Romero R, Yoon BH, Mazor M, et al. The diagnostic and prognostic value of amniotic fluid white blood cell count, glucose, interleukin-6 and Gram stain patients with preterm labor and intact membranes. *Am J Obstet Gynecol*. 1993;169:805.

132. Romero R, Quintero R, Oyarzun E, et al. Intra-amniotic infection and the onset of labor in preterm premature rupture of membranes. *Am J Obstet Gynecol*. 1988;159:661.

133. Feinstein S, Vintzileos A, Lodeiro J, et al. Amniocentesis with premature rupture of membranes. *Obstet Gynecol*. 1986;68:147.

134. Romero R, Yoon BH, Mazor M, et al. A comparative study of the diagnostic performance of amniotic fluid glucose, white blood cell count, interleukin-6, and gram stain in the detection of microbial invasion in patients with preterm premature rupture of membranes. *Am J Obstet Gynecol*. 1993;169:839.

135. Gomez R, Romero R, Ghezzi F, et al. The fetal inflammatory response syndrome. *Am J Obstet Gynecol*. 1998;179:194.

136. Romero R, Gomez R, Ghezzi F, et al. A fetal systemic inflammatory response is followed by the spontaneous onset of preterm parturition. *Am J Obstet Gynecol*. 1998;179:186.

137. Yoon BH, Romero R, Jun JK, et al. An increase in fetal plasma cortisol but not dehydroepiandrosterone sulfate is followed by the onset of preterm labor in patients with preterm premature rupture of the membranes. *Am J Obstet Gynecol*. 1998;179:1107.

138. Carroll SG, Papaioannou S, Davies ET, et al. Maternal assessment in the prediction of intrauterine infection in preterm prelabor amniorrhexis. *Fetal Diagn Ther*. 1995;10:290.

139. Rainaut M, Pagniez M, Hercent T, et al. Characterization of mononuclear cell subpopulations in normal fetal peripheral blood. *Hum Immunol*. 1987;18:331.

140. Linch DC, Beverley PCL, Levinsky RJ, et al. Phenotypic analysis of fetal blood leukocytes: Potential for prenatal diagnosis of immunodeficiency disorders. *Prenat Diagn*. 1982;2:211.

141. Durandy A, Oury C, Griscelli C, et al. Prenatal testing for inherited immune deficiencies by fetal blood sampling. *Prenat Diagn*. 1982;102:995.

142. Hirschhorn R. Prenatal diagnosis of adenosine deaminase deficiency and selected other immunodeficiencies. In: Milunsky A, ed. *Genetic Disorders and the fetus: Diagnosis, Prevention, and Treatment,* vol 3. Baltimore: Johns Hopkins University Press; 1992:453.

143. Diukman R, Tanigawara S, Cowan MJ, et al. Prenatal diagnosis of Chediak–Higashi syndrome. *Prenat Diagn*. 1992;12:877.

144. Durandy A, Cerf-Bensussan N, Dumez Y, et al. Prenatal diagnosis of severe combined immunodeficiency with

defective synthesis of HLA molecules. *Prenat Diagn.* 1987; 7:27.

145. Linch DC, Beverley CL, Levinsky R, et al. Prenatal diagnosis of three cases of severe combined immunodeficiency: Severe T cell deficiency during the first half of gestation in fetuses with adenosine deaminase deficiency. *Clin Exp Immunol.* 1984;56:223.

146. Newburger PE, Cohen HJ, Rothchild SB, et al. Prenatal diagnosis of granulomatous disease. *N Engl J Med.* 1979;300:178.

147. Borregaard N, Bang J, Berthelsen JG, et al. Prenatal diagnosis of chronic granulomatous disease. *Lancet.* 1982;1:114.

148. Matthay KK, Golbus MS, Wara DW, et al. Prenatal diagnosis of chronic granulomatous disease. *Am J Med Genet.* 1984;17:731.

149. Bussel J. Minutes of the Neonatal Subcommittee of the International Committee of Thrombosis and Hemostasis Working Party on Neonatal Alloimmune Thrombocytopenia. Brussels, Belgium; 1987.

150. Rosendaal FR, Brocker-Briends AHJT, van Houwelingen JC, et al. Sex ratio of the mutation frequencies in haemophilia A: Estimation of meta-analysis. *Hum Genet.* 1990;86:139.

151. Peake IR, Lillicrap DP, Boulyjenkov V, et al. Hemophilia: Strategies for carrier detection and prenatal diagnosis. *Bull WHO.* 1993;71:429.

152. Kazazian HH. The molecular basis of hemophilia A and the present status of carrier and antenatal diagnosis of the disease. *Thromb Haemost.* 1993;70:60.

153. Goodeve AC, Preston FE, Peake IR. Factor VIII gene rearrangements in patients with severe haemophilia A. *Lancet.* 1994;343:329.

154. Sacchi E, Randi AM, Tagliavacca L, et al. Carrier detection and prenatal diagnosis of hemophilia A: 5 Years' experience at a hemophilia center. *Int J Clin Lab Res.* 1992;21:310–313.

155. Kemahli S, Goldman E, McCraw A, et al. Value of DNA analysis with multiple DNA probes for the detection of hemophila A carriers. *Pediatr Hematol Oncol.* 1994;11:55.

156. Aseev M, Curin V, Baboev K, et al. Allele frequencies and molecular diagnosis in haemophilia A and B patients from Russia and from some Asian republics of the former USSR. *Prenat Diagn.* 1994;14:513.

157. Ljung RCR. Prenatal diagnosis of haemophilia. *Bailliere Clin Haematol.* 1996;9:243.

158. Ljung RCR. Prenatal diagnosis of haemophilia. *Haemophilia.* 1999;5:84.

159. Firshein SI, Hayer LW, Lazarchick J, et al. Prenatal diagnosis of classic hemophilia. *N Engl J Med.* 1979;300:937.

160. Mibashan RS, Rodeck CH, Thumpstaon JK, et al. Plasma assay of fetal factors VIIIC and IX for prenatal diagnosis of hemophilia. *Lancet.* 1979;2:1309.

161. Peake IR, Bloom AL, Giddings JC, et al. An immunoradiometric assay for procoagulant factor VIIIAg: Results in hemophilia, von Willebrand's disease and fetal plasma and serum. *Br J Haematol.* 1979;42:269.

162. Mibashan RS, Rodeck CH. Haemophilia and other genetic defects of haemostatis. In: Rodeck CH, Nicolaides KH, eds. *Prenatal Diagnosis. Proceedings of the Eleventh Study Group of the Royal College of Obstetricians and Gynaecologists.* Chichester, England;1984;179.

163. Kasper CK, Osterud B, Minami J, et al. Hemophilia B: Characterization of genetic variants and detection of carriers. *Blood.* 1977;50:351.

164. Tagliavacca L, Sacchi E, Mannucci PM. Carrier detection and feasibility of prenatal diagnosis of hemophila B by multiplex polymerase chain reaction. *Int J Clin Lab Res.* 1993;23: 169.

165. Caprino D, Acquila M, Mori PG. Carrier detection and prenatal diagnosis of hemophilia B with more advanced techniques. *Ann Hematol.* 1993;67:289.

166. Holmberg L, Gustavi B, Cordesius E, et al. Prenatal diagnosis of hemophilia B by an immunoradiometric assay of factor IX. *Blood.* 1980;56:397.

167. Young JH, Wang JC, Gau JP, Hu HT. Prenatal and molecular diagnosis of hemophilia B. *Am J Hematol.* 1996;52:243.

168. Hoyer LW, Lindsten J, Blomback RM, et al. Prenatal evaluation of a fetus at risk for von Willebrand's disease. *Lancet.* 1979;2:191.

169. Cook RL, Miller RC, Katz VL, et al. Immune thrombocytopenic purpura in pregnancy: A reappraisal of management. *Obstet Gynecol.* 1991;78:578.

170. Scioscia AL, Grannum PA, Copel JA, et al. The use of percutaneous umbilical blood sampling in immune thrombocytopenic purpura. *Am J Obstet Gynecol.* 1988;72:346.

171. Moise KJ Jr, Carpenter RJ Jr, Cotton DB, et al. Percutaneous umbilical cord blood sampling in the evaluation of fetal platelet counts in pregnant patients with autoimmune thrombocytopenic purpura. *Obstet Gynecol.* 1988;72:346.

172. Weiner C. Cordocentesis and immune thrombocytopenia. *Am J Obstet Gynecol.* 1990;163:1371.

173. Kelton JG. Management of the pregnant patient with idiopathic thrombocytopenic purpura. *Ann Intern Med.* 1983;99:796.

174. Ayromlooi J. A new approach to the management of immunologic thrombocytopenic purpura in pregnancy. *Am J Obstet Gynecol.* 1978;130:235.

175. Berry S, Leonardi MR, Wolfe HM, et al. Maternal thrombocytopenia: Predicting neonatal thrombocytopenia with cordocentesis. *J Reprod Med.* 1997;42:276.

176. DeVries LS, Connell J, Bydder GM, et al. Recurrent intracranial hemorrhages *in utero* in an infant with alloimmune thrombocytopenia. *Br J Obstet Gynaecol.* 1988;985:299.

177. Burrows RR, Caco CC, Kelton JG. Neonatal alloimmune thrombocytopenia: Spontaneous *in utero* intracranial hemorrhage. *Am J Hemotol.* 1988;28:98.

178. Kaplan C, Daffos F, Forestier F, et al. Management of alloimmune thrombocytopenia: Antenatal diagnosis and *in utero* transfusion of maternal platelets. *Blood.* 1988;72:340.

179. Bussel JB, Berkowitz RL, McFarland JG, et al. Antenatal treatment of neonatal alloimmune thrombocytopenia. *N Eng J Med.* 1988;319:1374.

180. Herman HJ, Jumbelic MI, Ancona RJ, et al. *In utero* cerebral hemorrhage in alloimmune thrombocytopenia. *Am J Pediatr Hematol Oncol.* 1985;8:312.

181. Porcelijn L, Kanhai HH. Fetal thrombocytopenia. *Curr Opin Obstet Gynecol.* 1998;10:117.

182. Seventh International Conference on Fetal Physiology and Fetal Blood Sampling. Philadelphia; October 1992.

183. Giovangrandi Y, Daffos F, Kaplan C, et al. Very early intracranial haemorrhage in alloimmune fetal thrombocytopenia. *Lancet.* 1990;336:310.

184. Nicolini U, Rodeck CH, Kochenour NK, et al. *In utero* platelet transfusion for alloimmune thrombocytopenia. *Lancet.* 1988;2:506.

185. Kay HH, Hage ML, Kurtzberg J, et al. Alloimmune

thrombocytopenia may be associated with system disease. *Am J Obstet Gynecol.* 1992;166:110.

186. Lynch L, Bussel JB, McFarland JG, et al. Antenatal treatment of alloimmune thrombocytopenia. *Obstet Gynecol.* 1992;80:67.

187. Donnenfeld AE, Wiseman B, Lavi E, et al. Prenatal diagnosis of thrombocytopenia absent radius syndrome by ultrasound and cordocentesis. *Prenat Diagn.* 1990;19:29.

188. Rothschild C, Forestier F, Daffos F, et al. Prenatal diagnosis in type IIA von Willebrand disease. *Nouv Rev Fr Hematol.* 1990;32:125.

189. Gruel Y, Boizard B, Daffos F, et al. Determination of platelet antigens and glycoproteins in the human fetus. *Blood.* 1987;68:488.

190. Eady RAJ, Gunner DB, Tidman MT, et al. Prenatal diagnosis of oculocutaneous albinism by electron microscopy of fetal skin. *J Invest Dermatol.* 1983;80:210.

191. Shimizu H, Ishiko A, Kikuchi A, et al. Prenatal diagnosis of tyrosinase-negative oculocutaneous albinism. *Lancet.* 1992;340:739.

192. Schwartz M, Mibashan RS, Nicolaides KH, et al. First trimester diagnosis of Wiskott-Aldrich by DNA markers. *Lancet.* 1989;2:1405.

193. Durandy A, Breton-Gorius J, Guy-Grand D, et al. Prenatal diagnosis of syndromes associating albinism and immune deficiencies. *Prenat Diagn.* 1993;13:13.

194. Lebo RV, Saiki RK, Swanson K, et al. Prenatal diagnosis of α-thalassemia by polymerase chain reaction and dual restriction enzyme analysis. *Hum Genet.* 1990;85:293.

195. Alter BP. Prenatal diagnosis of hemoglobinopathies: Development of methods for study of fetal red cells and fibroblasts. *Am J Pediatr Hematol.* 1985;5:378.

196. Old JM. Haemoglobinopathies. Community clues to mutation detection. In: Elles R, ed. *Methods in Molecular Medicine, Molecular Diagnosis of Genetic Diseases.* Totowa, NJ: Humana Press; 1996:169.

197. Weatherall DJ, Old JM, Thein SL, et al. Prenatal diagnosis of the common haemoglobin disorders. *J Med Genet.* 1985;22:422.

198. Steinberg M. DNA diagnosis for the detection of sickle hemoglobinopathies. *Am J Hematol.* 1993;43:110.

199. Kazazian HH, Boehm C. Molecular basis and prenatal diagnosis of beta-thalassemia. *Blood.* 1988;72:1107.

200. Kazazian HH. Prenatal diagnosis of beta-thalassemia. *Semin Perinatol.* 1991;15:15.

201. Lindeman R, Hu SP, Volpato F, et al. Polymerase chain reaction (PCR) mutagenesis enabling rapid non-radioactive detection of common beta-thalassaemia mutations in Mediterraneans. *Br J Haematol.* 1991;78:100.

202. Bilardo CM, Nocolaides KH. Cordocentesis in the assessment of the small-for-gestational age fetus. *Fetal Ther.* 1988;3:24.

203. Weiner CP, Williamson RA. Evaluation of severe growth retardation using cordocentesis—Hematologic and metabolic alterations by etiology. *Obstet Gynecol.* 1989;73:225.

204. Economides DL, Crook D, Nicolaides KH. Hypertriglyceridemia and hypoxemia in small for gestational age fetuses. *Am J Obstet Gynecol.* 1990;162:382.

205. Nicolini U, Nicolaidis P, Fisk NM, et al. Limited role of fetal blood sampling in prediction of outcome in intrauterine growth retardation. *Lancet.* 1990;336:768.

206. Pardi G, Cetin I, Marconi AM, et al. Diagnostic value of blood sampling in fetuses with growth retardation. *N Engl J Med.* 1993;328:692.

207. Cetin I, Corbetta C, Sereni LP, et al. Umbilical amino acid concentrations in normal and growth-retarded fetuses sampled in utero by cordocentesis. *Am J Obstet Gynecol.* 1990;162:253.

208. Bernardini I, Evans MI, Nicolaides KH, et al. The fetal concentrating index as a gestational age-independent measure of placental dysfunction in intrauterine growth retardation. *Am J Obstet Gynecol.* 1991;164:1481.

209. Economides DL, Nicolaides KH, Gahl WA, et al. Plasma amino acids in appropriate-and small-for-gestational-age fetuses. *Am J Obstet Gynecol.* 1989;161:1219.

210. Cox WL, Daffos F, Forestier F, et al. Physiology and management of intrauterine growth retardation: A biologic approach with fetal blood sampling. *Am J Obstet Gynecol.* 1988;159:36.

211. Maier RF, Bohme K, Dudenhausen JW, et al. Cord blood erythropoietin in relation to different markers of fetal hypoxia. *Obstet Gynecol.* 1993;81:575.

212. Economides DL, Nicolaides KH, Campbell S. Metabolic and endocrine findings in appropriate and small for gestational age fetuses. *J Perinat Med.* 1991;19:97.

213. Westgren M, Lingman G, Persson B. Cordocentesis in IUGR fetuses. *Clin Obstet Gynecol.* 1997;40:755.

214. Ostlund E, Bang P, Hagenas L, Fried G. Insulin-like growth factor I in fetal serum obtained by cordocentesis is correlated with intrauterine growth retardation. *Hum Reprod.* 1997;12:1840.

215. Thrope-Beeston JG, Nicolaides KH, Snijders RJM, et al. Thyroid function in small for gestational age fetuses. *Obstet Gynecol.* 1991;77:701.

216. Van den Hof N, Nicolaides KH. Platelet count in normal, small, and anemic fetuses. *Am J Obstet Gynecol.* 1990;172:735.

217. Nicolaides KH, Economides DL, Soothill PW. Blood gases, pH, and lactate in appropriate-and small-for gestational age fetuses. *Am J Obstet Gynecol.* 1989;151:996.

218. Soothill PW, Nicolaides KH, Bilardo CM, et al. Relation of fetal hypoxia in growth retardation to mean blood velocity in the fetal aorta. *Lancet.* 1987;2:1118.

219. Bilardo CM, Nicolaides KKH, Campbell S. Doppler measurements of fetal and uteroplacental circulations: Relationship with umbilical venous blood gases measured at cordocentesis. *Am J Obstet Gynecol.* 1990;162:115.

220. Visser GHA, Sadovsky G, Nicolaides KH. Antepartum heart rate patterns in small-for-gestation-age third-trimester fetuses: Correlations with blood gas values obtained at cordocentesis. *Am J Obstet Gynecol.* 1990;162:698.

221. Ribbert LSM, Snijders RJM, Nicolaides KH, et al. Relationship of fetal biophysical profile and blood gas values at cordocentesis in severely growth-retarded fetuses. *Am J Obstet Gynecol.* 1990;153:569.

222. Manning FA, Snijders R, Harman CR, et al. Fetal biophysical profile score. *Am J Obstet Gynecol.* 1993;1169:755.

223. Nicolaides KH, Soothill PW, Rodeck CH, et al. Ultrasound guided sampling of umbilical cord and placental blood to assess fetal well-being. *Lancet.* 1987;1:1065.

224. Pardi G, Guscaglia M, Ferrazzi E, et al. Cord sampling for the evaluation of oxygenation and acid–base in growth-retarded human fetuses. *Am J Obstet Gynecol.* 1987;157:1221.

225. Nicolini U, Rodeck CH. Fetal blood and tissue sampling. In: Brock DJH, Rodeck CH, Ferguson-Smith MA, eds. *Prenatal*

Diagnosis and Screening. New York: Churchill-Livingstone; 1992:39.

226. Shalev E, Blondheim O, Peleg D. Use of cordocentesis in the management of preterm or growth-restricted fetuses with abnormal monitoring. *Obstet Gynecol Surv*. 1995;50:839.

227. Shah DM, Boehm FH. Fetal blood gas analysis from cordocentesis for abnormal fetal heart rate patterns. *Am J Obstet Gynecol*. 1989;161:374.

228. Soothill PW, Ajayi RA, Campbell S, et al. Relationship between fetal acidemia at cordocentesis and subsequent neurodevelopment. *Ultrasound Obstet Gynecol*. 1992;2:80.

229. Cox WL, Forestier F, Capella-Pavlovsky M, et al. Fetal blood sampling in twin pregnancies. *Fetal Ther*. 1987;2:101.

230. Robertson EG, Neer KJ. Placental injection studies in twin gestation. *Am J Obstet Gynecol*. 1983;147:170.

231. Blickstein I. The twin–twin transfusion syndrome: What are appropriate diagnostic criteria? *Am J Obstet Gynecol*. 1989;161:365.

232. Rausen AR, Seki M, Strauss L. Twin transfusion syndrome. *J Pediatr*. 1965;66:613.

233. Danskin FH, Neilson JP. Twin-to-twin transfusion syndrome: What are appropriate diagnostic criteria? *Am J Obstet Gynecol*. 1989;161:365.

234. Saunders NJ, Snijders RJM, Nicolaides KH. Twin–twin transfusion syndrome during the 2nd trimester is associated with small intertwin hemoglobin differences. *Fetal Diagn Ther*. 1991;6:34.

235. Bruner JP, Rosemond RL. Twin-to-twin transfusion syndrome: A subset of the twin oligohydramnios-polyhydramnios sequence. *Am J Obstet Gynecol*. 1993;169:925.

236. Puder KS, Berry SM, Bottoms SF, et al. Intrauterine hematologic findings in twins with normal and abnormal growth (abstract). *Am J Obstet Gynecol*. 1990;170:400.

237. Fisk NM, Borrell A, Hubinont C, et al. Fetofetal transfusion syndrome: Do the neonatal criteria apply in utero? *Arch Child Dis*. 1990;65(suppl 7):657.

238. Lemery DR, Santolaya-Forgas J, Serre AF, et al. Fetal erythropoietin in twin pregnancies with discordant growth. *Fetal Diagn Ther*. 1995;10:86.

239. Berry SM, Puder KS, Bottoms SF, et al. Comparison of intrauterine hematologic and biochemical values between twin pairs with and without stuck twin syndrome. *Am J Obstet Gynecol*. 1995;172:1403.

240. Saunders NJ, Snijders RJM, Nicolaides KH. Twin–twin transfusion syndrome during the 2nd trimester is associated with small intertwin hemoglobin differences. *Fetal Diagn Ther*. 1991;6:34.

241. Okamura K, Murotsuki J, Kosuge S, et al. Diagnostic use of cordocentesis in twin pregnancy. *Fetal Diagn Ther*. 1994;9:385.

242. Quintero RA, Reich H, Puder KS, et al. Operative fetoscopy: A new frontier in fetal medicine (abstract). *Am J Obstet Gynecol*. 1994;170:297.

243. Evans MI, Golberg JD, Dommergues M, et al. Efficacy of second trimester selective termination for fetal abnormalities: International collaborative experience among the world's largest centers. *Am J Obstet Gynecol*. 1994;171:90.

244. Aberg A, Metelman F, Cantz M, et al. Cardiac puncture of fetus with Herler's disease avoiding abortion of unaffected co-twin. *Lancet*. 1978;2:990.

245. Chitkara U, Berkowitz RL, Wilkins IA, et al. Selective second-trimester termination of the anomalous fetus in twin pregnancies. *Obstet Gynecol*. 1989;73:690.

246. Kerenyi TD, Chitkara U. Selective birth in twin pregnancy with discordancy for Down syndrome. *N Engl J Med*. 1981; 304:1525.

247. Rodeck CH. Fetoscopy in the management of twin pregnancies discordant for a severe abnormality. *Acta Genet Med Gemmellol*. 1985;33:57.

248. Wittman BK, Farquharson DF, Thomas WDS, et al. The role of feticide in the management of severe twin transfusion syndrome. *Am J Obstet Gynecol*. 1987;155:1023.

249. Skupski DW, Wolf CF, Bussel JB. Fetal transfusion therapy. *Obstet Gynecol Surv*. 1996;51:181.

250. Weiner CP. Diagnosis and treatment of twin to twin transfusion in the mid-second trimester of pregnancy. *Fetal Ther*. 1987;2:71.

251. Peters MT, Nicolaides KH. Cordocentesis for the diagnosis and treatment of human fetal parvovirus infection. *Obstet Gynecol*. 1990;75:501.

252. Schild RL, Bald R, Plath H, et al. Intrauterine management of fetal parvovirus B19 infection. *Ultrasound Obstet Gynecol*. 1999;13:161.

253. Irons MB, Nores J, Stewart TL, et al. Antenatal therapy of Smith–Lemli–Opitz syndrome. *Fetal Diagn Ther*. 1999;14:133.

254. Fung TY, Lau TK, Tam WH, Li CK. In utero exchange transfusion in homozygous alpha-thalassemia: A case report. *Prenat Diagn*. 1998;18:838.

255. Weinblatt M, Petrikovsky B, Bialer M, et al. Prenatal evaluation and in utero platelet transfusion for thrombocytopenia absent radii syndrome. *Prenat Diagn*. 1994;14: 892.

256. Noia G, DeSantis M, Toci A, et al. Early prenatal diagnosis and therapy of fetal hypothyroid goiter. *Fetal Diagn Ther*. 1992;7:138.

257. Abuhamad AZ, Fisher DA, Warsof SL, et al. Antenatal diagnosis and treatment of fetal goitrous hypothyroidism: Case report and review of the literature. *Ultrasound Obstet Gynecol*. 1995;6:368.

258. Hadi HA, Strickland D. In utero treatment of fetal goitrous hypothyroidism caused by maternal Graves' disease. *Am J Perinatol*. 1995;12:455.

259. Vicens-Calvet E, Potau N, Carreras E, et al. Diagnosis and treatment in utero of goiter with hypothyroidism caused by iodide overload. *J Pediatr*. 1998;133:147.

260. Crombleholme TM, Langer JC, Harrison MR, et al. Transplantation of fetal cells. *Am J Obstet Gynecol*. 1991;175:218.

261. Linch DC, Rodeck CH, Nicolaides K, et al. Attempted bone-marrow transplantation in a 17-week fetus. *Lancet*. 1987;2: 1453.

262. Touraine JL, Raudrant D, Royo C, et al. In-utero transplantation of stem cells in bare lymphocyte syndrome. *Lancet*. 1989;1:1382.

30

Ultrasound-Guided Fetal Invasive Therapy:

Current Status

Frank A. Manning

The rapid development of high-quality dynamic fetal imaging methods now permits the recognition of discrete developmental anomalies of fetal organ systems at an even earlier gestational age. It is now possible to monitor the progression of such anomalies in concert to determine their structural and functional sequelae. The observation of the "natural" history of anomalies has prompted the development of innovative, if largely unproven, invasive methods for averting the otherwise inevitable outcome.

Invasion of the fetal environment with therapeutic intent, although not a new concept in perinatal medicine (having been successfully practiced in alloimmunization syndromes since the landmark reports of Liley and Bowman),[1,2] has undergone a resurgence in interest and application. There are now many forms of invasive fetal therapy yielding a range of proven and unproven benefits. The most well-established form of invasive fetal therapy is fetal intravascular transfusion: This treatment of the alloimmunized anemic fetus has yielded an amazing reduction in mortality and morbidity (see Chap. 25). An extension of this principle to replace missing or abnormal cell lines (stem cell therapy), gene products, or genes themselves is an area of active and promising research but falls outside the scope of this summary.

Invasive intrauterine maneuvers designed to overcome intrinsic anomalous obstruction of fluid dynamics have been the object of intensive clinical study. In some conditions, such as simple obstructive uropathies, these therapies have yielded results that strongly suggest a true therapeutic benefit. In other instances, such as obstructive hydrocephalus, the benefits, if any, of *in utero* diversion therapies are much more obscured. The bulk of this chapter deals with these two sets of obstructive disorders, the data being derived from the International Fetal Medicine and Surgery Society Registry.[3] In other conditions, such as to menigomyelocoele aggressive, *in utero* surgical repair has been attempted; the number of cases to date is so few that comment on efficacy is currently unwarranted.

FETAL UROPATHY: FREQUENCY AND PATHOPHYSIOLOGY (FIG. 30–1)

Developmental anomalies of the fetal urinary tract are among the most commonly recognized congenital anomalies.[4,5] The incidence of lethal renal anomalies in the Manitoba study population is between 0.3 and 0.7 per 1000 live births. Dynamic ultrasound imaging allows for assessment of both the structural and functional characteristics of the developing fetal urinary tract. Ultrasound assessment of the spectrum of congenital disease of the fetal urinary tract is neither simple nor direct, and diagnostic accuracy depends to a large degree on the experience of the ultrasonographer and the quality of the equipment used. Serious diagnostic errors with this method have been reported.[6–8] Fortunately, the risk of diagnostic error is least with lower tract (outlet) obstructive uropathies,[6,7] which is the area of major concern to fetal surgeons.

In the normal fetus, the kidneys may be seen from as early as 12 weeks' gestation. As gestational age advances, renal mass and internal architecture become progressively well defined. With newer high-resolution ultrasound equipment,

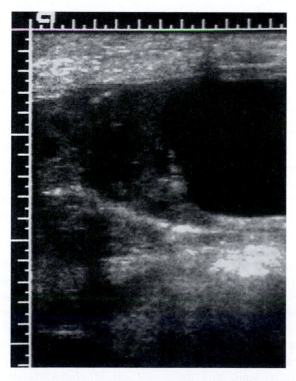

Figure 30–1. A sonogram of the thorax and abdomen in the parasagittal plane in a fetus with lower obstructive uropathy secondary to posterior urethral valves. The fetal bladder is massively enlarged (megalocystis), distending the fetal abdomen and compressing the intraabdominal organ. Note the inverse curve of the diaphragm and the compression of the heart and lungs. A fetus with these findings should be considered a candidate for *in utero* chronic vesicoamniotic shunting.

the renal arteries and arcuate arteries may be seen after 20 weeks of gestation, and renal blood flow patterns can be assessed. The fetal bladder is seen from as early as 14 weeks of gestation, and micturition pattern may be recorded as an indirect means of assessing fetal urine production rates.[9] In the male fetus, the external genitalia are usually recognized with certainty at about 16 to 20 weeks of gestation, and turbulence created by fetal voiding is often observed. Because fetal urine production is a major contributor to amniotic fluid volume in later pregnancy,[10] ultrasound assessment of amniotic fluid adequacy provides an important insight into the adequacy of renal function.

There is a very wide spectrum of congenital fetal uropathies ranging from complete absence of functioning renal tissue (renal agenesis) to minor and often transient dilation of the renal pelvis. Although undetermined with certainty at present, it theoretically seems that few of these urinary tract diseases would benefit from *in utero* therapeutic maneuvers. At the time of writing, the diseases deemed amenable to fetal surgical diversion are restricted to those that produce bladder outlet obstruction, primarily urethral valve syndromes, urethral atresia, or possibly persistent cloacal syndromes.

It is evident from ovine fetal experiments that obstruction of the outflow tract produces pathologic renal changes, the extent and nature of which vary with the fetal age at obstruction. Ureteral ligation late in pregnancy in fetal sheep (22 weeks is the human equivalent) produces simple hydronephrosis, whereas earlier obstruction (13 to 19 weeks is the human equivalent) produces changes suggestive of renal dysplasia.[11,12] Ureteral occlusion in late gestation (29 weeks is the human equivalent) causes simple hydronephrosis; in earlier gestation (16 weeks is the human equivalent), it causes unequivocal renal dysgenesis. Lethal pulmonary hypoplasia may be a complication with obstruction at either age.[13–16] Of major importance is the observation that subsequent release of experimental obstruction halts the progression of both the renal and pulmonary effects.[14,15] These are landmark experiments because they provide insight into the pathogenesis of renal lesions and provide a rational basis for consideration of *in utero* urinary diversion therapy in the affected human fetus.

The spectrum of outcomes in human fetuses with outlet obstruction fits reasonably well with these experimental models. When total obstruction occurs in very early human pregnancy, the most common result may be renal dysgenesis/agenesis and pulmonary hypoplasia, a uniformly lethal fetal condition. Lethal renal dysgenesis secondary to outlet obstruction in early human pregnancies has been reported.[8] The obstruction also can be either anatomically partial or anatomically complete but rendered functionally partial due to gross dilation of the fetal bladder, ureters, and urachus, producing a less severe effect on the developing kidneys and lungs. Spontaneous cure of total obstructive uropathy can occur *in utero* by a pressure effect at the site of obstruction (e.g., type I mucosal hypertrophy posterior urethral valve), by bladder rupture and urinary ascites,[17] or by urachal cyst formation and subsequent rupture into the amniotic space. We have observed spontaneous resolution of outlet obstruction uropathy due to persistent cloacal syndrome by the latter mechanism (F. A. Manning, C. R. Harman, and S. Menticoglou, unpublished data, 1986). These experiments of nature appear to confirm that release of obstruction of the outflow tract can halt the natural progression of the renal and pulmonary effects of such obstruction.

OBSTRUCTIVE UROPATHY: NATURAL HISTORY

The natural history of bladder outlet obstruction remains the critical and key unanswered question. Persistent absence of renal function *in utero* as may occur with anatomic (renal agenesis) or functional (severe renal dysgenesis) defects frequently results in fetal death. The mechanisms are assumed to be cord compression secondary to gross oligohydramnios. What proportion of any fetuses with outlet obstruction present in this manner is unknown, but it is probably relatively high. The outcome of fetuses with outlet obstruction of either later onset or a less severe functional form appears to be highly variable. Many of these fetuses die *in utero*, again most likely a consequence of oligohydramnios, but some will deliver alive, often prematurely. The natural (untreated) outcome of fetal lower urinary tract obstructive uropathy can be estimated from 79 cases submitted to the International Fetal Surgery Registry or reported in the literature (Table 30–1). Only 5 of these 79 fetuses (6.3%) survived. The survival rate of neonates born with posterior urethral valves differs from that reported for fetuses with the same condition. Nakayama et al.[18] identified 11 neonates in whom the diagnosis of posterior urethral valves was made *at birth*. Because these neonates were subjected to aggressive resuscitative measures, it may be assumed that this population represents only a portion of those perinates born with the condition. Others may have been denied the resuscitative measures because of the observed anomalies at birth. Five of these anomalous fetuses died (45%), either within hours (three cases) or days (two cases), from respiratory insufficiency due to proven (four cases) or assumed (one case) pulmonary hypoplasia. All of the infants who perished exhibited extreme oligohydramnios.

TABLE 30–1. FETAL OBSTRUCTIVE UROPATHY: NATURAL HISTORY

No. of cases	79
Average age at diagnosis	23 weeks (18–29)
Average age at delivery	34 weeks (19–40)
PN mortality	93.7% (*n* = 74)
Therapeutic abortion	6.5% (10%)
Survivors	6.3% (*n* = 5)

PN, postnatal.
Source: International Fetal Medicine and Surgery Society Registry, 1994.

These data, when compared with outcome data of similar fetuses treated *in utero,* reveal a nearly twofold difference in mortality (45 to 22.8% mortality, respectively).[3]

The survival rates for posturethral valve syndrome in both treated fetuses and neonates are much lower than those reported among older children with this condition.[19] The powerful influence of natural selection in the prenatal period no doubt accounts for these differences.[18] The long-term morbidity among survivors in the two groups also differs sharply. All untreated survivors with this condition exhibited serious morbidity. Four of six survivors had prolonged respiratory insufficiency suggestive of sublethal pulmonary hypoplasia, and five of six survivors had signs of chronic renal impairment, as shown by azotemia, defects in fixed acid excretion, and growth failure. In contrast, none of the 16 survivors of *in utero* therapy exhibited clinical signs of respiratory insufficiency, and only one has developed chronic renal failure. The long-term outcomes of these cases are, of course, unknown and must be determined because late-onset renal disease has been described with this condition.[19]

Comparison of outcome data between these somewhat similar groups presents a powerful argument for the benefits of *in utero* surgery for this specific condition, posterior urethral valve syndrome. It may be argued that in view of the serious nature of the condition of the newborn, the disease *in utero* is unlikely to be less severe. Whether or not such comparisons establish the benefit of *in utero* therapy beyond a reasonable doubt remains debatable. Definitive scientific evidence can only be garnered by a prospective trial in which diagnosed *in utero* cases are randomly assigned to a treated or nontreated category. However, the rather clear experimental evidence in animals delineating the pathophysiology of the condition, the observed differences in perinatal outcome between treated fetuses and neonates born with the condition, and the anecdotal reports of successful outcome in treated fetuses all suggest the therapy is beneficial among selected cases.

A second critical natural selection process becomes operative in the immediate postnatal period. The successful transition from fetal to neonatal life depends critically on the rapid establishment of adequate pulmonary function. Pulmonary hypoplasia, a common sequela of severe obstruction uropathy, prevents this successful transition. What proportion of liveborns with obstructive uropathy are lost at birth as a result of this lethal natural selection process is also unknown, but two separate observations suggest this proportion may be high. The International Fetal Surgery Registry report described the outcome of 79 liveborn infants with obstructive uropathy treated *in utero*; 34 of these 79 (43%) died in the immediate newborn period from pulmonary hypoplasia.[3] Nakayama et al.[18] described the outcome in 11 liveborn infants with obstructive uropathy (posterior urethral valve syndrome) evident at birth; 5 of the 11 (45%) died in the immediate neonatal period from pulmonary hypoplasia.[18] The prognosis for those affected perinates who survive these two powerful selection periods, the fetal and immediate neonatal, improves dramatically. Survival rates of up to 95% have been reported for infants with obstructive uropathy (posterior urethral valve syndrome) who survive the immediate neonatal period.[19]

It is this range of outcomes created by natural selection that accounts for much of the controversy surrounding indications for and efficacy of fetal surgical diversion therapy for obstructive uropathy. There is experimental and serendipitous clinical evidence that release of fetal urinary tract obstruction can halt the progression of renal and pulmonary sequelae. The major challenge for fetal surgeons lies in case selection, specifically in the differentiation of those perinates who will die from disease in the fetal and immediate neonatal periods from those perinates who will survive to benefit from postnatal therapy. The secondary challenge is to devise effective therapeutic maneuvers to ensure maximal continued benefit to the selected at-risk fetus with minimal risk to the mother.

FETAL SURGERY: CASE SELECTION CRITERIA AND METHODS

Selection of the fetuses who will benefit from *in utero* surgical urinary tract diversion procedures is achieved by application of rigid exclusion criteria. The working guidelines are discussed in the following paragraphs.

First, the affected fetus must be immature. Despite the optimistic enthusiasm of the fetal surgeon, there can be little doubt that neonatal repair of obstructive uropathies will almost always be a safer and more definitive procedure. Therefore, as the first principle, the fetus of sufficient age and maturity to sustain extrauterine survival should never be a candidate for *in utero* surgery.

Second, the obstruction must be sustained and associated with deterioration and damage. Therapy should only be considered in the fetus with bladder outlet obstruction and bilateral progressive renal disease. The primary aim of therapy is to prevent both renal and pulmonary sequelae. Penetrating the fetus with a needle, even when done by an experienced operator using the most sophisticated ultrasound guidance systems, is not without risk. Obstetricians have accumulated a great deal of experience with needle penetration of the fetal peritoneal cavity and less experience with bladder puncture. For either method, the fetal death rate directly attributable to the procedure is about 5%.[3,20] Therefore, the issues must not be whether or not therapy is possible, for it nearly always is, but rather if such therapy will benefit the fetus and if the potential benefit outweighs any real fetal risk. Against this background, the justification for prenatal therapy for unilateral disease as has been reported[21,22] may be lacking, although in some cases an apparent amelioration of associated maternal disease has been described.[22]

Third, the fetus must be otherwise normal. The fetus with both obstructive uropathy and some other organ system(s) structural anomaly or karyotypic anomaly should not be considered a candidate for prenatal therapy. Such an association is not uncommon; of 98 treated cases reported to the International Fetal Surgery Registry, 8 (8.1%) had multiple organ system anomalies and 8 (8.1%) had karyotypic anomalies. Thus, 16 of 98 fetuses (16.3%) had lethal anomalies, a rate that is 15 to 30 times higher than that of the general population. Although maternal morbidity has not been described as a complication of *in utero* therapy for obstructive uropathy, severe maternal morbidity or death has been caused by other invasive intrauterine procedures, such as amniocentesis[23] and intrauterine transfusion.[24] Serious and potentially life-threatening maternal infection (chorioamnionitis) can occur as a consequence of diagnostic or therapeutic maternal percutaneous placement of a fetal bladder catheter.[25] Therefore, it follows that a detailed and complete ultrasound fetal organ system review should be a prerequisite to any therapeutic efforts. In theory, such a review should detect all associated structural anomalies; in practice, the detection rate is about 90%.[26] Confirmation that the affected fetus being considered for therapy has a normal karyotype has been a difficult problem because the traditional diagnostic method, amniocentesis for amniocyte culture, requires waiting up to 4 weeks for results. Further, in the presence of oligohydramnios, a frequent associated finding with obstructive uropathy, an amniotic fluid sample may not be obtainable. In such cases, fetal urine obtained by vesicocentesis may yield sufficient cells for culture,[27] but the reliability of this method is not uniform and considerable delay is involved. The new technique of direct fetal umbilical vein blood sampling,[28,29] yielding karyotype results as early as within 2 days, can most certainly circumvent these problems.

Fourth, amniotic fluid volume does not predict outcome. The relation between amniotic fluid volume, as estimated by ultrasound, and outcome in fetuses with obstructive uropathy is nuclear. Hence, the use of this variable for case selection remains controversial. Because fetal urine production is a major contributor to the dynamic amniotic fluid compartment in later pregnancy,[8] it follows that significant fetal obstructive disease should be associated with a reduction or absence of amniotic fluid (oligohydramnios). The data contained in the International Fetal Surgery Registry do not support this supposition. The majority of fetuses with obstructive uropathy do have oligohydramnios (78%), but the survival rates are similar among treated fetuses with or without oligohydramnios (41 and 40%, respectively).[3] Further, perinatal death due to pulmonary hypoplasia is observed among fetuses with obstructive uropathy and apparent normal amniotic fluid volume.

The discrepancy between the predicted and observed relationships of amniotic fluid volume to perinatal outcome in fetuses with obstructive uropathy may be due to a variety of factors. Amniotic fluid volume determination by ultrasound is often done by subjective assessment, and the use of objective criteria, such as the largest fluid pocket measurement, has not been uniform.[30] With such subjective conditions, the true relationship remains uncertain. Alternately, in fetuses with partial or incomplete obstruction, there may be sufficient outflow impedance to cause proximal dilation and damage even though urine efflux may be sufficient to maintain some amniotic fluid.

Fifth, adequate fetal lung tissue must be present. Pulmonary hypoplasia is by far the most common cause of perinatal death in obstructive uropathies, accounting for most deaths among treated pregnancies.[3] Chronic oligohydramnios, both in the experimental animal model and in the human, is associated with an increased incidence of lethal pulmonary hypoplasia.[31,32] It is tempting to suggest that the high incidence of pulmonary hypoplasia seen in fetuses with obstructive uropathy is, therefore, caused by this oligohydramnios. In the experimental animal model, reversal of experimental oligohydramnios restores lung growth and prevents pulmonary hypoplasia.[31] A similar recovery of lung growth is seen with corrected experimental obstructive uropathy.[12] The clinical human experience also clearly indicates that *in utero* diversion therapy, resulting in restoration of normal amniotic fluid volume, may be associated with intact survival, even in the presence of pretreatment extreme oligohydramnios.[27,33] Thus, despite reported opinions to the contrary,[34] there is simply no evidence that oligohydramnios is a contraindication to therapy; however, the observation of lethal pulmonary hypoplasia with obstructive uropathy even in the presence of normal amniotic fluid volume indicates there must be more than one etiologic factor for pulmonary hypoplasia. Intrinsic pulmonary compression due to bladder and urinary tract dilation may be another cause; diaphragmatic hernia, either experimental or clinical, is known to cause pulmonary hypoplasia by the same method.[35] In such circumstances, urinary tract decompression by *in utero* diversion therapy may be expected to enhance lung growth and, therefore, improve survival.

An alternate explanation for the association of lung and urinary tract anomalies is that the primary insult, the nature of which remains entirely unknown, affects the endodermal lung primordia and the mesodermal genitourinary primordia simultaneously. Such a mechanism, although possible, is viewed as highly unlikely because most teratogens affect either all germ cell layers or a single layer, but rarely, if ever, do they affect only two of the three layers. Nonetheless, if such a mechanism is indeed operant, then the theoretic arguments for urinary tract diversion to prevent pulmonary hypoplasia are without foundation.

Pulmonary Hypoplasia: Ultrasound Diagnosis

Determination of volume and functional capacity and the noninflated, fluid-filled fetal lung is difficult and lacks complete precision. The best contemporary method for diagnosis of pulmonary hypoplasia is measurement of chest circumference by ultrasound. Fetal chest circumference is measured at the level of the cardiac atrioventricular valves. There is a linear relationship between chest circumference and gestational age,[36] and an observed failure of normal chest growth portends pulmonary hypoplasia.[37] A fetal chest circumference that measures below the fifth percentile for gestational age predicts pulmonary hypoplasia in about 95% of cases (positive predictive accuracy) but will miss the diagnosis in about 7% of cases (negative predictive accuracy 93%).[38] The relation between the incidence and character of fetal breathing movements and pulmonary hypoplasia is controversial. In an initial study Blott et al. reported the absence of fetal breathing to be predictive of pulmonary hypoplasia.[39] In contrast, Moessinger et al. noted breathing movements to be present in fetuses with a subsequent autopsy diagnosis of pulmonary hypoplasia.[40] Our experience, which now includes more than 70 perinates with lethal pulmonary hypoplasia, has failed to demonstrate any predictive value of either fetal breathing or sustained apnea (F. A. Manning, unpublished observation, 1994).

EVALUATION OF RENAL FUNCTION

Fetal urine is produced from as early as 9 weeks of gestation and is an ultrafiltrate of fetal serum, made hypotonic by selective tubular reabsorption of sodium and chloride, in excess of free water loss.[41] In experimental urinary tract observation, fetal kidneys damaged by long-standing disease, are "salt wasters," producing isotonic or hypertonic urine.[42]

Evaluation of fetal renal function is becoming an integral part of individual case selection. Temporary external drainage of the fetal bladder permits direct measurement of fetal urine production rate and estimates of fetal glomerular filtration rate by creatinine or iothalamate excretion and ongoing electrolyte composition.[41] The degree of invasion and the potential risks of leaving a direct connection to the fetus open at the maternal skin level mean that this continuous monitoring is of limited application. The mainstay of direct evaluation of fetal renal function, however, remains transcutaneous, ultrasound-directed decompression of the fetal bladder with a single, simple needle puncture. This provides urine for analysis of electrolytes, osmolarity, protein electrophoresis (notably β_2-microglobulin), amino acid concentration, as well as a potential for retrograde urography.

In 20 human fetuses referred for treatment of bilateral congenital hydronephrosis, Harrison et al. assessed the prognostic value of various criteria used to assess fetal renal functional potential[42] (Table 30–2). This evaluation included temporary placement of fetal bladder catheters, with exterioration to measure fetal urine output and composition. Fetuses were divided retrospectively into two groups: 10 cases with "poor function" based on severe renal dysplasia and pulmonary hypoplasia at autopsy or biopsy, or renal and pulmonary insufficiency at birth, and 10 cases with "good function" based on nondysplastic kidney at autopsy or biopsy, or "normal"

TABLE 30–2. PROGNOSTIC CRITERIA FOR FETUSES WITH BILATERAL OBSTRUCTIVE UROPATHY

Good Prognosis	Poor Prognosis[a]
Normal amniotic fluid volume	Severe oligohydramnios
Normal kidneys	Cystic kidneys
Sodium ≤ 100 mEq/L	Sodium ≥ 100 mEq/L or >95th percentile
Chloride ≤ 90 mEq/L	Chloride ≥ 90 mEq/L or >95th percentile
Osmolarity ≤ 210 mOsm/L	Osmolarity ≥ 210 mOsm/L
Urea > 4 mmol/L	Urea < 4 mmol/L
Calcium 1.6 mmol/L	Calcium > 1.75 mmol/L
β_2-Microglobulin 0 or trace	β_2-Microglobulin strong band

[a] If one or more are abnormal.

renal and pulmonary function at birth. Fetuses with "good" renal function tended to have normal amniotic fluid volume, normal kidneys on ultrasound examination, and hypotonic urine, with urinary sodium less than 100 mmol, chloride below 90, and urine osmolarity less than 210 mOsm/L. Fetuses with "poor" renal function tended to have decreased amniotic fluid volume, abnormal kidneys on ultrasound examination, and isotonic urine with urinary sodium concentration of more than 100, chloride above 90, and osmolarity greater than 210 mOsm/L. In their retrospective study those prognostic criteria were accurate in almost 90% of cases; however, when applied prospectively, the predictive value of those prognostic criteria suggested by Harrison et al. varies between 50 and 100%.[43–46]

Observation of the fetal urinary tract after drainage may be highly revealing. Indirect evidence of renal function (bladder filling and emptying, resolution of dilation in upper collecting systems, objective changes in amniotic fluid volume) *after* bladder drainage is valuable in assigning prognosis. Successful drainage of the grossly distended urinary tract will provide an opportunity for detailed evaluation of other fetal intraabdominal structures and review of the decompressed renal anatomy. For example, ultrasonic demonstration of renal cortical cysts, which would not resolve with drainage of the urinary tract, has a specificity of 100% and a sensitivity of 44% in identifying lethal renal dysplasia. Overall, no parameter or combination of factors is presently satisfactory for evidence of long-term renal competence.

Treatment of Obstructive Uropathy

As indicated, only those fetuses with proven obstructive uropathy of a persistent and progressive nature and with known immaturity are considered candidates for *in utero* diversion therapy. At our center, in addition to informed consent from both parents, case review and approval by a Fetal Therapy Committee, composed of a neonatologist, obstetrician, ultrasonographer, and members of the community at large, is required before the procedure is attempted.

Preoperative medications are based on a protocol tested extensively in patients requiring intrauterine fetal transfusion.[24] Prophylactic antibiotics (ampicillin 500 mg, cloxacillin 500 mg po tid) are begun the day before surgery and continued for a total duration of 48 h. Morphine (10 to 15 mg IM) and scopolamine (0.67 mg IM) are given to the mother about 1 h before the procedure to produce maternal and fetal sedation and analgesia. The procedure is done in an operating room with full aseptic technique.

Initially the fetal lie and bladder position are confirmed using a sterile ultrasound head. A fetal target site in the lower abdominal quadrant is identified, and the maternal surface abdominal wall coordinates are noted and marked. Two different methods for catheter placement are available: an overload system in which the catheter is loaded over a trocar and a hollow needle system in which the catheter is threaded down the needle shaft. In our center, we have abandoned the overload system because offloading of the catheter may be very difficult and because the catheter may "accordian" along the trocar shaft with attempts to offload. Our system involves a thin-walled, 17-gauge Toughy needle with a 15-degree angulation at the distal end. This needle is advanced under continuous ultrasound guidance to enter the fetal bladder; the position is confirmed by flow of urine, usually under some pressure. Confirmation that the needle tip is free in the bladder is confirmed by injection of 0.25 to 0.5 mL of air down the needle, and ultrasound observation of air bubbles within the bladder. A precut 3-French single- or double-pigtail Teflon catheter with spiral side holes is threaded on a wire guide and advanced through the needle. The catheter is cut so that at least 5 cm of catheter will protrude from the fetal abdomen into the amniotic sac. With the distal end of the catheter in the fetal bladder, the wire guide is withdrawn, allowing the pigtail to coil. The needle is then slowly withdrawn from the fetal abdomen while the catheter and guide wire are stabilized. As the needle tip leaves the fetus, the needle is tilted to maximize the angle within the fetal abdominal wall, and the guide wire is withdrawn. The needle is then slowly withdrawn as the catheter is advanced with the introducer. The precut proximal end drops from the needle tip into the amniotic cavity, thereby creating a chronic vesicoamniotic shunt. The proximal end of the catheter is the most difficult to place; care must be taken not to place the entire catheter within the fetal bladder or the proximal end within the fetal abdomen, thereby creating vesicoperitoneal shunt and fetal urinary ascites. Proximal catheter end placement is more difficult when oligohydramnios is present, but it may be accomplished. In severe oligohydramnios, it may be reasonable to leave the proximal end of the catheter in the myometrium, allowing for fetal movement to draw the end into the amniotic space. We have observed one fetus in which proper proximal end placement was achieved by this method.

Ultrasound is used to confirm successful catheter placement, and the changes observed are usually immediate and dramatic. Rapid bladder decompression and an increase in amniotic fluid volume or, in the case of preoperative oligo-hydramnios, the appearance of amniotic fluid, occurs within minutes of shunt placement. The proximal and distal ends of the catheter should be visible, and the area of transabdominal passage should be noted. Failure to see those characteristics within the first 15 mins after shunt procedure indicates improper placement and is an indication to repeat the procedure. Once a shunt is placed properly, it is essential to monitor shunt function frequently (once a week) because with fetal growth and movement, the proximal end may become dislodged or blocked. We have also observed one instance where the fetus apparently pulled the shunt from his abdomen. In the ideal case, vesicoamniotic shunt placement is a single short procedure. In our experience, however, the procedure can be difficult, and in one case was impossible despite several attempts. The number of separate attempts at shunt placement before the procedure is abandoned varies among operators; at our center we agreed that no more than four attempts in an individual patient would occur.

INVASIVE THERAPY FOR OBSTRUCTIVE UROPATHY: CLINICAL OUTCOME (TABLE 30–3)

As of January 1999, 98 cases of obstructive uropathy treated by *in utero* chronic placement of a vesicoamniotic shunt have been reported. In total, 30 of 73 cases (41%) survived for at least the neonatal period (28 days) and up to 4 years after treatment. Survival was best among fetuses with proven posterior urethral valve syndrome (71%) (see Table 30–3). Fifty-eight perinates died, of which 19 were still-births and 39 were neonatal deaths (Table 30–4). In 15 of 58 cases (25.9%), the pregnancy was electively terminated after shunt placement. In 7 of the 15 cases, pregnancy was terminated because of an abnormal karyotype result obtained after treatment. The chromosomal abnormalities recorded were trisomy 13 (three cases), trisomy 18 (two cases), tetraploidy (92,XXXX), and deletion of the large arm of chromosome 2. Seven pregnancies were terminated because of suspected major renal

dysfunction, which is shown by ultrasound demonstration of renal dysplasia. In the remaining 83 cases, pregnancy was ongoing after shunt placement. Forty of these fetuses survived (48.2%). Five perinatal deaths (three stillbirths) occurred as a direct consequence of fetal therapy yielding a procedure-related mortality of 8.6%.

Most neonatal deaths (34 of 39) were due to pulmonary hypoplasia. Two neonates died from pulmonary immaturity: labor in these perinates occurred after shunt placement. In one of the cases, there was overt chorioamnionitis present, and the mother had a complicated febrile postpartum course and recovered. These neonates ultimately died from renal failure.

Chronic morbidity in survivors was infrequent and occurred in 3 of 40 survivors (7.5%). One child with posterior urethral valve syndrome has developed chronic renal failure that requires treatment with hemodialysis, and this child is waiting for a renal transplant. Another survivor has borderline renal function and chronic pulmonary insufficiency evident at 2 years of age. A third child, a female, has persistent cloacal syndrome.

No obvious relationship between gestational age, either at time of diagnosis or treatment, and perinatal survival was noted (Table 30–5). Similarly, survival was not related to a subjective evaluation of the amniotic fluid volume. The survival rate in cases in which amniotic fluid was judged as

TABLE 30–4. FETAL OBSTRUCTIVE UROPATHY: CLASSIFICATION BY DEATH BY TIME AND ETIOLOGY ($n = 58$)

Etiology of Death	Time of Death		% of Death
	Stillbirth	Newborn	
Elective termination	15	0	25.9
Associated anomalies	1	0	1.7
Procedure related	3	2	8.6
Pulmonary hypoplasia	0	34	38.6
Renal disease	0	3	5.2
Total	19	39	—

TABLE 30–3. FETAL OBSTRUCTIVE UROPATHY: PRIMARY DIAGNOSIS AND OUTCOME IN 98 CASES

Primary Diagnosis	No. of Cases	% of Total	No. of Survivors	% Survival by Diagnosis
Posterior urethral valve syndrome	31	31.6	22	71
Karyotype abnormality	7	7.14	0	0
Renal dysplasia by ultrasound	6	6.12	0	0
Urethral atresia	8	8.2	1	12.5
"Prune-belly" syndrome	5	5.10	4	80
Cloacal anomalies	1	1.00	0	0
Ureteropelvic function obstruction	2	2.04	2	100
Unspecified etiology	38	37.8	11	28
Total	98	100	40	41

TABLE 30–5. FETAL OBSTRUCTIVE UROPATHY: OUTCOME BY GESTATIONAL AGE AT DIAGNOSIS AND TREATMENT

	At Diagnosis		At Treatment	
Gestational Age	No.	% Survival	No.	% Survival
16 to <24 weeks	61	36	51	27
24 to <29 weeks	18	50	24	54
≥29 weeks	19	48	23	56
Total	**98**	**41**	**98**	**41**

normal was 40.9% (9 of 22 cases), and survival with subjective oligohydramnios was 40.8% (31 of 76 cases).

The cumulative experience with chronic vesicoamniotic shunt placement in selected fetuses with persistent lower tract obstructive uropathy strongly suggests the treatment is indicated and beneficial. The comparison of survival rate between the 98 treated cases (41%) and the 79 historical controls (6.3%) is impressive, yielding a more than sixfold difference. Further, the frequency of chronic morbidity among treated survivors (7.5%) is encouragingly low. These comparisons need be interpreted with some caution because a case selection bias may be operant. The definitive resolution of the true benefit of fetal surgery for obstructive uropathy will require a prospective randomized clinical trial. Pending such a trial, fetal treatment at the present time would appear to be warranted and is recommended for selected cases.

OBSTRUCTIVE HYDROCEPHALUS: INVASIVE FETAL TREATMENT (FIG. 30–2)

Case Selection
Unlike obstructive uropathy, for which there are markers to define disease severity and predict postnatal prognosis, obstructive hydrocephalus remains primarily an ultrasound, morphologic diagnosis without additional biochemical or biophysical tests that are useful in assigning long-term prognosis. Further, irreversible brain damage associated with or resulting from obstructive hydrocephalus may not be lethal but may cause severe sustained postnatal morbidity.

Chronic Ventriculoamniotic Shunting
The method for placement of a chronic ventriculoamniotic shunt is similar to that for placement of the vesicoamniotic shunt. Under direct and continuous ultrasound guidance, the carrier needle is placed through the parietal bone and advanced into the dilated posterior horn of the lateral ventricle. Off-loading of the shunt initially places the distal end into the ventricle; then the needle is withdrawn outside the fetal calvaria, and the proximal end of the shunt is dropped into the amniotic cavity. The ventriculoamniotic shunt contains a one-way membrane valve to prevent reflux of amniotic fluid into the ventricular circulation and contains retaining flanges of anchorage.

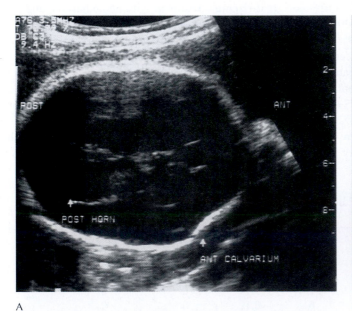

A

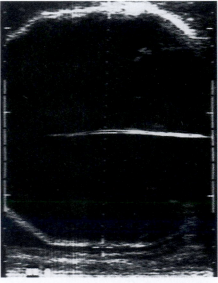

B

Figure 30–2. (A) Mild ventriculomegaly. This sonogram of the fetal head in the transverse plane demonstrates mild dilation of the ventricle (best seen in the far field) most evident in the posterior (occipital) horn. The presumed etiology was aqueductal stenosis. **(B)** Severe ventriculomegaly (hydrocephalus). In this sonogram of the fetal head in the transverse plane, there is overt enlargement and distortion (rounding) of the calvarium. The only recognizable structure is the falx. Note the separation of the folds of this structure. On dynamic scan the falx was noted to waver with fetal movement.

TABLE 30–6. FETAL OBSTRUCTIVE HYDROCEPHALUS: DISTRIBUTION BY PRIMARY DIAGNOSIS AND SURVIVAL IN 41 TREATED CASES

Primary Diagnosis (Postnatal)	No. of Cases	% of Total Cases	No. of Deaths	% Mortality by Diagnosis	No. of Survivors by Diagnosis	% Survival by Diagnosis
Aqueductal stenosis	32	76.9	4	13.3	28	87.5
Associated anomalies	5	12.7	2	40	3	60
Holoprosencephaly	1	2.6	1	100	0	0
Dandy–Walker syndrome	1	2.6	0	0	1	100
Porencephalic cyst	1	2.6	0	0	1	100
Arnold–Chiari malformation	1	2.6	0	0	1	100
Total	41	100	7		34	

Treatment of Fetal Obstructive Hydrocephalus: Clinical Data

Forty-one cases of fetal hydrocephalus treated by *in utero* surgical decompression have been reported.[3] Thirty-nine of these cases (95%) were treated by chronic ventriculoamniotic shunt placement, and two were treated by serial ventriculocentesis (three and six procedures per patient, respectively). The type of shunt used varied, but in most cases (39 of 44) a Silastic shunt with a one-way valve to prevent amniotic fluid reflux was used. In all cases, hydrocephalus was defined by progressive ventriculomegaly as determined by ultrasound monitoring of absolute ventricular size and the ventricular hemisphere size ratio. Distribution of cases by etiology of hydrocephalus as determined after delivery is listed in Table 30–6. The mean gestational age at the time of diagnosis was 25 ± 2.73 weeks (range 18 to 31 weeks). The mean gestational age at treatment was 27 ± 2.6 weeks (range 23 to 33 weeks). The duration of effective therapy cannot be determined because objective means of assessment of shunt function are not available.

Seven of 41 treated fetuses died (17%), one before birth and six after birth (see Table 30–6). The stillbirth occurred during attempts at shunt placement and was a direct result of needle trauma to the brainstem. Three of the six postnatal deaths were due to prematurity resulting from premature labor and delivery that occurred within 48 h of shunt placement. In each of these three cases, chorioamnionitis was suspected on clinical grounds but was confirmed by bacteriologic cultures in only one case (*Staphylococcus aureus,* coagulase negative). These four deaths (one stillbirth, three neonatal deaths) are considered a consequence of therapeutic attempts, giving a procedure-related mortality rate of 9.75%. The remaining three postnatal deaths were related to associated lethal anomalies, including one infant with holoprosencephaly, one infant with cranial–facial abnormalities and pulmonary hypoplasia, and one infant with arthrogryposis multiplex congenita.

The 34 surviving infants were followed for 8.2 ± 5.8 months (range 1 to 18 months) from the time of entry into the registry. Twelve of the 34 surviving fetuses (35.3%) had had aqueductal stenosis and were reported as normal at follow-up (mean follow-up duration 8.6 ± 6 months, range 1 to 18 months) (Table 30–7). The remaining 22 survivors exhibited different degrees of neurologic handicap. Four of the 34 survivors (11.76%) were classified as having mild to moderate handicap. In two of these infants, a delay in reaching developmental milestones was reported, and a developmental quotient was assessed as below 80. In the remaining child, the designation of mild to moderate handicap was due to a myelomeningocele-related lower limb paresis with apparent normal intellectual development at age 18 months. Eighteen of 34 surviving infants (52.9%) were classified as having severe handicap (mean follow-up duration 8 ± 5.7 months, range 3 to 18 months). All exhibited gross delay in reaching

TABLE 30–7. FETAL OBSTRUCTIVE HYDROCEPHALUS: OUTCOME IN 34 TREATED SURVIVING INFANTS

Primary Diagnosis (Postnatal)	No. Survivors	Normal n	Normal %	Mild/Moderate Handicap n	Mild/Moderate Handicap %	Severe Handicap n	Severe Handicap %
Aqueductal stenosis	28	12	42.8	2	7.2	14	50
Associated anomalies	3	0	0	0	0	3	100
Dandy–Walker syndrome	1	0	0	1	100	0	0
Porencephalic cyst	1	0	0	0	0	1	100
Arnold–Chiari malformation	1	0	0	1	100	0	0
Total	34	12	35.3	4	11.8	18	52.9

developmental milestones; in tested infants the developmental quotient was always less than 60. Five of these infants have cortical blindness, three have a seizure disorder, and two have spastic diplegia.

Outcome among survivors was related to the primary etiology of obstructive hydrocephalus. Aqueductal stenosis of uncertain etiology was the most common etiologic factor for obstructive hydrocephalus (28 of 41 cases, 68.3%). The only intact survivors were found in this group (see Table 30–7). Four fetuses had primary central nervous system lesions other than aqueductal stenosis. One of these fetuses had holoprosencephaly, exhibited gross functional anomalies, and died at 2 1/2 months of age. One infant had Dandy–Walker syndrome and exhibited moderate developmental delay at 18 months of age. One infant had a porencephalic cyst of unknown etiology and exhibited gross developmental delay by 6 months of age. The final infant in this group had Arnold–Chiari syndrome with normal intellectual development at age 18 months, but with lower limb paresis. In five infants, obstructive hydrocephalus was associated with other major organ system anomalies (12.7% of total cases). These anomalies included cranial–facial abnormalities with pulmonary hypoplasia, arthrogryposis multiplex congenita, multiple system anomaly, diaphragmatic hernia, and one case of trisomy 21. The incidence of associated karyotypic abnormalities in patients with obstructive hydrocephalus was low, being confined to the single case of trisomy 21 (2.6% of total cases).

No relationship between the duration of shunt placement and outcome could be determined.

The outcome data of human hydrocephalic fetuses treated *in utero* are difficult to interpret. *Hydrocephalus* is a broad clinical descriptive term referring to a constellation of pathologic findings, in which ventriculomegaly is invariable. *Obstructive hydrocephalus* describes a pathophysiologic process in which ventriculomegaly results from impedance of cerebrospinal fluid circulation due to an anatomic block at various sites and various other pathologic conditions. Adverse neurologic sequelae are presumed due to cerebral tissue compression with resultant dysfunction and atrophy.[47] The rationale for chronic ventricular decompression is to reduce ventricular pressure and pathologic enlargement, thereby preserving cerebral tissue and avoiding cephalomegaly.

The outcome of hydrocephalic perinates differs in accordance with the time of onset of disease and the underlying etiology. Because accurate prenatal diagnosis of hydrocephalus is a relatively recent development, most of the outcome data are derived from studies of infants born with overt hydrocephalus. In neonates born with overt hydrocephalus and not treated, the prognosis is grim; fewer than 15% survive, and almost all survivors exhibit some degree of neurologic impairment.[48] The outcome in treated hydrocephalic neonates is substantially better and continues to improve. In 1973, survival in neonates born with overt hydrocephalus and treated by chronic ventricular shunts was 44%; 15% of

survivors were normal at follow-up.[48] By 1982, survival in these neonates increased to 86% with nearly two thirds of survivors normal at follow-up.[49] Thus, postnatal therapy improves survival and reduces morbidity in these infants.

Applications of these postnatal data to the fetal condition may be neither simple nor direct. Prenatal selection, both natural and contrived, must be operant in these comparisons. The very fact that a fetus survives to the onset of labor, then survives the delivery process, may be a powerful prognostic indicator of more favorable neonatal outcome. Three reports regarding the natural history of fetal ventriculomegaly highlight potential inaccuracies in comparing neonatal and fetal data. In 1984, Glick et al.[50] reported outcome in 24 fetuses with ventriculomegaly; 10 fetuses survived (42%), and 6 of 10 survivors (25% of total cases) were normal at follow-up. In 1984, Chervenak et al.[51] described 50 affected fetuses, of which 14 survived (28%) and 6 were normal (12% of total cases). In 1985, Clewell et al.[52] provided an additional 13 cases, of which 3 survived (23%) and 2 were normal (15% of total cases). Considered collectively, 27 of these 87 fetuses (31%) survived and 17 were normal (19.5% of total cases). Thus, outcome for both nontreated fetal and neonatal hydrocephalus is considerably worse than that reported for treated neonatal hydrocephalus. Comparison of outcome in nontreated fetuses with the Registry data of outcome in treated fetuses can offer only partial insight into the value, if any, of treatment, because these groups are not carefully matched. Despite these caveats, it may be encouraging to note survival is better in the treated fetal group (83%) than in the nontreated group (31%), and it is now similar to survival in neonates born with overt hydrocephalus (86%). Further, the intact survival rate is higher in treated fetuses (34%) than that observed in nontreated fetuses (19.5%), but it is lower than the rate observed in treated neonates born with overt hydrocephalus (66%).

The primary etiology of the hydrocephalus will influence both mortality and morbidity rates. Detailed sonographic assessment of fetal intracranial architecture is a rapidly improving diagnostic modality, permitting ever more accurate definition of the etiology of fetal hydrocephalus. This advance may be expected to enhance greatly the selection of appropriate cases for *in utero* therapy. This point is illustrated in the data compiled in the Registry of treated hydrocephalic fetuses. Holoprosencephaly is associated with a very high mortality and a near-certain probability of severe retardation in survivors[53]; the prognosis is not improved by neonatal therapy. In the Registry, a single case of holoprosencephaly, unrecognized before delivery, was treated by *in utero* surgery; the infant was grossly retarded and died at 2 1/2 months of age. In retrospect, prenatal recognition of holoprosencephaly, now a diagnostic reality, would have precluded any attempts at therapy. Similarly, prenatal recognition of lethal anomalies and phenotypic or karyotypic defects that would assure a high probability of serious morbidity would preclude therapeutic intervention. In the Registry data, 5 of 41 cases (12.7%)

exhibited such anomalies. Forewarning in each of these cases would have prevented attempts at therapy. Four of these five anomalies may not be diagnosed using newer, high-resolution dynamic ultrasound methods, and the single karyotypic abnormality (trisomy 21) may be diagnosed by either amniocyte culture or the more rapid method of direct preparation from a pure fetal blood sample.

In other conditions, accurate prenatal diagnosis may not be as helpful in making decisions regarding fetal invasive therapy. In neonates born with hydrocephalus and myelomeningocele, mortality in untreated cases is high (70%)[54] and may be reduced with neonatal shunt procedures (52%).[55] Morbidity among treated survivors, however, remains a constant problem, with almost all (98%) exhibiting motor handicap and many (40%) exhibiting mental retardation.[56,57] In the Registry data, only a single case is reported of a treated fetus with ventriculomegaly secondary to aqueductal hydrocephalus–myelomeningocele. In this infant, the myelomeningocele was unrecognized before delivery; the child has apparent normal intellect but has major motor problems (lower limb paresis). Studies in a primate model of fetal hydrocephalus suggest *in utero* shunting of affected fetuses may improve neonatal survival and outcome. Michejda and Hodger[58] compared mortality and morbidity rates between nontreated and *in utero* shunted primate fetuses *(Macaca mulatta),* in which neural tube defects with associated hydrocephalus were induced using a point teratogen (triamcinolone). Neonatal mortality was a constant finding in nontreated cases, preceded by progressive hydrocephalus seizures and progressive gross abnormality of neuromuscular function. In contrast, in fetuses treated *in utero,* the perinatal survival was high (85%), and all survivors exhibited normal postnatal growth and normal neuromuscular development. Whereas comparison of survival rates between the fetal animal model and the human fetus may be valid, comparison of cognitive and intellectual morbidity is obviously limited by species differences. In short, fetal animal model experiments cannot answer the critical question of whether or not prenatal therapy can preserve intact intellectual development among survivors.

Evaluation of benefits, if any, of prenatal therapy for hydrocephalus secondary to posterior fossa cysts (Dandy–Walker syndrome) is equally difficult. The single treated case in the Registry resulted in a liveborn infant with moderate handicap evident at 18 months of age. Infants born with Dandy–Walker syndrome and left untreated usually die.[59] In treated newborns, survival is common (64%), and most survivors are reported as having normal intellectual development (77%).[60,61] When this condition is associated with other central nervous system malformations, however, most notably agenesis of the corpus callosum, survival is poor and major intellectual retardation of survivors is the rule.[61] Unfortunately, prenatal diagnosis of agenesis of the corpus callosum is not easily achieved using current ultrasound methods.

Aqueductal stenosis is the most commonly assigned clinical etiology of overt neonatal hydrocephalus (43 to 50% of cases), as well as the most common autopsy diagnosis (29.5%).[60] This clinical diagnosis was even more common among treated Registry cases, being assigned in 28 of 34 cases (82%). Although spontaneous arrest of hydrocephalus due to aqueductal stenosis may occur, most newborns with the condition will die if left untreated. Virtually all survivors with progressive disease will exhibit ultimate severe intellectual and motor retardation. Aggressive early neonatal shunting improves both survival rates and the prospect of intact survival. Survival in treated neonates is reported as 78%, and normal intellectual development is reported in 82% of survivors.[49] Both survival and intact survival are related to the inheritance pattern of this condition. Cases of X-linked recessive aqueductal stenosis account for up to 15% of the total and carry a high mortality rate (79.4%) and virtually no prospect for intact survival, even with aggressive neonatal surgery. The prognosis of aqueductal stenosis due to multifactorial inheritance patterns is not well described because most series describing outcome of treated neonates include cases of X-linked recessive disease.[62] It seems likely that the outcome of infants with disease of multifactorial inheritance would be enhanced if these cases were considered separately.

Series of prenatally diagnosed and untreated human fetal hydrocephalus include only 20 cases of proven or probable aqueductal stenosis.[50–52] Twelve of these 20 perinates died (60%), of which five died before or during labor as a direct result of intervention (two by elective pregnancy termination, three by intrapartum cephalocentesis). Eight perinates survived (40%), of which six (30% of total cases) were normal at follow-up. In contrast, in the Registry data, 26 of 32 fetuses with this condition survived (86.7%), and 12 survivors (37.5%) were normal at follow-up. These data may indicate that fetal survival is improved with *in utero* therapy but do not indicate any obvious improvement in survivor morbidity.

ISOLATED PLEURAL EFFUSIONS: FETAL PLEUROAMNIOTIC SHUNTING (FIG. 30–3)

Fetal pleural effusion can occur as a unilateral or bilateral condition, and it can occur in isolation, in association with cystic hygroma (including the karyotypic normal fetus), and in association with ascites and subcutaneous edema (nonimmune hydrops). In the normal state the small quantity of pleural fluid is not visualized by ultrasound examination of the fetal chest. The diagnosis of fetal pleural effusion is, therefore, simple and direct: The abnormal volume of accumulated pleural fluid is seen as an echolucent mass displacing and compressing the echogenic fetal lung (see Fig. 30–3).

The clinical features of 124 cases of fetal pleural effusion reported in the English-language literature have been

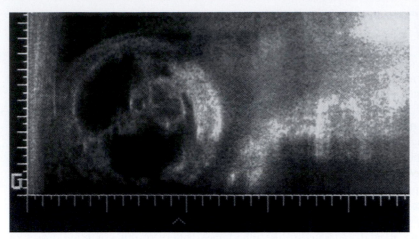
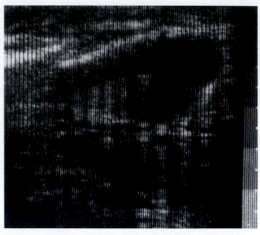

A   B

Figure 30–3. (A) Bilateral pleural effusion. This transverse scan of the fetal thorax at the level of the heart demonstrates overt bilateral lucencies in the thoracic cavity. Fetal lung tissue was compressed and difficult to visualize. Note the associated thoracic wall edema likely secondary to lymphatic obstruction. **(B)** Unilateral pleural effusion. This sonogram of the fetal thorax in the coronal plane demonstrates a large effusion in the right hemithorax. The fetal lung is easily visible and appears moderately compressed. The left hemithorax, not seen well in this image, was normal. There was a moderate degree of mediastinal shift. This fetus was proven to have chylothorax and survived with treatment (serial thoracocentesis).

summarized.[63] The diagnosis was established from as early as 14 weeks, but on average it was first made at 30 weeks. Other anomalies were present in nearly half (46%) of cases (Table 30–8) and included karyotypic anomalies (trisomies 21 and XO). The overall survival was 54% and included 11 cases with spontaneous resolution *in utero*. Perinatal survival was related to gestational age at delivery, improving as expected as fetal age advanced. Perinatal survival was 11% for fetuses with pleural effusions delivered before 31 weeks of gestation and was sharply increased to 61% in fetuses delivered at 32 weeks or after. The presence or absence of hydrops greatly influenced perinatal survival. In fetuses with pleural effusions associated with ascites and subcutaneous edema, the overall survival was 41%, whereas in fetuses in whom pleural effusion was an isolated finding, the survival rate was 80%. Perinatal outcome is also strongly related to whether the effusion is unilateral or bilateral. In a series of 32 cases reported by Longaker et al.[64] survival with a unilateral effusion was uniform (100%), whereas survival with a bilateral lesion was 52%.

TABLE 30–8. PERINATAL OUTCOME OF FETAL PLEURAL EFFUSION

Pleural Effusion: Fetal Therapy		
Procedure	*n*	Survival (%)
No. of treatments (postnatal)	52	53
Periodic aspiration	24	82
Thoracoamniotic shunt	68	78

CHRONIC PLEUROAMNIOTIC SHUNTING: TECHNICAL CONSIDERATIONS

The initial and crucial step in prenatal treatment of pleural effusion is case selection. Prenatal treatment is reserved for structurally normal fetuses with a bilateral effusion (without associated nonimmune hydrops) presenting at or before 32 weeks of gestation. The initial evaluation must include a detailed assessment of fetal morphometrics, morphology, and functional well-being, with treatment being reserved for those fetuses without associated anomalies or evidence of chronic asphyxial compromise. Invasive prenatal karyotype determination is indicated at the initial visit. The method used will differ but in most instances will be cordocentesis. The fetus should be observed repeatedly over an interval of 1 to 2 weeks to confirm the persistence of the effusion and to await the results of the karyotype. Treatment is considered only in the normal fetus with subjectively large persistent bilateral effusions. Treatment may be by one of two methods: serial thoracocentesis or placement of a chronic pleuroamniotic shunt. The choice of method will differ by fetal age, access, and the experience of the operator. In general, in the fetus at or near 32 weeks of gestation, thoracocentesis is the method of choice at least for the initial procedure. In the more immature fetus, chronic shunt placement is the usual choice.

Both procedures are done percutaneously using local anesthesia in the maternal skin and continuous ultrasound guidance. Thoracocentesis is done using either an 18- or 20-gauge spinal needle. Attempts should be made to avoid the placenta whenever possible and in the unsensitized Rh-negative patient, 150 μg of immune globulin should be given immediately after the procedure is completed. The needle is guided toward the lateral aspect of the fetal thorax. Care must be taken to avoid a central entry point, which may damage the fetal heart, and an inferior entry point, which may be associated with liver and spleen laceration and hemorrhage. The needle tip is observed to approach the thorax, adjusted toward an intercostal space, and advanced briskly through the chest wall into distended pleural space. There is little prospect of damaging lung tissue provided the depth of penetration is controlled. The stylet is removed, and the pleural fluid is aspirated under gentle suction until most or all of the fluid is removed. The amount of fluid present varies from about 50 to 150 mL. A fluid sample should be saved for cell and biochemical analysis. The observation of a nearly pure lymphocyte population in the pleural fluid is strong presumptive evidence of congenital chylothorax, a condition associated with an excellent perinatal prognosis. Pleural fluid is also an excellent source for cell culture for fetal karyotype determination. The needle is then removed from the abdomen. A separate needle is inserted at a site over the contralateral chest, and the procedure is repeated. An attempt to approach the contralateral pleural space via the mediastinum has been described but is generally not accepted as a safe procedure.

The technique for chronic shunt placement differs only slightly from that used for serial thoracocentesis. The modified needle used for shunt placement is considerable and is in the range of a 12 gauge. It is usually necessary, and preferable, to make a small incision in the maternal skin surface to facilitate the needle penetration. Once the needle tip is placed successfully in the fetal pleural space, the stylet is removed and a small sample of pleural fluid is aspirated. Care must be taken to prevent loss of the pleural fluid because such loss makes placement of the shunt much more difficult. A precut transverse double-pigtail catheter is threaded into the stylet and advanced until the distal end is seen under ultrasound to coil in the fetal pleural space. The needle is then slowly withdrawn until the level is about 0.5 cm outside of the chest wall and the remainder in the catheter is introduced and observed to coil in the amniotic cavity. The pleural space usually diminishes rapidly in size although complete drainage may not occur or may require several hours or even days to be effected. Once the shunt is placed satisfactorily, the procedure is repeated on the contralateral side. The description of shunt placement is done more easily than the actual procedure, and, in some cases, it may be difficult or impossible to get the shunt in the correct space. As a general working rule it seems best to limit the attempts to a maximum of two for either cavity. Failing at this point it is likely more prudent either to abandon the procedure entirely or to attempt it at a later date and rely subsequently on serial thoracocentesis. Fetal risks associated with chronic pleuroamniotic shunt placement are similar to those associated with other invasive fetal procedures, that is, a risk of fetal death of about 3 to 5% per procedure occurring mainly as a result of fetal hemorrhage either into the maternal circulation or at the site of needle trauma.

Outcome

Perinatal survival appears to be significantly improved as a result of prenatal treatment by either serial thoracocentesis or the placement of a chronic pleuroamniotic shunt(s). The overall survival in untreated cases was 50% as compared with 78% in shunted fetuses[65–67] (see Table 30–8). These observations strongly support the value of fetal treatment in selected cases of pleural effusion. Long-term outcome of survivors is not known.

BRONCHOGENIC CYST (FIG. 30–4)

Rarely segments of the premature foregut, the analogue of the bronchopulmonary tree, may become isolated and develop as fluid-filled intrathoracic cysts. These inclusion cysts are usually multiple with one or more dominant cysts located within either the lung parenchyma or the mediastinum.[68] The cyst wall is lined by ciliated columnar epithelium, and the cyst becomes filled with a serouslike fluid (see Fig. 30–4). On ultrasound these cysts appear as rounded echolucent structures commonly associated with compression of lung tissue and occasionally associated with displacement of the heart and mediastinum. There is usually a slow but progressive increase in cyst size with advancing gestation. Bronchogenic cysts are rarely associated with other fetal organ structures or with karyotypic malformation. The major clinical consequence of the cyst is compression of the lung and subsequent pulmonary hypoplasia, either segmented or generalized[69] compression of the esophagus with resultant hydramnios and compression of the intrathoracic great vessels and lymphatics, resulting in ascites and nonimmune hydrops.[70]

Management

The recognition of a bronchogenic cyst or other cystic masses within the fetal thorax is not an indication for any treatment per se, but rather treatment should be reserved for those fetuses in which there is either evidence of deleterious effects of compression or in which the rate of increase in the size of the cyst(s) portends a high probability of compression complication. In the mature fetus with these complications, delivery and postnatal corrective procedures are indicated. In the mature fetus, ultrasound-guided percutaneous decompression of the cyst either by repeated procedures (thoracocentesis) or placement of a shunt between the cyst and the amniotic cavity may be indicated. Decompression of these cysts have been associated with resolution of the compression complicated and long-term survival.[71–74]

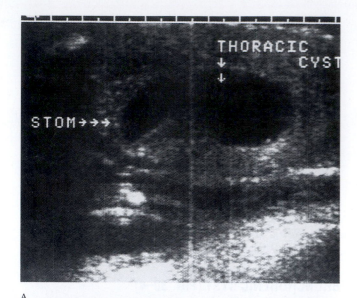

A

B

Figure 30–4. Bronchogenic cyst. **(A)** This sonogram of the fetal thorax/abdomen in the oblique transverse plane demonstrates a cystic mass in the left hemithorax contained within and compressing the left lung. The cystic mass was spherical and on serial scans was slowly enlarging. **(B)** The left hemithorax after ultrasound-guided percutaneous decompression of the cyst. The fluid in the cyst was under pressure at aspiration and 26 cc of straw-colored fluid was removed. The cyst did not reaccumulate fluid. Thoracotomy in the neonate confirmed a bronchogenic cyst. This perinate survived.

INVASIVE THERAPY FOR NEURAL TUBE DEFECTS

The concept of open fetal surgical repair of myelomenigocoele has recently been advanced by Bruner et al.[75] This treatment is based on experimental observations of surgically induced open spinal defects in the immature fetal lamb, in which in the absence of interval repair the newborn lambs exhibited severe loss of lower limb function, whereas after interval repair there appeared to be either prevention or amelioration of the lower limb paralysis.[76,77] However, the natural history of these experimental lesions in the fetal lamb has been recently reported by our group and raise doubt about the proported benifit of interval repair.[77] Nonetheless, the concept that repair might prevent functional loss has now been extended to the human fetus.[78] To date there have been neither random nor case control data available to substantiate any benifit of human repair of myelomeningocoele, and the case reports,[79] although provocative, are not conclusive in confirming a defined protective benefit. As of late 1999 this human fetal surgical procedure must be considered to be highly experimental with unproven benefits. Until such time as controlled data become available, the procedure should not be considered as part of the established spectrum of invasive fetal therapies.

SUMMARY

The concept of ultrasound-guided invasive fetal therapy for correction and amelioration of acquired and congenital defects has moved from the theoretical to the sporadic clinical case to routine application. In some areas, such as alloimmune anemia, such therapies have proven to be extremely beneficial, resulting in intact survival in nearly all cases. In other conditions, such as the lower obstructive uropathies and bilateral pleural effusions, fetal diversion therapy appears to be effective in reducing both mortality and morbidity. In contrast, in fetuses with obstructive hydrocephalus, one of the potential drawbacks of *in utero* invasive therapy, that of avoiding perinatal death at the expense of an increase in sustained debilitating handicap, appears to have been realized. All of these therapies have a proven risk to the fetus and at least a potential risk to its mother. In view of these risks, and in some instances nebulous benefits, it seems advisable to confine such therapeutic heroics to a few select medical centers to maximize operative experience and to facilitate collection of meaningful follow-up data.

REFERENCES

1. Liley AW. Intrauterine transfusion of fetus in haemolytic disease. *Br Med J.* 1963;2:1107–1109.
2. Bowman JM, Friesen RF. Multiple intraperitoneal transfusion of the fetus for erythroblastosis foetalis. *N Engl J Med.* 1964;271:703–707.
3. Manning FA, Harrison MR, Rodeck C. Catheter shunts for fetal hydrocephalus: Report of the International Fetal Surgery Registry. *N Engl J Med.* 1986;315:336–340.
4. Campbell S, Pearch JM. The prenatal diagnosis of fetal

structural anomalies by ultrasound. *Clin Obstet Gynecol.* 1983; 10:475–506.

5. Gruenewald SM, Crocker EF, Walker AG, et al. Antenatal diagnosis of urinary tract abnormalities: Correlation of ultrasound appearance with postnatal diagnosis. *Am J Obstet Gynecol.* 1984;148:278–283.

6. Pocock RP, Witcombe JB, Andrews HS, et al. The outcome of antenatally diagnosed urological abnormalities. *Br J Urol.* 1985;57:788.

7. Thomas DFM, Irving HC, Arthur RJ. Prenatal diagnosis: How useful is it? *Br J Urol.* 1985;57:784.

8. Avni EF, Rodesch F, Schulman CC. Fetal uropathies: Diagnostic pitfalls and management. *J Urol.* 1985;134:921.

9. Chamberlain PF, Manning FA, Morrison I, et al. Circadian rhythm in bladder volumes in the term human fetus. *Obstet Gynecol.* 1984;64:657–660.

10. Seeds AE. Current concepts of amniotic fluid dynamics. *Am J Obstet Gynecol.* 1980;138:575–586.

11. Beck AD. The effect of intra-uterine urinary obstruction upon the development of the fetal kidney. *J Urol.* 1971;105: 784–789.

12. Tanaghu EA. Surgically induced partial urinary obstruction in the fetal lamb. II: Urethral obstruction. *Invest Urol.* 1972; 10:25–34.

13. Harrison MR, Ross N, Noall R, et al. Correction of congenital hydronephrosis *in utero.* I: The model: Fetal urethral obstruction produces hydronephrosis and pulmonary hypoplasia in fetal lambs. *J Pediatr Surg.* 1983;18:247–256.

14. Harrison MR, Nakayama DK, Noall R, et al. Correction of congenital hydronephrosis *in utero.* II: Decompression measures the effects of obstruction on the fetal lung and urinary tract. *J Pediatr Surg.* 1982;17:965–974.

15. Glick PL, Harrison MR, Noall R, et al. Correction of congenital hydronephrosis *in utero.* III: Early mid-trimester ureteral obstruction produces renal dysplasia. *J Pediatr Surg.* 1983;18: 681–687.

16. Glick PL, Harrison MR, Adzick NS, et al. Correction of congenital hydronephrosis *in utero.* IV: *in utero* decompression prevents renal dysplasia. *J Pediatr Surg.* 1984;19:649–657.

17. Smythe AR. Ultrasonic detection of fetal ascites and bladder dilatation with resulting prune belly. *J Pediatr.* 1981;98: 978–980.

18. Nakayama DK, Harrison MR, de Lorimier AA. Prognosis of posterior urethral valve syndrome presenting at birth. *J Pediatr Surg.* 1986;21:43–45.

19. Williams DI. Urethral valves: A hundred cases with hydronephrosis. *Birth Defects.* 1977;13:55.

20. Bowman JM, Manning FA. Intrauterine transfusion: Winnipeg 1982. *Obstet Gynecol.* 1983;61:203–209.

21. Kirkinen P, Joupila P, Tuononen S, et al. Repeated transabdominal renocentesis in a case of fetal hydronephrotic kidney. *Am J Obstet Gynecol.* 1982;142:1049–1052.

22. Vintzileos AM, Nochimson DJ, Walzak MP, et al. Unilateral fetal hydronephrosis: Successful *in utero* surgical management. *Am J Obstet Gynecol.* 1983;145:885–886.

23. Hasaart TA, Essed GG. Amniotic fluid embolism after transabdominal amniocentesis. *Eur J Obstet Gynecol Reprod Biol.* 1983;16:25–30.

24. Bowman JM. Rh erythroblastosis foetalis 1975. *Semin Hematol.* 1975;12:189–193.

25. Glick PL, Harrison MR, Golbus MS, et al. Management of the fetus with congenital hydronephrosis. II: Prognostic criteria and selection for treatment. *J Pediatr Surg.* 1985;20:343–350.

26. Manning FA, Morrison I, Lange IR, et al. Fetal assessment based on fetal biophysical profile scoring: Experience in 12,620 referred high risk pregnancies. I: Perinatal mortality by frequency and etiology. *Am J Obstet Gynecol.* 1985;151:343–350.

27. Manning FA, Harman CR, Lange IR, et al. Antepartum chronic fetal vesicoamniotic shunts for obstructive uropathy: A report of two cases. *Am J Obstet Gynecol.* 1983;145:819–822.

28. Daffos F, Capella-Pavlovsky M, Forestier F. Fetal blood sampling during pregnancy with use of a needle guided by ultrasound. A study of 607 consecutive cases. *Am J Obstet Gynecol.* 1985;153:655–661.

29. Menticoglou S, Harman CR, Manning FA, et al. Percutaneous ultrasound guided direct fetal blood sampling for prenatal diagnosis. Charlottetown, P.E.I., Canada. *Proceedings of the Society for Obstetrics and Gynecology.* June 1986.

30. Chamberlain PF, Manning FA, Morrison I, et al. Ultrasound evaluation of amniotic fluid volume. I: The relationship of marginal and decreased amniotic fluid volume to perinatal outcome. *Am J Obstet Gynecol.* 1984;150:245–249.

31. Nakayama KD, Glick PL, Harrison MR, et al. Experimental pulmonary hypoplasia due to oligohydramnios and its reversal by relieving thoracic compression. *J Pediatr Surg.* 1983;18:347–353.

32. Nimrod CA, Varela-Gittings F, Machin G, et al. The effect of very prolonged membrane rupture on fetal development. *Am J Obstet Gynecol.* 1984;148:540–543.

33. Shalev E, Weiner E, Feldman E, et al. External bladder–amniotic fluid shunt for fetal urinary test obstruction. *Obstet Gynecol.* 1984;63(suppl):32–34.

34. Thomas DF, Irving HC, Arthur RJ. Prenatal diagnosis: How useful is it? *Br J Urol.* 1985;57:784–787.

35. Harrison MR, Adzick NS, Nakayama DK. Fetal diaphragmatic hernia: Pathophysiology, natural history and outcome. *Clin Obstet Gynecol.* 1986;29:490–495.

36. Chitkara U, et al. Prenatal sonographic assessment of the fetal thorax: Normal values. *Am J Obstet Gynecol.* 1987;157: 1069.

37. Fong K, Ohlsson A, Zalev A. Fetal thoracic circumference: A prospective cross-sectional study with real-time ultrasound. *Am J Obstet Gynecol.* 1988;158:1154.

38. Nimrod C, Nicholson S, Davies D, et al. Pulmonary hypoplasia testing in clinical obstetrics. *Am J Obstet Gynecol.* 1988;158:227.

39. Blott M, Greenough A, Nicolaides KH, et al. Fetal breathing movements as a predictor of favourable pregnancy outcome after oligohydramnios due to membrane rupture in the second trimester. *Lancet.* 1987;2:129.

40. Moessinger AC, Fox HE, Higgins A, et al. Fetal breathing movements are not a reliable predictor of continued lung development in pregnancies complicated by oligohydramnios. *Lancet.* 1987;2:1297.

41. Lumbers ER. A brief review of fetal renal function. *J Dev Physiol.* 1983;6:1–10.

42. Harrison MR, Filly RA. The fetus with obstructive uropathy: Pathophysiology, natural history, selection, and treatment. In: Harrison MR, Golbus MS, Filly FA, eds. *The Unborn Patient.* Philadelphia: Saunders; 1990;328–393.

43. Weiner C, Williamson R, Bonsib SM, et al. *in utero* bladder diversion—Problems with patient selection. *Fetal Ther.* 1986;1: 196–202.

44. Grannium PA, Ghidini A, Scioscia A, et al. Assessment of fetal renal reserve in low level obstructive uropathy (letter). *Lancet.* 1989;1:181–182.

45. Wilkins IA, Chitkara U, Lynch L, et al. The nonpredictive value of fetal urinary electrolytes: Preliminary report of outcomes and correlations with pathologic diagnosis. *Am J Obstet Gynecol.* 1987;157:694–698.

46. Watson AR, Readett D, Nelson CS, et al. Dilemmas associated with antenatally detected urinary tract abnormalities. *Arch Dis Child.* 1988;63:719–722.

47. Weller RO, Shulman K. Infantile hydrocephalus: Clinical, histological and ultrastructural study of brain damage. *J Neurosurg.* 1972;36:255–265.

48. Mealey J, Gilmore RL, Bubb MP. The prognosis of hydrocephalus overt at birth. *J Neurosurg.* 1973;39:248.

49. McCullough DC, Balzer-Martin LA. Current prognosis in overt neonatal hydrocephalus. *J Neurosurg.* 1982;57:378.

50. Glick PL, Harrison MR, Nakayama DK, et al. Management of ventriculomegaly in the fetus. *J Pediatr.* 1984;105:97.

51. Chervenak FA, Duncan C, Mert LR, et al. Outcome of fetal ventriculomegaly. *Lancet.* 1984;2:179.

52. Clewell WH, Meier PR, Manchester DK, et al. Ventriculomegaly: Evaluation and management. *Semin Perinatol.* 1985; 9:98.

53. Roach E, DeMyer W, Palmer K, et al. Holoprosencephaly: Birth data, genetic and demographic analysis of 30 families. *Birth Defects.* 1975;11:294.

54. Laurence KM. The survival of untreated spina bifida dystica. *Dev Med Child Neurol.* 1966;11(suppl):10.

55. Lorber J. Results of treatment of myelomeningocoele: An analysis of 524 unselected cases with special reference to possible selection for treatment. *Dev Med Child Neurol.* 1971;13: 279.

56. Raimondi AJ, Soare P. Intellectual development in shunted hydrocephalic children. *Am J Dis Child.* 1974;127:664.

57. Althouse R, Wald N. Survival and handicap of infants with spina bifida. *Arch Dis Child.* 1980;55:845.

58. Michejda M, Hodger GD. *in utero* diagnosis and treatment of non-human primate fetal skeletal anomalies. I: Hydrocephalus. *JAMA.* 1981;246:1093.

59. Carrier H, Tommasi T, Goutell A, et al. La malformation de Dandy–Walker. *Ann Anat Pathol.* 1973;18:405.

60. Vintzileos AM, Ingardia CJ, Nochimson DJ. Congenital hydrocephalus: A review and protocol for perinatal management. *Obstet Gynecol.* 1983;62:539.

61. Hirsch JF, Pierre-Kahn A, Renier D, et al. The Dandy–Walker malformation: A review of 40 cases. *J Neurosurg.* 1984;61:515.

62. Burton B. Recurrence risks of congenital hydrocephalus. *Clin Genet.* 1979;16:47.

63. Weber AM, Philipson EH. Fetal pleural effusion: A review and meta-analysis for prognostic indicators. *Obstet Gynecol.* 1992;79:218.

64. Longaker MT, Laberge JM, Dansereau J, et al. Primary fetal hydrothorax: Natural history and management. *J Pediatr Surg.* 1989;24:573.

65. Nicolaides KH, Azar G. Thoracoamniotic shunting. In: Chervenak FA, Isaacson GC, Campbell S, eds. *Ultrasound in Obstetrics and Gynecology.* Boston: Little, Brown; 1993;1289ff.

66. Rodeck CH, Fisk NM, Fraser DI, et al. Long-term *in utero* drainage of fetal hydrothorax. *N Engl J Med.* 1988;319:1135.

67. Manning FA, Harman CR. Unpublished observation, 1994.

68. Albright EB, Crane JP, Shackelford GD. Prenatal diagnosis of a bronchogenic cyst. *J Ultrasound Med.* 1988;7:91.

69. Young G, L'Heururx PR, Krueckenberg ST, et al. Mediastinal bronchogenic cyst: Prenatal sonographic diagnosis. *Am J Radiol.* 1989;152:125.

70. O'Mara CS, Baker RR, Jeyasingham K. Pulmonary sequestration. *Surg Obstet Gynecol.* 1978;147:609.

71. Nicolaides KH, Blott M, Greenough A. Chronic drainage of fetal pulmonary cyst. *Lancet.* 1987;1:618.

72. Berraschek G, Geutingen J, Gruber W, et al. Intrauterine treatment of a fetal pulmonary cyst by chorioamniotic shunt. *Arch Gynecol Obstet Gynecol.* 1993;169:1622.

73. Obwegeser R, Deutinger J, Berraschek G. Fetal pulmonary cyst treated by repeated thoracocentesis. *Am J Obstet Gynecol.* 1993;169:1622.

74. Kyle PM, Lange IR, Menticoglou SM, et al. Intrauterine thoracocentesis of fetal cystic lung malformation. *Fetal Ther.* 1994;9:84.

75. Talipan N, Bruner JP. Myelomenigocoele repair *in utero*: A report of three cases. *Pediatr Neurosurg.* 1998;28:177.

76. Meuli M, Meuli-Simmen C, Yingling CD, et al. Creation of a myelomenigocoele *in utero*: A model of functional damage from spinal cord exposure in fetal sheep. *J Pediatr Surg.* 1995;30:1021.

77. Meuli M, Meuli-Simmen C, Yingling CD, et al. *in utero* surgery repair of experimental myelomenigocoele saves neurological function at birth. *J Pediatr Surg.* 1996;31:397.

78. Manning FA, Bastide A, Harman CR. Surgical neural tube defect in the immature fetal lamb: The natural history of healing and spinal cord function. *Am J Obstet Gynecol.* 2000; in press.

79. Adzick NS, Sutton LN, Crombleholme TM, et al. Successful fetal surgery for spina bifida. *Lancet.* 1998;352:1675.

31

Ultrasound Examination of the Uterine Cervix During Pregnancy

Maria-Teresa Gervasi • *Roberto Romero* • *Eli Maymon* •
Percy Pacora • *Philippe Jeanty*

The uterine cervix plays a central role in the maintenance of normal pregnancy and in parturition. Midtrimester cervical ripening, clinical expression of which is often referred to as *cervical incompetence,* is a major diagnostic and therapeutic challenge and a subject of intense debate among clinicians.

During most of normal pregnancy, the cervix remains firm and closed, despite a progressive increase in the size of the fetus and, consequently, uterine distention. At the end of pregnancy and during labor, the cervix changes consistency (softens), shortens (effaces), and dilates to allow the expulsion of the conceptus. The term *cervical ripening* refers to the anatomic, biophysical, and biochemical processes that underlie the changes in cervical consistency, effacement, and dilatation that generally precede the onset of spontaneous labor.

Contrary to what was believed for many years, cervical ripening is an active metabolic process affecting the extracellular matrix components of the cervix. These changes increase cervical compliance. Untimely cervical ripening could result in complications of pregnancy. For example, failure of the cervix to ripen before myometrial activation at term (i.e., onset of increased uterine contractility) may be the cause of a prolonged latent phase of labor. Preterm premature cervical ripening may lead to midtrimester spontaneous abortion or spontaneous preterm labor and birth.

PHYSIOLOGY OF CERVICAL RIPENING

The uterine cervix is essentially a connective tissue organ, with smooth muscle cells accounting for less than 8% of the distal part of the cervix.[1] The ability of the cervix to retain the conceptus during pregnancy is unlikely to depend on a traditional sphincteric mechanism. Indeed, perfusion of strips of human cervix with vasopressin, a hormone that stimulates smooth muscle contraction, induces a very modest contractile response in comparison to that induced by vasopressin in strips from the uterine isthmus and the fundus, which contain more muscle.[2]

The normal function of the cervix during pregnancy depends largely on the regulation of connective tissue metabolism. This tissue is formed by an abundant extracellular matrix that surrounds individual cells. The major macromolecular components of the extracellular matrix are collagen, proteoaminoglycans, elastin, and various glycoproteins, such as fibronectins. Collagen is considered the most important component of the extracellular matrix because it determines the tensile strength of fibrous connective tissue. Changes in cervical characteristics during pregnancy have been attributed to changes in collagen content and metabolism.[3] Proteoaminoglycans have also been implicated in cervical physiology. The proteoaminoglycan decorin (PG-S$_2$) has a high affinity for collagen and can cover the surface of the collagen fibrils, stabilizing them and promoting the formation of thicker collagen bundles or fibers. In contrast, byglycan (PG-S$_1$) has no affinity for collagen and, therefore, can disorganize collagen fibrils. The predominant proteoglycan is PG-S$_2$ in the nonpregnant state and PG-S$_1$ in the pregnant state.[4]

The biochemical events that have been implicated in cervical ripening are: 1) decrease in total collagen content; 2) increase in collagen solubility (probably indicating degradation or newly synthesized weaker collagen); and 3) increase in collagenolytic activity (both collagenase and leukocyte elastase). Contrary to what is generally believed, extracellular matrix turnover in the cervix is very high;[5] thus, mechanical properties of the cervix can change very quickly.

Uldbjerg et al.[4] demonstrated the importance of collagen content in cervical dilatation. They reported a strong correlation between the collagen content (measured by hydroxyproline determination) of cervical biopsies obtained after delivery and the time required for the cervix to dilate from 2 to 10 cm.[6] Moreover, collagen concentration in the cervix of nonpregnant women is a function of parity: the higher the parity, the lower the collagen content.[7] This observation provides an explanation for the shorter labor in parous women.

The changes in extracellular matrix components during cervical ripening have been likened to an inflammatory response.[8] Indeed, during cervical ripening there is an influx of inflammatory cells, including macrophages, neutrophils, mast cells, and eosinophils into the cervical stroma. Considerable evidence supports a role for proinflammatory cytokines and chemokines in cervical ripening.[9–13] Interleukin-1 (IL-1), interleukin-8 (IL-8), and tumor necrosis factor-α can induce the morphologic and biophysical changes associated with cervical ripening when locally applied to the cervix.[14] Interleukin-8, a major chemokine capable of inducing chemotaxis and thus infiltration of the cervix by inflammatory cells, has been considered as a central mediator of cervical ripening. Increased concentrations of this chemokine have been demonstrated in biopsies of the cervix. Interleukin-8 concentrations increase six-fold in the cervix at term and show an additional 11-fold increase after cervical ripening associated with parturition.[15] Similar findings have been reported by Osmers et al. in biopsies obtained from the lower uterine segment.[16] Moreover, these investigators reported a strong correlation between the IL-8 concentrations and those of two metalloproteinases: MMP-8 and MMP-9.

Substantial evidence supports a role for matrix degrading enzymes in the process of cervical ripening. These enzymes are collectively known as *matrix metalloproteinases* (MMPs). Cervical dilatation is associated with an increase in collagenolytic activity (MMP-1) in tissue and serum.[17,18] However, studies conducted by Osmers et al. have demonstrated that most of the cervical collagenase activity in the cervix/lower uterine segment during parturition is attributable to collagenase derived from neutrophils and specifically from MMP-8 (neutrophil collagenase).[16] Uldbjerg et al. reported increases in leukocyte serine elastase associated with cervical ripening.[6]

Several lines of evidence support the participation of sex steroid hormones in cervical ripening. This evidence includes: 1) intravenous administration of 17 β-estradiol induces cervical ripening;[19] 2) estrogen stimulates collagen degradation *in vitro;*[17] 3) progesterone blocks the estrogen-induced collagenolysis *in vitro;*[17] and 4) administration of progesterone receptor antagonist induces cervical ripening in the first trimester of pregnancy.[20] However, recent experimental evidence indicates that the role of sex steroid hormones in cervical ripening is complex. For example, cervical ripening in the rat begins long before a decrease in progesterone serum concentrations, suggesting a progesterone-independent mechanism capable of inducing cervical ripening in this species.[21] With regard to the role of estrogens, the administration of estrogen to pregnant women does not consistently result in cervical ripening. Moreover, the administration of neither estradiol nor its precursor (androstenedione) induces cervical ripening in the presence of high concentrations of progesterone in guinea pigs.[22] Moreover, the administration of estradiol to guinea pigs treated with onapristone (a progesterone receptor antagonist that induces cervical ripening) attenuates the cervical ripening normally induced by that compound.[22] Therefore, more work is required to determine the precise role of sex steroids in cervical ripening.

Prostaglandins are used to induce cervical ripening prior to the induction of labor or abortion. Within hours of administration, PGE$_2$ can produce clinical and histologic changes resembling physiologic ripening that normally develops over several weeks of gestation. The mechanism of action of PGE$_2$ is thought to involve stimulation of collagenolytic activity and synthesis of PG-S$_1$ by cervical tissue.[6] However, the observation that neither indomethacin[23] nor the specific cyclooxygenase-II inhibitor, flosulide,[20] inhibits the physiologic and antiprogestin-induced cervical ripening raises questions about the central role attributed to prostaglandins in cervical ripening.

Nitric oxide (NO) has been implicated in cervical ripening. The evidence for this is that the local application of NO donors can induce cervical ripening in guinea pigs and humans[24,25] and that treatment of guinea pigs and rats with NO inhibitors NG-nitro-L-arginine-methyl ester (L-NAME) delays cervical ripening and results in prolonged delivery.[26] More studies are required to determine the precise role of this mediator in physiologic and pathologic cervical ripening.

PREMATURE CERVICAL RIPENING

Premature ripening of the cervix during the midtrimester, whose clinical expression is cervical shortening, is a frequent finding in patients with a history of one or more midtrimester spontaneous abortions and/or early preterm deliveries and is a major risk factor for early preterm delivery.[27–29]

Midtrimester ripening of the cervix can be secondary to a congenital disorder (i.e., congenital mullerian duct abnormalities, diethylstilbestrol [DES] exposure *in utero*), to a connective tissue disorder (i.e., Ehlers–Danlos syndrome), to surgical trauma (i.e., conization, resulting in substantial loss of connective tissue), or to traumatic damage to the structural integrity of the cervix (i.e., repeated cervical dilatation of the cervical canal associated with termination of pregnancy).[30–32] However, some patients will show the typical signs of advanced cervical dilatation (feeling of vaginal pressure caused by the protruding membranes, rupture of membranes in the midtrimester in the absence of prior uterine contractions) in their first pregnancy, without any apparent cause.

The prevalence of subclinical microbial invasion of the amniotic cavity in patients presenting with cervical dilatation of at least 2 cm between 14 and 24 weeks is 51.5%.[33] The high rate of microbial invasion may be due to premature dilatation of the cervix with exposure of the chorioamniotic membranes to the microbial flora of the lower genital tract, resulting in secondary infection. Alternatively, microbial invasion may be due to ascending intrauterine infection that induces premature cervical ripening as part of the activation of the common terminal pathway of human parturition (uterine contractions, cervical ripening, and membrane/decidual activation). Support for the association between premature cervical ripening and intrauterine infection or inflammation derives from an observation reported by Guzman et al. that progressive cervical shortening in the midtrimester (cervical length below 20 mm, either spontaneous or induced) is significantly associated with the presence of acute chorioamnionitis in the placentae of patients who had a preterm delivery.[34] Because uterine contractions are usually painless and are often undetected by patients at this stage of pregnancy, the clinical picture of an infection-induced spontaneous abortion may be indistinguishable from that of cervical shortening due to a primary cervical disease. In either case, shortening of the cervix in the midtrimester seems to indicate a process that is already advanced in the pathogenic cascade leading to spontaneous abortion or preterm delivery.

EVALUATION OF THE CERVICAL STATUS

Clinical Evaluation of Cervical Status

The traditional method used for evaluation of cervical ripening is the digital examination of the cervix, and several scoring systems have been developed to quantify cervical parameters. The most widely used is the pelvic score, frequently referred to as the Bishop score. In 1964, Bishop et al. described cervical changes associated with the successful induction of labor at term. They also noted that women with similar changes before term may be more likely to deliver prematurely than those without such changes.[35] Bishop et al. suggested that anatomic changes in the cervix may alert physicians that patients are at risk, thus allowing intervention. To determine the pelvic or Bishop score, a digital examination is performed and points are ascribed for the degree of cervical dilatation, effacement (cervical length), consistency, position of the cervix, and fetal station relative to the level of the ischial spines. The station, or level, is the only component of the score that is not related to the cervix but rather to the degree of descent of the presenting part. A low score indicates an unripe cervix, and a high score indicates a ripe cervix. A commonly used alternative scoring system has been proposed by Calder et al.[36] The most important differences between the two scoring systems relate to cervical dilatation and effacement. In the Calder score, the length of the cervix in centimeters, rather than effacement in percentages, is used. Also, cervical dilatation is scored with a different number of points. This modification has been introduced to take into account the fact that it is extremely rare to have a cervical dilatation of 5 cm or more in the absence of labor. A critical analysis of the single components of the Bishop score indicates that they do not have the same value and that cervical dilatation is the most important.

Bishop et al. were primarily concerned with predicting the initiation of spontaneous labor. They found that a higher pelvic score was associated with the impending onset of spontaneous labor. This observation is important because it indicates that cervical changes are gradual and that they precede the onset of labor by several weeks. Further evidence that the cervix is important in parturition is that the Bishop score predicts the likelihood of successful induction of labor at term. The higher the score, the greater the likelihood of spontaneous vaginal delivery.[37]

Do Changes in Cervical Status Precede Preterm Labor?

Cervical ripening is not a process unique to term labor; it also occurs in preterm labor. A short cervix is a risk factor for preterm labor and delivery, and several investigators have shown an increased risk of preterm delivery among women with cervical effacement detected on pelvic examination.[38–44]

The largest study examining the relationship between cervical ripening and the subsequent risk of preterm delivery published to date was conducted in France by Papiernik et al. Serial digital examinations were conducted in 8303 women, of whom 4430 had a gestational age of less than 37 weeks. Dilatation of the internal os of the cervix was the most important risk factor in predicting preterm delivery. Once dilatation of the internal os occurred, the interval to delivery was similar in patients who subsequently went into either spontaneous term or preterm labor.[38] This observation indicates that cervical ripening is a general feature of human parturition and that it has a similar timetable in preterm and term parturition.

What Is the Clinical Value of Changes in Dilatation and Effacement of the Uterine Cervix in the Prediction of Spontaneous Preterm Delivery?

While the study by Papiernik et al. demonstrated that a dilated internal os after the 25th week of gestation was the single most significant risk factor for preterm delivery, a short cervix (1 cm or less) also increases the risk, although to a lesser extent. Other investigators have reported similar findings.[45]

Problems with Digital Examination of the Cervix

Digital examination of the cervix is subjective, has limitations and potential risks. The subjective component is underscored by two studies that have examined inter-observer variability. Holcomb et al. addressed this issue in a study in which obstetricians were asked to estimate the length of an uneffaced cervix at term. The mean length was 2.47 cm (standard deviation of 0.64 cm). However, the range reported by different examiners differed from 1 to 4 cm; the coefficient of variation was 26%.[46] In another study, Phelps et al. constructed an *in vitro* model to examine interobserver variability among nurses, residents, and staff physicians. Polyvinyl chloride pipes ranging in width from 1 to 10 cm in diameter were mounted inside cardboard boxes. One hundred two examiners with different degrees of experience were asked to estimate the size of the pipes. The overall accuracy for determining the exact diameter was 56.3% and improved to 89.5% when an error of ±1 cm was tolerated. The intra-observer variability (the probability of a given examiner reporting different measurements on two separate occasions for the same pipe diameter) was 52% and improved to 10.5% if an error ±1 cm was allowed. Of interest is that no statistically significant difference was found in the accuracy of nurses, residents, and staff physicians.[47]

Digital examination has limitations in assessing the status of the internal os and cervical length. Determination of effacement (cervical length) requires placement of the examining finger through the endocervical canal and in close proximity to the fetal membranes. This poses potential risks. Leniham et al.[48] reported that premature rupture of membranes was more common in women who had repeated pelvic examinations than in the control group (18% [32 of 174] vs. 6% [10 of 175], $p < 0.01$).[48] This observation differs from that reported by Main et al. in a preterm delivery prevention program in which women at risk for preterm delivery were randomized to either bi-weekly pelvic examinations or standard obstetric care. No difference in the incidence of preterm premature rupture of membranes (PROM) was noted between

the two groups [50% (8 of 16) vs. 28.6% (4 of 14)].[49] Although these results have been confirmed by other studies, it is unclear whether pelvic examination in such studies required placing the examining finger into the endocervical canal, the only accurate way to determine cervical length. Sonek et al.[50] found that digital examination was poorly correlated with sonographic measurements of cervical length in pregnant women. The two methods were used in 83 pregnant women and the correlation coefficient was only 0.49.[50] The results of digital examinations underestimated the cervical length determined by sonography. The difference was attributed to the ability of ultrasound to evaluate the portion of the cervix which is above the vaginal fornices, and, therefore, inaccessible to the examiner's finger (if not placed within the endocervical canal).

SONOGRAPHIC EVALUATION OF THE UTERINE CERVIX

Sonographic imaging of the cervix is an objective, less invasive and more precise method than digital examination for assessing cervical status. Effacement (or cervical shortening), changes in the anatomy of the internal os (or funneling), endocervical dilatation with bulging of membranes, dynamic changes in cervical morphology, and cervical response to transfundal pressure can be determined by transabdominal, endovaginal, or transperineal scanning.

Technique: Cervical Assessment by Sonography

The cervix can be examined using a transabdominal, endovaginal, and transperineal approach. Transabdominal sonography requires a full bladder for adequate visualization of the cervix. Endovaginal scanning does not require a distended bladder. The transperineal technique can be used to image the cervix when an endovaginal transducer is not available[51,52] and does not require a full bladder. This is important, because overdistention of the bladder compresses and artificially lengthens the cervix.[53] Andersen[54] compared the results of transvaginal and transabdominal ultrasound measurements of cervical length in 186 pregnant women. The mean transvaginal cervical length was significantly shorter than that obtained by the transabdominal approach (5.2 mm on average). Transabdominal measurements obtained with mild degrees of bladder filling were quite similar to those reported by transvaginal examination.[54] The effect of an overdistended bladder is not detectable in non-pregnant women. The different behavior of the pregnant and nonpregnant cervix in response to the pressure exerted by the bladder is most likely due to the changes in extracellular matrix composition (collagen and glycosaminoglycans) during normal pregnancy.[55]

We prefer the endovaginal technique for optimal assessment of the cervix. The close proximity of the probe to the cervix and the use of a high-frequency transducer improves image quality. In addition, cervical funneling, a predictor of preterm delivery, may be detected by transvaginal sonography and missed by transabdominal sonography.

Before conducting the examination, patients are asked to empty their bladder. During the examination, the patient lies in the supine position with flexed knees and hips. The probe is covered with either a glove or an appropriate sheath. Gel is placed between the transducer and the cover and on the surface sheath. The operator introduces the vaginal probe, which is advanced in the anterior fornix until a midline sagittal view of the cervix and lower uterine segment and the internal os, external os, cervical canal, and endocervical mucosa, are identified (Fig. 31–1). We also identify the endocervical mucosa that is used to define the upper edge of the cervix. Otherwise, cervical length may erroneously include part of the lower uterine segment.

Excessive pressure with the probe may elongate the cervix. To avoid this, the probe is slowly withdrawn until the image blurs and is subsequently reapplied with an amount of pressure sufficient to restore the image. The cervical length is measured by freezing the screen three separate times. The reliability of measurements is increased when the variation between the measurements is not more than 2 to 3 mm; the average length of examination is 5 to 10 mins. For clinical purposes, the shortest cervical length is reported provided that the image is adequate. The examination is recorded on videotape and the presence of a funnel or dynamic cervical changes are noted in the report. A funnel is defined as dilatation of the upper portion of the cervical canal (Fig. 31–2). This can only be recognized by being certain that the walls of the funnel are formed by endocervical mucosa. Otherwise, the walls of the lower uterine segment can be erroneously considered as a funnel.

Several potential problems should be avoided: 1) The cervical canal is sometimes curved, therefore, cervical length

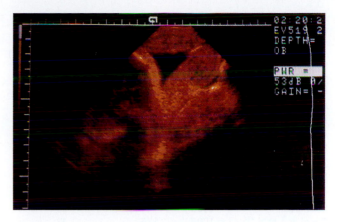

Figure 31–2. Transvaginal sonographic appearance of a cervix with a V-shaped funnel.

should be determined by tracing the length of the cervix or by adding the sum of two straight sections. 2) If the duration of the examination is too short and the patient has dynamic cervical changes, the cervical length and funnel may not represent the true baseline status of the cervix. This may be responsible for some observations in which patients gain cervical length over time. 3) The contours of the anterior and posterior lips of the ectocervix are usually clearly defined. However, in some instances, the boundaries of the ectocervix cannot be discerned. 4) In selected patients whose cervix cannot be adequately imaged, instillation of saline into the vagina allows precise recognition of the ectocervix.[56] 5) Standardized measurements of a funnel are difficult as a funnel can be obliterated by pressure from the transducer, it is often transient, and a distended bladder can obscure it. Because the longer the funnel, the shorter the remaining cervical length,[29,57] it has been argued that the endocervical length contains most of the information required for the prediction of preterm delivery. Cervical length is favored by many because it is far more reproducible than the assessment of funneling. A full discussion of the value of detecting funneling is available later in this chapter.

A rare pitfall in the examination of the cervix is the presence of a large endocervical polyp that can make identification of the correct plane difficult to image.[50] Although cervical examination may appear simple to the experienced sonographer, certain patients may present significant challenges. For example, a cervix with an unusual orientation may be difficult to find. In a recent study, Yost et al. reported that 27% of the scans performed in 60 women presented some anatomic or technical difficulty.[58]

Cervical Length in the Prediction of Preterm Delivery in Asymptomatic Patients

Several studies have addressed the biometry of the pregnant uterine cervix using transabdominal, endovaginal, and

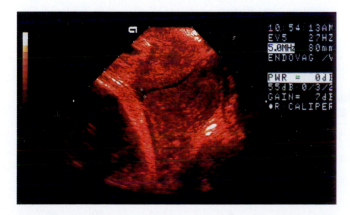

Figure 31–1. Transvaginal sonographic appearance of a normal uterine cervix; the internal os, the external os, and the endocervical canal can be easily visualized.

TABLE 31–1. CERVICAL LENGTH (MEAN OR MEDIAN) IN LOW-RISK POPULATIONS IN MIDTRIMESTER

Reference	Year	N	Cervical Length (mm)
Ayers et al.[109]	1988	150	52
Podobnik et al.[110]	1988	80	48
Andersen et al.[59]	1990	125	41
Kushnir et al.[60]	1990	24	48
Andersen et al.[54]	1991	77	42
Murakawa et al.[111]	1993	177	37
Zorzoli et al.[112]	1994	154	42
Iams et al.[85]	1995	106	37
Iams et al.[29]	1996	2915	35
Cook et al.[113]	1996	41	41
Tongsong et al.[114]	1997	175	42
Heath et al.[64]	1998	1252	38

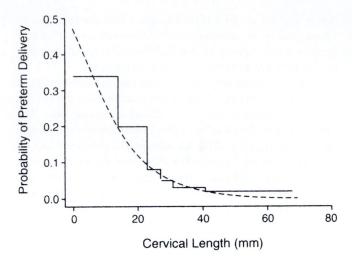

Figure 31–3. Estimated probability of spontaneous preterm delivery before 35 weeks of gestation from the logistic regression analysis *(dashed line)* and observed frequency of spontaneous preterm delivery *(solid line)* according to cervical length measured by transvaginal ultrasonography at 24 weeks. *(Reproduced with permission from Iams JD, et al. N Engl J Med. 1996;334:567–572.)*

perineal scanning. In most cases, cervical length is stable in the first 30 weeks of pregnancy both in nulliparous and in multiparous women who deliver at term, and a progressive, although not substantial, shortening of the cervix occurs in the third trimester of pregnancy.[59–61] Median or mean cervical lengths in low-risk populations in the midtrimester are shown in Table 31–1.

A short cervix is a significant risk factor for preterm delivery. Andersen et al.,[59] in a study of 113 women evaluated on one occasion before 30 weeks of gestation, reported that a cervical length of less than 39 mm is associated with a 25% risk of preterm delivery, whereas a long cervix (defined as a cervical length of 39 mm or more) decreases the risk of preterm birth (4.7%). Furthermore, the risk of spontaneous preterm birth was inversely related to the cervical length.[59] These findings have been confirmed by several other investigators in both low-risk and high-risk asymptomatic populations.[29,50,60,62–64]

Table 31–2 presents the details of some of the studies with adequate information to allow calculation of diagnostic indices and predictive values. Our review will focus on the highlights of studies that significantly contribute to the understanding of the value of cervical sonography in screening for spontaneous preterm birth.

The Maternal Fetal Medicine Network (MFMN) of the National Institute of Child Health and Human Development (NICHD) conducted a prospective cohort study entitled the Preterm Prediction Study. The value of clinical, demographic, microbiologic, biochemical, and sonographic parameters in the prediction of preterm birth were examined. Iams et al.[29] reported the cardinal observations of cervical sonography; 2915 low-risk asymptomatic patients were examined at 24 weeks and at 28 weeks of gestation by transvaginal sonography to evaluate the cervix and calculate the risk of delivering before 35 weeks. They found that the shorter the cervix, the greater the risk of preterm delivery (Fig. 31–3). An exponential increase in the relative risk of delivering before 35 weeks was described (Fig. 31–4). The diagnostic indices and predictive values for different cutoff values of cervical length, funneling, and Bishop score are displayed in Table 31–3.[29] This large study confirmed the results of Andersen et al., indicating that a short cervix increases the risk for preterm

TABLE 31–2. MEASUREMENT OF CERVICAL LENGTH BY ULTRASOUND IN LOW RISK ASYMPTOMATIC PREGNANT WOMEN AND PRETERM DELIVERY (PTD) RATE ACCORDING TO DIFFERENT CUTOFF VALUES

Reference	Year	N	Gestation (wks)	Cutoff (mm)	Definition of PTD	% Prevalence of PTD	% Sensitivity	% Specificity	% PPV	% NPV
Andersen et al.[59]	1990	113	<30	<39	<37 wks	15	76	59	25	93
Tongsong et al.[63]	1995	730	28–30	≤35	<37 wks	12	66	62	20	93
Iams et al.[29]	1996	2915	24	<20	<35 wks	4	23	97	26	97
Taipale et al.[67]	1998	3694	18–22	≤25	<37 wks	2	6	100	39	99
Heath et al.[66]	1998	2702	23	≤15	≤32 wks	1.5	58	99	52	99
Hassan et al.[65]	1999	6877	14–24	≤15	≤32 wks	3.6	8	99	47	97

PTD, preterm delivery; PPV, positive predictive value; NPV, negative predictive value.

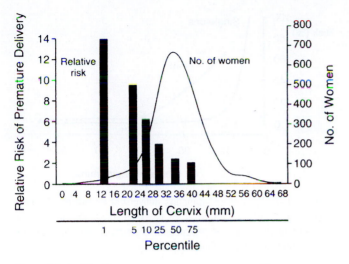

Figure 31–4. Distribution of subjects across percentiles for cervical length measured by transvaginal ultrasonography at 24 weeks of gestation *(solid line)* and relative risk of spontaneous preterm delivery before 35 weeks of gestation according to percentiles for cervical length *(bars)*. *(Reproduced with permission from Iams JD, et al. N Engl J Med. 1996;334:567–572.)*

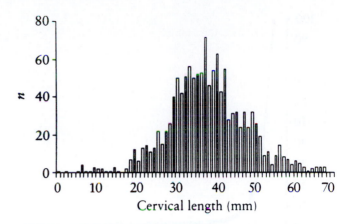

Figure 31–5. Distribution of cervical length at 23 weeks of gestation in 2702 low-risk patients. *(Reproduced with permission from Heath VCF, et al. Ultrasound Obstet Gynecol. 1998;12:312–317.)*

delivery and that a long cervix decreases such risk, and extended the observations by allowing discernment of the comparative value of cervical length with other predictors of preterm delivery (demographic, biochemical, microbiologic, and clinical).

An important series of studies reported by Heath et al. and conducted at King's College Hospital in London examined the value of cervical sonography in the screening of preterm birth. Cervical length was measured by transvaginal sonography in a low-risk population of 2702 patients (for the distribution of cervical length at 23 weeks of gestation, see Fig. 31–5). Patients with a history of preterm birth, of Afro-Caribbean origin, of young maternal age (younger than 20 years), and thin (low body mass index) had a shorter cervix than those without such risk factors. However, when logistic

regression analysis was used to examine the contribution of all these parameters to the prediction of preterm birth (before 32 weeks), a short cervix was the only predictor of outcome.[65] These findings suggest that clinical and demographic risk factors associated with preterm birth operate through a short cervix. In this study, a cervix of 15 mm or less at 23 weeks of gestation in 1.7% of the population identified 60% of patients who subsequently had a spontaneous preterm birth (before 32 weeks) and 80% of those who had a spontaneous preterm birth (before 28 weeks) (Fig. 31–6).

We conducted a retrospective cohort study of 6877 women with cervical sonography performed between 14 and 24 weeks. Examinations were conducted transabdominally and, in case of cervical length shorter than 30 mm or suboptimal visualization, transvaginally. A cervical length of 15 mm or less had a positive predictive value of 48%, a negative predictive value of 97%, a sensitivity of 8%, and a specificity of 99.7% for spontaneous preterm delivery at or before 32 weeks. A history of preterm delivery and African-American ethnicity were also associated with the occurrence

TABLE 31–3. SENSITIVITY, SPECIFICITY, AND PREDICTIVE VALUE OF CERVICAL LENGTH, FUNNELING, AND BISHOP SCORE FOR PRETERM DELIVERY BEFORE 35 WEEKS OF GESTATION

Variable	Cervix at 24 Weeks						Cervix at 28 Weeks					
	≤20 mm	≤25 mm	≤30 mm	Presence of Funnel	Bishop Score ≥ 6	Bishop Score ≥ 4	≤20 mm	≤25 mm	≤30 mm	Presence of Funnel	Bishop Score ≥ 6	Bishop Score ≥ 4
% Sensitivity	23.0	37.3	54.0	25.4	7.9	27.6	31.3	49.4	69.9	32.5	15.8	42.5
% Specificity	97.0	92.2	76.3	94.5	99.4	90.9	94.7	86.8	68.5	91.6	97.9	82.5
% Positive predictive value	25.7	17.8	9.3	17.3	38.5	12.1	16.7	11.3	7.0	11.6	25.6	9.9
% Negative predictive value	96.5	97.0	97.4	96.6	96.0	96.5	97.6	98.0	98.5	97.6	96.3	96.9

Reproduced with permission from Iams JD, et al., N Engl J Med. 1996;334:567–572.

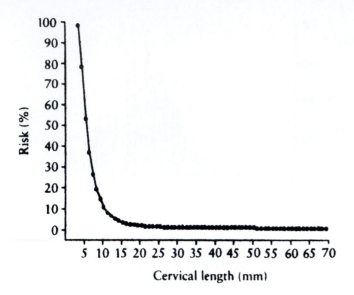

Figure 31–6. Risk for spontaneous delivery at or before 32 weeks according to cervical length at 23 weeks. *(Reproduced with permission from Heath VCF, et al. Ultrasound Obstet Gynecol. 1998;12:312–317.)*

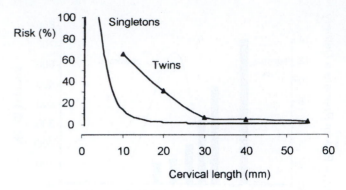

Figure 31–7. Rate of spontaneous delivery at or before 32 weeks according to cervical length at 23 weeks of gestation in twin and singleton pregnancies. *(Reproduced with permission from Souka AP, et al. Obstet Gynecol. 1999;94:450–454.)*

of spontaneous preterm birth, although the odds ratio was considerably lower than that of a short cervix.[66] The low sensitivity of a short cervix in this study is similar to that reported by Taipale and Hiilesmaa in a large study in Finland.[67] The apparent discrepancy among studies could be explained by the different gestational ages at which ultrasound examination was conducted. We have evidence that the later scan is more predictive for preterm delivery than the earlier scan. The study by Heath et al. includes examinations conducted at 23 weeks, whereas the studies by Hassan et al.[66] and by Taipale and Hiilesmaa included examinations performed at lower gestational ages.

In conclusion, a short cervix identifies a population at high risk for spontaneous preterm delivery. However, at least one-third and perhaps more patients who delivered preterm (before 32 weeks) will not have a short cervix in the midtrimester; therefore, cervical length with ultrasound is not a screening tool but rather a method for risk assessment. The high positive predictive value of a short cervix (nearly 50% for spontaneous preterm birth before 32 weeks) justi-

fies trials of intervention (see Cervical Cerclage to Prevent Preterm Birth).

Sonographic Evaluation of Cervical Length in Twin Pregnancies

Twin gestations occur in 1% of all pregnancies and they are at increased risk of preterm birth. Several studies have examined the value of endovaginal sonography for the prediction of preterm delivery in twin pregnancies.[68–73]

The Preterm Prediction Study of the MFMN, NICHD examined risk factors for preterm delivery in twin gestations. Goldenberg et al. reported that a short cervix, defined as a length of 25 mm or less, was more common in twin than in singleton gestations at 24 and 28 weeks. Moreover, at 24 weeks, a short cervix was the only factor predictive of preterm birth. At 28 weeks, a positive fetal fibronectin was significantly associated with spontaneous preterm birth before 32 weeks.[69] Souka et al.[73] performed scans in 215 twin pregnancies at 23 weeks of gestation. The sensitivities of a short cervix defined (as a length of ≤25 mm or less) in the prediction of spontaneous preterm delivery at 28, 30, 32, and 34 weeks were 100%, 80%, 47%, and 35%, respectively (Table 31–4). The rate of spontaneous delivery at or before 32 weeks increased exponentially with decreasing cervical length at 23 weeks (Fig. 31–7). An interesting observation was that the risk of preterm delivery for patients with a cervical length of

TABLE 31–4. RATE OF IATROGENIC AND SPONTANEOUS DELIVERY AT DIFFERENT GESTATIONAL AGES AND SENSITIVITY FOR SPONTANEOUS DELIVERY ACCORDING TO CERVICAL LENGTH IN TWIN GESTATIONS

Gestation (wks)	n	Iatrogenic Delivery	Spontaneous Delivery	Cervical Length			
				≤15 mm	≤25 mm	≤35 mm	≤45 mm
≤28	10	2 (0.9%)	8 (3.8%)	4 (50%)	8 (100%)	8 (100%)	8 (100%)
≤30	13	3 (1.4%)	10 (4.7%)	4 (40%)	8 (80%)	9 (90%)	10 (100%)
≤32	25	8 (3.8%)	17 (8.0%)	4 (24%)	8 (47%)	12 (71%)	16 (94%)
≤34	59	22 (10.4%)	37 (17.5%)	4 (11%)	13 (35%)	21 (57%)	34 (92%)

Reproduced with permission from Souka AP, et al., Obstet Gynecol. 1999;94:450–454.

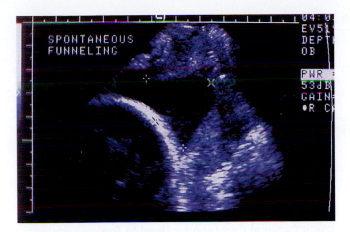

Figure 31–8. U-shaped funnel.

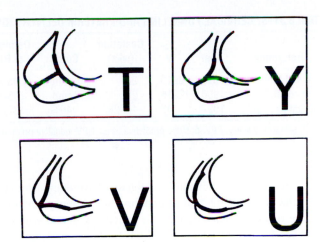

Figure 31–9. Schematic representation of the correlation between the length of the cervix and the changes of the internal cervical os; the letters T, Y, V, and U illustrate these changes graphically. *(Reproduced with permission from Zilianti M, et al. J Ultrasound Med. 1995;14:719–724.)*

≤25 mm or less in twin pregnancies was similar to the risk in singleton pregnancies with cervical length of 15 mm or less (52%). This has been interpreted as indicating that the cervical length required to confer protection against preterm delivery is greater in twin gestations than that of singleton gestations.[73]

A long cervix in twin gestations is reassuring. Imsesis et al. reported that 97% of twin gestations with a cervical length of 35 mm or more delivered after 34 weeks of gestation.[72]

One study has examined the value of cervical ultrasound in 32 triplet gestations. Progressive shortening of the cervix occurred with advancing gestational age. Cervical length in patients who delivered before 33 weeks was significantly shorter at 20, 29, and 31 weeks than in patients who delivered after 33 or more weeks.[74] Further studies in high-order multiple gestations are warranted.

Funneling in Screening for Subsequent Preterm Birth

Funneling is the dilatation of the internal cervical os. Funneling can be considered as effacement in progress.[75] Two types of funneling have been described: the V and the U shaped. In the V-shaped pattern, the membranes protrude into the cervical canal to form a triangular-shaped funnel. In the U-shaped pattern, the membranes protruding into the endocervical canal form a curvilinear image (Figs. 31–2 and 31–8). Zilianti et al. described the normal progression of the morphology of the upper cervix during the course of labor at term with transperineal sonography and coined the acronym of TYVU to describe the morphologic changes.[52] Figure 31–9 displays such an evolution. Similar findings can be demonstrated with endovaginal sonography. However, the work was conducted in term labor and it remains to be determined whether or not cervical changes in preterm labor follow the same pattern.

Figure 31–10 shows the morphology of the cervix, including the funnel length and funnel width, used to calculate the cervical index. The cervical index is equal to the sum of the funnel length plus 1 divided by the endocervical length.[28] This parameter was derived to take into account both remaining endocervical length and the length of the funnel, as they are both part of the original endocervical canal before

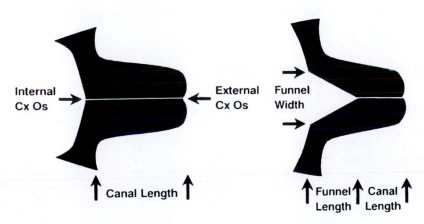

Internal Cx Os   External Cx Os   Funnel Width

Canal Length   Funnel Length   Canal Length

Figure 31–10. Morphology of the cervix, including the funnel length and funnel width. The cervical index is equal to the sum of the funnel length plus 1 divided by the endocervical length. *(Reproduced with permission from Gomez R, et al. Am J Obstet Gynecol. 1994;171:956–964.)*

TABLE 31–5. CERVICAL FUNNELING AND PRETERM DELIVERY RISK IN ASYMPTOMATIC PATIENTS

Reference	Year	N	Gestation (wks)	Cutoff	Definition of PTD	% Prevalence of PTD	% Sensitivity	% Specificity	% PPV	% NPV
Iams et al.[29]	1996	2915	24	3 mm	<35wks	4.3	25	94	17	97
Iams et al.[29]	1996	2915	28	3 mm	<35wks	4.3	32	92	12	98
Berghella et al.[57]	1997	43	16–28	≥40%	<37wks	42	78	76	70	83

PTD, preterm delivery; PPV, positive predictive value; NPV, negative predictive value.

effacement begins. Several investigators have demonstrated that the cervical index and funneling are strong predictors of the risk of preterm delivery in patients with and without preterm labor (Tables 31–5 and 31–6). Some investigators have described the dimensions of the funnel as a percentage of the endocervical length. This is fundamentally a concept similar to that of the cervical index. For example, a funnel representing 40 to 50% or more of the total cervical length has been associated with an increased risk of preterm birth when noted before 30 weeks in a population with a high prevalence of preterm delivery (42%).[57]

In the NICHD Preterm Prediction Study, Iams et al. reported that the value of funneling (defined as 3 mm in width) as a predictor of delivery was similar to the value of cervical length, but the data showed substantial variation across centers. The relative risk of funneling for preterm delivery before 35 weeks was 5.0 at 24 weeks and 4.78 at 28 weeks.[29] The diagnostic indices are displayed in Table 31–3. It is of interest that in the study by Taipale and Hiilesmaa, funneling, defined as dilatation of the internal os of 5 mm or greater, was a stronger predictor of preterm delivery before 35 weeks than was endocervical cervical length. This study enrolled 3694 patients between 18 and 22 weeks of gestation. A dilated internal os (funneling) had a relative risk of 28 for preterm delivery before 35 weeks, whereas a short cervix (defined as length of less than 30 mm) had a relative risk of only 8. Multiple logistic regression analysis demonstrated that the adjusted odds ratio for delivery before 35 weeks was 20 for funneling and 6.5 for a short cervix.[67] We believe that the most likely explanation for the better performance of funneling than to cervical length in this study is that the definition of a short cervix was less than 30 mm. Most studies have indicated that such cervical length has a low positive predictive value for preterm delivery. Results may be different if a cervical length of 15 mm or 20 mm is used for analysis.

Can a Cervical Cerclage be Used to Prevent Preterm Delivery in Patients with a Short Cervix or Funneling?

The interest in predicting spontaneous preterm birth derives from the hope that an intervention in patients at risk will prevent preterm delivery. Cervical cerclage may be such an intervention. This operation was introduced in 1950 by Lash et al. for the treatment of patients at risk for spontaneous midtrimester abortion because of a primary cervical disease, an "incompetent cervix."[76] Many uncontrolled studies and three randomized clinical trials have been reported thus far. The design and results of these studies will be discussed later in this chapter.

Heath et al. reported the results of a study in which a large population was screened with cervical ultrasound. Clinicians responsible for the care of the patients with a short cervix (defined as 15 mm or less) were informed of the results and allowed to use their preference for further management. Of the 43 patients with a short cervix, 22 were treated with the placement of Shirodkar cerclage and 21 were managed expectantly. Although there were no differences in the clinical characteristics of the two groups, the rate of preterm delivery (before 32 weeks) was 52% (11 of 21) in the group managed expectantly and only 5% (1 of 22) in the group managed with a cervical cerclage (Fig. 31–11).[77] These observations are the basis for a randomized clinical trial that has been organized by Nicolaides et al. and the Fetal Medicine Foundation of the United Kingdom which is in progress. The study aims to recruit 24,000 patients.

In contrast, Berghella et al. reported negative results when placing a McDonald cerclage in patients with an

TABLE 31–6. CERVICAL FUNNELING AND PRETERM DELIVERY RISK IN SYMPTOMATIC PATIENTS

Reference	Year	N	Gestation (wks)	Cutoff	Definition of PTD	% Prevalence of PTD	% Sensitivity	% Specificity	% PPV	% NPV
Okitsu et al.[61]	1992	77	12–30	5 mm	<37wks	17	69	72	33	92
Gomez et al.[28]	1994	59	20–35	≥9 mm	<36wks	37	71	91	83	83
Timor-Tritsch et al.[80]	1996	70	20–35	Wedging	<37wks	27	100	74	59	100
Rizzo et al.[107]	1996	108	24–36	>5 mm	<37wks	43.5	70	67	62	74

PTD, preterm delivery; PPV, positive predictive value; NPV, negative predictive value.

(a) Expectant management

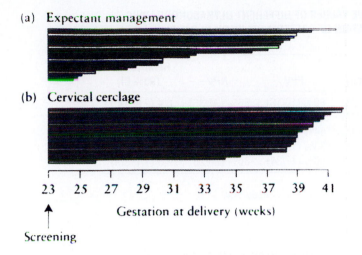

(b) Cervical cerclage

23 25 27 29 31 33 35 37 39 41

Gestation at delivery (weeks)

↑
Screening

Figure 31–11. Interval between gestational age at screening and gestational age at delivery in patients treated with expectant management and cervical cerclage. *(Reproduced with permission from Gomez R, et al.* Am J Obstet Gynecol. *1994;171:956–964.)*

abnormal cervix. In this study, 168 women at risk for preterm delivery underwent serial sonography between 14 and 23 weeks. Patients with a cervical length of less than 25 mm or funneling greater than 25% of the cervical length were offered either a McDonald cerclage or expectant management. Sixty-three patients had an abnormal cervix; 39 underwent cerclage and 24 were managed expectantly. Patients in the two groups were similar in clinical characteristics, cervical length, and funneling, but those who were treated with a cerclage had a lower gestational age when the cervical changes were identified (18 vs. 21 weeks) than did those in the control group. In this study, cervical cerclage did not reduce the rate of preterm delivery (27% with cerclage vs. 23% with expectant management) or the duration of pregnancy after the identification of abnormal cervical findings.[78] The different results reported by Heath et al. and those of Berghella et al. can be attributed to the definition of an abnormal cervix and the type of cerclage (McDonald vs.

Shirodkar) used. The sample size required to test the hypothesis in patients with a longer cervix (less than 25 mm rather than 15 mm) is also expected to be larger. The question of whether or not a cervical cerclage can reduce the rate of preterm birth can only be answered by a randomized clinical trial.

CERVICAL EXAMINATION IN PATIENTS WITH PRETERM LABOR

Meta-analysis of randomized clinical trials in which patients with preterm labor were treated with either a placebo or beta-adrenergic agents indicated that 47% of women treated with placebo deliver at term.[79] This has been interpreted as indicating that many patients are falsely diagnosed to have preterm labor. Assessment of the likelihood of preterm delivery is of clinical interest because it may influence important clinical decisions such as administration of tocolysis and steroids, transfer to a tertiary care center, and discharge from the hospital.

Examination of the cervix with ultrasound in patients presenting with preterm labor can assist in assessing the risk for preterm delivery. Table 31–7 summarizes the results of some of the studies published to date. In general, the shorter the cervix at presentation, the higher the risk for preterm delivery. An abnormal cervical index and the presence of funneling also increase the risk of preterm delivery, as demonstrated by Gomez et al.[28] (Table 31–8). Timor-Tritsch et al.[80] studied the clinical significance of funneling for the prediction of preterm delivery in a population with symptoms of preterm labor. In 70 patients admitted to the hospital for threatened preterm labor, "wedging" of the internal os was associated with preterm delivery, with a sensitivity of 100%, a specificity of 74%, a positive predictive value of 59%, and a negative predictive value of 100%.[80]

Another important observation on 60 singleton and twin pregnant women has been that all patients presenting with preterm labor and a cervix longer than 30 mm delivered at term.[75]

TABLE 31–7. MEASUREMENT OF CERVICAL LENGTH BY TRANSVAGINAL ULTRASOUND IN WOMEN WITH SYMPTOMS OF PRETERM LABOR

Reference	Year	N	Gestation (wks)	Cutoff	Definition of PTD	% Prevalence of PTD	% Sensitivity	% Specificity	% PPV	% NPV
Murakawa et al.[111]	1993	32	18–37	<20 mm	<37 wks	34	27	100	100	72
				≥35 mm			100	71	65	100
Iams et al.[75]	1994	60	24–35	<30 mm	<36 wks	40	100	44	55	100
Gomez et al.[28]	1994	59	20–35	≤18 mm	<36 wks	37	73	78	67	83
Rizzo et al.[107]	1996	108	24–36	≤20 mm	<37 wks	43	68	79	71	76
Rozenberg et al.[108]	1997	76	24–34	≤26 mm	<37 wks	26	75	73	50	89

PTD, preterm delivery; PPV, positive predictive value; NPV, negative predictive value.

TABLE 31–8. DIAGNOSTIC INDEXES AND PREDICTIVE VALUES OF DIFFERENT ULTRASONOGRAPHIC CERVICAL BIOMETRIC FINDINGS IN THE IDENTIFICATION OF PRETERM DELIVERY IN PATIENTS WITH ACUTE PRETERM LABOR

	Sensitivity	Specificity	PPV	NPV	Relative Risk (95% CI)
Cervical index ≥ 0.52	76% (16/21)	94% (31/33)	89% (16/18)	86% (31/36)	6.4 (2.8–14.7)
Cervical length ≤ 18 mm	73% (16/22)	78% (29/37)	67% (16/24)	83% (29/35)	3.9 (1.8–8.5)
Funnel width ≥ 6 mm	67% (14/21)	76% (25/33)	64% (14/22)	78% (25/32)	2.0 (1.4–6.0)
Funnel length ≥ 9 mm	71% (15/21)	91% (30/33)	83% (15/18)	83% (30/36)	5.0 (2.3–10.7)
Funneling present	77% (17/22)	54% (20/37)	50% (17/34)	80% (20/25)	2.5 (1.1–5.9)

PPV, positive predictive value; NPV, negative predictive value.
Reproduced with permission from Gomez R, et al., Am J Obstet Gynecol. 1994;171:956–964.

The high negative predictive value for preterm birth associated with a long cervix and with the absence of funneling has important clinical implications in symptomatic patients.

Can Sonography be Used for the Assessment of Cervical Dilatation?

Several investigators have examined the value of ultrasound in assessing cervical dilatation. Lim et al. compared digital examination and ultrasound assessment of cervical dilatation in 82 women before planned induction of labor.[81] Cervical dilatation by digital examination was found to be significantly greater than that derived by sonography. Mahony et al. found little correlation between digital and sonographic (transperineal) assessment of cervical dilatation.[82] The agreement of these two studies underscores the limitations of ultrasound in determining cervical dilatation.

In a recent study, the appearance of a sonographically undilated cervix was found in six of nine women who were evaluated for threatened preterm labor and who had dilation by digital examination at least equal to 2 cm. The investigators suggested that there might be a better correlation between digital and sonographic dilatation if the cervix was imaged in the transverse rather than in the sagittal plane.[58]

Dynamic Cervical Changes During Real-Time Examination

Dynamic cervical changes consist of spontaneous transient funneling of the internal os and shortening of the cervical canal during the course of an examination of the cervix. These modifications have been reported in patients with the diagnosis of an incompetent cervix[83] and in patients at risk for preterm delivery.[50] Because external uterine pressure can induce similar findings, dynamic changes have been attributed to the effect of uterine contractions on a compliant cervix.[83] Okitsu et al. report that the presence of dynamic cervical changes is associated with a 22% positive predictive value for preterm delivery.[61]

CERVICAL INCOMPETENCE

The ability of the cervix to retain the conceptus during pregnancy has been referred to as *cervical competence* and the condition in which the cervix fails to fulfill its physiologic role is designated by default as *cervical incompetence*. Obstetricians have traditionally made this diagnosis based on obstetric history.

The diagnosis is often applied to patients with a history of one or more midtrimester spontaneous abortions and/or early preterm deliveries in which the basic process is thought to be the failure of the cervix to remain closed during pregnancy. The basic assumption is that cervical dilatation and effacement have occurred in the absence of a significant increase in uterine contractility. The presenting symptom is often a feeling of vaginal pressure caused by the distention of this organ by the protruding membranes or rupture of membranes in the midtrimester of pregnancy. Typically, there is no vaginal bleeding, the fetus is born alive, and labor is short and pain free. A history of repeated midtrimester abortions at similar gestational ages is highly suggestive of the condition.

Cervical incompetence can be due to congenital müllerian duct abnormalities, DES exposure or be secondary to cervical surgical trauma (i.e., conization or cervical operations requiring dilatation of the canal). However, some patients will present with the typical picture in their first pregnancy without any apparent cause. Regrettably, there is no objective diagnostic test for this condition. Several methods have been proposed for the evaluation of a patient after a pregnancy loss (i.e., a hysterosalpingogram and passage of a no. 8 Hegar cervical dilatator). However, there is a paucity of scientific evidence to support the value of these tests.

It is noteworthy that cervical incompetence is thought to result in midtrimester spontaneous abortion. However, cervical disease (i.e., hypoplastic cervix, DES exposure, or a weakened cervix after conization) is also associated with an increased risk of preterm premature rupture of membranes and preterm labor. Therefore, there is a need to revisit the traditional definition of cervical incompetence.

We have proposed that parturition has a common terminal pathway characterized by increased myometrial contractility, cervical ripening, and membrane/decidual activation. These processes are required for both term and preterm parturition. Normal labor at term is characterized by coordinated activation of these three mechanisms; thus, patients will present with increased uterine contractility, cervical effacement, and dilatation and eventually rupture their membranes. However, premature activation of different components can occur in a coordinated or uncoordinated way. The premature coordinated activation of these mechanisms is observed in patients with classic preterm labor with progressive cervical dilation leading to preterm delivery. Preferential activation of cervical ripening in the midtrimester leads to the condition known as cervical incompetence. Later in pregnancy some patients will complain of vaginal pressure and will be recognized to have cervical dilatation and effacement out of proportion to the frequency and intensity of myometrial contractility. Although these patients are traditionally considered to have preterm labor, clearly cervical ripening is the main component of the terminal pathway activated in these particular cases.[84] This model of preterm parturition is important because it suggests that premature cervical ripening may result in a spectrum of disease ranging from midtrimester abortion, some forms of preterm labor, and precipitous labor at term. Figures 31–12 and 31–13 show these concepts.

The hypothesis that there is a spectrum of cervical competence has been examined by Iams et al.[85] A cross-sectional study was conducted in which cervical length was measured in patients from the following groups: 1) typical history of cervical incompetence; 2) previous preterm delivery at or before 26 weeks, 3) previous preterm delivery 27 weeks to 32 weeks; 4) previous preterm delivery before 33 weeks; and 5) a control group of women with previous term de-

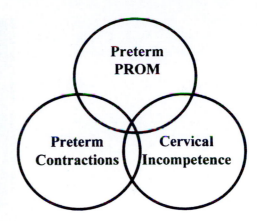

Figure 31−13. Clinical manifestations of the premature activation of the common terminal pathway of human parturition. *(Reproduced with permission from Romero R, et al. In: Elder MG, Lamont RF, Romero R, eds. Preterm Labor. New York: Churchill-Livingstone; 1997:29.)*

livery. A strong relation was found between cervical length in the index pregnancy and previous obstetric history. This relationship appears linear and patients considered to have a typical history of an incompetent cervix did not constitute a unique group.[85] Similar results have been observed by Guzman et al.[86] who observed a strong relation between previous obstetric history and cervical length in the subsequent pregnancy. Specifically, they reported that the frequency of a short cervix (cervical length less than 2 cm) or progressive shortening of the cervix to a length shorter than 2 cm was associated with the gestational age at delivery in the previous pregnancy.[86] Collectively, these studies suggest that there is a relation between a history of preterm delivery and the cervical length. Inasmuch as patients with a short cervix are at increased risk for a midtrimester pregnancy loss (clinically referred to as cervical incompetence) or spontaneous preterm delivery with intact or rupture of membranes, a short cervix must be considered as the expression of a spectrum of cervical disease. However, further investigation is required to determine the reason why some women with a short cervix have an adverse pregnancy outcome and others have an uncomplicated term delivery. Indeed, approximately 50% of women with a cervix of 15 mm or less deliver after 32 weeks without a cerclage.[77] This suggests that cervical length is only one of the factors determining the degree of cervical competence for a certain patient.

Sonographers have used the term *cervical incompetence* to refer to a midtrimester condition in which the cervix is open and the membranes bulge into the vagina. Figures 31–14 and 31–15 display the sonographic appearance of a grossly incompetent cervix. This diagnosis has clinical implications because its treatment consists of emergency cerclage. The standard management for such a patient in a subsequent pregnancy is to place a cerclage electively after 14 weeks.

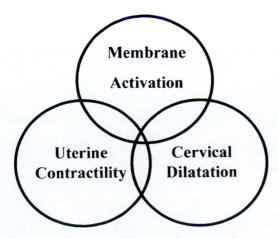

Figure 31−12. The common terminal pathway of preterm and term parturition. *(Reproduced with permission from Romero R, et al. In: Elder MG, Lamont RF, Romero R, eds. Preterm Labor. New York: Churchill-Livingstone; 1997:29.)*

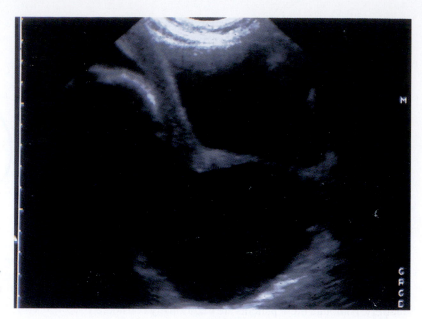

Figure 31–14. Sonographic appearance of a grossly incompetent cervix, with bulging of the membranes in the vagina.

A common clinical problem is the management of the patient with an equivocal history for cervical incompetence. Sonographic examination of the cervix is currently being used in clinical practice to monitor cervical changes in the midtrimester to determine the need for a cervical cerclage. Surveillance can be conducted by determining cervical length and detecting funneling before and after a cervical stress test. Under normal circumstances, the cervical length does not change between 12 and 24 weeks. However, in patients who eventually develop a short cervix, the rate of cervical shortening may vary dramatically. For example, Guzman et al. reported that the rate of cervical shortening in some patients is as much as 5 mm per week, as shown in Fig. 31–16.[87]

A "cervical stress test" is a method to identify a compliant cervix, that is, one that has prematurely ripened. The stress test consists of increasing intrauterine pressure while monitoring cervical length and the appearance of funneling. Intrauterine pressure can be increased by applying transfundal pressure, a Valsalva maneuver, or changing the position of the patient from supine to standing.[88,89] Guzman et al. concluded that transfundal pressure is the most sensitive stress test and also it is the most commonly used method (moderate pressure on the maternal abdomen in the direction of the uterine axis for about 15 seconds).[88] Under normal circumstances, application of fundal pressure does not affect cervical length or results in funneling. In contrast, if pressure results in

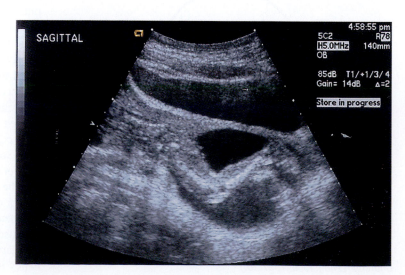

Figure 31–15. Sonographic appearance of a grossly incompetent cervix, with bulging of the membranes in the vagina. The fetal lower extremities protruded into the vagina.

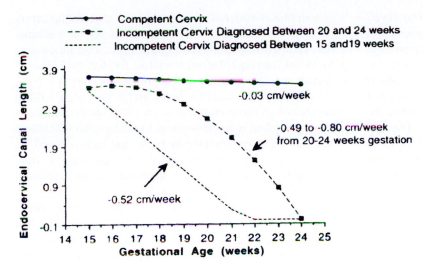

Figure 31-16. Multivariable linear regression models of the endocervical lengths of women at risk for pregnancy loss and preterm birth between 15 and 24 weeks of gestation in cases of competent and incompetent cervix. (*Reproduced with permission from Guzman ER, et al.* Obstet Gynecol. *1998;92:31–37.*)

funneling or shortening of the cervix, ripening of the cervix has occurred.

The basis for the utilization of a transfundal pressure stress test is a study conducted by Guzman et al., in which fundal uterine pressure was applied to 150 pregnant women without risk factors at 16 to 24 weeks. No changes in cervical length or funneling were detected. The rate of preterm delivery and midtrimester loss was 6% (9 of 150). Of the nine patients who had a normal response to transfundal pressure and had adverse pregnancy outcome, two had spontaneous midtrimester abortions at 22 and 23 weeks and the remainder had preterm deliveries. The same stress test was applied to 31 women at risk for cervical incompetence on the basis of history (i.e., midtrimester spontaneous abortions, early preterm labor, previous cone biopsy, DES exposure, uterine anomaly or requirement for emergency cerclage in previous pregnancy, etc.). Transfundal pressure resulted in opening of the internal os in 45% (14 of 31) of patients. All but one patient with a positive response were treated with a cervical cerclage. The patient managed expectantly had a spontaneous abortion, whereas 64% (9 of 14) of the treated patients delivered at term, 21% (3 of 14) had a preterm delivery, and 14% (2 of 14) had a spontaneous abortion (before 24 weeks).[88]

Subsequently, Guzman et al. followed prospectively 10 patients at risk for cervical incompetence who had a positive cervical stress test at the first examination in the midtrimester. A positive stress test was defined as a decrease in endocervical length equal to or greater than 2.0 mm. Nine of these 10 patients (one case was lost to follow-up) were followed with serial scans until the cervical length was less than 10 mm or a digital examination revealed a dilated cervix, at which point a cervical cerclage was placed. The patient with a positive stress test temporarily lost to follow-up had a spontaneous abortion at 23 weeks. All patients with a positive test

were treated with a cervical cerclage; 66% (6 of 9) delivered near term (<36 weeks), two patients delivered preterm (at 27 and 34 weeks); and one patient lost her pregnancy at the time of cerclage placement (18 weeks). This study shows that a positive response to transfundal pressure in the midtrimester is followed by progressive cervical changes.[91]

A frequent clinical question is whether patients with an equivocal history of cervical incompetence should have an elective cerclage placed at 14 to 16 weeks or be followed with serial measurements until there is evidence of increased cervical compliance. The literature suggests that the outcome of pregnancy is better in patients undergoing an elective cerclage rather than an emergency procedure. However, Guzman et al. compared the pregnancy outcome in 138 patients at risk for pregnancy loss who were treated with an elective cerclage ($n = 81$) or monitored with serial examinations and treated when ultrasound showed signs of cervical abnormalities ($n = 57$). No differences in outcome were observed.[92]

Ultrasound can be helpful in assisting in the intraoperative placement of a cerclage. Using continuous transabdominal ultrasound guidance, it is possible to monitor the precise placement of the cerclage to ensure placement of the stitch as close as possible to the internal cervical os.[93]

Ultrasound can also be used in the evaluation of the cervix after cerclage placement. Althuisius et al. demonstrated that the placement of an elective McDonald suture resulted in an increased mean endocervical length from 21 mm (95% confidence interval [CI], 19 to 23) to 34 mm (95% CI, 30 to 38).[94] Similar findings have been reported after the placement of Shirodkar procedures.[95] Guzman et al. reported that the risk for preterm delivery is six times greater if the difference between preoperative and postoperative cervical length is less than 10 mm.[96]

Transvaginal sonography may be used for the postoperative monitoring of patients who have undergone cervical cerclage. Quinn et al. reported that all patients who developed a dilated internal os and herniation of the membranes after placement of a Shirodkar cerclage had a preterm birth (between 5 and 7 weeks after the detection of sonographic abnormalities).[97] Similar findings were reported by Rana et al. with transabdominal sonography in a small number of patients.[98] Andersen et al. observed 32 patients with endovaginal sonography after cerclage placement. The risk of preterm delivery was significantly increased in those patients who developed shortening of the upper cervix (above the suture) to 10 mm or less as compared with patients whose upper cervical length was longer than 20 mm (58 vs. 10%, $p = 0.006$). A short upper cervix (10 mm) had a sensitivity, specificity, positive predictive value, and negative predictive value of 86%, 76%, 50%, and 95%, respectively, for the prediction of delivery before 34 weeks of gestation.[99]

Randomized Clinical Trials of Cervical Cerclage

The clinical value of cervical cerclage has been a subject of debate. Three randomized clinical trials have been conducted thus far in singleton gestations. Table 31–9 summarizes the details of the clinical trials. All studies were conducted before evaluation of the cervix with sonography became widespread. We summarize the highlights of the studies.

Rush et al. reported a study conducted in 194 women at high risk for late spontaneous abortion or preterm delivery. Patients were randomly allocated to either cerclage ($n = 96$) or expectant management ($n = 98$) between 15 and 21 weeks. The overall rate of preterm delivery was 33%, but there was no difference in the rate of preterm delivery between patients treated with McDonald cerclage or expectant management (preterm delivery before 37 weeks; expectant management, 32%, vs. cerclage, 34%). The duration of pregnancy was slightly longer in patients managed expectantly than in the cerclage group, but this difference was attributed to days gained after the 37th week. Rupture of membrane was more frequent in patients who had a cerclage than in the control group (18.7 % [18 of 96] vs. 12.3% [12 of 98]), but this difference did not reach statistical significance. There was no difference in neonatal outcome. However, fever during the puerperium was more common in patients managed with cerclage (cerclage: 9.6% [10 of 96] vs. expectant: 3% [3 of 98], $p = 0.07$).[100]

Lazar et al. reported a trial of 506 women considered to be at moderate risk for preterm delivery based on a scoring system that considered obstetric history, state of the cervix (i.e., open internal os, a short cervix at digital examination, etc.). Two hundred sixty-eight patients were allocated to McDonald cerclage placement with no. 3 nylon and 238 to expectant management. The rate of preterm delivery was 6.7% (18 of 268) in the cerclage group and 5.5% (13 of 238) in the control group (overall rate was 6.1%). Patients in the cerclage group had more admissions to the hospital (excluding hospitalization for cerclage or birth) and received oral tocolysis more frequently than did those in the control group ($p < 0.01$ for each). However, there were no differences in perinatal mortality between the two groups.[101]

The largest trial conducted to date was organized by the Medical Research Council of the United Kingdom and the Royal College of Obstetricians and Gynecologists. The criteria for enrollment was uncertainty on the part of the obstetricians as to whether to recommend a cerclage. The main reason for enrollment was a past history of one or more second-trimester spontaneous abortions or preterm deliveries (71% of patients) and a history of cervical operation. The type of operation and surgical material was left to the discretion of the caregiver, and the study was conducted in multiple countries. Of patients allocated to cerclage, only 92% had the suture inserted, whereas 8% of those in the control group had a cerclage. The mean gestational age at cerclage was 15.9 weeks (interquartile range was 14.3 to 18.4). The primary outcome was delivery at less than 33 completed weeks. The rate of delivery before 33 weeks (range of 20 to 33 weeks) was significantly lower in the cerclage group than in the control group (cerclage, 13%, vs. control group, 17%; odds ratio of 0.72; 95 CI, 0.53 to 0.97; $p = 0.03$). Fever attributed to uterine infection was more common in patients allocated to the cerclage group (6 vs. 3%; odds ratio, 2.12; 95% CI, 1.08 to 4.16; $p = 0.03$). The investigators estimated that 25 cerclages would need to be inserted to prevent one preterm delivery before 33 weeks. The overall rate of preterm delivery was 28% (before 37 weeks). A subgroup analysis suggested that patients with a history of three spontaneous midtrimester abortions or preterm deliveries seemed to benefit the most from the procedure.[102] The investigators called for research in methods to identify patients who may benefit from this operation.

One small study examined the value of cervical cerclage in twin gestation. There was no evidence of benefit in this condition.[103]

TABLE 31–9. RANDOMIZED STUDIES OF ELECTIVE CERVICAL CERCLAGE

Reference	Year	N	Indication	Weeks at Cerclage	Delivery < 37 Weeks	
					% Cerclage	% Controls
Rush et al.[100]	1984	194	High risk of cervical incompetence	18	34	32
Lazar et al.[101]	1984	506	Moderate risk of cervical incompetence	<28	6.7	5.5
MRC/RCOG[102]	1993	1292	Obstetrician uncertainty	16	26	31

TABLE 31–10. RISK OF SPONTANEOUS PRETERM BIRTH AT VARIOUS GESTATIONAL AGES WITH VARIOUS COMBINATIONS OF RISK FACTORS IN NULLIPARAS AND MULTIPARAS

Risk Factor	% Nulliparas				% Multiparas			
	n	<32 wks	<35 wks	<37 wks	n	<32 wks	<35 wks	<37 wks
All negative	103	.06	1.7	6.0	1190	0.5	1.5	7.3
Only FFN+	52	3.9	5.8	11.5	73	2.7	9.6	19.2
Only CL ≤ 25 mm	109	3.7	9.2	18.4	64	0	4.7	15.6
Only PSPB	—	—	—	—	278	1.8	8.6	17.6
FFN+ + CL ≤ 25 mm	17	35.3	58.8	64.7	16	18.8	25.0	43.8
FFN+ + PSPB	—	—	—	—	25	24.0	40.0	48.0
CL ≤ 25 mm + PSPB	—	—	—	—	48	8.3	29.2	35.4
All three	—	—	—	—	10	50.0	60.0	60.0

FFN+, fetal fibronectin positive; CL, cervical length; PSPB, prior spontaneous preterm birth.
Reproduced with permission from Goldenberg RL, et al., Am J Public Health. 1998;88:233–238.

In conclusion, results of randomized clinical trials suggest that cerclage either had a modest effect on reducing the rate of preterm delivery or no effect whatsoever. We believe that the fundamental problem is that preterm labor is a syndrome with multiple etiologies, and the operation can only benefit those patients who have a primary or important cervical process responsible for preterm delivery. It is clear that obstetrical history is insufficient to identify such patients. We believe that future studies in which patient selection for cerclage is based on results of cervical ultrasound or noninvasive determination of collagen content may identify a role for cerclage in modern obstetrics.

Noninvasive Assessment of Collagen Content

A decrease in total collagen content, an increase in collagen solubility and collagenolytic activity characterize cervical ripening during pregnancy. A quantitative method to determine cervical ripening that analyzes the collagen content of the cervix through fluorescence spectroscopy has been proposed by Garfield and Chwalitz. The collascope is an optical device that determines cervical collagen content by means of a fluorescent signal generated whenever collagen cross links are excited by light whose wavelength is about 340 nm. The system has been used in rats and in humans at different stages

of pregnancy and has shown that cervical ripening occurs progressively in the last trimester of pregnancy.[104] Further studies are required to determine the value of this technology in obstetrics and if it adds information not provided by ultrasound.

BIOCHEMICAL MARKERS TO PREDICT PRETERM BIRTH

The use of biochemical markers for the prediction of preterm birth has the potential advantage of providing direct evidence of changes in the extracellular matrix at the interface between fetal membranes and maternal decidua. There is clear evidence that the processes leading to the breakdown of the extracellular matrix of the cervix and to cervical ripening are detectable by the release in cervical and vaginal secretions of metalloenzymes, cytokines, and fetal fibronectin.

Fetal fibronectin is an extracellular matrix protein and its presence in the cervical or vaginal secretions after the 20th week of pregnancy has been found to be predictive of preterm delivery.[105] Other potential biochemical markers of cervical ripening (e.g., IL-6 and MMPs) can be expected to appear preceding the shortening of the cervix and preterm labor but their usefulness remains to be tested.

TABLE 31–11. DIAGNOSTIC INDICES AND PREDICTIVE VALUES OF FETAL FIBRONECTIN DETERMINATION AND ULTRASONOGRAPHIC CERVICAL MEASUREMENT FOR PREDICTION OF PRETERM DELIVERY

	% Sensitivity	% Specificity	% PPV	% NPV
Cervical fetal fibronectin ≥ 60 ng/mL	80.85	83.61	79.17	85.00
Vaginal fetal fibronectin > 50 ng/mL	74.47	86.89	81.40	81.54
Cervical index ≥ 0.50	70.21	80.33	73.33	77.78
Cervical length ≤ 20 mm	68.09	78.69	71.11	76.19
Funneling present	70.2	67.2	62.2	74.5

PPV, positive predictive value; NPV, negative predictive value.
Reproduced with permission from Rizzo G, et al., Am J Obstet Gynecol. 1996;175:1146–1151.

TABLE 31–12. RISK OF PRETERM DELIVERY ACCORDING TO TEST USED IN PATIENTS WITH ACUTE PRETERM LABOR

	Abnormal Test Result[a]	Normal Test Result	Odds Ratio (95% CI)
*f*FN	45.2% (14/31)	13.3% (6/45)	5.3 (1.9–15.5)
TVS	50.0% (15/30)	10.9% (5/46)	8.2 (2.8–24.4)
*f*FN or TVS	45.0% (18/40)	5.5% (2/36)	13.9 (3.7–52.2)
*f*FN and TVS	52.4% (11/21)	16.4% (9/55)	5.6 (1.9–16.2)

CI, confidence interval; *f*FN, fetal fibronectin; TVS, transvaginal ultrasonographic measurement of cervical length.
[a]Abnormal test result = *f*FN > 50 ng/mL, cervical length ≤ 26 mm.
Reproduced with permission from Rozenberg P, et al., Am J Obstet Gynecol. 1997;176:196–199.

Fetal Fibronectin

Fetal fibronectin is a high-molecular-weight glycoprotein (45 kDa) normally expressed by chorion cells. Fibronectins are extracellular cement that have been implicated in the normal process of adhesion of the membranes to the decidua. As part of the process of parturition, matrix degrading enzymes are thought to digest macromolecular components of the matrix including fibronectins. These proteins leak into the cervical and vaginal secretions, where they can be detected as an indirect index of "membrane activation."[84,105] Therefore, increased concentrations of fibronectin in vaginal fluid are present in patients with both term and preterm labor.

The detection of fetal fibronectin in vaginal fluid has been studied to identify asymptomatic patients who may be at risk for preterm delivery and also in patients presenting in preterm labor. The largest study to date examining the relation between fetal fibronectin and cervical length was the MFMN NICHD Preterm Prediction Study. Goldenberg et al. reported that the risk of preterm delivery before 32 weeks for an asymptomatic nulliparous with a positive fetal fibronectin test is 3.9% and that the risk for an isolated short cervix (equal to or less than 25 mm) is 3.7%. However, a patient with both risk factors had a risk of 35%. A similar synergistic effect was demonstrable in multiparous women. Table 31–10 displays the risk of preterm delivery for nulliparous and parous women.[106] Thus, patients with a short cervix and a positive fetal fibronectin are at particularly increased risk for preterm delivery. We believe that a patient with a short cervix and a positive fibronectin represents a group in which activation of two of the components of the common terminal pathway of parturition have already occurred (cervical ripening and membrane activation). Some of these cases may represent cases of subclinical ascending intrauterine infection.

Several studies have addressed the question of whether biochemical markers add significant information to that provided by sonographic examination of the cervix in patients presenting with preterm labor. Rizzo et al. studied 108 patients with preterm labor and intact membranes with fetal fibronectin and sonographic examination of the cervix. The prevalence of preterm delivery was 43%. A fetal fibronectin of 60 ng/mL or more had the highest diagnostic performance

in predicting preterm delivery (81% sensitivity, 84% specificity, 79% positive predictive value, and 85% negative predictive value). The diagnostic indices and predictive values are presented in Table 31–11. However, logistic regression analysis indicated that a fetal fibronectin of 60 ng/mL was the strongest predictor of preterm delivery. Also, patients with positive fibronectin and an abnormal cervical index (equal to or greater than 0.50) had a shorter interval to delivery.[107] These data suggest that ultrasound can add some information to that provided by fetal fibronectin. We believe that the most important observation of this study is that the diagnostic value of sonography, which is immediately available, is almost equivalent to that of fetal fibronectin, which is expensive and requires a laboratory assay.

Rozenberg et al. reported a prospective study of 76 patients with signs of preterm labor between 24 and 34 weeks of gestation. The prevalence of preterm birth (before 37 weeks) was 26%. Table 31–12 presents the diagnostic and predictive values of fetal fibronectin and cervical length by transvaginal sonography. The investigators did not find a difference in the performance of both tests and concluded that fetal fibronectin adds little additional information to that provided by sonography.[108]

REFERENCES

1. Schwalm H, Dubrauszky V. The structure of the musculature of the human uterus—Muscles and connective tissue. *Am J Obstet Gynecol.* 1966;94:391.
2. Danforth D. The distribution and functional activity of the cervical musculature. *Am J Obstet Gynecol.* 1954;68:1261.
3. Yu SY, Tozzi CA, Babiarz J, et al. Collagen changes in rat cervix in pregnancy-polarized light microscopic and electron microscopic studies. *PSEBM.* 1995;209:360.
4. Uldbjerg N, Forman A, Peterson LK, et al. Biochemical changes of the uterus and cervix during pregnancy. In: Reece EA, Hobbins JC, Mahoney MJ, et al, eds. *Medicine of the Fetus and of the Mother.* Philadelphia: JB Lippincott; 1992:849.
5. Leppert PC. Proliferation and apoptosis of fibroblasts and smooth muscle cells in rat uterine cervix throughout gestation and the effect of the antiprogesterone onapristone. *Am J Obstet Gynecol.* 1998;178:713.

6. Uldbjerg N, Ekman G, Malmstrom A, et al. Ripening of the human uterine cervix related to changes in collagen, glycosaminoglycans, and collagenolytic activity. *Am J Obstet Gynecol.* 1983;147:662.

7. Petersen LK, Uldbjerg N. Cervical hydroxyproline concentration in relation to age and parity. In: Leppert P, Woessner F, eds. *Extracellular Matrix of the Uterus, Cervix and Fetal Membranes.* Ithaca: Perinatology Press; 1991.

8. Liggins GC. Cervical ripening as an inflammatory reaction. In: Ellwood DA, Anderson ABM, eds. *The Cervix in Pregnancy and Labour: Clinical and Biochemical Investigations.* Edinburgh: Churchill-Livingstone; 1981.

9. Ito A, Hiro D, Ojima Y, et al. The role of leukocyte factors in uterine cervical ripening and dilatation. *Biol Reprod.* 1987; 37:511.

10. Ito A, Hiro D, Ojima Y, et al. Spontaneous production of interleukin-1 factors from pregnant rabbit uterine cervix. *Am J Obstet Gynecol.* 1988;159:261.

11. Ito A, Leppert PC, Mori Y. Human recombinant interkeukin-1 increases elastase-like enzyme in human uterine cervical fibroblasts. *Gynecol Obstet Invest.* 1990;30:239.

12. Osmers RG, Adelmann-Grill BC, Rath W, et al. Biochemical events in cervical ripening dilatation during pregnancy and parturition. *J Obstet Gynaecol.* 1995;21:185.

13. Kelly RW. Pregnancy maintenance and parturition: The role of prostaglandin in manipulating the immune and inflammatory response. *Endocr Rev.* 1994;15:684.

14. Chwalisz K, Benson M, Scholz P, et al. Cervical ripening with the cytokines interleukin 8, interleukin 1beta and tumor necrosis factor alpha in guinea pigs. *Hum Reprod.* 1994;9: 2173.

15. Sennstrom MK, Brauner A, Lu Y, et al. Interleukin-8 is a mediator of the final cervical ripening in humans. *Eur J Obstet Gynecol Reprod Biol.* 1997;74:89.

16. Osmers RG, Blaser J, Kuhn W. Interleukin-8 synthesis and the onset of labor. *Obstet Gynecol.* 1995;86:223.

17. Rajabi MR, Dodge GR, Soloman S, et al. Immunochemical and immunohistochemical evidence of estrogen-mediated collagenolysis as a mechanism of dilatation in the guinea pig at parturition. *Endocrinology.* 1991;128:371.

18. Granström L, Ekman GE, Malmstrom A, et al. Serum collagenase levels in relation to the state of the human cervix during pregnancy and labor. *Am J Obstet Gynecol.* 1992;167: 1284.

19. Pinto RM, Raboa W, Votta RA. Uterine cervix ripening in term pregnancy due to the action of estradiol-17. *Am J Obstet Gynecol.* 1965;92:319.

20. Chwalisz K, Shi S, Neef G, et al. The effect of antigestagen ZK 98 299 on the uterine cervix. *Acta Endocrinol.* 1987;283: 113.

21. Shi S-Q, Beier HM, Garfield RE, et al. The specific cyclooxygenase inhibitor flosulide inhibits antiprogestin-induced preterm birth. *J Soc Gynecol Invest.* 1996;3(suppl):540.

22. Chawlisz K, Kosub B, Garfield RE. Estradiol inhibits the onapristone (ZK 98 299) induced preterm parturition in guinea pigs by blocking cervical ripening. *J Soc Gynecol Invest.* 1995;2:267.

23. Chwalisz K, Garfield RE. Antiprogesterones in the induction of labor. *Ann NY Acad Sci.* 1994;734:387.

24. Chawlisz K, Shao-Qing S, Garfield RE, et al. Cervical ripening in guinea pigs after a local application of nitric oxide. *Hum Reprod.* 1997;12:2093.

25. Thomson AJ, Lunan CB, Cameron AD, et al. Nitric oxide donors induce ripening of the human cervix: A randomized controlled trial. *Br J Obstet Gynecol.* 1997;104:1054.

26. Chwalisz K, Buhimschi I, Garfield RE. Role of nitric oxide in obstetrics. *Prenat Neonat Med.* 1996;1:292.

27. Romero R, Mazor M, Gomez R, et al. Cervix, incompetence and premature labor. *Fetus.* 1993;545:1.

28. Gomez R, Galasso M, Romero R, et al. Ultrasonographic examination of the uterine cervix is better than cervical digital examination as a predictor of the likelihood of premature delivery in patients with preterm labor and intact membranes. *Am J Obstet Gynecol.* 1994;171:956.

29. Iams JD, Goldenberg RL, Meis PJ, et al. The length of the cervix and the risk of spontaneous premature delivery. *N Engl J Med.* 1996;334:567.

30. Abramovici H, Faktor JH, Pascal B. Congenital uterine malformations as indication for cervical suture (cerclage) in habitual abortion and premature delivery. *Int J Fertil.* 1983;28: 161.

31. Singer MS, Hochman M. Incompetent cervix in a hormone-exposed offspring. *Obstet Gynecol.* 1978;51:625.

32. Rudd NL, Nimrod C, Holbrook KA, et al. Pregnancy complications in type IV Ehlers–Danlos syndrome. *Lancet.* 1983; 8:50.

33. Romero R, Gonzalez R, Sepulveda W, et al. Microbial invasion of the amniotic cavity in patients with suspected cervical incompetence: Prevalence and clinical significance. *Am J Obstet Gynecol.* 1992;167:1085.

34. Guzman ER, Shen-Schwartz S, Benito C, et al. The relationship between placental histology and cervical ultrasonography in women at risk for pregnancy loss and spontaneous preterm birth. *Am J Obstet Gynecol.* 1999,181.793.

35. Bishop EH. Pelvic scoring for elective induction. *Obstet Gynecol.* 1964;24:266.

36. Calder AA, Embrey MP, Hillier K. Extra-amniotic prostaglandin—E2 for the induction of labor at term. *J Obstet Gynaecol Br Commonw.* 1974;81:39.

37. Weekes AR, Flynn MJ. Engagement of the fetal head in primigravidae and its relationship to duration of gestation and time of onset of labor. *Br J Obstet Gynecol.* 1975;82:7.

38. Papiernik E, Bouyer J, Collin D, et al. Precocious cervical ripening and preterm labor. *Obstet Gynecol.* 1986;67:238.

39. Bouyer J, Papiernik E, Dreyfus J, et al. Maturation signs of the cervix and prediction of preterm birth. *Obstet Gynecol.* 1988;68:209.

40. Anderson A, Turnbull AC. Relationship between length of gestation and cervical dilatation, uterine contractility, and other factors during pregnancy. *Am J Obstet Gynecol.* 1969;105:1207.

41. Stubbs TM, Van Dorsten JP, Miller MC 3rd. The preterm cervix and preterm labor: Relative risks, predictive values, and change over time. *Am J Obstet Gynecol.* 1986;155:829.

42. Leveno KJ, Cox K, Roark ML. Cervical dilatation and prematurity revisited. *Obstet Gynecol.* 1986;68:434.

43. Holbrook RH Jr., Falcon J, Herron M, et al. Evaluation of the weekly cervical examination in a preterm birth prevention program. *Am J Perinatol.* 1987;4:240.

44. Catalano PM, Ashikaga T, Mann LI. Cervical change and

uterine activity as predictors of preterm delivery. *Am J Perinatol.* 1989;6:185.

45. Copper R, Hauth R, Goldenberg R, et al. Cervical changes and tocodynanometry vs. spontaneous preterm delivery in nulliparas (abstract 267). Presented at the Annual Meeting of the Society of Perinatal Obstetricians, San Francisco, February 8–13, 1993.

46. Holcomb W Jr., Smeltzer JS. Cervical effacement: Variations in belief among clinicians. *Obstet Gynecol.* 1991;78:4347.

47. Phelps JY, Higby K, Smyth MH, et al. Accuracy and intraobserver variability of simulated cervical dilatation measurements. *Am J Obstet Gynecol.* 1995;173:942.

48. Lenihan JP Jr. Relationship of antepartum pelvic examination to premature rupture of membranes. *Obstet Gynecol.* 1984;63:33.

49. Main DM, Richardson DK, Hadley CB, et al. Controlled trial of a preterm labor detection program: Efficacy and costs. *Obstet Gynecol.* 1989;74:873.

50. Sonek JD, Iams JD, Blumenfeld M, et al. Measurement of cervical length in pregnancy: Comparison between vaginal ultrasonography and digital examination. *Obstet Gynecol.* 1990;76:172.

51. Jeanty P, D'Alton M, Romero R, et al. Perineal scanning. *Am J Perinatol.* 1986;3:289.

52. Zilianti M, Azuaga A, Calderon F, et al. Monitoring the effacement of the uterine cervix by transperineal sonography: A new perspective. *J Ultrasound Med.* 1995;14:719.

53. Mason GC, Maresh MJ. Alterations in bladder volume and the ultrasound appearance of the cervix. *Br J Obstet Gynaecol.* 1990;97:457.

54. Andersen HF. Transvaginal and transabdominal ultrasonography of the uterine cervix during pregnancy. *J Clin Ultrasound.* 1991;19:77.

55. Jackson GM, Ludmir J, Bader TJ. The accuracy of digital examination and ultrasound in the evaluation of cervical length. *Obstet Gynecol.* 1992;79:214.

56. O'Brien JM, Allen AA, Barton JR. Intravaginal saline as a contrast agent for cervical sonography in the obstetric patient. *Ultrasound Obstet Gynecol.* 1999;13:137.

57. Berghella V, Kuhlman K, Weiner S, et al. Cervical funneling: Sonographic criteria predictive of preterm delivery. *Ultrasound Obstet Gynecol.* 1997;10:161.

58. Yost NP, Bloom SL, Twickler DM, et al. Pitfalls in ultrasonic cervical length measurements for predicting preterm birth. *Obstet Gynecol.* 1999;93:510.

59. Andersen HF, Nugent CE, Wanty SD, et al. Prediction of risk for preterm delivery by ultrasonographic measurement of cervical length. *Am J Obstet Gynecol.* 1990;163:859.

60. Kushnir O, Vigil DA, Izquierdo L, et al. Vaginal ultrasonographic assessment of cervical length changes during normal pregnancy. *Am J Obstet Gynecol.* 1990;162:991.

61. Okitsu O, Mimura T, Nakayama T, et al. Early prediction of preterm delivery by transvaginal ultrasonography. *Ultrasound Obstet Gynecol.* 1992;2:402.

62. Riley L, Frigoletto FD Jr., Benacerraf BR. The implications of sonographically identified cervical changes in patients not necessarily at risk for preterm birth. *J Ultrasound Med.* 1992;11:75.

63. Tongsong T, Kamprapanth P, Srisomboon J, et al. Single transvaginal sonographic measurement of cervical length early

in the third trimester as a predictor of preterm delivery. *Obstet Gynecol.* 1995;86:184.

64. Heath VC, Southall TR, Souka AP, et al. Cervical length at 23 weeks of gestation: Prediction of spontaneous preterm delivery. *Ultrasound Obstet Gynecol.* 1998;12:312.

65. Heath VC, Southall TR, Souka AP, et al. Cervical length at 23 weeks of gestation: Relation to demographic characteristics and previous obstetric history. *Ultrasound Obstet Gynecol.* 1998:304.

66. Hassan SS, Romero R, Berry SM, et al. Patients with a sonographic cervical length ≤15 mm have a 50% risk of early spontaneous preterm delivery (abstract 4). Presented at the 6th Annual Meeting of the Central Association of Obstetricians and Gynecologists, Maui, Hawaii, October 24–27, 1999.

67. Taipale P, Hiilesmaa V. Sonographic measurement of uterine cervix at 18–22 weeks' gestation and the risk of preterm delivery. *Obstet Gynecol.* 1998;92:902.

68. Michaels WH, Schreiber FR, Padgett RJ, et al. Ultrasound surveillance of the cervix in twin gestations: Management of cervical incompetency. *Obstet Gynecol.* 1991;78:739.

69. Goldenberg RL, Iams JD, Miodovnik M, et al. The preterm prediction study: Risk factors in twin gestations. *Am J Obstet Gynecol.* 1996;175:1047.

70. Kushnir O, Izquierdo LA, Smith JF, et al. Transvaginal sonographic measurement of cervical length: Evaluation of twin pregnancies. *J Reprod Med.* 1995;40:380.

71. Crane JM, Van den Hof M, Armson BA, et al. Transvaginal ultrasound in the prediction of preterm delivery: Singleton and twin gestations. *Obstet Gynecol.* 1977;90:357.

72. Imseis HM, Albert TA, Iams JD. Identifying twin gestations at low risk for preterm birth with a transvaginal ultrasonographic cervical measurement at 24–26 weeks' gestation. *Am J Obstet Gynecol.* 1997;177:1149.

73. Souka AP, Heath V, Flint S, et al. Cervical length at 23 weeks in twins in predicting spontaneous preterm delivery. *Obstet Gynecol.* 1999;94:450.

74. Ramin KD, Ogburn PL Jr., Mulholland TA, et al. Ultrasonographic assessment of cervical length in triplet pregnancies. *Am J Obstet Gynecol.* 1999;180:1442.

75. Iams JD, Paraskos J, Landon MB, et al. Cervical sonography in preterm labor. *Obstet Gynecol.* 1994;84:40.

76. Lash AF, Lash SR. Habitual abortion; the incompetent internal os of the cervix. *Am J Obstet Gynecol.* 1950;59:68.

77. Heath VC, Souka AP, Erasmus I, et al. Cervical length at 23 weeks of gestation: The value of Shirodkar suture for the short cervix. *Ultrasound Obstet Gynecol.* 1998;12:318.

78. Berghella V, Daly SF, Tolosa JE, et al. Prediction of preterm delivery with transvaginal ultrasonography of the cervix in patients with high-risk pregnancies: Does cerclage prevent prematurity? *Am J Obstet Gynecol.* 1999;181:809.

79. King JF, Grant A, Keirse MJ, et al. Betamimetics in preterm labor: An overview of the randomized controlled trials. *Br J Obstet Gynaecol.* 1988;5:211.

80. Timor-Tritsch IE, Boozarjomehri F, Masakowski Y, et al. Can a snapshot sagittal view of the cervix by transvaginal ultrasonography predict active preterm labor? *Am J Obstet Gynecol.* 1996;174:990.

81. Lim BH, Mahmood TA, Smith NC, et al. A prospective comparative study of transvaginal ultrasonography and

digital examination for cervical assessment in the third trimester of pregnancy. *J Clin Ultrasound.* 1981;20:599.

82. Mahony BS, Nyberg DA, Luthy DA, et al. Translabial ultrasound of the third trimester uterine cervix: Correlation with digital examination. *J Ultrasound Med.* 1990;9:717.

83. Parulekar SG, Kiwi R. Dynamic incompetent cervix uteri: Sonographic observations. *J Ultrasound Med.* 1988;7:481.

84. Romero R, Gomez R, Mazor M, et al. The preterm labor syndrome. In: Elder MG, Lamont RF, Romero R, eds. *Preterm Labor.* New York: Churchill-Livingstone; 1997:29.

85. Iams JD, Johnson FF, Sonek J, et al. Cervical competence as a continuum: A study of ultrasonographic cervical length and obstetrical performance. *Am J Obstet Gynecol.* 1995; 172:1097.

86. Guzman ER, Mellon R, Vintzileos AM, et al. Relationship between endocervical canal length between 15–24 weeks gestation and obstetric history. *J Matern Fetal Med.* 1998;7:269.

87. Guzman ER, Mellon C, Vintzileos AM, et al. Longitudinal assessment of endocervical canal length between 15 and 24 weeks' gestation in women at risk for pregnancy loss or preterm birth. *Obstet Gynecol.* 1998;92:31.

88. Guzman ER, Rosenberg JC, Houlihan C, et al. A new method using vaginal ultrasound and transfundal pressure to evaluate the asymptomatic incompetent cervix. *Obstet Gynecol.* 1994; 83:248.

89. Arabin B, Aardenburg R, van Eyck J. Maternal position and ultrasonic cervical assessment in multiple pregnancy. *J Reprod Med.* 1997;42:719.

90. Guzman ER, Pisatowski DM, Vintzileos AM, et al. A comparison of ultrasonographically detected cervical changes in response to transfundal pressure, coughing, and standing in predicting cervical incompetence. *Am J Obstet Gynecol.* 1997;177:660.

91. Guzman ER, Vintzileos AM, McLean DA, et al. The natural history of a positive response to transfundal pressure in women at risk for cervical incompetence. *Am J Obstet Gynecol.* 1997;176:634.

92. Guzman ER, Forster JK, Vintzileos AM, et al. Pregnancy outcomes in women treated with elective versus ultrasound-indicated cervical cerclage. *Ultrasound Obstet Gynecol.* 1998; 12:323.

93. Ludmir J, Jackson GM, Samuels P. Transvaginal cerclage under ultrasound guidance in cases of severe cervical hypoplasia. *Obstet Gynecol.* 1991;78:1067.

94. Althuisius SM, Dekker GA, van Geijn HP, et al. The effect of therapeutic McDonald cerclage on cervical length as assessed by transvaginal ultrasonography. *Am J Obstet Gynecol.* 1999;180:366.

95. Funai EF, Paidas MJ, Rebarber A, et al. Change in cervical length after prophylactic cerclage. *Obstet Gynecol.* 1999;94: 117.

96. Guzman ER, Lazarou G, Ananth CV, et al. The relationship of peri-operative cervical ultrasound parameters with pregnancy outcome in women treated with ultrasound-indicated cerclage (abstract 77). *Ultrasound Obstet Gynecol.* 1998;12:S1.

97. Quinn MJ. Vaginal ultrasound and cervical cerclage: A prospective study. *Ultrasound Obstet Gynecol.* 1992;2:410.

98. Rana J, Davis SE, Harrigan JT. Improving the outcome of cervical cerclage by sonographic follow-up. *J Ultrasound Med.* 1990;9:275.

99. Andersen HF, Karimi A, Sakala EP, et al. Prediction of cervical cerclage outcome by endovaginal ultrasonography. *Am J Obstet Gynecol.* 1994;171:1102.

100. Rush RW, Isaacs S, McPherson K, et al. A randomized controlled trial of cervical cerclage in women at high risk of preterm delivery. *Br J Obstet Gynaecol.* 1984;91:724.

101. Lazar P, Gueguen S, Dreyfus J, et al. Multicenter controlled trial of cervical cerclage in women at moderate risk of preterm delivery. *Br J Obstet Gynaecol.* 1984;91:731.

102. MRC/RCOG Working Party on Cervical Cerclage. Final report of the Medical Research Council/Royal College of Obstetricians and Gynaecologists Multicentre Randomized Trial of Cervical Cerclage. *Br J Obstet Gynaecol.* 1993;100:516.

103. Dor J, Shalev J, Mashiach S, et al. Elective cervical suture of twin pregnancies diagnosed ultrasonically in the first trimester following induced ovulation. *Gynecol Obstet Invest.* 1982;13:55.

104. Garfield RE, Saade G, Buhimschi C, et al. Control and assessment of the uterus and cervix during pregnancy and labour. *Hum Reprod Update.* 1998;4:637.

105. Lockwood CJ, Senyei AE, Dische MR, et al. Fetal fibronectin in cervical and vaginal secretions as a predictor of preterm delivery. *N Engl J Med.* 1991;325:669.

106. Goldenberg RL, Iams JD, Mercer BM, et al. The preterm prediction study: the value of new vs. standard risk factors in predicting early and all spontaneous preterm births. *Am J Public Health.* 1998;88:233.

107. Rizzo G, Capponi A, Arduini D, et al. The value of fetal fibronectin in cervical and vaginal secretions and of ultrasonographic examination of the uterine cervix in predicting premature delivery for patients with preterm labor and intact membranes. *Am J Obstet Gynecol.* 1996;175:1146.

108. Rozenberg P, Goffinet F, Malagrida L, et al. Evaluating the risk of preterm delivery: A comparison of fetal fibronectin and transvaginal ultrasonographic measurement of cervical length. *Am J Obstet Gynecol.* 1997;176:196.

109. Ayers JW, DeGrood RM, Compton AA, et al. Sonographic evaluation of cervical length in pregnancy: Diagnosis and management of preterm cervical effacement in patients at risk for premature delivery. *Obstet Gynecol.* 1988;71:939.

110. Podobnik M, Bulic M, Smiljanic N, et al. Ultrasonography in the detection of cervical incompetence. *J Clin Ultrasound.* 1988;13:383.

111. Murakawa H, Utumi T, Hasegawa I, et al. Evaluation of threatened preterm delivery by transvaginal ultrasonographic measurement of cervical length. *Obstet Gynecol.* 1993;82: 829.

112. Zorzoli A, Soliani A, Perra M, et al. Cervical changes throughout pregnancy as assessed by transvaginal sonography. *Obstet Gynecol.* 1994;84:960.

113. Cook CM, Ellwood DA. A longitudinal study of the cervix in pregnancy using transvaginal ultrasound. *Br J Obstet Gynaecol.* 1996;103:16.

114. Tongsong T, Kamprapanth P, Pitaksakorn J. Cervical length in normal pregnancy as measured by transvaginal sonography. *Int J Gynaecol Obstet.* 1997;58:313.

32

Sonography of Trophoblastic Diseases

Arthur C. Fleischer • Howard W. Jones, III

Sonography is important in the evaluation of patients with gestational trophoblastic diseases (GTDs). Gestational trophoblastic diseases are a group of disorders that are thought to originate through fertilization of the ovum by one or more spermatozoa in either a normal or abnormal manner. This is in contrast to the nongestational forms of choriocarcinoma that can arise in the ovary or testicle and do not involve fertilization or a prior gestational event. The trophoblastic neoplasms arise from the trophoblastic elements of the developing blastocyst and, therefore, retain certain inherent characteristics, such as the ability to invade underlying tissues and the ability to synthesize human chorionic gonadotropin (hCG).

The role of sonography in gestational trophoblastic disease is greatest in establishing the diagnosis of hydatidiform mole.[1] A characteristic sonographic appearance of hydropic villi occurs with most molar pregnancies. Sonography is also considered an important adjunctive test to serial β-hCG assays in malignant trophoblastic disease. With sonography, it is possible to demonstrate uterine invasion by trophoblastic tissue.[2] It can also be used to monitor the response of the tumor to therapy, and the presence of other metastatic sites can be ascertained.[3] Color Doppler sonography affords detection in areas of abnormal blood flow within the myometrium and can be used as a means to monitor the effectiveness of chemotherapy (see Fig. 32–8).[4]

Gestational trophoblastic disease has been classified in a variety of ways (Table 32–1). Initial attempts at classification were based on histopathologic criteria. Currently, with the use of hCG monitoring, patients have been classified according to a clinical staging system. The use of different classification systems has probably contributed to confusion among obstetricians and sonologists concerning the sonographic categorization of these diseases. In this chapter, the sonographic features of the various forms of GTD are presented relative to both the pathologic and clinical classifications.

Because the sonographic features of an invasive mole and choriocarcinoma are similar, they are presented under the same heading. Accordingly, the discussion portion of the chapter is divided into two major categories of GTD: molar pregnancies and malignant GTDs. Although it may be difficult to differentiate the various pathologic types of gestational trophoblastic disorders by their sonographic features alone, the combination of clinical, laboratory, and sonographic findings can usually specify the type and extent of trophoblastic disease that is present.

TABLE 32–1. CLASSIFICATION SCHEMAS FOR GESTATIONAL TROPHOBLASTIC DISEASE

Pathologic	Clinical
Hydatidiform mole	Molar pregnancy
Complete	Complete
Partial	Partial
With coexistent fetus	With coexistent fetus
Invasive mole (chorioadenoma destruens)	Malignant, nonmetastatic trophoblastic disease
Choriocarcinoma	Malignant, metastatic trophoblastic disease

Adapted with permission from Jones H III. In: Jones H Jr, Jones S, eds. Novak's Textbook of Gynecology, 10th ed. Baltimore: Williams & Wilkins; 1981;659–689.

CLASSIFICATION SCHEMES

Histopathologic

This classification divides trophoblastic diseases into hydatidiform mole, invasive mole (chorioadenoma destruens), and choriocarcinoma based on histopathologic criteria.

Hydatidiform mole is characterized by marked edema and enlargement of the chorionic villi, producing vesicular structures. The vesicles are the characteristic that allows sonographic identification. These changes are accompanied by disappearance of the villus blood vessels and proliferation of the trophoblast (cytotrophoblast and syncytiotrophoblast) that line the villi (Fig. 32–1). Although moles with an abundantly proliferative trophoblast may have a greater likelihood of being malignant, it is not possible to accurately predict the malignant potential of a given mole based on the histologic appearance. Approximately 20% of complete moles are followed by additional malignant sequelae of invasive mole or choriocarcinoma.[5] Further classification of hydatidiform mole based on histopathologic criteria has not proven to be an accurate prognostic indication to select the 20% of patients

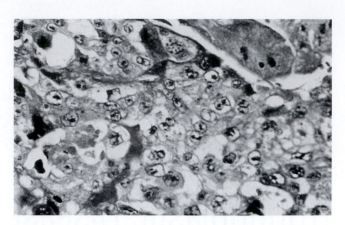

Figure 32–2. Choriocarcinoma. Under high magnification sheets of pleomorphic trophoblastic cells are seen. There are no villi.

with a molar pregnancy who will subsequently develop malignant disease.[6]

Invasive mole (chorioadenoma destruens) is the term used to describe trophoblastic disease where there has been invasion into the myometrium of the uterus. Grossly, a vesicular structure is preserved (Fig. 32–2). Microscopic examination will reveal edematous villi invading the myometrium. There is often abundant trophoblastic proliferation of the remaining villi. Where the villi invade the underlying myometrium, some hemorrhage is produced. Necrosis, however, is absent. Hysterectomy is rarely used in the treatment of trophoblastic disease today. Therefore, the diagnosis of invasive mole is rarely made based on surgical pathology.

Choriocarcinoma is characterized by the lack of any remaining villus structure. Microscopic examination will reveal sheets of highly malignant trophoblast with proliferation of both cytotrophoblast and syncytial trophoblast (Fig. 32–3). There is associated hemorrhage and necrosis, which is the other hallmark of choriocarcinoma. Choriocarcinoma accounts for approximately 5% of all GTDs.[6] Local pelvic metastases and lung metastases are the most common, but liver, brain, kidney, and bowel metastases may occur as well.

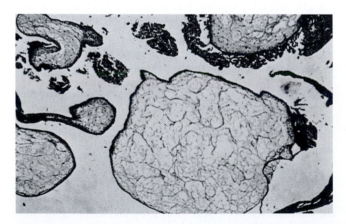

Figure 32–1. Microscopic appearance of hydatidiform mole. Note the enlarged avascular edematous villi with a thin rim of proliferative trophoblastic cells.

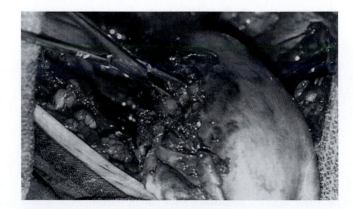

Figure 32–3. Invasive mole with perforation through myometrium of vesicular tissue.

Clinical

Careful follow-up of patients with hCG monitoring and the use of chemotherapy as the main mode of therapy rather than surgery has led to a replacement of the histopathologic classification by a more practical clinical classification of GTD. This clinical classification still recognizes hydatidiform moles, both the complete and partial types.

Any patient with a pathologic diagnosis of choriocarcinoma or invasive mole is considered to have malignant GTD, as are patients who develop rising hCG levels. Patients are not classified as having malignant GTD solely by a pathologic diagnosis of hydatidiform mole; such patients may or may not follow a malignant clinical course.[3] Patients with malignant GTD are further subdivided into nonmetastatic or metastatic groups. Clinical experience in treating patients with trophoblastic disease has further identified a group of patients with metastatic disease that is considered to be at high risk.[7,8] This includes patients with liver or brain metastasis, β-hCG levels above 40,000 mIU/mL before therapy, an interval of more than 4 months between pregnancy and initiation of therapy, failure of previous chemotherapy, and trophoblastic disease that develops after a full-term pregnancy.[9] These high-risk patients require especially diligent radiologic and sonographic evaluation in their follow-up.

MOLAR PREGNANCIES

Pathogenesis and Clinical Aspects

The pathogenesis of hydatidiform mole has remained a subject of considerable speculation for many years. The work of Kajii and Ohama,[10] however, demonstrated that hydatidiform mole results from the fertilization of an "empty egg," that is, an ovum without any active chromosomal material. The chromosomes of the sperm, finding no chromosomal complement from the ovum, reduplicate themselves, resulting in a 46,XX molar pregnancy. This has also been called a *complete mole* or *classic mole*. In complete mole, there is complete lack of fetal development, so there are no identifiable fetal parts or fetal membranes that can be seen in this situation. Complete moles are associated with different degrees of trophoblastic proliferation and may follow either a benign or malignant clinical course. Only about 20% of cases will eventually pursue a malignant course.[5]

Some cases of hydatidiform mole are found to contain a small complement of fetal structure, such as a placenta with membranes, or even a developed fetus. This is referred to as a *partial mole*. These cases usually involve some edema of the villi but relatively little trophoblastic proliferation. Hydropic degeneration is present, but with some elements associated with fetal structures, the designation *partial mole* has been made.[11] Although subsequent malignancy has been reported, partial moles are almost always benign.[12] In a partial mole, the fetus usually has significant congenital anomalies and a

triploid karyotype.[13] Two sets of chromosomes are of paternal origin, and the third set is of maternal origin.

A fetus with a coexisting molar pregnancy can occur. This is much less common than a partial molar pregnancy; however, it can grossly appear similar to the partial mole. This disorder is thought to result from a dizygotic pregnancy, with one fetus resulting from a normal fertilization and the other being a complete molar pregnancy.[14] In these patients, a fetus and normal placenta can usually be identified, in contrast to a partial molar pregnancy where a normal placenta is not present.

Hydropic degeneration of the placenta may give a similar sonographic appearance to complete and partial mole, but, histologically, it is not associated with trophoblastic proliferation. The villi and hydropic degeneration of the placenta are swollen and edematous and thus may resemble abnormal trophoblastic tissue. Microscopic examination will usually reveal the absence of cisternal formation; only hydropic swelling is seen. Hydropic degeneration may be seen in 20 to 40% of placentas from abortuses.[5]

The most common presenting clinical sign of molar pregnancy is vaginal bleeding, which may be seen in 89 to 97% of cases; in approximately half of the cases, the bleeding may be severe enough to produce anemia.[15]

A uterus that is enlarged beyond what is expected based on gestational age is considered "classic" for molar pregnancy; however, this is only seen in 33 to 51% of cases.[15] In approximately 50% of cases, patients will present with what is easily recognized as a molar pregnancy based on the passage of vesicular tissue via the vagina.[16] If there has been significant expulsion of molar tissue before presentation, the uterus may appear normal for size or even small for dates, both clinically and sonographically.

Molar pregnancies should always be considered in the differential diagnosis of a patient presenting with severe preeclampsia before 24 weeks of gestation without underlying renal disease. Although this presentation is considered classic for hydatidiform mole, it is only seen in 6 to 12% of cases of molar pregnancy.[15]

Theca-lutein cysts are often encountered in patients with molar pregnancies. The actual incidence of these cysts in association with molar pregnancy has been reported in various series to range from 18 to 37%.[17,18] Compared with clinical examination, sonography can more accurately assess the presence or absence of theca-lutein cysts (Figs. 32–4 and 32–5).[19] In one large series, theca-lutein cysts were detected clinically in 10% of patients with molar pregnancy, compared with 37% of patients when examined by sonography.[18] The presence or absence of theca-lutein cysts does not seem to be an accurate predictor of later development of an invasive mole or choriocarcinoma.[18] A review of a series at the University of Southern California has suggested, however, that patients with theca-lutein cysts have a twofold increase of malignant sequalae.[20] In most patients who undergo spontaneous resolution of hCG levels, the cysts also regress spontaneously;

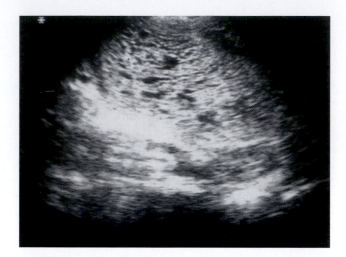

Figure 32–4. Typical sonographic appearance of hydatidiform mole with small vesicular cystic spaces.

however, they may occasionally undergo torsion and, therefore, require surgical intervention.

The laboratory findings for molar gestation are usually diagnostic. Measurement of hCG, specifically the beta subunit, is almost always abnormally elevated in molar gestations. The assay is not foolproof, because it can be spuriously elevated in twin gestations or may occasionally fail to show significant elevation in a molar pregnancy.[21]

As soon as the diagnosis of molar pregnancy is confirmed, the uterus should be evacuated. This typically involves suction curettage (dilation and evacuation, or D&E). Before evacuation, a chest x-ray should be obtained to exclude metastatic disease that might already be present. The

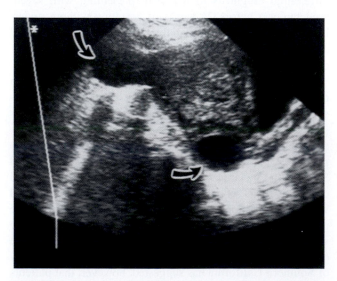

Figure 32–5. Complete hydatidiform mole demonstrating two theca-lutein cysts *(curved arrows),* one superior to the fundus and one in the cul-de-sac.

patient should also be evaluated as to her pulmonary status, cardiac status, thyroid status, and to be sure that adequate coagulation factors are present.[15] After D&E, serial β-hCGs are obtained weekly to assess the status of any remaining trophoblastic tissue. The level of this glycoprotein hormone should return to normal approximately 10 to 12 weeks after evacuation; however, it may occasionally take longer.[22] As previously mentioned, theca-lutein cysts will usually regress after successful treatment of molar pregnancy. Their presence or absence should not be taken as absolute indication of the presence or activity of residual trophoblastic disease.[23]

Sonography has an important role in evaluating those patients in whom the β-hCG subsequently rises. It can detect the presence or absence of intrauterine pregnancies that may occur after the initial evacuation. It can also detect the small number of patients with molar gestation who have a coexisting normal pregnancy.[24] It may also detect the presence of residual trophoblastic disease and can detect invasion of the myometrium by this residual trophoblastic tissue.[2]

Sonographic Features

The sonographic appearance of a hydatidiform mole is quite distinctive.[1] In most cases, a sonographic pattern arising from molar tissue consists of echogenic intrauterine tissue that is interspersed with numerous punctuate sonolucencies (see Fig. 32–4). Irregular sonolucent areas may occur secondary to internal hemorrhage or an area of unoccupied uterine lumen.

The sonographic appearance of a hydatidiform mole differs according to its gestational duration and the size of the hydropic villi.[25] For instance, hydatidiform moles that occur from 8 to 12 weeks typically appear as homogeneously echogenic intraluminal tissue, because the villi at this stage have a maximum diameter of 2 mm (see Fig. 32–5). As the hydatidiform mole matures to 18 to 20 weeks, the vesicles have a maximum diameter of 10 mm, which is readily delineated as cystic spaces on sonography (Fig. 32–6).

In contrast to the complete mole, partial molar pregnancy, hydatidiform mole coexistent with fetus, and hydropic degeneration of the placenta are associated with the presence of a fetus or fetal parts. Although it may be difficult to differentiate between a partial molar pregnancy and a complete mole with a coexistent fetus on the basis of sonography, these two entities can be differentiated from a complete mole when an identifiable fetus is present.[14,17] In addition, the complete mole with a coexistent fetus typically has a fetus with a separate normal placenta as well as the molar mass. This contrasts with a partial mole in which only a portion of the placenta is normal and most of it has a vesicular pattern.

Sonography can also delineate the theca-lutein cyst that enlarges under the influence of high levels of β-hCG elaborated by the trophoblasts. These cysts appear as multiloculated cystic masses that are usually located superior to the

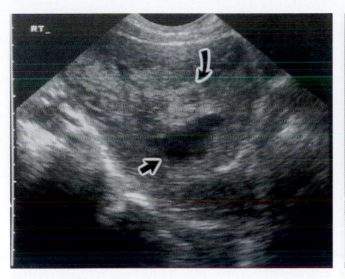
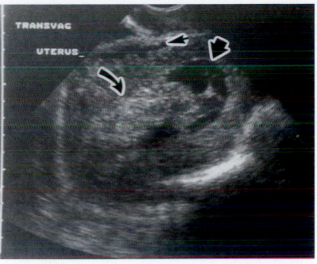

A   B

Figure 32–6. Hydatidiform mole with cystic spaces. **(A)** Transabdominal longitudinal scan demonstrating echogenic material *(curved arrow)* within the enlarged uterus, and irregular cystic region along the lower uterine lumen *(straight arrow).* **(B)** Semicoronal transvaginal sonogram demonstrating echogenic material *(curved arrow)* within the uterine lumen, representing trophoblastic tissue and irregular cystic space inferiorly. A myometrial vein is distended *(arrowhead).*

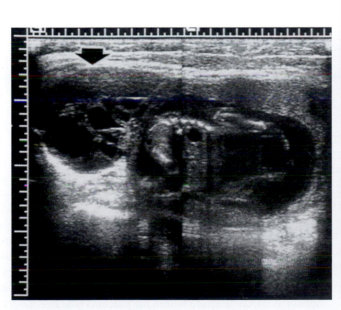
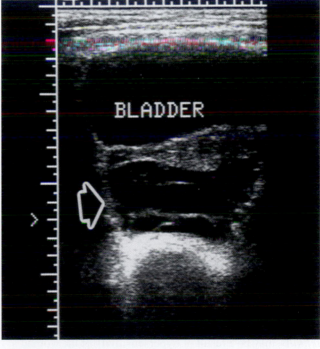

A   B

Figure 32–7. Hypereactio luteinalis. **(A)** Composite obstetric sonogram demonstrating multiloculated cystic mass *(arrow)* superior to the uterine fundus. **(B)** Same patient demonstrating a second multiloculated cystic mass *(arrow)* in the cul-de-sac. At surgery, massively enlarged ovaries that contained multiple luteinized cysts were found. *(Courtesy of Bill Wilson, MD.)*

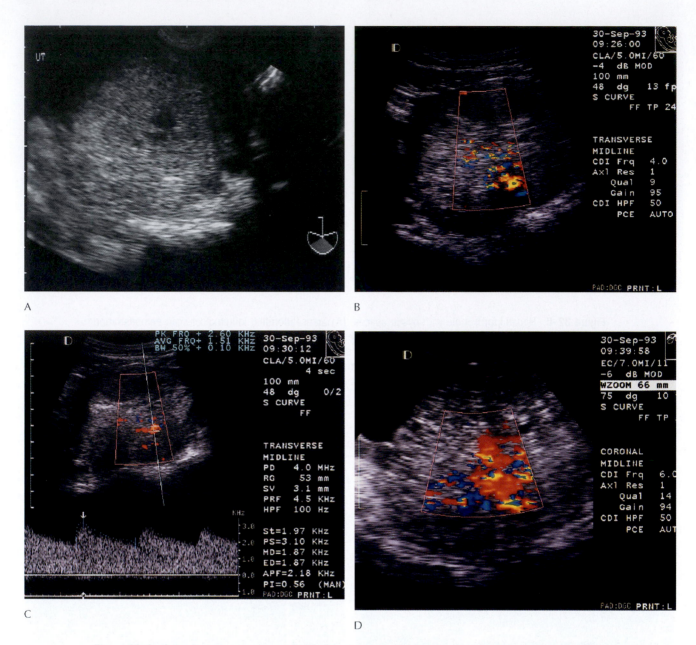

Figure 32–8. Color Doppler sonogram (CDS) of partial mole. **(A)** Transvaginal sonogram showing diffuse thickening of placenta with punctuate hypoechoic areas. **(B)** Transabdominal CDS of the same patient as in **A** showing increased flow within molar tissue. **(C)** Transabdominal CDS showing low-impedance, high-diastolic flow within the same areas as **B**. **(D)** Transvaginal CDS of the same area seen in **B** and **C**.

uterine fundus or, less commonly, in the cul-de-sac (see Fig. 32–5).

Rarely, there can be massive enlargement of the ovaries with luteinization of several follicles in apparently normal pregnancies. This condition, which is termed *hypereactio luteinalis,* may be a result of hypersensitivity of the woman's ovary to high circulating levels of hCG (Fig. 32–7).

Invasive trophoblastic disease can be diagnosed with color Doppler sonography by demonstration of enlarged vessels within the myometrium that usually exhibit low-impedance, high-diastolic flow[4] (Fig. 32–8).

Sonographic Differential Diagnosis

Hydropic degeneration of the placenta associated with incomplete or missed abortions is the most common condition that can simulate the appearance of a molar pregnancy (Fig. 32–9). The hydropic areas may be focal or diffuse and appear as anechoic space within the placenta (see Fig. 32–9). This is due to the sonographic similarity of a hydropic placenta with marked swelling of the villi to molar tissue. A fetus may or may not be present with hydropic degeneration of the placenta. Serum β-hCG levels are generally lower in hydropic degeneration than in partial or complete moles, probably due

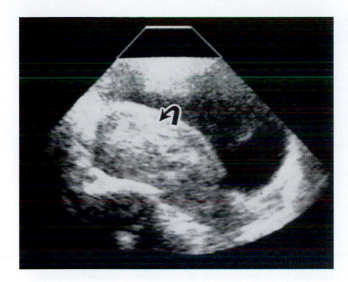

Figure 32–9. Choriocarcinoma appearing as an echogenic area *(arrow)* within myometrium of the anterior corpus.

to the reduced number of functioning trophoblasts. Hydropic changes in the placenta can be associated with triploidy.[26]

Technical factors that may be used to improve the ability to distinguish partial from complete moles or hydropic degeneration have been described.[3] Specifically, detailed examination of the entire intrauterine contents with transducers that are optimally focused to a particular region within the uterus has been stressed. Transvaginal scanning may be helpful in some cases in which the molar tissue cannot be adequately delineated transabdominally. Using this technique, the typical vesicular texture arising from molar tissue can be correctly distinguished from tissue texture emanating from retained products of conception or leiomyomata.[3]

Pulsed and color Doppler sonography have been used to assess the presence of invasive trophoblastic disease.[27] This technique is discussed in greater detail in the section devoted to invasive trophoblastic diseases.

Occasionally, the sonographic appearance of a uterine leiomyoma may mimic that of a hydatidiform mole. However, as described in Chapter 37, uterine leiomyomata typically have a whorled internal consistency that is distinctly different from the vesicular pattern encountered in the hydatidiform mole. They may also contain areas of hyaline and myxomatous degeneration that can simulate the sonographic appearance of hemorrhage within a hydatidiform mole. We have also encountered some partially solid ovarian tumors that simulate the appearance of a hydatidiform mole. Patients with this type of mass can usually be distinguished from those with molar pregnancies by clinical and laboratory methods because the β-hCG is not elevated in nonpregnant conditions.

Finally, patients with retained products of conception with hemorrhage can simulate the sonographic appearance of molar pregnancies. One is usually not able to demonstrate a vesicular pattern of tissue associated with retained products, however.

Although absolute distinction between the various trophoblastic disorders may not always be possible on the basis of sonography, the sonographic evaluation of these disorders may have clinical importance. Specifically, it is known that the malignant potential of a complete mole is greater than that of a partial mole or hydropic degeneration. Thus, the sonographic findings can have a significant clinical impact on the treatment and management of these disorders.

INVASIVE MOLE AND CHORIOCARCINOMA

Pathogenesis and Clinical Aspects

The majority of patients who develop malignant trophoblastic disease will have a history of an antecedent molar pregnancy. In a series of patients reported by Duke University, 86% of patients who developed malignant trophoblastic disease did so after a hydatidiform molar pregnancy.[25] Approximately 10% of patients had a history of a previous full-term pregnancy, and another 5% had an abortion or some other form of pregnancy event. In patients who presented with high-risk disease, there was a larger proportion of patients presenting after full-term pregnancy, abortions, and other types of pregnancy events.

Histologically, invasive moles differ from choriocarcinoma. A villous structure is maintained in invasive mole and is always absent in choriocarcinoma. Both disorders are associated with excessive trophoblastic proliferation and invasion of the myometrium. In general, choriocarcinoma is associated with a great deal of hemorrhage and necrosis.

Generally, an invasive mole is first suspected in a patient with a history of evacuation of a hydatidiform mole who subsequently presents with continued uterine bleeding, a persistently elevated hCG level, persistently enlarged theca-lutein cysts, or a combination of these. This clinical picture, however, can also be seen in patients who histologically are found to have choriocarcinoma. Because hysterectomy is rarely performed in the current management of trophoblastic diseases, these entities are not recognized separately in the clinical staging system. Patients with choriocarcinoma that extends outside the uterus can present for the first time with manifestations of metastatic spread to the lungs, liver, or brain. In the lungs, metastatic choriocarcinoma has a rather specific radiographic appearance of radiodense masses with hazy borders, due to the hemorrhage around the metastases. The metastases may undergo rapid regression after therapy has been instituted. Because these diseases are very responsive to chemotherapeutic agents, their early clinical and sonographic recognition is imperative for institution of appropriate therapy.

The sonographic appearance of invasive trophoblastic tissue is that of a focal irregular echogenic region within the uterine myometrium (Figs. 32–9 and 32–10). Irregular

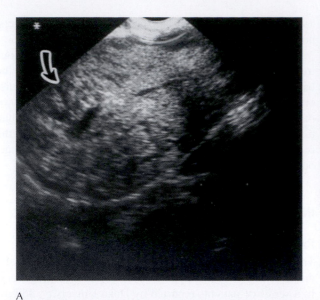

A

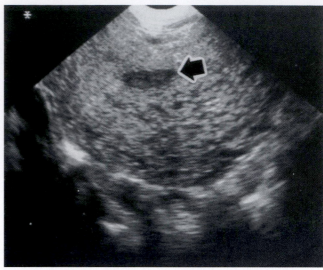

B

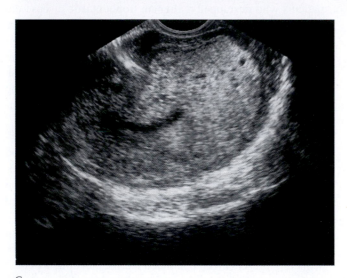

C

Figure 32–10. Locally invasive trophoblastic disease. **(A)** Long-axis transvaginal sonogram, demonstrating irregular area in the right side of the uterine fundus *(curved arrow)*. **(B)** Transvaginal semiaxial sonogram showing a hypoechoic tumor focus *(arrow)* measuring approximately 3 X 7 mm. **(C)** Transvaginal sonogram showing trophoblastic tissue containing punctate cystic areas within the myometrium.

hypoechoic areas may surround the more echogenic tropho-blastic tissue corresponding to areas of myometrial hemor-rhage.

Due to its proximity to the uterus, myometrial implants may be best delineated with transvaginal scanning (see Fig. 32–10). Pulsed Doppler sonography has been used to assess the presence and relative aggressiveness of myometrial im-plants by depicting increased and typically turbulent flow to these tumors through the uterine arteries.[27] Color Doppler sonography of invasive trophoblastic disease usually exhibits low-impedance, high-diastolic velocity flow within the myo-metrium (Fig. 32–11).[4]

In addition to the echogenic intrauterine areas, sonogra-phy is helpful in the detection of theca-lutein cysts associated with trophoblastic disease. These cysts are typically bilateral, multiloculated cystic masses that characteristically measure between 4 and 8 cm in diameter. Sonography has been shown

to be more sensitive than physical examination in the detec-tion of these cysts because it may be difficult to palpate a cyst that is displaced high in the pelvis by an enlarged uterus. The presence of theca-lutein cysts may be an indication of per-sistent trophoblastic activity because it has been shown that malignant trophoblastic disease develops more commonly in patients with persistent theca-lutein cysts.[20] Because it can take up to 4 months for these cysts to regress after evacua-tion of a molar pregnancy, their presence or absence during the period of follow-up cannot be taken as an accurate indi-cation of the presence or activity of remaining trophoblastic tissue.

Sonography and pulsed Doppler analysis of the uterus can be useful, when used in combination with serial β-hCG assays, in the evaluation of tumor response to chemo-therapy.[25] Serial evaluation of tumor volume can be accom-plished using sonography; reduced volume follows closely

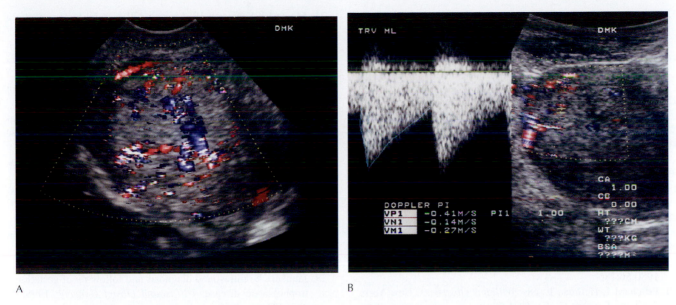

Figure 32–11. Color Doppler sonogram of invasive trophoblastic disease. **(A)** Color Doppler sonogram showing a hypervascular, echogenic mass within the myometrium that represented invasive trophoblastic disease. **(B)** Same patient as in **A** in coronal scan plane showing low-impedance, high-velocity flow.

the diminution in β-hCG values in successfully treated patients. Preliminary reports also describe the sensitivity of pulsed Doppler techniques for detection of tumor growth or regression.[27] Transvaginal color Doppler sonography can demonstrate changes in blood flow, which correlate to a decrease in β-hCG in successfully treated choriocarcinoma or no change in nonresponders. The changes in flow seem to parallel changes in β-hCG in both responders and nonresponders.[28] The presence of tumor is implied when the Doppler waveforms obtained from the uterine arteries show increased systolic and diastolic flow with low resistance similar to that typically seen in third-trimester pregnancy.

Sonography also is helpful in evaluation of the liver for metastatic disease in patients with malignant, metastatic trophoblastic disease.[14] Typically, the metastases associated with choriocarcinoma appear as echogenic foci within the liver. The kidneys can also be evaluated for the presence of obstructive uropathy, which is important not only to rule out metastatic involvement but also because effective chemotherapy often requires adequate renal function.

SUMMARY

As discussed and illustrated in this chapter, sonography has an important role in the evaluation of patients with benign and malignant GTD. The sonographic features of hydatidiform mole and its variants are usually diagnostic. If malignant trophoblastic disease is suspected clinically, sonography can be used to establish the presence and extent of disease, as well as in the serial evaluation of patients undergoing treatment.

REFERENCES

1. Fleischer A, James A, Krause D, et al. Sonographic patterns in trophoblastic disease. *Radiology*. 1978;126:215.
2. Berkowitz RS, Birnholz J, Goldstein DP, et al. Pelvic ultrasonography and the management of gestational trophoblastic disease. *Gynecol Oncol*. 1983;15:403.
3. Requard C, Mettler F. Use of ultrasound in the evaluation of trophoblastic disease and its response to therapy. *Radiology*. 1980;135:419.
4. Desai RK, Desberg AL. Diagnosis of gestational trophoblastic disease: Value of endovaginal color flow Doppler sonography. *AJR*. 1991;157:787–788.
5. Reid M, McGohan JO. Sonographic evaluation of hydatidiform mole and its look-alike. *AJR*. 1983;140:307.
6. Jones H III. Gestational trophoblastic disease. In: Jones H Jr, Jones S, eds. *Novak's Textbook of Gynecology*, 10th ed. Baltimore: Williams & Wilkins; 1981;659–689.
7. Hertz R, Lewis JL Jr, Lipsett MB. Five years experience with the chemotherapy of metastatic choriocarcinoma and related trophoblastic tumors in women. *Am J Obstet Gynecol*. 1961; 82:631.
8. Hammond CB, Borchert LG, Tyrey L, et al. Treatment of metastatic trophoblastic disease: Good and poor prognosis. *Am J Obstet Gynecol*. 1973;115:451.
9. Surwit EA, Hammond CB. Treatment of metastatic trophoblastic disease with poor prognosis. *Obstet Gynecol*. 1980;55:565.
10. Kajii T, Ohama K. Androgenetic origin of hydatidiform mole. *Nature*. 1977;168:633.
11. Vassilakos P, Riotton G, Kajii T. Hydatidiform mole: Two entities. A morphologic and cytogenetic study with some clinical considerations. *Am J Obstet Gynecol*. 1977;127:167.
12. Szulman A, Surti J, Berman M. Patient with partial mole requiring chemotherapy. *Lancet*. 1978;1:1099.

13. Szulman A, Surti N. The syndromes of hydatidiform mole. I: Cytogenic and morphologic correlations. *Am J Obstet Gynecol*. 1978;131:665.

14. Szulman A, Surti N. The syndromes of hydatidiform mole. II: Morphologic evaluation of the complete and partial mole. *Am J Obstet Gynecol*. 1978;132:20.

15. Munyer T, Callen P, Filly R, et al. Further observations on the sonographic spectrum of gestational trophoblastic disease. *J Clin Ultrasound*. 1981;9:349.

16. Gordon AN. Gestational trophoblastic disease. In: Kase NG, Weingold AB, eds. *Principles and Practice of Clinical Gynecology*, 2nd ed. New York: Wiley; 1988.

17. Szulman AE, Surti V. The clinicopathologic profile of the partial hydatidiform mole. *Obstet Gynecol*. 1982;59:597.

18. Kobayashi M. Use of diagnostic ultrasound in trophoblastic neoplasms and ovarian tumors. *Cancer*. 1978;38:441.

19. Santos-Rasmos A, Forney J, Schwartz B. Sonographic findings and clinical correlations in molar pregnancies. *Obstet Gynecol*. 1980;56:186.

20. Pritchard J, Hellman L, eds. *Williams Obstetrics*. New York: Appleton-Century-Crofts; 1971;578.

21. Montz FJ, Schlaerth JB, Morrow CP. Natural history of theca lutein cysts. *Gynecol Oncol*. 1987;26:414.

22. Callen P. Ultrasonography in evaluation of gestational trophoblastic disease. In: Callen P, ed. *Ultrasonography in Obstetrics and Gynecology*. Philadelphia: Saunders; 1983;259–270.

23. Goldstein D, Berkowitz R, Cohen S. The current management of molar pregnancies. *Curr Probl Obstet Gynecol*. 1979;3:1.

24. MacVicar J, Donald I. Sonar in the diagnosis of early pregnancy and its complications. *J Obstet Gynaecol Br Commonw*. 1968;70:387.

25. Jones W, Lauerson N. Hydatidiform mole with coexistent fetus. *Am J Obstet Gynecol*. 1975;122:267.

26. Taylor KJW, Schwartz PE, Kohorn EI. Gestational trophoblastic neoplasia: Diagnosis with Doppler US. *Radiology*. 1987;165:445–448.

27. Hammond CB, Weed JC, Currie JL. The role of operation in the current therapy of gestational trophoblastic disease. *Am J Obstet Gynecol*. 1980;136:844.

28. Jauniaux E. Ultrasound diagnosis and follow-up of gestational trophoblastic disease. *Ultrasound Obstet Gynecol*. 1998;11:367–377.

Postpartum Ultrasound

J. Patrick Lavery • Kathleen A. Gadwood

The puerperium is the 6-week period after delivery. During this time physical recovery from the events of labor and delivery takes place. There is a regression from the dramatic physiologic changes that developed throughout the course of pregnancy. It is during the puerperium that the female organs, as well as other systems in the body, are attempting to regain their prepregnancy function and size.

Robinson[1] was the first to use diagnostic ultrasound to investigate puerperal changes in 1972. Malvern and Campbell availed themselves of this diagnostic modality to evaluate the basis for postpartum bleeding in 1973.[2] Thus, from near the time of its introduction into clinical medicine, sonography has been a valuable adjunct to the clinician in evaluating puerperal pathology and affording the investigator a better understanding of the normal anatomic changes occurring during this time. With the vastly improved resolution and sensitivity found in currently available equipment, it can be anticipated that diagnostic ultrasound will play an increasingly prominent role in the assessment of puerperal dynamics, both normal and abnormal.

Although the postpartum period is a time of physiologic resolution, the events surrounding delivery, both vaginal and by cesarean section, often lead to complications in a significant number of patients. These adverse sequelae of delivery are most often related to hemorrhage or infection.[3] Conditions such as endomyometritis, postpartum hemorrhage, wound abscess or hematoma formation, and urinary tract infection are but some of the diagnoses accounting for the 5 to 10% morbidity seen following childbirth.[4]

This chapter reviews normal and pathologic findings that may be seen sonographically during the puerperium. Major emphasis will be placed on changes within the genital tract. Other systems, which are occasionally the site of clinically significant complications, will also be described and discussed. Normal variations and common pathologic findings will be highlighted to acquaint the reader with the spectrum of use that sonography affords in the understanding and management of clinical conditions occurring during the puerperium.

NORMAL ANATOMY

The Uterus

In the nonpregnant state, the uterus occupies a midline position and measures approximately 8 cm in length.[5] Uterine size may be influenced by gravidity and pathologic conditions, such as leiomyomata or adenomyosis.[6] Physiologically, the uterus grows from a pregravid weight of approximately 140 g to a final term weight of 1 kg.[7] Blood flow to the uterus increases during pregnancy from 50 cc/min to 500 cc/min at term. During the puerperium the uterus regresses to nearly its pregravid weight. Factors such as parity, breast or bottle feeding, and route of delivery have not been demonstrated to influence the rate of uterine involution.[8–10]

The process of uterine involution is perhaps the most dramatic aspect of the anatomic changes occurring during the puerperium. It is a rapid reversal of the growth changes

TABLE 33–1. THE UTERUS DURING INVOLUTION: MEAN MEASUREMENTS TAKEN DURING THE FIRST 2 WEEKS IN 37 NORMAL SINGLETON GESTATIONS[8]

Time After Delivery	Length	Width	AP Diameter	Endometrial Cavity (AP)
24 h	17.5	12.3	9.0	1.2
48 h	16.3	11.3	8.7	1.3
1 week	12.9	9.4	7.8	1.3
2 weeks	11.0	7.7	6.6	1.0

Measurements in centimeters. AP, anteroposterior.
Used with permission from Lavery JP, Shaw L. J Ultrasound Med. 1989;8:481.

that occurred during pregnancy. In this regression process, remarkably there is no cell destruction. Cell size is reduced with concomitant loss and reabsorption of tissue fluid and contractile proteins. Animal experiments have shown an orderly process of cellular restitution where cytoplasmic and collagen disintegration take place without tissue necrosis.[11]

The most rapid phase of uterine involution takes place during the first week postpartum, during which there is seen a nearly 50% reduction in size.[8–10,12] By this time the term-size gravid uterus will have come from its subxyphoid position to approximately halfway between the umbilicus and the pubic symphysis. The mean measurements of uterine size obtained sonographically in the first 2 postpartum weeks in a group of 37 normal parturients are shown in Table 33–1.[8] In a more recent study, Wachsberg et al.[10] also performed serial postpartum measurements in 100 women and found that the uterus resumed nongravid dimensions by 6 to 8 weeks postpartum. The investigators discussed the technical variability of measurements associated with the type of transducer used, the presence of uterine contractions, and the degree of uterine angulation, which is influenced by the degree of bladder distention. Because of this angulation they advocated use of a sector transducer and the taking of two measurements as the uterus may be angled over the sacrum (Fig. 33–1).

Measuring the size of the postpartum uterus with ultrasound is of physiologic interest but is seldom done with ultrasound in nonpathologic clinical settings because its size is readily assessed on physical examination. The process of uterine involution occurs more rapidly after preterm deliveries, when viewed both clinically and sonographically, than after deliveries that take place at term.

The myometrium will show a heterogeneous echo appearance on sonographic study that is related to the anatomic changes in the vascular structure and the changes in uterine blood flow, as well as the degree of resolution of tissue edema and fluid content that will take place during the time of postpartum evaluation. Variations will be seen among normal patients at different times after delivery depending on the respective stage of resolution when viewed. Significantly enlarged vascular channels mediating intramural blood flow

during pregnancy may be seen early in the puerperium only to disappear in subsequent evaluation as the vessels constrict and involute (Fig. 33–2). The temporary compression of these vascular channels can occur over a period of a few minutes secondary to contractions and is complete by 3 to 4 weeks postpartum.[10]

The endometrial cavity maintains a consistent size of less than 2 cm in anteroposterior (AP) diameter during the early puerperium. The appearance of the endometrium will differ even among clinically normal cases. It is not unusual to see some fluid within the canal. The interface of the endometrial cavity and the myometrium may be smooth and well defined or irregular and nonhomogeneous[8] (Fig. 33–3). On occasion small echogenic areas may be seen within the uterus representing residual clots or pieces of membrane not expelled at the time of delivery. An enlarged endometrial cavity (AP diameter > 2.5 cm) may be associated with a hypotonic uterus even without retained products. The length and width of the endometrial echo will also decrease in proportion to overall uterine involution.[9]

It is sometimes difficult to distinguish between the normal variations and the abnormal thickening seen with retained material or uterine hypotonia. Clinical correlation will be necessary to make this distinction in the practical setting (see section on postpartum hemorrhage).

The Broad Ligament

The broad ligament (Fig. 33–4) is a reflection of the parietal peritoneum extending medially from the bony pelvic side wall beneath the infundibulopelvic ligament to the lateral margin of the uterus bilaterally and extending inferiorly to the pelvic floor. It contains the vascular supply to the uterus and the fallopian tubes. Although difficult to visualize sonographically in the normal patient because of the homogeneous nature of the areolar tissue that acts as its supporting structure and the frequent shadowing of bowel gas above it, the broad ligament may be a location of significant pathologic findings. The minimally resistant loose areolar tissue encompassing the uterine vessels medially and the vascular supply to the fallopian tubes and ovaries superiorly increase the potential for this area in the broad ligament to be the site of hematoma, abscess, or phlegmon formation in the puerperal period (Fig. 33–5).

The Ovaries

The ovaries, normally found within the true pelvis in the nonpregnant state, are extrapelvic in location during much of the puerperium. They can be demonstrated approximately 50% of the time on routine scanning[8] (Fig. 33–6A). After the first trimester, when ovarian cysts are frequently found and substantially regress, the ovary does not undergo any other significant change in size or contour related to pregnancy. The characteristics of a luteoma of pregnancy have been described,[13] however. This represents a mostly cystic

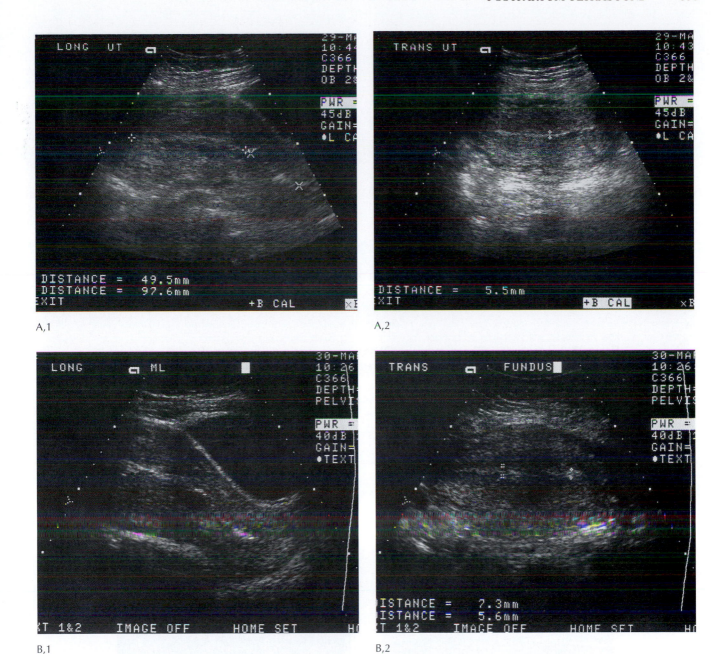

Figure 33–1. Sonograms of a normally regressing uterus at 12 (**A,1** and **2**) and 36 (**B,1** and **2**) hours after delivery. Longitudinal and transverse views are shown. The endometrial stripe (x's in **A,1**) shows some angulation that may be influenced by bladder size and the sacrum in the immediate postpartum period.

enlargement of the ovary due to stromal hypertrophy and fluid accumulation that represents an exaggerated luteinizing reaction to the hormonal stimulus of pregnancy (Fig. 33–6B and C). In this unusual condition, the ovary will regress in size during the puerperium as opposed to the case of a true neoplasm, which will persist even after the elevated levels of pregnancy-associated hormones have regressed. Virilization of a female fetus has been reported with this clinical entity.[13]

The Cul-de-sac

The cul-de-sac is a potential space posterior to the uterus created by the peritoneal reflection between the uterus and the rectum. Free intraperitoneal fluid in the abdomen may settle in this dependent recess. Ascites from any cause, including hypoalbuminemia or severe preeclampsia, will be visualized in this area. In the absence of free fluid, however, this area is not easily defined sonographically either during pregnancy or in the normal puerperium.

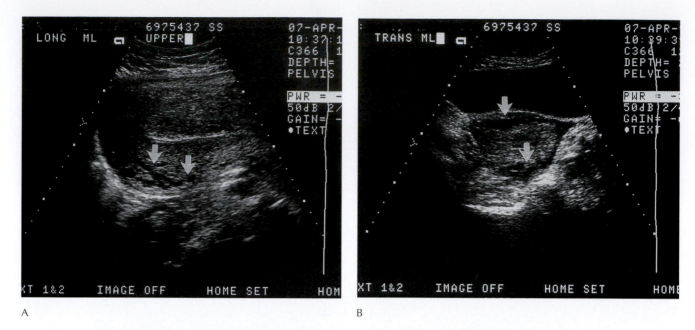

A

B

Figure 33–2. Longitudinal **(A)** and transverse **(B)** sonograms of an early involuting uterus showing large vascular channels *(arrows)*. These channels are obliterated over a short period of time.

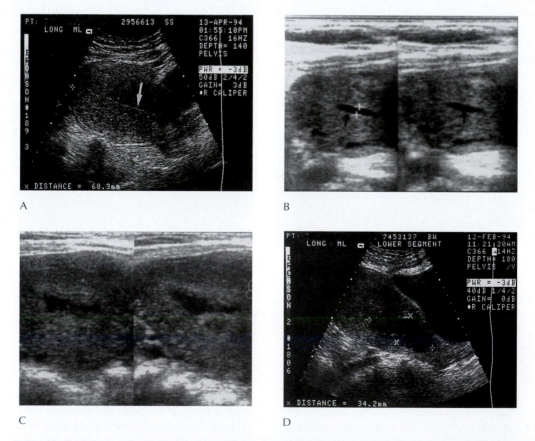

A

B

C

D

Figure 33–3. The normal variation see in the endometrial lining/cavity can be appreciated from the following series of cases, all of which had uncomplicated outcomes. **(A)** A well-defined linear "endometrial stripe" with no evident cavity *(arrow)*. **(B)** A small amount of fluid in the endometrial cavity. **(C)** An irregular fluid collection with shaggy borders for the endometrial lining. **(D)** A large fluid collection filling the hypotonic endometrial cavity. Anteroposterior diameter of the endometrial cavity is greater than 2.5 cm in this case of uterine hypotonia.

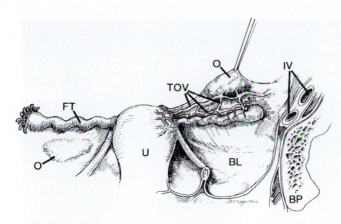

Figure 33–4. Schematic illustration of the broad ligament, the peritoneal sheet containing loose areolar tissue supporting the uterus and containing the vascular supply to the uterus and fallopian tubes. *(Reprinted with permission from Fleischer AC, Romero R, Manning FA, et al., eds. The Principles and Practice of Ultrasonography in Obstetrics and Gynecology, 4th ed. Norwalk, CT: Appleton & Lange; 1990.)*

Extraperitoneal Spaces

Pelvic extraperitoneal spaces are for the most part compressed potential spaces not easily visualized with ultrasound. The retropubic space of Retzius, pararectal, paravesical, and paravaginal areas are potential areas where blood accumulation or abscess formation can take place. In pathologic states (e.g., suspected retroperitoneal hemorrhage) computed tomography (CT) or magnetic resonance imaging (MRI) for hematoma identification would be more definitive than sonography.[14]

PATHOLOGY

Postpartum Hemorrhage

Hemorrhage represents one of the most significant causes of maternal morbidity following childbirth. Postpartum hemorrhage (PPH) is divided into two diagnostic entities according to the time of clinical presentation: primary and secondary.

Primary PPH occurs during the first 24 h after delivery and is associated with acute clinical problems, such as coagulopathies; dysfunctional and prolonged labors; chorioamnionitis; placental implantation abnormalities, such as placenta previa and accreta; the use of uterine relaxing agents, such as halothane or magnesium sulfate; and incomplete removal of the placenta. Clinical circumstances at the time of delivery usually point to the diagnosis and guide therapeutic endeavors.

Secondary PPH occurs more than 24 h after delivery and is seen in 1% of patients. It is caused by either retained placental tissue or subinvolution of the placental site (Fig. 33–7). At times it may be difficult to distinguish between clots, which in general tend to be homogeneous, and placental fragments, which have areas of increased echogenicity. The value of sonography in detecting retained material after spontaneous abortion has been demonstrated.[15] Surgical intervention by dilation and curettage (D&C) during the puerperal period will increase the probability of inducing uterine scar formation (synechiae) with the consequence of Asherman's syndrome and subsequent infertility.[16] In Dewhurst's series only 32% of 89 patients subjected to a D&C for secondary PPH had pathologically confirmed tissue obtained.[17] Lee et al. confirmed this observation in a study in which 56 patients underwent diagnostic ultrasound evaluation for PPH and only 14 (25%) required a D&C because of sonographic evidence of retained products of conception.[18] In the remaining 42 patients, where there was no ultrasound evidence of retained secundines, all patients responded satisfactorily to medical therapy. Hertzberg and Bowie[19] suggested five categories of diagnosis when evaluating the puerperal uterus for retained products by ultrasound. In their series the finding most commonly associated with retained placental tissue was an echogenic mass in the uterine cavity (see section on retained placenta). If a thin endometrial stripe or only endometrial fluid was seen, no patient had retained products,

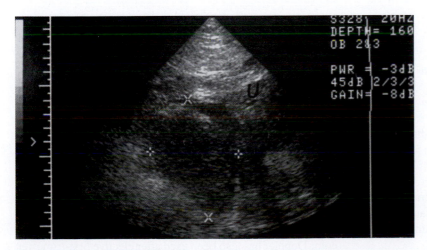

Figure 33–5. Hematoma (defined by *calipers*) of the broad ligament following cesarean section appearing as a heterogeneous mass lateral to the uterus (U).

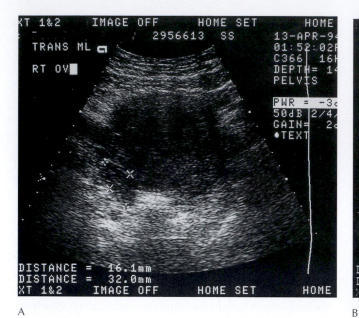

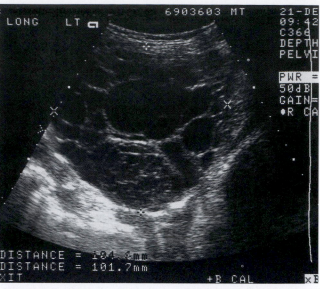

Figure 33–6. (A) Ovary (defined by *calipers*) appears as a pelvic mass adjacent to the uterus. **(B)** Enlarged cystic ovary (10 cm) compatible with a luteoma of pregnancy in another patient immediately postpartum. **(C)** The same ovary viewed 3 months later after spontaneous regression.

either on pathologic examination or clinical follow-up. These categories include

1. Normal uterine "stripe" — Likely benign
2. Endometrial fluid present — Likely benign
3. Echogenic masses often stippled/AP measurements exceed 1.5 cm — Probable products of conception
4. Hyperechoic foci/ no mass — Seen after intrauterine instrumentation
5. Heterogenous mass/ enlarged cavity — Probable retained products

Uterine instrumentation (i.e., D&C) can cause introduction of gas bubbles into the endometrial cavity. These can appear as bright echogenic foci, which may or may not shadow. A similar appearance could be seen in a case of endometritis with a gas-forming pathogenic organism (Fig. 33–8). The distinction is usually made historically.

The utility of Doppler ultrasound to evaluate for retained products in the postpartum period has never been thoroughly evaluated but theoretically may have potential merit. Trophoblastic tissue typically shows a low-impedance, high-diastolic flow pattern (Fig. 33–9). These characteristics have been shown to be useful in distinguishing early intrauterine pregnancies from pseudogestational sacs associated with ectopic pregnancies.[20] Vaginal ultrasound with color Doppler has also been used after elective first-trimester

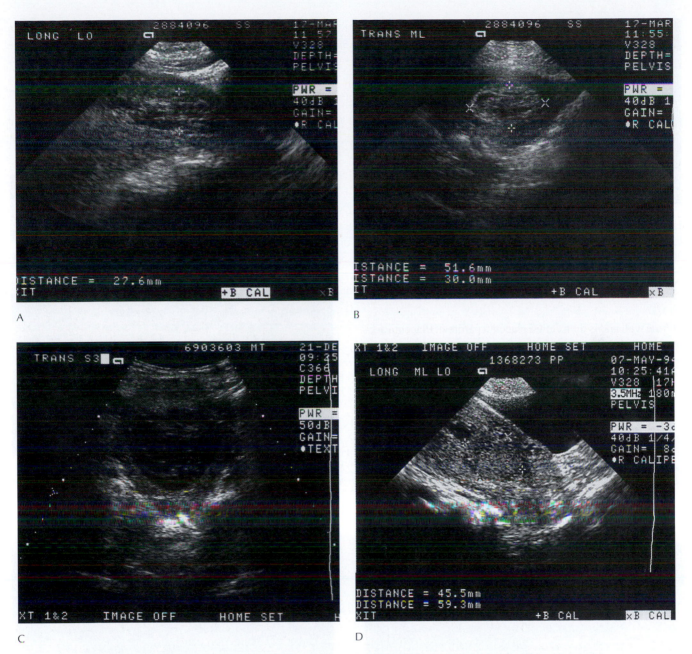

Figure 33–7. Retained products of conception can be difficult to distinguish from blood clot alone. **(A, B)** Longitudinal and transverse views showing complex echogenic material in the lower segment caused by placental fragments. **(C)** Transverse view from a different patient showing septated fluid collection in uterus with retained tissue found at dilation and curettage. **(D)** In another patient, there is uniformly echogenic material in lower segment confirmed clinically as only clot. Note similarity to **A**.

abortions when looking for retained tissue. The presence of intrauterine material and a typical peritrophoblastic flow pattern on Doppler do not necessarily imply clinically important retained products of conception in the first few days after abortion.[21] Additional research will be needed to determine if Doppler will aid in the diagnosis and management of the postpartum patient with prolonged bleeding.

The use of ultrasound and judicious patient assessment can thus minimize the need for operative intervention and subsequent reproductive complications in some patients experiencing PPH.

Retained Placenta

The problems of postpartum hemorrhage and retained products have already been discussed. Two unique facets of a retained placenta, however, deserve separate mention. Placenta accreta is the abnormal adherence of the placenta in whole or part to the uterine myometrium. It can at times invade the

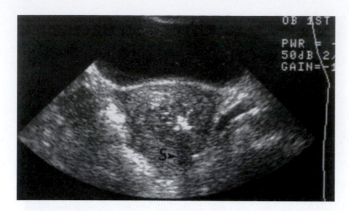

Figure 33–8. Clinically confirmed case of endomyometritis typified by poorly defined and thickened appearance of the endometrium and showing inferior shadowing (S) related to possible gas or retained material. A similar pattern may be seen following uterine instrumentation.

uterine wall and is then called placenta percreta. Placenta accreta occurs in about 1 in 1000 deliveries and usually warrants hysterectomy. The clinical condition has been diagnosed antepartum with the following sonographic characteristics:

1. Loss of normal hypoechoic retroplacental myometrial zone.
2. Thinning or disruption of the hyperechoic uterine serosa–bladder interface.
3. The presence of focal exophytic masses.[22]

Although for the obstetrician the more invasive forms of accreta, namely placenta increta and placenta percreta, re-

quire definitive surgical intervention, two reports attest to the value of conservative management of a partial accreta[23] and a complete accreta.[24] Sonography can be used to assist in the diagnosis and follow-up until final passage of all material. Figure 33–10 shows characteristic aspects of a retained degenerating fragment of placenta adherent to the uterine wall.

An abdominal pregnancy takes place when implantation and development occur within the abdomen but outside the

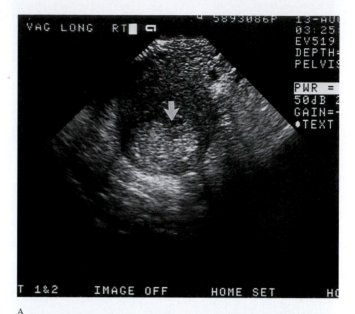

A

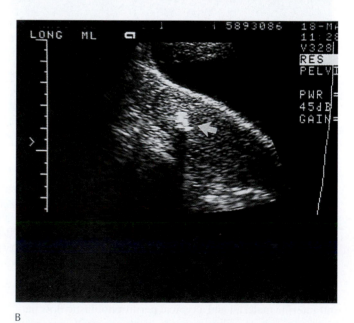

B

Figure 33–10. (A) A retained placental fragment from a patient with partial placenta accreta diagnosed at cesarean section who was followed up conservatively after delivery (arrow). The placenta is proximate to the serosal surface of the fundus. **(B)** Study of the same patient 7 months postdelivery who was asymptomatic. The retained placenta is smaller and calcified (arrow).

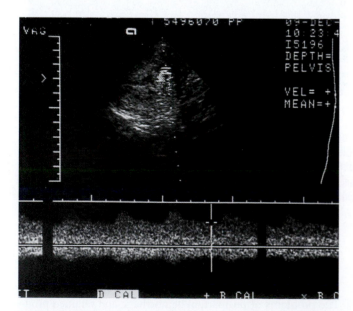

Figure 33–9. Retained trophoblastic tissue showing low-impedance, high-diastolic flow pattern. Vaginal probe used with sample volume cursor placed along endometrial stripe. The central blur is from color-encoded Doppler.

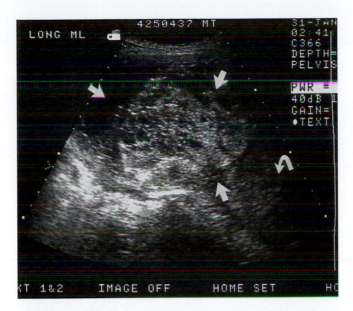

Figure 33–11. Total placenta *(straight arrows)* remaining in the abdomen superior to the uterus *(curved arrow)* 12 weeks after delivery by laparotomy of a 35-week gestation abdominal pregnancy.

uterus.[25] The likelihood of survival is small. Martin et al. cited a fetal survival of 17% in their series of 15 abdominal pregnancies.[26] If pregnancy is allowed to progress and laparotomy is performed for fetal delivery, the placenta is often left in place to naturally involute following the removal of the fetus.

Figure 33–11 depicts a placenta retained in the abdomen after an abdominal pregnancy was carried to 35 weeks of gestational age and delivered by laparotomy. The placenta had been observed to regress over a 12-week period after the delivery.

Uterine Inversion

Uterine inversion is an uncommon obstetric complication occurring after the passage of the placenta. The reported incidence varies but is probably seen no more frequently than 1 in 2000 deliveries and may be associated with excess fundal pressure and cord traction. Hsieh and Lee[27] described the sonographic findings in this condition. As the clinical circumstances are usually quite dramatic, with hemorrhage, pain, shock, and the inverted uterus presenting at the introitus, the diagnosis is evident. Delayed incomplete inversion was described by Gross and McGahan[28] where they noted the sonographic characteristics to be poor delineation of the endometrial stripe on longitudinal scanning, which instead of being linear had the central uterine echoes take on a Y-shaped configuration.

Postpartum Infection

Puerperal infectious morbidity will take place following 3 to 4% of vaginal births and after 10 to 15% of cesarean de-

TABLE 33–2. FACTORS ASSOCIATED WITH INCREASED RISK OF PUERPERAL INFECTION

Medical	Surgical
Premature membrane rupture	General anesthesia
Internal fetal monitoring	Operator expertise
Obesity	Intraoperative delay
Anemia	and complications
Multiple pelvic exams during labor	Classical uterine incision
Chorioamnionitis	
Prolonged labor	
Retained secundines	
Prolonged membrane rupture	

Social
Low socioeconomic status
Poor hygiene
Smoking, ethanol, and drug abuse

liveries, although significantly higher rates have been noted in certain populations at risk.[29,30] Factors that predispose to puerperal infectious morbidity are listed in Table 33–2. The most common source of puerperal sepsis is from organisms normally present in the vagina, including both aerobic and anaerobic species. *Escherichia coli, Bacteroides* species, aerobic and anaerobic streptococci, and enterococci are the most common organisms isolated in these infections.

Endomyometritis is a clinical diagnosis associated with fever, uterine tenderness, elevated white blood cell count, and often, foul-smelling lochia. Sonographically certain findings are associated with this condition and may support the clinical diagnosis. These include a dilated or irregular endometrial cavity occasionally containing fluid, shadowing echoes secondary to gas in the absence of intrauterine instrumentation, and often the presence of fluid in the cul-de-sac. Retained products of conception will predispose to infection and serve as a nidus for bacterial growth. Endomyometritis usually presents within the first 3 to 4 days after delivery. Streptococcal endomyometritis is often clinically evident within 24 h after delivery. Later (more than 4 days) febrile illness is more likely related to abscess formation, would infection, septic pelvic thrombophlebitis, or the development of a phlegmon, an indurated inflammatory mass often confluent with the uterus and the broad ligament[31] (Fig. 33–12). A phlegmon is a nonfluctuant inflammatory mass that on ultrasound appears to be of lower density and less well circumscribed or encapsulated than an abscess. It requires prolonged and intense antibiotic medical therapy as opposed to the surgical or percutaneous catheter drainage warranted with an abscess. Anticoagulation with heparin is often employed as adjunctive therapy. In one series phlegmon represented 19% of infectious complications following cesarean delivery.[32]

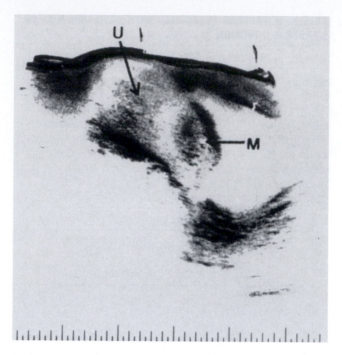

Figure 33–12. A phlegmon developing from the anterior wall of the uterus (U) following cesarean section. At laparotomy this nonfluctuant mass (M) was found to extend into the broad ligament. A bladder flap hematoma may have the same appearance. Management is dependent on the clinical condition.

Abscesses will appear as complex masses that are primarily cystic with internal echoes and have a wall or margin around them, the thickness of which depends on their stage of development. Rarely, acoustic shadowing from gas formation may be seen (Fig. 33–13). The presence of a wall or capsule distinguishes an abscess from a phlegmon. The reliable sonographic diagnosis of abscesses has been reported by Taylor et al.[33] in a series of 67 nonpuerperal patients.

Abscess formation can occur superficially in a wound, deep in the pelvis, in the broad ligament, in the uterus, at any point along the line of surgical incision, or even in the cul-de-sac. An abscess or an infected hematoma is indistinguishable from a sterile hematoma when viewed sonographically, and, if clinically questioned, needle aspiration may be useful for diagnosis and in some cases therapy. Sonography can aid in the localization of the fluid collection and thus expedite surgical or percutaneous drainage as warranted.

Cesarean Section Delivery

Special note should be made about the role of ultrasound in evaluating complications after cesarean deliveries because this mode of delivery now accounts for approximately 25% of all births in the United States.[34] The rate of uterine involution is no different after cesarean birth or vaginal delivery.[8] The area immediately under the abdominal incision may be the site for hematoma formation, and more difficult to assess is the area under the fascia, a site prone to hematoma formation

particularly with Pfannenstiel's incisions (Fig. 33–14). On scanning, the uterine incision line may show an edematous appearance with an inhomogeneous swelling in the lower uterine segment. Hyperechoic areas along the incision line are related to the suture material employed in the uterine closure. Coated material, such as Vicryl (Ethicon, Somerville, NJ, USA), is more echogenic than the chromic suture material now used less frequently (Fig. 33–15). Abnormal echogenicity may also be seen under the anterior peritoneal reflection between the uterus and the urinary bladder due to the development of a bladder flap hematoma as described by Baker et al.[35] (Fig. 33–16). Such hematomas are generally associated with venous bleeding and may show some lateralization as they expand. On ultrasound, these generally complex masses may be cystic or solid depending on the degree of organization that has taken place in the hematoma and on the presence or absence of superimposed infection. When anechoic areas are seen along the incision line and are greater than 2 cm in diameter (some edema may be normal), hematoma formation should be suspected and clinical correlation sought.[36] Such echo-free areas, described by Faustin et al.,[37] were found in 29% of patients in their series often after excess blood loss at surgery. For these investigators, an anechoic area of 3.5 cm or greater was associated with subsequent postoperative morbidity.

In addition to bladder flap and broad ligament hematomas, fluid collections may occur in extraperitoneal locations such as the space of Retzius.[14] Intraperitoneal bleeding from a uterine vessel can also lead to a hemoperitoneum.

Efforts are being made to discourage the practice of routine "repeat" cesarean sections. Investigational work with ultrasound has attempted to correlate patterns seen after cesarean section birth with subsequent wound healing and the status of the uterine incision. Burger et al.[38] reviewed the sonographic appearance of 48 puerperal patients. While describing several "patterns" related to degree of thickening and fluid containing cystic areas, no correlation could be made with the clinical outcome or longterm status of the wound. Because the frequency of uterine dehiscence and rupture approaches 1% with low transverse uterine incisions, greater numbers would be required and longer follow-up would be necessary before a definitive statement could be made about such observations. Michaels et al.[39] observed sonographic changes in the antepartum period in the lower uterine segment including thinning (<5 mm) of the uterine wall, ballooning, and wedge defects. Although the study was not designed to test the performance of the uterus in labor, there did appear to be anatomic differences that can be appreciated before delivery and that may influence labor management.

Transperineal sonography has been shown to complement transabdominal scanning for the identification of postoperative complications, such as hematomas and abscesses.[40] This technique does not require a full bladder and may be of less discomfort to the patient who has a recent abdominal incision.

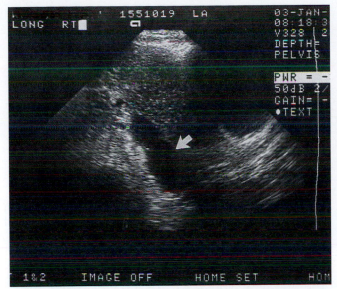

A

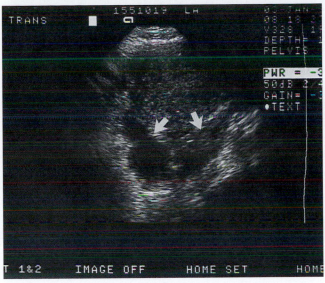

B

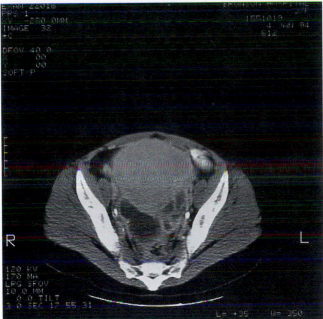

C

Figure 33–13. Longitudinal **(A)** and transverse **(B)** views show focal fluid collection *(arrows)* in the cul-de-sac in a febrile patient. Abscesses were successfully drained through the vagina. **(C)** Comparative computed tomogram similar in plane to **B**.

THE GENITOURINARY SYSTEM

During pregnancy the urinary tract undergoes major physiologic and anatomic changes. These changes persist for some time into the puerperal period. Ureteral dilation and concomitant hydronephrosis, related to hormonal factors from early pregnancy, may be seen even before uterine enlargement takes place. Peake prospectively studied 159 gravid women and found hydronephrosis developing as early as 11 to 15 weeks of gestation.[41] Two-thirds of all patients were affected. Hydronephrosis in pregnancy will achieve maximum dilation at 24 to 28 weeks, with the renal pelvic diameter achieving a 63% enlargement over nonpregnant controls.[42] Sonographic assessment may be warranted to evaluate some renal symptoms, particularly in the antepartum period, but radiographic evaluation is generally more definitive, especially when searching for calculi.

Fetal evaluation occasionally demonstrates congenital malformations, specifically agenesis and dysgenesis.[43] Because of the high (9%) association of renal anomalies in the parents of such infants, sonography is a valuable adjunct to be employed as a simple noninvasive method of assessment of maternal renal anatomy even before delivery. The recommendation has been made that all first-degree relatives

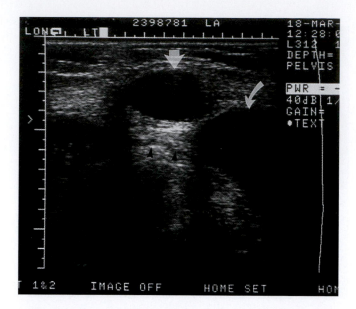

Figure 33–14. Subfascial hematoma seen postpartum after cesarean delivery. Hematoma fluid collection *(solid arrow)*, urinary bladder *(curved arrow)*, and peritoneal reflection *(arrowheads)* are identified.

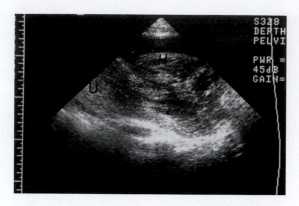

Figure 33–16. Large bladder flap hematoma (H) appearing as an enlarged heterogeneous area above the uterus (U), the border of which is poorly defined.

(parents and siblings) of affected infants (fetuses) should be screened for asymptomatic malformations when such fetal renal anomalies are diagnosed.[44]

Complete resolution of pregnancy-related urinary tract changes does not occur until 6 to 8 weeks postpartum. Symptoms that may have been present secondary to the pressure-induced hydronephrosis are usually obviated in the immediate time after delivery. In assessing the postpartum pelvis, for

any problem, the occasional pelvic kidney must be appropriately identified (Fig. 33–17).

THE HEPATOBILIARY SYSTEM

Biliary tract disease can occur at any time during gestation, but there appears to be a predisposition for some aspects of pathology in this system to present more frequently in the third trimester and postpartum.[45] Pregnancy is associated with an elevation of serum lipids and cholesterol. Gallstone formation is fostered in such a chemical environment. Cholelithiasis is a condition that affects women four times more frequently than men. Glenn and McSherry[46] reported that in a majority of 300 women studied with gallstones, the

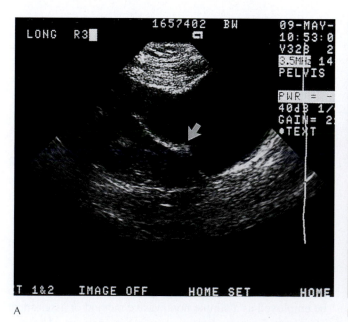

A

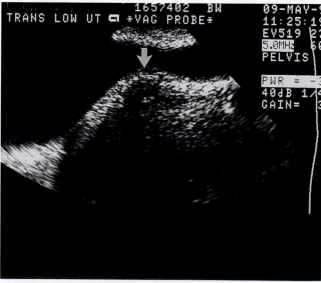

B

Figure 33–15. Transvesical **(A)** and endovaginal **(B)** scans show commonly seen edematous swelling *(arrows)* along the uterine incision line beneath the bladder reflection following cesarean section.

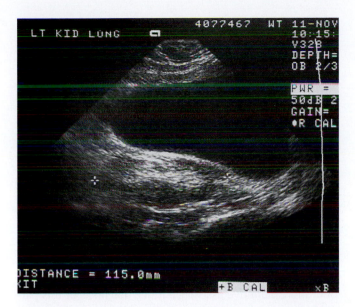

Figure 33–17. Pelvic kidney *(calipers)* appears as a solid mass behind the urinary bladder.

onset of their symptoms was associated with a pregnancy. Braverman et al.[47] and Stauffer et al.[48] both demonstrated a significant increase in gallbladder volume occurring during pregnancy. With enlargement, changes in bile salt concentration and the stasis that occurs secondary to progesterone, it is not surprising that Williamson and Williamson[49] reported that 11% of gravid patients had cholelithiasis most often presenting in the third trimester. A lesser frequency of this same pathologic finding was seen in an unselected series where 4.2% of 338 gravid patients had gallbladder disease.[48]

Edematous change was reported in the gallbladder wall of two severely preeclamptic patients by Gadwood et al.[50] The normal gallbladder wall measures less than 3 mm in thickness. A thickened gallbladder wall can be seen in patients with cholecystitis and other causes unrelated to intrinsic gallbladder pathology. Patients with preeclampsia frequently have low serum albumin, which causes increased extracellular fluid and can be manifest in the gallbladder as mural thickening. In these reported patients this finding as well as the maternal disease resolved within 1 week of delivery (Fig. 33–18).

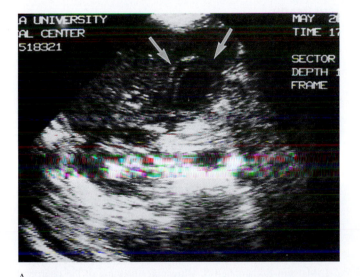

A

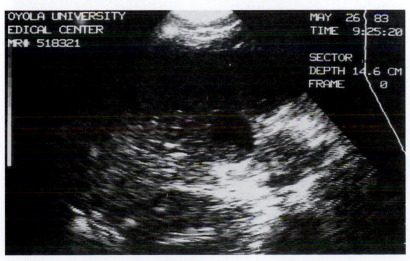

B

Figure 33–18. (A) Gallbladder wall edema *(arrows)* in a severely preeclamptic patient. **(B)** The same patient 1 week postpartum with normal wall thickness and small amount of sludge within gallbladder. Preeclampsia had resolved.

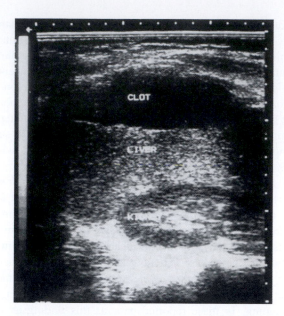

Figure 33–19. Subcapsular hematoma of the liver (CLOT) in a patient with severe coagulopathy. Symptoms, drop in hemoglobin, and sonogram occurred 3 days after delivery. A four-unit blood transfusion was required. Complete resolution on follow-up took 12 weeks.

Vascular changes occur throughout the body during pregnancy with increased flow and vasodilation. The hepatobiliary system is no exception. Kaemmerer et al.[51] studied the portal vascular system during the puerperium and noted that it took some 3 weeks to return to normal.

Clinically critical coagulopathies may occur with severe preeclampsia or eclampsia and with abnormalities of placental implantation (e.g., abruptio placentae). These coagulation disturbances usually take several days to resolve. With the preeclampsia–eclampsia syndrome in particular, liver swelling and subcapsular hemorrhage may take place.[52] Surveillance of the liver is warranted in the puerperal period to rule out a subcapsular hematoma of the liver in the presence of unexplained blood loss, particularly when associated with such a coagulopathy, and in the presence of chest or upper abdominal discomfort in such patients[53] (Fig. 33–19).

Acute pancreatitis is a medical complication rarely associated with pregnancy, but when it is found it usually has a predilection for the third trimester and the 5 months postpartum.[54] Clinical associations include hyperlipidemia, hyperparathyroidism, thiazide ingestion, collagen vascular disease, and chronic alcoholism. Presenting symptoms include nausea, fever, midepigastric pain with spread to the lower abdomen, and radiation to the back. An elevated serum amylase is diagnostic. Sonographically, with acute pancreatitis the gland is enlarged and shows diminished echogenicity. Pancreatic pseudocysts and fluid collections can easily be evaluated with ultrasound. In the puerperal period, as at other times, conservative management is recommended.

VASCULAR RISKS AND COMPLICATIONS

Thrombotic and thromboembolic complications, such as pulmonary emboli, are increased in frequency during pregnancy and particularly in the puerperal period. These events occur in 2 to 5 of 1000 births.[55] Particularly relevant to this discussion is the complication of ovarian vein thrombosis.[56,57] This problem may be manifest by pelvic pain, tachycardia, leukocytosis, and fever. Clinically, the diagnosis is usually made by a process of exclusion, and sonography has then been employed to support the clinical suspicion. Sonography may demonstrate a mass with internal echoes consistent with a thrombus contained within a dilated vein.[58] In a review of various imaging modalities, however, Savader and associates felt that CT scanning was the superior modality to diagnose puerperal ovarian vein thrombosis.[59] Newer techniques in duplex Doppler and MRI may be more sensitive and might offer more definitive assistance in the diagnosis of this particular puerperal complication.[60,61]

SUMMARY

Nearly from its inception into clinical practice ultrasound has been used to evaluate physiologic and pathologic changes during the puerperal period. Normal changes that are seen in the puerperium must be appreciated by the clinician and sonologist to enable them to correlate unusual ultrasound findings with the condition of the patient to establish appropriate diagnoses and to implement appropriate therapeutic regimens.

REFERENCES

1. Robinson HP. Sonar in the puerperium. *Scott Med J.* 1972; 17:364.
2. Malvern J, Campbell S. Ultrasonic scanning of the puerperal uterus following secondary postpartum hemorrhage. *J Obstet Gynaecol Br Commonw.* 1973;80:320.
3. Cunningham FG, Macdonald PC, Gant NF, et al., eds. *Williams Obstetrics,* 19th ed. Norwalk, CT: Appleton & Lange; 1993; Chapters 26, 28.
4. Emmons SL, Krohn N, Jackson M, et al. Development of wound infections among women undergoing cesarean section. *Obstet Gynecol.* 1988;72:559.
5. Piiroinen O, Kaihola HL. Uterine size measured by ultrasound during the menstrual cycle. *Acta Obstet Gynecol Scand.* 1975;54:247.
6. Siedler D, Laing FC, Jeffrey RB, et al. Uterine adenomyosis. *J Ultrasound Med.* 1987;6:345.
7. Hytten FE, Chamberlain G. *Clinical Physiology in Obstetrics.* London: Blackwell Scientific; 1981:221.
8. Lavery JP, Shaw L. Sonography of the puerperal pelvis. *J Ultrasound Med.* 1989;8:481.
9. Rodeck CH, Newton JR. Study of the uterine cavity by

ultrasound in the early puerperium. *Br J Obstet Gynaecol.* 1976; 83:795.

10. Wachsberg RH, Kurtz AB, Levine CD, et al. Real-time ultrasonographic analysis of the normal postpartum uterus. *J Ultrasound Med.* 1994;13:215–221.

11. Parakkal PF. Macrophages: The time course and sequence of their distribution in the postpartum uterus. *J Ultrastruct Res.* 1972;40:284.

12. Van Rees D, Bernstine RL, Crawford W. Involution of the postpartum uterus: An ultrasonic study. *J Clin Ultrasound.* 1981; 9:55.

13. Cunningham FG, Macdonald PC, Gant NF, et al., eds.*Williams Obstetrics*, 19th ed. Norwalk, Conn: Appleton & Lange; 1993: 214.

14. Yamashita Y, Torashima M, Harada M, et al. Postpartum extraperitoneal pelvic hematoma: Imaging findings. *AJR.* 1993; 161:805.

15. Kurtz AB, Shlansky-Goldberg RD, Choi HY, et al. Detection of retained products of conception following spontaneous abortion in the first trimester. *J Ultrasound Med.* 1991;10:387.

16. Buttram VC. What sets the stage for IUA? *Contemp Ob-Gyn.* 1978;11:33.

17. Dewhurst CJ. Secondary postpartum hemorrhage. *J Obstet Gynaecol Br Commonw.* 1966;73:53.

18. Lee CY, Madrazo B, Drukker BH. Ultrasonic evaluation of the postpartum uterus in the management of postpartum bleeding. *Obstet Gynecol.* 1981;58:227.

19. Hertzberg BS, Bowie JD. Ultrasound of the postpartum uterus. *J Ultrasound Med.* 1991;10:451.

20. Dillon EH, Feyock AL, Taylor KJW. Pseudogestational sacs: Doppler US differentiation from normal or abnormal intrauterine pregnancies. *Radiology.* 1990;176:359.

21. Dillon EH, Case CQ, Ramos IM, et al. Endovaginal US and Doppler findings after first trimester abortion. *Radiology.* 1993; 186:87.

22. Finberg HJ, Williams JW. Placenta accreta: Prospective sonographic diagnosis in patients with placenta previa and prior cesarean section. *J Ultrasound Med.* 1992;11:333.

23. Petrovic O, Zupanic M, Rukavina B, et al. Placenta accreta: Postpartum diagnosis and a potentially new mode of management using real-time ultrasonography. *J Clin Ultrasound.* 1984; 22:204.

24. Gibb DMF, Soothill PW, Ward KJ. Conservative management of placenta accreta. *Br J Obstet Gynaecol.*1994;101:79.

25. Costa SD, Presley J, Basert G. Advanced abdominal pregnancy. *Obstet Gynecol. Surv.* 1991;46:515.

26. Martin JN, Sessums JK, Martin RW, et al. Abdominal pregnancy: Current concepts and management. *Obstet Gynecol.* 1988;71:549.

27. Hsieh TT, Lee JD. Sonographic findings in acute puerperal uterine inversion. *J Clin Ultrasound.* 1991;19:306.

28. Gross RC, McGahan JP. Sonographic detection of partial uterine inversion. *AJR.* 1985;144:761.

29. Gibbs RS, Rodgers PJ, Castaneda YS, et al. Endometritis following vaginal delivery. *Obstet Gynecol.* 1988;72:519.

30. Willison JR. The conquest of cesarean section related infections. *Obstet Gynecol.* 1988;72:519.

31. Lavery JP, Howell RS, Shaw L. Ultrasonic demonstration of a phlegmon following cesarean delivery. *J Clin Ultrasound.* 1985;13:134.

32. DePalma RL, Leveno KJ, Cunningham FG, et al. Identification and management of women at high risk for pelvic infection following cesarean section. *Obstet Gynecol.* 1980;55:185s.

33. Taylor KJ, Worsen JF, DeGraff C, et al. Accuracy of gray scale ultrasound diagnosis of abdominal and pelvic abscesses in 220 patients. *Lancet.* 1978;I:83.

34. Shiono PH, McNellis D, Rhoads GG. Reasons for the rising cesarean delivery rates. *Obstet Gynecol.* 1987;69:696.

35. Baker ME, Bowie JD, Killam AP. Sonography of post cesarean section bladder flap hematoma. *AJR.* 1985;144:75.

36. Baker ME, Kay H, Mahoney BS, et al. Sonography of the low transverse incision—Cesarean section. *J Ultrasound Med.* 1988;7:389.

37. Faustin D, Minkoff H, Schaffer R, et al. Relationship of ultrasound findings after cesarean section to operative morbidity. *Obstet Gynecol.* 1985;66:915.

38. Burger NF, Darazs P, Boes EGM. An echogenic evaluation during the early puerperium of the uterine wound after cesarean section. *J Clin Ultrasound.* 1982;10:271.

39. Michaels WH, Thompson HO, Boutt A, et al. Ultrasound diagnosis in the scarred lower uterine segment during pregnancy. *Obstet Gynecol.* 1988;71:112.

40. Hertzberg BS, Bowie JD, Kliewer MA. Complications of cesarean section: Role of transperineal US. *Radiology.* 1993;188:533.

41. Peake SL, Roxburgh HB, Langlois SLEP. Ultrasonic assessment of hydronephrosis of pregnancy. *Radiology.* 1983;1146:167.

42. Erickson LM, Nicholson SF, Lewall DB, et al. Ultrasound evaluation of hydronephrosis of pregnancy. *J Clin Ultrasound.* 1979;7:128.

43. Romero R, Cullen M, Grannum P, et al. Antenatal diagnosis of renal anomalies with ultrasound. *Am J Obstet Gynecol.* 1985;151:38.

44. Roodhooft AM, Birnholz JC, Holmes LB. Familial nature of congenital absence and severe dysgenesis of both kidneys. *N Engl J Med.* 1984;310:1341.

45. Hiatt JR, Hiatt JCG, Williams RA, et al. Biliary disease in pregnancy: Strategy for surgical management. *Am J Surg.* 1986;151: 263.

46. Glenn F, McSherry CK. Gallstones and pregnancy among 300 young women treated by cholecystectomy. *Surg Gynecol Obstet.* 1968;127:1067.

47. Braverman DZ, Johnson ML, Kern F. Effects of pregnancy and contraceptive steroids on gall bladder function. *N Engl J Med.* 1980;302:362.

48. Stauffer RA, Adams A, Wygal J, et al. Gallbladder disease in pregnancy. *Am J Obstet Gynecol.* 1982;144:661.

49. Williamson SL, Williamson MR. Cholecystosonography in pregnancy. *J Ultrasound Med.* 1984;3:329.

50. Gadwood KA, Reynes CJ, Flisak ME, et al. Gallbladder wall thickening in preeclampsia. *JAMA.* 1985;253:71.

51. Kaemmerer H, Rapp K, Wagner HH. Ultrasound study of the portal vascular system in the puerperium. *Roentgen Bl.* 1985;38:244.

52. Manas KJ, Welsh JD, Rankin RA, et al. Hepatic hemorrhage without rupture in preeclampsia. *N Engl J Med.* 1985;312:424.

53. Lavery JP, Berg J. Subcapsular hematoma of the liver in pregnancy. *South Med J.* 1989;82:1568.

54. Present DH. Diseases of the biliary tract and pregnancy. In: Cherry SH, Berkowitz R, Kase N, eds. *Medical, Surgical*

and Gynecological Complications of Pregnancy. Baltimore: Williams & Wilkins; 1985:203–219.

55. Hathaway WE, Bonnar J. *Hemostatic Disorders of the Pregnant Woman and Newborn Infant.* New York: Elsevier; 1987.

56. Munsick RA, Gillanders LA. A review of the syndrome of puerperal ovarian vein thrombophlebitis. *Obstet Gynecol Surv.* 1981;36:57.

57. Bahnson RR, Wendel EF, Vogelzang RL. Renal vein thrombosis following puerperal ovarian vein thrombophlebitis. *Am J Obstet Gynecol.* 1985;152:290.

58. Rooholamini SA, Au AH, Hansen GC, et al. Imaging of pregnancy-related complications. *Radiographics.* 1993;13: 753.

59. Savader SJ, Otero RR, Savader BL. Puerperal ovarian vein thrombosis: Evaluation with CT, US, and MR imaging. *Radiology.* 1988;167:637.

60. Martin B, Mulopulus GP, Bryan PJ. MRI of puerperal ovarian vein thrombosis. *AJR.* 1986;147:291.

61. Baran GW, Frisch KM. Duplex Doppler evaluation of puerperal ovarian vein thrombosis. *AJR* 1987;149:321.

Sonographic Evaluation of Maternal Disorders During Pregnancy

Arthur C. Fleischer • Thomas C. Wheeler

Because of its ability to evaluate the uterus, placenta, and fetus, and because it does not use ionizing radiation, sonography is the diagnostic modality of choice for several maternal disorders that occur during pregnancy. The disorders discussed in this overview include pelvic masses, cholecystitis, and renal disorders.

PELVIC MASSES DURING PREGNANCY

The pregnant patient who has a pelvic mass palpated or delineated sonographically presents a special management problem for the obstetrician. Factors that affect obstetric management include the size of the mass, its internal consistency, its most likely histologic composition, the possibility of its becoming torsed or incarcerated, and whether or not it could hinder vaginal delivery. Sonography has an important role in documenting enlargement or regression of a mass. Sonographic delineation of the internal contents of a pelvic mass assists in narrowing its differential diagnosis. Masses that contain irregular septae, papillary excrescences, or large solid areas are more suspicious for malignancy than simple cysts.

Sonography will frequently detect adnexal pathology that previously would have gone unrecognized. Properly used, however, sonography will actually decrease the number of unnecessary laparotomies performed during pregnancy.

This chapter discusses the role of sonography in the evaluation of pelvic masses that can be encountered in a pregnant patient. An attempt will be made to differentiate those masses that may require immediate surgical intervention from those that usually do not.

Clinical Aspects

Sonography provides important clinical information in the evaluation of a patient with a pelvic mass. In fact, with routine use of sonography in obstetric care, pelvic masses are often discovered by the initial sonographic examination. A pelvic mass may become clinically manifest during pregnancy if it is palpated during physical examination or produces abdominal pain. Adnexal pathology also may be detected in the later stages of pregnancy if it impedes the conduct of labor. Fifty percent of ovarian masses remain asymptomatic throughout gestation.[1] When symptomatic, patients typically present with vague complaints of abdominal distention and discomfort. These symptoms are often attributed to pregnancy itself so it is understandable that many symptomatic adnexal masses are unsuspected.

Detection of pelvic masses by palpation can be limited during pregnancy because of the difficulty of distinguishing a pelvic mass from an enlarged uterus. This problem is particularly encountered in large or obese patients. Because it is often difficult to establish the size, extent, and nature of a pelvic mass during pregnancy by physical examination alone, sonography is particularly helpful.

In general, conservative management is followed in a gravid patient who has a pelvic mass that is smaller than 5 cm, is not painful, and does not enlarge on serial examinations.[2] If the mass is larger than 5 cm and appears to be enlarging or causing significant pain, however, surgical intervention may be indicated. Surgical intervention is indicated if there is a possibility of torsion or rupture of an adnexal mass. The incidence of torsion complicating adnexal pathology in the nonpregnant state is about 2%, but this may increase to levels as high as 11 to 50% during pregnancy.[3] Torsion is more likely to occur in pedunculated masses and during periods of rapid change in uterine size or position.[4] The probability of rupture of the mass may also be increased if it is tethered in the posterior cul-de-sac.

Sonographic demonstration of the internal structure of a pelvic mass may enter into the decision of whether or not to perform surgery. Demonstration of a simple cyst, for example, may preclude immediate surgery. If a mass contains solid irregular areas, the chance of malignancy is increased, and surgery prior to delivery may be indicated. Whether malignant or benign, the vast majority of adnexal masses complicating pregnancy are unilateral. Even malignant tumors of epithelial origin are unilateral 90% of the time.[5] This may prove to be clinically important as bilateral masses prove most often to be benign processes, such as endometriomas or luteomas of pregnancy.

Ovarian malignancies are fortunately rare in pregnancy with an incidence variably reported to be between 1 in 12,000 and 1 in 50,000 live births.[6] The preoperative diagnosis depends largely on sonographic assessment because oncofetal antigens provide little additional information as tumor markers. Maternal serum α-fetoprotein, human chorionic gonadotropin, carcinoembryonic antigen, and even CA-125 are all elevated in uncomplicated pregnancies.[7]

In addition to establishing the parameters of a pelvic mass, sonography has an important role in establishing the exact gestational age of the pregnancy. This is helpful because laparotomies and manipulation of the gravid uterus are preferably performed during the second trimester. Open laparoscopy has even been described as useful at this juncture in pregnancy.[8] Such timing decreases the possibility of spontaneous abortion in the first trimester and avoids the potential problems in the third trimester of preterm labor and limited surgical access to the abdomen due to an enlarged uterus. When an asymptomatic mass is diagnosed at term, cesarean section should be considered. This allows for timely surgical exploration and may avoid complications related to torsion and rupture with rapid uterine involution.

SONOGRAPHIC EVALUATION OF PELVIC MASSES

This discussion covers pelvic masses that are cystic, complex, and solid. Although some types of pelvic masses can demonstrate a variety of sonographic appearances, one can usually narrow the differential diagnosis down to one or two of the most probable diagnoses based on sonographic features of a pelvic mass.

The role of color Doppler sonography (CDS) in the evaluation of the adnexal mass in pregnant patients awaits further experience. Preoperative CDS may indicate which masses are more likely to be malignant by demonstration of low-impedance, high-diastolic velocity flow (Fig. 34–1). The decrease in vascular resistance attributed to angiogenesis in a growing tumor may be paralleled by low impedance in the ovarian vessels previously described in uncomplicated pregnancies.[9] Masses that have undergone torsion or infarction may have little or no flow demonstrable by CDS.

Color Doppler sonography provides a means to distinguish possibly malignant masses from those that are probably benign. In our series of 34 pregnant patient with complex masses, low impedance flow [pulsatility index (PI) < 1.0] was found to have a positive predictive value of 0.48 but, more importantly, a negative predictive value of 0.93.[24]

Cystic Masses

The most common cystic mass that occurs during pregnancy is a corpus luteum cyst. During the first few weeks of pregnancy, the corpus luteum produces progesterone that sustains the decidualized endometrium. Typically, corpora lutea appear as 2- to 3-cm anechoic masses located within the ovary (Fig. 34–2). They can enlarge up to 5 to 10 cm. Most corpus luteum cysts are asymptomatic, nonpalpable, and primarily detected by sonography rather than by palpation (Fig. 34–3). They usually do not require intervention because they regress prior to 16 to 18 weeks.[10] Occasionally, they can contain internal echoes and septae secondary to internal hemorrhage or separation of the luteinized lining from the wall of the cyst. Uncomplicated parovarian or peritoneal inclusion cysts may have a similar sonographic appearance to corpus luteum cysts.

Theca-lutein cysts represent an exaggerated corpus luteum response in patients with high levels of human chorionic gonadotropin. Occasionally, theca-lutein cysts can undergo marked enlargement, resulting in multiloculated pelvoabdominal cystic masses associated with pregnancy. These masses typically contain uniformly sized 2- to 3-cm anechoic spaces representing the cystic portions of the mass (Fig. 34–4). Theca-lutein cysts are frequently present with hydatidiform moles and other forms of gestational trophoblastic diseases, as well in some isoimmunized pregnancies.

In addition to corpus luteum cysts, there are several other types of pelvic masses that may appear as anechoic adnexal structures on sonography. These include a hydrosalpinx,

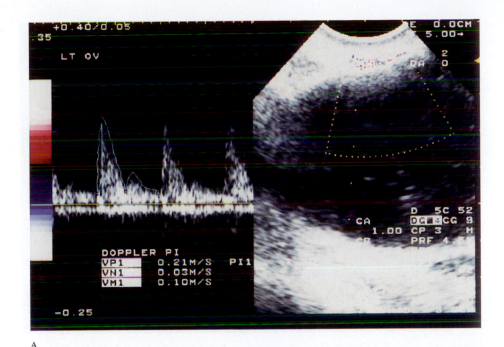

A

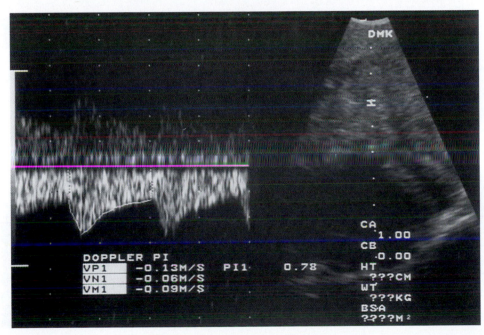

B

Figure 34–1. Transvaginal color Doppler sonogram (TV-CDS) of benign and malignant ovarian masses in pregnant patients. **(A)** Mostly cystic mass with high-impedance flow within the wall. This was a cystadenoma at surgery. **(B)** Complex predominantly solid mass with low-impedance flow found at cesarean section to represent an ovarian carcinoma. *(Figure continued.)*

peritoneal inclusion cysts, and developmental or remnant cyst (parovarian) cyst. Peritoneal inclusion cysts typically are irregularly shaped because they form between the peritoneal surfaces of organs and may not have a true wall. Usually, there is a history of pelvic surgery in patients with peritoneal inclusion cysts. Hydrosalpinges typically occur as sequelae to pelvic inflammatory disease. When small, their fusiform configuration and origin from the cornual areas of the uterus can usually be depicted on transvaginal sonography. When they enlarge, however, they can assume

a rounded configuration similar to other ovarian cysts. Parovarian cysts arise from the mesovarium in remnants of the Gartner's duct.[11] They can remain adnexal in location or, when enlarged, can project superior to the uterine fundus. Rarely, these masses may have thin internal septations similar to ovarian epithelial tumors. Most of these masses are asymptomatic and do not require surgical intervention during pregnancy.

There are several types of ovarian neoplasms that appear as predominantly cystic pelvic masses (Figs. 34–5 through

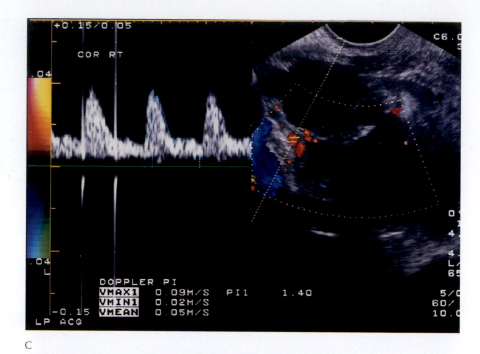

C

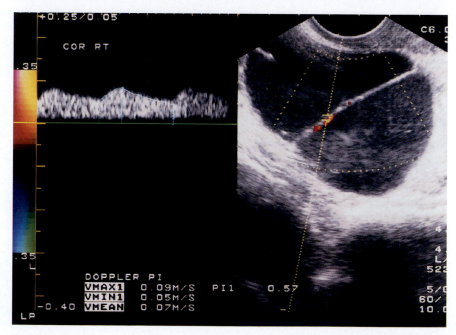

D

Figure 34–1. *(continued)* Three TV-CDSs showing high- **(C)** and low-impedance **(D,E)** flow within a mucinous cystadenoma appearing as a septated, mostly cystic mass. *(Figure continued.)*

34–7). In general, ovarian epithelial neoplasms are the most common cystic tumor to demonstrate significant enlargement during pregnancy.[12] As in the nongravid patient, mucinous or serous cystadenomas can contain various amounts of internal septation (see Fig. 34–6). Multiple thick septations are typically found in mucinous cystadenomas, whereas serous tumors tend to be unilocular (see Fig. 34–7). Cystic masses that contain irregular solid components, papillary excrescences, or both should be distinguished from those that are unilocular.

In general, masses that contain internal septations or papillary excrescences are more likely to have borderline or malignant histology (Fig. 34–8). The presence of maternal ascites with a cystic pelvic mass increases the likelihood of a malignant lesion.

Torsion of a cystic mass may be suggested if there is unusual thickening of the wall of the mass. Usually, torsion of a pelvic mass is associated with severe pelvoabdominal pain. Torsion of an ovarian mass is typically associated with

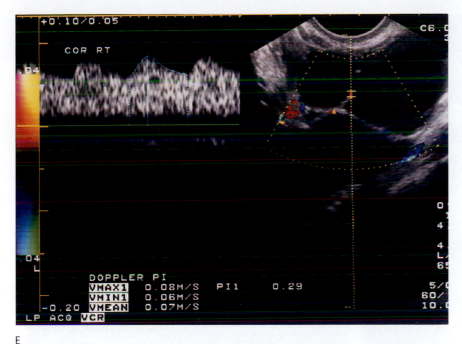

E

Figure 34–1. *(continued)* See legend on facing page.

intraperitoneal fluid related to obstruction of venous and lymphatic drainage.[4] Over the course of a pregnancy, a torsed ovary can be observed to enlarge significantly, probably due to vascular engorgement within the affected ovary. Often, the affected ovary is lodged within the cul-de-sac.

Complex Masses

The term *complex* implies that the mass contains both cystic and solid components. Complex masses can be further cat-egorized into those that are predominantly cystic and those that are predominantly solid. Complex masses can be cystic and contain echogenic components or solid masses that contain areas of cystic degeneration.

The most common complex mass encountered during pregnancy is a dermoid cyst. Ten percent of dermoids are initially diagnosed during pregnancy, and they are the most common tumor in the reproductive age group.[13] These masses are thought to arise parthenogenetically from germ cells within

Figure 34–2. Transvaginal sonogram of 5-week pregnancy with two corpora luteum cysts *(between + 's)* associated with ovulation introduction.

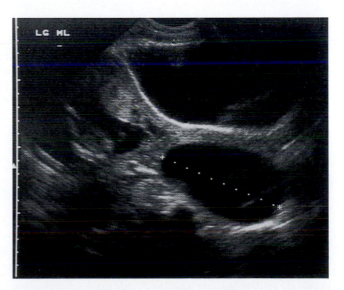

Figure 34–3. Transabdominal sonogram demonstrating cystic mass *(between + 's)* posterior to the lower uterine segment. On a follow-up exam 4 weeks later, the mass had completely regressed. Most likely this represented a corpus luteum cyst.

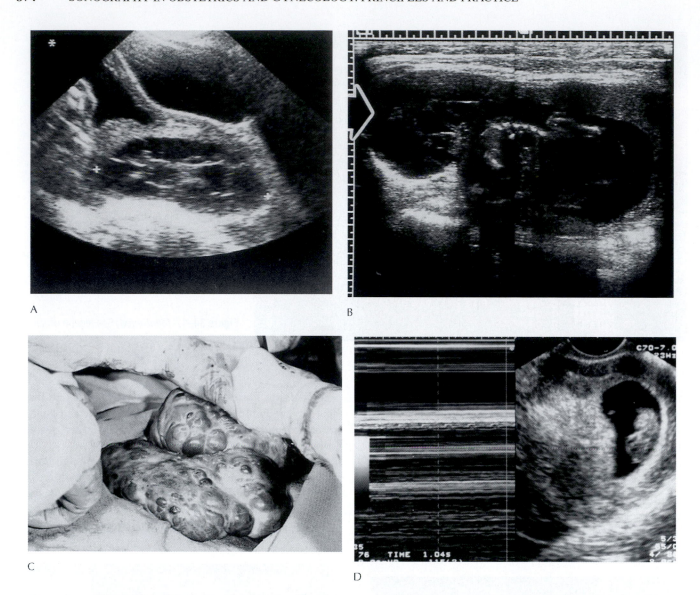

A

B

C

D

Figure 34–4. Enlarged ovaries contaiing theca-luteum cysts. **(A)** Enlarged ovary *(between +'s)* within the cul-de-sac containing several cystic spaces. **(B)** Composite scan demonstrating an enlarged ovary *(arrow)* superior to the fundus, containing several cystic spaces. **(C)** At surgery, massively enlarged ovaries that contained multiple theca-lutein cysts were found. Hyperstimulated ovaries seen in early pregnancy. *(Courtesy of Bill Wilson, MD, and Lonnie Burnett, MD.)* **(D)** Transvaginal sonography showing a living 9-week fetus. *(Figure continued.)*

the ovary. As a consequence of this method of development, dermoid cysts usually contain heterologous tissue elements including teeth, hair, skin, and fat in various proportions. Tooth elements can usually be recognized by their dense echogenicity with distal shadowing. Fat, hair, and skin elements usually produce a moderately echogenic appearance (Fig. 34–9). Some dermoid cysts that contain sebaceous material can demonstrate layering of this material above that of serous fluid.

Because most benign teratomas arise within the ovary, they are prone to undergoing torsion. They typically present as masses superior to the uterine fundus. Slow leakage

from a dermoid cyst can result in granulomatous peritonitis, whereas sudden rupture can lead to an acute abdominal crisis.

Occasionally, solid masses secondary to uterine fusion abnormalities may simulate the appearance of a solid mass or fibroid. It may be difficult to delineate the nongravid uterine horn in the later stages of pregnancy. In the first trimester, the nongravid bicornuate horn typically has a rounded solid structure with an echogenic central interface related to the decidual reaction that occurs in the nonpregnant horn. As the uterus enlarges, however, it may be more difficult to delineate this nongravid horn due to compression and axial rotation by the gravid uterus.